AF659950

GATE PREP SERIES

GATE

Graduate Aptitude Test in Engineering

2022

Life Sciences

Solved Papers

(2000-2021)

by

Dr. Prabhanshu Kumar
Ph.D.

Er. Preeti T. Kumar
M.Tech.

G. K. PUBLICATIONS (P) LTD.

Title : GATE 2022 - Life Sciences - Solved Papers 2000-2021

Language : English

Author's Name : Dr. Prabhanshu Kumar and Er. Preeti T. Kumar

Typeset & Published by :

Career Launcher Infrastructure (P) Ltd.

A-45, Mohan Cooperative Industrial Area, Near Mohan Estate Metro Station, New Delhi - 110044

Marketed by :

G.K. Publications (P) Ltd.

Plot No. 9A, Sector-27A, Mathura Road, Faridabad, Haryana-121003

ISBN : **978-93-91061-30-2**

Printer's Details : Made in India, New Delhi.

For product information :

Visit ***www.gkpublications.com*** or email to ***gkp@gkpublications.com***

Contents

GATE

Graduate Aptitude Test in Engineering

IIT Institutes

GATE 2021 will be conducted by
Indian Institute of Technology, Mumbai

Indian Institute of Technology, Kharagpur

GATE 2020 conducted by
Indian Institute of Technology, Delhi

Indian Institute of Technology, Chennai

Indian Institute of Technology, Guwahati

Indian Institute of Technology, Roorkee

Indian Institute of Technology, Kanpur

Preface

The Graduate Aptitude Test in Engineering (GATE) is an online exam conducted by the IITs for admissions to PG courses in IITs, IISc Bangalore, NITs and many state run universities as well as private universities. Also there are more than 37 PSUs that use GATE score for recruitments. A large number of corporates are also using GATE score as a tool to screen students for placements.

GK Publications is well known as the "publisher of choice" to students preparing for GATE and other technical examinations in the country. We published the first set of books in 1994 when GATE exam, both objective and conventional, was conducted in the paper and pencil environment, and used as a check point for entry to post graduate courses in IITs and IISCs. At that time, students had little access to technology and relied mainly on instructor led learning followed by practice with books available for these examinations.

A lot has changed since then!

Today, GATE is conducted in an online only mode with multiple choice and numerical based questions. The score is valid for three years and is used not only for post graduate courses but is also used by major PSUs for recruitment. Today's students have easy access to technology and the concept of a monologue within the classroom has changed to dialogue where students come prepared with concepts and then discuss topics. They learn a lot of things on the go with their mobile devices and practice for mock tests online.

We, as a leading publisher of GATE books, have also embraced change. Today, our books are no more guides and papers only but come with a fully supported mobile app and a web portal. The mobile app provides access to video lectures, short tests and regular updates about the exam. The web portal in additional to what is available on the app provides full length mock tests to mimic the actual exam and help you gauge your level of preparedness. The combination of practice content in print, video lectures, and short and full length tests on mobile and web makes this product a complete courseware for GATE preparation.

This book includes previous years GATE questions along with detailed solution of each question for better understanding. It will help the GATE aspirants to know an idea about the pattern of questions asked in GATE examination.

We also know that improvement is a never ending process and hence we welcome your suggestions and feedback or spelling and technical errors if any. Please write to us at gkp@gkpublications.com

We hope that our small effort will help you prepare well for the examination.

We wish you all the best!

GK Publications Pvt. Ltd.

About GATE

The Graduate Aptitude Test in Engineering (GATE) conducted by IISc and IITs has emerged as one of the bench mark tests for engineering and science aptitude in facilitating admissions for higher education (M.Tech./Ph.D.) in IITs, IISc and various other Institutes/Universities/ Laboratories in India. With the standard and high quality of the GATE examination in 27 disciplines of engineering and science, Humanities and Social Sciences subjects, it identifies the candidate's understanding of a subject and aptitude and eligibility for higher studies. During the last few years, GATE score is also being used as one of the criteria for recruitment in Government Organizations such as Cabinet Secretariat, and National/State Public Sector Undertakings in India. Because of the importance of the GATE examination, the number of candidates taking up GATE exams has increased tremendously. GATE exams are conducted by the IITs and IISc as a computer based test having multiple choice questions and numerical answer type questions. The questions are mostly fundamental, concept based and thought provoking. From 2017 onwards GATE Exam is being held in Bangladesh, Ethiopia, Nepal, Singapore, Sri Lanka and United Arab Emirates. An Institute with various nationalities in its campus widens the horizons of an academic environment. A foreign student brings with him/ her a great diversity, culture and wisdom to share. Many GATE qualified candidates are paid scholarships/assistantship, especially funded by Ministry of Human Resources Development, Government of India and by other Ministries. IIT, Kharagpur is the Organizing Institute for GATE 2022.

Why GATE?

Admission to Post Graduate and Doctoral Programmes

Admission to postgraduate programmes with MHRD and some other government scholarships/ assistantships in engineering colleges/institutes is open to those who qualify through GATE. GATE qualified candidates with Bachelor's degree in Engineering/Technology/Architecture or Master's degree in any branch of Science/Mathematics/Statistics/Computer Applications are eligible for admission to Master/Doctoral programmes in Engineering/Technology/Architecture as well as for Doctoral programmes in relevant branches of Science with MHRD or other government scholarships/assistantships. Candidates with Master's degree in Engineering/ Technology/Architecture may seek admission to relevant Ph.D programmes with scholarship/ assistantship without appearing in the GATE examination.

Financial Assistance

A valid GATE score is essential for obtaining financial assistance during Master's programs and direct Doctoral programs in Engineering/Technology/Architecture, and Doctoral programs in relevant branches of Science in Institutes supported by the MHRD or other Government agencies. As per the directives of the MHRD, the following procedure is to be adopted for admission to the post-graduate programs (Master's and Doctoral) with MHRD scholarship/ assistantship. Depending upon the norms adopted by a specific institute or department of the Institute, a candidate may be admitted directly into a course based on his/her performance in GATE only **or** based on his/her performance in GATE **and** an admission test/interview conducted by the department to which he/she has applied **and/or** the candidate's academic record. If the candidate is to be selected through test/interview for post-graduate programs, a minimum of 70% weightage will be given to the performance in GATE and the remaining 30% weightage will be given to the candidate's performance in test/interview and/or academic record, as per MHRD guidelines. The admitting institutes could however prescribe a minimum passing percentage of marks in the test/interview. Some colleges/institutes specify GATE qualification as the mandatory requirement even for admission without MHRD scholarship/assistantship. To avail of the financial assistance (scholarship), the candidate must first secure admission to a program in these Institutes, by a procedure that could vary from institute to institute. Qualification in GATE is also a minimum requirement to apply for various fellowships awarded by many Government organizations. Candidates are advised to seek complete details of admission procedures and availability of MHRD scholarship/assistantship from the concerned admitting institution. The criteria for postgraduate admission with scholarship/assistantship could be different for different institutions. The management of the post-graduate scholarship/assistantship is also the responsibility of the admitting institution. Similarly, reservation of seats under different categories is as per the policies and norms prevailing at the admitting institution and Government of India rules. *GATE offices will usually not entertain any enquiry about admission, reservation of seats and / or award of scholarship / assistantship*.

PSU Recruitments

As many as 37 PSUs are using GATE score for recruitment. It is likely that more number of PSUs may start doing so by next year. Below is the list of PSUs:

MDL, BPCL, GAIL, NLC LTD, CEL, Indian Oil, HPCL, NBPC, NECC, BHEL, WBSEDCL, NTPC, ONGC, Oil India, Power Grid, Cabinet Secretariat, Govt. of India, BAARC, NFL, IPR, PSPCL, PSTCL, DRDO, OPGC Ltd., THDC India Ltd., BBNL, RITES, IRCON, GHECL, NHAI, KRIBHCO, Mumbai Railway Vikas Corporation Ltd. (MRVC Ltd.), National Textile Corporation, Coal India Ltd., BNPM, AAI, NALCO, EdCIL India.

Important :

1. Admissions in IITs/IISc or other Institutes for M.Tech./Ph.D. through GATE scores shall be advertised separately by the Institutes and GATE does not take the responsibility of admissions.
2. Cabinet Secretariat has decided to recruit officers for the post of Senior Field Officer (Tele) (From GATE papers of EC, CS, PH), Senior Research Officer (Crypto) (From GATE papers of EC, CS, MA), Senior Research Officer (S&T) (From GATE papers EC, CS, CY, PH, AE, BT) in the Telecommunication Cadre, Cryptographic Cadre and Science & Technology Unit respectively of Cabinet Secretariat. The details of the scheme of recruitment shall be published in National Newspaper/Employment News by the concerned authority.
3. Some PSUs in India have expressed their interest to utilize GATE scores for their recruitment purpose. The Organizations who intend to utilize GATE scores shall make separate advertisement for this purpose in Newspapers etc.

Who Can Appear for GATE?

Eligibility for GATE

Before starting the application process, the candidate must ensure that he/she meets the eligibility criteria of GATE given in Table.

Eligibility Criteria for GATE 2022

Degree/Program	Qualifying Degree/Examination	Description of Eligible Candidates	Expected Year of Completion
B.E. / B.Tech. / B.Pharm.	Bachelor's degree in Engineering / Technology (4 years after 10+2 or 3 years after B.Sc. / Diploma in Engineering / Technology)	Currently in the 3rd year or higher grade or already completed	2022
B. Arch.	Bachelor's degree of Architecture (5- year course) / Naval Architecture (4- year course) / Planning (4- year course)	Currently in the 3rd year or higher grade or already completed	2023 (for 5-year program), 2022 (for 4-year program)
B.Sc. (Research) / B.S.	Bachelor's degree in Science (Post-Diploma/4 years after 10+2)	Currently in the 3rd year or higher grade or already completed	2022
Pharm. D. (after 10+2)	6 years degree program, consisting of internship or residency training, during third year onwards	Currently in the 3rd/4th/5th/6th year or already completed	2024
M.B.B.S.	Degree holders of M.B.B.S. and those who are in the 5th/6th/7th semester or higher semester of such programme.	5th, 6th, 7th or higher semester or already completed	2022
M. Sc. / M.A. / MCA or equivalent	Master's degree in any branch of Arts/Science/Mathematics/Statistics/ Computer Applications or equivalent	Currently in the first year or higher or already Completed	2022
Int. M.E./ M.Tech. (Post-B.Sc.)	Post-B.Sc Integrated Master's degree programs in Engineering/ Technology (4-year program)	Currently in the 1st / 2nd/3rd/4th year or already completed	2024
Int. M.E./ M.Tech. or Dual Degree (after Diploma or 10+2)	Integrated Master's degree program or Dual Degree program in Engineering/Technology (5-year program)	Currently in the 3rd /4th/5th year or alreadycompleted	2023
B.Sc. / B.A. / B.Com.	Bachelor degree in any branch of Science / Arts / Commerce (3 years program)	Currently in the 3rd year or already completed	2021
Int. M.Sc. / Int. B.S. / M.S.	Integrated M.Sc. or 5-year integrated B.S.-M.S. program	Currently in the 3rd year or higher or already completed	2022
Professional Society Examinations (equivalent to B.E. / B.Tech. / B.Arch.)	B.E./B.Tech./B.Arch. equivalent examinations of Professional Societies, recognized by MoE/UPSC/AICTE (e.g. AMIE by Institution of Engineers-India, AMICE by the Institute of Civil Engineers-India and so on)	Completed Section A or equivalent of such professional courses	NA

In case a candidate has passed one of the qualifying examinations as mentioned above in 2020 or earlier, the candidate has to submit the degree certificate / provisional certificate / course completion certificate / professional certificate / membership certificate issued by the society or institute. In case, the candidate is expected to complete one of the qualifying criteria in 2022 or later as mentioned above, he/she has to submit a certificate from Principal or a copy of marks card for section A of AMIE.

Certificate From Principal

Candidates who have to submit a certificate from their college Principal have to obtain one from his/her institution beforehand and upload the same during the online submission of the application form.

Candidates With Backlogs

Candidates, who have appeared in the final semester/year exam in 2022, but with a backlog (arrears/failed subjects) in any of the papers in their qualifying degree should upload a copy of any one of the mark sheets of the final year,

OR

obtain a declaration from their Principal along with the signature and seal beforehand and upload the same during the online submission of the application form.

GATE Structure

Structure of GATE

GATE 2022 will be conducted on 27 subjects (papers). Table below shows the list of papers and paper codes for GATE 2022. A candidate is allowed to appear in ANY ONE or UP TO TWO papers of the GATE examination. However, note that the combination of TWO papers in which a candidate can appear MUST be from the pre-defined list as given in Table. Also note that for a paper running in multiple sessions, a candidate will be mapped to appear for the examination in one of the sessions ONLY.

List of GATE Papers and Corresponding Codes

GATE Paper	Code	GATE Paper	Code
Aerospace Engineering	AE	Instrumentation Engineering	IN
Agricultural Engineering	AG	Mathematics	MA
Architecture and Planning	AR	Mechanical Engineering	ME
Bio-medical Engineering	BM	Mining Engineering	MN
Biotechnology	BT	Metallurgical Engineering	MT
Civil Engineering	CE	Petroleum Engineering	PE
Chemical Engineering	CH	Physics	PH
Computer Science and Information Technology	CS	Production and Industrial Engineering	PI
Chemistry	CY	Statistics	ST
Electronics and Communication Engineering	EC	Textile Engineering and Fibre Science	TF
Electrical Engineering	EE	Engineering Sciences	XE*
Environmental Science & Engineering	ES	Humanities & Social Sciences	XH**
Ecology and Evolution	EY	Life Sciences	XL***
Geology and Geophysics	GG		

Note: *Environmental Science and Engineering (ES) and Humanities and Social Sciences (XH) are two new papers introduced in GATE 2022.*

*XE Paper Sections	Code	**XH Paper Sections	Code	***XL Paper Sections	Code
Engineering Mathematics (Compulsory) (15 marks)	A	Reasoning and Comprehension (Compulsory) (25 marks)	B1	Chemistry (Compulsory) (25 marks)	P
Any TWO optional Sections (2x35 = 70 marks)		Any ONE optional Section (60 marks)		Any TWO optional Sections (2x30 = 60 marks)	
Fluid Mechanics	B	Economics	C1	Biochemistry	Q
Materials Science	C	English	C2	Botany	R
Solid Mechanics	D	Linguistics	C3	Microbiology	S
Thermodynamics	E	Philosophy	C4	Zoology	T
Polymer Science and Engineering	F	Psychology	C5	Food Technology	U
Food Technology	G	Sociology	C6		
Atmospheric and Oceanic Sciences	H				

*XE (Engineering Sciences), **XH (Humanities & Social Sciences), ***XL (Life Sciences), papers are of general nature and will be comprised of Sections listed in the above table

Note: *Each subject / paper is of total 100 marks. General Aptitude (GA) section of 15 marks is common for all papers. Hence remaining 85 marks are for the respective subject / paper code.*

Combination of Two Papers Allowed to Appear in GATE 2022 (subject to availability of infrastructure and schedule)

Code of The First (Primary) Paper	Codes of Papers Allowed as The Second Paper
AE	XE
AG	ES
AR	CE
BM	BT / XL
BT	BM / XL
CE	AR / ES
CH	CY / PE / XE
CS	MA
CY	CH / XL
EC	IN / PH
EE	IN
ES	AG / CE
EY	XL
GG	MN / PE / PH
IN	EC / EE / PH
MA	CS / PH / ST
ME	XE
MN	GG / XE
MT	PH / XE
PE	CH / GG / XE
PH	EC / GG / IN / MA / MT / ST
PI	XE
ST	MA / PH
TF	XE
XE	AE / CH / ME / MN / MT / PE / PI / TF
XH	----
XL	BM / BT / CY / EY

General Aptitude Questions

All the papers will have a few questions that test the General Aptitude (Language and Analytical Skills), apart from the core subject of the paper.

Duration and Examination Type

All the papers of the GATE 2022 examination will be for 3 hours duration and they consist of 65 questions for a total of 100 marks. Since the examination is an ONLINE computer based test (CBT), at the end of the stipulated time (3-hours), the computer screen will automatically close the examination inhibiting any further action.

Candidates will be permitted to occupy their allotted seats 40 minutes before the scheduled start of the examination. Candidates can login and start reading the instructions 20 minutes before the start of examination. The late login time (if any) recorded by the computer system MUST NOT be beyond 30 minutes from the actual starting time of the examination. Under NO circumstances, will a candidate be permitted to login after 30 minutes from the actual examination starting time. Candidates will NOT be permitted to leave the examination hall before the end of the examination.

Pattern of Question Papers

GATE 2022 may contain questions of THREE different types in all the papers:

(i) **Multiple Choice Questions (MCQ)** carrying 1 or 2 marks each, in all the papers and sections. These questions are objective in nature, and each will have choice of four answers, out of which ONLY ONE choice is correct.

Negative Marking for Wrong Answers: For a wrong answer chosen in a MCQ, there will be negative marking. For 1-mark MCQ, 1/3 mark will be deducted for a wrong answer. Likewise, for 2-mark MCQ, 2/3 mark will be deducted for a wrong answer.

(ii) **Multiple Select Questions (MSQ)** carrying 1 or 2 marks each in all the papers and sections. These questions are objective in nature, and each will have choice of four answers, out of which ONE or MORE than ONE choice(s) is / are correct.

Note: There is NO negative marking for a wrong answer in MSQ questions. However, there is NO partial credit for choosing partially correct combinations of choices or any single wrong choice.

(iii) **Numerical Answer Type (NAT)** Questions carrying 1 or 2 marks each in most of the papers and sections. For these questions, the answer is a signed real number, which needs to be entered by the candidate using the virtual numeric keypad on the monitor (keyboard of the computer will be disabled). No choices will be shown for these types of questions. The answer can be a number such as 10 or –10 (an integer only). The answer may be in decimals as well, for example, 10.1 (one decimal) or 10.01 (two decimals) or –10.001 (three decimals). These questions will be mentioned with, up to which decimal places, the candidates need to present the answer. Also, for some NAT type problems an appropriate range will be considered while evaluating these questions so that the candidate is not unduly penalized due to the usual round-off errors. Candidates are advised to do the rounding off at the end of the calculation (not in between steps). Wherever required and possible, it is better to give NAT answer up to a maximum of three decimal places.

Note: *There is NO negative marking for a wrong answer in NAT questions. Also, there is NO partial credit in NAT questions.*

Marking Scheme – Distribution of Marks and Questions

General Aptitude (GA) Questions

In all papers, GA questions carry a total of 15 marks. The GA section includes 5 questions carrying 1-mark each (sub-total 5 marks) and 5 questions carrying 2-marks each (sub-total 10 marks).

Question Papers other than GG, XE, XH and XL

These papers would contain 25 questions carrying 1-mark each (sub-total 25 marks) and 30 questions carrying 2-marks each (sub-total 60 marks) consisting of some MCQ type questions, while the remaining may be MSQ and / or NAT questions.

GG (Geology and Geophysics) Paper

Apart from the General Aptitude (GA) section, the GG question paper consists of two parts: Part A and Part B. Part A is compulsory for all the candidates. Part B contains two sections: Section 1 (Geology) and Section 2 (Geophysics). Candidates will have to attempt questions in Part A and questions in either Section 1 or Section 2 of Part B. The choice of Section 1 OR Section 2 of Part B has to be made at the time of online registration in GOAPS. At the examination hall, candidate cannot request for change of section.

Part A consists of 25 questions carrying 1-mark each (sub-total 25 marks and some of these will be MSQ and/or numerical answer type questions while remaining questions will be MCQ type). Either section of Part B (Section 1 and Section 2) consists of 30 questions carrying 2-marks each (sub-total 60 marks and some of these will be MSQ and/or numerical answer type questions while remaining questions will be MCQ type).

XE Paper (Engineering Sciences)

A candidate appearing in the XE paper has to answer the following:

- GA – General Aptitude carrying a total of 15 marks.
- Section A – Engineering Mathematics (Compulsory): This section contains 11 questions carrying a total of 15 marks: 7 questions carrying 1-mark each (sub-total 7 marks), and 4 questions carrying 2-marks each (sub-total 8 marks). Some questions will be of numerical answer type while remaining questions will be MCQ type.
- Any two of XE Sections B to H: The choice of two sections from B to H can be made during the examination after viewing the questions. Only TWO optional sections can be answered at a time. A candidate wishing to change midway of the examination to another optional section must first choose to deselect one of the previously chosen optional sections (B to H). Each of the optional sections of the XE paper (Sections B through H) contains 22 questions carrying a total of 35 marks: 9 questions carrying 1-mark each (sub-total 9 marks) and 13 questions carrying 2-marks each (sub-total 26 marks). Some questions will be of MSQ and/or numerical answer type while remaining questions will be MCQ type.

XH Paper (Humanities and Social Sciences)

A candidate appearing in the XH paper has to answer the following:

- **GA – General Aptitude** carrying a total of 15 marks.
- **Section B1 – Reasoning and Comprehension (Compulsory):** This section contains

15 questions carrying a total of 25 marks: 5 questions carrying 1-mark each (sub-total 5 marks) and 10 questions carrying 2-marks each (sub-total 20 marks). Some questions will be of MSQ and/or numerical answer type while remaining questions will be MCQ type.

- **Any ONE of XH Sections C1 to C6:** The ONE choice of section from C1 to C6 has to be made at the time of online registration in GOAPS. At the examination hall, candidate cannot request for change of section. Each of the optional sections of the XH paper (Sections C1 through C6) contains 40 questions carrying a total of 60 marks: 20 questions carrying 1-mark each (sub-total 20 marks) and 20 questions carrying 2-marks each (sub-total 40 marks). Some questions will be of MSQ and/or numerical answer type while remaining questions will be MCQ type.

XL Paper (Life Sciences)

A candidate appearing in the XL paper has to answer the following:

- **GA – General Aptitude** carrying a total of 15 marks.
- **Section P–Chemistry (Compulsory):** This section contains 15 questions carrying a total of 25 marks: 5 questions carrying 1-mark each (sub-total 5 marks) and 10 questions carrying 2-marks each (sub-total 20 marks). Some questions will be of MSQ and/or numerical answer type while remaining questions will be MCQ type.
- **Any two of XL Sections Q to U:** The choice of two sections from Q to U can be made during the examination after viewing the questions. Only TWO optional sections can be answered at a time. A candidate wishing to change midway of the examination to another optional section must first choose to deselect one of the previously chosen optional sections (Q to U). Each of the optional sections of the XL paper (Sections Q through U) contains 20 questions carrying a total of 30 marks: 10 questions carrying 1-mark each (sub-total 10 marks) and 10 questions carrying 2-marks each (sub-total 20 marks). Some questions will be of MSQ and/or numerical answer type while remaining questions will be MCQ type.

GATE Score

After the evaluation of the answers, the actual (raw) marks obtained by a candidate will be considered for computing the GATE Score. For multi-session papers (subjects), raw marks obtained by the candidates in different sessions will be converted to Normalized marks for that particular subject. Thus, raw marks (for single session papers) or normalized marks (for multi-session papers) will be used for computing the GATE Score, based on the qualifying marks.

Calculation of Normalized Marks for Multi-Session Papers

In GATE 2022 examination, some papers may be conducted in multi-sessions. Hence, for these papers, a suitable normalization is applied to take into account any variation in the difficulty levels of the question papers across different sessions. The normalization is done based on the fundamental assumption that "in all multi-session GATE papers, the distribution of abilities of candidates is the same across all the sessions". This assumption is justified since the number of candidates appearing in multi-session papers in GATE 2022 is large and the procedure for allocation of session to candidates is random. Further, it is also ensured that for the same multi-session paper, the number of candidates allotted in each session is of the same order of magnitude.

Based on the above, and considering various normalization methods, the committee arrived at the following formula for calculating the normalized marks for the multi-session papers.

Nsormalization mark of jth candidate in the ith session $\widehat{M_{ij}}$ is given by

$$\widehat{M_{ij}} = \frac{\bar{M}_t^g - M_q^g}{\bar{M}_{ti} - M_{iq}} (M_{ij} - M_{iq}) + M_q^g$$

where

M_{ij} : is the actual marks obtained by the jth candidate in i^{th} session

$\bar{M}_t^g$: is the average marks of the top 0.1% of the candidates considering all sessions

M_q^g : is the sum of mean and standard deviation marks of the candidates in the paper considering all sessions

$\bar{M}_{ti}$: is the average marks of the top 0.1% of the candidates in the ith session

M_{iq} : is the sum of the mean marks and standard deviation of the ith session

Calculation of GATE Score for All Papers

For all papers for which there is only one session, actual marks obtained by the candidates will be used for calculating the GATE 2022 Score. For papers in multi-sessions, normalized marks will be calculated corresponding to the raw marks obtained by a candidate and the GATE 2022 Score will be calculated based on the normalized marks.

The GATE 2022 score will be computed using the formula given below.

$$\text{GATE Score} = S_q + (S_t - S_q)\frac{(M - M_q)}{(\bar{M}_t - M_q)}$$

where

M : marks obtained by the candidate (actual marks for single session papers and normalized marks for multi-session papers)

M_q : is the qualifying marks for general category candidate in the paper

$\bar{M}_t$: is the mean of marks of top 0.1% or top 10 (whichever is larger) of the candidates who appeared in the paper (in case of multi-session papers including all sessions)

S_q : 350, is the score assigned to M_q

S_t : 900, is the score assigned to $\bar{M}_t$

In the GATE 2022 the qualifying marks (M_q) for general category student in each subject will be 25 marks (out of 100) or $\mu + \sigma$, whichever is larger. Here μ is the mean and σ is the standard deviation of marks of all the candidates who appeared in the paper.

After the declaration of results, GATE Scorecards can be downloaded by the GATE qualified candidates ONLY.

The GATE 2022 Committee has the authority to decide the qualifying mark/score for each GATE paper. In case of any claim or dispute with respect to GATE 2022 examination or score, the Courts and Tribunals in Mumbai alone will have the exclusive jurisdiction to entertain and settle them.

GATE Syllabus

GENERAL APTITUDE (GA)

Verbal Aptitude

Basic English Grammar: tenses, articles, adjectives, prepositions, conjunctions, verb-noun agreement, and other parts of speech.

Basic Vocabulary: words, idioms, and phrases in context, Reading and comprehension, Narrative sequencing.

Quantitative Aptitude

Data Interpretation: data graphs (bar graphs, pie charts, and other graphs representing data), 2-and 3-dimensional plots, maps, and tables.

Numerical Computation and Estimation: ratios, percentages, powers, exponents and logarithms, permutations and combinations, and series, Mensuration and geometry, Elementary statistics and probability.

Analytical Aptitude

Logic: Deduction and induction, Analogy, Numerical relations and reasoning.

Spatial Aptitude

Transformation of shapes: translation, rotation, scaling, mirroring, assembling, and grouping Paper folding, cutting, and patterns in 2 and 3 dimensions.

XL - P CHEMISTRY (COMPULSORY FOR ALL XL CANDIDATES)

Section 1: Atomic Structure and Periodicity

Planck's quantum theory, wave particle duality, uncertainty principle, comparison between Bohr's model and quantum mechanical model of hydrogen atom, electronic configuration of atoms and ions. Hund's rule and Pauli fs exclusion principle.

Periodic table and periodic properties: ionization energy, electron affinity, electronegativity and atomic size.

Section 2: Structure and Bonding

Ionic and covalent bonding, MO and VB approaches for diatomic molecules, VSEPR theory and shape of molecules, hybridization, resonance, dipole moment, structure parameters such as bond length, bond angle and bond energy, hydrogen bonding and van der Waals interactions. Ionic solids, ionic radii and lattice energy (Born-Haber cycle). HSAB principle.

Section 3: s, p and d Block Elements

Oxides, halides and hydrides of alkali, alkaline earth metals, B, Al, Si, N, P, and S. General characteristics of 3d elements. Coordination complexes: valence bond and crystal field theory, color, geometry, magnetic properties and isomerism.

Section 4: Chemical Equilibria

Osmotic pressure, elevation of boiling point and depression of freezing point, ionic equilibria in solution, solubility product, common ion effect, hydrolysis of salts, pH, buffer and their applications. Equilibrium constants (Kc, Kp and Kx) for homogeneous reactions.

Section 5: Electrochemistry

Conductance, Kohlrausch law, cell potentials, EMF, Nernst equation, thermodynamic aspects and their applications.

Section 6: Reaction Kinetics

Rate constant, order of reaction, molecularity, activation energy, zero, first and second order kinetics, catalysis and elementary enzyme reactions. Reversible and irreversible inhibition of enzymes.

Section 7: Thermodynamics

Qualitative treatment of state and path functions, First law, reversible and irreversible processes, internal energy, enthalpy, Kirchoff equation, heat of reaction, Hess's law, heat of formation. Second law, entropy and free energy. Gibbs-Helmholtz equation, free energy change and spontaneity, Free energy changes from equilibrium constant.

Section 8: Structure-Reactivity Correlations and Organic Reaction Mechanisms

Acids and bases, electronic and steric effects, Stereochemistry, optical and geometrical isomerism, tautomerism, conformers and concept of aromaticity. Elementary treatment of SN1, SN2, E1, E2 and radical reactions, Hoffmann/Saytzeff rules, addition reactions, Markownikoff rule and Kharasch effect. Elementary hydroboration reactions. Grignard's reagents and their uses. Aromatic electrophilic substitutions, orientation effect as exemplified by various functional groups. Identification of common functional groups by chemical tests.

Section 9: Chemistry of Biomolecules

Amino acids, proteins, nucleic acids and nucleotides. Peptide sequencing by chemical and enzymatic proteolytic methods. DNA sequencing by chemical and enzymatic methods. Carbohydrates (upto hexoses only). Lipids (triglycerides only). Principles of biomolecule purification-Ion exchange and gel filtration chromatography. Identification of these biomolecules and BeerLambert's law.

XL - Q BIOCHEMISTRY

Section 1:

Organization of life; Importance of water; Structure and function of biomolecules: Amino acids, Carbohydrates, Lipids, Proteins and Nucleic acids; Protein structure, folding / misfolding and function; Myoglobin, Hemoglobin, Lysozyme, Ribonuclease A, Carboxypeptidase and Chymotrypsin.

Section 2:

Enzyme kinetics, regulation and inhibition; Vitamins and Coenzymes; Bioenergetics and metabolism; Generation and utilization of ATP; Metabolic pathways and their regulation: glycolysis, TCA cycle, pentose phosphate pathway, oxidative phosphorylation, gluconeogenesis, glycogen and fatty acid metabolism; Metabolism of Nitrogen containing compounds: nitrogen fixation, amino acids and nucleotides. Photosynthesis, Calvin cycle.

Section 3:

Biochemical separation techniques: ion exchange, size exclusion and affinity chromatography, centrifugation; Characterization of biomolecules by electrophoresis; DNA- protein and protein . protein interactions; UV-visible and fluorescence spectroscopy; Mass spectrometry.

Section 4:

Cell structure and organelles; Biological membranes; Action potential; Transport across membranes; Membrane assembly and Protein targeting; Signal transduction; Receptor-ligand interaction; Hormones and neurotransmitters.

Section 5:

DNA replication, transcription and translation; DNA damage and repair; Biochemical regulation of gene expression; Recombinant DNA technology and applications: PCR, site directed mutagenesis, DNA-microarray; Next generation sequencing; Gene silencing and editing.

Section 6:

Immune system: Innate and adaptive; Cell of the immune system; Active and passive immunity; Complement system; Antibody structure, function and diversity; B cell and T Cell receptors; B cell and T cell activation; Major histocompatibilty complex; Immunological techniques: Immunodiffusion, immune-electrophoresis, RIA and ELISA, flow cytometry; monoclonal antibodies and their applications.

XL - R BOTANY

Section 1: Plant Systematics

Botanical nomenclature, history of plant taxonomy, diversity and classification of plants, APG system of plant classification; phylogenetics and cladistics, molecular taxonomy and DNA barcoding; Centers for plant taxonomy and herbaria in India.

Section 2: Plant Anatomy

Anatomy of root, stem and leaves, floral organs, embryo and young seedlings, Primary and secondary meristems, stellar organization, vascular system and their ontogeny, xylem and phloem structure, secondary growth in plants and wood anatomy, plant cell structure and differences from animal cells.

Section 3: Plant development; cell and tissue morphogenesis

Life cycle of an angiosperm, development of male and female gametophyte; cell fate determination and tissue patterning; spacing mechanisms in trichomes and stomata. Embryogenesis, organization and function of shoot and root apical meristems. Transition to flowering: photoperiodism and vernalization, ABC model of floral organ patterning, pollen germination, double fertilization, seed development; Xylem and phloem cell differentiation, photomorphogenesis; phytochrome, cryptochrome, phototropin. Role of auxin, cytokinin, gibberellins, and brassinosteroids on plant development.

Section 4: Plant physiology and biochemistry

Plant water relations, mechanisms of uptake and transport of water, ions, solutes from soil to plants, apoplastic and symplastic transport mechanisms. Mechanism of stomatal movements, nitrogen metabolism, photosynthesis; C3, C4 and CAM cycles, photorespiration, respiration: glycolysis, TCA cycle and electron transport chain. Plant responses and mechanisms of abiotic stresses including drought, salinity, freezing and heat stress, metal toxicity; role of abscisic acid in abiotic stresses. Structure and function of biomolecules (proteins, carbohydrates, lipids, nucleic acid), enzyme kinetics. Structure and biosynthesis of major plant secondary metabolites (alkaloids, terpenes, phenylpropanoids, flavonoids). Biosynthesis, mechanism of action and physiological effects of auxin, cytokinin, gibberellic acids, brassinosteroid, ethylene, strigolactone, abscisic acid, salicylic and jasmonic acid. Senescence and programmed cell death.

Section 5: Genetics and genomics

Cell cycle and cell division. Principles of Mendelian inheritance, linkage, recombination, genetic mapping; extra chromosomal inheritance; Introduction to epigenetics; gene silencing- transgene silencing, post transcriptional gene silencing, miRNA and siRNA; evolution and organization of eukaryotic genome structure, gene expression, gene mutation and repair, chromosomal aberrations (numerical: euploidy and aneuploidy and structural: deletion, duplication, inversion, translocation), transposons. Model organisms for functional genetics and genomics; Introduction to transcriptomics, proteomics and metabolomics.

Section 6: Plant Breeding, Genetic Modification, Genome Editing

Principles, methods-selection, hybridization, heterosis; male sterility, genetic maps and molecular markers, embryo rescue, haploid and doubled haploids, plant tissue culture: micropropagation, embryo culture and in vitro regeneration, somatic embryogenesis, artificial seed, cryopreservation, somaclonal variation, somatic cell hybridization, marker-assisted selection, gene transfer methods viz. direct and vector-mediated, generation of transgenic plants; Introduction to genome editing: CRISPR/Cas9, Cre-Lox system to generate chimeras; plastid transformation; chemical mutagenesis.

Section 7: Economic and applied Botany

A general account of economically and medicinally important plants- cereals, pulses, plants yielding fibers, timber, sugar, beverages, oils, rubber, pigments, dyes, gums, drugs and narcotics. Economic importance of algae, fungi, lichen and bacteria. Major Indian cash crops. Effect of industrialization on agricultural botany such as plastic on fiber economy. Genetically modified crops and its regulation eg. Bt cotton, Bt brinjal golden rice etc.

Section 8: Plant Pathology

Nature and classification of plant diseases, diseases of important crops caused by fungi, bacteria, nematodes and viruses, and their control measures (chemical and biological) mechanism(s) of pathogenesis, resistance: basal, systemic, induced systemic resistance, gene for gene concept. Molecular detection of pathogens; plant-microbe interactions: symbionts and mycorrhiza, pathogens and pests. Signaling pathways in plant defence response; salicylic acid (SA) and jasmonic acid (JA) in plant-pathogen and plant-herbivore interaction, necrosis; host-parasitic plant interaction (such as Cuscuta).

Section 9: Ecology and Environment

Ecosystems-types, dynamics, degradation, biogeochemical cycles, ecological succession; food webs and energy flow through ecosystem; vegetation types of the world, Indian vegetation types and biogeographical zones, climate and flora endemism; pollution and global climate change, speciation and extinction, biodiversity and conservation strategies, ecological hotspots, afforestation, habitat restoration; plant interactions with other organisms; epiphytes, parasites and endophytes.

XL - S MICROBIOLOGY

Section 1: Historical Perspective

Discovery of microbial world; Landmark discoveries relevant to the field of microbiology; Controversy over spontaneous generation; Role of microorganisms in transformation of organic matter and in the causation of diseases.

Section 2: Methods in Microbiology

Pure culture techniques; Principles of microbial nutrition; Enrichment culture techniques for isolation of microorganisms; antigen and antibody detection methods for microbial diagnosis; Light-, phase contrast-, fluorescence- and electron-microscopy; PCR, real-time PCR for quantitation of microbes; Next generation sequencing technologies in microbiology.

Section 3: Microbial Taxonomy and Diversity

Bacteria, Archea and their broad classification; Eukaryotic microbes: Yeasts, molds and protozoa; Viruses and their classification; Molecular approaches to microbial taxonomy and phylogeny.

Section 4: Prokaryotic Cells: Structure and Function

Prokaryotic Cells: cell walls, cell membranes and their biosynthesis, mechanisms of solute transport across membranes, Flagella and Pili, Capsules, Cell inclusions like endospores and gas vesicles; Bacterial locomotion, including positive and negative chemotaxis.

Section 5: Microbial Growth

Definition of growth; Growth curve; Mathematical expression of exponential growth phase; Measurement of growth and growth yields; Synchronous growth; Continuous culture; Effect of environmental factors on growth; Bacterial biofilm and biofouling.

Section 6: Control of Micro-organisms

Disinfection and sterilization: principles, methods and assessment of efficacy.

Section 7: Microbial Metabolism

Energetics: redox reactions and electron carriers; Electron transport and oxidative phosphorylation; An overview of metabolism; Glycolysis; Pentose-phosphate pathway; Entner-Doudoroff pathway; Glyoxalate pathway; The citric acid cycle; Fermentation; Aerobic and anaerobic respiration; Chemolithotrophy; Photosynthesis; Calvin cycle; Biosynthetic pathway for fatty acids synthesis; Common regulatory mechanisms in synthesis of amino acids; Regulation of major metabolic pathways.

Section 8: Microbial Diseases and Host Pathogen Interaction

Normal microbiota; Classification of infectious diseases; Reservoirs of infection; Nosocomial infection; Opportunistic infections; Emerging infectious diseases; Mechanism of microbial pathogenicity; Nonspecific defense of host; Antigens and antibodies; Humoral and cell mediated immunity; Vaccines; passive immunization; Immune deficiency; Human diseases caused by viruses, bacteria, and pathogenic fungi.

Section 9: Chemotherapy/Antibiotics

General characteristics of antimicrobial drugs; Antibiotics: Classification molecular mechanism of mode of action and resistance; Antifungal and antiviral drugs.

Section 10: Microbial Genetics

Types of mutation; UV and chemical mutagens; Selection of mutants; Ames test for mutagenesis; Bacterial genetic system: transformation, conjugation, transduction, recombination, plasmids, transposons; DNA repair; Regulation of gene expression: repression and induction; Operon model; Bacterial genome with special reference to E.coli; Phage λ and its life cycle; RNA ; mutation in virus genomes, virus recombination and reassortment; Basic concept of microbial genomics.

Section 11: Microbial Ecology

Microbial interactions; Carbon, sulphur and nitrogen cycles; Soil microorganisms associated with vascular plants; Bioremediation; Uncultivable microorganisms; basic concept of metagenomics and metatranscriptomics.

XL - T ZOOLOGY

Section 1: Animal Diversity

Distribution, systematics and classification of animals, phylogenetic relationships (based on classical and molecular phylogenetic tools).

Section 2: Evolution

Origin and history of life on earth, theories of evolution, natural selection, adaptation, speciation.

Section 3: Genetics

Basic Principles of inheritance, molecular basis of heredity, sex determination and sex-linked characteristics, cytoplasmic inheritance, linkage, recombination and mapping of genes in eukaryotes, population genetics, genetic disorders, roles of model organisms in understanding genetic principles.

Section 4: Biochemistry and Molecular Biology

Nucleic acids, proteins, lipids and carbohydrates; replication, transcription and translation, Krebs cycle, glycolysis, enzyme catalysis, hormones and their actions, roles of vitamins and minerals.

Section 5: Cell Biology

Basic principles of cellular microscopy, structure of cell, cytoskeletal organization, cellular organelles and their structure and function, cell cycle, cell division, chromosomes and chromatin structure.

Section 6: Gene expression in Eukaryotes

Eukaryotic genome organization and regulation of gene expression, transposable elements.

Section 7: Animal Anatomy and Physiology

Comparative physiology, the respiratory system, Muscular system, circulatory system, digestive system, the nervous system, the excretory system, the endocrine system, the reproductive system, the skeletal system.

Section 8: Parasitology and Immunology

Nature of parasite, host-parasite relation, protozoan and helminthic parasites, the immune response, cellular and humoral immune response.

Section 9: Development Biology

Gametogenesis, Embryonic development, cellular differentiation, organogenesis, metamorphosis, Model organisms used in developmental biology, genetic and molecular basis of development, stem cells.

Section 10: Ecology

The ecosystem, Animal distribution, ecological niche and its contribution to ecological diversity, the food chain, population dynamics, species diversity, zoogeography, biogeochemical cycles, conservation biology, ecotoxicology.

Section 11: Animal Behaviour

Type of behaviours, courtship, mating and territoriality, instinct, learning and memory, social behaviour across the animal taxa, communication, pheromones, evolution of behavior in animals.

XL - U FOODTECHNOLOGY

Section 1: Food Chemistry and Nutrition

Carbohydrates: structure and functional properties of mono-, oligo-, & poly- saccharides including starch, cellulose, pectic substances and dietary fibre, gelatinization and retrogradation of starch. Proteins: classification and structure of proteins in food, biochemical changes in post mortem and tenderization of muscles. Lipids: classification and structure of lipids, rancidity, polymerization and polymorphism. Pigments: carotenoids, chlorophylls, anthocyanins, tannins and myoglobin. Food flavours: terpenes, esters, aldehydes, ketones and quinines. Enzymes: specificity, simple and inhibition kinetics, coenzymes, enzymatic and non- enzymatic browning. Nutrition: balanced diet, essential amino acids and essential fatty acids, protein efficiency ratio, water soluble and fat soluble vitamins, role of minerals in nutrition, co-factors, anti-nutrients, nutraceuticals, nutrient deficiency diseases. Chemical and biochemical changes: changes occur in foods during different processing.

Section 2: Food Microbiology

Characteristics of microorganisms: morphology of bacteria, yeast, mold and actinomycetes, spores and vegetative cells, gram-staining. Microbial growth: growth and death kinetics, serial dilution technique. Food spoilage: spoilage microorganisms in different food products including milk, fish, meat, egg, cereals and their products. Toxins from microbes: pathogens and non-pathogens including Staphylococcus, Salmonella, Shebelle, Escherichia, Bacillus, Clostridium, and Aspergillums genera. Fermented foods and beverages: curd, yoghurt, cheese, pickles, soya-sauce, sauerkraut, idly, dose, vinegar, alcoholic beverages and sausage.

Section 3: Food Products Technology

Processing principles: thermal processing, chilling, freezing, dehydration, addition of preservatives and food additives, irradiation, fermentation, hurdle technology, intermediate moisture foods. Food pack aging and storage: packaging materials, aseptic packaging, controlled and modified atmosphere storage. Cereal processing and products: milling of rice, wheat, and maize, parboiling of paddy, bread, biscuits, extruded products and ready to eat breakfast cereals. Oil processing: expelling, solvent extraction, refining and hydrogenation. Fruits and vegetables processing: extraction, clarification, concentration and packaging of fruit juice, jam, jelly, marmalade, squash, candies, tomato sauce, ketchup, and puree, potato chips, pickles. Plantation crops processing and products: tea, coffee, cocoa, spice, extraction of essential oils and oleoresins from spices. Milk and milk products processing: pasteurization and sterilization, cream, butter, ghee, ice- cream, cheese and milk powder. Processing of animal products: drying, canning, and freezing of fish and meat; production of egg powder. Waste utilization: pectin from fruit astes, uses of by-products from rice milling. Food standards and quality maintenance: FPO, PFA, A-Mark, ISI, HACCP, food plant sanitation and cleaning in place (CIP).

Section 4: Food Engineering

Mass and energy balance: Momentum transfer: Flow rate and pressure drop relationships for Newtonian fluids flowing through pipe, Reynolds number. Heat transfer: heat transfer by conduction, convection, radiation, heat exchangers. Mass transfer: molecular diffusion and Flick's law, conduction and convective mass transfer, permeability through single and multilayer films. Mechanical operations: size reduction of solids, high pressure homogenization, filtration, centrifugation, settling, sieving, mixing & agitation of liquid. Thermal operations: thermal sterilization, evaporation of liquid foods, hot air drying of solids, spray and freeze-drying, freezing and crystallization. Mass transfer operations: psychometric, humidification and dehumidification operations.

GATE - 2021

XL : LIFE SCIENCES

Time : 3 Hours | ***Maximum Marks : 100***

GENERAL APTITUDE

Q. 1 – Q. 5 carry one mark each

1. Gauri said that she can play the keyboard ______ her sister.

(a) as well as (b) as better as

(c) as nicest as (d) as worse as

2. A transparent square sheet shown above is folded along the dotted line. The folded sheet will look like ______.

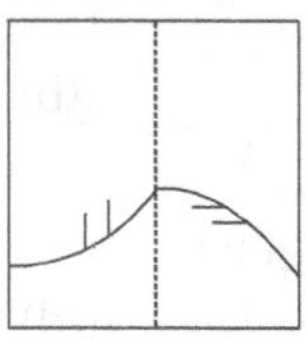

(a) 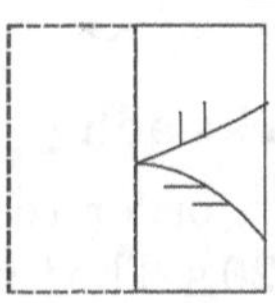 (b) 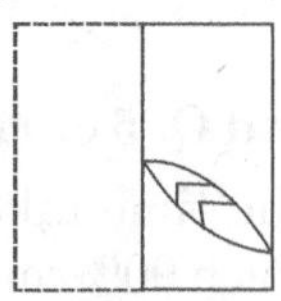

(c) 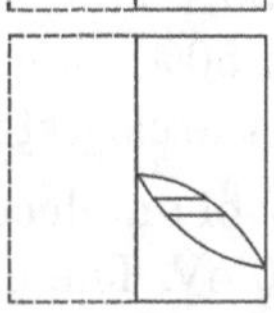 (d) 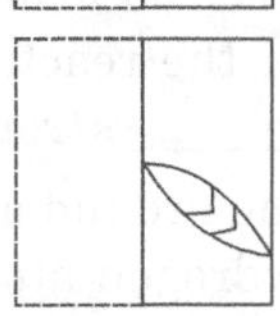

3. If θ is the angle, in degrees, between the longest diagonal of the cube and any one of the edges of the cube, then, cos θ =

(a) $\frac{1}{2}$ (b) $\frac{1}{\sqrt{3}}$

(c) $\frac{1}{\sqrt{2}}$ (d) $\frac{\sqrt{3}}{2}$

4. If $\left(x-\frac{1}{2}\right)^2-\left(x-\frac{3}{2}\right)^2 = x+2$, then the value of x is:

(a) 2 (b) 4

(c) 6 (d) 8

5. Pen : Write :: Knife : ______

Which one of the following options maintains a similar logical relation in the above?

(a) Vegetables (b) Sharp

(c) Cut (d) Blunt

Q. 6 – Q. 10 carry two marks each

6. Listening to music during exercise improves exercise performance and reduces discomfort. Scientists researched whether listening to music while studying can help students learn better and the results were inconclusive. Studens who needed external stimulation for studying fared worse while students who did not need any external stimulation benefited from music.

Which one of the following statements is the CORRECT inference of the above passage?

(a) Listening to music has no effect on learning and a positive effect on physical exercise.

(b) Listening to music has clear positive effect both on physical exercise and on learning.

(c) Listening to music has a clear positive effect on physical exercise. Music has a positive effect on learning only in some students.

(d) Listening to music has clear positive effect on learning in all students. Music has a positive effect only in some students who exercise.

7. A jigsaw puzzle has 2 pieces. One of the pieces is shown above. Which one of the given options for the missing piece when assembled will form a rectangle? The piece can be moved, rotated or flipped to assemble with the above piece.

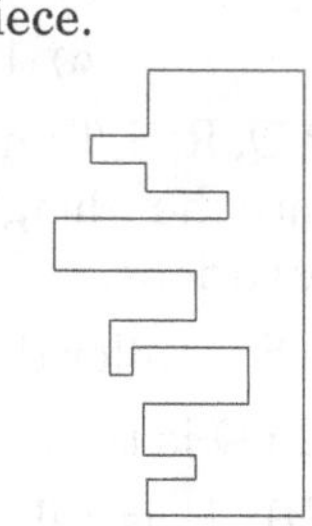

(a) 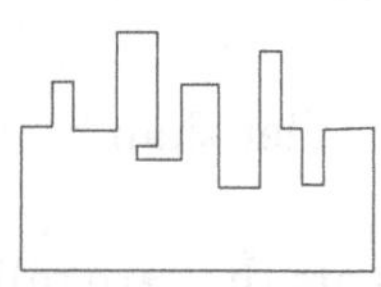 (b) 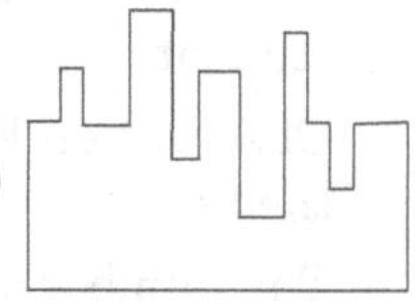

(c) 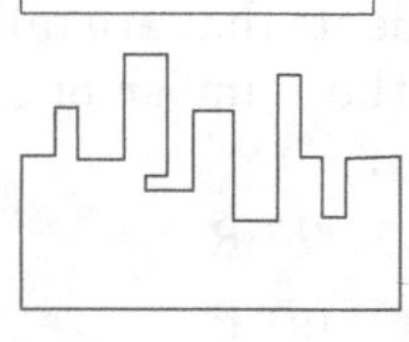 (d) 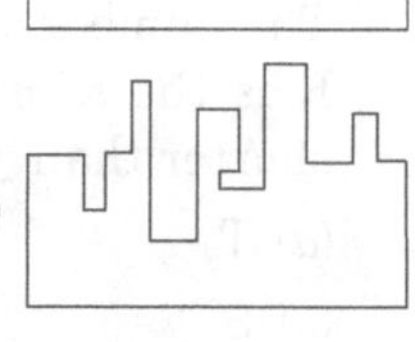

8. The number of students in three classes is in the ratio 3:13:6. If 18 students are added to each class, the ratio changes to 15:35:21.

The total number of students in all the three classes in the beginning was:

(a) 22 (b) 66

(c) 88 (d) 110

9. The number of units of a product sold in three different years and the respective net profits are presented in the figure below. The cost/unit in Year 3 was ₹ 1, which was half the cost/unit in Year 2. The cost/unit in Year 3 was one-third of the cost/unit in Year 1. Taxes were paid on the selling price at 10%, 13% and 15% respectively for the three years. Net profit is calculated as the difference between the selling price and the sum of cost and taxes paid in that year.

The ratio of the selling price in Year 2 to the selling price in Year 3 is _____.

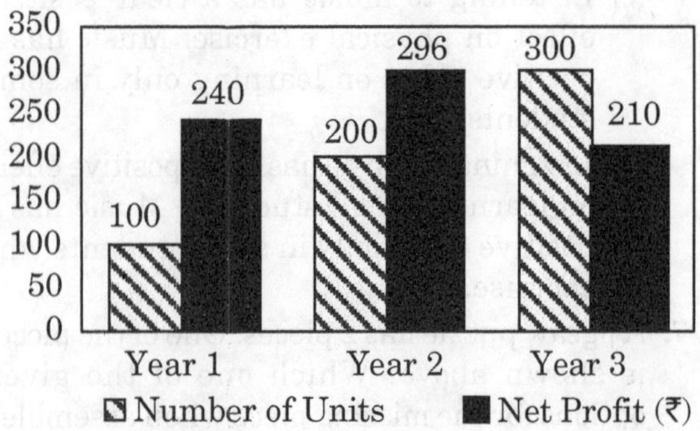

(a) 4:3 (b) 1:1

(c) 3:4 (d) 1:2

10. Six students P, Q, R, S, T and U, with distinct heights, compare their heights and make the following observations.

Observation I: S is taller than R.

Observation II : Q is the shortest of all.

Observation III: U is taller than only one student.

Observation IV: T is taller than S but is not the tallest.

The number of students that are taller than R is the same as the number of students shorter than _____.

(*a*) T (*b*) R

(*c*) S (*d*) P

CHEMISTRY

Q. 1 and Q. 2 carry one mark each

1. The geometry of $Fe(CO)_5$ is

(Given: Atomic number of Fe = 26)

(a) pentagonal planar

(b) square pyramidal

(c) trigonal bipyramidal

(d) trigonal pyramidal

2. The structure of the major product Q of the following reaction is

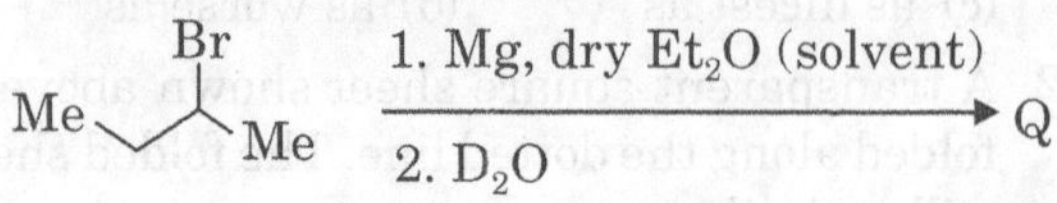

(a) 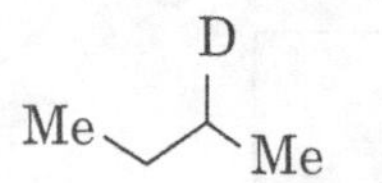

(b) 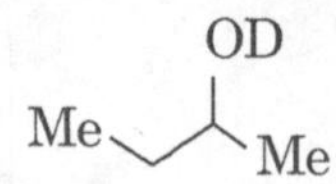

(c) 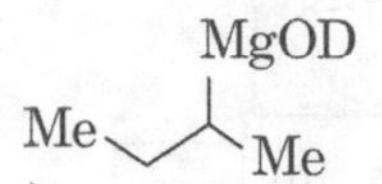

(d) 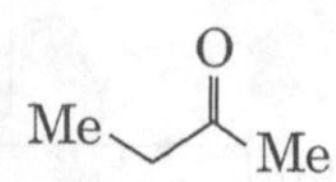

Q. 3 and Q. 5 carry one mark each

3. The time taken by a first order reaction to reach 90% completion is 20 s. The time taken for the reaction to reach 50% completion is _______s (rounded off to the closest integer).

4. The ground state energy of an electron in a hydrogen atom is –13.60 eV. The energy of the electron in the third excited state is _____ eV (rounded off to two decimal places).

5. A solution of a compound shows an absorbance of 0.42 at 275 nm in a cuvette with 0.1dm light path. The molar absorptivity of the compound is $\varepsilon_{275} = 8.4 \times 10^3\ M^{-1}\ cm^{-1}$. The concentration of the compound is _______ × 10^{-5} M(rounded off to the closest integer).

Q. 6 and Q. 9 carry two marks each

6. The CORRECT order of acidity of the following compounds is

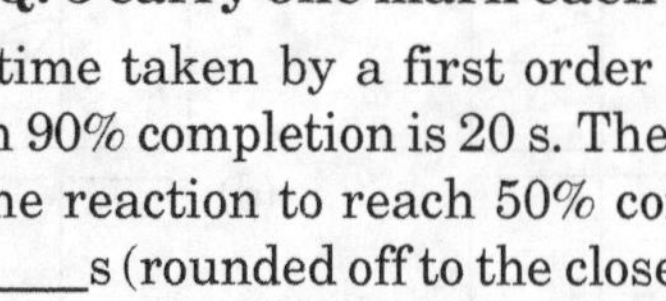

I II III

(a) II > I > III (b) II > III > I

(c) III > II > I (d) III > I > II

7. The O–O bond order in O_2^{2-} species is

(a) 0.5 (b) 1.0

(c) 1.5 (d) 2.0

8. For a reaction X → Products

Group I contains three plots of reactant concentrations as function of time, where x = concentration of reactant X at time t; $x0$ = concentration of reactant X at initial time, t = 0. Group II gives a list of different orders of reaction. Match the plots with the order of the reaction.

Group I	Group II
(P) 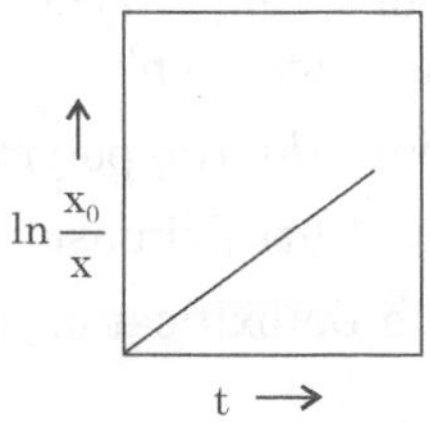	(1) Zero order
(Q) 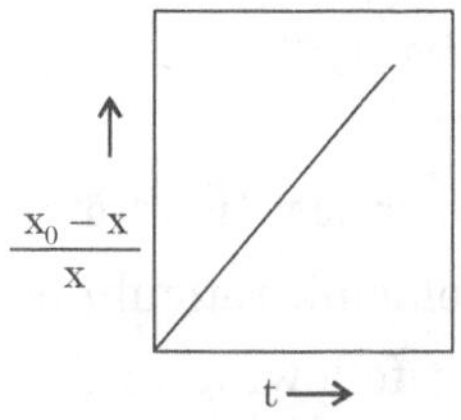	(2) First order
(R) 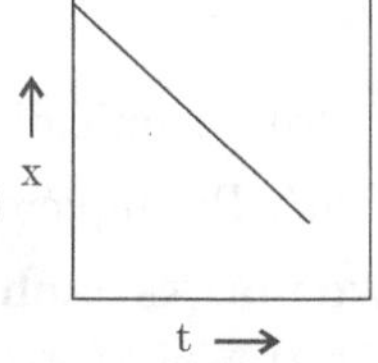	(3) Second order

(a) (P) - (1), (Q) - (2), (R) - (3)

(b) (P) - (3), (Q) - (2), (R) - (1)

(c) (P) - (2), (Q) - (3), (R) - (1)

(d) (P) - (2), (Q) - (1), (R) - (3)

9. The structure of the major product S of the following reaction is

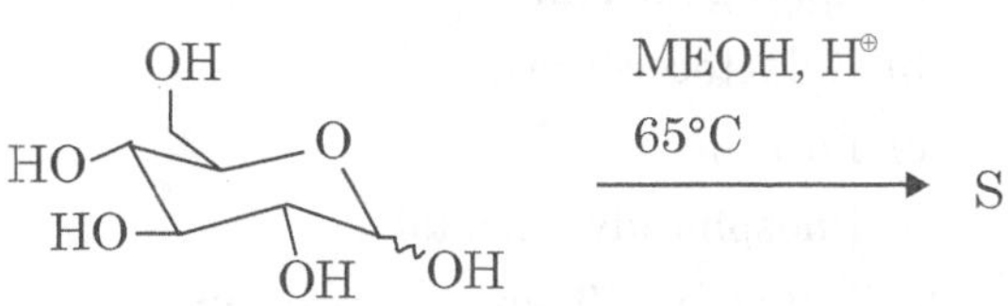

(a) 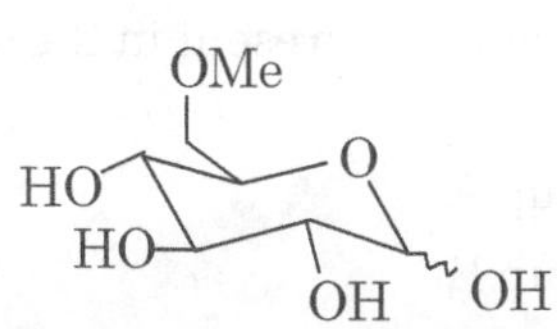

(b) 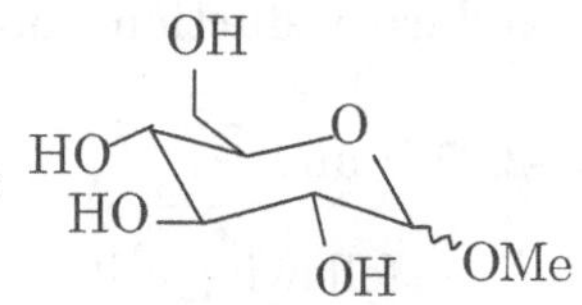

(c) 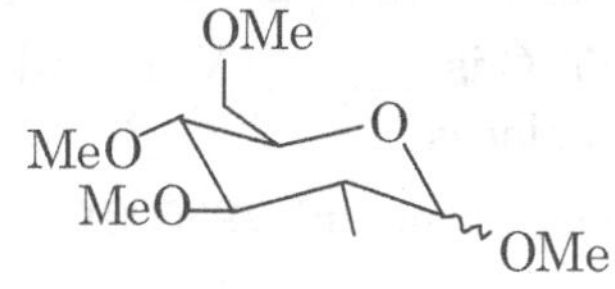

(d) 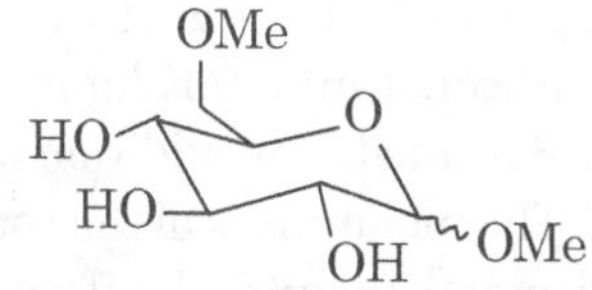

Q. 10 and Q. 11 carry two marks each

10. The CORRECT combination(s) of Y and T for the following elimination reaction is(are)

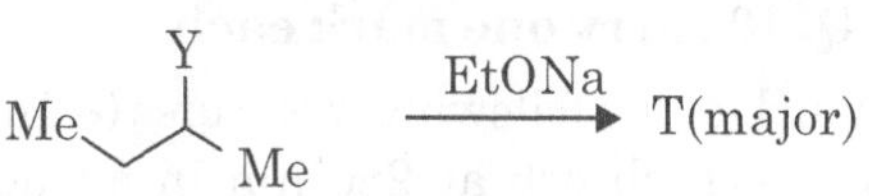

(a) $Y = \overset{\oplus}{N}Me_3$ and T = 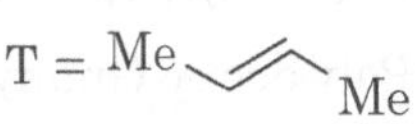

(b) $Y = \overset{\oplus}{N}Me_3$ and T = 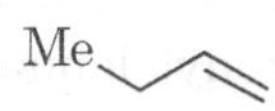

(c) Y = Br and T = 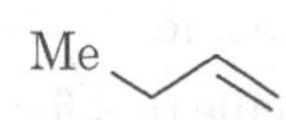

(d) Y = Br and T = 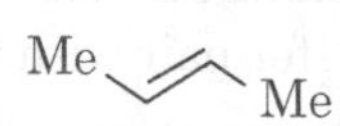

11. Among the following, the diamagnetic species is(are)

(Given: Atomic number of fe = z6, Co = 27 and Ni = 28)

(a) $[CoF_6]^{3-}$ (b) $[Ni(H_2O)_6]^{2+}$

(c) $[Fe(CN)_6]^{4-}$ (d) $[Co(NH_3)_6]^{3+}$

Q. 12 – Q. 15 carry two mark each

12. Given the following standard heats of formation, $\Delta_f H^{\ominus}(P, g) = 314.6$ kJ mol^{-1}, $\Delta_f H^{\ominus}(PH_3, g) = 5.4$ kJ mol^{-1}, and $\Delta_f H^{\ominus}(H, g) = 218.0$ kJ mol^{-1}, the average bond enthalpy of a P-H bond in $PH_3(g)$ is _____ kJ mol^{-1}, (rounded off to one decimal place).

13. The total number of possible geometrical isomer(s) for $[PtBrCl(NH_3)(py)]^0$ is _____.

(Given: py = Pyridine and atomic number of Pt = 78)

14. Given the standard reduction potentials,

$E^{\ominus}_{Mg^{2+}/Mg} = -2.37$ V and $E^{\ominus}_{Ag^{+}/Ag} = 0.80$ V,

the potential of the following cell

Ag^+ (aq. 1, mM) + Mg(s) $\rightleftharpoons$ Ag(s) + Mg^{2+} (aq., 0.2 M) at 25° C is ______ V (rounded off to two decimal places).

(Given: Faraday constant = 96500 C mol^{-1}, Gas constant R = 8.314J K^{-1} mol^{-1})

15. The freezing point of 80 g of acetic acid (freezing point constant 3.9 K kg mol^{-1}) was lowered by 7.8 K due to the addition of 20 g of a compound. The molar mass of the compound is ______g mol^{-1} (rounded off to closest integer).

BIOCHEMISTRY

Q. 1 – Q. 10 carry one mark each

1. Which of the following molecules (~ 1mg/mL) do NOT absorb at 280 nm in an aqueous solution of pH 7.00 at room temperature?

(*a*) Poly deoxy-Guanylate (poly dG)

(*b*) Adenosine triphosphate

(*c*) Phenylalanine

(*d*) Tyrosine

2. A molecule that forms a donor-acceptor energy transfer pair with the *dansyl* group is ____

(*a*) Aspartate (*b*) Histidine

(*c*) Lysine (*d*) Tryptophan

3. The stationary phase used in gel filtration chromatography is composed of ____

(*a*) Blue dextran

(*b*) Carboxymethyl (CM) cellulose

(*c*) Diethylaminoethyl (DEAE) cellulose

(*d*) Sepharose

4. According to the "*wobble hypothesis*" inosine at the third position of the anticodon cannot form hydrogen bonds with ____

(*a*) Adenine (*b*) Cytidine

(*c*) Guanine (*d*) Uracil

5. pKa value of the guanidinium group of Arginine is ____

(*a*) 4.30 (*b*) 7.40

(*c*) 9.20 (*d*) 12.50

6. The non-coenzyme vitamine is ____

(*a*) Ascorbic acid

(*b*) Folic acid

(c) Nicotinic acid

(*d*) Thiamine

7. Telomerase has a function similar to ____

(*a*) DNA dependent DNA polymerase

(*b*) RNA polymerase

(*c*) DNA gyrase

(*d*) Reverse transcriptase

8. Which one of the following enzymes is used in Polymerase Chain Reaction?

(*a*) *Klenow* fragment (*b*) *Taq* polymerase

(*c*) *T7* polymerase (*d*) Primase

9. In hepatocytes, the detoxification of drugs occurs in ____

(*a*) Golgi apparatus

(*b*) Nucleolus

(*c*) Rough endoplasmic reticulum

(*d*) Smooth endoplasmic reticulum

10. Which one of the following antibiotics can form an ion channel in the bacterial membrane?

(*a*) Ampicillin (*b*) Gramicidin A

(*c*) Gentamicin (*d*) Rifampicin

Q. 11 and Q. 12 carry Two marks each

11. Which one of the following cells lack hypoxanthine-guanine Phosphoribosyt transferase (HGPRT)

(a) B Cell (b) T Cell

(c) Macrophage (d) Myeloma Cell

12. Which of the following lipids is non-ionic?

(a) Sphingomyelin

(b) Galactocerebroside

(c) Lecithin

(d) Phosphatidyl inositol

Q. 13 – Q. 20 carry Two marks each

13. Anti-B antibodies are present in the serum of ____

(*a*) Blood group A

(*b*) Blood group B

(c) Blood group AB

(*d*) Blood group O

14. Which of the following are energy requiring processes?
   (*a*) Facilitated diffusion
   (*b*) Active transport
   (*c*) Nonmediated transport
   (*d*) $\frac{Na^+}{K^+}$ transport

15. Which of the following are correctly paired?
   (*a*) Replication: DnaA
   (*b*) Recombination: RecA
   (c) DNA repair : Rho factor
   (*d*) Transcription: Sigma factor

16. The high energy compound(s) is/are:
   (a) Phosphoenol pyruvate
   (b) Adenosine monophosphate
   (c) 1, 3-Bisphosphoglycerate
   (d) Vitamin K

17. Given below are four plots obtained from separate experiments on enzyme inhibition kinetics. The velocity (v) of the reaction is plotted at varying concentrations of substrate (s) and inhibitor (I). The plot(s) corresponding to competitive inhibition is/are

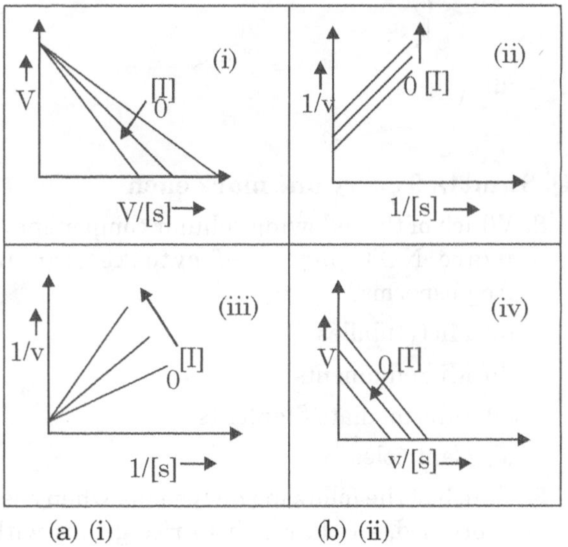

   (a) (i) (b) (ii)
   (c) (iii) (d) (iv)

18. With respect to sodium dodecyl sulphate - polyacrylamide gel electrophoresis (SDS-PAGE), which of these statement(s) is/are true?
   (a) Ethidium bromide is used to track the progress of electrophoretic mobility
   (b) β-mercaptoethanol is used to reduce disulphide bonds
   (c) The protein migrates towards the anode
   (d) The lower molecular weight protein migrates slower than the larger molecular weight protein

19. In the plot given below, the solid line represents oxygen binding to hemoglobin under physiological conditions. The broken line represents the condition(s) of

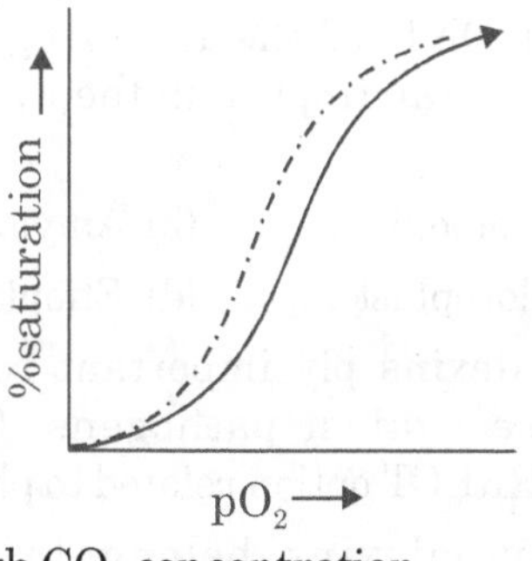

   (a) High CO_2 concentration
   (b) Increase in 2, 3-Bisphosphoglycerate concentration
   (c) High pH
   (d) Loss of cooperativity

20. Considering the open chain forms, which of the following pair(s) represent/s an epimer?
   (a) D-mannose and D-fructose
   (b) D-glucose and D-mannose
   (c) D-glucose and D-fructose
   (d) D-galactose and D-glucose

BOTANY

Q. 1 – Q. 7 carry one mark each

1. Wheat plants treated with prolonged cold temperature at the seedling stage flower eariler than the untreated control. Seeds collected from these treated individuals, however, give rise to plants that do not flower early. This phenomenon is called
   (a) vernalization
   (b) temperature acclimation
   (c) photoperiodism
   (d) adaptation

2. Which ONE of the following plant taxa contains vascular tissue (xylem and phloem) but not woody tissue?
   (a) Oak (b) Moss
   (c) Pine (d) Fern

3. Which ONE of the following statements regarding spores and gametes is CORRECT?
(a) Spores can directly undergo mitosis whereas gametes cannot.
(b) Gametes can directly undergo mitosis whereas spores cannot.
(c) Neither spores nor gametes can directly undergo mitosis
(d) Both spores and gametes can directly undergo mitosis.

4. Which ONE of the following organelles controls gravitropism in the roots of higher plants?
(a) Chromoplast (b) Amyloplast
(c) Chloroplast (d) Etioplast

5. Phytoalexins ply important role in plant defense against pathogens. Choose the INCORRECT option related to phytoalex ins.
(a) Phytoalexins belong to secondary metabolites
(b) Phytoalexins have antifungal activity.
(c) Phytoalexins are abundant in plants under normal condition.
(d) Different hosts produce phyallexins of varying chemical nature.

6. The figure shows the germination percentage of imbibed seeds treated with the given sequence of red (R) and far-red (F) light (each exposure lasting 5 min). The percentage of germination was scored after 72 hours in darkness at 25°C. Based on this, which ONE of the following options is CORRECT?

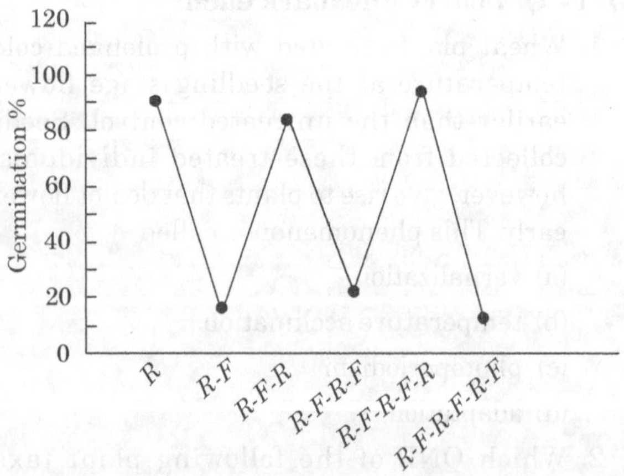

(a) Red light induces seed germination whereas far-red light inhibits it.
(b) Red light inhibits seed germination whereas far-red light induces it.
(c) Both red and far-red light inhibit seed germination.
(d) Both red and far-red light induce seed germination.

7. The structure of four plant hormones are shown. Identify the CORRECT hormone that is responsible for bending of coleoptiles of canary grass in response to unidirectional white light.

(a) 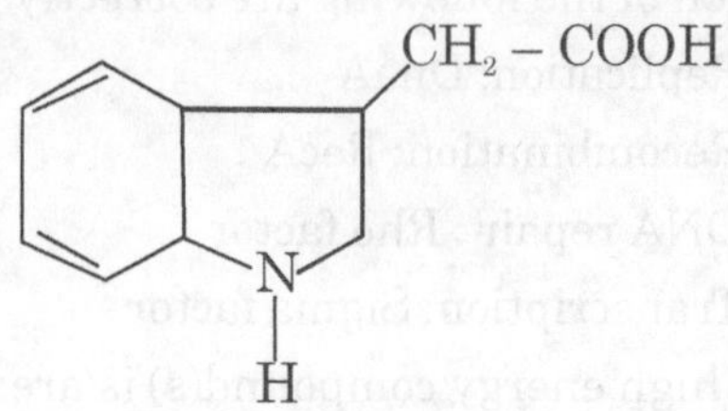

(b) 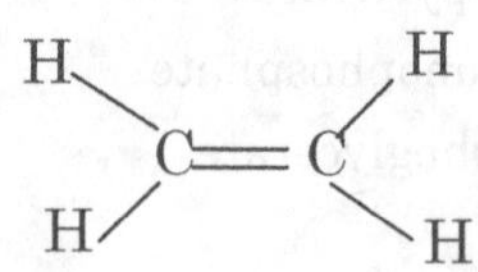

(c) 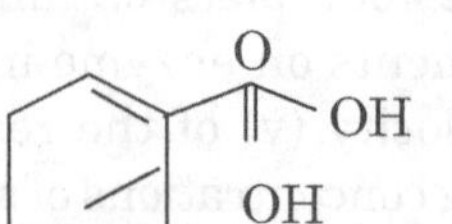

(d) 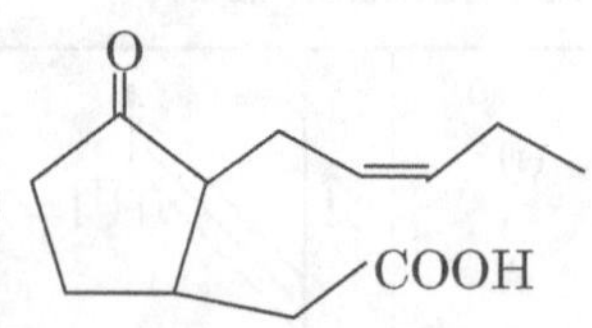

Q. 8 and Q. 9 carry one mark each

8. Which of the following cellular component(s) is/are NOT part(s) of cytoskeleton in Angiosperms?
(a) Microtubules
(b) Microfilaments
(c) Intermediate filaments
(d) Centrioles

9. Which of the following enzyme(s), when over expressed, would result in rice grains with increased β-carotene content?
(a) Phytoene synthase
(b) Carotene desaturase
(c) β-glucoronidase
(d) Enolpyruvalshikimate-3-phosphate synthase (EPSPS)

10. In spiral phyllotaxis, leaves are initiated sequentially on the meristem with two successive primordia being separated by golden angle. If a plant follows right-handed spiral phyllotaxis when looked down the meristem, then the angle between two successive leaves would be _____degrees (with correct sign, round off to one decimal place).

Q. 11 – Q. 15 carry two marks each

11. Match the cell/tissue types in GROUP I with their corresponding total DNA content in GROUP II of a typical diploid Angiosperm species and choose the CORRECT option (C denotes DNA content in haploid genome).

GROUP I	GROUP II
(P) Pollen tube	(1) 1C
(Q) Megaspore mother cell	(2) 2C
(R) Synergid	(3) 3C
(S) Embryo sac prior to fertilization	(4) 4C
	(5) 8C

(a) P-1,Q-2, R-3, S-5 (b) P-2, Q-2, R-1, S-5
(c) P-1, Q-2, R-1, S-5 (d) P-2, Q-1, R-2, S-4

12. Match the modified organs in GROUP I with their corresponding prototypic forms in GROUP II and choose the CORRECT option.

Group I	Group II
P. Tendrils in grape wine	1. Modified stem
Q. Tendrils in garden pea	2. Modified leaf
R. Spines	
S. Thorns	

(a) P-1, Q-2, R-2, S-1
(b) P-2, Q-1, R-1, S-2
(c) P-1, Q-2, R-1, S-2
(d) P-1, Q-1, R-2, S-1

13. The diagram describes the ABC model of flower patterning in Arabidopsis where the A, B and C functions are operational in the whorls (1+2), (2+3) and (3+4), respectively, in the wild-type flower. Removal of A or C function results in the floral organ arrangements as (carpel; stamen; stamen; carpel) or (sepal; petal; petal; sepal), respectively. Based on these observations, which ONE of the following molecular pathways is CORRECT for floral organ pattern generation? Arrow indicates activation and bar indicates inhibition.

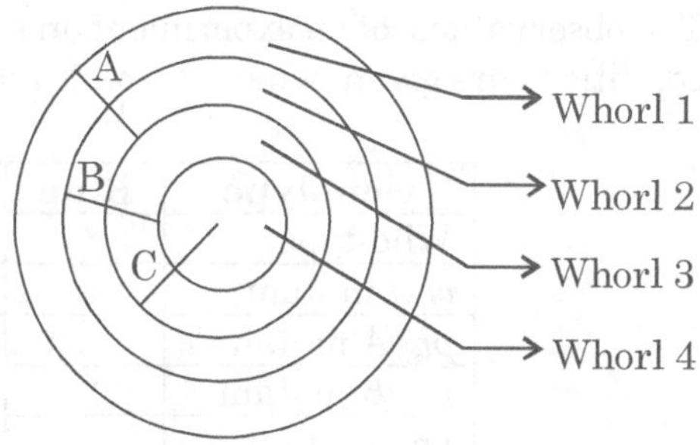

(a)
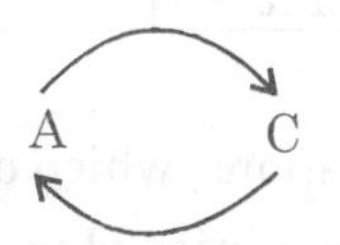

(b)
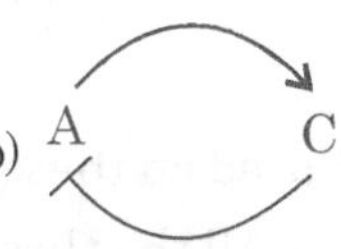

(c)
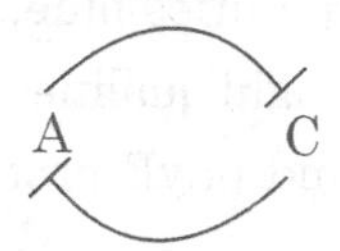

(d)
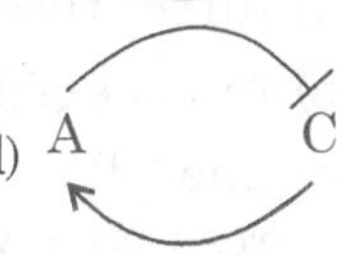

14. Find the CORRECT match among the plant species in GROUP I, the predominant phytochemical in GROUP II and the economic/medical use in GROUP III.

	GROUP I		GROUP II		GROUP III
P.	*Syzygium aromaticum*	i.	Vincristine	1.	Toothache relief
Q.	*Gracillaria sp.*	ii.	Eugenol	2.	Dessert jelly
R.	*Catharanthus roseus*	iii.	Agar	3.	Leukaemia treatment
S.	*Theobroma cacao*	iv.	Morphine	4.	Analgesic
T.	*Papaver somniferum*	v.	Flavonols	5.	Beverage

(a) P-i-1, Q-ii-3, R-iii-4, S-v-5, T-iv-2
(b) P-ii-1, Q-iii-2, R-i,3, S-v-5, T-iv-4
(c) P-ii-1, Q-iii-2, R-v,4, S-i-3, T-iv-5
(d) P-i-2, Q-ii-3, R-iv,1, S-iii-5, T-v-4

15. Match the genetically modified crop in GROUP I with the corresponding genetic element in GROUP II.

GROUP I	GROUP II
P. Tomato with delayed fruit ripening	1. EPSP synthase
Q. Herbicide-resistant soybean	2. Δ1 2-Desaturase-
R. Insect-resistant cotton	3. Polygalacturonase
S. Soybean with modified oil content	4. Bt-Cry protein

(a) P-3,Q-1, R-4, S-2
(b) P-1, Q-3, R-2, S-4
(c) P-2, Q-1, R-4, S-3
(d) P-3, Q-2, R-4, S-1

Q. 16 – Q. 18 carry two marks each

16. To understand the mechanism of systemic acquired resistance (SAR), a team of researchers isolated a mutant with reduced SAR response. Sequencing of this mutant revealed homozygous mutations in two genes, X and Y. Which of the following experiment(s) would test whether the mutant phenotype is caused by mutation in either or both the genes?

(a) Complement the mutant with X or Y and analyze the phenotype in each case.
(b) Complement the mutant with both X and Y and analyze the phenotype.
(c) Cross the mutant with wild-type and analyze the segregation pattern of the phenotype.
(d) Compare the expression of X and Y in mutant and wild-type plants.

17. The observations of an experiment on seed germination in various genotypes under different light conditions are given, where ✓ and X indicate germination and the lack of it, respectively.

Genotype	Blue	Red	Far-red	White	Dark
Wild-type	✓	✓	✓	✓	X
cryl mutant	X	✓	✓	✓	X
phyA mutant	✓	✓	X	✓	X
phyB mutant	✓	X	✓	✓	X
vp1 mutant	✓	✓	✓	✓	✓

Based on these observations, which of the following option(s) is/are CORRECT?

(a) All the three light qualities-blue, red and far-red – are required for seed germination.
(b) Any one of the three light qualities - blue, red and far-red – is sufficient to induce seed germination.
(c) The CRY1, phyA and phyB proteins are required for flue, red and far-red light perception, respectively.
(d) The VP1 protein is unlikely to be involved in light perception.

18. Which of the following option(s) is/are CORRECT in the context of hybrid plant generation using Barnase/Barstar-based male sterile lines?

(a) Barnase inhibits Barstar.
(b) Barstar inhibits Barnase.
(c) Barnase and Barstar are used to generate the male sterile line and the restorer line, respectively.
(d) Barnase and Barstar are used to generate the restorer line and the male sterile line, respectively.

Q. 19 and Q. 20 carry two marks each

19. In a diploid plant species, the *T* allele produces tall individuals and is completely dominant over the *t* allele that produces short individuals. Similarly,the *W* allele produces round seeds and is completely dominant over the w allele that produces wrinkled seeds (assume *T* and *W* loci not linked). If a parent with *TTWW* genotype is crossed to another parent with ttww genotype, the fraction of the F_2 population produced by the fusion of both recombinant gametes would be ______. (Round-off to two decimal places.)

20. In a population of a diploid plant species obeying Hardy-Weinberg equilibrium a locus regulating flower colour has two alleles R and r. Individuals with *RR*, *Rr* and *rr* genotypes produce red, pink and white flowers, respectively. If the ratio of red, pink and white flower-producing individuals in the population is 6:3:1, then frequency of r allele in the population would be ________%. (Round-off to two decimal places.)

MICROBIOLOGY

Q. 1 – Q. 5 carry one mark each

1. Antonie van Leeuwenhoek observed several microscopic organisms under his hand-made microscope. He described them as
   (a) Bacteria (b) Fungi
   (c) Animalcules (d) Bacteriophages.
2. Which ONE of the following pathways oxidizes 1 mole of glucose to 2 moles of pyruvic acid along with one mole each of ATP, NADH and NADPH, in *Pseudomonas* spp., but not in *Bacillus* spp.?
   (a) Gluconeogenesis
   (b) Embden-Meyerhoff Pathway (EMP)
   (c) Entner-Doudoroff (ED) Pathway
   (d) Pentose Phosphate Pathway (PPP)
3. Water balance in extreme halophiles such as *Halobacterium* is maintained by cell surface glycoproteins consisting of
   (a) glycine and lysine
   (b) lysine and histidine
   (c) glycine
   (d) aspartate and glutamate
4. *Nocardia* spp. are not amenable to the classical method of Gram staining due to the presence of
   (a) N-acetyltalosaminuronic acid in the cell wall.
   (b) thick peptidoglycan
   (c) mycolic acid.
   (d) keto-deoxy-octulosonic acid.
5. Protists belonging to the genus *Trichonympha* thrive in the gut of termites. They help the termites use wood as a food source. This relationship is an example of
   (a) parasitism (b) competition
   (c) commensalism (d) mutualism

Q. 6 – Q. 9 carry one mark each

6. Which of the following is/are used as electron donor/s for CO_2 reduction during photosynthasis in purple sulfur bcateria?
   (a) Hydrogen sulfide (b) Thiosulfates
   (c) Methane (d) Sulfates
7. Which of the following catalyze(s) substrate-level phosphorylation?
   (a) ATP synthase
   (b) Succinate thiokinase
   (c) Phosphofructokinase
   (d) Pyruvate kinase
8. Which of the following method(s) can be applied to identify a bacterial species?
   (a) Fluorescent in situ hybridization (FISH)
   (b) Polymerase chain reaction (PCR) followed by sequencing of the amplicon
   (c) Gram staining
   (d) Acid-fast staining
9. Which of the following event(s) would contribute to the induction of *lac* operon in a wild-type strain of *E.* **coli**?
   (a) Accumulation of allolactose in the cell
   (b) Direct binding of cAMP to the promoter DNA
   (c) Binding of cAMP to a specific protein leading to its interaction with the promoter
   (d) Elimination of cAMP from the cell

Q. 10 carry one mark

10. One mole of a circular bacterial plasmid was digested with a high-fidelity restriction enzyme. The plasmid has five restriction sites for the enzyme used. The number of moles of fragments released upon cleavage at all sites is ______.

Q. 11 – Q. 16 carry two marks each

11. Under anaerobic fermentative growth conditions, one mole of glucose yields 22 grams of *streptococcus faecalis* or 8.6 grams of *Zymomonas mobilis*. The molar growth yield (Y_{ATP}) for (i) S. *faecalis* and (ii) *Z. mobilis* will be
   (a) (i) 11 and (ii) 4.3 (b) (i) 22 and (ii) 4.3
   (c) (i) 22 and (ii) 8.6 (d) (i) 11 and (ii) 8.6

12. The order of abundance of quinones (ubiquinone [UQ], menaquinone [MQ] and demethylmenaquinone [DMQI]) in *E. coli* growing anaerobically on fumarate is

(a) UQ > DMQ > MQ

(b) MQ > DMQ > UQ

(c) MQ = DMQ > UQ

(d) MQ > UQ > DMQ

13. What is the number of ATPs generated per molecule of NADH during oxidative phosphorylation in *E.coli* via (i) NDH-1 and cytochrome bo complex or (ii) the NDH-2 and cytochrome bd complex?
(Assume $H^+/ATP = 3$)

(a) (i) 2.00 and (ii) 3.67

(b) (i) 3.00 and (ii) 2.67

(c) (i) 2.70 and (ii) 0.67

(d) (i) 2.50 and (ii) 0.50

14. Match the Immunoglobulin classes with their function

Immunoglobulin	Function
(i) IgE	(p) protects the fetus
(ii) IgG	(q) first antibody to be produced in response to infection
(iii) IgM	(r) provides localized protection of mucosal surfaces
(iv) IgA	(s) mediates allergic reaction
	(t) directly lyses the target cells

(a) (i) - (s), (ii) - (p), (iii) - (q), (iv) - (r)

(b) (i) - (p), (ii) - (t), (iii) - (q), (iv) - (r)

(c) (i) - (q), (ii) - (p), (iii) - (t), (iv) - (r)

(d) (i) - (r), (ii) - (p), (iii) - (t), (iv) - (s)

15. The figure shows the profiles of quantitative real-time PCR (qRT-PCR) tests for SARS-CoV-2 conducted on the throat swab samples of three individuals (X, Y and Z). Tests were carried out under identical conditions. Dotted line represents the threshold fluorescent value. Identify the correct statement on the status of the COVID-19 tests of the individuals based on their qRT-PCR profiles.

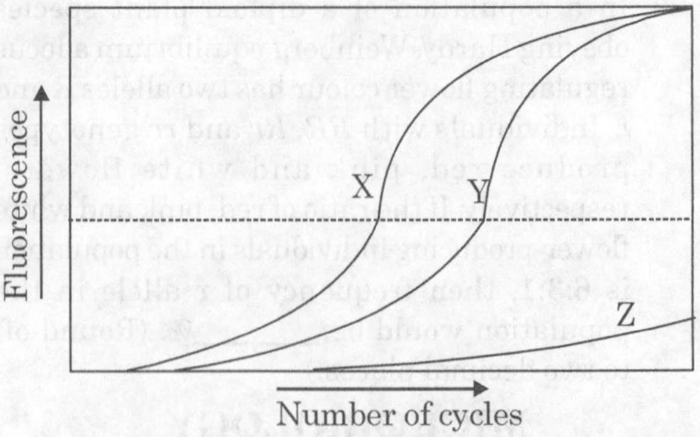

(a) X and Y are negative; Z is positive

(b) X and Y are positive; There is no apparent difference in their viral load

(c) X and Y are positive; X has the highest viral load

(d) X and Y are positive; Y has the highest viral load

16. The rate of appearance of recombinant *E.coli* strains containing different genes after a mating between Hfr and F^- strains is shown in the graph (left). The approximate location of different genes (p, q, r, s, t, x, and y) along the Hfr chromosome is also shown (right). Based on this information, identify the recombinants X, Y and Z.

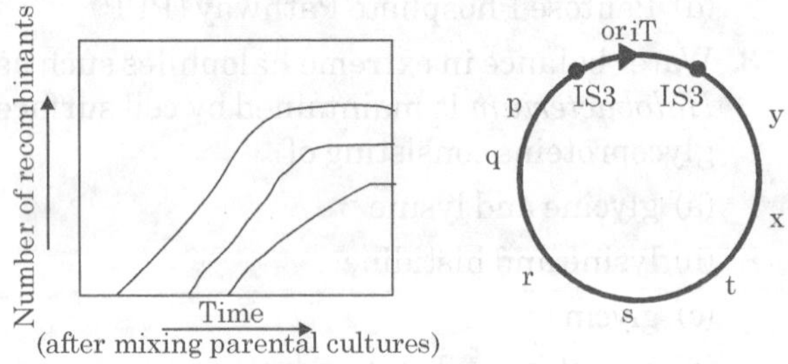

(a) X is x^+, Y is r^+ and Z is p^+.

(b) X is p^+, Y is r^+ and Z is x^+.

(c) X is x^+, Y is p^+ and Z is r^+.

(d) X is p^+, Y is x^+ and Z is r^+.

Q. 17 – Q. 20 carry two mark each

17. The genome of a bacterium encodes for 10 different surface antigens, whose expression can be turned 'ON' or 'OFF' randomly and independently. The number of possible antigenic combinations is ______.

18. Suppose the mRNAs in a newly discovered bacteria are composed of only two distinct nucleotides (as opposed to four found in all known organisms). Considering that the organism has no nucleotide modification systems, the number of nucleotides required per codon to encode at least 20 distinct amino acids will be ______.

19. The decimal reduction time (D) for reducing 10^{12} spores of *Clostridium botulinum* to 1 spore at 111°C will be______ min (in integer). The D value is 0.2 min at 121°C. The increase in temperature required to change D to $\frac{1}{10^{th}}$ of its initial value (Z value) is 10°C.

20. The generation time of E. coli is 30 minutes. For an exponentially growing culture, the initial number of bacteria required to reach a number of 10^9 in 2 hours is________$\times 10^7$ (round off to two decimal places).

ZOOLOGY

Q. 1 – Q. 7 carry one mark each

1. Ichthyophis belongs to which of the following Class?

(a) Mammalia (b) Reptilia
(c) Amphibia (d) Aves

2. The two homologous genes occurring in different species are called

(a) paralogous (b) orthologous
(c) pseudologous (d) prologous

3. The expression of holandric genes causes which of the following genetic trait in humans?

(a) Haemophilia
(b) Sickle cell anaemia
(c) Down's Syndrome
(d) Hypertrichosis

4. Assume that the anticodon for an unknown amino acid is 3′ AUG 5′. The corresponding code on DNA sequence would be

(a) 3′ TAC 5′ (b) 5′ TAG 3′
(c) 3′ ATG 5′ (d) 5′ ATG 3′

5. The Organ of Corti is found in which of the following parts of human body?

(a) Heart (b) Inner ear
(c) Kidney (d) Nasal cavity

6. In adult athletes, muscles grow larger when exercised and are capable of regeneration after injury. This is due to proliferation and differentiation of

(a) satellite cells (b) myelin sheath
(c) oxyntic cells (d) choanocytes

7. The term innate behavior is a sort of animal behavior that is

(a) triggered by an environmental change
(b) learnt by hit-and-trial approach
(c) trained and taught by the parent
(d) fixed developmentally at the genetic level

Q. 8 – Q. 10 carry one mark each

8. A man, whose mother and father had blood groups A and O respectively, marries a woman with blood group AB. If the man has blood group A, then the number of different blood groups possible among their children will be ________ (in integer).

9. A population of snakes in an isolated island is in Hardy – Weinberg equilibrium for a gene with only two alleles (A and a). If the allelic frequency of A is 0.6, then the genetic frequency of Aa is ________ (round off to 2 decimal places).

10. In the structure of a polypeptide, one α-helix (3.6_{13} helix) contains 32 intra-chain hydrogen bonds. The number of turns in the helix will be ________ (in integer).

Q. 11 – Q. 16 carry two marks each

11. Match the terms in Column I with the specific descriptions in Column II

Column I	Column II
P. Zygote	(i) A hollow sphere of cells
Q. Morula	(ii) A newly born offspring
R. Blastocyst	(iii) A cell that results from fertilization
S. Ovum	(iv) An embryo
T. Neonate	(v) An unfertilized egg
U. Fetus	(vi) A compact mass of cells

(a) P-(iii), Q-(vi), R-(i), S-(v), T-(ii), U-(iv)
(b) P-(v), Q-(ii), R-(iii), S-(vi), T-(i), U-(iv)
(c) P-(ii), Q-(iv), R-(vi), S-(v), T-(i), U-(iii)
(d) P-(iii), Q-(vi), R-(ii), S-(v), T-(iv), U-(i)

12. Match the autoimmune diseases in Column I for the self-antigens in Column II

Column I	Column II
P. Rheumatoid arthritis	(i) Myelin
Q. Systemic lupus erythematosus	(ii) Connective tissue
R. Myasthenia gravis	(iii) DNA
S. Multiple sclerosis	(iv) Acetylcholine receptors

(a) P-(i), Q-(ii), R-(iii), S-(iv)
(b) P-(ii), Q-(iii), R-(iv), S-(i)
(c) P-(iii), Q-(i), R-(iv), S-(ii)
(d) P-(iv), Q-(i), R-(ii), S-(iii)

13. Match the types of cell movements during gastrulation in Column I with the descriptions in Column II

Column I	Column II
P. Invagination	(i) Migration of individual cells from the surface into the embryo's interior
Q. Involution	(ii) Infolding of a sheet (epithelium) of cells during the formation of endoderm in sea urchin
R. Ingression	(iii) Splitting of one cellular sheet into two nearly parallel sheets
S. Delamination	(iv) Inward movement of an expanding outer layer of cells so that it spreads over the internal surface of the remaining external cells

(a) P-(ii), Q-(iii), R-(iv), S-(i)
(b) P-(iv), Q-(i), R-(iii), S-(ii)
(c) P-(ii), Q-(iv), R-(i), S-(iii)
(d) P-(iii), Q-(ii), R-(iv), S-(i)

14. Match the therapeutic factors in Column I with the applications in Column II

Column I	Column II
P. Humulin	(i) Cancer therapy
Q. Erythropoietin	(ii) Diabetes
R. Plasminogen activator	(iii) Osteoporosis
S. Cathepsin K inhibitor	(iv) Anaemia
T. Leptin	(v) Myocardial infraction
	(vi) Obesity

(a) P-(ii), Q-(iv), R-(v), S-(iii), T-(vi)
(b) P-(ii), Q-(v), R-(i), S-(iv), T-(iii)
(c) P-(v), Q-(vi), R-(iv), S-(iii), T-(i)
(d) P-(iii), Q-(iv), R-(ii), S-(v), T-(vi)

15. Match the cell organelles in Column I with the appropriate functions in Column II

Column I	Column II
P. Peroxisome	(i) Conversion of lipid to carbohydrate
Q. Endoplasmic reticulum	(ii) Oxidation of fatty acids
R. Glyoxysome	(iii) *N*-linked glycosylation
S. Golgi complex	(iv) Microtubule organization center
T. Centrioles	(v) *O*-linked glycosylation

(a) P-(ii), Q-(iii), R-(v), S-(i), T-(iv)
(b) P-(iv), Q-(v), R-(i), S-(ii), T-(iii)
(c) P-(iv), Q-(v), R-(iii), S-(i), T-(ii)
(d) P-(ii), Q-(iii), R-(i), S-(v), T-(iv)

16. Cohesin and Condensin proteins of eukaryotes belong to which one of the following groups?
(a) Structural maintenance of chromosomes (SMC) proteins
(b) Histones
(c) DNA polymerases
(d) Topoisomerases

Q. 17 – Q. 18 carry two marks each

17. Which of the following options represent the animals as Endemic to India?
(a) Pygmy Hog (b) Mountain Bongo
(c) Hirola (d) Purple Frog

18. Which of the following amino acids contain more than one chiral center?
(a) Leucine (b) Isoleucine
(c) Serine (d) Threonine

Q. 19 – Q. 20 carry two marks each

19. An enzyme catalyzes the conversion of 30 μM of a substrate to product at reaction velocity of 9.0 μM s^{-1}. When $[E_t]$ = 30 nM and K_m = 10 μM, K_{cat}/K_m of enzyme will be n × 10^7 $M^{-1}s^{-1}$. The value of n is _________ (in integer).

20. A cross is made between two animals of genotypes *AaBb x AaBb*, where loci *A* and loci *B* assort independently. The progeny of this dihybrid cross was then allowed to self-cross. The proportion of the progeny that showed segregation for loci *A* (i.e., produce *A*- and *aa* progeny) in % will be _________ (in integer).

FOOD TECHNOLOGY

Q. 1 – Q. 10 carry one mark each

1. In a typical bacterial growth curve, the first order kinetics for growth rate is observed in
(a) Lag phase (b) Log phase
(c) Stationary phase (d) Decline phase

2. Which of the following microorganisms is NOT a causative agent for food borne diseases?
(a) *Campylobacter jejuni*
(b) *Clostridium perfingens*
(c) *Norovirus*
(d) *Borrelia burgdorferi*

3. Which one of the following is NOT a fermented food product?
(a) Tofu (b) Vinegar
(c) Sauerkraut (d) Tempeh

4. The Protein Efficiency Ratio (PER) is defined as
(a) Percentage of absorbed nitrogen retained in the body
(b) Weight gain in body mass (in gram) per gram protein intake
(c) Ratio of essential and non-essential amino acids in a protein
(d) Percent *in vitro* digestibility of a protein

5. Which one of the following enzymes sequentially releases maltose from starch?
(a) α-Amylase (b) β-Amylase
(c) Glucoamylase (d) Pullulanase

6. Highest mole % of amino acid mixture present in glutenin of wheat gluten are
(a) Glutamine and glutamic acid
(b) Serine and lysine
(c) Alanine and tryptophan
(d) Proline and glycine

7. Which one of the following compounds is present in soybean and acts as phytoesterogen?
(a) Tangeretin (b) Lutin
(c) Quercetin (d) Genistein

8. Which one of the followings is an oligosaccharide?
(a) Xanthan (b) Alginate
(c) Raffinose (d) Gellan

9. Bittering agent in grape fruit formed after juice extraction under acidic conditions is
(a) Quinine (b) Theobromine
(c) Isohumulone (d) Limonin

10. Difference between adsorption and desorption isotherms is known as
(a) Hysteresis (b) Dryness
(c) Evaporation (d) Dehydration

Q. 11 – Q. 13 carry two marks each

11. The conversion of pyruvate to lactic acid in homolactic fermentation is catalyzed by
(a) Lactate dehydrogenase
(b) Pyruvate dehydrogenase
(c) Lactase
(d) Pyruvate decarboxylase

12. Which one of the following statement is INCORRECT with respect to Controlled Atmosphere Package (CAP) and Modified Atmosphere Package (MAP) of agro-produce?
(a) CAP and MAP limit microbial as well as biochemical activities.
(b) Gas composition inside a MAP during the storage is continuously monitored and regulated.
(c) CAP implies a greater degree of precision than MAP in maintaining specific levels of the gas composition.

(d) Modification of the atmosphere inside a MAP is achieved by natural interplay between respiration of products and permeation of gases through the packaging film.

13. Match unit operation in Column I with its application in food processing in Column II.

Column I	**Column II**
P. Hydrogenation	1. Removal of soft wax
Q. Blanching	2. Shortening of fat
R. Leaching	3. Inactivation of enzyme
S. Winterization	4. Separation of dye

(a) P-2, Q-4, R-2, S-1 (b) P-2, Q-3, R-4, S-1
(c) P-4, Q-1, R-2, S-3 (d) P-4, Q-2, R-1, S-3

Q. 14 – Q. 19 carry two marks each

14. Which of the followings are correct pair of GRAS chemical food preservative affected organism and given food matrix?

(a) Sodium lactate-Bacteria-Pre-cooked meat
(b) Caprylic acid-Insects-Cheese wraps
(c) Dehydroacetic acid-Molds-Squash
(d) Sodium nitrite-Clostridia-Meat curing preparations

15. Choose the correct pair of pigment and their corresponding color in plant Products

(a) Carotene-Yellow-orange-Peppers
(b) Betanin-Purple/red-Cactus pear
(c) Lycopene-Red-Red beets
(d) Flavanols-Orange-red-Cauliflowers

16. Which of the following compounds act as anti-nutritional factors?

(a) Phytate
(b) Isoflavones
(c) Trypsin Inhibitor
(d) Resveratrol

17. Which of the following is/are commonly used medium/media in the supercritical fluid extraction of spices and tea?

(a) Water
(b) Carbon dioxide
(c) Dichloromethane
(d) Carbon dioxide with Ethanol

18. Which of the following expressions represent the Reynolds number of a a fluid flowing through a uniform circular cross section pipe?

(a) $\dfrac{(\text{density of the fluid}) \times (\text{average velocity of the fluid}) \times (\text{internal diameter of the pipe})}{(\text{dynamic viscosity of the fluid})}$

(b) $\dfrac{(\text{average velocity of the fluid}) \times (\text{int ernal diameter of the pipe})}{(\text{kinematic viscosity of the fluid})}$

(c) $\dfrac{(\text{dynamic viscocity of the fluid})}{(\text{average velocity of the fluid}) \times (\text{density of the fluid}) \times (\text{int ernal diameter of the pipe})}$

(d) $\dfrac{(\text{kinematic vis cos ity of the fluid})}{(\text{average velocity of the fluid}) \times (\text{int ernal diameter of the pipe})}$

19. Which of the following combinations of analytical equipment, property measured and food property are correct?

(a) Particle size analyzer - particle size distribution - span value
(b) Texture profile analyzer - morphology - chewiness
(c) Differential scanning calorimeter - glass transition temperature - degree of caking
(d) Capillary viscometer - viscosity - sensory

Q. 20 carry two marks

20. Dry air is fed into a tray dryer. The percentage relative humidity of the air leaving the dryer is 60% at 70°C and 101.35 kPa. If saturated vapour pressure of water at 70°C is 31.2 kPa the humidity of the air leaving the dryer in kg water per kg dry air (round off to 3 decimal places) will be ______.
(Given : Molecular weight of water and air are 18.02 g mol^{-1} and 28.97 g mol^{-1} respectively)

ANSWERS

General Aptitude

1. (*a*)	**2.** (*b*)	**3.** (*b*)	**4.** (*b*)	**5.** (*c*)	**6.** (*c*)
7. (*a*)	**8.** (*c*)	**9.** (*a*)	**10.** (*c*)		

Chemistry

1. (*c*)	**2.** (*a*)	**3.** (6 to 6)	**4.** (-0.86 to -0.84)	**5.** (5 to 5)	**6.** (b)
7. (b)	**8.** (*c*)	**9.** (*b*)	**10.** (b, d)	**11.** (c, d)	
12. (321.0 to 321.2)		**13.** (3 to 3)	**14.** (3.00 to 3.02)	**15.** (125 to 125)	

Biochemistry

1. (*c*)	**2.** (*d*)	**3.** (*d*)	**4.** (*c*)	**5.** (*d*)	**6.** (*a*)
7. (*d*)	**8.** (*b*)	**9.** (*d*)	**10.** (*b*)	**11.** (*d*)	**12.** (*b*)
13. (*a*, *d*)	**14.** (*b*, *d*)	**15.** (*a*, *b*, *d*)	**16.** (*a*, *c*)	**17.** (*a*, *c*)	**18.** (*b*, *c*)
19. (*c*)	**20.** (*b*, *d*)				

Botany

1. (*a*)	**2.** (*d*)	**3.** (*a*)	**4.** (*b*)	**5.** (*c*)	**6.** (*a*)
7. (*a*)	**8.** (*c*, *d*)	**9.** (*a*, *b*)	**10.** (137.4 to 137.6 or -137.6 to -137.4)		
11. (*b*)	**12.** (*a*)	**13.** (*c*)	**14.** (*b*)	**15.** (*a*)	**16.** (*a*, *b*, *c*)
17. (*b*, *d*)	**18.** (*b*, *c*)	**19.** (0.25 to 0.25)	**20.** (25 to 25)		

Microbiology

1. (*c*)	**2.** (*c*)	**3.** (*d*)	**4.** (*c*)	**5.** (*d*)	**6.** (*a*, *b*)
7. (*b*, *d*)	**8.** (*a*, *b*)	**9.** (*a*, *c*)	**10.** (5 to 5)	**11.** (*d*)	**12.** (*b*)
13. (*c*)	**14.** (*a*)	**15.** (*c*)	**16.** (*b*)	**17.** (1024 to 1024)	
18. (5 to 5)	**19.** (24 to 24)	**20.** (6.20 to 6.30)			

Zoology

1. (*c*)	**2.** (*b*)	**3.** (*d*)	**4.** (*c*)	**5.** (*b*)	**6.** (*a*)
7. (*d*)	**8.** (3 to 3)	**9.** (0.48 to 0.48)	**10.** (10 to 10)	**11.** (*a*)	**12.** (*b*)
13. (*c*)	**14.** (*a*)	**15.** (*d*)	**16.** (*a*)	**17.** (*a*, *d*)	**18.** (*b*, *d*)
19. (4 to 4)	**20.** (50 to 50)				

Food Technology

1. (*b*)	**2.** (*d*)	**3.** (*a*)	**4.** (*b*)	**5.** (*b*)	**6.** (*a*)
7. (*d*)	**8.** (*c*)	**9.** (*d*)	**10.** (*a*)	**11.** (*a*)	**12.** (*b*)
13. (*b*)	**14.** (*a*, *d*)	**15.** (*a*, *b*)	**16.** (*a*, *c*)	**17.** (*a*, *b*, *d*)	**18.** (*a*, *b*)
19. (*a*, *c*)	**20.** (0.135 to 0.150)				

EXPLANATIONS

GENERAL APTITUDE

1. 'As well as' is used in positive degree.
2. The folded sheet is look like option (b).

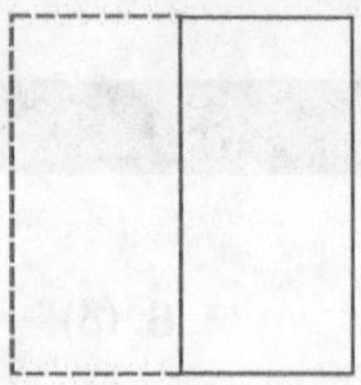

3.

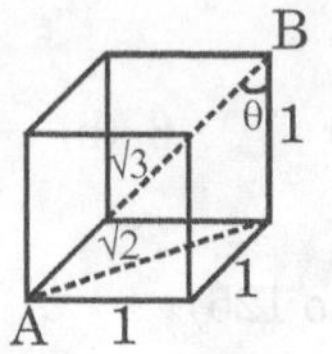

$$\cos\theta = \frac{BX}{AB} = \frac{1}{\sqrt{3}}$$

4. As we know that

$(a-b)^2 = a^2 + b^2 - 2ab$

As given expression

$$\left(x-\frac{1}{2}\right)^2 - \left(x-\frac{3}{2}\right)^2 = (x+2)$$

So,

$$\Rightarrow \left[x^2 + \left(\frac{1}{2}\right)^2 - 2(x)\left(\frac{1}{2}\right)\right] - \left[x^2 + \left(\frac{9}{4}\right) - 2(x).\left(\frac{3}{2}\right)\right]$$

$= [x + 2]$

$$\Rightarrow \left[x^2 + \frac{1}{4} - x - x^2 - \frac{9}{4} + 3x\right] = [x+2]$$

$\Rightarrow [-2 + 2x] = [x + 2]$

$x = 4$

5. Pen is to write just as knife is to cut.
6. Listening to music improves exercise performance and reduces discomfort. Music as positive effort only on few students during learning.
7. When the piece can be moved, rotated or flipped to assemble with the given piece is option (a)
8. The total number of students in three classes in the beginning.

Let us consider:

$3a + 13a + 6a = 22a = n$

after addition of 18 student total number of students.

$15b + 35b + 21b = 71b$

$3a + 18 + 13a + 18 + 6a + 18 = 22a + 54$

$22a + 54 = 71b$

$n + 54 = 71b$

$n = 71b - 54$

Let $(b = 2)$

So, $n = 71 \times 2 - 54 = 88$

9. Let us consider, the selling price in year '2' be 'x'.

$\therefore$ Net profit = Selling price – (Cost + Taxes)

$296 = x - (400 + 0.13x)$

$296 = 0.87x - 400$

$$x = \frac{696}{0.87} = 800$$

So, selling price in year '2' = Rs.800

In year 3, total cost = 300 × 1 = Rs.300

Taxes paid = 0.15% of selling price.

Now, let us consider, the selling price in year 3 be 'y'

$\therefore 210 = y - (300 + 0.15y)$

$\Rightarrow 210 = (0.85y - 300)$

$$y = \frac{510}{0.85} = 600$$

$\therefore$ Selling price in year '3' = 600

$$\text{So, } \frac{x}{y} = \frac{800}{600} = \frac{4}{3}.$$

10. I: S > R

II: Q < P, R, S, T, U

From III & IV observation

P > T > S > R > U > Q

The number of students that are taller than 'R' is same as the number of students shorter than S.

CHEMISTRY

1. In Fe $(CO)_5$, oxidation no. of Fe is 0

CO is strong field ligand.

Fe. (Z = 26) (Ground state)

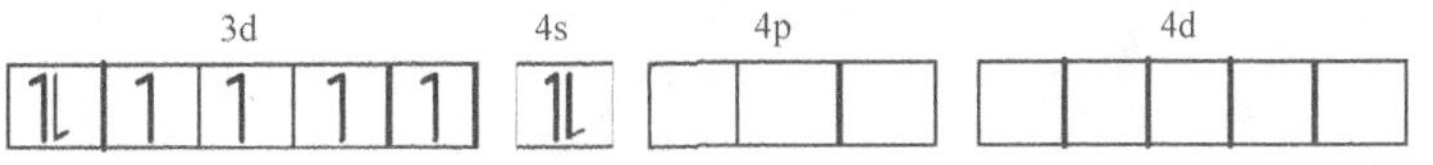

Fe in Oxidation complex (oxidation no. of Fe is 0)

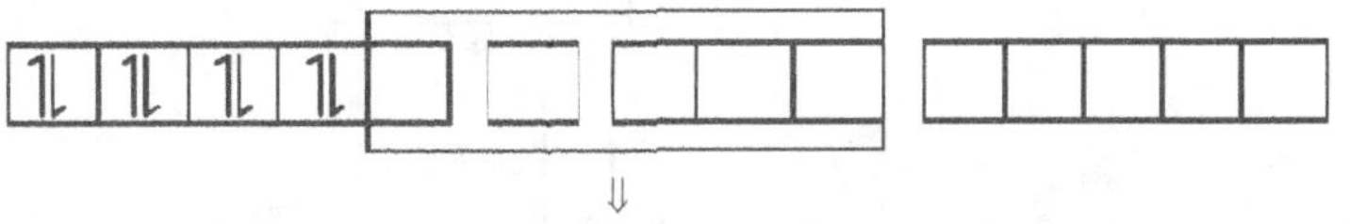

This orbital is involve in hybridisation.

∴ Hybridisation will be dsp^3 & Structure will be trignonal bipyramidal.

2.

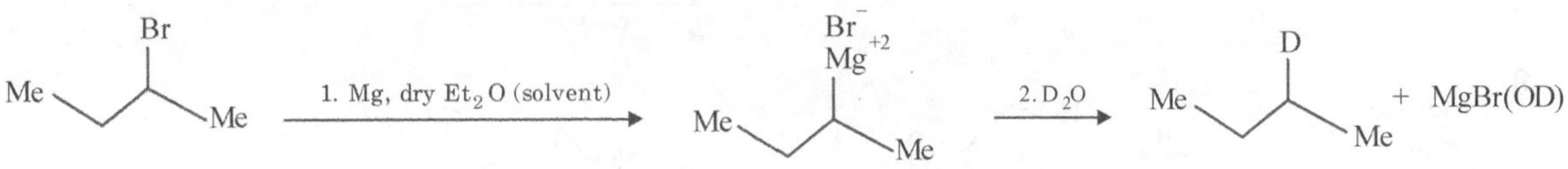

3. $K = \dfrac{2.303}{t}\log\left(\dfrac{A_0}{A}\right) = \dfrac{2.303}{t}\log\dfrac{A_0}{A_0/10}$

$K = \dfrac{2.303}{20} = 0.115\,\text{sec}^{-1}$

50% completion = $t_{1/2}$

$t_{1/2} = \dfrac{0.693}{K} = \dfrac{0.693}{0.115} \simeq 6\,\text{sec}$

4. $E_{nm} = -13.6\dfrac{Z^2}{n^2}\,eV$

in 3rd excited state, n = 4, z = 1

$E_3 = -13.6 \times \dfrac{1^2}{4^2}\,eV = -0.85\,eV$

5. Using Beer's law

$A = \in l C$

$A = 0.42$

$\in = 8.4 \times 10^3\ M^{-1}\,cm^{-1}$

$l = 0.1\ dm = 1cm$

Putting value

$0.42 = 8.4 \times 10^3 \times 1 \times C$

$C = 5 \times 10^{-5}\ M$

6. Acidity is related to tendency to loose/give H^+ ions easily

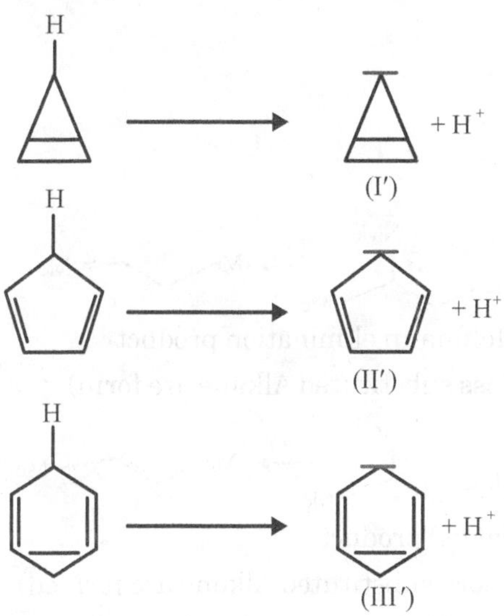

II is Aromatic & is most stable.

∴ Stability order II′ > III′ > I′.

7. $^-O—O^-$

B.O = 1 & can also be solved using molecular orbital theory.

as O_2^{2-} have 18 e^-

$$B.O = \frac{\text{no. of } e^- \text{ bonding molecular orbital} - \text{no. of } e^- \text{ in antibonding molecular orbital}}{2}$$

$$= \frac{10-8}{2} = 1$$

8. I[st] order $\Rightarrow \ln \frac{x_0}{x} = kt$:

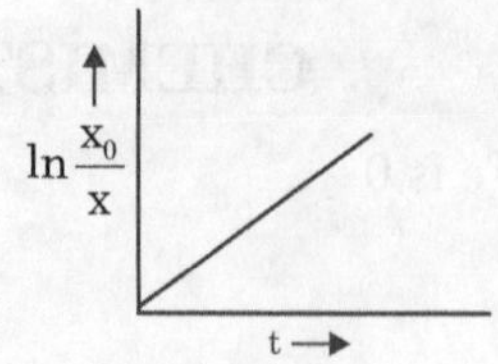

Zero order $\Rightarrow x_0 - x = kt$:

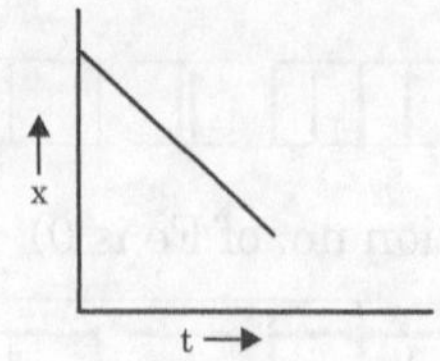

IInd order $\Rightarrow \frac{1}{x} = \frac{1}{x_0} + kt$:

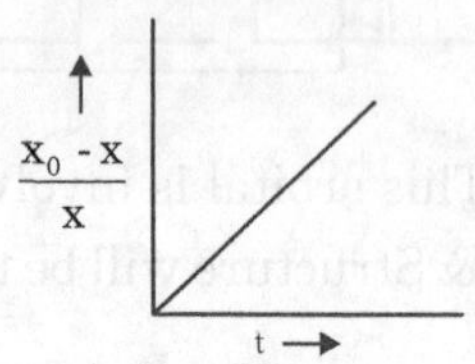

9.

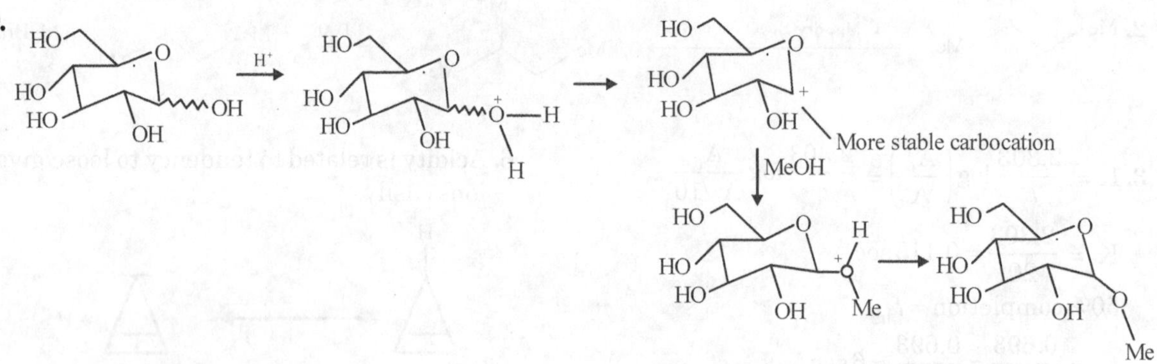

10.

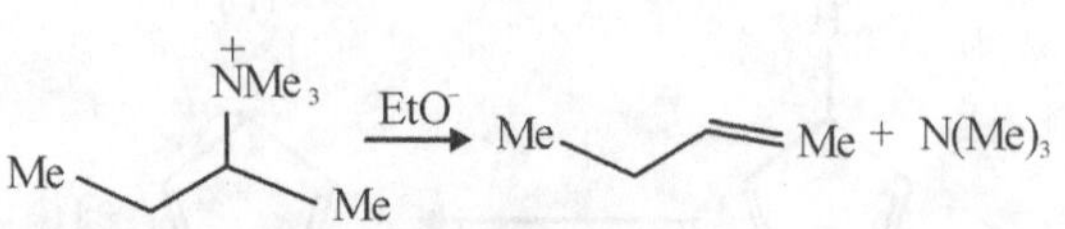

Holfmann elimination product.
(less substituted Alkane are form)

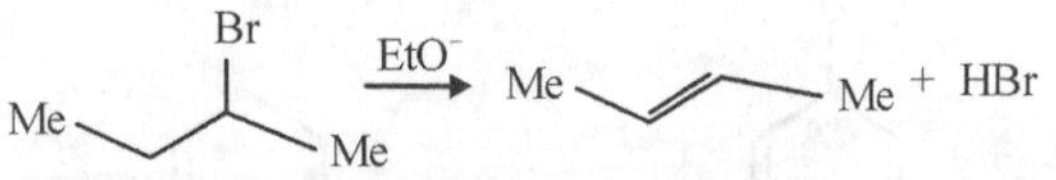

Satzeff product
(more substituted Alkene are formed)

11. F^- & H_2O are weak field liganed.

In this case pairing of e^- in inner d orbital will not occur.

In CN^- & NH_3 pairing of e^- in inner d orbital will occur.

12. $PH_{3(g)} \longrightarrow P_{(g)} + 3H_{(g)}$

$$\Delta H_r^\circ = \Delta_f H^\circ(P,g) + 3 \times \Delta_f H^\circ(H,g) - \Delta_f H^\circ(PH_3 g)$$

$= 314.6$ KJ $+ 3 \times 218.0$ KJ $- 5.4$ KJ

$= 963.2$ KJ

$\therefore$ Average band enthalpy of P–H $= \frac{\Delta H_r}{3}$

$= \frac{963.2}{3}$ KJ $\simeq 321$ KJ

13.

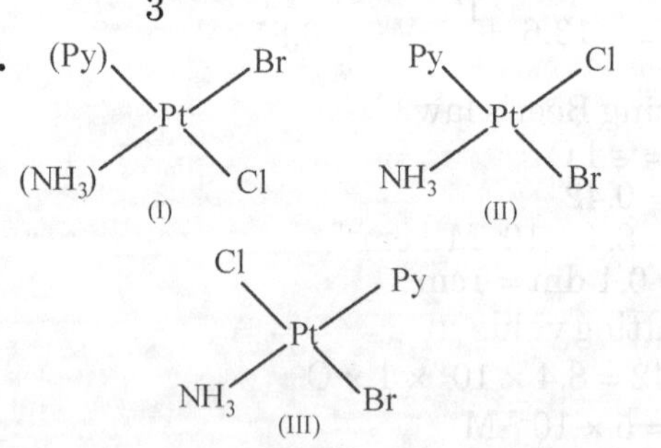

14. $E_{cell} = E^\circ_{cell} - \frac{0.0529}{n} \log Q$

$$\underset{(ag,\ 1\ mM)}{2Ag^+} + Mg_{(b)} \longrightarrow 2Ag_{(s)} + \underset{(ag,\ 0.2\ M)}{Mg^{+2}}$$

$n = 2$

$$Q = \frac{Mg^{+2}}{(Ag^+)^2} = \frac{0.2}{(0.001)^2}$$

$$E^{\circ}_{cell} = E^{\circ}_{Ag^{+}/Ag} + E^{\circ}_{Mg/Mg^{+2}} = 0.80 + 2.37$$
$$= 3.17\ V$$

$$E = 3.17 - \frac{0.0529}{2}\log\frac{0.2}{(0.001)^2} \simeq 3.00$$

15. $\Delta T_f = K_f\, m$

$\Delta T_f = 7.8\ K$

$K_f = 3.9\ K\ Kg$

$$m = \frac{\text{no. of moles of solute}}{\text{mass of solvent (in kg)}} = \frac{\frac{20}{M}}{\frac{80}{1000}}$$

$$= \frac{20 \times 1000}{M \times 80} = \frac{250}{M}$$

$\Delta T_f = K_f\, m$

$$\frac{768}{10} = \frac{369}{10} \times \frac{250}{M}$$

$$M = \frac{250}{2} = 125g$$

BIOCHEMISTRY

1. Phenylalanine molecules (~ 1mg/mL) do NOT absorb at 280 nm in an aqueous solution of pH 7.00 at room temperature. Only the amino acids tryptophan (Trp, W) and tyrosine (Tyr, Y) and to a lesser extent cysteine (Cys, C) contribute significantly to peptide or protein absorbance at 280nm. Phenylalanine (Phe, F), which was mentioned above, absorbs only at lower wavelengths (240-265nm).

2. A molecule that forms a donor-acceptor energy transfer pair with the *dansyl* group is Tryptophan

3. The stationary phase used in gel filtration chromatography is composed of Sepharose. Typically, when an aqueous solution is used to transport the sample through the column, the technique is known as **gel-filtration chromatography**, versus the name gel permeation chromatography, which is used when an organic solvent is used as a mobile phase. The chromatography column is packed with fine, porous beads which are composed of dextran polymers (Sephadex), agarose (Sepharose), or polyacrylamide (Sephacryl or BioGel P). The pore sizes of these beads are used to estimate the dimensions of macromolecules.

4. According to the "*wobble hypothesis*" inosine at the third position of the anticodon cannot form hydrogen bonds with Guanine.

The wobble hypothesis, can explain two events: 1) formation of the uracil-guanine pair as a result of codon-anticodon interaction in the third position and 2) encoding of isoleucine by three codons (for the universal genetic code). This hypothesis is based on two statements: in the third position of the codon nucleotides can ¯wobble , and inosine can form pairs with uracil, cytosine, and adenine.

5. Arginine, also known as L-arginine, is an α-amino acid. The amino acid side-chain of arginine consists of a 3-carbon aliphatic straight chain, the distal end of which is capped by a guanidinium group, which has a pK_a of 12.48, and is therefore always protonated and positively charged at physiological pH. However, using complementary approaches of potentiometry and NMR spectroscopy, the equilibrium acid dissociation constant (pKa value) of the arginine guanidinium group is 13.8 ± 0.1. This is substantially higher than that of ~ 12 often used in structure-based electrostatics calculations and cited in biochemistry textbooks.

6. The non-coenzyme vitamin is Ascorbic acid. Ascorbic acid (Vitamin C) was recognized as a vitamin in 1933. No coenzyme form is identified. It is required for hydroxylation reactions in collagen synthesis and neurotransmitter synthesis. It is also functioning as an antioxidant. Ascorbic acid can be synthesized from glucose by all mammals except primates and guinea pigs.

7. Telomerase is a reverse transcriptase enzyme that carries its own RNA molecule (e.g., with the sequence 32´-CCCAAUCCC-5´ in *Trypanosoma brucei*) which is used as a template when it elongates telomeres. Telomerase is active in gametes and most cancer cells, but is normally absent from, or at very low levels in, most somatic cells.

8. *Taq* DNA polymerase is the most common enzyme used for PCR amplification. This enzyme is extremely heat resistant with a half-life of 40 minutes at 95°C. At its optimal temperature (72°C), nucleotides are incorporated at a rate of 2–4 kilobases per minute. However, polymerases are active over a broad temperature range

9. Smooth endoplasmic reticulum in liver cells of vertebrates helps in detoxification. Hepatocytes have the ability to metabolize, detoxify, and inactivate exogenous compounds such as drugs, insecticides, and endogenous compounds such as steroids. One of the detoxifying functions of hepatocytes is to modify ammonia into urea for excretion. The most abundant organelle in liver cells is the smooth endoplasmic reticulum.

10. Gramicidin A antibiotic can form an ion channel in the bacterial membrane. Gramicidins are ionophores. Their dimers **form ion channel** - like pores in cell **membranes** and cellular organelles of **bacteria** and animal cells. Inorganic monovalent **ions**, such as **potassium** (K^+) and **sodium** (Na^+), **can** travel through these pores freely via diffusion.

11. Most myeloma cell lines are deficient in the enzyme hypoxanthine guanine phosphoribosyl transferase (**HGPRT**) although there are also others deficient in thymidine kinase (TK) and ouabain. HGPRT is essential for DNA and RNA synthesis. Lack of this enzyme prevents survival of myelomas in hypoxanthine-aminopterin-thymidine (HAT) medium, the culture medium in which post-fusion cell mixtures are grown, whereas fused cells are able to survive because they inherit the enzyme from the lymphocyte parent.

12. Galactocerebroside is a non-ionic lipid component that occurs in appreciable amounts in mammalian brain tissues, particularly myelin, and appears to have primarily a structural role in myelin formation and integrity. A galactosylceramide, or **galactocerebroside** is a type of cerebroside consisting of a ceramide with a galactose residue at the 1-hydroxyl moiety. The galactose is cleaved by galactosylceramidase. Galactosylceramide is a marker for oligodendrocytes in the brain, whether or not they form myelin.

13. Naturally occurring **Antibodies** produced against ABO **blood group** antigens - Anti-A is found in the serum of people with blood groups O and B. Anti-B is found in the serum of people with blood groups O and A. **Anti**-A and **anti-B** bind to RBCs and activate the complement cascade, which lyses the RBCs while they are still in the circulation (intravascular hemolysis).

14. **Active transport** is the **energy-requiring process** of pumping molecules and ions across membranes "uphill" - against a concentration gradient. An example of this type of active transport system, is the **sodium-potassium pump,** which exchanges sodium ions for potassium ions across the plasma membrane of animal cells.

15. Correctly paired terms are (*a*) Replication: DnaA , (*b*) Recombination: RecA and (*d*) Transcription: Sigma factor.

16. The high energy compound(s) are: (a) Phosphoenol pyruvate (c) 1, 3-Bisphosphoglycerate. Glycolysis takes place in 10 steps, five of which are in the preparatory phase and five are in the pay-off phase. Phosphofructokinase is the rate-limiting enzyme. ATP is generated by substrate-level phosphorylation by high-energy compounds, such as 1,3-bisphosphoglycerate and phosphoenol pyruvate.

17. Four plots obtained from separate experiments on enzyme inhibition kinetics. The velocity (v) of the reaction is plotted at varying concentrations of substrate (s) and inhibitor (I). The plot(s) corresponding to competitive inhibition are (a) (i) and (c) (iii).

18. **SDS-PAGE** is a discontinuous electrophoretic system which is commonly used as a method to separate proteins with molecular masses between 5 and 250 kDa. The combined use of sodium dodecyl sulfate and polyacrylamide gel allows to eliminate the influence of structure and charge, and proteins are separated solely on the basis of differences in their molecular weight. With respect to sodium dodecyl sulphate - polyacrylamide gel electrophoresis (SDS-PAGE), the true statement(s) are - (b) β-mercaptoethanol is used to reduce

disulphide bonds and (c) The protein migrates towards the anode.

19. In the plot given, the solid line represents oxygen binding to hemoglobin under physiological conditions. The broken line represents the condition(s) of High pH.

20. Epimers are optical isomers that differ in the configuration of a single carbon atom. For example, D-galactose and D-mannose are epimers of D-glucose. D-Galactose is an epimer of D-glucose because the two sugars differ only in the configuration at C-4. D-Mannose is an epimer of D-glucose because the two sugars differ only in the configuration at C-2. Hence Considering the open chain forms, following pair(s) represent an epimer (b) D-glucose and D-mannose and (d) D-galactose and D-glucose.

BOTANY

1. **Vernalization** is the induction of a plant's flowering process by exposure to the prolonged cold of winter, or by an artificial equivalent. After vernalization, plants have acquired the ability to flower, but they may require additional seasonal cues or weeks of growth before they will actually flower. This is sometimes used to refer to herbal (non-woody) plants requiring a cold dormancy to produce new shoots and leaves[1] but this usage is discouraged.

2. Fern plant taxa contains vascular tissue (xylem and phloem) but not woody tissue. The ferns, gymnosperms, and flowering plants are all vascular plants. Because they possess vascular tissues, these plants have true stems, leaves, and roots. Fern stems never become woody (composed of secondary tissue containing lignin), because all tissues of the plant body originate at the stem apex.

3. The CORRECT statement regarding spores and gametes is Spores can directly undergo mitosis whereas gametes cannot. In haplodiplontic life cycles, gametes are not the direct result of a meiotic division. Diploid sporophyte cells undergo meiosis to produce haploid **spores**. Each spore goes through mitotic divisions to yield a multicellular, haploid gametophyte. Mitotic divisions within the gametophyte are required to produce the gametes. The diploid sporophyte results from the fusion of two gametes. Among the Plantae, the gametophytes and sporophytes of a species have distinct morphologies (in some algae they look alike). How a single genome can be used to create two unique morphologies is an intriguing puzzle.

4. Amyloplast organelles controls gravitropism in the roots of higher plants. Gravitropism is the directional control of plant organ growth in response to gravity. Specialized gravity-sensing cells contain amyloplasts that can change their position according to the direction of gravity. Gravity signaling, which is elicited by the relocation of amyloplasts, is a key process that redirects auxin transport from gravity-sensing cells to the lower flank of gravity-responsive organs.

5. Phytoalexins ply important role in plant defense against pathogens. The INCORRECT option related to phytoalexins is (c) Phytoalexins are abundant in plants under normal condition. **Phytoalexins** are antimicrobial and often antioxidative substances synthesized de novo by **plants** that accumulate rapidly **at** areas of pathogen infection.

6. Based on the given statement, the CORRECT options is Red light induces seed germination whereas far-red light inhibits it.

7. The CORRECT hormone that is responsible for bending of coleoptiles of canary grass in response to unidirectional white light is option (a)

8. (c) Intermediate filaments and (d) Centrioles cellular component(s) are NOT parts of cytoskeleton in Angiosperms

9. (a) Phytoene synthase and (b) Carotene desaturase enzyme(s), when over expressed, would result in rice grains with increased β-carotene content. To increase the beta-carotene (provitamin A) content and thus the nutritional value of Golden Rice, the optimization of the enzymes employed, phytoene synthase (PSY) and the Erwinia uredovora carotene desaturase, must be considered.

10. In spiral phyllotaxis, leaves are initiated sequentially on the meristem with two successive primordia being separated by golden angle. If a plant follows right-handed

spiral phyllotaxis when looked down the meristem, then the angle between two successive leaves would be 137.4 or -137.4 degrees.

11. Correct match of the cell/tissue types in GROUP I with their corresponding total DNA content in GROUP II of a typical diploid Angiosperm species (C denotes DNA content in haploid genome) is:

GROUP I	GROUP II
P. Pollen tube	2C
Q. Megaspore mother cell	2C
R. Synergid	1C
S. Embryo sac prior to fertilization	8C

12. Correct match of the modified organs in GROUP I with their corresponding prototypic forms in GROUP II is:

Group I	Group II
P. Tendrils in grape wine	1. Modified stem
Q. Tendrils in garden pea	2. Modified leaf
R. Spines	2. Modified leaf
S. Thorns	1. Modified stem

13. (b) 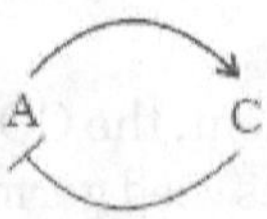

14. The CORRECT match among the plant species in GROUP I, the predominant phytochemical in GROUP II and the economic/medical use in GROUP III is as –

Group I	Group II	Group III
Syzygium aramaticum	Eugenol	Toothache relief
Gracillaria sp.	Agar	Desert jelly
Catharantghus reseus	Vincristine	Leukaemia treatment
Theobroma cacao	Flavonols	Beverage
Papaver somniferum	Morphine	Analgesic

15. Correct match of the genetically modified crop in GROUP I with the corresponding genetic element in GROUP II is:

GROUP I	GROUP II
P. Tomato with delayed fruit ripening	3. Polygalactu-ronase
Q. Herbicide resistant soybean	1. EPSP synthase
R. Insect-resistant cotton	4. Bt-Cry protein
S. Soybean with modified oil content	2. Δ1 2-Desaturase

16. To understand the mechanism of systemic acquired resistance (SAR), a team of researchers isolated a mutant with reduced SAR response.

Sequencing of this mutant revealed homozygous mutations in two genes, X and Y. Following experiment(s) i.e. -:

(a) Complement the mutant with X or Y and analyze the phenotype in each case.

(b) Complement the mutant with both X and Y and analyze the phenotype.

(c) Cross the mutant with wild-type and analyze the segregation pattern of the phenotype.

would test whether the mutant phenotype is caused by mutation in either or both the genes.

17. The observations of an experiment on seed germination in various genotypes under different light conditions are given, where ✓ and X indicate germination and the lack of it, respectively.Based on these observations, the following options are CORRECT:

(b) Any one of the three light qualities - blue, red and far-red – is sufficient to induce seed germination.

(d) The VP1 protein is unlikely to be involved in light perception.

18. The CORRECT options in the context of hybrid plant generation using Barnase/Barstar-based male sterile lines are:

(b) Barstar inhibits Barnase.

(c) Barnase and Barstar are used to generate the male sterile line and the restorer line, respectively.

19. In a diploid plant species, the *T* allele produces tall individuals and is completely dominant over the *t* allele that produces short individuals. Similarly,the *W* allele produces round seeds and is completely dominant over the w allele that produces wrinkled seeds (assume *T* and *W* loci not linked). If a parent with *TTWW* genotype is crossed to another parent with ttww genotype, the fraction of the F_2 population produced by the fusion of both recombinant gametes would be 0.25.

20. In a population of a diploid plant species obeying Hardy-Weinberg equilibrium a locus regulating flower colour has two alleles R and *r*. Individuals with *RR*, *Rr* and *rr* genotypes produce red, pink and white flowers, respectively. If the ratio of red, pink and white flower-producing individuals in the population is 6:3:1, then frequency of r allele in the population would be 25 %

There are two equations necessary to solve a Hardy-Weinberg Equilibrium question:

$p + q = 1$

$p^2 + 2pq + q^2 = 1$

p is the frequency of the dominant allele. q is the frequency of the recessive allele. p^2 is the frequency of individuals with the homozygous dominant genotype. $2pq$ is the frequency of individuals with the heterozygous genotype. q^2 is the frequency of individuals with the homozygous recessive genotype.

According to Hardy – Weinberg law

p^2	+	$2pq$	+	q^2	= 1
↓		↓		↓	
RR		*Rr*		*rr*	
↓		↓		↓	
6	:	3	:	1	

Frequency of *r* alleles will be

(*Rr*) (*rr*)

1.5 + 1 = 2.5/10

Therefor the = 25 %

MICROBIOLOGY

1. Antonie van Leeuwenhoek observed several microscopic organisms under his hand-made microscope. He described them as Animalcules. Using single-lensed microscopes of his own design and make, van Leeuwenhoek was the first to observe and to experiment with microbes, which he originally referred to as *dierkens*, *diertgens* or *diertjes* (Dutch for "small animals" [translated into English as *animalcules*, from Latin *animalculum* = "tiny animal"]). He was the first to relatively determine their size. Most of the "animalcules" are now referred to as unicellular organisms, although he observed multicellular organisms in pond water. He was also the first to document microscopic observations of muscle fibers, bacteria, spermatozoa, red blood cells, crystals in gouty tophi, and among the first to see blood flow in capillaries. Although van Leeuwenhoek did not write any books, he described his discoveries in letters to the Royal Society, which published many of his letters, and to persons in several European countries.

2. Entner-Doudoroff (ED) Pathway pathways oxidizes 1 mole of glucose to 2 moles of pyruvic acid along with one mole each of ATP, NADH and NADPH, in Pseudomonas spp., but not in Bacillus spp. Glucose catabolism of Pseudomonas putida is carried out exclusively through the Entner–Doudoroff (ED) pathway due to the absence of 6-phosphofructokinase.

3. Water balance in extreme halophiles such as *Halobacterium* is maintained by cell surface glycoproteins consisting of aspartate and glutamate

4. *Nocardia* spp. are not amenable to the classical method of Gram staining due to the presence of mycolic acid. *Nocardia* colonies have a variable appearance, but most species appear to have aerial hyphae when viewed with a dissecting microscope, particularly when they have been grown on nutritionally limiting media. *Nocardia* grow slowly on nonselective culture media, and are strict aerobes with the ability to grow in a wide temperature range. Some species are partially acid-fast (meaning a less concentrated solution of sulfuric or hydrochloric acid should be used during the staining procedure) due to the presence of intermediate-length mycolic acids in their cell wall. Majority of strains possess the cord factor (trehalose 6-6' dimycolate), an important virulence factor.

5. Protists belonging to the genus *Trichonympha* thrive in the gut of termites. They help the termites use wood as a food source. This relationship is an example of mutualism. Mutualism is defined as an interaction between individuals of different species that results in positive (beneficial) effects on per capita reproduction and/or survival of the interacting populations

6. Hydrogen sulfide and Thiosulfates are used as electron donors for CO_2 reduction during photo-synthasis in purple sulfur bcateria. The purple sulfur bacteria (PSB) are part of a group of Proteobacteria capable of photosynthesis, collectively referred to as purple bacteria. They are anaerobic or microaerophilic Unlike plants, algae, and cyanobacteria, purple sulfur bacteria do not use water as their reducing agent, and therefore do not produce oxygen. Instead, they can use sulfur in the form of sulfide, or thiosulfate (as well, some species can use H_2, Fe^{2+}, or NO_2^-) as the electron donor in their photosynthetic pathways. The sulfur is oxidized to produce granules of elemental sulfur. This, in turn, may be oxidized to form sulfuric acid.

7. Succinate thiokinase and Pyruvate kinase catalyze substrate-level phosphorylation. In glycolysis, the second substrate-level phosphorylation occurs by dephosphorylating phosphoenolpyruvate, catalyzed by pyruvate kinase, producing pyruvate and ATP In glycolysis. Succinate thiokinase, is a Krebs cycle enzyme that catalyzes the conversion of succinyl CoA to succinic acid. During this step, CoA is released and one molecule of GTP is formed from GDP. This is a substrate level phosphorylation.

8. Fluorescent in situ hybridization (FISH) and Polymerase chain reaction (PCR) followed by sequencing of the amplicon can be applied to identify a bacterial species. Fluorescence in situ hybridization (FISH) is a molecular technique that provides identification and visualization of bacteria in situ. Polymerase chain reaction, or PCR, is a technique to make many copies of a specific DNA region *in vitro*. Genetic marker is known gene or DNA sequence (with a known location on the chromosome) used to identify individual or species.

9. Accumulation of allolactose in the cell and Direct binding of cAMP to the promoter DNA would contribute to the induction of *lac* operon in a wild-type strain of *E.* coli.

10. One mole of a circular bacterial plasmid was digested with a high-fidelity restriction enzyme. The plasmid has five restriction sites for the enzyme used. The number of moles of fragments released upon cleavage at all sites is 5.

11. Under anaerobic fermentative growth conditions, one mole of glucose yields 22 grams of *streptococcus faecalis* or 8.6 grams of *Zymomonas mobilis*.

As we know that

$$Y_{ATP} = \text{gram cell produced /mole ATP.}$$

We also know that 2 mole ATP are generated per mol glucose in case of anaerobic fermentation of *streptococcus faecalis* and 1 mole ATP are generated per mol glucose in case of anaerobic fermentation of *Zymomonas mobilis. Therefore,* the molar growth yield (Y_{ATP}) for (i) S. *faecalis* and (ii) *Z. mobilis* will be (i) 11 and (ii) 8.6:

12. The order of abundance of quinones (ubiquinone [UQ], menaquinone [MQ] and demethylmenaquinone [DMQI]) in *E. coli* growing anaerobically on fumarate is MQ > DMQ > UQ.

13. The number of ATPs generated per molecule of NADH during oxidative phosphorylation in *E.coli* via (i) NDH-1 and cytochrome bo complex or (ii) the NDH-2 and cytochrome bd complex will be (i) 2.70 and (ii) 0.67

14. Correct match of the Immunoglobulin classes with their function

Immunoglobulin		Function	
(i)	IgE	(s)	mediates allergic reaction
(ii)	IgG	(p)	protects the fetus
(iii)	IgM	(q)	first antibody to be produced in response to infection
(iv)	IgA	(r)	provides localized protection of mucosal surfaces

15. The figure shows the profiles of quantitative real-time PCR (qRT-PCR) tests for SARS-CoV-2 conducted on the throat swab samples of three individuals (X, Y and Z). Tests were carried out under identical conditions. Dotted line represents the threshold fluorescent value. The correct statement on the status of the COVID-19 tests of the individuals based on their qRT-PCR profiles is (c) X and Y are positive; X has the highest viral load.

16. Based on given information, the recombinants X, Y and Z. are:

(b) X is p^+, Y is r^+ and Z is x^+.

17. The genome of a bacterium encodes for 10 different surface antigens, whose expression can be turned 'ON' or 'OFF' randomly and independently. The number of possible antigenic combinations is 1024.

18. Suppose the mRNAs in a newly discovered bacteria are composed of only two distinct nucleotides (as opposed to four found in all known organisms). Considering that the organism has no nucleotide modification systems, the number of nucleotides required per codon to encode at least 20 distinct amino acids will be 5.

19. Given ; As per Second Condition D = 0.2 min. at 121 °C.

Then at this condition

$N_t = 1$ & $N_o = 10$ when t= D

As we know that from thermal death kinetics;

ln $(N_o/N_t) = Kt$;

or $\ln (10/1) = 0.2K$

or $2.303 \log 10 = 0.2K$

or $K = 2.303/0.2 = 11.515$

But as per first condition,

$No = 10^{12}$

and $N_t = 1$

and $t = ?$

we know that from thermal death kinetics;

ln $(No/N_t) = Kt$;

Therefore

$2.303 \log (10^{12}/1) = 11.515\,t$

Therefore $t = (2.303 \times 12)/11.515$

Or $t = 2.4$ minutes

20. Given;

(1) The generation time (td) of E. coli is 30 minutes.

(2) Initial number of bacteria (X_o) required to reach a number of 10^9 i.e. $(X_t) = 10^9$

(3) Total time (t) = 2 hours = 120 minutes

As we know that for an exponentially growing culture;

$X_t = X_o 2^n$;

where $n = t / td$,

Hence $n = 120/30 = 4$

Therefore, $10^9 = X_o 2^4$;

or $X_o = 10^9/16 = 6.25 \times 10^7$

Hence, Initial number of bacteria

$= 6.25 \times 10^7$

The decimal reduction time (D) for reducing 10^{12} spores of *Clostridium botulinum* to 1 spore at 111°C will be_______ min (in integer). The D value is 0.2 min at 121°C. The increase in temperature required to change D to of its initial value (Z value) is 10°C.

ZOOLOGY

1. Ichthyophis belongs to Amphibia Class

Kingdom :	Animalia
Phylum :	Chordata
Class :	Amphibia
Order :	Gymnophiona
Clade :	Apoda
Family :	Ichthyophiidae
Genus :	Ichthyophis

2. The two homologous genes occurring in different species are called orthologous.

Homologous sequences are orthologous if they were separated by a speciation event: when a species diverges into two separate species, the copies of a single gene in the two resulting species are said to be orthologous. Homologous sequences are paralogous if they were separated by a gene duplication event: if a gene in an organism is duplicated to occupy two different positions in the same genome, then the two copies are paralogous.

3. Holandric genes mean the genes present on Y-chromosome.

Hypertrichosis:
Y-chromosome inheritance pattern.

4. Assume that the anticodon for an unknown amino acid is 3 AUG 5. The corresponding code on DNA sequence would be 3 ' ATG 5.

5. The Organ of Corti is an organ of the inner ear located within the cochlea which contributes to audition.

6. In adult athletes, muscles grow larger when exercised and are capable of regeneration after injury. This is due to proliferation and differentiation of satellite cells. Skeletal muscle satellite cells are considered to play a crucial role in muscle fiber maintenance, repair and remodeling. Satellite cells proliferate following muscle traumaand form new myofibers through a process similar to fetal muscle development. After several cell divisions, the satellite cells begin to fuse with the damaged myotubes and undergo further differentiations and maturation, with peripheral nuclei as in hallmark. Satellite cell activation is measured by the extent of proliferation and differentiation.

7. An innate behaviour is an instinctive response that is developmentally fixed - it is independent of environmental context. Innate behaviours have a genetic basis and are hence inherited from parents.

8. A man, whose mother and father had blood groups A and O respectively, marries a woman with blood group AB. If the man has blood group A, then the number of different blood groups possible among their children will be 3 i.e. A, B and AB.

9. In the simplest case of a single locus with two alleles denoted A and a with frequencies $f(A) = p$ and $f(a) = q$, respectively, the expected genotype frequencies under random mating are $f(AA) = p^2$ for the AA homozygotes, $f(aa) = q^2$ for the aa homozygotes, and $f(Aa) = 2pq$ for the heterozygotes. In the absence of selection, mutation, genetic drift, or other forces, allele frequencies p and q are constant between generations, so equilibrium is reached.

As given the allelic frequency ($f(A)$) of A, i.e. $p = 0.6$, hence the frequency of another allele $f(a)$ i.e. q will be $= 0.4$.

Therefore, the genetic frequency of Aa i.e. $f(Aa) = 2pq = 2 \times 0.6 \times 0.4 = 0.48$.

10. An α-helix (radius = 2.3 Å) is a right-handed helix that has 3.6 amino acids per helical turn (100° turn/residue), and the structure is stabilized by H-bonds formed between the C=O of residue n and the N_H of residue n+4; both these groups are part of the helical backbone and not the side chains (R groups) that protrude out of the backbone.

Every main chain C=O and N-H group is hydrogen-bonded to a peptide bond 4 residues away (i.e. O_i to N_{i+4}). This gives a very regular, stable arrangement. Therefore, in the structure of a polypeptide, one α-helix (3.6_{13} helix) contains 32 intra-chain hydrogen bonds will have 36 amino acids. Hence the number of turns in the helix will be 36/3.6 = 10 turns.

11. The correct match of Column I with the specific descriptions in Column II :

Column I	Column II
P. Zygote	(iii) A cell that results from fertilization
Q. Morula	(vi) A compact mass of cells
R. Blastocyst	(i) A hollow sphere of cells
S. Ovum	(v) An unfertilized egg
T. Neonate	(ii) A newly born offspring
U. Fetus	(iv) An embryo

12. Correct match of the autoimmune diseases in Column I for the self-antigens in Column II :

Column I	Column II
P. Rheumatoid arthritis	(ii) Connective tissue
Q. Systemic lupus erythematosus	(iii) DNA
R. Myasthenia gravis	(iv) Acetylcholine receptors
S. Multiple sclerosis	(i) Myelin

13. Match the types of cell movements during gastrulation in Column I with the descriptions in Column II:

(c) P-(ii), Q-(iv), R-(i), S-(iii)

Column I	Column II
P. Invagination	(ii) Infolding of a sheet (epithelium) of cells during the formation of endoderm in sea urchin
Q. Involution	(iv) Inward movement of an expanding outer layer of cells so that it spreads over the internal surface of the remaining external cells
R. Ingression	(i) Migration of individual cells from the surface into the embryo 's interior

S. Delamination (iii) Splitting of one cellular sheet into two nearly parallel sheets

14. Match the therapeutic factors in Column I with the applications in Column II

Column I	Column II
P. Humulin	(ii) Diabetes
Q. Erythropoietin	(iv) Anaemia
R. Plasminogen activator	(v) Myocardial infraction
S. Cathepsin K inhibitor	(iii) Osteoporosis
T. Leptin	(vi) Obesity

(a) P-(ii), Q-(iv), R-(v), S-(iii), T-(vi)

15. Correct match of the cell organelles in Column I with the appropriate functions in Column II :

Column I	Column II
P. Peroxisome	(ii) Oxidation of fatty acids
Q. Endoplasmic	(iii) N-linked glycosylation
R. Glyoxysome reticulum	(i) Conversion of lipid to carbohydrate
S. Golgi complex	(v) O-linked glycosylation
T. Centrioles	(iv) Microtubule organization

(d) P-(ii), Q-(iii), R-(i), S-(v), T-(iv)

16. Chromosome cohesion and condensation are essential prerequisites of proper segregation of genomes during mitosis and meiosis, and are supported by two structurally related protein complexes, cohesin and condensin, respectively. At the core of the two complexes lie members of the structural maintenance of chromosomes (SMC) family of ATPases. Structural maintenance of chromosomes (SMC) proteins are also found in most bacterial and archaeal species, implicating the existence of an evolutionarily conserved theme of higher-order chromosome organization and dynamics. SMC dimers adopt a two-armed structure with an ATP-binding cassette (ABC)-like domain at the distal end of each arm.

17. (a) Pygmy Hog and Purple Frog represent the animals as Endemic to India. The purple frog, also known as the Pignose frog, is only found in the rainforests of western ghats in India. It spends most of its life underground. Pygmy Hog, found in Assam in India. The mountain bongo is only found in the wild in a few mountain regions of central Kenya. The hirola, Hunter's hartebeest or Hunter's antelope, is a critically endangered antelope species found on the border between Kenya and Somalia.

18. All amino acids except glycine have at least one chiral center at C^{α} (the alpha carbon is a chiral centre). Threonine and isoleucine have an additional chiral center at C^{β}. The β carbon of isoleucine is optically active, just as the β carbon of threonine. These two amino acids, isoleucine and threonine, have in common the fact that they have two chiral centers.Nucleic acids also have chiral centers. For example, in DNA the atoms C1', C3', and C4' are chiral, while RNA has an additional chiral center at C2'. Chirality is central to all molecular interactions in biological systems.

19. We know that,

$$V_o = \frac{K_{cat}[E][S]}{K_m + [S]}$$

Given,

1. $V = 9.0\ \mu MS^{-1}$
   or $V = 9 \times 10^{-6}\ MS^{-1}$
2. $[S] = 30\ \mu M$
   or $[S] = 30 \times 10^{-6}\ M$
3. $[E_o] = 30\ nM$
   or $[E_o] = 30 \times 10^{-9}\ M$
4. $K_{cat}/K_m = n \times 10^7\ M^{-1}S^{-1}$
5. $K_m = 10\ \mu M$
   or $K_m = 10 \times 10^{-6} M$
   Hence, $K_{cat} = n \times 10^7 \times 10 \times 10^{-6}\ M$
   or $K_{cat} = n \times 10^2$

Putting all the values in the equation the

$$9 \times 10^{-6} = \frac{n \times 10^2 \times 30 \times 10^{-9} \times 30 \times 10^{-6}}{10 \times 10^{-6} + 30 \times 10^{-6}}$$

By solving this we will get $\boxed{n = 4}$

20. The heterozygous population which is showing segregation is Aa which comes to be 50%. Therefore this genotype only will segregate, others are homozygous and do not segregate.

GATE - 2020

XL : LIFE SCIENCES

Time : 3 Hours *Maximum Marks : 100*

GENERAL APTITUDE

Q. 1 – Q. 5 carry one mark each

1. Rajiv Gandhi Khel Ratana Award was conferred _____ Mary Kom, a six time world champion in boxing, recently in ceremony ____ the Rashtrapati Bhawan (the President's official residence) in New Delhi.
   (*a*) with, at (*b*) on, in
   (*c*) to, at (*d*) on, at

2. Despite a string of poor performances, the chances of K.L Rahul's selection in the team are _____
   (*a*) Slim (*b*) Bright
   (*c*) Obvious (*d*) Uncertain

3. Select the word that fits the analogy:
   Cover: Uncover:: Associate: _____
   (*a*) Unassociate (*b*) Inassociate
   (*c*) Misassociate (*d*) Dissociate

4. Hit by floods, the kharif (summer sown) crops in various parts of the country have been affected. Officials believe that the loss in production of the kharif crops can be recovered in the output of the rabi (winter sown) crops so that the country can achieve its food-grain production target of 291 million tons in the crop year 2019-20 (July-June). They are hopeful that good rains in July-August will help the soil retain moisture for a longer period, helping winter sown crops such as wheat and pulses during the November-February period. Which of the following statements can be inferred from the given passage?
   (*a*) Officials declared that the food grain production target will be met due to good rains
   (*b*) Officials want the food grain production target to be met by the November-February period.
   (*c*) Officials feel that the food grain production target cannot be met due to floods
   (*d*) Officials hope that the food grain production target will be met due to a good rabi produce

5. The difference between the sum of the first 2n natural numbers and the sum of the first n odd numbers is _____
   (*a*) $n^2 - n$
   (*b*) $n^2 + n$
   (*c*) $2n^2 - n$
   (*d*) $2n^2 + n$

Q. 6 – Q. 10 carry two marks each

6. Repo rate is the rate at which Reserve Bank of India (RBI) lends commercial banks, and reverse repo rate at which RBI borrows money from commercial banks.
   Which of the following statements can be inferred from the above passage?
   (*a*) Decrease in repo-rate will increase cost of borrowing and decrease lending by commercial banks
   (*b*) Decrease in repo-rate will decrease cost of borrowing and increase lending by commercial banks
   (c) Increase in repo-rate will decrease cost of borrowing and decrease lending by commercial banks
   (*d*) Increase in repo-rate will decrease cost of borrowing and increase lending by commercial banks

7. P,Q,R,S,T,U,V and W are seated around a circular table
   I. S is seated opposite to W
   II. U is seated at the second place to the right of R
   III. T is seated at the third place to the right of R
   IV. V is a neighbour of S
   Which of the following must be true?
   (*a*) P is a neighbour of R
   (*b*) Q is a neighbour of R
   (*c*) P is not seated opposite to Q
   (*d*) R is the left neighbour of S

8. The distance between Delhi and Agra is 233 km. A car P started travelling from Delhi to Agra and another car Q started from Agra to Delhi along the same road 1 hour after the car P started. The two cars crossed each other 75 minutes after the car Q started. Both cars

were travelling at constant speed. The speed of car P was 10km/hr more than the speed of car Q. How many kilometres the car Q had travelled when the cars crossed each other?

(*b*) 75.2 (*a*) 66.6

(*d*) 116.5 (*c*) 88.2

9. For a matrix $M = [m_{ij}]$: i, j = 1, 2, 3, 4: the diagonal elements are all zero and $m_{ij} = -m_{ji}$. The minimum number of elements required to fully specify the matrix is ______.

(*a*) 0 (*b*) 6

(*c*) 12 (*d*) 16

10. The profit shares of two companies P and Q are shown in the figure. If the two companies have invested a fixed and equal amount every year, then the ratio of the total revenue of company P to the total revenue of company Q, during 2013-2018 is ______.

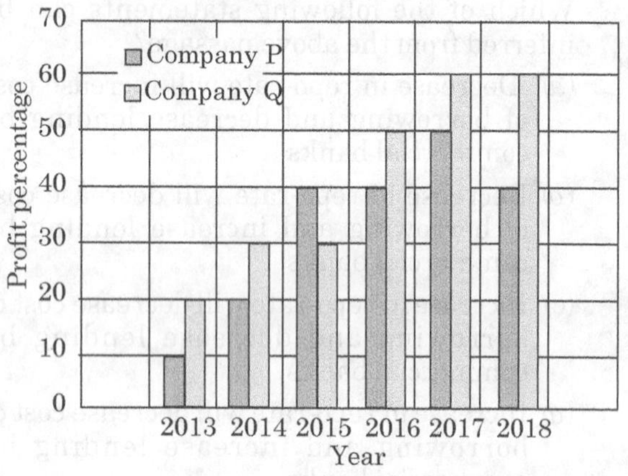

(*a*) 15 : 17 (*b*) 16 : 17

(*c*) 17 : 15 (*d*) 17 : 16

P: CHEMISTRY (COMPULSORY)

Q. 1 – Q. 5 carry one mark each

1. An aqueous solution contains a mixture of 10^{-8} M NaCl and 10^{-8} M HCl.

Choose the correct statement about this solution.

(a) The solution is a buffer with pH less than 7.00

(b) The solution is a buffer with pH greater than 7.00

(c) The solution is not a buffer but has its pH less than 7.00

(d) The solution is not a buffer but has its pH greater than 7.00

2. The coordination complex which has a distorted octahedral structure is

(Given: Atomic numbers of V: 23; Mn: 25; Ni: 28; Cu: 29)

(a) $[Ni(H_2O)_6]^{2+}$ (b) $[Mn(H_2O)_6]^{2+}$

(c) $[V(H_2O)_6]^{2+}$ (d) $[Cu(H_2O)_6]^{2+}$

3. In naphthalene, the value of the integer "n" according to Huckel's rule of aromaticity is ______.

4. The azimuthal quantum number (*l*) of an electron in the d_{z^2} orbital of a copper atom (atomic number: 29)is ______.

5. The standard enthalpy of reaction (in kJ mol^{-1}) for obtaining three moles of H_2 (g) from atomic hydrogen in gas phase is ______. (Given: Standard enthalpy of formation of atomic hydrogen in gas phase is 218 kJ mol^{-1})

Q. 6 – Q. 15 carry two marks each

6. The **correct** order of the first ionization energies of He, B, N and O in their corresponding ground state is

(a) He > N > O > B (b) O > N > B > He

(c) He > B > N > O (d) N > O > B > He

7. Based on the molecular orbital theory, which one of the following statements with respect to N_2, N_2^+, O_2 and O_2^+ is correct?

(a) Bond orders of N_2 and O_2 are higher than their corresponding cations.

(b) Bond energy of N_2^+ is higher than that of N_2, whereas bond energy of O_2^+ is lower than that of O_2.

(c) The unpaired electrons in N_2^+ and O_2^+ are present in σ and π* orbitals, respectively.

(d) The bond in N_2^+ is shorter than that in N_2, whereas bond in O_2 is shorter than that in O_2^+.

8. Which one of the following statements is incorrect about the diborane molecule?

(a) B-Ht bond is a 2-centre-2-electron bond (H^t: terminal hydrogen).

(b) BH^bB bond is a 3-centre-2-electron bond (H^b: bridged hydrogen).

(c) The bond angle H^tBH^t is 122° (H^t: terminal hydrogen).

(d) The B-H^t bond distance is longer than B-H^b bond distance (H^t: terminal hydrogen, H^b: bridged hydrogen).

9. Given below are Newman projections of ethylene glycol and 1,2-difluoroethane about their respective C-C bonds. The most stable conformations (lowest energy) of ethylene glycol and 1,2-difluoroethane are

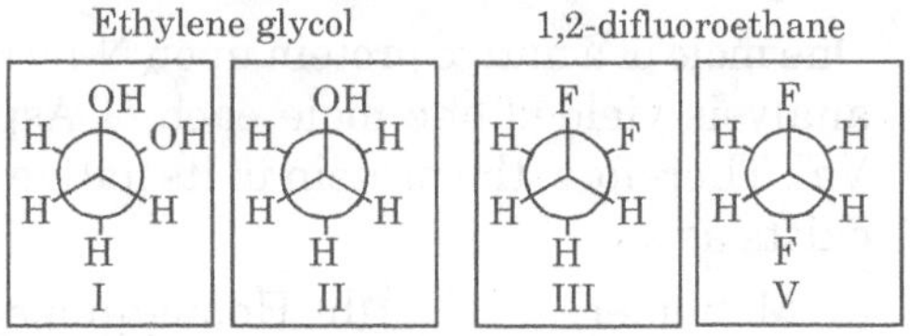

(a) I and III respectively.
(b) I and IV respectively.
(c) II and III respectively.
(d) II and IV respectively.

10. In the reaction given below, choose the condition that gives an anti-Markovnikov's product.

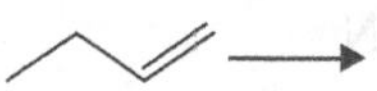

(a) Peroxide/HCl
(b) Aqueous mercuric acetate treatment
(c) Diborane addition
(d) Sulfuric acid addition

11. Which one of the following hexoses will give an osazone that has a different melting point from that of the osazone obtained from D (+) glucose?

(a)

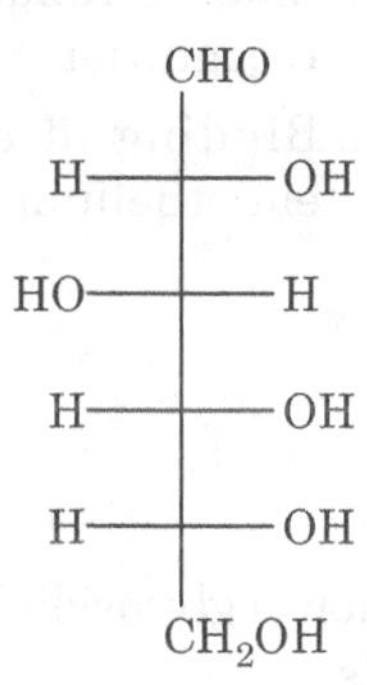

(b)

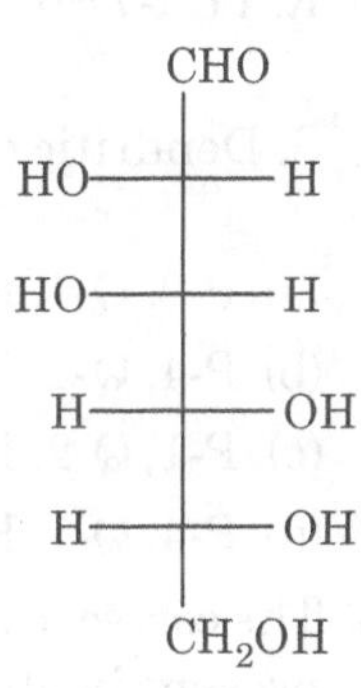

(c)

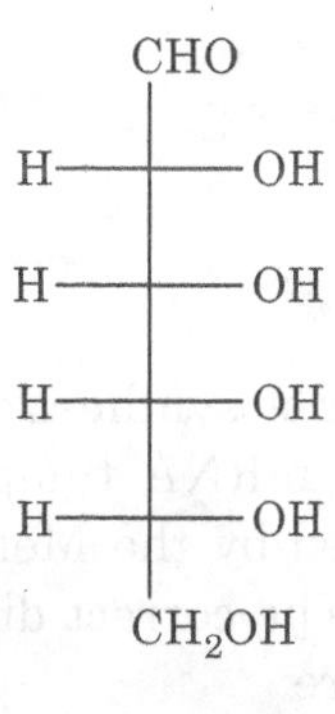

(d)

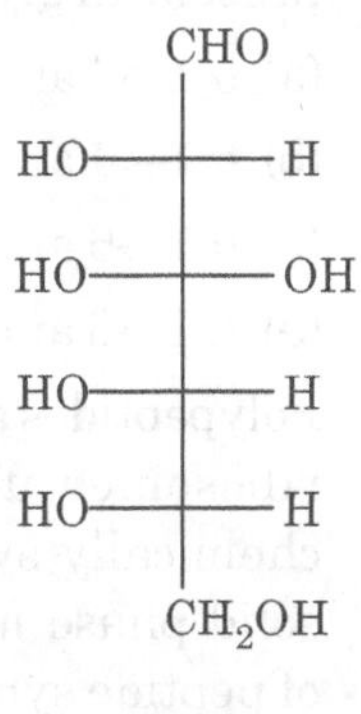

12. A molecule in solution crystallizes into two different crystal forms with rate constants of 0.02 s^{-1} and 0.13 s^{-1}. If the crystallization is assumed to be under kinetic control, then the half-life (in seconds, rounded off to one decimal place) of the molecule is _____.

13. The standard potential $\left(E^{o}_{cell}\right)$ for a cell reaction given below is +0.7 V. The standard reaction free energy ($\Delta_r G^o$) for this cell is _____ kJ mol^{-1} (correct up to two decimal places). (Given: Faraday constant. F = 96500 C mol^{-1})

$$Au^{3+}(aq) + 3\,Ag(s) \longrightarrow Au(s) + 3Ag^{+}(aq)$$

14. The activation energy (E_a) estimated for a reaction from the Arrhenius equation is 21 kJ mol^{-1}. If the frequency factor is assumed to be independent of temperature, then the ratio of the rate constants determined at 298 K and 260 K is _____ (rounded off to two decimal places). (Given: Gas constant, R = 8.315J K^{-1} mol^{-1})

15. At a given pressure, a substance is heated from 2000 K to 2600 K. If the entropy of the substance is 60 JK^{-1} mol^{-1}, and is assumed to be constant over the given temperature range, then the change in the chemical potential (in kJ mol^{-1}) of the substance is ____.

Q: BIOCHEMISTRY

Q. 1 – Q. 10 carry one mark each

1. Which one of the following hormones initiates a signaling cascade by directly binding to an intra-cellular receptor?

(a) Insulin (b) Gonadotropin
(c) Progesterone (d) Epinephrine

2. Which one of the following bonds is NOT present in ATP?

(a) Phosphoester
(b) Phosphoanhydride
(c) N-Glycosidic
(d) α-Glycosidic

3. The reaction involved in the direct conversion of L-phenylalanine to L-tyrosine is

(a) Hydroxylation (b) Decarboxylation
(c) Transamination (d) Reduction

4. The human major histocompatibility complex (MHC) is
(a) Polygenic and monomorphic
(b) Polygenic and polymorphic
(c) Monogenic and polymorphic
(d) Monogenic and monomorphic

5. Har Gobind Khorana and Marshall Nirenberg elucidated the genetic code by using a cell-free protein synthesizing system. It was found that poly (U) and poly (C) result in the synthesis of poly(L-Phe) and poly(L-Pro) respectively. Based on these observations, which one of the following conclusions is correct?
(a) Codon GGG specifies L-Phe and codon AAA specifies L-Pro
(b) Codon CCC specifies L-Phe and codon UUU specifies L-Pro
(c) Codon AAA specifies L-Phe and codon GGG specifies L-Pro
(d) Codon UUU specifies L-Phe and codon CCC specifies L-Pro

6. Binding of an antibody to its cognate antigen does NOT involve
(a) Covalent bonds
(b) Electrostatic forces
(c) Van der Waals forces
(d) Hydrogen bonds

7. A globular protein of molecular weight 50 kDa exists as a mixture of monomers and dimers in solution. The most appropriate technique for the separation of these two forms of the protein is
(a) Thin layer chromatography
(b) Ion exchange chromatography
(c) Gel filtration chromatography
(d) Paper chromatography

8. Choose the correct order of molecules, according to their ability to diffuse across a lipid bilayer.
(a) $CO_2 > H_2O >$ Glucose > RNA
(b) $CO_2 >$ Glucose $> H_2O >$ RNA
(c) RNA > Glucose $> CO_2 > H_2O$
(d) $H_2O > CO_2 >$ RNA > Glucose

9. When one glucose unit from glycogen gets converted to lactate in the muscle, the net number of ATP molecules produced is ______.

10. Considering that the three pK_as of histidine are $pK_1 = 1.8$, $pK_2 = 9.2$ and $pK_R = 6.0$, its isoelectric point will be ______ (rounded off to one decimal place).

Q. 11 – Q. 20 carry two marks each

11. One mole of a native protein upon N-terminal analysis yielded one mole each of Asp and Val. Therefore, the protein in its native state exists as a
(a) Monomer (b) Homo-dimer
(c) Hetero-dimer (d) Tetramer

12. The prosthetic groups/cofactors involved in both $1e^-$ and $2e^-$ transfer in the mitochondrial electron transport chain are
(a) NAD and NADP
(b) NAD and FAD
(c) Heme and FMN
(d) Coenzyme Q and FMN

13. Match the items in **Group I** with the most appropriate items in **Group II** and choose the correct option.

Group I	**Group II**
P. Integrin	1. Phagocytosis in the neural tissue
Q. Microglial cell	2. Antigen processing by cross-presentation
R. TLR-7	3. Single stranded RNA recognition
S. Dendritic cell	4. Binding of cells to endothelium

(a) P-2, Q-1, R-3, S-4
(b) P-4, Q-1, R-3, S-2
(c) P-1, Q-2, R-3, S-4
(d) P-4, Q-1, R-2, S-3

14. The correct combination of glycosidic linkages present in glycogen is
(a) α 1→4 and α 1→6
(b) α 1→4 and β 1→6
(c) α 1→6 and β 1→4
(d) α 1→6 and β 1→6

15. Polypeptides are either biosynthesized on the ribosomes using an mRNA template or chemically synthesized by the Merrifield's solid phase method. The correct directions of peptide synthesis are

(a) C→N direction on the ribosomes and N→C direction on the solid phase

(b) N→C direction on the ribosomes and C→N direction on the solid phase

(c) N→C direction in both cases

(d) C→N direction in both cases

16. A solution absorbs 20% of the incident light in a cuvette of path length 1.0 cm. The amount of light transmitted by the same solution in a cuvette of 3.0 cm path length is ______ % (rounded off to one decimal place).

17. The second pKa of phosphoric acid is 6.8. The ratio of Na_2HPO_4 to NaH_2PO_4 required to obtain a buffer of pH 7.0 is ______ (rounded off to two decimal places).

18. A PCR in a 1 00 μL reaction volume, containing two primers at a concentration of 0.2 μM each, is set up to amplify a 250 base pair DNA fragment. Consider the average molecular weight of one base pair as 660 Da. If the primers are fully consumed by the end of the reaction, the amount of the final PCR product formed is ______ μg (rounded off to one decimal place).

19. An enzyme obeying Michaelis-Menten kinetics shows a reaction velocity (v) of 10 μmol/min when the substrate concentration [S] equals its K_M. The maximal velocity V_{max} for this enzyme is ________ μmol/min (correct to integer number). (K_M is Michaelis-Menten constant)

20. The enzyme glucose isomerase catalyzes the inter-conversion of glucose and fructose as shown.

$$\text{Glucose} \rightleftarrows \text{Fructose}$$

The $\Delta G_0'$ for this reaction is zero kcal/mol. After adding glucose isomerase to a 0.12 M glucose solution and allowing the reaction to attain equilibrium, the final concentration of fructose in the reaction mixture will be ________ mM.

R: BOTANY

Q. 1 – Q. 10 carry one mark each

1. Indefinite stamen is a characteristic feature of which of the following plant families?

(a) Malvaceae

(b) Apocynaceae

(c) Poaceae

(d) Brassicaceae

2. In natural condition, which of the following plants **DOES NOT** exhibit anomalous secondary growth?

(a) Rice (b) Aloe

(c) Yucca (d) Dracaena

3. In a typical angiosperm under natural condition, primary meristems are usually established during

(a) Gametogenesis

(b) Embryogenesis

(c) Vegetative phase development

(d) Secondary growth

4. 2-Methoxy-3,6-dichlorobenzoic acid belongs to which class of plant growth regulators?

(a) Synthetic auxin

(b) Synthetic cytokinin.

(c) Strigolactone

(d) Brassinosteroid

5. In a typical green plant, the first stable product of Calvin cycle is

(a) Oxaloacetic acid

(b) Succinic acid

(c) Maleic acid

(d) 3-Phosphoglyceric acid

6. Among the following, which best describes an organism that lives at the expense of other organisms, harmful but usually not killing?

(a) Predator (b) Symbiotic

(c) Prey (d) Parasite

7. The oleo-gum resin asafoetida (hing) is obtained from the cut surface of

(a) Stem (b) Root

(c) Leaf (d) Fruit

8. 'Bakanae" disease or 'foolish seedling' disease is caused by

(a) Fungus (b) Bacterium

(c) Virus (d) Mycoplasma

9. Which of the following chemicals is used for doubling of chromosome numbers during production of 'doubled haploids' in crop plants?

(a) Hygromycin (b) Kanamycin

(c) Colchicine (d) Glufosinate

10. An mRNA of a nuclear encoded plant gene, DSH20 has an ORF of 1353 nucleotides. Provided that average molecular weight of amino acid is 110 Dalton (Da), calculated molecular weight of DSH20 protein in kDa (round off to 1 decimal place) is ______ .

Q. 11 – Q. 20 carry two marks each

11. **Group I, Group II** and **Group III** represent enzyme, product of the enzymatic reaction, and metabolic process, respectively.

Group I	Group II	Group III
P. Hexokinase	i. Malate	1. Glycolysis
Q. Fumarase	ii. Glucose 6-P	2. Photorespiration
R. PEP Carboxylase	iii. Hydrogen peroxide	3. TCA cycle
S. Glycolate oxidase	iv. Cinnamic acid	4. Photosynthesis
	v. Oxaloacetic acid	

The **CORRECT** combination for **Group I, Group II** and **Group III** is

(a) P-ii-1, Q-iv-3, R-v-2, S-iii-4

(b) P-ii-1, Q-i-3, R-v-4, S-iii-2

(c) P-ii-2, Q-v-3, R-i-4, S-iii-1

(d) P-iii-1, Q-i-3, R-iv-4, S-ii-2

12. Match the following in **CORRECT** combination between **Group I** and **Group II** with reference to the agents that interfere with oxidative phosphorylation

Group I	Group II
P. Cyanide	(i) Blocks electron transfer from cyt b to cyt c_1
Q. Antimycin A	(ii) Inhibits F_1
R. Aurovertin	(iii) Uncoupling of phosphorylation from electron transfer
S. 2,4-Dinitrophenol	(iv) Inhibits cytochrome oxidase
	(v) Inhibits K^+ ionophore

(a) P-iv, Q-i, R-ii, S-iii (b) P-v, Q-i, R-iii, S-iv

(c) P-iv, Q-iii, R-ii, S-v (d) P-v, Q-ii, R-iii, S-iv

13. In relation to Agrobacterium mediated genetic engineering in plants, match the following in **CORRECT** combination

Gene name	Function
P. *virA*	(i) Acetosyringone receptor
Q. *virB*	(ii) Conjugal tube formation
R. *virDl*	(iii) Topoisomerase
S. *virG*	(iv) Inducer of all *vir* operons
	(v) Octopine synthesis

(a) P-iv, Q-iii, R-ii, S-v

(b) P-ii, Q-i, R-iii, S-v

(c) P-i, Q-ii, R-iii, S-iv

(d) P-iii, Q-i, R-ii, S-iv

14. Match the plant part **(Group I)** with the product obtained **(Group II)** and the representative plant species (**Group III**) in **CORRECT** combination

Group I	Group II	Group III
P. Bark	(i) Tannins	1. Papaver somniferum
Q. Leaf	(ii) Saffron	2. Camellia sinensis
R. Flower	(iii) Codeine	3. Cinnamomum zeylanicum
S. Fruit	(iv) Aromatic oil	4. Crocus sativus

(a) P-ii-1, Q-i-3, R-iv-2, S-iii-4

(b) P-ii-1, Q-i-2, R-iv-4, S-iii-3

(c) P-ii-2, Q-iv-3, R-i-4, S-iii-1

(d) P-iv-3, Q-i-2, R-ii-4, S-iii-1

15. Select the **CORRECT** combination by matching the disease, causal organism and the affected plant.

Disease	Causal organism	Affected plant
P. Stem rust	(i) Cercospora personata	1. Wheat
Q. Wart disease	(ii) Plasmopara viticola	2. Ground nut
R. Tikka/leaf spot	(iii) Synchytrium endobioticum	3. Potato
S. Downey mildew	(iv) Puccinia graminis	4. Grape
		5. Apple
		6. Rice

(a) P-iv-1, Q-iii-3, R-i-2, S-ii-4

(b) P-ii-1, Q-i-6, R-iv-4, S-iii-2

(c) P-iii-1, Q-iv-3, R-i-5, S-ii-4

(d) P-iv-1, Q-ii-3, R-iii-2, S-i-5

16. Match the following alkaloids with their uses and source plants in **CORRECT** combination

Alkaloid	Use	Source plant
P. Morphine	(i) Anti-cancer	1. Cinchona officinalis
Q. Quinine	(ii) Analgestic	2. Catharanthus roseus
R. Atropine	(iii) Anti-cholinergic	3. Papaver somniferum
S. Vinblastine	(iv) Anti-malarial	4. Hyoscyamus niger

(a) P-ii-3, Q-iv-1, R-iii-4, S-i-2

(b) P-ii-1, Q-i-3, R-iv-4, S-iii-2

(c) P-ii-2, Q-iv-1, R-i-4, S-iii-3

(d) P-iii-4, Q-ii-1, R-iv-3, S-i-2

17. Match the following ecological terms with their appropriate definitions

Term	Definition
P. Niche	(i) Position of a species in food chain
Q. Biotas	(ii) Place of a living organism in the biotic environment and its relations to food and enemies

R. Trophic level (iii) Physical environment of an organism

S. Habitat (iv) Totality of organisms (flora and fauna) in a given place or region

(a) P-i, Q-ii, R-iv, S-iii (b) P-ii, Q-iv, R-i, S-iii
(c) P-iv, Q-iii, R-i, S-ii (d) P-iii, Q-i, R-ii, S-iv

18. Arrange the following 'water reservoirs of Earth' in decreasing order of water volume

P. Streams

Q. Groundwater

R. Glaciers

S. Lakes and inland seas

(a) R-Q-S-P (b) P-Q-R-S
(c) S-P-R-Q (d) R-P-Q-S

19. Selection markers and the corresponding genes used in plant genetic engineering are given below:

Selection Marker	Gene
P. Kanamycin	(i) *hptIV*
Q. Hygromycin	(ii) *bar*
R. Bialaphos	(iii) *pmi*
S. Mannose	(iv) *nptII*

Choose the **CORRECT** combination

(a) P-ii, Q-i, R-iv, S-iii (b) P-iv, Q-ii, R-i, S-iii
(c) P-iv, Q-i, R-ii, S-iii (d) P-iii, Q-iv, R-ii, S-i

20. A double homozygous mutant develops green and wrinkled seeds. When it was crossed with a true-breeding plant having yellow and round seeds, all the F1 plants developed yellow and round seeds. After self-fertilization of F1, the calculated percentage probability of plants with green and wrinkled seeds in the F2 population (round off to 2 decimal places) is ______

S: MICROBIOLOGY

Q. 1 – Q. 10 carry one mark each

1. The technique of microbial "pure culture" was pioneered by

(a) Edward Jenner

(b) Louis Pasteur

(c) Robert Hooke

(d) Robert Koch

2. The antibacterial trimethoprim is an inhibitor of

(a) dihydrofolate reductase

(b) dihydropteroate synthetase

(c) N^5, N^{10}-methenyl tetrahydrrofolate synthetase

(d) serine hydroxymethyl transferase

3. Choose the correct taxonomical hierarchy among the following:

(a) Species, Genus, Family, Order, Class, Phylum, Domain

(b) Species, Genus, Order, Class, Family, Phylum, Domain

(c) Species, Genus, Order, Family, class, Phylum, Domain

(d) Species, Genus, Family, Class, Order, Phylum, Domain

4. Shifting a *Saccharomyces cerevisiae* culture from fermentative to aerobic respiratory mode will

(a) decrease carbon dioxide production

(b) increase alcohol production

(c) increase glucose consumption

(d) decrease ATP generation per mole of glucose

5. Which one of the following diseases is treated by a neuraminidase inhibitor?

(a) Chickenpox

(b) Polio

(c) Influenza

(d) Japanese encephalitis

6. Which one of the following does NOT provide three-dimensional images?

(a) Atomic force microscopy

(b) Confocal scanning laser microscopy

(c) Diferential interference contrast microscopy

(d) Phase-contrast microscopy

7. Which one of the following will increase the resolution of a light microscope?

(a) Decreasing the numerical aperture of the objective lens

(b) Using objective lens with a longer working distance

(c) Using a medium of higher refractive index

(d) Increasing the wavelength of light

8. Which one of the following conditions favors maximum expression of *lac* operon genes in *E. coli?*

(a) Glucose-low, lactose-low, cAMP-high

(b) Glucose-high, lactose-low, cAMP-high

(c) Glucose-low, lactose-high, cAMP-high

(d) Glucose-high, lactose-high, cAMP-low

9. Match the cellular organelle in **Group I** with its function in **Group II**

Group I	Group II
P. Golgi apparatus	1. Lipid degradation
Q. Nucleolus	2. Protein degradation
R. Peroxisome	3. Protein sorting
S. Proteasome	4. Ribosomal RNA synthesis

(a) P-3, Q-2, R-1, S-4

(b) P-3, Q-4, R-1, S-2

(c) P-1, Q-2, R-4, S-3

(d) P-3, Q-1, R-4, S-2

10. A 250 μl of bacteriophage stock containing 8×10^8 phages/ml is added to 500 μl of *E. coil* culture containing 4×10^8 cells/ml. The multiplicity of infection is ______.

Q. 11 – Q. 20 carry two marks each

11. Digestion of an immunoglobulin G (IgG) molecule with pepsin will NOT

(a) generate a bivalent antigen binding fragment

(b) generate monovalent antigen binding fragments

(c) destroy the complement binding site

(d) cleave the heavy chain of IgG molecule

12. Match the process involved in nitrogen or sulfur cycle in **Group I** with the corresponding microbe in **Group II**.

Group I	Group II
P. Denitrification	1. *Azotobacter*
Q. Nitrogen fixation by free-living microbe	2. *Beggiatoa*
R. Oxidation of H_2S to sulfur	3. *Pseudomonas*
S. Nitrogen fixation by a symbiotic microbe	4. *Rhizobium*

13. Determine the correctness or otherwise of the following Assertion [a] and the Reason [r].

Assertion [a]: Diphtheria exotoxin is an example of A-B type toxin.

Reason [r]: The A component of the toxin is released from the host cell while the B component inhibits protein synthesis and kills the host cell.

(a) Both [a] and [r] are true and [r] is the correct reason for [a]

(b) Both [a] and [r] are true but [r] is not the correct reason for [a]

(c) Both [a] and [r] are false

(d) [a] is true but [r] is false

14. Which one of the following statements about control of microbial growth is NOT correct?

(a) Nonionizing radiation leads to thymine dimers formation is DNA

(b) Spirochetes and mycoplasma can pass through membrane filters (0.22-0.45 μm)

(c) Use of high concentration of salts and sugars to preserve food is a chemical method of microbial control

(d) Thermoduric bacteria can survive pasteurization

15. An example of a differential and selective medium in which colonies of Gram-negative bacteria produce large amounts of acidic products and appear green with a metallic sheen is

(a) Blood agar (b) EMB agar

(c) MacConkey agar (d) Mannitol salt agar

16. Which one of the following is an example of substrate level phosphorylation?

(a) Glucose to Glucose 6-phosphate

(b) Fructose 6-phosphate to Fructose 1, 6-bisphosphate

(c) 1-3-bisphosphoglycerate to 3-phosphoglycerate

(d) 2-phosphoglycerate to Phosphoenolpyruvate

17. A bacterial culture containing 3×10^5 live cells was exposed to a newly developed sterilizing agent. After 30 minutes of exposure, 3 live cells remained in culture. The decimal reduction time (in minutes) for the new agent is ______.

18. A bacterial culture has a generation time of 34 minutes. The time taken (in minutes, rounded off to two decimal places) for the OD_{550} of this exponentially growing culture to increase from 0.25 to 0.85 is _____.

    Assume that OD_{550} has a linear relationship with the cell density.

19. A 100 μl aliquot (10^{-4} dilution) of the bacterial culture plated on the nutrient agar gave 4 colonies. The bacterial stock concentration (in million cells/ml, rounded, off to one decimal place) is ________ .

20. A continuous bacterial culture carried out in a chemostat is set to a flow rate of 40 ml/hr. The culture volume is equivalent to that of a cubical container having 10 cm sides. The dilution rate (in hr^{-1}, rounded off to two decimal places) of this system is ___.

T: ZOOLOGY

Q. 1 – Q. 10 carry one mark each

1. Which ONE of following leucocytes is phagocytic and has clear cytoplasm?

   (a) Eosinophil (b) Monocyte

   (c) T_H-lymphocyte (d) Basophil

2. Which ONE of the following techniques can be used for detecting the subcellular localization of serotonin receptor in intact cells?

   (a) Immunoelectron microscopy

   (b) SDS-PAGE

   (c) Fluorescence in-situ hybridization

   (d) Differential centrifugation.

3. Which ONE of the following is NOT a site for *in situ* conservation?

   (a) Biosphere reserve

   (b) Wild life sanctuary

   (c) Zoological garden

   (d) Biodiversity hotspot

4. Which ONE of the following is the precursor molecule for corticosteroids?

   (a) Androgen

   (b) Estrogea

   (c) Pregnenolone

   (d) Mineralocorticoids

5. Transitional epithelia is found in which ONE of the following organs?

   (a) Liver (b) Lung

   (c) Brain (d) Urinary bladder

6. Visual signal transduction cascade is activated by rhodopsin and involves degradation rather than synthesis of which ONE of the following second messenger molecules?

   (a) cAMP (b) IP3

   (c) cGMP (d) DAG

7. The genomes of both human and Drosophila code for an amylase that acts on the same substrate. However, the sequence of nucleotides in the genes encoding the two is dissimilar. This is an example of which ONE of the following types of evolution?

   (a) Neutral (b) Directional

   (c) Convergent (d) Divergent

8. "Round dance" is performed by forager bees to indicate the distance between a food source and their colony. Which ONE of the following best represents this distance?

   (a) 45 meters

   (b) 450 meters

   (c) 1000 meters

   (d) More than 2000 meters

9. Which ONE of the following phyla have choanocytes?

   (a) Ctenophora (b) Nematoda

   (c) Cnidaria (d) Porifera

10. Which ONE of the following glial cells is NOT derived from the ectoderm?

    (a) Astrocytes

    (b) Microglial cells

    (c) Oligodendrocytes

    (d) Ependyma

Q. 11 – Q. 20 carry two marks each

11. Tarantulas and mosquitoes both belong to the phylum Arthropods. Which ONE of the following represents the correct number of legs in them respectively?

    (a) 6 and 6

    (b) 6 and 8

    (c) 8 and 8

    (d) 8 and 6

12. Match the following subcellular organelles in **Column I** with associated functions in **Column II**

Column I	**Column II**
P. Nucleolus	(i) Glycoprotein biosynthesis
Q. Peroxisomes	(ii) Oxidation of fatty acids and amino acids
R. Endoplasmic reticulum	(iii) Protein trafficking
S. Golgi bodies	(iv) Ribosome biogenesis

(a) P-(iii), Q-(ii), R-(i), S-(iv)
(b) P-(i), Q-(ii), R-(iii), S-(iv)
(c) P-(iv), Q-(ii), R-(i), S-(iii)
(d) P-(ii), Q-(iii), R-(i), S-(iv)

13. Match the following genetic disorders in **Column I** with associated typical. chromosomal changes mentioned in **Column II**

Column I	**Column II**
P. Klinefelter syndrome	(i) 45,XO
Q. Down syndrome	(ii) 5p minus
R. Turner syndrome	(iii) 47,XXY
S. Cri du chat syndrome	(iv) Trisomy 21

(a) P-(iv), Q-(iii), R-(ii), S-(i)
(b) P-(iv), Q-(ii), R-(i), S-(iii)
(c) P-(iii), Q-(iv), R-(ii), S-(i)
(d) P-(iii), Q-(iv), R-(i), S-(ii)

14. Match the following components listed in **Column I** with their respective organs in **Column II**

Column I	**Column II**
P. Endolymph	(i) Testes
Q. Vitreous humour	(ii) Ear
R. Vas deferens	(iii) Ovary
S. Corpus luteum	(iv) Eye

(a) P-(ii), Q-(iv), R-(i), S-(iii)
(b) P-(ii), Q-(i), R-(iv), S-(iii)
(c) P-(iii), Q-(iv), R-(i), S-(ii)
(d) P-(iii), Q-(iv), R-(ii), S-(i)

15. Match the following digestive enzymes in **Column I** with their respective functions in **Column II.**

Column I	**Column II**
P. Erepsin	(i) converts proteins to peptides
Q. Steapsin	(ii) activates trypsinogen to trypsin
R. Pepsin	(iii) converts fat into fatty acid and glycerol
S. Enterokinase	(iv) converts polypeptides to amino acids

(a) P-(iv), Q-(iii), R-(ii), S-(i)
(b) P-(iv), Q-(iii), R-(i), S-(ii)
(c) P-(iii), Q-(iv), R-(i), S-(ii)
(d) P-(iii), Q-(iv), R-(ii), S-(i)

16. Which ONE of the following graphs represents the relationship between ventricular end-diastolic volume and cardiac output in a healthy adult individual. at rest (solid line) and upon exercise (dotted line)?

(a)
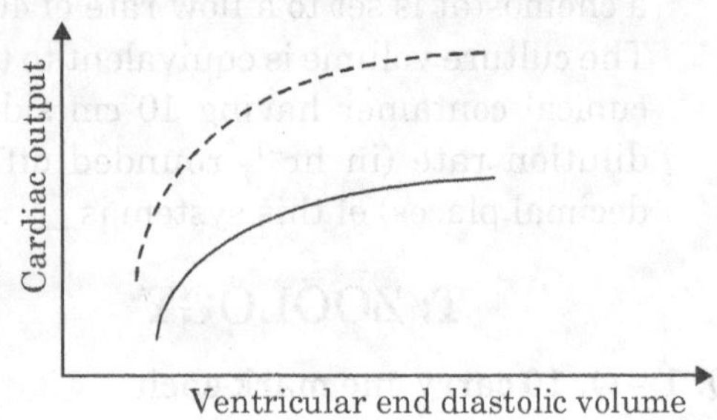

(b)
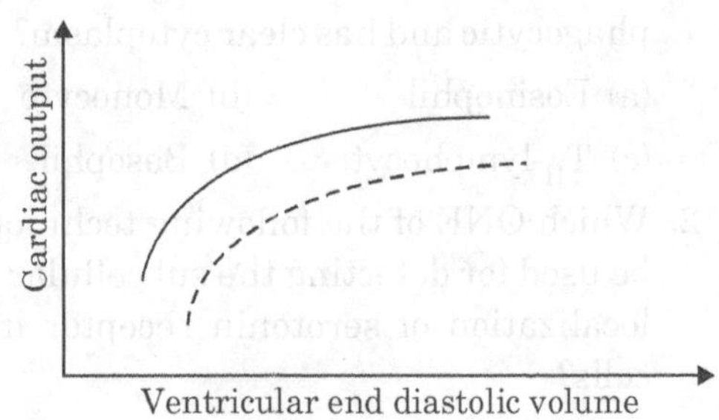

(c)
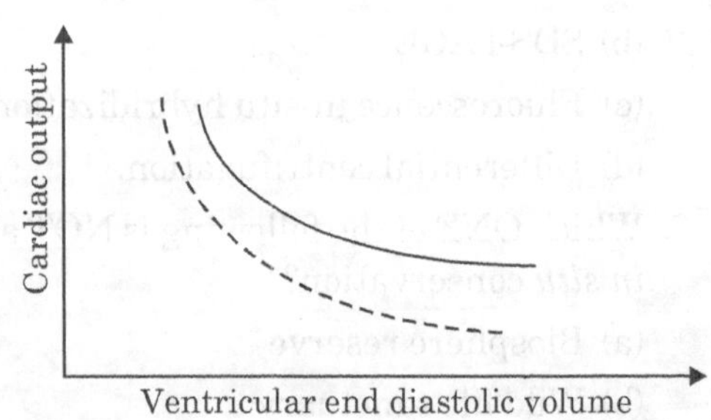

(d)
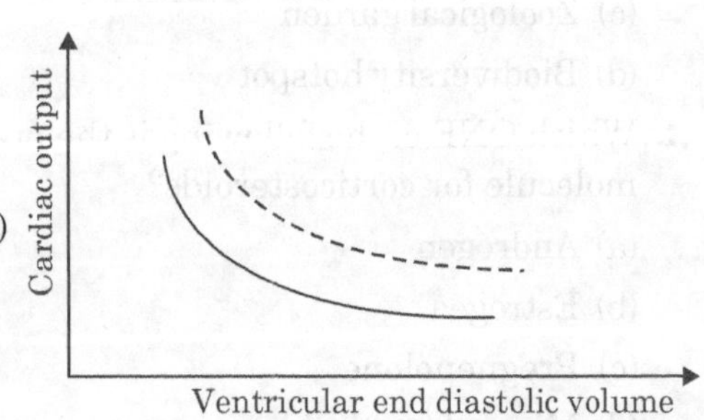

17. Match the household insect vectors in **Column I** with their associated diseases in **Column II**.

Column I	Column II
P. Kissing bug (Hemiptera)	(i) Bubonic plague
Q. Sand fly (Diptera)	(ii) Tularemia
R. Deer fly (Diptera)	(iii) Chagas disease
S. Oriental rat flea (Siphoneptera)	(iv) Kala azar

(a) P-(iv), Q-(iii), R-(ii), S-(i)
(b) P-(iii), Q-(ii), R-(i), S-(iv)
(c) P-(i), Q-(iv), R-(iii), S-(ii)
(d) P-(iii), Q-(iv), R-(ii), S-(i)

18. Match the proteins in **Column I** with the organs in which they are maximally expressed in **Column II**.

Column I	Column II
P. Keratin	(i) Liver
Q. Surfactants	(ii) Pancreas
R. Pro-carboxypeptidase	(iii) Lung
S. Albumin	(iv) Skin

(a) P-(iv), Q-(i), R-(iii), S-(ii)
(b) P-(iii), Q-(iv), R-(ii), S-(i)
(c) P-(iv), Q-(iii), R-(ii), S-(i)
(d) P-(i), Q-(ii), R-(iii), S-(iv)

19. The graph below shows the activity of enzyme pepsin in the presence of inhibitors aliphatic alcohols (P) or N-acetyl-1-phenylalanine (Q). Which ONE of the following represents the nature of inhibition by P and Q, respectively?

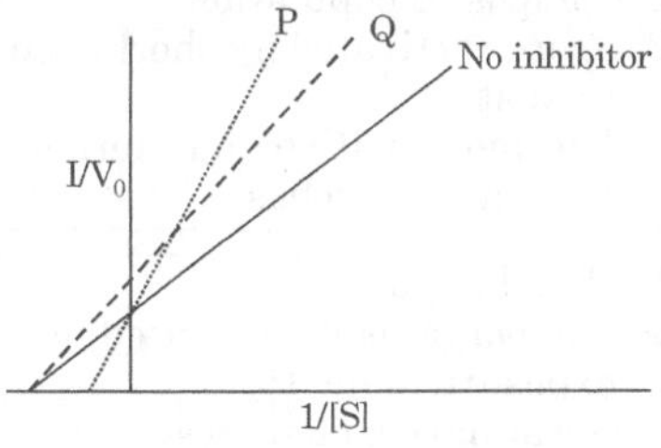

(a) Non-competitive and competitive
(b) Competitive and non-competitive
(c) Non-competitive and uncompetitive
(d) Competitive and uncompetitive

20. In Drosophila, the red eye phenotype (W) is dominant over the recessive white eye mutant (w). In a mixed population of red and white eye flies of 10,000 individuals, 3,600 flies were white eyed. The percentage of the heterozygous red eye flies in this population is ________.

U: FOOD TECHNOLOGY

Q. 1 – Q. 10 carry one mark each

1. The enzyme majorly involved in postmortem degradation of muscle proteins is
(a) Trypsin (b) Calpin
(c) Transglutaminase (d) Pepsin

2. Which of the following is the correct pair of essential fatty acids?
(a) Oleic acid and Lenoleic acid
(b) Lenoleic acid and Linolenic acid
(c) Linolenic acid and Lauric acid
(d) Linolenic acid and Oleic acid

3. Nisin A is produced by
(a) Aspergillus niger
(b) Acetobacter aceti
(c) Lactobacillus lactis
(d) Clostridium perfringens

4. Which of the following bacteria will stain purple color after Gram staining?
(a) Bacillus subtilis
(b) Pseudomonas
(c) Pseudomonas aeruginaosa
(d) Yersinia pestis

5. The enzyme system used for removal of glucose from egg white prior to its drying consists of
(a) Glucose oxidase and Catalase
(b) Ghicosidase and Glucoisomerase
(c) Glucoisomerase and Catalase
(d) Glucoarnylase and Glucose oxidase

6. The INCORRECT pair of food borne illness and its causative microorganism is
(a) Brucellosis - Brucella Sp.
(b) Peptic ulcers - Bacillus subtilis
(c) Bubonic plague - Yersinia pestis
(d) Q fever - Coxiella burnatii

7. Which of the following is commonly used as a preservative in the tomato sauce?
(a) Sodium sulphite (b) Potassium sorbate
(c) Potassium sulphite (d) Sodium benzoate

8. A fluid with flow behaviour index less than one ($n < 1$) is
(a) Dilatant (b) Pseudoplastic
(c) Bingham plastic (d) Newtonian

9. The velocity of 2.2 uni diameter fat particles inside a centrifuge, running at 6000 rpm and 20°C, is 0.25 mm s^{-1}. The velocity of 1.5 μm diameter fat particles inside the same centrifuge running at 7500 rpm and same temperature (round off to 2 decimal places) will be ________ mm s^{-1}.

10. The initial population of a bacterial strain increases from 1×10^4 cells per mL to 1×10^6 cells per mL in 120 minutes. The generation time for this strain (round off to 2 decimal places) is ____________ minutes.

Q. 11 – Q. 20 carry two marks each

11. Match the protein in **Column I** with its food source in **Column II**.

Column I	Column II
P. Zein	1. Soybean
Q. Gluten	2. Maize
R. Glycinin	3. Egg
S. Ovalbumin	4. Wheat

(a) P-4, Q-1, R-2, S-3 (b) P-4, Q-3, R-1, S-2
(c) P-2, Q-3, R-1, S-4 (d) P-2, Q-4, R-1, S-3

12. Match the carbohydrate in **Column I** with corresponding enzyme used for its hydrolysis in **Column II**.

Column I	Column II
P. Pectin	1. Xylanase
Q. Lactose	2. β-galactosidase
R. Hemicellulose	3. Polygalacturonase
S. Inulin	4. β-fructofuranosidase

(a) P-3, Q-2, R-1, S-4 (b) P-2, Q-4, R-1, S-3
(c) P-1, Q-2, R-3, S-4 (d) P-4, Q-3, R-1, S-2

13. Match the edible oil refining stage in **Column I** with its purpose in **Column II**.

Column I	Column II
P. Degumming	1. Separation of triglycerides
Q. Neutralization	2. Removal of pigments
R. Bleaching	3. Removal of phosphatides
S. Winterization	4. Removal of free fatty acids

(a) P-3, Q-1, R-2, S-4 (b) P-1, Q-4, R-2, S-3
(c) P-4, Q-3, R-1, S-2 (d) P-3, Q-4, R-2, S-1

14. Match the food material in **Column I** with iis related term in **Column II**.

Column I	Column II
P. Coffee	1. Wort
Q. Cocoa	2. Must
R. Beer	3. Arabica
S. Wine	4. Theobroma

(a) P-4, Q-2, R-1, S-3 (b) P-3, Q-4, R-1, S-2
(c) P-3, Q-4, R-2, S-1 (d) P-1, Q-3, R-4, S-2

15. Match the component/system in **Column I** with the peeling method for fruits and vegetables in **Column II**.

Column I	Column II
P. Lye solution	1. Flash peeling
Q. Carborundum rollers	2. Flame peeling
R. Pressure vessel	3. Abrasion peeling
S. Conveyor belt	4. Caustic peeling

(a) P-4, Q-3, R-2, S-1 (b) P-3, Q-4, R-1, S-2
(c) P-3, Q-3, R-1, S-2 (d) P-3, Q-4, R-2, S-1

16. Which among the given options correctly explains the nature of the microhial culture represented by lines 1, 2 and 3 in the following figure?

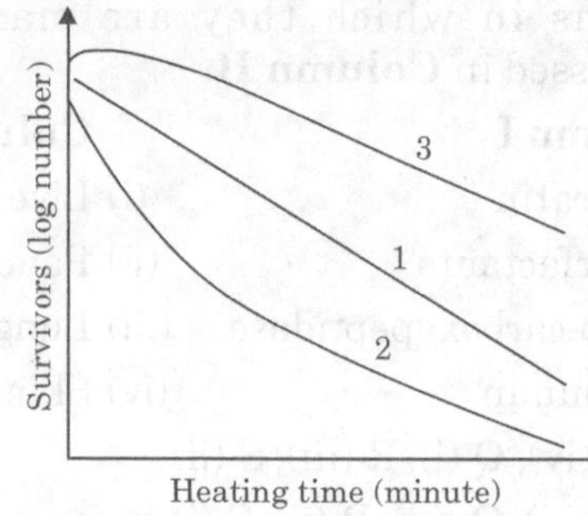

(a) 1. Germination of spores
2. Homogeneous population
3. Mixed population of spores and vegetative cells

(b) 1. Homogeneous population
2. Mixed population of heat sensitive and heat resistant microbes
3. Germination of spores

(c) 1. Composite population
2. Spores activated by short exposure to heat
3. Thermo sensitive and thermo resistant microbes

(d) 1. Mixed population
2. Microorganisms activated by short exposure to heat
3. Germination of spores

17. Match the equation/law in **Column I** with its application in **Column II**.

Column I	Column II
P. Plank's equation	1. Terminal velocity
Q. Arrhenius equation	2. Freezing time
R. Guggenheim-Anderson-de Boer equation	3. Abrasion peeling
S. Stoke's law	4. Monolayer moisture content

(a) P-1, Q-3, R-4, S-2 (b) P-2, Q-3, R-1, S-4
(c) P-2, Q-3, R-4, S-1 (d) P-4, Q-3, R-1, S-2

18. Match the absorber used in modified atmosphere packaging and storage in **Column I** with the scavenger in **Column II**.

Column I	Column II
P. Oxygen absorber	1. Calcium chloride
Q. Carbon dioxide absorber	2. Magnesium oxide
R. Ethylene absorber	3. Ferric oxide
S. Moisture absorber	4. Potassium permanganate

(a) P-3, Q-2, R-4, S-1
(b) P-1, Q-2, R-4, S-3
(c) P-2, Q-3, R-4, S-1
(d) P-3, Q-2, R-1, S-4

19. During extrusion cooking, food materials are generally subjected to a combination of
(a) high shear and low pressure
(b) high temperature and high shear
(c) low shear and high temperature
(d) low shear and low pressure

20. An orange juice flowing at 0.80 kg s^{-1} enters a counter current double pipe heat: exchanger at 20°C and leaves at 72°C. Inlet and outlet temperatures of the hot water used as heating medium in the exchanger are 81°C and 74°C, respectively. The specific heat of the orange juice is 3.74 kJ kg^{-1} K^{-1} and overall heat transfer coefficient is 492 W m^{-2} K^{-1}. The heat transfer surface area (round off to 2 decimal places) will be ______ m^2.

ANSWERS

General Aptitude

1. (*c*) **2.** (*b*) **3.** (*d*) **4.** (*d*) **5.** (*b*) **6.** (*d*) **7.** (*c*) **8.** (*b*) **9.** (*b*)
10. (*b*)

P: Chemistry (Compulsory)

1. (*c*) **2.** (*d*) **3.** (2 to 2) **4.** (2 to 2) **5.** (-1308 to -1308)
6. (*a*) **7.** (*c*) **8.** (*d*) **9.** (*a*) **10.** (*c*) **11.** (*c*)
12. (4.5 to 4.7) **13.** (-202.66 to -202.64) **14.** (3.44 to 3.46) **15.** (-36 to -36)

Q: Biochemistry

1. (*c*) **2.** (*d*) **3.** (*a*) **4.** (*b*) **5.** (*d*) **6.** (*a*)
7. (*c*) **8.** (*a*) **9.** (3 to 3) **10.** (7.5 to 7.7) **11.** (*c*) **12.** (*d*)
13. (*b*) **14.** (*a*) **15.** (*b*) **16.** (51.1 to 51.3) **17.** (1.58 to 1.60)
18. (3.2 to 3.4) **19.** (20 to 20) **20.** (60 to 60)

R: Botany

1. (*a*) **2.** (*a*) **3.** (*b*) **4.** (*a*) **5.** (*d*) **6.** (*d*)
7. (*b*) **8.** (*a*) **9.** (*c*) **10.** (49.5 to 49.5) **11.** (*b*) **12.** (*a*)
13. (*c*) **14.** (*d*) **15.** (*a*) **16.** (*a*) **17.** (*b*) **18.** (*a*)
19. (*c*) **20.** (6.25 to 6.25)

S: Microbiology

1. (*d*) **2.** (*a*) **3.** (*a*) **4.** (*a*) **5.** (*c*) **6.** (*d*)
7. (*c*) **8.** (*c*) **9.** (*b*) **10.** (1 TO 1) **11.** (*b*) **12.** (*d*)
13. (*d*) **14.** (*c*) **15.** (*b*) **16.** (*c*) **17.** (6 to 6)
18. (58.50 to 61.50) **19.** (0.4 to 0.4) **20.** (0.04 to 0.04)

T: Zoology

1. (*b*) **2.** (*a*) **3.** (*c*) **4.** (*c*) **5.** (*d*) **6.** (*c*)
7. (*c*) **8.** (*a*) **9.** (*d*) **10.** (*b*) **11.** (*d*) **12.** (*c*)
13. (*d*) **14.** (*a*) **15.** (*b*) **16.** (*a*) **17.** (*d*) **18.** (*c*)
19. (*b*) **20.** (48 to 48)

U: Food Technology

1. (*b*) **2.** (*b*) **3.** (*c*) **4.** (*a*) **5.** (*a*) **6.** (*b*)
7. (*d*) **8.** (*b*) **9.** (0.15 to 0.21) **10.** (17.00 to 19.00) **11.** (*d*)
12. (*a*) **13.** (*d*) **14.** (*b*) **15.** (*c*) **16.** (*b*) **17.** (*c*)
18. (*a*) **19.** (*b*) **20.** (11.00 to 14.00)

EXPLANATIONS

GENERAL APTITUDE

1. Rajiv Gandhi Khel Ratana Award was conferred on Mary Kom, a six time world champion in boxing, recently in ceremony at the Rashtrapati Bhawan (the President's official residence) in New Delhi.
2. Despite means without being affected by something.
3. Dissociate is the opposite of Associate.
4. Officials hope that the food grain production target will be met due to a good rabi produce.
5. Sum of first n natural numbers

$$= \frac{[n(n+1)]}{2}$$

Sum of first 2n natural numbers

$$= \frac{[2n(2n+1)]}{2} \quad ....(1)$$

Sum of first n odd numbers $= n^2$ ...(2)

Difference of (1) and (2)

$D = 2n^2 + n - n^2 = n^2 + n$

6. Decrease in repo-rate will decrease cost of borrowing and increase lending by commercial banks is the correct inference.
7. 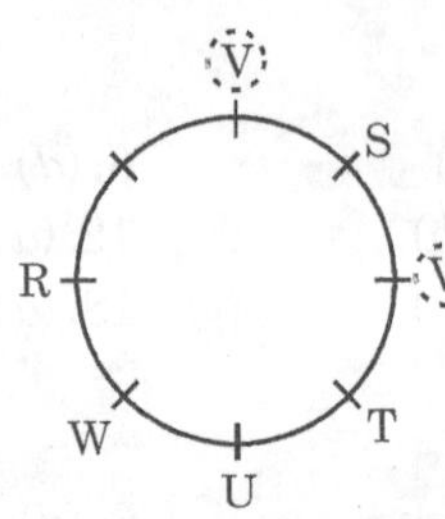

V can take any of the two positions.

In above diagram, P can not be seated opposite to Q.

8. 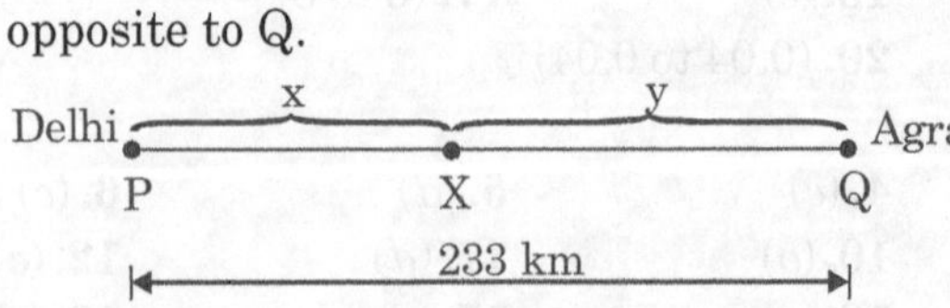

$V_P = V_Q + 10$ ...(i)

$x = V_P \times 2.25$

$y = V_Q \times 1.25$

$x + y = 233$

$V_P \times 2.25 + V_Q \times 1.25 = 233$ ...(ii)

$$V_P = \frac{491}{7} \text{ km/hr}$$

$$V_Q = \frac{421}{7} \text{ km/hr}$$

Distance travelled by Q

$\Rightarrow y = V_Q \times 1.25$

$$= \frac{421}{7} \times 1.25$$

$y = 75.17$ km

9. Total no. of elements in in 4 × 4 matrix is 16; of which four diagonal elements are zero. Remaining 12 elements can be divided in to two equal groups of 6 elements each. Both groups are opposite signed elements to meet the given condition.
10. Let the fixed investment annually be 'A'.

Total revenue of company P (2013 to 2018) = 1.1A + 1.2A + 1.4A + 1.4A + 1.5A + 1.4A = 8A

Total revenue of Company Q (2013 to 2018) = 1.2A + 1.3A + 1.3A + 1.5A + 1.6A + 1.6A = 8.5 A

P: CHEMISTRY (COMPULSORY)

1. Strong acid or strong base does not from buffer solution

10^{-8}M Nacl and 10^{-8}M HCl

This solution will be simple like 10^{-8}MHCl

$PH = -\log[H^+]$

$H^+ = 10^{-8}$M (from HCl) + 10^{-7}M (appro) from water

$\therefore$ pH < 7 ($\approx$6.9)

Correct answer (c) : Solution is not a buffer but has its pH less than 7.00

2. $[Ni(H_2O)_6]^{2+}$ → d^8 with two unpaired e^- Hybridisation → sp^3d^2.

$[V(H_2O)_6]^{2+}$ → d^3 with three unpaired e^- Hybridisation → d^2sp^3.

$[Mn(H_2O)_6]^{2+}$ → d^5 with five unpaired e^- Hybridisation → sp^3d^2.

(Above three symmetical structure because of unpaired e^-)

$\left[Cu(H_2O)_6\right]^{2+}$ → d^9 with one unpaired e^- & Hybridisar is sp^3d^2.

(This is unsymmetical structure e^-)

Correct answer : $\left[Cu(H_2O)_6\right]^{2+}$

3. 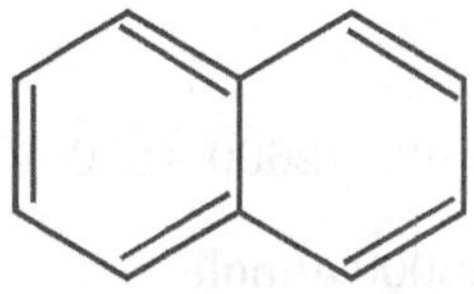 → naphthalene 10 π e^-

Huded Rule

$(4n + 2)\pi = 10$

$n = 2$

Correction Answer : Value of integer n is 2.

4. Cu(z = 29)

dz^2 $l = 2$

Answer is 2.

5. $\frac{1}{2}H_{2(g)} \rightarrow H$ $\Delta h = 218$ KJ/mol.

$H \rightarrow \frac{1}{2}H_{2(g)}$ $\Delta h = -218$ KJ/mol.

$6 \times \left(H \rightarrow \frac{1}{2}H_2\right)$ $\Delta h = -6 \times 218$

$6H \rightarrow 3H_{2(g)} = -1308$ KJ

∴ Answer is –1308 KJ

(for 3 mole of H_2 formax)

6. First Ionisation energy × radius of atom × Stability of atom (Half filled efilly field)

$He \rightarrow 1s^2$

$B \rightarrow 1s^2\,2s^2\,2p^1 \rightarrow B^+ (1s^2\,2s^2) + 1e^-$

(noble gas confignation)

$N \rightarrow 1s^2\,2s^2\,2p^3$

(half filled stable) $\rightarrow N^+ (1s^2\,2s^2\,2p^2) + e^-$

$O \rightarrow 1s^2\,2s^2\,2p^4 \rightarrow O^+ (1s^2\,2s^2\,2p^3) + e^-$

(half filled)

∴ He > N > O > B

Correction Anser : (a)

7. Bond Order (B.O.)

$N_2 = 3$

$N_2^+ \rightarrow 2.5$

$O_2 \rightarrow 2$

$O_2^+ \rightarrow 2.5$

Bond order × Stabno;otu × Bond strength

$\times \frac{1}{\text{Bond}}$ length.

N_2^+ $\overset{\sigma 2}{1s} < \overset{\sigma 2}{1s} < \overset{\sigma 2}{2s} < \overset{\sigma 2}{2s} < \pi 2p_x^2$

$= \pi 2py^2 < \sigma \frac{1}{2p_z}$

O_2^- $\overset{\sigma 2}{1s} < \overset{\sigma 2}{1s} < \overset{\sigma 2}{2s} < \overset{\sigma 2}{2s} < \overset{\sigma 2}{2P_2} < \pi 2p_x^2$

$= \pi 2py^2 < \pi 2p_x^2 = \pi \frac{1}{2py} < \sigma 2p_z$

Answer is (c)

8. 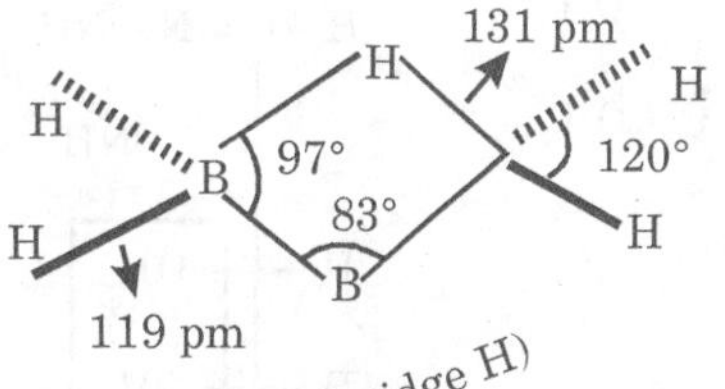

(Bridge H)

B – H – B → 3 - Center 2 - electron band

3 centre but only $2e^-$

B–H (terminal) → 2 center 2 - electron

Answer (d)

9. In ethyline glucol there will be intramolecular H-Bonding

∴ Gauche > Anti (Stablitys)

In 1,2 - difluoroethane

(Ani > Guache > Stability order)

I > II, IV > III } Stability order

Answer : (b)

10. In Alpene

Aqueoes mercuric acclate give morponikoff product

Sulfuric acid additia

Perodie HCl does not give anti-morkonipoff product because in chain reaction same steps are endothermic

∴ Answer is (c)

11.

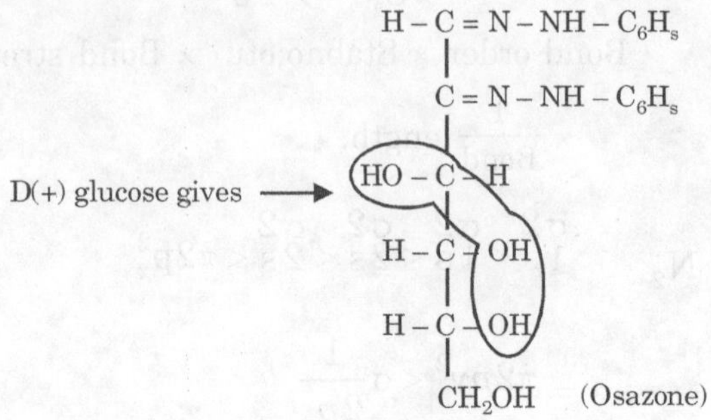

All other optin except 'c' option gives same physical arrangement.

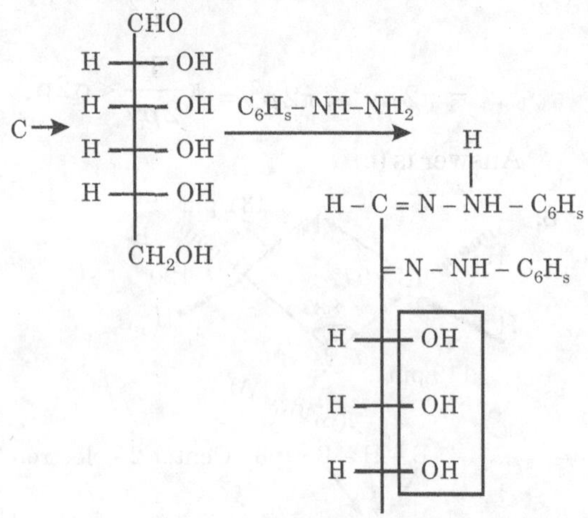

12.

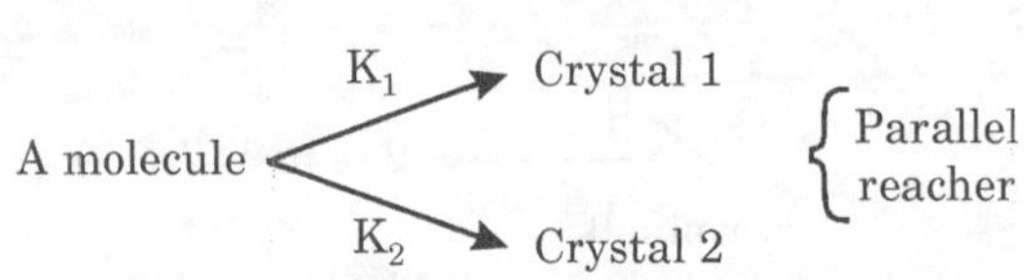

K (rate constant) = K_1 + K2

$= 0.02\ s^{-2} + 0.13\ s^{-1} = 0.15 s^{-1}$

Order of reaction is 1 as unit of rate content is 8–1

$$t_{\frac{1}{2}} = \frac{0.693}{K} = \frac{0.693}{0.15} = 4.5$$

13. $\Delta G° = -nE°F$

$= -3 \times 0.7 \times 96500 \times 10^{-3}$ KJ/mole

= –1308 KJ/mole

Answer is –1308 KJ/mole

14. $$\log\frac{K_2}{K_1} = \frac{Eo}{2.303R}\left(\frac{1}{T_1} - \frac{1}{T_1}\right) \begin{cases} K_2 = K_{298} \\ K_1 = K_{260} \end{cases}$$

$$\log\frac{K_2}{K_1} = \frac{21 \times 10^3}{2.303 \times 8.315}\left(\frac{1}{260} - \frac{1}{298}\right)$$

Anser is $\frac{K_{298}}{K_{260}} = 3.44$

15. $\Delta H = \int sdT = S\Delta T = 60 \times (2600 - 2000)$

= 36000 J/mole

= 36 KJ /mole

Answer is 36 KJ/mole

Q: BIOCHEMISTRY

1. The **progesterone receptor** (**PR**), also known as **NR3C3** or nuclear receptor subfamily 3, group C, member 3, is a protein found inside cells. It is activated by the steroid hormone progesterone.

   In humans, PR is encoded by a single *PGR* gene residing on chromosome 11q22, it has two isoforms, PR-A and PR-B, that differ in their molecular weight. The PR-B is the positive regulator of the effects of progesterone, while PR-A serve to antagonize the effects of PR-B.

2. **A glycosidic bond** or **glycosidic linkage** is a type of covalent **bond** that joins a carbohydrate (sugar) molecule to another group, which may or may not be another carbohydrate. a-Glycosidic bond is NOT present in ATP.

3. Hydroxylation of proteins occurs on three residues, most commonly proline at either the 3- or 4-position, lysine at the 5-position, and asparagine at the 3-position. Hydroxylation reaction is involved in the direct conversion of L-phenylaknine to L-tyrosine.

4. Major histocompatibility complex (MHC) is a cell-surface molecule encoded by a large gene family in all vertebrates. MHC molecules display a molecular fraction called an epitope and mediate interactions of leukocytes with other leukocytes or body cells.

The MHC gene family is divided into three subgroups—class I, class II, and class III. Diversity of antigen presentation, mediated by MHC classes I and II, is attained in multiple ways:

i. The MHC's genetic encoding is polygenic,
ii. MHC genes are highly polymorphic and have many variants,
iii. Several MHC genes are expressed from both inherited alleles (variants).

5. Bar Gobind Khorana and Marshall Nirenberg elucidated the genetic code by using a cell-free protein synthesizing system. It was found that pol (U) and poly (C) result in the synthesis of poly(L-Phe) and poly(L-Pro) respectively. Based on these observations, the correct conclusions is : Codon UUU specifies L-Phe and codon CCC specifies L-Pro.

6. **Antibodies bind antigens** through weak chemical interactions, and **bonding is** essentially **non-covalent**. Electrostatic interactions, hydrogen **bonds**, van der Waals forces, and hydrophobic interactions **are** all known to be **involved** depending on **the** interaction sites.

7. Gel filtration chromatography, a type of size exclusion chromatography, can be used to either fractionate molecules and complexes in a sample into fractions with a particular size range, to remove all molecules larger than a particular size from the sample, or a combination of both operations. Gel filtration chromatography can be used to separate compounds such as small molecules, proteins, protein complexes, polysaccharides, and nucleic acids when in aqueous solution. When an organic solvent is used as the mobile phase, the process is instead referred to as gel permeation chromatography. proteins are eluted from the GF column in decreasing order of size.

8. CO2 > H2O > Glucose > RNA is the correct order of molecules, according to their ability to diffuse across a lipid bilayer.

9. The conversion of glucose to lactate in muscle is given by cori cycle also known as lactic acid cycle.

   The complete reaction is given by

   $$\text{Glucose} + 2P_i + 2\text{ADP} \rightarrow 2 \text{ lactate} + 2\text{ ATP} + 2H_2O$$

   So, one glucose will produce net 2 ATP when converted into lactate.

10. The 3 Pka per histidine are $Pk_1 = 1.8$, $Pk_2 = 9.2$ & $Pk_R = 60$

    So, pr Histidine α-COOH $Pk_1 = 1.8$

    α-NH_3 $Pk_2 = 9.2$

    & side chain $Pk_R = 6.0$

    Here, additional acidic or basic group is present as side-chain functions and the PI is the average of the Pk_a's of two most similar acids.

    So,

    $$\text{PI of Histiding} = \frac{1}{2}(Pk_R + Pk_2) = \frac{1}{2}(9.2 + 6.0)$$
    $$= 7.6$$

11. A protein **homodimer** is formed by two identical proteins. A protein **heterodimer** is formed by two different proteins. ***Heterodimer is*** a protein composed of two polypeptide chains differing in composition in the order, number, or kind of their amino acid residues. Most protein dimers in biochemistry are not connected by covalent bonds. An example of a non-covalent heterodimer is the enzyme reverse transcriptase, which is composed of two different amino acid chains.

12. The prosthetic groups/cofactors involved in both 1e– and 2e– transfer in the mitochondrial electron transport chain are Coenzyme Q and FMN.

    Initiation of Electron Transport Chain: Once the NADH has been made from a metabolite in the citric acid cycle inside of the mitochondria, it interacts with the first complex 1 enzyme, known as NADH reductase. This complex 1 contains a coenzyme flavin mononucleotide (FMN) which is similar to FAD.

    The sequence of events is that the NADH, plus another hydrogen ion enter the enzyme complex and pass along the 2 hydrogen ions, ultimately to an interspace in the mitochondria. These hydrogen ions, acting as a pump, are utilized by ATP synthetase to produce an ATP for every two hydrogen ions produced. Three complexes (1, 3, 4) act in this manner to produce 2 hydrogen ions each, and thus will produce 3 ATP for every use of the complete electron transport chain.

In addition, NADH passes along 2 electrons to first FMN, then to an iron-sulfur protein (FeS), and finally to coenzyme Q. The net effect of these reactions are to regenerate coenzyme NAD^+. This regeneration of reactants occurs in many of the reactions so that a cycling effect occurs. The NAD^+ is ready to react further with metabolites in the citric acid cycle.

Coenzyme Q, which also picks up an additional 2 hydrogen ions to make $CoQH_2$, is soluble in the lipid membrane and can move through the membrane to come into contact with enzyme complex 3.

13. Match of the items in Group I with the most appropriate items in Group II

Items in Group I	Items in Group II
P. Integrin	4. Binding of cells to endothelium
Q. Microglial cell	1. Phagocytosis in the neural tissu
R. TLR-7	3. Single stranded RNA recognition
S. Dendritic cell	2. Antigen processing by cross-presentation

14. Glycogen is a very large, branched polymer of glucose residues. Most of the glucose units in glycogen are linked by á-1,4-glycosidic bonds. The branches are formed by á-1,6-glycosidic bonds, present about once in 10 units.

Two chains of glucose molecules joined by á-1,4-glycosidic bonds are linked by an á-1,6-glycosidic bond to create a branch point. Such an á-1,6-glycosidic bond forms at approximately every 10 glucose units, making glycogen a highly branched molecule.

15. Each ***mRNA*** molecule is simultaneously translated by many ***ribosomes***, all synthesizing protein in the same ***direction***: reading the ***mRNA*** from 52 to 32 and synthesizing the ***polypeptide*** from the ***N*** terminus to the ***C*** terminus. The complete ***mRNA***/poly-***ribosome*** structure is called a polysome.

In the early 1960s, Merrifield proposed the use of a polystyrene-based solid support for peptide synthesis. Peptides could be assembled stepwise from the C to N terminus using Ná-protected amino acids. ***Solid phase peptide synthesis*** is traditionally carried out in the ***C '! N direction***.

Therefore, Polypeptides are either biosynthesized on the ribosomes using an mRNA template or chemically synthesized by the Merrifield's solid phase method. The correct directions of peptide synthesis are N'!C direction on the ribosomes and C'!N direction on the solid phase.

16. Solution absorbs 20% per curvetle of path length 1 cm.

Now, we know that A = εcl

for 1st condition = $A_1 = 0.2, l = 1$ cm

2nd condition = $A_2 = ?, l = 3$ cm

$\therefore \quad A_2 = 3 \times A_1 = 0.6$

Now, the relation between absorbance & transmitance is given by

$$A = 2 - \log_{10} \%T$$

$$\therefore \quad \log_{10}\%T = 2 - A = 2 - 0.6 = 1.4$$

$$\therefore \quad \%T = 25.12$$

17. Pka of phosphuric acid = 6.8

Now, we know that PH

$$= PK_A + \log\frac{[Na_2HPO_4]}{[NaH_2PO_4]}$$

Now, required $P^H = 7$

$$7 = 6.8 + \log\frac{[Na_2HPO_4]}{[NaH_2PO_4]}$$

$$\therefore \frac{[Na_2HPO_4]}{[NaH_2PO_4]} = 10^{0.2} = 1.585$$

So, the ratio of Na_2HPO_4 to NaH_2PO_4 is 1.585.

18. MW of DNA flagment = $\frac{250 \times 660}{1000} = 165$

PCR Reaction Volume = 100 µl.

Concentration of each primer = 0.2 µm

Now, Final conc. of PCR Product/ml

= Primer conc. × MW of DNA

= 0.2 × 165 = 33 µg/ml

but the PCR reaction volume = 100 µl

So, final conc. of PCR product = 33 × 100 = 3.3 µg

19. Reaction velocity, v = 10 µ ml/min

Now, according to M·M limetics the reaction velocity is given by following equation.

$$v = \frac{V_{max}[S]}{K_m + [S]}$$

Now, substituting v = 10 μ ml/min & [S] = K_m

$$\therefore \quad 10 = \frac{V_{max} K_m}{K_m + K_m}$$

$$\Rightarrow \quad V_{max} = 20 \ \mu \text{ ml/min}$$

20. The equilibrium reaction is given by following

glucose → Fructose

$\Delta G° = 0$ kcal/mgl

$$\text{Now,} \quad K_{eq} = \frac{[\text{Fructose}]}{[\text{Glucose}]}$$

$$\text{Now,} \quad K_{eq} = e^{-\frac{\Delta G°}{RT}}$$

$$\therefore \quad K_{eq} = 1$$

So, [Fructose] = [Glucose]

Now, at equilibrium the concentration of glucose and fructose is equal in the solution.

So, the conc. of fructose in the reaction mix is $\frac{1}{2}$ of the conc. of glucose solution.

$$\text{i.e.,} \quad \frac{0.12}{2} = 0.06 \text{ M}$$

So, fructose conc. = 0.06 M

= 0.06 × 1000 mm = 60 mm

R: BOTANY

1. Malvaceae family shows indefinite stamens with united filaments in a tube. This condition is called as monadelphous. **Malvaceae**, or the **mallows**, is a family of flowering plants. Well-known members of economic importance include okra, cotton, cacao and durian.
2. In monocotyledons, vascular bundles are closed. The secondary growth is absent due to lack of cambium but in some plants like *Dracena* and *Yucca* secondary growth takes place. Anomolous secondary growth occurs in *Dracena* and absent in maize, wheat and rice.
3. The primary meristem, as a meristematic tissue, is comprised of undifferentiated (others, partially differentiated), embryonic cells. They are actively dividing cells, with thin walls and large nuclei. These cells do not form secondary cell wall thickenings, and therefore have only primary cell walls. An example of a primary meristem is the apical meristem. Apical meristems are meristematic tissues located in the apices of plant, e.g. root apex and shoot apex.
4. Dicamba (2-Methoxy-3,6-dichlorobenzoic acid) is a methoxybenzoic acid that is O-methylsalicylic acid substituted by chloro groups at positions 3 and 6. It has a role as a xenobiotic, an environmental contaminant, a herbicide, a synthetic auxin and an agrochemical. It is a methoxybenzoic acid and a dichlorobenzene. It is a conjugate acid of a 3,6-dichloro-2-methoxybenzoate.
5. The **first stable** compound produced in **Calvin cycle** is a **3** carbon compound, that is **3 phosphoglyceric acid** (PGA). Due to this, the **Calvin cycle** is also called as C3 **cycle.** In C4 plant, the **first stable product** is a 4 carbon compound, that is Oxaloacetic **Acid** (OAA).
6. **parasitism** is a symbiotic relationship between species, where one organism, the **parasite**, lives on or in another organism, the host, causing it some harm, and is adapted structurally to this way of life. Parasitism means relationship between two species of plants or **animals** in which one benefits at the **expense** of the **other**, sometimes **without killing** the host **organism**.
7. Ferula **asafoetida** is herbaceous plant of the umbelliferae family. It is **oleo gum resin obtained** from the rhizome and **root** of plant. This spice is used as a digestive aid, in food as a condiment and in pickles.
8. Bakanae disease is also called as foolish seedling disease. It affects the rice plant through the roots or crowns. It is caused by the fungus *Gibberella fujikuroi*. Affected seedlings show abnormal elongation and in severe cases may lead to death. This disease helped in discovery of hormone gibberellin produced by fungus *Gibberella fujikuroi.*
9. Artificial chromosomal doubling is achieved by treating the haploid seedlings with chemicals that exhibit anti-mitotic activity. Colchicine is widely used for chromosomal doubling in Doubled haploid (DH) line production pipelines.

11. The CORRECT combination for Group I, Group II and Group III is:

Group I (enzyme)	Group II (product of the enzymatic reaction)	Group III (metabolic process)
P. Hexokinase	ii. Glucose 6-P	1. Glycolysis
Q. Fuirarase	i. Malate	3. TCA cycle
R. PEP Carboxylase	v. Oxaloacetic acid	4. Photosynthesis
S. Glycolate oxidase	iii. Hydrogen peroxide	2. Photorespiration

12. CORRECT MATCH of Group I and Group II with reference to the agents that interfere with oxidative phosphorylation:

Group I	Group II
P. Cyanide	iv. Inhibits cytochrome oxidase
Q. Antimycin A	i. Blocks electron transfer
R. Aurovertin	ii. Inhibits F1
S. 2,4-Dinitrophenol	iii. Uncoupling of phosphorylation from electron transfer

13. CORRECT combination in relation to Agrobacterium mediated genetic engineering in plants is

Gene name	Function
P. vir A	i. Acetosyringone recepto
Q. vir B	ii. Conjugal tube formatio
R. vir Dl	iii. Topoisomerase
S. virG	iv. Inducer of all vir operons

14. CORRECT combination of the plant part (Group I) with the product obtained (Group II) and the representative plant species (Group III) is:

Group I (plant part)	Group II (product obtained)	Group III (plant species)
P. Bark	iv. Aromatic oi	3. Cinnamomum zeylanicum
Q. Leaf	i. Tannins	2. Camellia sinensis
R. Flower	ii. Saffron	4. Crocus sativu
S. Fruit	iii. Codeine	1. Papaver somniferum

15. The CORRECT match of the disease, causal organism and the affected plant is:

Disease	Causal organism	Affected plan
P. Stem rust	iv. Puccinia gramini	1. Wheat
Q. Wart diseas	iii. Synchytrium endobioticum	3. Potato
R. Tikkal/leaf spot	i. Cercospora personata	2. Ground nut
S. Downey mildew	ii. Plasmopara viticola	4. Grape

16. CORRECT match of alkaloids with their uses and source plants :

Alkaloid	Use	Source plant
P. Morphine	ii. Analgestic	3. Papaver somniferum
Q. Quinine	iv. Anti-malarial	1. Cinchona officinali
R. Atropin	iii. Anti-cholinergic	4. Hyoscyamus niger
R. Atropin	i. Anti-cancer	2. Catharanthus roseus

17. Correct match of the ecological terms with their appropriate definitions:

Term	Definition
P. Niche	ii. Place of a living organism in the biotic environment and its relations to food and enemies
Q. Biotas	iv. Totality of organisms (flora and fauna) in a given place or region
R. Trophic level	i. Position of a species in food chain
S. Habitat	iii. Physical environment of an organism

18. 'water reservoirs of earth' as per decreasing order of water volume is:

Ocean > Glaciers > Groundwater > Lakes and inland sea > Streams

19. CORRECT combination of selection markers and the corresponding genes used in plant genetic engineering are:

Selection Marker	Gene
P. Kanamycin	iv. nptII
Q. Hygromycin	i. hptIV
R. Bialaphos	ii. bar
S. Mannose	iii. pmi

20. Please type the matter given bellow

Yellow Round YYRR × Green Wrinkled yyrr

↓

Yellow Round YyRr

YyRr × YyRr

↓

9 : 3 : 3 : 1

Yellow Round, Yellow Wrinkled, Green Round, Green Wrinkled $\left(\frac{1}{16}\right)$

↓

$$\text{Probability} = \frac{1}{16} = 0.625$$

Percentage probability = 0.625 × 106 = 6.25

S: MICROBIOLOGY

1. The existence of microorganisms was predicted many centuries before they were first observed, for example by the Jains in India and by Marcus Terentius Varro in ancient Rome. The first recorded microscope observation was of the fruiting bodies of moulds, by Robert Hooke in 1666, but the Jesuit priest Athanasius Kircher was likely the first to see microbes, which he mentioned observing in milk and putrid material in 1658. Antonie van Leeuwenhoek is considered a father of microbiology as he observed and experimented with microscopic organisms in 1676, using simple microscopes of his own design. Scientific microbiology developed in the 19th century through the work of Louis Pasteur and in medical microbiology Robert Koch. The technique of microbial "pure culture" was pioneered by Robert Koch.

2. Trimethoprim inhibits dihydrofolate reductase, the enzyme that catalyzes the last step of bacterial folic acid synthesis. Instead, trimethoprim is nearly always used in combination with sulfamethoxazole for synergistic effects. This antibacterial also possesses antimalarial properties. When used alone, trimethoprim is bacteriostatic, but it is bactericidal when combined with sulfonamides. Trimethoprim is used in combination with sulfonamides to treat urinary tract infections, prostatic infections, otitis media in children, elimination of *Shigella*, and treatment of *Pneumocystis carinii* pneumonia.

3. The correct taxonomical hierarchy is as : (a) Species, Genus, Family, Order, Class, Phylum, Domain

4. More carbon dioxide production occurs during alcohol production i.e. anaerobic fermentation and shifting a Saccharomyces cerevisiae culture from fermentative to aerobic respiratory mode will decrease carbon dioxide production as aerobic fermentation support biomass growth rather than alcohol production.

5. Neuraminidase inhibitors are a new class of **antiviral drugs** that inhibit influenza A and B viruses.

6. Phase-contrast microscopy does NOT provide three-dimensional images. Phase-contrast microscopy is a technique used for gaining contrast in a translucent specimen without staining the specimen. One major advantage is that phase-contrast microscopy can be used with high-resolution objectives, but it requires a specialized condenser and more expensive objectives. Specimens for phase-contrast microscopy should be as small as possible, and they must be mounted in a fluid or gel for an even grey background in the image.

7. Using a medium of higher refractive index will increase the resolution of a light microscope.

In order to ***increase the resolution*** (d=ë/2 NA), the specimen must be viewed ***using*** either shorter wavelength (ë) ***light*** or ***through*** an imaging ***medium with*** a relatively high ***refractive index*** or ***with*** optical components which have ***a high*** NA (or, indeed, a combination of all of these factors).

8. The repressor is encoded by the lacI gene under control of its own promoter. In the presence of glucose and/or the absence of lactose in wild-type Escherichia coli cells, the operon is down-regulated and considered to be "off." The operon is activated in the presence of lactose or synthetic lactose analogs under conditions where glucose levels are low, which activates CAP-cAMP [3]. Thus, high levels of transcription of the lac operon occur only under the appropriate conditions of lactose availability and the absence of glucose. Therefore Glucose-low, lactose-high, cAMP-high conditions favors maximum expression of lac operon genes in E. coli.

9. Correct match of the cellular organelle in Group I with its function in Group II:

Group I (cellular organelle)	**Group II** (function)
P. Golgi apparatus	3. Protein sorting
Q. Nucleolus	4. Ribosomal RNA synthesis
R. Peroxisome	1. Lipid degradation
S. Proteasome	2. Protein degradation

10. Amt. of Bactero phage stock = 250 μl

Conc. of Bactero phage = 8×10^8 phages/ml

So, conc. of bacterio phage in 250 μl.

$$= \frac{8\times10^8}{4} = 2\times10^8 \text{ phages/250 μl}$$

Now, E.coli culture contains 4×10^8 cells/ml

So, 500 μl E.coli culture contains = $\frac{4\times10^8}{2}$

$= 2 \times 10^8$ cells/500 μl

So, the multiplicity of infection

$$= \frac{\text{No. of E.coli cells}}{\text{No. of phages cells}}$$

$$= \frac{2\times10^8}{2\times10^8} = 1$$

11. Digestion of an immunoglobulin G (1gG) molecule with pepsin will NOT generate monovalent antigen binding fragments. Pepsin is a nonspecific endopeptidase that is active only at acid pH. It is irreversibly denatured at neutral or alkaline pH. Digestion by the enzyme pepsin normally produces one F(ab')2 fragment and numerous small peptides of the Fc portion. The resulting F(ab')2 fragment is composed of two disulfide-connected Fab units. The Fc fragment is extensively degraded, and its small fragments can be separated from F(ab')2 by dialysis, gel filtration or ion exchange chromatography.

12. Correct match of the process involved in nitrogen or sulfur cycle in Group I with the corresponding microbe in Group II:

Group I

(process involved in nitrogen or sulfur cycle)

P. Denitrification

Q. Nitrogen fixation by free-living microbe

R. Oxidation of H2S to sulfur

S. Nitrogen fixation by symbiotic microbe

Group II (corresponding microbe)

3. *Pseudomonas*

1. *Azotobacter*

2. *Beggiatoa*

4. *Rhizobium*

13. Assertion [a]: Diphtheria exotoxin is an example of A-B type toxin is true but **Reason [r]:** The A component of the toxin is released from the host cell while the B component inhibits protein synthesis and kills the host cell is false.

14. The statement about control of microbial growth i.e. "Use of high concentration of salts and sugars to preserve food is a chemical method of microbial control" is NOT correct

15. Eosin methylene blue agar (**EMB**) is a selective and differential **medium** used to isolate fecal coliforms. Eosin Y and methylene blue (6:1) are pH indicator dyes which combine to form a dark purple precipitate at low pH; they also serve to inhibit the growth of most Gram-positive organisms. colonies of Gram-negative bacteria produce large amounts of acidic products and appear green with a metallic sheen is EMB agar.

16. Substrate-level phosphorylation is a metabolic reaction that results in the formation of ATP or GTP by conversion of a higher energy substrate (whether phosphate group attached or not) into lower energy product and a using some of the released chemical energy, the Gibbs free energy, to transfer a phosphoryl (PO_3) group to ADP or GDP from another phosphorylated compound.

Glycolysis: The first substrate-level phosphorylation occurs after the conversion of 3-phosphoglyceraldehyde and Pi and NAD+ to 1,3-bisphosphoglycerate via glyceraldehyde 3-phosphate dehydrogenase. 1,3-bisphosphoglycerate is then dephosphorylated via phosphoglycerate kinase, producing 3-phosphoglycerate and ATP through a substrate-level phosphorylation.

The second substrate-level phosphorylation occurs by dephosphorylating phosphoenolpyruvate, catalyzed by pyruvate kinase, producing pyruvate and ATP.

17. Bacterial culture containing 3×10^5 live cells

So, initial no. of live cells $N_0 = 3 \times 10^5$

Sterilizing time t = 30 min

Final no. of live cells $N_t = 3$

$\therefore$ We know that, $\ln\frac{N_0}{N_t} = kt$

$$\therefore \quad k = \frac{\ln(N_0/N_t)}{t} = \frac{\ln(3\times10^5/3)}{30}$$

$$= \frac{11.513}{30}$$

$$k = 0.384\ \text{min}^{-1}$$

Now, decimal reduction time $(D_r) = \frac{2.303}{K}$

$$\therefore \quad D_r = \frac{2.303}{0.384}$$

$$\therefore \quad D_r = 6.00\ \text{min}$$

18. Bacterial culture generation time = 34 min

OD_{550} is increase from 0.25 + 0.85

So, the no. of times the concentration of cells from initial culture

$$= \frac{0.85}{0.25} \quad (\because \text{According to OD reading})$$

$$= 3.4$$

So, we can say that, $N_t = 3.4$ No.

Now, the cell generation equation is given by

$$N_t = \text{No. } 2^{t/Td}$$

t = time required

T_d = generation time

= 34 min

$$\therefore \quad 3.4\ \text{No.} = \text{No. } 2^{t/Td}$$

$$\therefore \quad \ln 3.4 = \frac{t}{T_d}\ln 2$$

$$\therefore \quad t = \frac{\ln 3.1}{\ln 2}\times 34$$

$$= 60.02\ \text{min}$$

19. Let x is the no. of cells/ml in stock solution.

Now, Dilution is 10^{-4}.

So, the no. of cells after dilution

$= 10^{-4}$ x cells/ml

Now, after dilution 100 μl adjust gave 4 colonias.

So, 1 ml of Aliquot gave 40 colonies.

and this 40 colonies = 10^{-4} x

$$\therefore \quad x = \frac{40}{10^{-4}} = 4\times10^5 \ \text{cells/ml}$$

$$\therefore \quad x = \frac{4\times10^5}{10^6}\ \text{million cells/ml}$$

$$= 0.4\ \text{million cells/ml}$$

So, the bacterial stock concentration is 0.4 million cells/ml

20. Flow rate F = 40 ml/hr

Vol. of cubical container

$$= 0.1 \times 0.1 \times 0.1\ m^3 \quad \left(\because \frac{10\text{cm}}{100} = 0.1\text{m}\right)$$

$$= 10^{-3}\ m^3$$

So, culture volume (V) = Vol. of cubical container

$$= 10^{-3}\ m^3$$

$$= 10^{-3} \times 1000\ \text{lit.} \quad (\because 1\ m^3 = 1000\ \text{lit})$$

$$= 1\ \text{lit}$$

$$V = 1000\ \text{ml}$$

$$\therefore \quad \text{Dilution rate} = \frac{F}{V} = \frac{40}{1000}\frac{\text{ml/hr}}{\text{ml}}$$

$$= 0.04\ \text{hr}^{-1}$$

T: ZOOLOGY

1. Monocytes are cells capable of ingesting bacteria and particulate matter, and act as 'scavenger cells' at the site of infections. They are larger than other leucocytes, measuring between 16 and 22 µm in diameter. Monocytes have one large nucleus, which is usually centrally placed within the cell and often kidney shaped (reniform). This nucleus has a stranded appearance, like a skein of wool, and when stained, is a pale violet colour. The copious cytoplasm, staining a pale greyish-blue, contains innumerable dust-like granules of reddish-blue. It may also possess vacuoles, which appear as clear spaces in the cytoplasm.
2. Immunoelectron microscopy technique can be used for detecting the subcellular localization of serotonin receptor in intact cells. Immunoelectron microscopy is an essential tool for evaluating subcellular localization of molecules within cells at nanometre resolution. This technique is especially useful for colocalization studies involving two or more proteins.
3. Zoological garden is NOT a site for in situ conservation. In-situ conservation is the on-site conservation or the conservation of genetic resources in natural populations of plant or animal species. It is the process of protecting an endangered plant or animal species in its natural habitat, either by protecting or restoring the habitat itself or by defending the species from predators. Examples - Sanctuaries and National Parks.

   Ex situ conservation literally means, "off-site conservation". It is the process of protecting an endangered species, variety or breed, of plant or animal outside of its natural habitat; for example, by removing part of the population from a threatened habitat and placing it in a new location, which may be a wild area or within the care of humans. Examples - Zoological Park and Botanical Garden.
4. A 21-carbon **steroid**, derived from cholesterol and found in **steroid** hormone-producing tissues. **Pregnenolone is the precursor** to gonadal **steroid** hormones and the adrenal **corticosteroids**.
5. Transitional epithelium is a layer of **cells** that forms the mucosal lining of your **ureters**, a portion of your **urethra**, and your **urinary bladder**. These **cells** are called transitional because they can undergo a change in their shape and structure.
6. The product of light activation, Metarhodopsin II, initiates the visual phototransduction pathway by stimulating the G protein transducin (G_t), resulting in the liberation of its á subunit. This GTP-bound subunit in turn activates cGMP phosphodiesterase. cGMP phosphodiesterase hydrolyzes (breaks down) cGMP, lowering its local concentration so it can no longer activate cGMP-dependent cation channels. This leads to the hyperpolarization of photoreceptor cells, changing the rate at which they release transmitters.
7. In **evolutionary** biology, **convergent evolution** is the process whereby organisms not closely related (not monophyletic), independently **evolve** similar traits as a result of having to adapt to similar environments or ecological niches. Therefore the genomes of both human and Drosophila code for an amylase that acts on the same substrate. However, the sequence of nucleotides in the genes encoding the two is dissimilar. This is an example of convergent evolution.
8. If a foraging honey bee (*Apis mellifera*) locates a profitable food source, she returns to the hive and performs a round dance to communicate its location. The forager bee moves in close circles over the comb, alternating directions. The round dance is performed by the forager bee when the food source is located in the immediate vicinity of the hive. Karl von Frisch determined that the critical distance for switching between the round dance and the waggle dance exists at 50 meters away from the hive. The scent attached to the forager bee's body communicates the type of food source in question to the follower bees. However, the scent of the food source alone is not sufficient information to guide the follower bees to said food source.
9. The group of organisms that comprise the phylum Porifera are known as the **sponges**. Sponges are often bright in color and found along coral reefs. Many people don't even realize that sponges are animals, not plants. Sponges are an example of an organism that don't have hands, a mouth, or a stomach.

Instead, these organisms have specialized cells called **choanocytes** that help them survive.

10. **Glia**, also called **glial cells** or **neuroglia**, are non-neuronal cells in the central nervous system (brain and spinal cord) and the peripheral nervous system that do not produce electrical impulses. They maintain homeostasis, form myelin, and provide support and protection for neurons. In the central nervous system, glial cells include oligodendrocytes, astrocytes, ependymal cells, and microglia, and in the peripheral nervous system glial cells include Schwann cells and satellite cells. Most glia are derived from ectodermal tissue of the developing embryo, in particular the neural tube and crest. The exception is **microglia**, which are derived from hemopoietic stem cells. In the adult, microglia are largely a self-renewing population and are distinct from macrophages and monocytes, which infiltrate an injured and diseased CNS.

11. Tarantulas and mosquitoes both belong to the phylum Arthropods. The correct number of legs in them are 8 and 6 respectively.

A **tarantula** has four pairs of **legs** and two additional pairs of appendages. Each **leg** has seven segments, which from the prosoma out are: coxa, trochanter, femur, patella, tibia, tarsus and pretarsus, and claw.

Mosquitoes have **six** legs and a pair of translucent wings. The mosquito's head contains **two** compound eyes and a pair of long antennae. The antennae are used by the mosquito to smell.

12. Correct match of the subcellular organelles in Column I with associated functions in Column II

Column I (subcellular organelles)

P. Nucleolus

Q. Peroxisomes

R. Endoplasmic reticulum

S. Golgi bodies

Column II (associated functions)

(iv) Ribosome biogenesis

(ii) Oxidation of fatty acids and amino acids

(i) Glycoprotein biosynthesis

(iii) Protein trafficking

13. Correct match of the genetic disorders in Column I with associated typical chromosomal changes mentioned in Column II

Column I (genetic disorders)	Column II (typical chromosomal changes)
P. Klinefelter syndrom	(iii) 47, XXY
Q. Down syndrome	(iv) Trisomy 21
R. Turner syndrome	(i) 45, XO
S. Cri du chat syndrome	(ii) 5p minus

14. Correct match of the components listed in Column I with their respective organs in Column II

Column I (Components)	Column II (respective organs)
P. Endolymph	(ii) Ear
Q. Vitreous humour	(iv) Eye
R. Vas deferens	(i) Testes
S. Corpus luteum	(iii) Ovary

15. Correct match of the digestive enzymes in Column I with their respective functions in Column. II.

Column I (digestive enzymes)

P. Erepsin

Q. Steapsin

R. Pepsin

S. Enterokinase

Column II (respective functions)

(iv) converts polypeptides lo amino acids

(iii) converts fat into fatty acid and glycerol

(i) converts proteins to peptides

(ii) activates trypsinogen to trypsin

16. Graph (a) represents the relationship between ventricular end-diastolic volume and cardiac output in a healthy adult individual at rest (solid line) and upon exercise (dotted line as cardiac output increases with ventricular end-diastolic volume. Both parameters follow same pattern with respect to a healthy adult individual at rest and at exercise state however at exercise state values of both the parameters remains high.

17. Correct match of the household insect vectors in Column I with their associated diseases in Column II

Column I (household insect vectors)	Column II (associated diseases)
P. Kissing bug (Hemiptera)	(iii) Chagas disease
Q. Sand fly (Diptera)	(iv) Kala azar
R. Deer fly (Diptera)	(ii) Tularemia
S. Oriental rat flea (Siphoneptera)	(i) Bubonic plague

18. Correct match of the proteins in Column I with the organs in which they are maximally expressed in Column II

Column I (proteins)	Column II (organs)
P. Keratin	(iv) Skin
Q. Surfactants	(iii) Lung
R. Pro-carboxypeptidase	(ii) Pancreas
S. Albumin	(i) Liver

19. The Lineweaver-Burk plots for inhibition

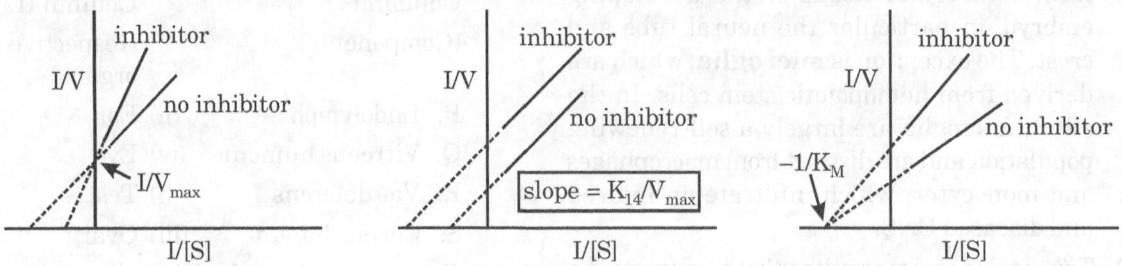

Competitive inhibition K_M increased V_{max} unaffected

Uncompetitive inhibition K_M reduced V_{max} reduced

Noncompetitive inhibition K_M unaffected V_{max} reduced

20. Red > White

Red = 10,000

White = 3600

Heterozygote Rr = ?

% of white = 3600/10000 = 0.36 or 36%

Therefore, , For heterozygote

$$Rr = 2pq = 2 \times 0.6 \times 0.4$$

$$Rr = 0.48$$

GATE 2019

XL : LIFE SCIENCES

Time : 3 Hours — *Maximum Marks : 100*

GENERAL APTITUDE

Q. 1 – 5 carry one mark each

1. A final examination is the _____ of a series of evaluations that a student has to go through.

(A) culmination (B) consultation
(C) desperation (D) insinuation

2. Once the team of analysts identify the problem, we _____ in a better position to comment on the issue.

Which one of the following choices CANNOT fill the given blank?

(A) are going to be (B) might be
(C) were to be (D) will be

3. Are there enough seats here? There are _____ people here than I expected.

(A) most (B) least
(C) many (D) more

4. If IMHO = JNIP; IDK = JEL; and SO = TP, then IDC =

(A) JDC (B) JED
(C) JCD (D) JDE

5. The product of three integers X, Y and Z is 192. Z is equal to 4 and P is equal to the average of X and Y. What is the minimum possible value of P?

(A) 6 (B) 9.5
(C) 7 (D) 8

Q. 6 – 10 carry two marks each

6. While teaching a creative writing class in India, I was surprised at receiving stories from the students that were all set in distant places: in the American West with cowboys and in Manhattan penthouses with clinking ice cubes. This was, till an eminent Caribbean writer gave the writers in the once-colonised countries the confidence to see the shabby lives around them as worthy of being "told".

The writer of this passage is surpised by the creative writing assignments of his students because________.

(A) None of the students had written about ice cubes and cowboys

(B) Some of the students had written about ice cubes and cowboys

(C) None of the students had written stories set in India

(D) Some of the students had written stories set in foreign places

7. X is an online media provider. By offering unlimited and exclusive online content at attractive prices for a loyalty membership, X is almost forcing its customers towards its loyalty membership. If its loyalty membership continues to grow at its current rate, within the next eight years more housholds will be watching X than cable television.

Which one of the following statements can be inferred from the above paragraph?

(A) Most households that subscribe to X's loyalty membership discontinue watching cable television

(B) Non-members prefer to watch cable television

(C) The X is cancelling accounts of non-members

(D) Cable television operators don't subscribe to X's loyalty membership

8. Fiscal deficit was 4% of the GDP in 2015 and that increased to 5% in 2016. If the GDP increased by 10% from 2015 to 2016, the percentage increase in the actual fiscal deficit is

(A) 25.00 (B) 37.50
(C) 35.70 (D) 10.00

9. Two pipes P and Q can fill a tank in 6 hours and 9 hours respectively, while a third pipe R can empty the tank in 12 hours. Initially, P and R are open for 4 hours. Then P is closed. The total time taken to fill the tank (in hours) is _____.

(A) 13.50 (B) 16.50
(C) 14.50 (D) 15.50

10. Mola is a digital platform for taxis in a city. It offers three types of rides – Pool, Mini and Prime. The table below presents the number of rides for the past four months. The platform earns one US dollar per ride. What is the percentage share of revenue contributed by Prime to the total revenues of Mola, for the entire duration?

	Month			
Type	January	February	March	April
Pool	170	320	215	190
Mini	110	220	180	70
Prime	75	180	120	90

(A) 23.97 (B) 16.24
(C) 38.74 (D) 25.86

CHEMISTRY

Q. 1 - Q. 5 carry one mark each & Q. 6 - Q. 15 carry two marks each

1. The compound that provides a carboxylic acid, upon treatment with Br_2/NaOH followed by acidification, is.

(A) 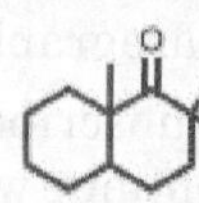 (B) 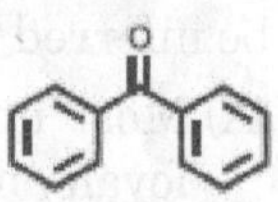

(C) 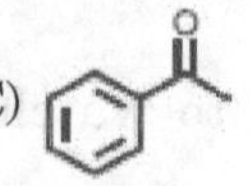 (D) 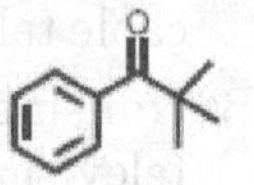

2. The boiling point of halogens from F_2 to I_2 increases due to

(A) decrease in electron affinity
(B) decrease in ionization potential
(C) dipole-dipole interaction
(D) induced dipole - induced dipole interaction

3. According to VSEPR theory, the species that has the smallest F-X-F angle (where X = central atom) is

(A) BF_3 (B) PF_3
(C) BF_4^- (D) IF_4^-

4. The total number of tautomers for the following molecule (including the structure provided below) is ______.

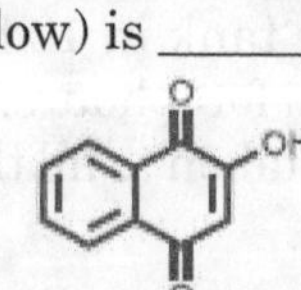

5. The total number of stereoisomers possible for the following structure is ______

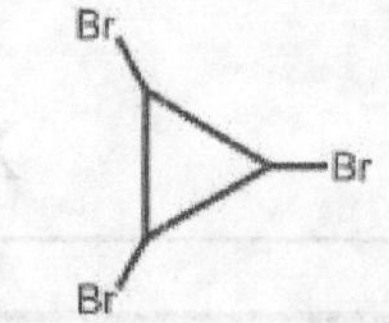

6. For the reaction mechanism,

$2X \rightleftharpoons Y$ For this step, assume $K_{eq} = [Y]/[X]^2$

$Y \longrightarrow P$ k: rate constant for this step

the rate law is

(A) $\frac{d[P]}{dt} = K_{eq}[Y]$ (B) $\frac{d[P]}{dt} = \kappa[X]^2$

(C) $\frac{d[P]}{dt} = \kappa K_{eq}[Y]$ (D) $\frac{d[P]}{dt} = \kappa K_{eq}[X]^2$

7. Match the type of reaction in Group-1 with the most appropriate description in Group-2

Group 1

P Hydroboration-oxidation
Q Nucleophilic aromatic substitution
R Wittig reaction
S Friedel-Crafts reaction

Group 2

1 Electrophilic aromatic substitution
2 Oxaphosphetane intermediate
3 Meisenheimer complex
4 Anti-Markownikoffs product

(A) P-2, Q-4, R-1, S-3 (B) P-4, Q-3, R-1, S-2
(C) P-4, Q-3, R-2, S-1 (D) P-2, Q-1, R-4, S-3

8. The reactants P and Q in the following reaction are

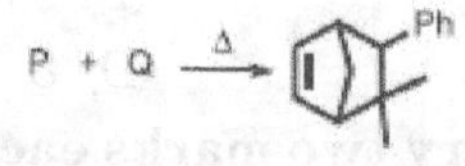

(A) 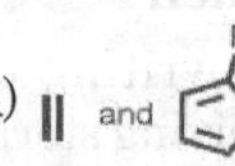

(B) 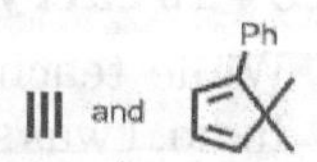

(C) 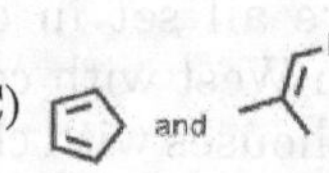

(D) 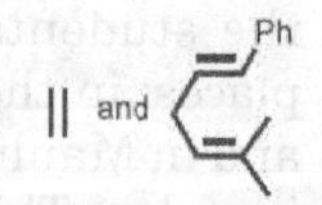

9. The major product formed in the following reaction is

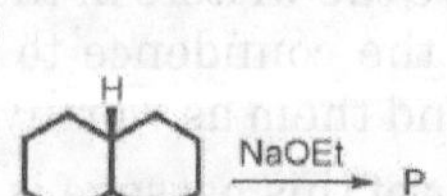

(A) 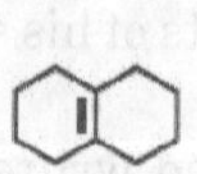 (B) 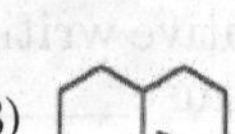

(C) 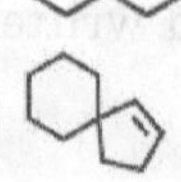 (D) 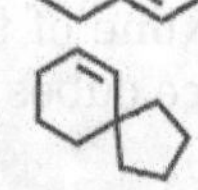

10. The most stable coordination complexes P and Q formed in the following reaction are

$$Fe^{3+} + Hg^{2+} + SCN^{-} \rightarrow P + Q$$

(A) 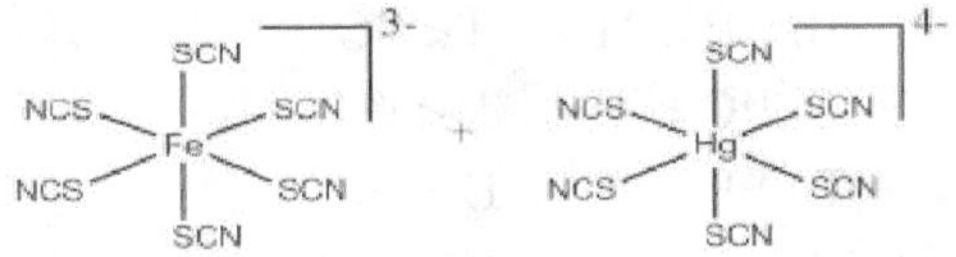

(B) 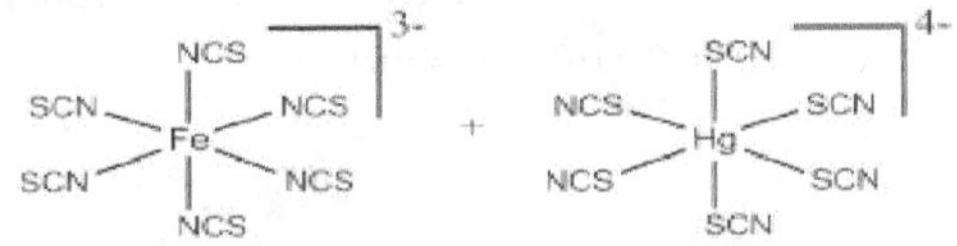

(C) 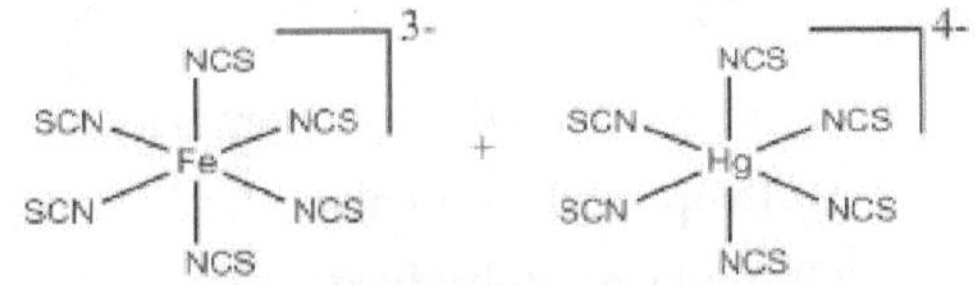

(D) 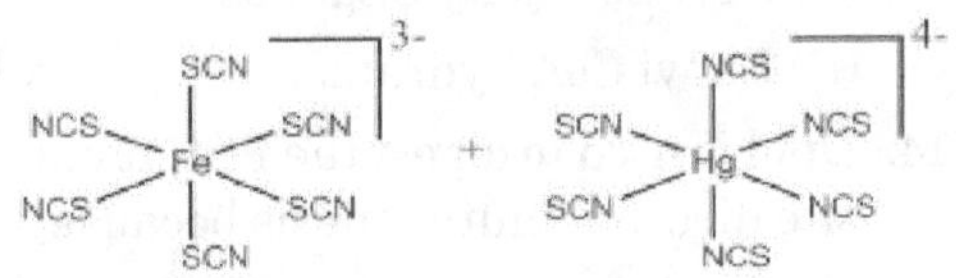

11. A coordination complex **Y** upon reaction with $AgNO_3$ solution does **NOT** give any precipitation. Complex **Y** possesses two isomers, of which one has zero dipole moment. The crystal field stabilization energy of **Y** is either $-0.8\ \Delta_o$ or $-0.8\ \Delta_t$. The magnetic moment for **Y** is found to be 3.9 Bohr Magneton. The coordination complex **Y** is

(A) $[Ti(NH_3)_4(Cl)_2]$

(B) $[Co(NH_3)_4(H_2O)_2]Cl_2$

(C) $[Co(NH_3)_2(Cl)_2]$

(D) $[Co(NH_3)_4(Cl)_2]$

12. A protein in denatured state (D) is in equilibrium with native state (N).

$$D \rightleftharpoons N$$

At 360 K, both N and D states are equally populated. If the standard entropy change for the reaction at this temperature $\Delta S^0 = -139$ J K^{-1} mol^{-1}, then the corresponding standard enthalpy change ΔH^0 for the reaction in kJ mol^{-1} **(rounded off to one decimal place)** is _______ .

13. The pH of a 1.0 L buffer solution containing 0.2 mol of acetic acid (CH_3COOH) and 0.3 mol of sodium acetate (CH_3COONa) is 5.0. The K_a of acetic acid is $P \times 10^{-5}$, where the numerical value of P **(rounded off to one decimal place)** is_____

14. Based on molecular orbital theory, the number of paramagnetic species in the following list N_2, N_2^{+}, N_2^{2-}, O_2, O_2^{+}, O_2^{-} and O_2^{2-} is _______ (assume that there is no change in energy of the orbitals upon addition/removal of electrons in a molecule)

15. Given the standard reduction potentials,

$E^0_{Cu^{+2}/Cu} = 0.34V$ and $E^0_{Ag^{+}/Ag} = 0.80V$,

the standard free energy change (ΔG^0) for the reaction

$Cu\,(s) + 2Ag^{+}\,(aq) \rightarrow Cu^{+2}\,(aq) + 2Ag\,(s)$

in kJ mol^{-1} **(rounded off to one decimal place;** $F = 96500$ C mol^{-1}), is _____

BIOCHEMISTRY

XL (Q to U): Q. 1 - Q. 10 carry one mark each & Q. 11 - Q. 20 carry two marks each.

1. Catalase is found exclusively in

(A) Lysosomes (B) Golgi apparatus

(C) Peroxisomes (D) Mitochondria

2. RAG recombinase is responsible for the formation of specific immune receptors. This process occurs in

(A) T cells &B cells

(B) Natural killer cells

(C) Macrophages

(D) Neutrophils

3. The example of substrate level phosphorylation in glycolysis is

(A) Conversion of Glucose to Glucose-6-phosphate

(B) Conversion of Glyceraldehyde-3-phosphate to 1,3-Bisphosphoglycerate

(C) Conversion of 1,3-Bisphosphoglycerase to 3-Phosphoglycerate

(D) Conversion of Dihydroxyacetone phosphate to Glyceraldehyde-3-phosphate

4. The dipeptide with least rotational barrier in the peptide bond is

(A) 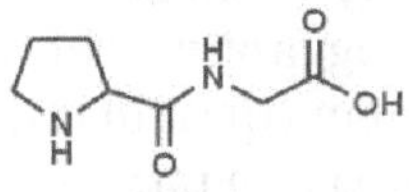

(B) 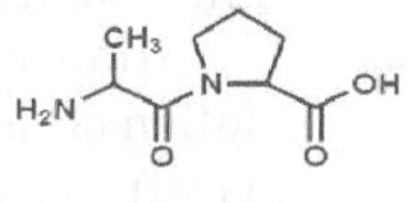

(C) 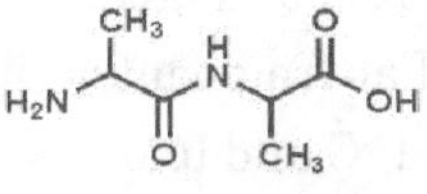

(D) 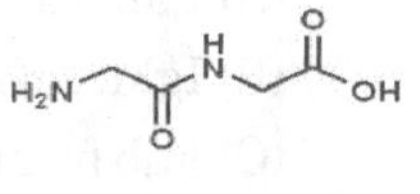

5. The light-harvesting pigment NOT used by Cyanobacteria for photosynthesis is
(A) Rhodopsin (B) Phycobilin
(C) Phycoerythrobilin (D) Phycocyanobilin

6. Slow intravenous infusion of ethanol is a therapy to treat methanol poisoning. The underlying chemical reaction is an example of
(A) Competitive inhibition
(B) Non-competitive inhibition
(C) Mixed inhibition
(D) Enzyme activation

7. Nitric oxide synthase is responsible for generation of Nitric oxide, an important signaling molecule. The substrate for this enzyme is
(A) Glycine
(B) Lysine
(C) Histidine
(D) Arginine

8. Allergies are due to a hyper immune response. Drugs given to counter allergies target
(A) Glycine (B) Histamine
(C) Insulin (D) Cellulose

9. The electrostatic interaction energy between a positively charged atom A and negatively charged atom B separated by 3 Å in water is -6 kJ/mol. Considering the relative permittivity of water to be 80, the electrostatic interaction energy in kJ/mol (rounded off to one decimal place) between atoms A and B in vacuum is ______.

10. You are given a 0.1M solution of Glucose (stock solution). The stock solution required to make 0.5 ml of 0.005M Glucose solution (rounded off to three decimal places) in ml is

11. A mixture of the following purified proteins, IgG, IgM and Fab fragment of immunoglobulins, is separated using gel filtration chromatography. The order of elution of these proteins (first to last) is
(A) Fab fragment, IgM and IgG
(B) IgM, IgG and Fab fragment
(C) Fab fragment, IgG and IgM
(D) IgG, IgM and Fab fragment

12. The ascending order of half-life for the radioactive isotopes, ^{125}I, ^{3}H, ^{14}C and ^{32}P, is
(A) $^{14}C < ^{125}I < ^{3}H < ^{32}P$
(B) $^{32}P < ^{3}H < ^{125}I < ^{14}C$
(C) $^{14}C < ^{3}H < ^{32}P < ^{125}I$
(D) $^{32}P < ^{125}I < ^{3}H < ^{14}C$

13. The enzyme **NOT** involved in oxidation of the molecule shown below is

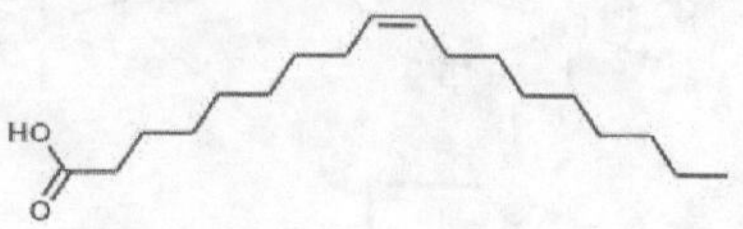

(A) Δ^3, Δ^2 - Enoyl -CoA isomerase
(B) Propionyl-CoA caboxylase
(C) Acyl CoA dehydrogenase
(D) Enoyl CoA hydratase

14. Dpnl is used to digest the PCR product during site directed mutagenesis because
(A) Dpnl digests irrespective of methylation status of DNA
(B) Dpnl digests only unmethylated DNA
(C) Dpnl digests only methylated DNA
(D) Dpnl digests GC-rich sequences

15. Which one of the following is an **incorrect** biomolecule-modification pair?
(A) Lipid- Palmitoylation
(B) DNA and Protein - Methylation
(C) Protein - Glycosylation
(D) RNA - Polyadenylation

16. The crystal structure of a peptide has an ordered structural repeat of amino acids with a distance of ~ 6.5 Å between the alternate Cα atoms. Which one of the following pair of dihedral angles (Φ and Ψ) accurately represents the peptide structure?
(A) $\Phi \approx -60°, \Psi \approx -50°$
(B) $\Phi \approx -120°, \Psi \approx -50°$
(C) $\Phi \approx -60°, \Psi \approx +120°$
(D) $\Phi \approx -120°, \Psi \approx -120°$

17. Absence of detectable protein expression upon blunt-ended mutation-free cloning of an *E.coli* gene with its own promoter in *E. coli* cells can be due to
(A) Cloning occurred in reverse orientation
(B) Cloning occurred out of frame
(C) Codon bias
(D) Rapid degradation of expressed protein

18. The C-terminal carboxyl group and the N-terminal amino group in amino acids have a dissociation constant (pK_a) of 2.2 and 9.2, respectively. The pK_a of side chain carboxyl group in glutamic acid is 4.2 and side chain amino group in lysine is 10.2. The difference in isoelectric point (pi) of lysine and glutamic acid (rounded off to two decimal places) is ______

19. X different sized DNA fragments can be observed upon incomplete EcoRI digestion of identical DNA molecules with two EcoRI sites as shown below. The maximum value of X is ______.

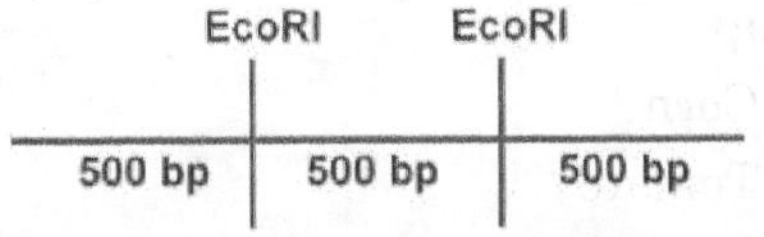

20. An uncharged protein (P) has an Asp in position 23 with a molecular weight of 6501 Da, as determined by mass spectrometry. The uncharged mutant of this protein (P') contains a single amino acid substitution with Asn at position 23. The molecular weight of P', as determined by mass spectrometry (rounded off to one decimal place) is ______ Da.

BOTANY

Q. 1 - Q. 10 carry one mark each

1. Which one of the following ecosystems is represented by an inverted pyramid of numbers?
   (A) Grassland (B) Pond
   (C) Desert (D) Parasitic forest

2. Raphides are deposits of
   (A) calcium oxalate
   (B) calcium carbonate
   (C) silica bodies
   (D) protein bodies

3. Which one of the following families shows bicollateral vascular bundle in the transverse section of the stem?
   (A) Rutaceae (B) Asteraceae
   (C) Cucurbitaceae (D) Malvaceae

4. Arbuscules are highly branched structures, formed by
   (A) ectomycorrhizae
   (B) endomycorrhizae
   (C) arbutoid mycorrhizae
   (D) monotropoid mycorrhizae

5. Which one of the following combinations of polysaccharides is present in plant cell wall?
   (A) Only cellulose, hemicellulose and fibroin
   (B) Only cellulose, hemicellulose and lignin
   (C) Only cellulose, hemicellulose and pectin
   (D) Only cellulose, pectin and lignin

6. Which one of the following statements is INCORRECT?
   (A) Nitrogen fixation is aerobic process
   (B) Dinitrogenase catalyzes reduction of nitrogen to ammonia
   (C) Root nodules are found in *Glycine max*
   (D) Nitrogen fixation is anaerobic process

7. Which one of the following statements is INCORRECT with respect to cyclic photophosphorylation?
   (A) ATP is generated without concomitant formation of NADPH
   (B) Electron flows from Photosystem I to cytochrome *bf* complex
   (C) Photosystem II does not participate in cyclic photophosphorylation
   (D) Cyclic photophosphorylation occurs when $NADP^+$/NADPH ratio is high

8. The plant cells are considered totipotent. The phenomenon of a mature cell reverting to the meristematic state and forming undifferentiated callus tissue is called
   (A) redifferentiation (B) dedifferentiation
   (C) organogenesis (D) recalcitrancy

9. Glyphosate is a broad spectrum herbicide. Upon application to leaves, it is translocated to meristematic areas and underground rhizomes by
   (A) phloem (B) xylem
   (C) border pits (D) tracheids

10. If a species has 2n = 16 chromosomes, the number of chromosomes per cell in a double monosomic individual would be ______

Q. 11 - Q. 20 carry two marks each.

11. Rubisco catalyzes conversion of ribulose 1, 5-bisphosphate to
    P. two molecules of stable 3-phosphoglycerate
    Q. one molecule of 3-phosphoglycerate and one molecule of phosphoglycolate
    R. one molecule of ribulose 5-phosphophate
    S. one molecule of ribose 5-phosphate
    Choose only the correct combination
    (A) P and S (B) Q and S
    (C) P and Q (D) R and S

12. Select correct combination of molecules given in **Group I** with their functions in **Group II**

Group I

P. Ubiquitin
Q. Phytotropins
R. Extensins
S. DELLA proteins

Group II

1. Cell wall loosening enzymes
2. Repressors in gibberellin signaling
3. Mediator of protein degradation
4. Noncompetitive inhibitors of polar transport of auxin

(A) P-3, Q-4, R-1, S-2 (B) P-3, Q-1, R-2, S-4
(C) P-4, Q-3, R-1, S-2 (D) P-1, Q-2, R-4, S-3

13. Match the plant species and their corresponding families with their economically important products:

Plant species

P. *Cannabis sativa*
Q. *Corchorus olitorius*
R. *Ocimum sanctum*
S. *Ricinus communis*

Family

1. Lamiaceae
2. Cannabaceae
3. Euphorbiaceae
4. Tiliaceae

Plant product

i. Oil from seeds
ii. Eugenol from leaves
iii. Fibre from stem
iv. Marijuana from leaves

(A) P-2-iv, Q-3-ii, R-4-iii, S-1-i
(B) P-3-iv, Q-2-i, R-1-ii, S-4-iii
(C) P-1-iii, Q-4-iii, R-2-i, S-3-ii
(D) P-2-iv, Q-4-iii, R-1-ii, S-3-i

14. Cybrids may arise through the
(A) fusion of a normal protoplast with another nucleated protoplast of different origin
(B) fusion between a normal protoplast and a protoplast containing viable nucleus
(C) elimination of one of the nuclei from heterokaryon formed from two protoplasts of different origin
(D) fusion of a normal cell with another nucleated cell

15. Match the disease with causative organism and affected crop

Disease

P. Powdery mildew
Q. White rust
R. Downy mildew
S. Late blight

Causative organism

1. *Albugo Candida*
2. *Phytophthora infestans*
3. *Erysiphe orontii*
4. *Peronoscleropora phillippinensis*

Crop

i. Corn
ii. Tomato
iii. Potato
iv. Mustard

(A) P-3-i, Q-1-iv, R-2-iii, S-4-ii
(B) P-3-ii, Q-1-iv, R-4-i, S-2-iii
(C) P-4-ii, Q-1-i, R-3-iv, S-2-iii
(D) P-2-iii, Q-3-ii, R-1-iv, S-4-i

16. Match the options in **Group I** with that of **Group II** with respect to steps in signal transduction mechanism in plants

Group I	Group II
P. Phospholipase C	1. stimulates release of calcium from intracellular stores
Q. Inositol triphosphate	2. regulates ion channels/ activates various enzymes
R. Diacylglycerol	3. hydrolyzes posphatidylinositol bisphosphate (PIP2)
S. Phosphatidic acid	4. phosphorylated to phosphatidic acid

(A) P-3, Q-4, R-2, S-1 (B) P-4, Q-3, R-2, S-1
(C) P-2, Q-3, R-1, S-4 (D) P-3, Q-1, R-4, S-2

17. Which one of the following statements is **CORRECT** with respect to endosperm development? It originates
(A) from the fusion product of three haploid nuclei - one from male gametophyte and two from the female gametophyte
(B) from the fusion product of three haploid nuclei - two from male gametophyte and one from the female gametophyte
(C) from the fusion product of two haploid nuclei - one from male gametophyte and one from the female gametophyte
(D) by a phenomenon called apomixis

18. Which one of the following methods is **INCORRECT** with respect to haploid plant production? It can be produced
(A) from an unfertilized egg cell
(B) from nucellar tissue
(C) from isolated pollen culture
(D) by distant hybridization, followed by selective elimination of chromosomes of one of the parents

19. Plant weight is determined by a pair of alleles at each of the two independently assorting loci (**Aa** and **Bb**) that are additive and equal in their effects. The recessive alleles do not contribute towards plant weight. Plants with genotype **aa bb** are 1 g in weight, whereas plants with genotype **AA BB** weigh 3.4 g. Plant with genotype **aa bb** is crossed with a plant of genotype AA BB. The weight (in g, round off to one decimal place) of an individual plant in F_1 progeny of this cross would be ________

20. A cell in G_1 of Interphase has 12 chromosomes. In Anaphase-I of meiosis, the number of DNA molecules per cell will be ________

MICROBIOLOGY

Q. 1 - Q. 10 carry one mark each & Q. 11 - Q. 20 carry two marks each.

1. Chloramphenicol and tetracycline are broad spectrum antibiotics which inhibit bacterial growth by targeting ______.
(A) cell wall synthesis (B) protein synthesis
(C) RNA synthesis (D) DNA synthesis

2. Which of the following radiation methods is used in preserving food from spoilage by microorganisms?
(A) Radio waves
(B) Microwaves
(C) Non-ionizing
(D) Ionizing

3. Which part of the lipopolysaccharides has toxic properties that make some bacterial infections a potentially serious medical problem?
(A) Polysaccharide side-chains
(B) Lipid A portion
(C) Repeat carbohydrate units
(D) Core region of polysaccharides

4. Microbes make up about ______ of earth's living material by weight.
(A) $1/4^{th}$
(B) $2/3^{rd}$
(C) $3/4^{th}$
(D) $4/5^{th}$

5. The highly contagious viral disease measles is caused by a
(A) double-stranded DNA virus
(B) single-stranded DNA virus
(C) single-stranded RNA virus
(D) double-stranded RNA virus

6. Secondary metabolites such as penicillin from mold are produced during the ______.
(A) lag phase
(B) idiophase
(C) log phase
(D) decline phase

7. Dick test is used to assess the susceptibility to ____ .
(A) diphtheria
(B) scarlet fever
(C) typhoid fever
(D) tuberculosis

8. Which of the following is a symbiotic bacterial genus that converts nitrogen into nitrogen containing compounds that are utilized by legume plants to synthesize amino acids?
(A) *Spirillum*
(B) *Azotobacter*
(C) *Rhizobium*
(D) *Clostridium*

9. What is the enzyme involved in the following reaction?
Triglyceride + $3H_2O \rightarrow$ Glycerol + fatty acids
(A) Glycerol phosphate denydrogenase
(B) Glycerol kinase
(C) Lipase
(D) Zymase

10. A bacterial culture contains 500 organisms / mL in the exponential growth phase at 8 am in the morning. If you consider a generation time of 20 minutes, the total number of organisms / mL (round off to the nearest integer) after three hours (i.e. at 11 am in the morning) will be ______

11. Folic acid synthesis in bacteria is competitively inhibited by sulfonamides. Which of the following essential components is replaced by sulfonamides during the process of folic acid synthesis?
(A) Pteridine
(B) Glutamic acid
(C) Para-amino benzoic acid
(D) Sulfamethaxazole

12. Which of the following cellular structures are absent in eukaryotes and are present at least in some prokaryotic organisms?
(i) Respiratory enzymes
(ii) Ribosomes
(iii) Nucleoid
(iv) Internal membranes
(v) Pili
(A) (iii) and (v) (B) (i) and (iv)
(C) (i), (iii) and (v) (D) (iii), (iv)

13. Granules are inclusion bodies found in bacteria. Which of the following statements are true about ganules?
(i) Granules can be storage vessels for carbohydrates/lipids
(ii) Some granules supply substances for a variety of metabolic processes
(iii) Granules are dissolved in cytoplasm
(iv) Granules are membrane-enclosed structures
(A) (ii) and (iii) (B) (iii) and (iv)
(C) (i) and (ii) (D) (i) and (iii)

14. Match the culture media to their uses

Culture Media
(i) Complex media
(ii) Selective media
(iii) Differential media
(iv) Enriched media

Uses
(p) identifying certain bacteria from mixed culture
(q) chemically undefined media for growing bacteria
(r) cultivating fastidious bacteria
(s) distinguishing one bacteria from another
(A) (i)-(s), (ii)-(r), (iii)-(q), (iv)-(p)
(B) (i)-(q), (ii)-(p), (iii)-(s), (iv)-(r)
(C) (i)-(q), (ii)-(r), (iii)-(p), (iv)-(s)
(D) (i)-(p), (ii)-(s), (iii)-(q), (iv)-(r)

15. Among the following characteristics listed below, select those that are the most appropriate for archaebacteria.
(i) Peptidoglycan containing muramic acid and D-amino acids are present in cell wall
(ii) Long chain branched alcohols (phytanols) bound to glycerol by ether linkages are found in the lipids of cytoplasmic membrane
(iii) First amino acid to initiate new polypeptide chain is N-Formylmethionine
(iv) Translation process is sensitive to the action of diphtheria toxin
(A) (i), (iii) (B) (ii), (iii), (iv)
(C) (ii), (iv) (D) (i), (ii), (iv)

16. Which of the following processes are involved in horizontal gene transfer (HGT)?
(i) Conjugation
(ii) Transduction
(iii) Binary fission
(iv) Transformation
(v) Translesion synthesis (vi) Transversion
(A) (i), (iii), (iv) (B) (i), (iv), (vi)
(C) (ii), (iv), (v) (D) (i), (ii), (iv)

17. Match the class of antibodies to appropriate description or function

Antibodies
(i) IgA
(ii) IgG
(iii) IgD
(iv) IgE

Description / function
(p) Mucosal immunity
(q) Immunity to parasitic infections
(r) Most abundant antibody in the blood
(s) Found on the B cell membranes
(A) (i)-(s), (ii)-(r), (iii)-(q), (iv)-(p)
(B) (i)-(p), (ii)-(q), (iii)-(s), (iv)-(r)
(C) (i)-(p), (ii)-(r), (iii)-(s), (iv)-(q)
(D) (i)-(p), (ii)-(s), (iii)-(q), (iv)-(r)

18. Match the diseases with the appropriate causative agents

Disease
(i) Rheumatic heart disease
(ii) Syphilis
(iii) Genital warts
(iv) Oral thrush

Causative agent

(p) *Candida albicans*

(q) Group A *Streptococcus*

(r) Human papilloma virus

(s) *Treponema pallidum*

(A) (i)-(p), (ii)-(q), (iii) -(s), (iv)-(r)

(B) (i)- (q), (ii)- (s), (iii)-(r), (iv)-(p)

(C) (i)-(r), (ii)-(s), (iii)-(p), (iv)-(q)

(D) (i)-(s), (ii)-(q), (iii)- (p), (iv) -(r)

19. Consider a spherical bacterial cell with diameter 2 μm and a eukaryotic cell of spherical shape with a diameter of 20 μm. The surface area to volume (in μm^{-1}) ratio of the bacterial cell (round off to 1 decimal place) is _______ times more than that of the eukaryotic cell.

20. When grouping bacteria using numerical taxonomy approach, many characteristics are determined for each strain. If all characteristics are same, then the % similarity is 100. When comparing two bacterial strains, if 72 characteristics are the same and 44 characteristics are different, the % similarity (round off to 2 decimal places) between the two strains is _____.

ZOOLOGY

Q. 1 - Q. 10 carry one mark each & Q. 11 - Q. 20 carry two marks each.

1. Which one of the following animals possesses two chambered heart?

(A) Chameleon (B) Peacock

(C) Gold fish (D) Blue whale

2. In eukaryotic chromatin organization, which one of the histones seals off the nucleosome at the location at which linker DNA enters and leaves the nucleosome?

(A) H1

(B) H2A-H2B

(C) H3

(D) H4

3. Which one of the following parasites does NOT cause lymphatic filariasis?

(A) *Brugia malayi*

(B) *Brugia timori*

(C) *Wuchereria bancrofti*

(D) *Mansonella streptocerca*

4. A species adapted to a specific habitat is called

(A) Biome (B) Ecotone

(C) Ecotype (D) Niche

5. The phylum that is characterized by the animals having a "water vascular system" is

(A) Cnidaria

(B) Annelida

(C) Mollusca

(D) Echinodermeta

6. The finches on the Galapagos Islands have widely differing beaks adapted according to their diets. This is an example of

(A) Adaptive radiation

(B) Parallel evolution

(C) Adaptive convergence

(D) Co-adaptation

7. Which one of the following animals is named as a "living fossil", where the animal is persisting above 400 million years without further major morphological evolution?

(A) King crabs (B) Porcelain crabs

(C) Horseshoe crabs (D) Hermit crabs

8. Consider the given peptide, A la-Glu-Val-Asn-Ile-Asp-Pro-Asp-Gln-Gly-Asp. The net charge on the peptide at pH 1.0 will be ______

9. The total number of complementary determining regions (CDRs) in the functional form of an IgM antibody is ______

10. In a 1500 base pair double stranded B-DNA, 70% of purines are adenine bases. The total number of hydrogen bonds (Watson-Crick base pairing) in the DNA will be _______

11. Match the given vitamins in **Column I** with the related proteins in **Column II**

Column I	**Column II**
a) Vitamin C	(1) Thrombin
b) Vitamin J	(2) Rhodopsin
c) Vitamin A	(3) Pyruvate dehydrogenase
d) Vitamin B_1	(4) Prolyl hydroxylase

(A) a-4; b-1; c-2; d-3

(B) a-4; b-1; c-3; d-2

(C) a-2; b-1; c-4; d-3

(D) a-3; b-4; c-2; d-1

12. Match the following terms in **Column I** with the appropriate explanation in **Column II**

Column I

a) Spliceosome

b) Peroxisome

c) Lysosome

d) Centrosome

Column II

1) Cell scavengers

2) Metabolism of long chain fatty acids

3) Microtubules

4) Post transcriptional modifications

(A) a-3; b-1; c-4; d-2 (B) a-4; b-2; c-1; d-3

(C) a-3; b-2; c-1; d-4 (D) a-4; b-3; c-1; d-2

13. Match the respective behaviour given in **Column I** with the appropriate explanation in **Column II**

Column I

a) Agonistic behaviour

b) Hierarchical behaviour

c) Altruistic behaviour

d) Cooperative behaviour

Column II

1) Individual behaviour where fitness of other increases at the expense of self

2) Individuals contribute towards enhancement of mutual fitness

3) Aggressive behaviour of individuals within a population

4) Existence of different levels of dominance within a population

(A) a-4; b-1; c-2; d-3 (B) a-3; b-4; c-1; d-2

(C) a-4; b-2; c-1; d-3 (D) a-3; b-4; c-2; d-1

14. Closure of neural tube during neurulation is the process in which neural tube eventually forms a closed cylinder that separates from surface ectoderm. Which one of the following terms is linked to the failure in the closure of entire neural tube i.e. brain and spinal cord, over the body axis?

(A) Craniorachischisis

(B) Spina bifida

(C) Anencephaly

(D) Cleft palate

15. Which one of the following factors does NOT contribute to "allopatric speciation"?

(A) The isolated population is exposed to different selection pressure as compared to parent population

(B) A population become geographically isolated from the parent population

(C) There is a gene flow between the two separated populations

(D) Genetic drift occurs between the two separated populations

16. Match the hormones in **Column I** to their respective physiological effects in **Column II**

Column I

a) Melatonin

b) Oxytocin

c) Cholecystokinin

d) Prolactin

e) Somatostatin

Column II

1) Inhibition of secretion of growth hormone

2) Synthesis of milk in mammary gland

3) Secretion of milk and uterine contraction

4) Secretion of enzymes from pancreatic acinar cells

5) Regulation of circadian rhythms

(A) a-5; b-4; c-2; d-3; e-1

(B) a-3; b-5; c-4; d-2; e-1

(C) a-5; b-1; c-2; d-3; e-4

(D) a-5; b-3; c-4; d-2; e-1

17. The molecular weight of a double stranded DNA fragment present in mitochondria is 7.92×10^8 g mol^{-1}. A pair of nucleotide contributes 0.34 nm to the length of DNA and the average molecular weight of a nucleotide is 330 g mol^{-1}. The number of protein molecules, consisting of 200 amino acids each, coded by this mitochondrial DNA is ______

18. An enzyme that follows Michaelis-Menten kinetics catalyzes the conversion of 35 μM substrate into product with a reaction velocity of 10 μM s^{-1}. The K_m and k_{cat} for the substrate are 14 μM and 500 s^{-1} respectively. The total amount of enzyme taken for the enzyme reaction is ______ nM.

19. A distinctly large population of randomly mating laboratory mice contains 36% albino mice, which is caused by a double recessive genotype (aa). The black coloured mice in the population is due to dominant genotype (AA/Aa). Considering the fact that this population is in Hardy-Weinberg equilibrium, the frequency of heterozygous alleles (Aa) in this population is _____

(round off to 2 decimal places).

20. A genetic cross was made between homozygous wild-type males ($a^+a^+b^+b^+c^+c^+$) and triple-mutant females (aabbcc) of *Drosophila melanogaster.* Then the Fi males ($a^+ab^+bc^+c$) were back crossed to the triple-mutant females which resulted in the following F_2 progenies:

a^+bc	16
ab^+c	115
abc	311
a^+b^+c	64
abc^+	61
$a^+b^+c^+$	317
a^+bc^+	99
ab^+c^+	17
Total	= 1000

The order of genes as determined from the above data was found to be "b a c" *{note that the order is equivalent to "c ab" and the order of outside makers are arbitrary).*

The map distance between "b and c" is _______ centiMorgan *(round off to 1 decimal place).*

FOOD TECHNOLOGY

Q. 1 - Q. 10 carry one mark each & Q. 11 - Q. 20 carry two marks each.

1. Colloidal stability of milk casein is because of the highly hydrated carbohydrate residues in _______.

(A) α_{s1} casein (B) α_{S2} casein
(C) β casein (D) κ casein

2. Rice bran is stabilized prior to oil extraction to protect it from the activity of ______.

(A) Polyphenol oxidase (B) Peroxidase
(C) Lipase (D) Lipoxygenase

3. Sticking of powder to wall of the chamber during spray drying of fruit juice is due to _______.

(A) Low glass transition temperature of the compounds in juice
(B) High glass transition temperature of the compounds in juice
(C) Improper processing parameters of spray dryer
(D) Presence of gums in feed material

4. Thearubigins and theaflavins in black tea are formed by the oxidation and dimerization of ____

(A) Quercetin
(B) Catechins
(C) Gallic acid
(D) Kaempferol

5. Ratio of Schmidt number to Lewis number is ____.

(A) Prandtl number
(B) Reynolds number
(C) Nusselt number
(D) Sherwood number

6. 'Red dog' is one of the byproducts during milling of _______.

(A) Corn
(B) Rice
(C) Ragi
(D) Wheat

7. a) **Assertion:** Ash content is one of the quality indicators of the flour to be used for bread making.

r) **Reason:** Higher ash content indicates better quality of the bread flour.

Choose the correct answer from the following:

(A) Both a) and r) are true and r) is the correct reason for a)
(B) Both a) and r) are true but r) is not the correct reason for a)
(C) Both a) and r) are false
(D) a) is true but r) is false

8. An ice cream mix of 870 g L^{-1} has been used to prepare ice cream which yielded a finished product of 490 g L^{-1}. The per cent over run is ______ *(round off to 1 decimal place).*

9. Impeller in a fruit juice mixing tank is rotating at 200 rpm with a Reynolds number $>10^4$. Density of juice is 1045 kg m^{-3}. If diameter of the impeller is doubled and other conditions remained constant, the power requirement of mixing will increase by a factor of ________.

10. Paddy consisting of 20% husk has been milled to remove 6% bran during polishing.
Assuming no other losses, yield (per cent) of polished rice from the paddy is ______ *(round off to 1 decimal place).*

11. Match the following laws in Column I with corresponding phenomenon in Column II.

Column I

P. Newton's law
Q. Hertz constant stress theory
R. Fick's law
S. Bond's law

Column II

1. Size reduction
2. Substance cooling
3. Damage of fruits and vegetables
4. Molecular diffusion

(A) P-2, Q-3, R-4, S-1
(B) P-3, Q-2, R-4, S-1
(C) P-3, Q-1, R-4, S-2
(D) P-4, Q-3, R-2, S-1

12. Match the mold in Column I with its asexual/sexual spore shown in Column II.

Column I	Column II
P. *Aspergillus*	1. Arthrospore
Q. *Geotrichum*	2. Oospores
R. *Rhizopus*	3. Conidia
S. *Oomycetes*	4. Sporangiospores

(A) P-3, Q-1, R-4, S-2 (B) P-1, Q-4, R-3, S-2
(C) P-4, Q-3, R-1, S-2 (D) P-4, Q-1, R-2, S-3

13. Match the foods given in Column I with their specific usage given in Column II.

Column I	Column II
P. Egg yolk	1. Ice cream
Q. Pregelatinised starch	2. Mayonnaise
R. Gum	3. Baking powder
S. Starch	4. Baby food

(A) P-2, Q-4, R-1, S-3 (B) P-4, Q-1, R-2, S-3
(C) P-2, Q-3, R-1, S-4 (D) P-1, Q-4, R-1, S-3

14. Match the bioactive compounds in Column I with their botanical source given in Column II.

Column I	Column II
P. Isoflavones	1. Corn
Q. Resistant starch	2. Grapes
R. Xanthophyll	3. Soybean
S. Resveratrol	4. Plantain (culinary banana)

(A) P-2, Q-4, R-1, S-3 (B) P-3, Q-4, R-1, S-2
(C) P-4, Q-1, R-2, S-3 (D) P-4, Q-3, R-2, S-1

15. Match the following microbial species in Column I with related disease caused by them as shown in Column II.

Column I	Column II
P. *Vibrio sp.*	1. Gastroenteritis
Q. *Shigellasp.*	2. Typhoid
R. *E. coli*	3. Cholera
S. *Salmonella typhi*	4. Bacillary dysentery

(A) P-1, Q-3, R-4, S-2
(B) P-2, Q-3, R-4, S-1
(C) P-3, Q-1, R-4, S-2
(D) P-3, Q-4, R-1, S-2

16. Buffalo milk having density of 1030 kg m^{-3} is homogenized with a pressure of 30 MPa. Given, acceleration due to gravity as 9.81 m s^{-2} and assuming no pressure loss, the velocity (m s^{-1}) of the milk flowing through the homogenizer valve will be *(round off to 2 decimal places).*

17. Potato slices have been dehydrated from an initial solid content of 12% to a final solid content of 94%. If the peeling and other losses are to the tune of 10%, final yield (per cent) of the dried chips per ton of fresh potato taken is *(round off to 2 decimal places).*

18. A mixed fruit beverage with 12 °Brix having specifc heat of 4298 J kg^{-1} K^{-1} is being heated from 30 °C to 95 °C for pasteurization at a flow rate of 1000 L h^{-1} in a tubular heat exchanger. Steam at 100 °C is used as heating medium which is converted into condensate at 100 °C. If the density of beverage is 1075 kg m^{-3} and the latent heat of steam at the given tempearture is 2257 kJ kg^{-1}, the mass flow rate of steam (kg min^{-1}) is *(round off to 2 decimal places).*

19. Room air is at 40 °C with 60% relative humidity. Saturated vapour pressure of water at 40 °C is 7.375 kPa. Humid volume of air (m^3 per kg of dry air) is ______ *(round off to 3 decimal places).*

20. Freezing of 100 mm spherical meat ball with 60% moisture at 35 °C is being done in an air blast freezer maintained at –45 °C. Given, latent heat of fusion for water is 333.2 kJ kg^{-1}, thermal conductivity of meat is 1.5 W m^{-1} °C^{-1}, convective heat transfer coefficient is 40 W m^{-2} °C^{-1}, density of frozen meat is 980 kg m^{-3} and initial freezing temperature of meatball is -10 °C. Using Plank's equation, freezing time (h) is ______ *(round off to 2 decimal places).*

ANSWERS

General Aptitude (GA)

1. *(A)* 2. *(C)* 3. *(D)* 4. *(B)* 5. *(C)*
6. *(D)* 7. *(A)* 8. *(B)* 9. *(C)* 10. *(A)*

Chemistry

1. *(C)* 2. *(C)* 3. *(D)* 4. (3 to 3) 5. (2 to 2)
6. *(D)* 7. *(C)* 8. *(C)* 9. *(A)* 10. *(B)*
11. *(D)* 12. (–51.0 to –49.0) 13. (1.4 to 1.6) 14. (5 to 5)
15. (–89.8 to – 87.8)

Biochemistry

1. *(C)* 2. *(A)* 3. *(C)* 4. *(B)* 5. *(A)*
6. *(A)* 7. *(D)* 8. *(D)* 9. (–480.1 to –479.9)
10. (0.024 to 0.026) 11. *(B)* 12. *(D)* 13. *(B)* 14. *(C)*
15. *(A)* 16. *(D)* 17. *(D)* 18. (6.49 to 6.51) 19. (3 to 3)
20. (6499.9 to 6500.1)

Botany

1. *(D)* 2. *(A)* 3. *(C)* 4. *(B)* 5. *(C)*
6. *(A)* 7. *(D)* 8. *(B)* 9. *(A)* 10. (14 to 14)
11. *(C)* 12. *(A)* 13. *(D)* 14. *(C)* 15. *(B)*
16. *(D)* 17. *(A)* 18. *(B)* 19. (2.2 to 2.2) 20. (24 to 24)

Microbiology

1. *(B)* 2. *(D)* 3. *(B)* 4. *(B)* 5. *(C)*
6. *(B)* 7. *(B)* 8. *(C)* 9. *(C)*
10. (255999 to 256001) 11. *(C)* 12. *(A)* 13. *(C)*
14. *(B)* 15. *(C)* 16. *(D)* 17. *(C)* 18. *(B)*
19. (9.9 to 10.1) 20. (61.50 to 62.50)

Zoology

1. *(C)* 2. *(A)* 3. *(D)* 4. *(C)* 5. *(D)*
6. *(A)* 7. *(C)* 8. (1 to 1) 9. (60 to 60)
10. (3450 to 3450) 11. *(A)* 12. *(B)* 13. *(B)* 14. *(A)*
15. *(C)* 16. *(D)* 17. (2000 to 2000) 18. (28 to 28)
19. (0.48 to 0.48) 20. (40.5 to 40.5)

Food Technology

1. *(D)* 2. *(C)* 3. *(A)* 4. *(B)* 5. *(D)*
6. *(D)* 7. *(D)* 8. (77.4 to 77.6) 9. (32 to 32)
10. (74.8 to 75.6) 11. *(A)* 12. *(A)* 13. *(A)* 14. *(B)*
15. *(D)* 16. (240.00 to 242.00) 17. (11.45 to 11.55) 18. (2.16 to 2.25)
19. (0.924 to 0.930) 20. (1.06 to 1.09)

EXPLANATIONS

GENERAL APTITUDE

4. For IMHO = JNIP
   I + 1 = J
   M + 1 = N
   H + 1 = I
   O + 1 = P
   For
   SO = TP
   S + 1 = T
   O + 1 = P
   Similarly, for
   IDC = JED
   I + 1 = J
   D + 1 = E
   C + 1 = D

5. Given product of three integers,
   X.Y.Z = 192
   Given : Z = 4
   $\therefore X.Y = \frac{192}{4} = 48$
   $\because \ P = \frac{X+Y}{2}$
   Now, Possible value of (X, Y) are
   (48, 1), (24, 2), (16, 3), (12, 4), (8, 6)
   So, $(P)_{min} = \frac{8+6}{2} = 7$
   So, min value of P is 7.

8. Let GDP in 2015 be x
   Now, in 2016, GDP will be 1.1x
   Fiscal deficit in 2015 = 0.04 × x
   Fiscal deficit in 2016 = 0.05 × 1.1 x
   Here percentage increase in the actual fiscal deficit
   $= \left(\frac{0.05 \times 1.1x - 0.04 \times x}{0.04x}\right) \times 100 = 37.5\%$

9. Here,
   In 1 hr, part of tank filled by P alone is = $\frac{1}{6}$
   In 1 hr, part of tank filled by Q alone is = $\frac{1}{9}$
   In 1 hr, part of tank emptied by R is = $\frac{1}{12}$
   Initially, P and R opened for 4 hr,
   So, part of tank filled = $4\left(\frac{1}{6} - \frac{1}{12}\right) = \frac{4}{12} = \frac{1}{3}$
   After 4 hr, P is closed and for 6 more hr Q and R are opened.
   So, part of tank filled = $6\left(\frac{1}{9} - \frac{1}{12}\right) = \frac{1}{6}$
   So, total tank filled in 10 hr
   $= \frac{1}{6} + \frac{1}{3} = \frac{2+4}{12} = \frac{1}{2}$
   So, remaining 1/2 part of the tank is filled by Q alone
   Now, Q will take 9/2 = 4.5 hr to fill remaining half of the tank.
   Hence, total time taken = 4 + 6 + 4.5
   = 14.5 hr

10. Here, Revenue shared by pool
    = 170 + 320 + 215 + 190 = 895$
    Similarly, Revenue shared by mini
    = 110 + 220 + 180 + 70 = 580$
    and, Revenue shared by prime
    = 75 + 180 + 120 + 90 = 465$
    Now, percentage share of revenue contributed by prime
    $= \frac{465}{895 + 580 + 465}$
    = 23.97%

CHEMISTRY

1. (c) As per the cannizzaro reaction and product is primary alcohol & carboxylic acid. The starting compound of cannizzaro reaction is C_6H_5CHO, which has the following structure.

The above structure is given in option c

2. (d) The boiling point of halogen are given as

(1) F $\rightarrow$ –188°C

Cl $\rightarrow$ –35°C

Br $\rightarrow$ 58.8°C

I $\rightarrow$ 184°C

(2) The boiling points increase down the group because of the Vander waal's force increases. This X is due to more electrons are there when you descend in the group. This vander waals force caused the induced dipole-dipole interaction. Thus the correct options is (D).

3. Following species are given,

BF_3, PF_3, BF_4^- , IF_4^-

- The central Atom (X) is B in BF_3 & BF_4^- ; P in PF_3 & I in IF_4^-
- All these from the angle F - X - F, where F is the rest of the element other than central atom (X).
- The electron pairs around central atom are represented by a formula XF_n E_m.

Where X = central Atom & has subscript one

F = represent a ligand (an atom bonded to X)

E = each E represent a lone pair of electron on the central atom X.

Component	Configuration ($X F_n E_m$)	Shape	Approximate F-X-F agnle
BF_3	XF_3E_0	Trigonal planner	120°
PF_3	XF_3E_1	Trigonal pyramidal	96.3°
BF_4^-	XF_4E_0	Tetrahedral	109.5°
IF_4^-	XF_6E_0	Octahedral	90°

So, as seen for IF_4^- , the F-X-F angle is minimum. Hence Answer is (D).

4. Tautomers are constitutional isomers of compound that are interconvertible.

This will result due to relocation or movement of proton.

Now, for a given molecule total 3 tautomers are there.

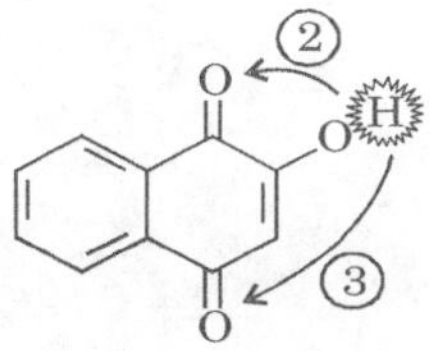

(1)

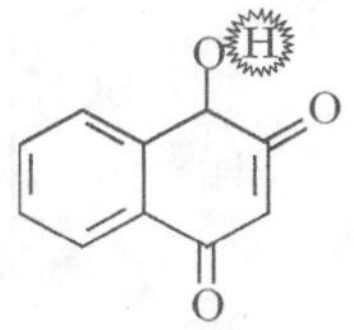

(2)

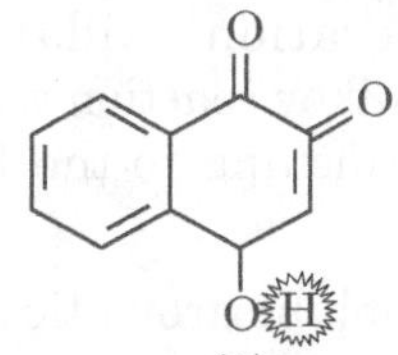

(3)

As Proton molecule (H) is relocate at different O molecule gives total 3 tautomers.

5. The structure given

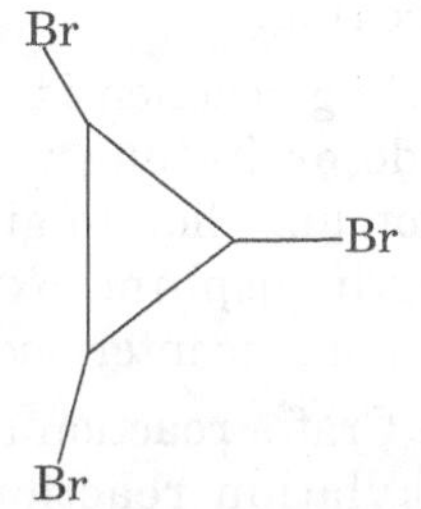

Now, stereoisomers contain Diastereomers and Enantiomers. Now the given structure has 2 Dia stereomers namely Cis & trans isomers & 1 Eantiomers, but this 1 Enantiomers resemble the same structure of Cis isomers.

So, total number of stereoisomers for the given structure is 2.

6. Given:-

(1) $2X \rightleftarrows Y; K_{eq} = \dfrac{[Y]}{[X]^2}$

(2) $Y \xrightarrow{K} P.$

(3) Now, as per rate law ,

$$\frac{dP}{dt} = KC_Y.$$

Now, $C_Y = [Y]$

$$\therefore \frac{dP}{dt} = K[Y] \qquad ...(1)$$

We had, $K_{eq} = \dfrac{[Y]}{[X]^2} \Rightarrow [Y] = K_{eq}[X]^2$

Substituting value of $[Y] = K_{eq}[X]^2$ in equation (1)

$$\therefore \frac{dP}{dt} = K\ K_{eq}[X]^2$$

Hence the answer is (D).

7. (1) Hydroboration oxidation is an anti Markovnikov reaction with the hydroxyl group attaching to the less substituted carbon.

(2) A nucleophilic aromatic substitution is a reaction in which nucleophile displaces a group like halide on an aromatic ring, which resemble to the meisenheimer complex in which nonbonded electrons of the carbanion become bonded to the aromatic ring.

(3) The witting reaction is a reaction of an aldehyde or Ketone with a triphenyl phosphonium ylide to give an alkene & triphenylphosphine oxide which is a oxaphosphetane intermediate

(4) Friedel Crafts reaction are of two types one alkylation reaction and another acylation reactions. Both proceed by electrophilic aromatic substitution.

So, as per the options given option C match with the above.

8. Given reaction

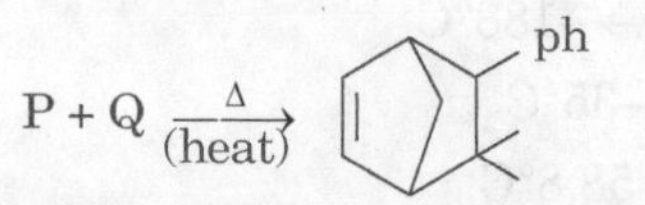

This is simple Diels - Alder reaction of type Pericyclic reaction which occurred between a conjugated diene & a substituted alkene.

So, P is amine 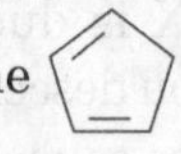 and Q will be diene

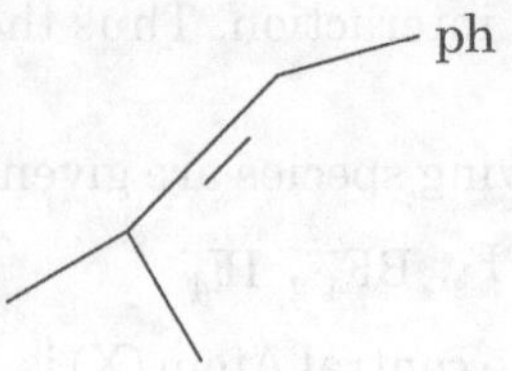

So, option (C) only match with this P & Q hence correct answer is option (C)

9. Given problem is transform of decalin when an elimination reaction is carried out with strong base sodium ethoxide (NaOEt) gives two trans trans & Cis which follow' Zaitsev's rule.

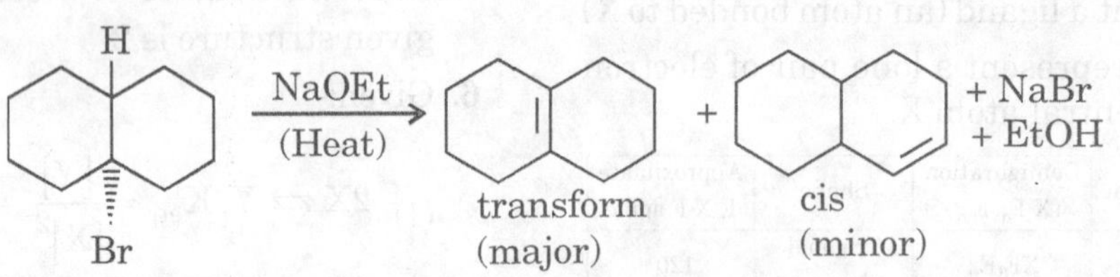

So option (A) is correct

10. Given reaction:

$Fe^{+3} + Hg^{+2} + 5CN^{-} \longrightarrow P + Q.$

In the above equation, Fe^{+3} is the hard atom with following configuration $1s^2\ 2s^2\ 2P^6\ 3s^2\ 3P^6\ 3d^5$; and Hg^{+2} is the soft atom with following configuration $1s^2\ 2s^2\ 2P^6\ 3s^2\ 3P^6\ 3d^{10}\ 4s^2\ 4P^6\ 4d^{10}\ 5s^2\ 5P^6\ 4f^{14}\ 5d^{10}$

Now, the electronic configuration of S is $1s^2\ 2s^2\ 2p^6\ 3s^2\ 2p^4$ & of N is $1s^2\,2s^2\ 2P^3$

Now, Fe^{+3} has the strong charge and thus it will bind with N Hg^{+2} has the affinity to bind with S, and thus following stable coordination complexes will formed.

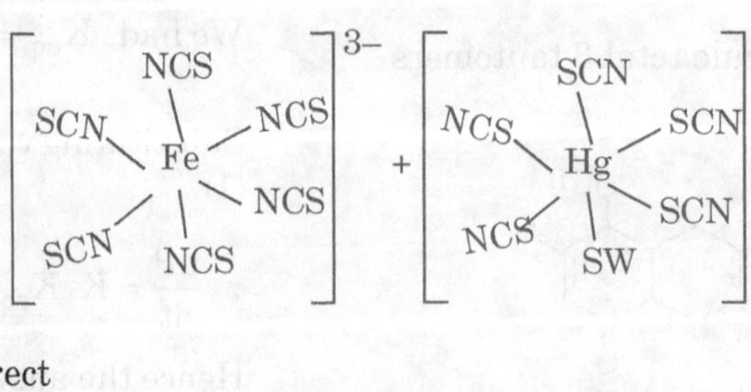

So, the option (B) is correct

11. Given: Coordination complex Y have two isomers,

- One isomer has zero dipole moment.
- The crystal field stabilization energy of Y is $-0.8\ \Delta_0$ or $-0.8\ \Delta_t$.
- The magnetic moment $\mu = 3.9$ Bohr magneton (B.M.).

∴ for give complex Y, $\mu = 3.9$ B.M.

Now, crystal field stabilized energy (CFSE)

$= -0.8\ \Delta_0$

$$\text{CFSE} = -\frac{4}{5}\Delta_0$$

This will be possible with high spin d^7 $\left(t_{2g}5e_g2\right)$ and $d^2\left(t_{2g}2e_g0\right)$ configuration.

Now, $\mu = \sqrt{n(n+2)} = 3.9$

Now, for d^2 configuration

$\mu = \sqrt{2(4)} = \sqrt{8} = 2.83$

for d^7 configuration $\mu = \sqrt{3(5)} = \sqrt{15} = 3.9$.

- So, the complex Y has configuration $d^7\left(t_{2g}5e_g^2\right)$ only.
- From the given four complex, the $[CO\ (NH_3)_4\ CCl_2)]$ has $d^7\left(t_{2g}5e_g^2\right)$ configuration with CO(11) element.

So, Answer is, the coordination complex Y = $[CO(NH_3)_4(Cl_2)]$

12. given $T = 360$ K, $\Delta S° = -139$ JK^{-1} mol^{-1}.

Now, we know that, $\Delta G° = \Delta H° - T\Delta°S$.

Now, for a system at equilibrium, $\Delta G° = 0$.

Thus, for a given problem $\Delta H° = T\Delta°S$

∴ $\Delta°H = 360 \times (-139)$

$= -50040$ J mol^{-1}

$= -50.04$ KJ mol^{-1}

13. Given:,

Conc. of Acetic Acid = 0.2 mol/lit

Conc. of sodium Acetate (conjugate base) = 0.3 mol/lit.

The relationship between pH, pKa is given by following eq.

Now, $\text{pH} = \text{pKa} + \log\frac{[\bar{A}]}{[\bar{H}A]}$. pH = 5.

Conc. of Acid $[^-HA] = 0.2$

Conc. of conjugate base $[A^-] = 0.3$

$$5 = \text{pKa} + \log\frac{0.3}{0.2} = \text{pKa} + 0.17609$$

∴ $\text{pKa} = 5 - 0.17609 = 4.8239$.

Now, pKa = –log Ka.

∴ $-\log \text{Ka} = 4.8239, \Rightarrow \log \text{Ka} = -4.8239$

∴ $\text{Ka} = 1.4 \times 10^{-5}$. So, P = 1.4

14. An element is considered to the paramagnetic when it contains at least one paramagnetic electron.

- Electrons that are alone in an orbital called paramagnetic electron and thus has a net spin because the spin of the lone electron does not get cancelled out.
- And if one orbital has not spin than entire atom will have a net spin and called paramagnetic.
- Now, Following species are paramagnetic as their sub shell is not filled N_2, N_2^{-2}, O_2^+, O_2, O_2^{-2} So total = species are 5

15. Given:

$E°_{\frac{Cu^{+2}}{Cu}} = 0.34V, E°_{\frac{Ag^{-1}}{Ag}} = 0.80V;$

$F = 96500\,C/mol$

Reaction: $Cu(s) + 2Ag_{(aq)} + \rightarrow Cu^{+2}_{(aq)} + 2Ag(s)$

Now, E° for given reaction.

$$E° = -E°_{\frac{Cu^{+2}}{Cu}} + E°_{\frac{Ag^+}{Ag}} = -0.34 + 0.80$$

$= +0.46$ V

Now, Free energe changy ($\Delta G°$) given by $\Delta G° = -nFE°$, where n = no. of moles of electron = 2 for given reaction.

∴ $\Delta G° = -2 \times 96500 \times 0.46 = -88780$ J/mol

$\Delta G° = -88.78$ KJ/mol

BIOCHEMISTRY

1. Peroxisomes contain at least 50 different enzymes, which are involved in a variety of biochemical pathways in different types of cells. Peroxisomes originally were defined as organelles that carry out oxidation reactions leading to the production of hydrogen peroxide. Because hydrogen peroxide is harmful to the cell, peroxisomes also contain the enzyme catalase, which decomposes hydrogen peroxide either by converting it to water or by using it to oxidize another organic compound.
2. During B cell and T cell development, the lymphoid-specific proteins RAG-1 and RAG-2 (The recombination-activating gene(RAG) endonuclease or RAG recombinase composed of the RAG1 and RAG2proteins) act together to initiate the assembly of antigen receptor genes through a series of site-specific somatic DNA rearrangements that are collectively called variable-diversity-joining(V(D)J) recombination.
3. Substrate-level phosphorylation refers to the formation of ATP from ADP and a phosphorylated intermediate, rather than from ADP and inorganic phosphate, Pi, as is done in oxidative phosphorylation.

   In Glycolysis, the first substrate-level phosphorylation occurs after the conversion of 3-phosphoglyceraldehyde and Pi and NAD+ to 1,3-bisphosphoglycerate via glyceraldehyde 3-phosphate dehydrogenase.

   1,3-bisphosphoglycerate is then dephosphorylated via phosphoglycerate kinase, producing 3-phosphoglycerate and ATP through a substrate-level phosphorylation.
4. The dipeptide with least rotational barrier in the peptide bond is:

   B) 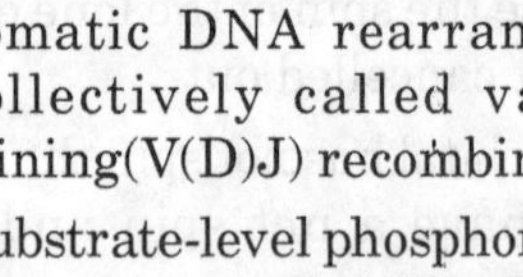

   Peptide bonds have a planar *trans* configuration and undergo very little rotation or twisting around the amide bond that links the ∝-amino nitrogen of one amino acid to the carbonyl carbon of the next amino acid. The planarity and rigidity of the peptide bond are accounted for by the fact that free rotation cannot occur around double bonds.
5. **Rhodopsin**, also called **visual purple**, pigment-containing sensory protein that converts light into an electrical signal. Rhodopsin is found in a wide range of organisms, from vertebrates to bacteria. In many seeing animals, including humans, it is required for vision in dim light and is located in the retina of the eye—specifically, within the tightly packed disks that make up the outer segment of the retina's photoreceptive.

   Cyanobacteria perform photosynthesis through the green pigment chlorophyll-a. They are, however, commonly referred to as blue-green algae because they produce accessory photosynthetic blue pigments, called phycobilins or phycocyanins, that play a role in photon capture for photosynthesis. Red to brown accessory photosynthetic pigments, called phycoerythrins, may also be produced.
6. Methanol poisoning can be treated with fomepizole, or if unavailable, ethanol. Both drugs act to reduce the action of alcohol dehydrogenase on methanol by means of competitive inhibition.
7. **Nitric oxide synthases** are a family of enzymes catalyzing the **production of nitric oxide** (NO) from L-arginine. NO is an **important** cellular **signaling molecule**. It helps modulate vascular tone, insulin secretion, airway tone, and peristalsis, and is involved in angiogenesis and neural development.
8. Antihistamines are effective medications used mainly for allergic rhinitis and other allergies. These medications counter the effects of histamines, a substance made by the body to help the immune system fight invading substances.
9. given : $\Delta E_1 = -6$ kJ/mol.

   (Electrostatic interaction energy between +ve charged A & –ve. Charged B in water)

   $r = 3 \times 10^{-10}$ mt (Distance between Atom A & B)

   ε_1 = relative permittivity of water = 80

   Now, electrostatic interaction energy is given by

   $$\Delta E = \frac{Kaq_1a_2}{\varepsilon r} \quad ...(1)$$

   a = Avogadro's No. = 6.023×10^{23}

$q = -1.602 \times 10^{-19}$ coulombs for –ve charge & $+ 1.602 \times 10^{-19}$ C for +ve charge

∴ Now finding k for given data.

$$\Delta E_1 = \frac{kaq_1q_2}{\varepsilon_1 r} \Rightarrow k = \frac{\Delta E_1 \varepsilon_1 r}{aq_1q_2}$$

$$= \frac{-6 \times 80 \times 3 \times 10^{-10}}{-6.023 \times 10^{23} \times (1.602 \times 10^{-19})^2}$$

∴ $k = 9.3159 \times 10^5$ N m^2c^{-2}

(Now, to find ΔE for Vacuum)

for Vacuum ε = 1.

$$\therefore \Delta E_{vacuum} = \frac{kaq_1q_2}{\varepsilon r}$$

$$= \frac{9.3159 \times 10^5 \times 6.023 \times 10^{23} \times (-1.602^2 - 366 \times 10)}{1 \times 3 \times 10^{-10}}$$

= –480.00 kJ/ml

10. given data:

0.1M glucose solution.

MW of glucose = 180

To make 0.5 ml of 0.005 M glucose solution.

$N_1 = 0.1$ $N_2 = 0.005$

$V_1 = ?$ ml $V_2 = 0.5$

$$\therefore N_1V_1 = N_2V_2 \Rightarrow V_1 = \frac{N_2V_2}{N_1}$$

$$\therefore V_1 = \frac{0.005 \times 0.5}{0.1}$$

$V_1 = 0.025$ ml.

11. A mixture of the following purified proteins, IgG, IgM and Fab fragment of immunoglobulins, is separated using gel filtration chromatography. The order of elution of these proteins (first to last) is IgM, IgG and Fab fragment. Gel filtration chromatography seprarates proteins, peptides, and oligonucleotides on the basis of size. Molecules move through a bed of porous beads, diffusing into the beads to greater or lesser degrees. Smaller molecules diffuse further into the pores of the beads and therefore move through the bed more slowly, while larger molecules enter less or not at all and thus move through the bed more quickly.

12. The ascending order of half-life for the radioactive isotopes, (^{125}I, ^3H, ^{14}C and ^{32}P) is $^{32}P < ^{125}I < ^3H < ^{14}C$. The rate at which a radioactive isotope decays is measured in half-life. The term half-life is defined as the time it takes for one-half of the atoms of a radioactive material to disintegrate.

13. **Propionyl-CoA carboxylase (PCC)** catalyses the carboxylation reaction of propionyl CoA in the mitochondrial matrix. The enzyme is biotin-dependent. The product of the reaction is (S)-methylmalonyl CoA. Propionyl CoA is the end product of metabolism of odd-chain fatty acids, and is also a metabolite of most methyl-branched fatty acids.

14. DpnI is used to digest the PCR product during site directed mutagenesis because DpnI digests only methylated DNA.

15. Palmitoylation is a reversible post-translational process by which eukaryotic and viral proteins are covalently linked to the C16 saturated fatty acid of palmitic acid.

Glycosylation mainly refers in particular to the enzymatic process that attaches glycans to proteins, or other organic molecules.

DNA methylation is a process by which methyl groups are added to the DNA molecule. **Protein methylation** is a type of post-translational modification featuring the addition of methyl groups to proteins.

Polyadenylation is the addition of a **poly(A) tail** to a messenger RNA.

Therefore, Lipid - Palmitoylation is an **incorrect** biomolecule-modification pair.

16. (d) A Dihedral angle of a protein is the internal angle of polypeptide backbone at which two adjacent planes meet.

Now, ϕ angle involves $C - N - C_\alpha - C$ or $(C_\alpha - C - N - C_\alpha)$ ψ angle involve $N - C_\alpha - C - N$.

Further, for an ordered structural repeat of amino acid the dihedral angle between $C - N - C_\alpha - C$ is –120° & the dihedral angle between $N - C_\alpha - C - N$ is +120°.

Now, dihedral angle between $C - N - C_\alpha - C$ = ϕ = –120° & dihedral angle between $N - C_\alpha - C - N$ = ψ = +120°.

17. Absence of detectable protein expression upon blunt-ended mutation-free cloning of an *E.coli* gene with its own promoter in *E. coli* cells can be due to rapid degradation of expressed protein.

18. Given: for lysine $pk_1 = 10.2, pk_2 = 9.2$

$$\therefore p_{i\ lysine} = \frac{1}{2}(pk_1 + pk_2) = \frac{1}{2}(10.2 + 9.2) = 9.7$$

for glutamic Acid $pk_1 = 4.2, pk_2 = 2.2$

$$\therefore p_{i\ glutamic\ Acid} = \frac{1}{2}(pk_1 + pk_2) = \frac{1}{2}(4.2 + 2.2) = 3.2$$

$\therefore$ Difference in isoelectronic point (P_I) of lysine & glutamic Acid = 9.7 – 3.2 = 6.50

19. Given:

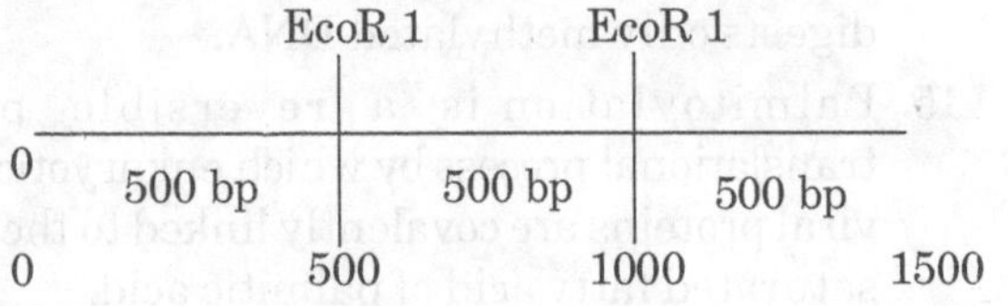

As per given data the initial size of single DNA is 1500 bp.

Now, ECORI digest at 2 sites 500bp each,

So, 3 DNA fragments of 500bp will be formed.

20. mol. wt. of Asp = 133.1027 g/mol

= 133.1027 Da.

mol. wt. of Asp = 132.12 g/mol = 132.12 Da.

Now, molecular wt. of uncharged protein is determined by mass spectrometry and will be given by following equation.

$$P = \frac{Mr + (z_1 - 1)}{(z_1 - 1)} \quad ...(1)$$

Now, P = 6501 Da for a uncharged protein (P) with Asp in 23 position.

Mr′ of Asp = 133.1027 g/ml. (MW of Asp)

Mr of Asn = 132.12 g/mol. (MW of Asn)

Now, to find MW of uncharged mutant of protein P′ we need to find z_1 using given data on equation (1)

$$6501 = \frac{132.12 + (z_1 - 1)}{z_1 - 1.}$$

$$\therefore \quad z_1 = 1.02048$$

$$\therefore \quad \text{MW. of } P' = \frac{133.1027 + (1.02048 - 1)}{(1.02048 - 1)}$$

$P' = 6500.12$ Da.

BOTANY

1. Ecological pyramids are visual representations of energy flow, biomass accumulation, and number of individuals at different trophic levels. There is also pyramid of numbers which represent the number of organisms in each trophic level. They may be upright (e.g. Grassland ecosystem), inverted (Parasitic ecosystem) or dumbbell shaped (forest ecosystem).

2. Raphides are needle-shaped crystals of calcium oxalate as the monohydrate or calcium carbonate as aragonite, found in more than 200 families of plants. Both ends are needle-like, but raphides tend to be blunt at one end and sharp at the other.

3. Bicollateral vascular bundle is a kind of a conjoint vascular bundle present in the stem that has only one xylem strand and two phloem strands. In such vascular bundle, the phloem is found both on the outer side and the inner side of the xylem. It is an open vascular bundle generally found in the stems of plants Cucurbita or Cephalandra.

4. An arbuscular mycorrhiza is a type of mycorrhiza in which the symbiont fungus penetrates the cortical cells of the roots of a vascular plant forming arbuscules. Once inside the parenchyma, the fungus forms highly branched structures for nutrient exchange with the plant called arbuscules.

5. Only cellulose, hemicellulose and pectin combinations of polysaccharides is present in plant cell wall.

6. Both anaerobic bacteria as well as the aerobic bacteria do biological nitrogen fixation however, the process occurs in absence of Oxygen and thus is anaerobic process. Further, biological nitrogen fixation is done by both free living and symbiotic bacteria.

7. Cyclic photophosphorylation is driven by photosystem I, which returns electrons to itself through the site of proton translocation and ATP synthesis. In cyclic photophosphorylation, electrons follow a different, circular path and only ATP (no NADPH) is produced. Therefore the statement Cyclic photophosphorylation occurs when NADP+/NADPH ratio is high is INCORRECT.

8. The phenomenon of a mature cell reverting to the meristematic state and forming undifferentiated callus tissue is termed 'dedifferentiation'. The phenomenon of conversion of component cells of callus tissue to whole plant or plant organs is called as 'redifferentiation'.

9. Glyphosate is a broad - spectrum herbicide that prevents the synthesis of aromatic amino acids. It is highly mobile in phloem thus when applied to leaves it is rapidly translocated to meristematic areas and underground rhizomes for effective control of weeds.

10. A double monosomic individual lacks one chromosome each from two different pairs of chromosomes. They are designated as 2n-1-1.

Therefore, as given, 2n = 16 individual who is double monosomic will have

= 16-1-1

= 14 number of chromosomes per cell

11. Rubisco catalyzes conversion of ribulose 1, 5-bisphosphate to : (P) two molecules of stable 3-phosphoglycerate; & (Q) one molecule of 3-phosphoglycerate and one molecule of phosphoglycolate.

12. Correct combination of molecules with their functions are:

Group I (Molecules)	Group II (Function)
P. Ubiquitin	3. Mediator of protein degradation
Q. Phytotropins	4. Noncompetitive inhibitors of polar transport of auxin
R. Extensins	1. Cell wall loosening enzymes
S. DELLA proteins	2. Repressors in gibberellin signaling

13. Correct match of the plant species and their corresponding families with their economically important products are:

Plant species	Family	Plant product
P. Cannabis sativa	2. Cannabaceae	iv. Marijuana from leaves
Q. Corchorus olitorius	4. Tiliaceae	iii. Fibre from stem
R. Ocimum sanctum	1. Lamiaceae	ii. Eugenol from leaves
S. Ricinus communis	3. Euphorbiaceae	i. Oil from seeds

14. **Cybrids** are produced in variable frequencies in normal protoplast fusion experiments due to one of the following methods:

I. Fusion of normal protoplast with an enucleated protoplast. The enucleated protoplast can be produced by high speed centrifugation (20,000-40,000xg) for 60 min with 5-50% percoll.

II. Fusion between a normal protoplast and another protoplast with a non-viable nucleus or suppressed nucleus.

III. Elimination of one of the nuclei after heterokaryons formation.

IV. Selective elimination of chromosomes at a later stage.

V. Irradiating (with X-rays or gamma rays) the protoplasts of one species prior to fusion in order to inactivate their nuclei.

VI. By preparing enucleate protoplasts (cytoplasts) of one species and fusing them with normal protoplasts of the other species.

15. Correct match of the diseases with causative organisms and affected crops are:

Disease	Causative organism	Crop
P. Powdery mildew	3. *Erysiphe orontii*	ii. Tomato
Q. White rust	1. *Albugo candida*	iv. Mustard
R. Downy mildew	4. *Peronosclerospora phillippinensis*	i. Corn
S. Late blight	2. *Phytophthora infestans*	iii. Potato

16. Correct match of the options in **Group I** with **Group II** with respect to steps in signal transduction mechanism in plants are:

Group I	Group II
P. Phospholipase C	3. hydrolyzes posphatidylin-ositol bisphosphate (PIP2)
Q. Inositol triphosphate	1. stimulates release of calcium from intracellular stores
R. Diacylglycerol	4. phosphorylated to phosphatidic acid
S. Phosphatidic acid	2. regulates ion channels/activates various enzymes

17. The CORRECT statements with respect to endosperm development is as - It originates from the fusion product of three haploid nuclei - one from male gametophyte and two from the female gametophyte.

18. The INCORRECT statements with respect to haploid plant production is as - It can be produced from Nuclear tissue.

19. As given contribution of ab = 0.5; and contribution of AB = 1.7 in the heterozygous individual (AaBb). Therefore the weight of an individual plant in F1 progeny of this cross would be = 2.2

20. The number of chromosomes at Anaphase-1 is double of the number of chromosomes at Interphase due to DNA replication. Each chromosomes is a single DNA molecule, hence the number of DNA molecules (or chromosomes) per cell will be 24.

MICROBIOLOGY

1. Tetracycline antibiotic. Mechanism of action of tetracyclines is to bind to 30S ribosomal subunit and inhibit protein synthesis. Chloramphenicol is a broad-spectrum antibiotic that interferes with mitochondrial protein synthesis and is active against a variety of organisms including salmonelloses not responsive to ampicillin.

2. **Food irradiation** is the process of exposing food and food packaging to ionizing radiation. Ionizing radiation, such as from gamma rays, x-rays, or electron beams, is energy that can be transmitted without direct contact to the source of the energy (radiation) capable of freeing electrons from their atomic bonds (ionization) in the targeted food. Food irradiation primarily extends the shelf-life of irradiated foods by effectively destroying organisms responsible for spoilage and foodborne illness and inhibiting sprouting.

3. **Lipopolysaccharide** is pyrogenic (responsible for fever), and also causes endotoxic shock. The **LPS is** composed of three distinct units; A phospholipid called Lipid A; It embeds Lipolysaccharide layer in the outer leaflet. Also known as endotoxin, it **is** responsible for **toxic effects** (fever and shock).

4. Microbes make up about 2/3rd of earth's living material by weight.

5. **Measles is caused** by the **measles virus,** a **single-stranded**, negative-sense, enveloped **RNA virus** of the genus Morbillivirus within the family Paramyxoviridae. The **virus** is **highly contagious** and is spread by coughing and sneezing via close personal contact or direct contact with secretions.

6. Secondary metabolites usually accumulate during the later stage of fermentation, known as the idiophase, which follows the active growth phase called the trophophase.

7. **Dick test** is method of determining susceptibility to scarlet fever by injection into the skin of 0.1 cubic centimetre of scarlet fever toxin.

8. *Rhizobium* is a symbiotic bacterial genus that converts nitrogen into nitrogen containing compounds that are utilized by legume plants to synthesize amino acids.

9. The enzyme involved in the following reaction is Lipase.

   Triglyceride + $3H_2O \rightarrow$ Glycerol + fatty acids

10. (a) given data:

    Culture in exponential phase at 8 A.M.

    Density of microorganism = 500/ml

    generation time = 20 min.

    $\therefore$ Density of microorganism at 11 A.M. i.e. after 3 hr = ?

    Now, No. of generations $= \frac{3 \times 60}{20} = 9$

    $\therefore$ Total No. of organism/ml after three hours

    $= 500 \times 2^9$

    = 256000.

11. Folic acid synthesis in bacteria is competitively inhibited by sulfonamides Para-amino benzoic acid (essential components) is replaced by sulfonamides during the process of folic acid synthesis.

12. Nucleoid and Pili are cellular structures absent in eukaryotes and are present at least in some prokaryotic organisms.

13. As per the given quote "Granules are inclusion bodies found in bacteria", the true statements about granules are: (i) Granules can be storage vessels for carbohydrates/ lipids and (ii) Some granules supply substances for a variety of metabolic processes.

14. Correct match of the culture media to their uses:

Culture Media	Uses
(i) Complex media	(q) chemically undefined media for growing bacteria
(ii) Selective media	(p) identifying certain bacteria from mixed culture
(iii) Differential media	(s) distinguishing one bacteria from another
(iv) Enriched media	(r) cultivating fastidious bacteria

15. Most appropriate characteristics for archaebacterial are: (ii) Long chain branched alcohols (phytanols) bound to glycerol by ether linkages are found in the lipids of cytoplasmic membrane (iv) Translation process is sensitive to the action of diphtheria toxin.

16. Horizontal gene transfer, also known as lateral gene transfer, is a process in which an organism transfers genetic material to another organism that is not its offspring. The ability of *Bacteria* and *Archaea* to adapt to new environments as a part of bacterial evolution most frequently results from the acquisition of new genes through horizontal gene transfer rather than by the alteration of gene functions through mutations. (It is estimated that as much as 20% of the genome of *Escherichia coli* originated from horizontal gene transfer.)

There are three mechanisms of horizontal gene transfer in bacteria: transformation, transduction, and conjugation. The most common mechanism for horizontal gene transmission among bacteria, especially from a donor bacterial species to different recipient species, is conjugation. Although bacteria can acquire new genes through transformation and transduction, this is usually a more rare transfer among bacteria of the same species or closely related species.

17. Correct match of the class of antibodies to appropriate description or function :

Antibodies	Description /function
(i) IgA	(p) Mucosal immunity
(ii) IgG	(r) Most abundant antibody in the blood
(iii) IgD	(s) Found on the B cell membranes
(iv) IgE	(q) Immunity to parasitic infections

18. Correct match of the diseases with the appropriate causative agents:

Disease	Causative agent
(i) Rheumatic heart disease	(q) Group A *Streptococcus*
(ii) Syphilis	(s) *Treponema pallidum*
(iii) Genital warts	(r) Human papilloma virus
(iv) Oral thrush	(p) *Candida albicans*

19. (a) Given data:

Dia of Spherical bacterial cell $d_1 = 2\ \mu m$.

Dia of Spherical eukaryotic cell $d_2 = 20\ \mu m$.

Now, surface Area of Spherical cell(s) $= 4\pi r^2 = \pi D^2$

Volume of Spherical cell (v) $= \frac{4}{3}\pi r^3 = \frac{\pi}{6}D^3$

Now, for Bacterial cell ratio of $\left(\frac{S}{V}\right)$

$$= \frac{\pi d_1^2}{\frac{\pi}{6}d_1^3} = \frac{6}{d_1} = \frac{6}{2} = 3\mu m^{-1}$$

For Eukaryotic cell ratio of $\left(\frac{S}{V}\right)$

$$= \frac{\pi d_2^2}{\frac{\pi}{6}d_2^3} = \frac{6}{d_2} = \frac{6}{20} = 0.3\mu m^{-1}$$

$\therefore \left(\frac{S}{V}\right)$ of Bacterial cell $= \frac{3}{0.3} = 10$

$\therefore$ i.e. 10 times of Eukaryotic cell $\left(\frac{S}{V}\right)$

20. Given data:

Same characteristics = 72

Different characteristics = 44.

$\therefore$ Total characteristics = 72 + 44 = 116

Now, % Similarity between two strain

$$= \frac{\text{No. of Same characteristics}}{\text{Total characteristics}} \times 100$$

$$= \frac{72}{116} \times 100 = 62.07\%$$

ZOOLOGY

1. Some animals like fishes, have only a two chambered heart. Their heart consists of one auricle or atrium, and one ventricle. However all reptiles, with the exception of crocodiles, have a three chambered heart – two auricles and one ventricle. Therefore Gold fish possesses two chambered heart.
2. In eukaryotic chromatin organization, H1 histones seals off the nucleosome at the location at which linker DNA enters and leaves the nucleosome. ***H1*** and its isoforms are involved ***in chromatin*** compaction and sit at the base of the ***nucleosome*** near the ***DNA*** entry and ***exit*** binding to the ***linker*** region of the ***DNA***.
3. *Mansonella streptocerca,* is the scientific name of a human parasitic roundworm causing the disease streptocerciasis. It is a common parasite in the skin of humans in the rain forests of Africa, where it is thought to be a parasite of chimpanzees, as well. This parasite does NOT cause lymphatic filariasis.
4. In evolutionary ecology, an **ecotype**, sometimes called **ecospecies**, describes a genetically distinct geographic variety, population or race within a species, which is genotypically adapted to specific environmental conditions.
5. The **water vascular system** is a hydraulic system used by echinoderms, such as sea stars and sea urchins, for locomotion, food and waste transportation, and respiration. The system is composed of canals connecting numerous tube feet. Echinoderms move by alternately contracting muscles that force water into the tube feet, causing them to extend and push against the ground, then relaxing to allow the feet to retract.
6. **Adaptive radiation** is a process in which organisms diversify rapidly from an ancestral species into a multitude of new forms, particularly when a change in the environment makes new resources available, creates new challenges, or opens new environmental niches. "The finches on the Galapagos Islands have widely differing beaks adapted according to their diets". This is an example of Adaptive radiation.
7. A **living fossil** is an extant taxon that closely resembles organisms otherwise known only from the fossil record. To be considered a living fossil, the fossil species must be old relative to the time of origin of the extant clade. Living fossils commonly are species-poor lineages, but they need not be. Horseshoe crab is named as a "living fossil", where the animal is persisting above 400 million years without further major morphological evolution.
8. (a) given:

Peptide : Ala – Glu– Val – Asn – Ile – Asp – Pro– As – Gln Gly – Asp.

pka (for side chain R-group) values :

Ala = 1 = 0

Glu = 1 = 4.25 (–COOH)

Val = 1 = 0

Asn = 1 = 13.2

Ile = 1 = 0

Asp = 3 = 3.65 (–COOH)

Pro = 1 = 0

Gln = 1 = 0

Gly = 1 = 0

N terminus P ka ≈ 8.5 ($-NH_3^+$)

C terminus P ka ≈ 3.2 (–COOH)

Now, net charge of Peptide

$$Q_{Peptide} = \Sigma Q^- + \Sigma Q^+$$

$$Q^- = \frac{(-1)}{1+10^{-(pH-p_{ka})}},\ Q^+ \frac{(+1)}{1+10^{+(PH-p_{ka})}}$$

$$\therefore Q_{Peptide} = \underset{\text{N – terminess}}{\frac{+1}{1+10^{+(1-8.5)}}} + \underset{\text{Glu}}{\frac{1}{1+10^{-(1-4.25)}}}$$

$$+ \underset{\text{Asn}}{\frac{1}{1+10^{+(1-13.2)}}}$$

$$- \underset{\text{Asp}}{\frac{3}{1+10^{-(1-3.65)}}} + \underset{\text{C terminess}}{\frac{1}{1+10^{-(1-3.2)}}} = 0.998$$

9. I_gM Antibody is Pentameric.

Now, there are 3 CDR_s (CDR_1, CDR_2 + CDR_3). Arranged on an amino acid sequence of variable domain of antigen recepter,

CDR_s are Part of the Variable chain in immgnoglobalin's.

Now, There are 3 CDR loops per variable domain in antibody.

Now, IgM is Pentameric.

i.e. it has 10 Antigen. receptors.

each Antigen receptors has 6 CDR_s (3 × 2 for 2 variable domain)

So, total No. of CDR_s is IgM = 10 × 6 = 60

10. Given : 1500 base pairs double stranded B-DNA;

There are 2 purines - adenine and Guanine

As given 70 % of purines are Adenines and rest are Guanines;

Therefore 70% of 1500 = 1050 Adenines

They will make double bonds i.e. (1050 × 2) = 2100 hydrogen bonds

However 30% of 1500 = 450 will be Guanines

Therefore they will make triple bonds i.e. (450 × 3) = 1350 hydrogen bonds

Hence total number of hydrogen bonds in the DNA = 2100 + 1350 = 3450

11. Correct match of the given vitamin with the related protein:

Column I	Column II
a) Vitamin C	4) Prolyl hydroxylase
b) Vitamin K	1) Thrombin
c) Vitamin A	2) Rhodopsin
d) Vitamin B1	3) Pyruvate dehydrogenase

12. Correct match of the term with the appropriate explanation is:

Column I	Column II
a) Spliceosome	4) Post transcriptional modifications
b) Peroxisome	2) Metabolism of long chain fatty acids
c) Lysosome	1) Cell scavengers
d) Centrosome	3) Microtubules

13. Correct match of the respective behaviour with the appropriate explanation is:

Column I	Column II
a) Agonistic behaviour	3) Aggressive behaviour of individuals within a population
b) Hierarchical behaviour	4) Existence of different levels of dominance within a population
c) Altruistic behaviour	1) Individual behaviour where fitness of other increases at the expense of self
d) Cooperative behaviour	2) Individuals contribute towards enhancement of mutual fitness

14. Closure of neural tube during neurulation is the process in which neural tube eventually forms a closed cylinder that separates from surface ectoderm. Craniorachischisis is linked to the failure in the closure of entire neural tube i.e. brain and spinal cord, over the body axis. Craniorachischisis is the most severe form of neural tube defect in which both the brain and spinal cord remain open to varying degrees. It is a very rare congenital malformation of the central nervous system.

15. Allopatric speciation is thus **speciation** that occurs **through** geographic isolation of **two populations** or groups of **populations**. In this scenario, a **population** is **split** by some geographic barrier, such as a mountain range or river for terrestrial organisms, or a land mass for aquatic organisms. Therefore the factor does NOT contribute to allopatric speciation is – "there is a gene flow between the two separated populations"

16. Correct match of the hormones to their respective physiological effects are:

Column I	Column II
a) Melatonin	5) Regulation of circadian rhythms
b) Oxytocin	3) Secretion of milk and uterine contraction
c) Cholecystokinin	4) Secretion of enzymes from pancreatic acinar cells
d) Prolactin	2) Synthesis of milk in mammary gland
e) Somatostatin	1) Inhibition of secretion of growth hormone

17. MW of DNA fragment = 7.92×10^8 g/mol

MW of 1 nucleotide = 330 g/mol

Hence MW of 1 nucleotide pair = 660 g/mol

Therefore Number of nucleotide pairs in the DNA molecule

$= 7.92 \times 10^8 \div 660 = 1.2 \times 10^6$

For a 200 amino acids long protein, the number of nucleotides pairs required = 200 × 3 = 600

Therefore total number of such proteins that can be coded by this DNA fragment

$= 1.2 \times 10^6 \div 600 = 2000$

18. Given : Substrate conc. = 35 μM. = [s]

Reaction Velocity = $10\ \mu MS^{-1}$ = V

Km = 14μm, $k_{cat} = 500\ S^{-1}$

Now, Enzymatic reaction Velocity is given by.

$$v = k_{cat}E_o \frac{S}{k_M + S}$$

$$\therefore\ E_o = \frac{v(k_M + S)}{k_{cat} \times S} = 0.028\mu M$$

$\therefore$ E_O = 28 nM (nano molar)

$\therefore$ Total Amount of enzyme used = 28 nM.

19. Given: Mouse Population which are albino mice = 36%

These mice have double recessive genotype (aa).

The black coloured mice have dominant genotype (AA/Aa)

$\therefore$ $f(aa) = q^2 = 0.36 \Rightarrow q = 0.6$

Now $p + q = 1 \Rightarrow p = 0.4$.

Now, frequency of heterozygove alleles (Aa) is given by f(Aa) = 2 pq = 2 × 0.6 × 0.4 = 0.48

20. Given: (1) F_2 Progenies are as follows

(2) $a^+b\ c$	16
$ab^+\ c$	115
abc	311
$a^+\ b^+\ c$	64
$a\ b\ c^+$	61
$a^+b^+c^+$	317
$a^+\ bc^+$	99
ab^+c^+	17
Total =	1000

(3) Now, I map unit (m.v.) = 1% recombination = 1 centi morgan.

we know that:

Map distance = % recombination.

$$= \frac{\text{(No. in SCO phenotypes + No. in DCO phenotypes)}}{\text{Total No. Progenies.}} \times 100$$

Now, map distance between b & c

= (map distance between b & a) + (map distance between b & c)

$\therefore\ b \longleftrightarrow c = b \longleftrightarrow a + a \longleftrightarrow c$

Now, SCO = Single cross over = $b^+ac(115)$, ba^+c^+ (99) between b & a = $b^+a^+c(64)$, $bac^+(61)$

DCO = Double cross over = $a^+bc(16)$, $a\ b^+c^+(17)$ = least frequent.

Now, $b \leftrightarrow a$ map distance

$$= \frac{115 + 99 + 16 + 17}{1000} \times 100 = 24.7\%$$

= 24.7 centi morgon.

$a \leftrightarrow c$ map distance

$$= \frac{64 + 61 + 16 + 17}{1000} \times 100 = 15.8\%$$

= 15.8 centi morgon.

$\therefore$ $b \leftrightarrow c$ map distance = 24.7 + 15.8 = 40.5 centi morgon

■■

GATE 2018

XL : LIFE SCIENCES

Time : 3 Hours *Maximum Marks : 100*

GENERAL APTITUDE

Q. 1 – Q. 5 carry one mark each.

1. Going by the ______ that many hands make light work, the school ______ involved all the students in the task."
   (*a*) principle, principal
   (*b*) principal, principle
   (*c*) principle, principle
   (*d*) principal, principal

2. "Her _____ should not be confused with miserliness; she is ever willing to assist those in need."
   The word that best fills the blank in the above sentence is
   (*a*) cleanliness (*b*) punctuality
   (*c*) frugality (*d*) greatness

3. Seven machines take 7 minutes to make 7 identical toys. At the same rate, how many minutes would it take for 100 machines to make 100 toys?
   (*a*) 1 (*b*) 7
   (*c*) 100 (*d*) 700

4. A rectangle becomes a square when its length and breadth are reduced by 10 m and 5 m, respectively, during this process, the rectangle loses 650 m^2 of area. What is the area of the original rectangle in square meters?
   (*a*) 1125 (*b*) 2250
   (*c*) 2924 (*d*) 4500

5. A number consists of two digits. The sum of the digits is 9. If 45 is subtracted from the number, its digits are interchanged. What is the number?
   (*a*) 63 (*b*) 72
   (*c*) 81 (*d*) 90

Q. 6 – Q. 10 carry two marks each

6. For integers a, b and c, what would be the minimum and maximum values respectively of a + b + c if log |a| + log |b| + log |c| = 0
   (*a*) –3 and 3 (*b*) –1 and 1
   (*c*) –1 and 3 (*d*) 1 and 3

7. Given that a and b are integers and $a + a^2b^3$ is odd, which one of the following statements is correct?
   (*a*) a and b are both odd
   (*b*) a and b are both even
   (*c*) a is even and b is odd
   (*d*) a is odd and b is even

8. From the time the front of train enters a platform, it takes 25 seconds for the back of the train to leave the platform, while travelling at a constant speed of 54 km/h. At the same speed, it takes 14 seconds to pass a man running at 9 km/h in the same direction as the train. What is the length of the train and that of the platform in meters, respectively?
   (*a*) 210 and 140 (*b*) 162.5 and 187.5
   (*c*) 245 and 130 (*d*) 175 and 200

9. Which of the following functions describe the graph shown in the below figure.

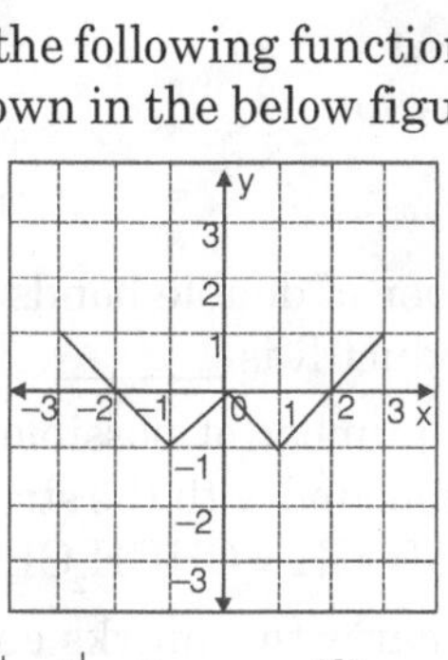

   (*a*) $y = ||x| + 1| - 2$ (*b*) $y = ||x| - 1| - 1$
   (*c*) $y = ||x| + 1| - 1$ (*d*) $y = ||x - 1| - 1|$

10. Consider the following three statements:
    (i) Some roses are red
    (ii) All red flowers fade quickly
    (iii) Some roses fade quickly
    Which of the following statements can be logically inferred from the above statements?
    (*a*) If (i) is true and (ii) is false, then (iii) is false.
    (*b*) If (i) is true and (ii) is false, then (iii) is true.
    (*c*) If (i) and (ii) are true, then (iii) is true.
    (*d*) If (i) and (ii) are false, then (iii) is false.

CHEMISTRY

Q. 1 – Q. 5 carry one mark each.

1. For the complete combustion of graphite and diamond in oxygen individually, the standard enthalpy change (ΔH^0_{298}) values are –393.5 kJ mol^{-1} and –395.4 kJ mol^{-1}, respectively.

   Then, the ΔH^0_{298} for the conversion of graphite into diamond is

   (*a*) +1.9 kJ mol^{-1} (*b*) –1.9 kJ mol^{-1}

   (*c*) +3.8 kJ mol^{-1} (*d*) –3.8 kJ mol^{-1}

2. For a 4s orbital of hydrogen atom, the magnetic quantum number (m) is

   (*a*) 4 (*b*) 3

   (*c*) 1 (*d*) 0

3. Hybridization of xenon in XeF_2 is

   (*a*) sp (*b*) sp^2

   (*c*) sp^3 (*d*) sp^3d

4. Two equivalents of P react with one equivalent of Q to produce a major product R.

   P = 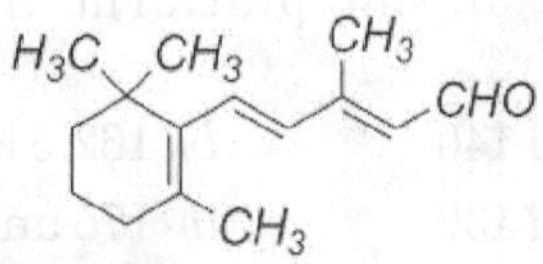

   Q = 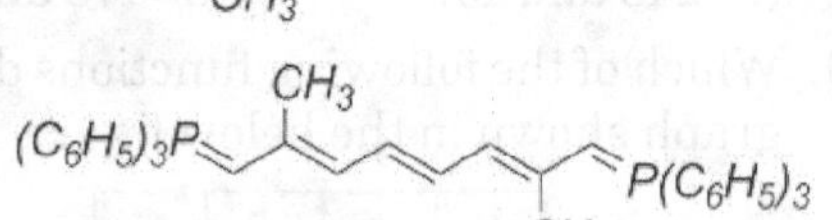

   The number of double bonds present in the major product R is ______.

5. The total number of possible stereoisomers for the compound with the structural formula $CH_3CH(OH)CH = CHCH_2CH_3$ is ______.

Q. 6 – Q. 15 carry two marks each

6. Among B–H, C–H, N–H and Si–H bonds in BH_3, CH_4, NH_3 and SiH_4, respectively, the polarity of the bond which is shown INCORRECTLY is

   (*a*) $B^{\delta+}-H^{\delta-}$ (*b*) $C^{\delta-}-H^{\delta+}$

   (*c*) $N^{\delta-}-H^{\delta+}$ (*d*) $Si^{\delta-}-H^{\delta+}$

7. Among the following statements,

   (i) $[NiCl_4]^{2-}$ (atomic number of Ni = 28) is diamagnetic

   (ii) Ethylamine is a weaker Lewis base compared to pyridine

   (iii) $[NiCl_2\{P(C_6H_5)_3\}_2]$ has two geometrical isomers

   (iv) Bond angle in H_2O is greater than that in H_2S the CORRECT one is

   (*a*) (i) (*b*) (ii)

   (*c*) (iii) (*d*) (iv)

8. In $[Mn(H_2O)_6]^{2+}$ (atomic number of Mn = 25), the d-d transitions according to crystal field theory (CFT) are

   (*a*) Laporte forbidden and spin forbidden

   (*b*) Laporte allowed and spin allowed

   (*c*) Laporte forbidden and spin allowed

   (*d*) Laporte allowed and spin forbidden

9. The major product M in the reaction

   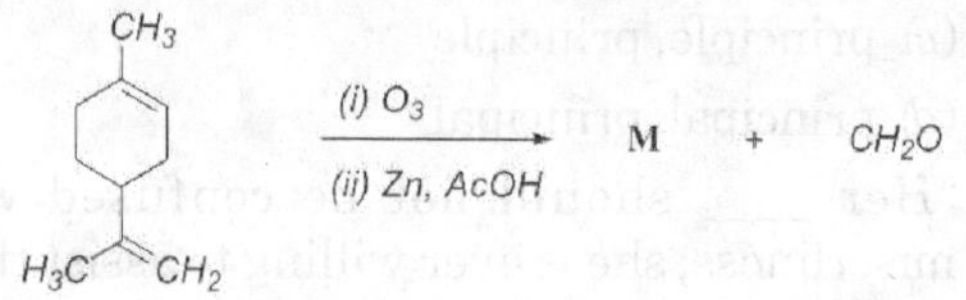

   (*a*) 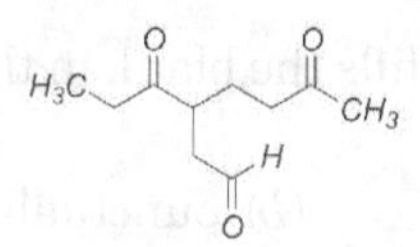 (*b*) 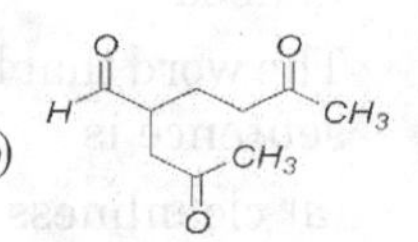

   (*c*) 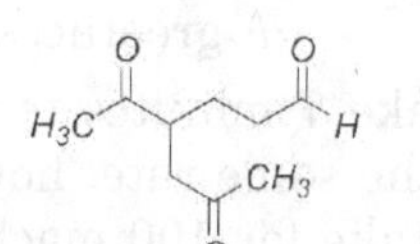 (*d*) 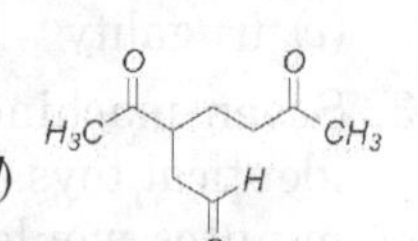

10. The two major products of the reaction

    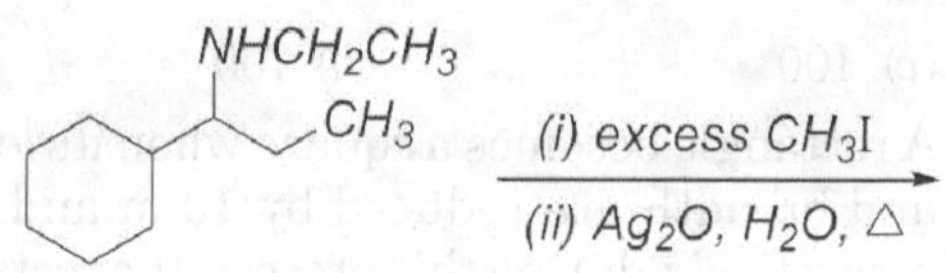

    are

    (*a*) 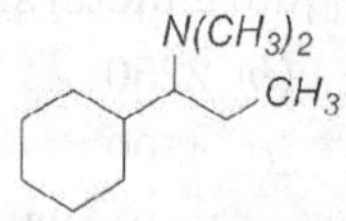 and $CH_2{=}CH_2$

    (*b*) 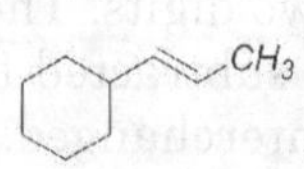 and $N(CH_3)_2CH_2CH_3$

    (*c*) 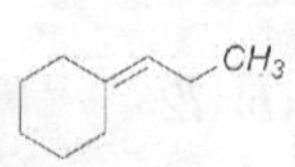 and $N(CH_3)_2CH_2CH_3$

    (*d*) 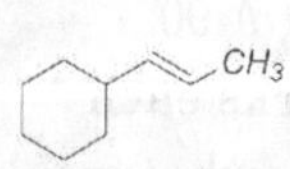 and $HN(CH_3)CH_2CH_3$

11. The compound, which upon mono-nitration using a mixture of HNO_3 and H_2SO_4, does NOT give the *meta*-isomer as the major product, is

(a) 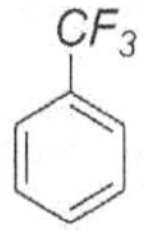 (b) 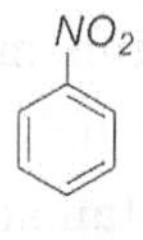

(c) 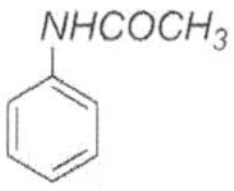 (d) 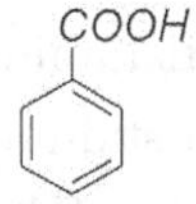

12. The standard reduction potential (E°) for the conversion of $Cr_2O_7^{2-}$ to Cr^{3+} at 25°C in an aqueous solution of pH 3.0 is 1.33 V. The concentrations of $Cr_2O_7^{2-}$ and Cr^{3+} are 1.0 × 10^{-4} M and 1.0 × 10^{-3} M, respectively. Then the potential of this half-cell reaction is (Given: Faraday constant = 96500 C mol^{-1}, Gas constant R = 8.314 J K^{-1} mol^{-1})
   (a) 1.04 V (b) 0.94 V
   (c) 0.84 V (d) 0.74 V

13. The solubility product (K_{sp}) of $Mg(OH)_2$ at 25°C is 5.6 × 10^{-11}. Its solubility in water is S × 10^{-2} g/L, where the value of S is ______ (up to two decimal places). (Given: Molecular weight of $Mg(OH)_2$ = 58.3 g mol^{-1})

14. The activation energy (E_a) values for two reactions carried out at 25°C differ by 5.0 kJ mol^{-1}. If the pre-exponential factors (A_1 and A_2) for these two reactions are of the same magnitude, the ratio of rate constants (k_1/k_2) is _____ (up to two decimal places).
   (Given: Gas constant R = 8.314 J K^{-1} mol^{-1})

15. One mole of helium gas in an isolated system undergoes a reversible isothermal expansion at 25°C from an initial volume of 2.0 liters to a final volume of 10.0 liters. The change in entropy (ΔS) of the surroundings is ______ J K^{-1} (up to two decimal places). (Given: Gas constant R = 8.314 J K^{-1} mol^{-1})

BIOCHEMISTRY

Q. 1 – Q. 10 carry one mark each.

1. To which one of the following classes of enzymes does chymotrypsin belong?
   (a) Oxidoreductase (b) Hydrolase
   (c) Transferase (d) Isomerase

2. The substrate saturation profile of an enzyme that follows Michaelis-Menten kinetics is depicted in the figure. What is the order of the reaction in the concentration range between 0.8 to 1.4 M?

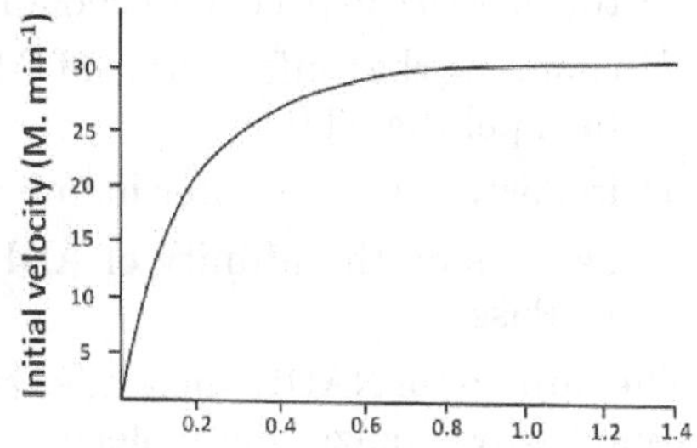

   (a) Zero (b) Fraction
   (c) First (d) Second

3. Which one of the following conformations of glucose is most stable?
   (a) Boat (b) Half Chair
   (c) Chair (d) Planar

4. Which one of the following profiles represent the phenomenon of cooperativity?

(a) 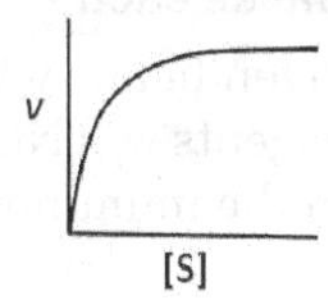

(b) 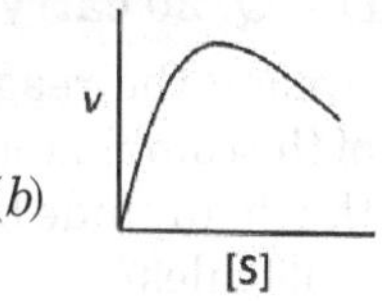

(c) 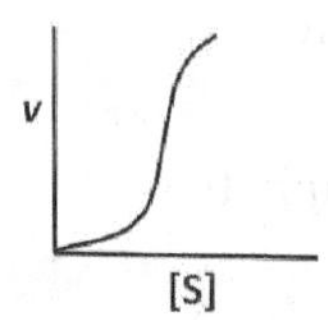

(d) 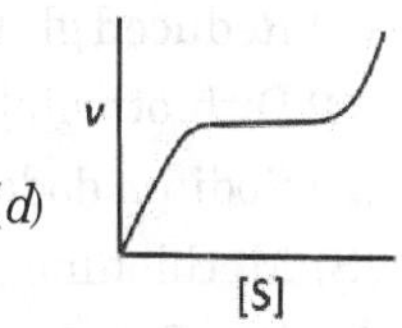

5. Which one of the following amino acids is responsible for the intrinsic fluorescence of proteins?
   (a) Pro (b) Met
   (c) His (d) Trp

6. The glycosylation of the proteins occurs in_____.
   (a) glyoxysomes (b) lysosomes
   (c) Golgi apparatus (d) plasma membrane

7. Which one of the following properties of the myeloma cells is used in the hybridoma technology to generate monoclonal antibody?
   (a) lack of thymidylate synthase
   (b) over-expression of hypoxanthine-guanine phosphoribosyl transferase
   (c) over-expression of inosine 5′-monophosphate cyclohydrolase
   (d) lack of hypoxanthine-guanine phosphoribosyl transferase

8. The movement of protons through the F_oF_1-ATPase during mitochondrial respiration is required for ____

(*a*) the increase in pH of mitochondrial matrix

(*b*) changing the conformation of F_oF_1-ATPase to expel the ATP

(*c*) importing P_i from inter membrane space

(*d*) decreasing the affinity of ADP to F_oF_1-ATPase

9. The number of $NADP^+$ molecules required to completely oxidize one molecule of glucose to CO_2 through pentose phosphate pathway is ____ (correct to integer number).

10. Measurement of the absorbance of a solution containing NADH in a path length of 1cm cuvette at 340 nm shows the value of 0.31. The molar extinction coefficient of NADH is 6200 M^{-1} cm^{-1}. The concentration of NADH in the solution is ____ M (correct to integer number).

Q. 11 – Q. 20 carry two marks each.

11. Among the reagents given below which one of the combination of reagents will NOT break the disulphide bonds in the immunoglobulin molecules?

(P) Reduced glutathione

(Q) Dithiothritol

(R) Sodium dodecyl sulphate

(S) Methionine

(*a*) R & S (*b*) P & R

(*c*) P & S (*d*) Q & R

12. Match the protein elution condition given in Group I with the appropriate chromatography matrices from Group II.

	Group I		Group II
P	Increasing concentration of sodium chloride	i	Phenyl-Sepharose
Q	Increasing concentration of histidine	ii	Chromatofocusing
R	Decreasing concentration of ammonium sulphate	iii	DEAE-Sephacryl
S	Decreasing concentration of H^+	iv	Ni-NTA

(*a*) P-iii; Q-iv; R-i; S-ii

(*b*) P-ii; Q-iv; R-i; S-iii

(*c*) P-i; Q-ii; R-iii; S-iv

(*d*) P- iv; Q-ii; R-iii; S-i

13. Which one of the following is NOT a neurotransmitter?

(*a*) Adrenaline

(*b*) Glutamate

(*c*) Histamine

(*d*) Histidine

14. The type-II hypersensitivity reaction is mainly mediated by____.

(*a*) IgE

(*b*) IgM

(*c*) IgA

(*d*) T cells

15. Which one the following reaction mechanisms drives the conversion of low energy 3-phosphoglyceral-dehyde to high energy 1,3-bisphosphoglycerate?

(*a*) Oxidation without anhydride bond formation

(*b*) Oxidation coupled with anhydride bond formation

(*c*) Substrate level phosphorylation

(*d*) Formation of carboxylate

16. A polymerase reaction is carried out for 10 cycles in a volume of 1 ml with 5 molecules of template DNA. Assuming that the efficiency of the reaction is 100 %, the number of molecules of DNA present in 100 μl at the end of the reaction is ___ (correct to integer number).

17. The secondary structure topology diagram of 400 amino acid long "Protein-X" is depicted in the figure. The start and end amino acid residue numbers of each α-helix are marked. The percentage (correct to integer number) of residues forming α-helix is____.

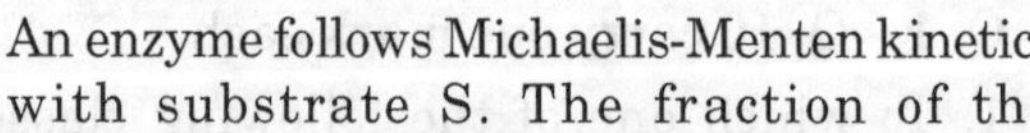

18. An enzyme follows Michaelis-Menten kinetics with substrate S. The fraction of the maximum velocity (V_{max}) will be observed with the substrate concentration [S] = $4K_m$ is ____ (correct to one decimal place). (K_m is Michaelis-Menten constant)

19. The mass spectrum of benzoic acid will generate the fragment as a base peak (100% relative abundance) of m/z (mass to charge ratio) at ____ (correct to integer number).

20. The standard free energy ($\Delta G'$) values of reactions catalyzed by citrate lyase and citrate synthetase are –670 and –8192 cal/mol, respectively.

$$\text{Citrate} \xrightleftharpoons{\text{Citrate lyase}} \text{Acetate} + \text{Oxaloacetate}$$

$\Delta G_1' = -670$ cal/mole

$$\text{Acetyl-CoA} + \text{Oxaloacetate} + H_2O \xrightleftharpoons{\text{Citrate synthetase}} \text{Citrate} + \text{CoA}$$

$\Delta G_2' = -8192$ cal/mole

The standard free energy (in cal/mol) of acetyl-CoA hydrolysis is ___ (correct to integer number).

BOTANY

Q. 1 – Q. 10 carry one mark each.

1. Which of the following genera produces dimorphic seeds that help to broaden the time of germination in a variable habitat?
   (*a*) Xanthium
   (*b*) Pisum
   (*c*) Magnifera
   (*d*) Linum

2. The genes for microRNA (miRNA) in plants are usually transcribed by
   (*a*) RNA polymerase I
   (*b*) RNA polymerase II
   (*c*) RNA polymerase III
   (*d*) RNA polymerase IV

3. Which of the statements is TRUE for transposable elements Ac and Ds?
   (*a*) Both Ac and Ds are autonomous because they encode their own transposase
   (*b*) Both Ac and Ds are non-autonomous because they do not encode their own transposase
   (*c*) Only Ac is autonomous because it encodes its own transposase
   (*d*) Only Ds is autonomous because it encodes its own transposase

4. Identify the CORRECT statement.
   (*a*) Receptor-like kinases play role in gametophytic self-incompatibility in Brassicaceae
   (*b*) Receptor-like kinases play role in sporophytic self-incompatibility in Solanaceae
   (*c*) Ribonucleases play role in sporophytic self-incompatibility in Brassicaceae
   (*d*) Ribonucleases play role in gametophytic self-incompatibility in Solanaceae

5. Which of the following statements is TRUE for an ecotone?
   (*a*) An ecotone is the synonym of an ecosystem
   (*b*) An ecotone is an interface zone of two or more ecosystems
   (*c*) An ecotone is a special feature of land biomes
   (*d*) An ecotone is exclusively characterized by decreased biodiversity

6. Acid rain with a pH of 4.0 is more acidic than the rain with a pH of 6.0 by
   (*a*) 2 times (*b*) 10 times
   (*c*) 100 times (*d*) 1000 times

7. Which of the following plants produces Ylang-ylang oil?
   (*a*) Cananga odorata
   (*b*) Carcum copticum
   (*c*) Pandanus odoratissimus
   (*d*) Pimenta racemosa

8. Identify the INCORRECT statement in connection with polar transport of auxin.
   (*a*) The putative influx carrier AUX1 is a cytosolic protein
   (*b*) Polar auxin transport in root tends to be both acropetal and basipetal in direction
   (*c*) Naphthylphthalamic acid (NPA) is an inhibitor of polar auxin transport
   (*d*) AUX1 and PIN1 proteins are located in the opposite ends of a cell for polar transport

9. Which of the following stains is used to visualize callose under the microscope?
   (*a*) Alcian blue (*b*) Aniline blue
   (*c*) Toluidine blue (*d*) Thymol blue

10. The coding sequence of a gene XLR18 has the single ORF of 783 bp. The approximate molecular weight of the XLR18 protein in kDa is ______.

Q. 11 – Q. 20 carry two marks each.

11. Statements given below are either TRUE (T) or FALSE (F). Select the CORRECT combination.

P. Mitosis occurs exclusively in diploid mother cell

Q. Mitosis occurs both in diploid and haploid mother cells

R. Meiosis occurs exclusively in diploid mother cell

S. Meiosis occurs both in diploid and haploid mother cells

(*a*) P-T, Q-F, R-T, S-F (*b*) P-F, Q-T, R-F, S-T

(*c*) P-T, Q-F, R-F, S-T (*d*) P-F, Q-T, R-T, S-F

12. You are asked to design a genetic construct for high-level expression of a gene encoding the therapeutic protein 18 (TP18) via plastid transformation. Select the CORRECT set of genetic elements for this construct.

(*a*) Actin1 promoter → TP18 coding sequence → Actin1 transcription terminator

(*b*) Ubiquitin1 promoter → TP18 coding sequence → Ubiquitin1 transcription terminator

(*c*) rbcS promoter → TP18 coding sequence → rbcS transcription terminator

(*d*) rbcL promoter → TP18 coding sequence → rbcL transcription terminator

13. Select the CORRECT combination of the following statements.

P. The cyclic electron transport chain involving PSI results in net production of both ATP and NADPH

Q. The cyclic electron transport chain involving PSI results in net production of ATP

R. Rubisco enzyme usually converts RuBP and CO_2 into 2-phosphoglycolate and 3-phosphoglycerate

S. Rubisco enzyme usually converts RuBP and O_2 into 2-phosphoglycolate and 3-phosphoglycerate

(*a*) P, Q

(*b*) R, S

(*c*) Q, S

(*d*) P, R

14. Match the fruit characters with their families and representative plant species.

Fruit character	Family	Plant species
P. Syconus	1. Moraceae	i. Canavalia ensiformis
Q. Capsule, opening by apical pores or valves	2. Fabaceae	ii. Artabotrys odoratissimus
R. Legume	3. Papaveraceae	iii. Ficus religiosa
S. An etaerio of drupe	4. Annonaceae	iv. Papaver somniferum
		v. Pistacia vera
		vi. Citrus aurantium

(*a*) P-2-iv, Q-3-ii, R-1-vi, S-4-v

(*b*) P-1-iii, Q-3-iv, R-2-i, S-4-ii

(*c*) P-3-i, Q-2-iii, R-4-ii, S-1-vi

(*d*) P-4-v, Q-1-ii, R-2-v, S-3-i

15. Select the CORRECT combination by matching the disease, affected plant and the causal organism.

Disease	Affected Plant	Causal organism
P. Black rot	1. Corn	i. Fusarium oxysporum f.sp. cubense
Q. Loose smut	2. Banana	ii. Acidovorax avenae subsp. citrulli
R. Panama wilt	3. Watermelon	iii. Botrysophaeria obtusa
S. Bacterial fruit blotch	4. Apple	iv. Ustilago maydis
		v. Plasmopara viticola
		vi. Venturia inaequalis

(*a*) P-2-v, Q-1-iv, R-3-iii, S-4-vi

(*b*) P-2-ii, Q-1-i, R-4-iii, S-3-i

(*c*) P-4-iii, Q-1-iv, R-2-i, S-3-ii

(*d*) P-4-vi, Q-1-iii, R-3-ii, S-2-v

16. Select the CORRECT combination by matching Group-I with Group-II.

Group-I	Group-II
P. Photorespiration	1. Glutamate → 2-Oxglutarate
Q. Respiration	2. Acetyl-CoA → Malonyl-CoA
R. Amino acid degradation	3. 2-Oxglutarate → Succinyl-CoA
S. Fatty acid synthesis	4. Glycine → Serine

(*a*) P-1, Q-2, R-3, S-4 (*b*) P-2, Q-1, R-4, S-1

(*c*) P-3, Q-4, R-2, S-3 (*d*) P-4, Q-3, R-1, S-2

17. Match the plant alkaloids with their uses and source species.

Alkaloid	Use	Source species
P. Codeine	1. Stimulant	i. Hyoscyamus niger
Q. Caffeine	2. Analgesic	ii. Catharanthus roseus
R. Scopolamine	3. Antineoplastic	iii. Cola nitida
S. Vinblastine	4. Anticholinergic	iv. Papaver somniferum
		v. Coptis japonica
		vi. Senecio jacobaea

(*a*) P-2-iv, Q-1-iii, R-4-i, S-3-ii
(*b*) P-4-iii, Q-2-v, R-1-vi, S-3-i
(*c*) P-2-v, Q-1-vi, R-3-iv, S-4-ii
(*d*) P-3-ii, Q-4-iii, R-1-iv, S-2-i

18. Identify the CORRECT combination of statements with respect to chemical defense in plants.

P. Pisatin, a phytoalexin produced by *Ricinus communis* is a constitutive defense compound

Q. *Phaseolus vulgaris* produces Phaseolus agglutinin I, which is toxic to the cowpea weevil

R. A single step non-enzymatic hydrolysis of cyanogenic glycoside releases the toxic hydrocyanic acid (HCN) to protect plant against herbivores and pathogens

S. Avenacin, a triterpenoid saponin from oat prevents infection by *Gaeumannomyces graminis*, a major pathogen of cereal roots

(*a*) P, Q (*b*) Q, S
(*c*) R, S (*d*) P, S

19. In garden pea, dwarf plants with terminal flowers are recessive to tall plants with axial flowers. A true-breeding tall plant with axial flowers was crossed with a true-breeding dwarf plant with terminal flowers. The resulting F_1 plants were testcrossed, and the following progeny were obtained:

Tall plants with axial flowers = 320
Dwarf plants with terminal flowers = 318
Tall plants with terminal flowers = 79
Dwarf plants with axial flowers = 83

The map distance between the genes for plant height and flower position is______cM.

20. Two true-breeding snapdragon (*Antirrhinum majus*) plants, one with red flowers and another with white flowers were crossed. The F_1 plants were all with pink flowers. When the F_1 plants were selfed, they produced three kinds of F_2 plants with red, pink and white flowers in a 1 : 2 : 1 ratio. The probability that out of the five plants picked up randomly, two would be with pink flowers, two with white flowers and one with red flowers is _____%.

MICROBIOLOGY

Q. 1 – Q. 10 carry one mark each.

1. David Baltimore's classification of viruses is based on differences in

(*a*) host cell receptors used by viruses
(*b*) the pathways required to synthesize virus mRNA
(*c*) the modes of transmission of viruses
(*d*) the envelope proteins on the surface of viruses

2. Which of the following immune system components can function as an opsonin?

(*a*) Antibodies (*b*) T-cell receptors
(*c*) Histamines (*d*) Interferons

3. The oral polio vaccine (OPV) consists of

(*a*) live attenuated virus
(*b*) killed virus
(*c*) viral toxin
(*d*) viral capsid subunit

4. Which of the following eukaryotic cellular components carries out intracellular degradation during autophagy?

(*a*) Nucleus
(*b*) Golgi bodies
(*c*) Ribosomes
(*d*) Lysosomes

5. Analysis of DNA sequences suggest that eukaryotic mitochondrial genomes primarily originated from

(*a*) fungi (*b*) protozoa
(*c*) algae (*d*) bacteria

6. Binomial nomenclature has NOT yet been adopted for

(*a*) bacteria (*b*) fungi
(*c*) viruses (*d*) protozoa

7. Which of the following is NOT an accepted method for sterilization?
(*a*) Autoclaving (*b*) X-rays
(*c*) Gamma rays (*d*) UV rays

8. The primary product of nitrogen fixation is
(*a*) N_2 (*b*) NH_4^+
(*c*) NH_2^- (*d*) NO_3

9. In humans, the key stages in the life cycle of malarial parasites occur in
(*a*) red blood cells and the liver
(*b*) red blood cells and platelets
(*c*) red blood cells and the pancreas
(*d*) red blood cells and the gut

10. You have a 50 mg/mL stock solution of arginine. To prepare 1 liter of growth medium for an arginine auxotroph that requires 70 g/mL of arginine, the volume of this stock solution that should be added is _____ mL (up to 1 decimal point).

Q. 11 – Q. 20 carry two marks each.

11. Accumulating evidence suggest that Domain Archaea is more closely related to Domain Eukarya than to Domain Bacteria. Which of the following properties are shared between eukaryotes and archaea?
(i) Protein biogenesis
(ii) Presence of sterol containing membranes
(iii) Ribosomal subunit structures
(iv) Adaptation to extreme environmental conditions
(v) Fatty acids with ester linkages in the cell membrane
(*a*) (ii), (iii) and (v) (*b*) (i), (ii), (iv), and (v)
(*c*) (i) and (iii) (*d*) (iii) and (iv)

12. Match the antimicrobial agents in group I with their category/mode of action in group II.

Group I		Group II
(i) Fluoroquinolones	(p)	beta lactam antimicrobial
(ii) Amphotericin B	(q)	inhibition of protein synthesis
(iii) Tetracycline	(r)	inhibition of nucleic acid synthesis
(iv) Amoxicillin	(s)	antifungal agent

(*a*) (i)-(q), (ii)-(s), (iii)-(r), (iv)-(p)
(*b*) (i)-(s), (ii)-(r), (iii)-(p), (iv)-(q)
(*c*) (i)-(r), (ii)-(s), (iii)-(q), (iv)-(p)
(*d*) (i)-(s), (ii)-(r), (iii)-(q), (iv)-(p)

13. Match the microorganisms to their predominant modes of transmission.

Microorganism	Mode of Transmission
(i) Bordetella pertussis	(p) Vector-borne
(ii) Dengue virus	(q) Blood-borne
(iii) Entamoeba histolytica	(r) Droplet infection
(iv) Hepatitis B virus	(s) Contaminated food

(*a*) (i)-(r), (ii)-(p), (iii)-(s), (iv)-(q)
(*b*) (i)-(s), (ii)-(q), (iii)-(p), (iv)-(r)
(*c*) (i)-(q), (ii)-(p), (iii)-(s), (iv)-(r)
(*d*) (i)-(s), (ii)-(r), (iii)-(p), (iv)-(q)

14. Match the precursors/intermediates with the corresponding metabolic pathways.

Precursor /Intermediates	Metabolic pathway
(i) Inosine monophosphate	(p) L-methionine biosynthesis
(ii) Ornithine	(q) L-tryptophan biosynthesis
(iii) Chorismate	(r) Purine biosynthesis
(iv) Homocysteine	(s) L-arginine biosynthesis

(*a*) (i)-(q), (ii)-(r), (iii)-(s), (iv)-(p)
(*b*) (i)-(p), (ii)-(r), (iii)-(s), (iv)-(q)
(*c*) (i)-(r), (ii)-(p), (iii)-(s), (iv)-(q)
(*d*) (i)-(r), (ii)-(s), (iii)-(q), (iv)-(p)

15. Match the scientists to their area of major contribution

Scientists	Area of major contribution
(i) Antonie van Leeuwenhoek	(p) Taxonomy
(ii) Carl Linnaeus	(q) Antimicrobial agents
(iii) Sir Alexander Fleming	(r) Vaccination
(iv) Louis Pasteur	(s) Microscopy

(*a*) (i)-(s), (ii)-(q), (iii)-(p), (iv)-(r)
(*b*) (i)-(s), (ii)-(p), (iii)-(q), (iv)-(r)
(*c*) (i)-(p), (ii)-(s), (iii)-(r), (iv)-(q)
(*d*) (i)-(q), (ii)-(p), (iii)-(r), (iv)-(s)

16. Which of the following combinations would improve the resolution of a microscope?
(i) Increasing the half aperture angle of the objective lens
(ii) Decreasing the wavelength of the illumination source
(iii) Decreasing the numerical aperture of the objective lens
(iv) Decreasing the refractive index of immersion medium
(*a*) (i) and (ii) (*b*) (ii) and (iii)
(*c*) (ii) and (iv) (*d*) (i) and (iii)

17. Active transport involves the movement of a biomolecule against a concentration gradient across the cell membrane using metabolic energy. If the extracellular concentration of a biomolecule is 0.005M and its intracellular concentration is 0.5M, the least amount of energy that the cell would need to spend to transport this biomolecule from the outside to the inside of the cell is ________ kcal/mol (up to 2 decimal points).

(Temperature T = 298K and universal gas constant R = 1.98 cal/mol.K)

18. A continuous cell culture being carried out in a stirred tank reactor is described in terms of its cell mass concentration X and substrate concentration S. The concentration of the substrate in the sterile feed stream is $S_F = 10$ g/L and yield coefficient $Y_{x/s} = 0.5$. The flow rates of the feed stream and the exit stream are equal (F = 5 mL/min) and constant. If the specific growth rate (h^{-1}) $\mu = \dfrac{0.3\ S}{(1+S)}$, the steady state concentration of S is ____ g/L (up to 1 decimal point).

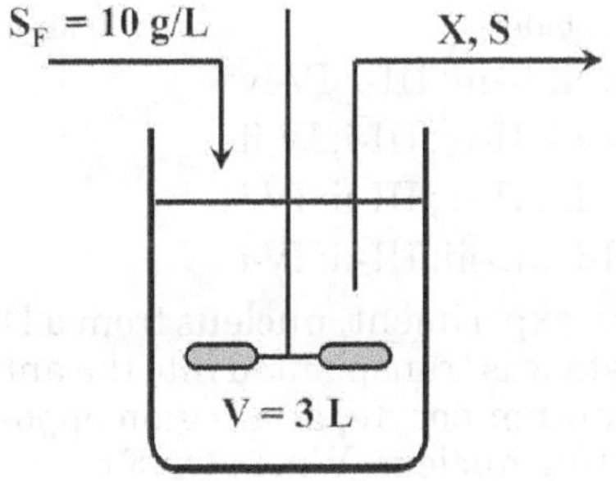

19. The initial concentration of cells (N_0) growing unrestricted in a culture is 1.0×10^6 cells/mL. If the specific growth rate (μ) of the cells is 0.1 h^{-1}, the time required for the cell concentration to become 1.0×10^8 cells/mL is ________ hours (up to 2 decimal points).

20. The following stoichiometric equation represents the conversion of glucose to lactic acid in a cell:

Glucose + 2Pi + 2ADP → 2Lactate + 2ATP + $2H_2O$ If the free energy of conversion of glucose to lactic acid only is $\Delta G° = -47000$ cal/mol, the efficiency of energy transfer is ______ % (up to 1 decimal point). ($\Delta G°$ for ATP hydrolysis is –7.3 kcal/mol)

ZOOLOGY

Q. 1 – Q. 10 carry one mark each.

1. Animals belonging to phylum Echinodermata are closer to chordates than other invertebrate phyla. Which ONE of the following reasons can account for this relatedness?
   (*a*) Highly evolved nervous system
   (*b*) Radially symmetric body plan
   (*c*) Deuterostomic development
   (*d*) Well-developed muscles

2. A zoologist recovered some tissue from preserved skin of a woolly mammoth. Further genetic analysis requires DNA isolation and increasing its amount. Which ONE of the following techniques would be most useful for increasing the amount of DNA?
   (*a*) RFLP analysis
   (*b*) Polymerase chain reaction (PCR)
   (*c*) Electroporation
   (*d*) Chromatography

3. In a chemical reaction where the substrate and product are in equilibrium in solution, what will occur if an enzyme is added?
   (*a*) The equilibrium of the reaction will not change.
   (*b*) There will be a decrease in product formed.
   (*c*) Additional substrate will be formed.
   (*d*) The free energy of the system will change

4. Tay-Sachs disease is a human genetic disorder that is associated with defects in which ONE of the following cellular organelles?
   (*a*) Endoplasmic reticulum
   (*b*) Mitochondria
   (*c*) Golgi apparatus
   (*d*) Lysosome

5. Increase in the existent population of grey peppered moth, *Biston betularia* during industrial revolution in Britain is an example of which ONE of the following evolutionary processes?
   (*a*) Neutral selection
   (*b*) Disruptive selection
   (*c*) Directional selection
   (*d*) Stabilizing selection

6. Which ONE of the following is NOT a characteristic of a cancer cell?
(*a*) Increase in cell motility
(*b*) Loss of contact inhibition
(*c*) Decrease in apoptosis
(*d*) Uncontrolled meiosis

7. Cardiac and cerebral tissues are derived from the following germ layers respectively
(*a*) Ectoderm and mesoderm
(*b*) Mesoderm and ectoderm
(*c*) Mesoderm and endoderm
(*d*) Endoderm and ectoderm

8. An animal's ability to escape from a predator by using the explored knowledge of home area is an example of
(*a*) Latent learning (*b*) Insight learning
(*c*) Mimicry (*d*) Imprinting

9. Bowman's capsules are present in which ONE of the following organs/ tissues?
(*a*) Renal cortex (*b*) Urinary bladder
(*c*) Renal medulla (*d*) Ureter

10. Which ONE of the following is the primary function of lung surfactants?
(*a*) Remove dust particles from bronchi
(*b*) Provide immunity to respiratory tract
(*c*) Prevent alveoli from collapsing by decreasing surface tension
(*d*) Aid in carbon dioxide exchange

Q. 11 – Q. 20 carry two marks each.

11. Match the disorders/diseases listed in Column I to their respective causative agents listed in Column II.

Column I	Column II
I. African tick bite fever	i. Trypanosoma gambiense
II. Yellow fever	ii. Zika virus
III. Microcephaly	iii. Rickettsia sp.
IV. Sleeping sickness	iv. Flavivirus

(*a*) I-iv, II-iii, III-ii, IV-i
(*b*) I-iii, II-iv, III-ii, IV-i
(*c*) I-iii, II-iv, III-i, IV-ii
(*d*) I-iii, II-i, III-iv, IV-ii

12. Glucose monomers are joined together by glycosidic linkages to form a cellulose polymer. During this process, changes in the free energy, total energy, and entropy respectively are represented correctly by which ONE of the following options?
(*a*) $+\Delta G$, $+\Delta H$, $+\Delta S$ (*b*) $+\Delta G$, $-\Delta H$, $-\Delta S$
(*c*) $-\Delta G$, $+\Delta H$, $+\Delta S$ (*d*) $+\Delta G$, $+\Delta H$, $-\Delta S$.

13. In *Drosophila melanogaster*, a mutation in *Ultrabithorax* which defines the third segment of the thorax or T3 leads to development of four winged flies, as the halteres develop into a second pair of wings. Which ONE of the following phenotypes in fly will result from overexpression of *Ultrabithorax* in the second thoracic segment?
(*a*) Four winged flies
(*b*) Two wings and two halteres flies
(*c*) Flies with four halteres
(*d*) Flies with two halteres

14. Which ONE of the following is TRUE in case of respiratory acidosis?
(*a*) Increased rate of ventilation is a cause of respiratory acidosis
(*b*) Blood pH more than 7
(*c*) Increased levels of carbon dioxide in blood
(*d*) Acidosis can be compensated through reduction of bicarbonate levels in plasma

15. Match the proteins / molecules listed in column I with the cellular location mentioned in the column II.

Column I	Column II
I. Galactosyl transferase	(i) Vesicles
II. Cytochrome oxidase	(ii) Cytosol
III. Clathrin	(iii) Golgi complex
IV. Tubulin	(iv) Mitochondria

(*a*) I-ii; II-iii; III-i; IV-iv
(*b*) I-iii; II-iv; III-i; IV-ii
(*c*) I-iii; II-iv; III-ii; IV-i
(*d*) I-iv; II-iii; III-ii; IV-i

16. In an experiment, nucleus from a Drosophila oocyte was transplanted into the anterior part of another oocyte, at a region opposite to the existing nucleus. Which ONE of the following phenotypes will the developing egg show?
(*a*) A ventralized egg with no dorsal appendages
(*b*) A dorsalized egg with two dorsal appendages
(*c*) A ventralized egg with two dorsal appendages
(*d*) A dorsalized egg with four dorsal appendages

17. Match the organisms listed in Column I with the features listed in Column II

Column I	Column II
I) Tapeworm	(i) Bioluminescence
II) Jellyfish	(ii) Viviparous
III) Trichinella	(iii) Lateral heart
IV) Earthworm	(iv) Microvilli on the body surface

(a) I-iii; II-i; III-iv; IV-ii
(b) I-ii; II-iv; III-i; IV-iii
(c) I-iv; II-i; III-ii; IV-iii
(d) I-iv; II-iii; III-ii; IV-i

18. Which ONE of the following statements is NOT part of the classical Darwinian theory of evolution by natural selection?
(a) A trait which is constantly used will get inherited by next generation.
(b) Phenotypic variations exist among the individuals of a population of a species
(c) Individuals that best fit into a given environment are more likely to survive
(d) Each population can randomly acquire a distinct and separate suite of variations.

19. A population of rabbits was determined to have a birth rate of 200 and mortality rate of 50 per year. If the initial population size is 4000 individuals, after 2 years of non-interfered breeding the final population size will be ________.

20. In a population which is in Hardy-Weinberg equilibrium, the frequency of occurrence of a disorder caused by recessive allele (q) is 1 in 1100. The frequency of heterozygotes in the population will be ________. (Give the answer to three decimal places).

FOOD TECHNOLOGY

Q. 1 – Q. 10 carry one mark each.

1. Which of the following is an oil soluble pigment present in fruits and vegetables?
(a) Flavonoids (b) Carotenoids
(c) Anthocyanins (d) Tannins

2. Which of the following represent the group of saturated fatty acids?
(a) Lauric, Myristic, Arachidic
(b) Palmitic, Linoleic, Linolenic
(c) Capric, Stearic & Oleic
(d) Behenic, Caprylic, Arachidonic

3. The anti-nutritional factor present in fava bean is
(a) Gossypol
(b) Curcine
(c) Vicine
(d) Cyanogen

4. Which of the following is a Gram positive bacteria?
(a) Listeria monocytogenes
(b) Proteus vulgaris
(c) Salmonella typhi
(d) Shigella dysenteriae

5. Irradiation carried out to reduce viable non-spore forming pathogenic bacteria using a dose between 3 to 10 kGy is
(a) Radurization
(b) Thermoradiation
(c) Radappertization
(d) Radicidation

6. Identify the correct statement related to the viscosity of Newtonian fluids from the following.
(a) It is not influenced by temperature
(b) It increases with shearing rate
(c) It decreases with shearing rate
(d) It is not influenced by shearing rate

7. Adult male Wistar rats were fed with a protein based diet. Total 150 g of protein was ingested per animal. If the average weight increased from 110 g to 350 g after the end of experiment, the Protein efficiency ratio of the given protein would be ______. (up to two decimal points).

8. The initial moisture content of a food on wet basis is 50.76%. Its moisture content (%) on dry basis is ______. (up to two decimal points)

9. The oxygen transmission rate through 2.54×10^{-3} cm thick low density polyethylene film with air on one side and inert gas on the other side is 3.5×10^{-6} mL cm^{-2} s^{-1}. Oxygen partial pressure difference across the film is 0.21 atm. The permeability coefficient of the film to oxygen is ______ $\times 10^{-11}$ mL (STP) cm cm^{-2} s^{-1} $(cm\ Hg)^{-1}$.

10. Ambient air at 30°C dry bulb temperature and 80% relative humidity was heated to a dry bulb temperature of 80°C in a heat exchanger by indirect heating. The amount of moisture gain (g kg^{-1} dry air) during the process would be _____.

Q. 11 – Q. 20 carry two marks each.

11. Match the commodity in Group I with the bioactive constituent in Group II

Group I	Group II
P. Ginger	1. Lutein
Q. Green tea	2. Gingerol
R. Spinach	3. Curcumin
S. Turmeric	4. Epigallocatechin gallate

(*a*) P-1, Q-2, R-3, S-4

(*b*) P-2, Q-4, R-1, S-3

(*c*) P-4, Q-1, R-3, S-2

(*d*) P-2, Q-3, R-1, S-4

12. Match the process operation in Group I with the separated constituent in Group II

Group I	Group II
P. Extraction	1. Phospholipids
Q. Degumming	2. Free fatty acids
R. Neutralization	3. Pigments
S. Bleaching	4. Crude oil

(*a*) P-3, Q-2, R-4, S-1 (*b*) P-4, Q-3, R-1, S-2

(*c*) P-4, Q-1, R-2, S-3 (*d*) P-4, Q-1, R-3, S-2

13. Match the spoilage symptom in Group I with the causative microorganism in Group II

Group I	Group II
P. Green rot of eggs	1. Micrococcus spp.
Q. Putrid swell in canned fish	2. Serretia Marcescens
R. Red bread	3. Pseudomonas fluorescens
S. Yellow discoloration of meat	4. Clostridium sporogens

(*a*) P-4, Q-3, R-2, S-1 (*b*) P-2, Q-1, R-4, S-3

(*c*) P-3, Q-4, R-2, S-1 (*d*) P-1, Q-4, R-3, S-2

14. Match the fermented product in Group I with the base material in Group II

Group I	Group II
P. Sake	1. Milk
Q. Chhurpi	2. Cabbage
R. Natto	3. Rice
S. Sauerkraut	4. Soybean

(*a*) P-3, Q-1, R-4, S-2 (*b*) P-1, Q-3, R-4, S-2

(*c*) P-4, Q-1, R-3, S-2 (*d*) P-2, Q-4, R-1, S-3

15. Match the operation in Group I with the process in Group II

Group I	Group II
P. Cleaning	1. Quality separation
Q. Grading	2. Clarification
R. Size reduction	3. Screening
S. Filtration	4. Comminution

(*a*) P-1, Q-3, R-4, S-2 (*b*) P-4, Q-1, R-3, S-2

(*c*) P-2, Q-4, R-1, S-3 (*d*) P-3, Q-1, R-4, S-2

16. Out of 7 principles of HACCP system, 4 are listed below. Arrange these principles in the order in which they are applied.

(P) Conduct a hazard analysis

(Q) Establish monitoring process

(R) Establish critical limit

(S) Establish record keeping and documentation process

(*a*) P, R, Q, S (*b*) Q, R, P, S

(*c*) P, Q, R, S (*d*) R, S, P, Q

17. Identify an example of a classical diffusional mass transfer process without involving heat, among the following.

(*a*) Drying of food grains

(*b*) Carbonation of beverages

(*c*) Distillation of alcohol

(*d*) Concentration of fruit juice

18. For an enzyme catalyzed reaction $S \rightarrow P$, the kinetic parameters are:

$[S] = 40$ M, $V_0 = 9.6$ M s^{-1} and $V_{max} = 12.0$ Ms^{-1}.

The K_m of the enzyme in M will be _______.(up to one decimal points)

19. A microbial sample taken at 10 AM contained 1×10^5 CFU/mL. The count reached to 1×10^{10} CFU/mL at 8 PM of the same day. The growth rate (h^{-1}) of the microorganism would be ______. (up to two decimal points)

20. The rate of heat transfer per unit area from a metal plate is 1000 W m^{-2}. The surface temperature of the plate is 120°C and ambient temperature is 20°C. The convective heat transfer coefficient (W m^{-2} °C^{-1}) using the Newton's law of cooling will be ______.

ANSWERS

General Aptitude (GA)

1. (*a*) 2. (*c*) 3. (*b*) 4. (*b*) 5. (*b*) 6. (*a*) 7. (*d*) 8. (*d*) 9. (*b*) 10. (*c*)

Chemistry

1. (*a*) 2. (*d*) 3. (*d*) 4. (11 to 11) 5. (4 to 4)
6. (*d*) 7. (*d*) 8. (*a*) 9. (*d*) 10. (*a*)
11. (*c*) 12. (*b*) 13. (1.39 to 1.43) 14. (7.39 to 7.54)
15. (–13.40 to – 13.36)

Biochemistry

1. (*b*) 2. (*a*) 3. (*c*) 4. (*c*) 5. (*d*)
6. (*c*) 7. (*d*) 8. (*b*) 9. (12 to 12) 10. (50 to 50)
11. (*a*) 12. (*a*) 13. (*d*) 14. (*b*) 15. (*b*)
16. (512 to 512) 17. (20 to 20) 18. (0.8 to 0.8) 19. (77 to 77)
20. (– 8862 to – 8862)

Botany

1. (*a*) 2. (*b*) 3. (*c*) 4. (*d*) 5. (*b*)
6. (*c*) 7. (*a*) 8. (*a*) 9. (*b*)
10. (28.00 to 31.00) 11. (*d*) 12. (*d*) 13. (*c*) 14. (*b*)
15. (*c*) 16. (*d*) 17. (*a*) 18. (*b*)
19. (20.25 to 20.25) 20. (11.00 to 12.00)

Microbiology

1. (*b*) 2. (*a*) 3. (*a*) 4. (*d*) 5. (*d*)
6. (*c*) 7. (*d*) 8. (*b*) 9. (*a*)
10. (1.38 to 1.42) 11. (*c*) 12. (*c*) 13. (*a*) 14. (*d*)
15. (*b*) 16. (*a*) 17. (2.60 to 2.80) 18. (0.5 to 0.5)
19. (45.50 to 46.50) 20. (30.5 to 31.5)

Zoology

1. (*c*) 2. (*b*) 3. (*a*) 4. (*d*) 5. (*c*)
6. (*d*) 7. (*b*) 8. (*a*) 9. (*a*) 10. (*c*)
11. (*b*) 12. (*d*) 13. (*c*) 14. (*c*) 15. (*b*)
16. (*d*) 17. (*c*) 18. (*a*) 19. (5270 to 5310)
20. (0.056 to 0.062)

Food Technology

1. (*b*) 2. (*a*) 3. (*c*) 4. (*a*) 5. (*d*)
6. (*d*) 7. (1.55 to 1.65) 8. (103.0 to 103.2) 9. (54 to 56) 10. (0 to 0)
11. (*b*) 12. (*c*) 13. (*c*) 14. (*a*) 15. (*d*)
16. (*a*) 17. (*b*) 18. (9.8 to 10.2) 19. (1.1 to 1.8) 20. (10 to 10)

EXPLANATIONS

GENERAL APTITUDE

3. $\frac{\text{Machine} \times \text{time}}{\text{Number of toys}} = \frac{M_1 \times t_1}{T_1} = \frac{M_2 \times t_2}{T_2}$

$\therefore \quad \frac{7 \times 7}{7} = \frac{100 \times t_2}{100}$

$\therefore \quad \boxed{t_2 = 7 \text{ min}}$

4. Let the initial length of rectangle is l and breath is b. Now if length is reduced by 10 m and breath is reduced by 5 m then it becomes square.

$\therefore \quad l - 10 = b - 5$

[$\because$ In square length = breadth]

$\therefore \quad l - b = 5$

Given, initial, Area (A) = $l \times b$

Now according to question,

$(l - 10)(b - 5) = A - 650$

$\therefore \quad lb - 10b - 5l + 50 = A - 650$

$\therefore \quad A - 10b - 5l = A - 700$

$\therefore \quad 10b + 5l = 700$

$\therefore \quad 10b + 5(b + 5) = 700$

$\therefore \quad 15b + 25 = 700$

$\therefore \quad 15b = 700 - 25$

$\therefore \quad 15b = 675$

$\Rightarrow \quad b = 45 \text{ m}$

$\therefore \quad l = 45 + 5 = 50 \text{ m}$

$\therefore$ Area of original rectangle (A) = $(45 \times 50)\text{m}^2$

$= 2250 \text{ m}^2.$

5. Let two digit number be xy.

Now sum of digit is 9

$\therefore \quad x + y = 9 \quad ....(i)$

and when '45' is subtracted from number then digit gets interchanged

$\therefore \quad 10x + y - 45 = 10y + x$

$\therefore \quad x - 5 = y$

$x - y = 5 \quad ....(ii)$

Now solving equation (*i*) and (*ii*) we get

$x = 7$ and $y = 2$

Hence the number is 72.

6. $\log|a| + \log|b| + \log|c| = 0$

It is possible only,

when $|a|$, $|b|$ and $|c|$ all are equal to 1.

$\therefore$ a, b, c may be $\pm 1, \pm 1, \pm 1$ respectively.

Now for minimum value of all three will be negative.

$\therefore$ minimum value = – 3

and maximum value of all three will be positive.

$\therefore$ maximum value = + 3

7. From option (*a*),

Let $\quad a = 1, b = 3$

$\therefore \quad a + a^2b^3 = 1 + 27$

$= 28$ (Even)

$\therefore$ Option (*a*) is wrong

From option (*b*)

Let $\quad a = 2, b = 4$

$\therefore \quad a + a^2b^3 = 2 + 4 \times 64$

$= 258$ (Even)

From option (*c*),

Let $\quad a = 2, b = 1$

From option (*d*),

for $x = 1$

$y = \big||x - 1| - 1\big|$

$= |-1| = 1$

$\therefore$ Option (*c*) is wrong.

Now from option (*b*),

for $\quad x = 1$

$y = \big||x| - 1\big| - 1$

$= |1 - 1| - 1 = -1$

$\therefore$ Option (*b*) is correct.

8. Train speed (S_T) = 54 km/h

Time = 25 sec for travelling length of train and length of platform

Man speed (S_M) = 9 km/h

Speed of train to man = 45 km/h

Time = 14 sec

So, length of train = time × speed

$= 14 \times 45 \times \frac{5}{18}$

Length of train (L_T) = $(35 \times 5 \text{ m}) = 175$ m

Length of platform (L) + length of train (L_T) = speed × time

$= 54 \times \frac{5}{18} \times 25 = 15 \times 25 = 375\text{m}$

$\therefore$ Length of platform (L) = 375 – 175 = 200 m

9. Here from graph for x = 1, y = – 1
Checking the same from options.
From option (*a*)
for $x = 1$

$$y = ||1| + 1| - 2$$
$$= 2 - 2 = 0$$

$\therefore$ Option (*a*) is wrong
From option (*c*)
for $x = 1$

$$y = ||x| + 1| - 1$$
$$= |1 + 1| - 1 = 1$$

$\therefore$ Option (*c*) is wrong.

10.

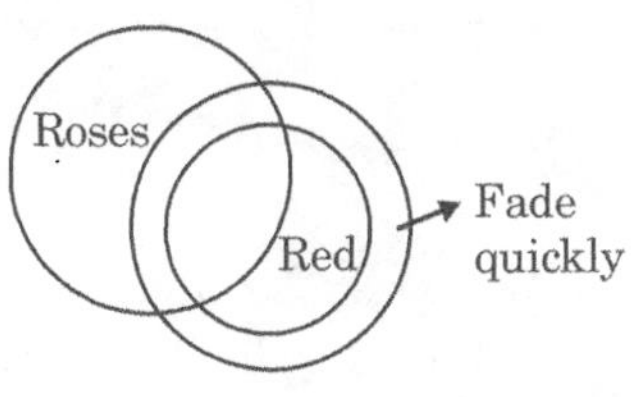

Case-I

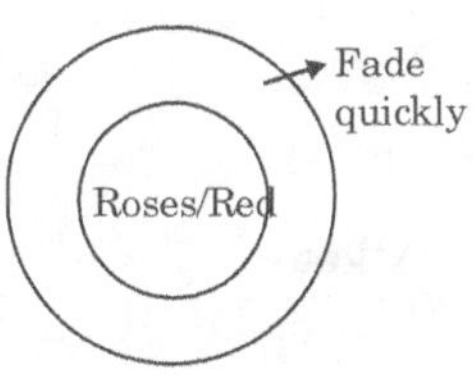

Case-II

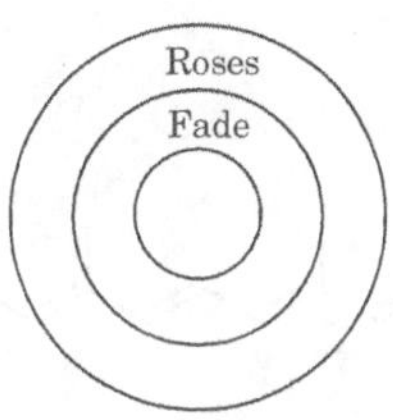

Case-III

CHEMISTRY

1. **Hess' Law** is:

If a chemical equation can be written as the sum of several other chemical equations, the enthalpy change of the first chemical equation equals to the sum of the enthalpy changes of the other chemical equations

C (s, graphite) —> C (s, diamond); $\Delta H° = +1.9$ kJ

In the common chemistry laboratory, this reaction cannot be examined directly. This is because, regardless of the low enthalpy, the reaction requires very, very high activation energy to get the reaction started. The consequence is that the enthalpy value cannot be determined directly in almost all labs.

However, Hess' Law offers a way out. If we had two (or more) reactions that could be added together, then we can add the respective enthalpies of the reactions to get what we want.

C (s, graphite) + O_2(g) —> CO_2(g) $\Delta H° = -393.5$ kJ
C (s, diamond) + O_2(g) —> CO_2(g) $\Delta H° = -395.4$ kJ

If we reverse the bottom equation, this will put the C (s, diamond) on the product side, where we need it. Also, when I add the two equations together, the oxygen and carbon dioxide will cancel out. This is, of course, what we want since those two substances are not in the final, desired equation. Here are the two equations again, with the second one reversed:

C (s, graphite) + O_2(g) —> CO_2(g); $\Delta H° = -393.5$ kJ
CO_2(g) —> C (s, diamond) + O_2(g); $\Delta H° = +395.4$ kJ
Or CO_2(g) + C (s, graphite) + O_2(g) —> CO_2(g) + C (s, diamond) + O_2(g); $\Delta H° = (-393.5\text{ kJ}) + (+395.4\text{ kJ})$
C (s, graphite) —> C (s, diamond; $\Delta H° =$ **+1.9 kJ.**

2. There are multiple orbitals within an atom. Each has its own specific energy level and properties. Because each orbital is different, they are assigned specific quantum numbers: 1s, 2s, 2p 3s, 3p,4s, 3d, 4p, 5s, 4d, 5p, 6s, 4f, 5d, 6p, 7s, 5f, 6d, 7p. The numbers, (n = 1,2,3, etc.) are called *principal quantum numbers* and can only be positive numbers. The letters (*s,p,d,f*) represent the *orbital angular momentum quantum number* (*l*) and the orbital angular momentum quantum number may be 0 or a positive number, but can never be greater than (n – 1). Each letter is paired with a specific *l* value:

s : subshell = 0
p : subshell = 1
d : subshell = 2
f : subshell = 3

An orbital is also described by its *magnetic quantum number* (m_l). The magnetic quantum number can range from – *l* to + *l*. This number indicates how many orbitals there are and thus how many electrons can reside in each atom.

For 4s orbital, or more specifically S subshell: l = 0, $m_l = 0$

3. **Xe (At. No. 54)** having three lone pairs and two bonds with each F, and alsototal steric number of 5. This also means that there are five orbitals present. The only possible **hybridization** with five orbitals is dsp^3 **hybridization** (1d + 1s + 3p = 5 dsp^3).
4. Two equivalents of P reacts with Q to form R(?)

P = 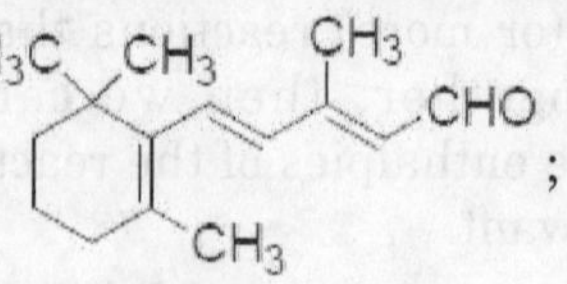 ; Q = 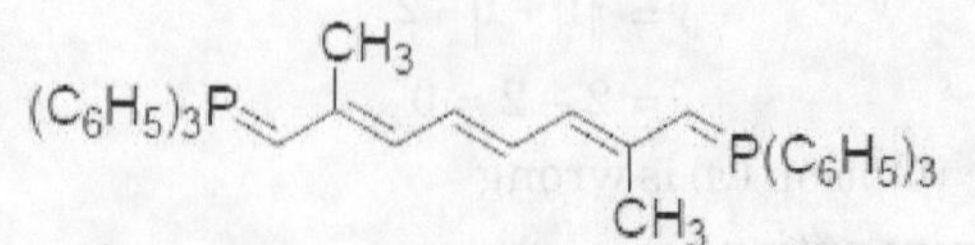

Organophosphorus ylides react with aldehydes or ketones to give substituted alkenes in a transformation called the **Wittig reaction**

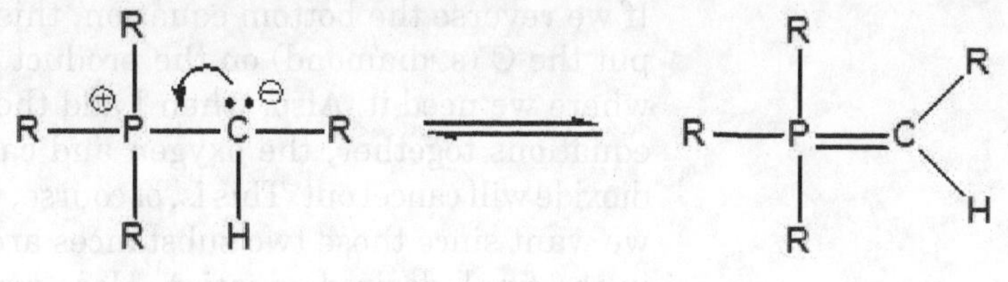

An Ylide

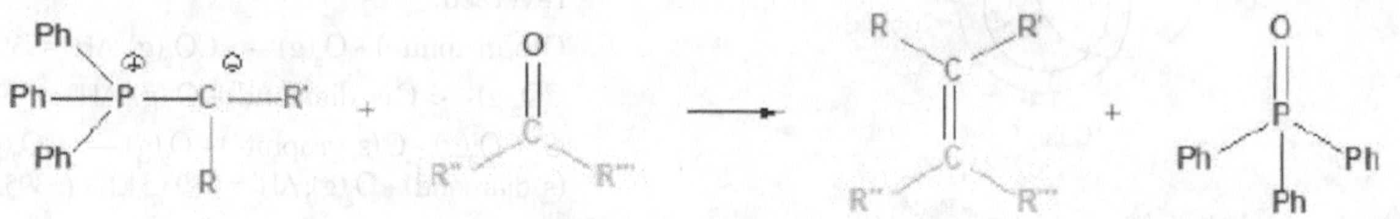

Ylide **Aldehyde or Ketone** **Alkene** **Triphenyl-phosphine oxide**

Similarly,

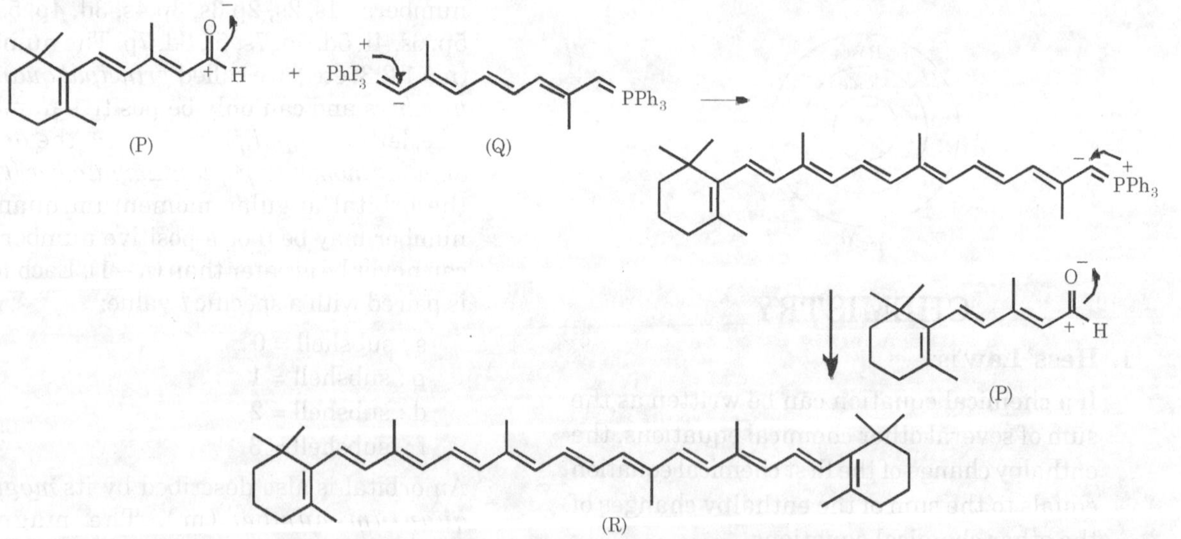

Therefore, number of double bonds present in the major product **R** is =11

5. There are 2 chiral centres (marked as bold carbon) in the given structural formula: CH_3**C**H(OH)**C**H=CHCH$_2$CH$_3$; As we know that the possible stereoisomers= 2^n; where n= no. of chiral centres. Since there are 2 chiral centres, therefore the possible stereoisomers = 2^2 = 4

6. Among B-H, C-H, N-H and Si-H bonds in BH_3, CH_4, NH_3 and SiH_4, respectively, the polarity of the bond which is shown **INCORRECTLY** is $Si^{\delta-}$—$H^{\delta+}$.

   Because of the electronegativity of **hydrogen** is greater than the **silicon**. So that the**Si–H bond polarity of** SiH_4 is the opposite of the C–**H bonds** of methane.

7. **Bond angle** is directly proportional to electronegativity of central atom. As electronegativity of O is **more than** S so **bond angle** of $\mathbf{H_2O}$ **more than** $\mathbf{H_2S}$. Due to **more** EN of oxygen, **bond** pair comes closer, which create **more** repulsion between **bond** pair.

   In $NiCl_4^{2-}$, there is Ni^{2+} ion, However, in presence of weak field Cl^- ligands, **NO** pairing of d-electrons occurs. Therefore, Ni^{2+} undergoes sp^3 hybridization to make bonds with Cl^- ligands in tetrahedral geometry. As there are unpaired electrons in the d-orbitals, $\mathbf{NiCl_4^{2-}}$ is **paramagnetic.**

   In a pyridine ring, for example, the nitrogen lone pair occupies an sp^2-hybrid orbital, and is *not* part of the aromatic sextet - it is essentially an imine nitrogen. Its electron pair is available for forming a bond to a proton, and thus the pyridine nitrogen atom is somewhat basic. So thatethylamines**are stronger bases than pyridine.**

8. **Spin Selection Rule:** The overall spin S of a complex must not change during an electronic transition, hence, $\Delta S = 0$.

   To be allowed, a transition must involve no change in spin state. This is because electromagnetic radiation usually cannot change the relative orientation of an electron spin.

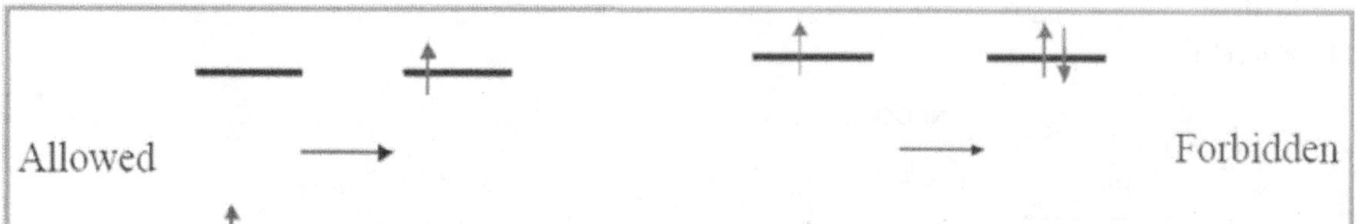

   $[Mn(H_2O)_6]^{2+}$ has a d^5 $[Mn^{+2}]$configuration [At no. Mn =25, d^7 configuration] and it is a high-spin complex. Electronic transitions are not only Laporte-forbidden, but also spin-forbidden. The dilute solutions of Mn^{2+} complexes are therefore colorles

9. Reaction is given as:

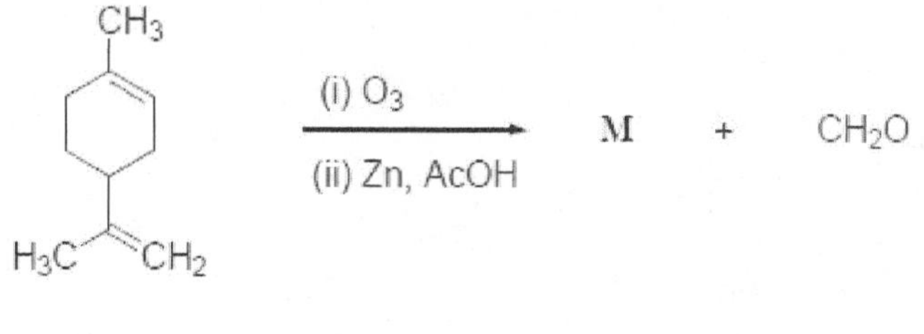

   The major product **M** in the above reactionwillbe :

(D) 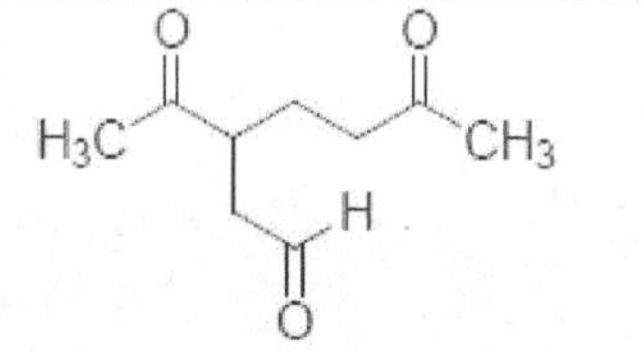

10. Hofmann elimination of amines to alkenes

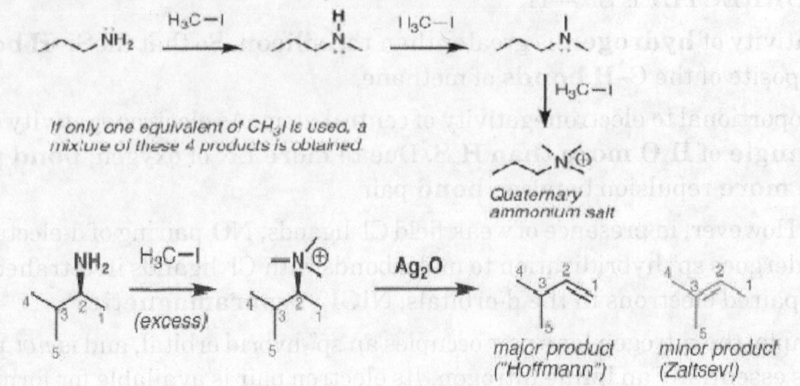

Therefore

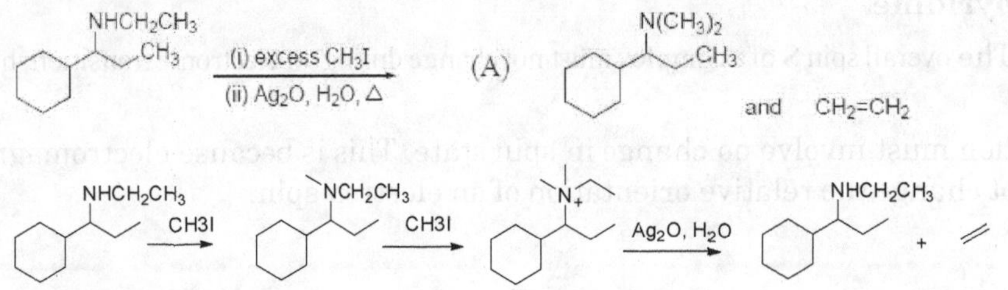

11. Fig (C):

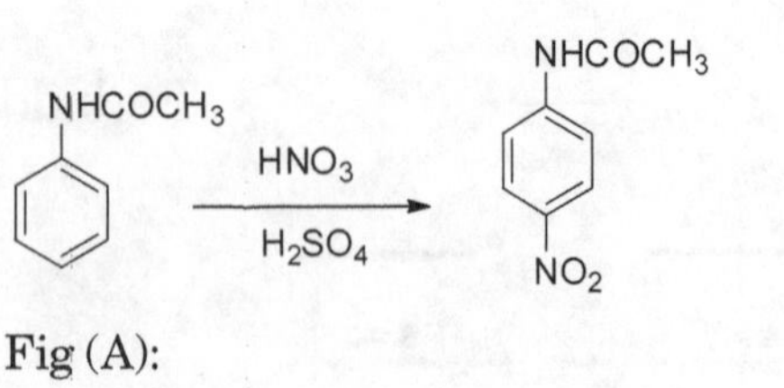

Fig (A):

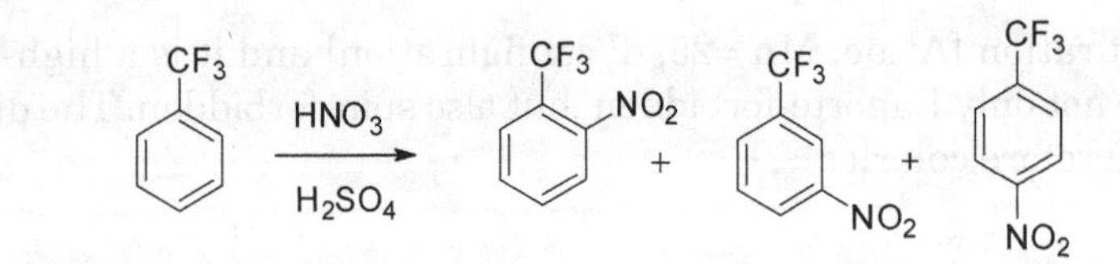

(trifluoromethyl)benzene 6% 91% 3%

Fig (B):

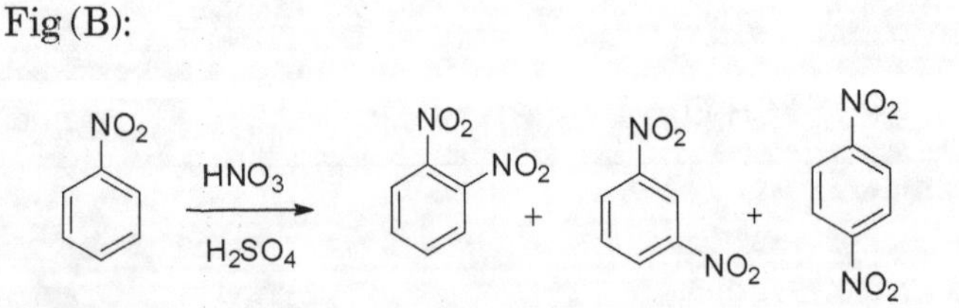

nitrobenzene 6% 92% 2%

Fig (D):

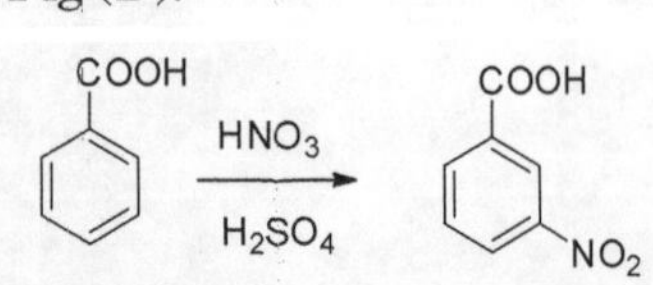

benzoic acid

Only acetanilide (Fig C) forms *p*-nitrroacetan-ilidehowever rest all other compounds (Fig A, B, &D) give the *meta*-isomer as the major product.

13. Given : Solubility product (Ksp) of $Mg(OH)_2$ at 25 °C = 5.6×10^{-11}. Its solubility in water is $S \times 10^{-2}$ g/L, where the value of S is = ?

As we know,

$$Mg(OH)^2 \text{ (s, satd. solution)} \rightleftharpoons Mg^{+2} \text{(aq.)} + 2OH^- \text{(aq.)}$$

Let the solubility of $Mg(OH)_2$ be A mol /l;

So the concentration of Mg^{+2} = Amol/l

But as per equation for each Mg^{+2} ions, two OH- ions are produced,

Hence conc. of OH^- ions = 2 Amol /l

But $K_{sp} = [Mg^{+2}][OH^-]^2$

Solubility product Ksp = Concentration of $(Mg^{+2}) \times [\text{Concentration of } (OH^-)]^2$

Then, $K_{sp} = A \times (2A)^2 = 4A^3$mol /l

But $K_{sp} = 5.6 \times 10^{-11}$(Given),

Therefore, $4A^3 = 5.6 \times 10^{-11}$ or $A^3 = 1.4 \times 10^{-11}$

or $A = 2.4 \times 10^{-4}$(mol/l)

As the Molecular weight of $Mg(OH)_2$

= 58.3 g mol^{-1}

Then $A = 2.4 \times 10^{-4} \times 58.3$(g/l)

But $A = S \times 10^{-2}$ g/L (Given)

Then, $S \times 10^{-2}$ g/L = $2.4 \times 10^{-4} \times 58.3$

or $S = 2.4 \times 10^{-2} \times 58.3$ (g/l) = 139×10^{-2} (g/l)

or S = 1.39 (g/l)

14. Given : Activation energy difference at 25°C i.e., $E_a1 - E_a2 = 5.0$ kJ mol^{-1} and $A_1 = A_2$.

As we know Arrhenius equation i.e.

$K = Ae^{-Ea/RT}$

Therefore, $K_1/K_2 = (A_1e^{-Ea1/RT})/(A_2e^{-Ea2/RT})$;

or $K_1/K_2 = (A_1/A_2)\exp[Ea1 - Ea2]/RT$;

Putting the given values in above equation, we get:

$$K_1/K_2 = A_1/A_2 \exp[5.0/8.314 \times 10^{-3} \times 298]$$

or $K_1/K_2 = \exp[2] = e^2$

But the value of e = approximately 2.718

or $e^2 = 7.389$,

Therefore; The ratio of rate constants (K_1/K_2) = 7.389

15. An **isothermal process** is a change of a system, in which the temperature remains constant: $\Delta T = 0$.

Isothermal processes are especially convenient for calculating changes in entropy. The formula for the entropy change, ΔS, is simply as:

ΔS = Qrev/T, where Qrev is heat transferred reversibly to the system and T is absolute temperature.This formula is valid only for a hypothetical reversible process; that is, a process in which equilibrium is maintained at all times.

If the surroundings are at a constant temperature, T, so that $\Delta S_{sur} = -Q/T$; the minus sign is used since the heat transferred to the surroundings is equal in magnitude and opposite in sign to the heat, Q, transferred to the system. In the reversible case, the change in entropy of the surroundings is equal and opposite to the change in the system, so the change in entropy of the universe is zero.

For the reversible process entropy change:

$\Delta S = -Qrev/T = -nR\ln(V_f/V_i) = 1 \times 8.314 \ln(10/2)$;

or $\Delta S = -8.314 \times 2.303 \times 0.0698 = -13.36$

BIOCHEMISTRY

1. Chymotrypsin is a **protease** enzyme that cleaves on the C-terminal phenylalanine (F), tryptophan (W) and tyrosine (Y) on peptide chains. Now A **protease** is an **enzyme** that performs proteolysis; protein catabolism by hydrolysis of peptide bonds. **Hydrolases** are hydrolytic **enzymes**, biochemical catalysts that use water to cleave chemical bonds, usually dividing a large molecule into two smaller molecules. Examples of common **hydrolases** include esterases, **proteases**, glycosidases, nucleosidases and lipases.

Oxidoreductase is an enzyme that catalyses the transfer of electrons from one molecule, the reductant, also called the electron donor, to another, the oxidant, also called the electron acceptor.

A **transferase** is any one of a class of enzymes that enact the transfer of specific functional groups (e.g. a methyl group) from one molecule (called the donor) to another (called the acceptor).

Isomerases are a general class of enzymes that convert a molecule from one isomer to another. **Isomerases** facilitate intramolecular rearrangements in which bonds are broken and formed.

2. 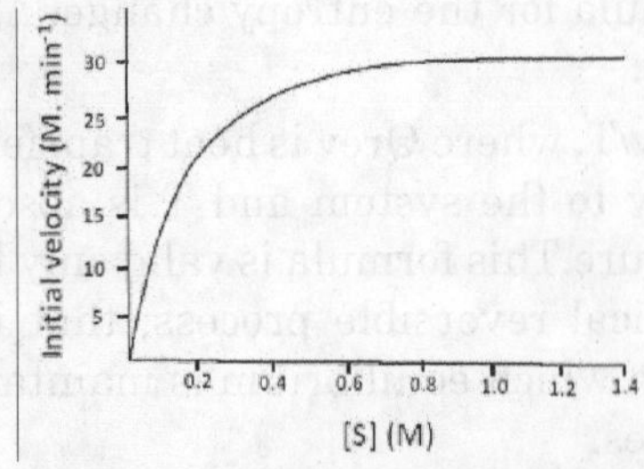

A plot of the reaction velocity (V_0) as a function of the substrate concentration [S] for an enzyme that obeys Michaelis-Menten kinetics shows that the maximal velocity (V_{max}) is approached asymptotically. The extent of product formation is determined as a function of time for a series of substrate concentrations. As expected, in each case, the amount of product formed increases with time, although eventually a time is reached when there is *no net change* in the concentration of S or P. The enzyme is still actively converting substrate into product and visa-versa but the reaction equilibrium has been attained.

Order of reaction is zero, when concentration increases from 0.8 to 1.4, as reaction rate is independent of concentration change i.e.reaction rate being constant.

3. Glucose can exist as a variety of different isomers. It can be linear or cyclic. Of the cyclic forms, it can be a 5 membered ring or a 6 membered ring. Each of the 5 and 6 membered rings can exist as 2 different stereoisomers. Finally, for the 5 and 6 membered rings, there are a variety of different conformations it can potentially exist in. In spite of all of the potential isomers it can exist as, under physiological pH it almost exclusively exists as **beta-glucopyranose** (see figure below) in the **chair conformation** with all of the large groups equatorial.

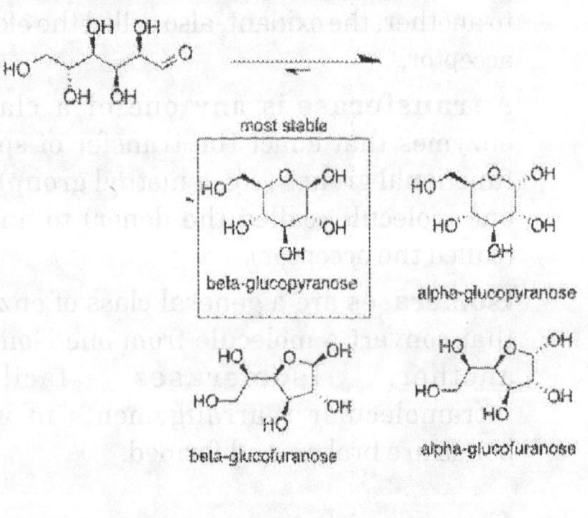

In nutshell, **beta-glucopyranose is most stable** conformation as

1. Its cyclic rather than linear, Enthalpically, two carbon oxygen single bonds are energetically more favourable than a carbon oxygen double bond
2. In a five membered ring, the bond angles are less than 109.5 degrees, which causes torsional strain. In the 6 membered ring,all of the atoms in the ring can form 109.5 degree bond angles so there isn't any torsional strain
3. The beta stereoisomer formed over the alpha stereoisomer. Alpha glucopyranose has 1,3 diaxial strain between a hydrogen and a hydroxyl group.The beta-glucopyranose isomer, one can see that the only groups that are axial are hydrogens, so 1,3diaxial strain is minimized.

4. Cooperativity can be seen in both enzymes and receptors, and describes the trends that occur when these structures contain multiple binding sites. Cooperativity describes the changes that occur when a binding site of one of these structures is activated or deactivated affecting the other binding sites in the same molecule.The activity of an enzyme can be graphed against the concentration of the substrate. For an enzyme that shows a cooperative behaviour, the relation between the two shows a sigmoidal curve instead of Michaelis and Menten behavior. The **graph** shows a **rapid increase in speed**. This reflects how **the binding on one subunit increases the chance that the other subunits will bind to a substrate**.

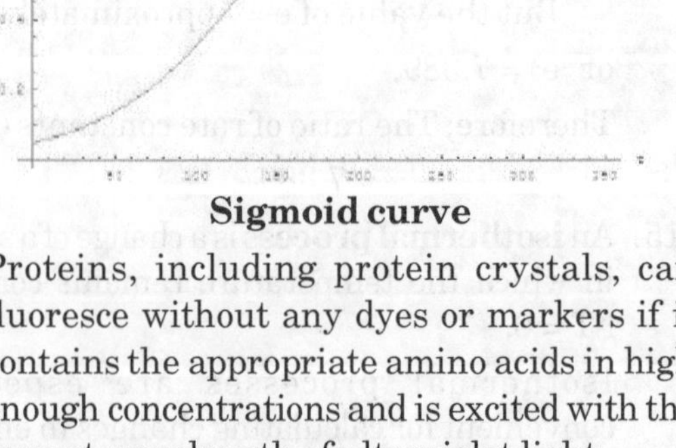

Sigmoid curve

5. Proteins, including protein crystals, can fluoresce without any dyes or markers if it contains the appropriate amino acids in high enough concentrations and is excited with the correct wavelength of ultraviolet light.

The amino acid **tryptophan** has the strongest fluorescence quantum yield of all of the amino acids found in proteins. The rest either do not fluoresce at all or only fluoresce weakly. Therefore **"Intrinsic Protein Fluorescence"** usually refers to the fluorescence emission of the tryptophan amino acid units.

Intrinsic protein fluorescence is caused by exciting the protein with 280 nm ultraviolet light and observing at approximately 350 nm. However, the actual emission wavelength can vary depending upon the polarity of the environment containing the tryptophan.

6. **Glycosylation** is a critical function of the biosynthetic-secretory pathway in the **endoplasmic reticulum** (ER) and **Golgi apparatus.** Approximately half of all proteins typically expressed in a cell undergo this modification, which entails the covalent addition of sugar moieties to specific amino acids. Most soluble and membrane-bound proteins expressed in the endoplasmic reticulum are glycosylated to some extent, including secreted proteins, surface receptors and ligands, and organelle-resident proteins. Additionally, some proteins that are trafficked from the Golgi to the cytoplasm are also glycosylated. Lipids and proteoglycans can also be glycosylated, significantly increasing the number of substrates for this type of modification.

7. Monoclonal antibodies are typically made by cell culture that involves fusing myeloma cells with mouse spleen cells immunized with the desired antigen. Rabbit B-cells can be used to form a rabbit hybridoma. Polyethylene glycol is used to fuse adjacent plasma membranes, but the success rate is low, so a selective medium in which only fused cells can grow is used. This is possible because myeloma cells have lost the ability to synthesize **hypoxanthine-guanine-phosphoribosyl transferase (HGPRT)**, an enzyme necessary for the salvage synthesis of nucleic acids. The absence of HGPRT is not a problem for these cells unless the de novo purine synthesis pathway is also disrupted. Exposing cells to aminopterin (a folic acid analogue, which inhibits dihydrofolate reductase, DHFR), makes them unable to use the de novo pathway and become fully auxotrophic for nucleic acids, thus requiring supplementation to survive

8. **F-ATPase**, also known as **F-Type ATPase** (also called ATP synthase), is an ATPase found in bacterial plasma membranes, in mitochondrial inner membranes (in oxidative phosphorylation, where it is known as Complex V), and in chloroplast thylakoid membranes. It uses a proton gradient to drive ATP synthesis by allowing the passive flux of protons across the membrane down their electrochemical gradient and using the energy released by the transport reaction to release newly formed ATP from the active site of F-ATPase.

   F-ATPase consists of two domains:

   - the F_o domain, which is integral in the membrane
   - the F_1, which is peripheral (on the side of the membrane that the protons are moving into).

   F_o-F_1 particles are mainly formed of polypeptides. As the protons bind to the subunits of the F_o domains, they cause parts of it to rotate. This rotation is propagated by a 'camshaft' to the F_1 domain. ADP and Pi (inorganic phosphate) bind spontaneously to the three β subunits of the F_1 domain, so that every time it goes through a 120° rotation ATP is released (rotational catalysis).

9. The breakdown of the simple sugar, glucose, in glycolysis provides the first 6-carbon molecule required for the pentose phosphate pathway. During the first step of glycolysis, glucose is transformed by the addition of a phosphate group, generating glucose-6-phosphate, another 6-carbon molecule. The pentose phosphate pathway can use any available molecules of glucose-6-phosphate, whether they are produced by glycolysis or other methods.

   In this case, glucose 6-phosphate is completely oxidized to CO_2. Three groups of reactions are active in this situation. First, the oxidative phase of the pentose phosphate pathway forms two molecules of NADPH and one molecule of ribose 5-phosphate. Then, ribose 5-phosphate is converted into fructose 6-phosphate and glyceraldehyde 3-phosphate by transketolase and transaldolase. Finally, glucose 6-phosphate is resynthesized from fructose 6-phosphate and glyceraldehyde 3-phosphate by the gluconeogenic pathway. The stoichiometries of these three sets of reactions are

6 Glucose 6-phosphate + 12 $NADP^+$ + 6 H_2O → 6 ribose 5-phosphate + 12 NADPH + 12 H^+ + 6CO_2

6 Ribose 5-phosphate → 4 fructose 6-phosphate + 2 glyceraldehyde 3-phosphate

4 Fructose 6-phosphate + 2 glyceraldehyde 3-phosphate + H_2O → 5 glucose 6-phosphate + P_i

The sum of the mode 3 reactions is

Glucose 6-phosphate + 12 $NADP^+$ + 7 H_2O → 6 CO_2 + 12 NADPH + 12 H^+ + P_i

Therefore, the number of NADP+ molecules required to completely oxidize one molecule of glucose to CO_2 through pentose phosphate pathway is 12.

10. The **Beer-Lambert law (or Beer's law)** is the linear relationship between absorbance and concentration of an absorbing species. The general Beer-Lambert law is usually written as

$$A = a(\lambda) \times b \times c$$

where A is the measured absorbance, a(λ) is a wavelength-dependent absorptivity coefficient, **b** is the path length, and **c** is the analyte concent-ration. When working in concentration units of molarity, the *Beer-Lambert law* is written as:

A = ε × b × c; Where ε is molar extinction coefficient (M^{-1} cm^{-1})

Given: Absorbance of a solution containing NADH in a path length of 1cm cuvette at 340 nm = 0.31, molar extinction coefficient of NADH = 6200 M^{-1} cm^{-1}

The concentration of NADH in the solution can be calculated as:

$$0.31 = 6200 \times 1 \times C$$

$$0.31/6200 = C$$

$$0.00005 = C$$

or C = 50 μM

11. Sodium dodecyl sulphate and methioninewill **NOT** break the disulphide bonds in the immunoglobulin molecules.

Reduced Glutathione (GSH) is an important antioxidant . Glutathione reduces disulfide bonds formed within cytoplasmic proteins to cysteines by serving as an electron donor. In the process, glutathione is converted to its oxidized form, glutathione disulfide (GSSG).

Dithiothreitol or DTT is also known as Cleland's Reagent. It contains two thiol groups and is commonly used to reduce disulfide bond in proteins. It can protect many thiol-containing biomolecules such as coenzyme A (Co-A), GSH from forming disulfide bonds.

Sodium dodecyl sulphate, synonymously **sodium lauryl sulphate** is a synthetic organic compound with the formula $CH_3(CH_2)_{11}SO_4Na$. It is an anionic surfactant used in many cleaning and hygiene products. The sodium salt is of an organosulphate class of organics. It consists of a 12-carbon tail attached to a sulphate group, that is, it is the sodium salt of *dodecyl hydrogen sulphate,* the ester of dodecyl alcohol and sulfuric acid.

Together with cysteine, methionine is one of two sulphur-containing proteinogenic amino acids. Excluding the few exceptions where methionine may act as a redox sensor (e.g.,), methionine residues do not have a catalytic role. This is in contrast to cysteine residues, where the thiol group has a catalytic role in many proteins.

12. Match of the protein elution condition given in **Group I** with the appropriate chromatography matrices from **Group II**.

Group-II	Group-I
DEAE-Sephacryl	Increasing concentration of sodium chloride
Phenyl-Sepharose	Separates molecules over a large molecular weight range. Decreasing concentration of ammonium sulphate
Chromatofocusing	Decreasing concentration of H+
Ni-NTA	Increasing concentration of histidine

13. Histidine is an aminoacid and all other options are neurotransmitter.

Histidine is a semi-essential amino acid (children should obtain it from food) needed in humans for growth and tissue repair; Histidine is important for maintenance of myelin sheaths that protect nerve cells and is metabolized to the neurotransmitter histamine.

14. Type II hypersensitivity results from antibodies of either IgG or **IgM** class binding to specific antigens on a cell surface or extracellular matrix, with subsequent activation of the classical complement cascade.

15. Oxidation coupled with anhydride bond formation reaction mechanisms drives the conversion of low energy 3- phosphoglyceraldehyde to high energy 1,3-bisphosphoglycerate

16. Number of molecules that will be formed at the end of 10 cycles = 5×2^{10}i.e. 5120 molecules. These molecules will be present in 1000 μl. In 100 μl the number of molecules will be 5120 / 10 = 512

17. From the given question

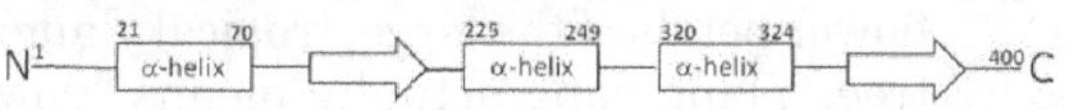

The percentage of residues forming α-helix is Then number of amino acid residues for each alfa -helix are:

(i) 21 to 70 = 50

(ii) 225 to 249 = 15

(iii)320 to 324 = 5

Therefore totals 83 amino acid residues forms all 3 alfa- helix. Then the percentage of residues forming alfa helix with total 400 amino acids = 80 × 100/400 = 20.0 %.

18. The fraction of themaximum velocity (V/ Vmax) with the substrate concentration [S] 4*K*m is

As per **Michaelis–Mentenkinetics** :

$V = V_{max}[S]/(K_M + [S])$

But $[S] = 4K_M$ is given;

Hence $V/V_{max} = 4K_M/(K_M + 4K_M)$

or $V/V_{max} = 4K_M/5K_M = 4/5$

or $V/V_{max} = \mathbf{0.8}$

19.

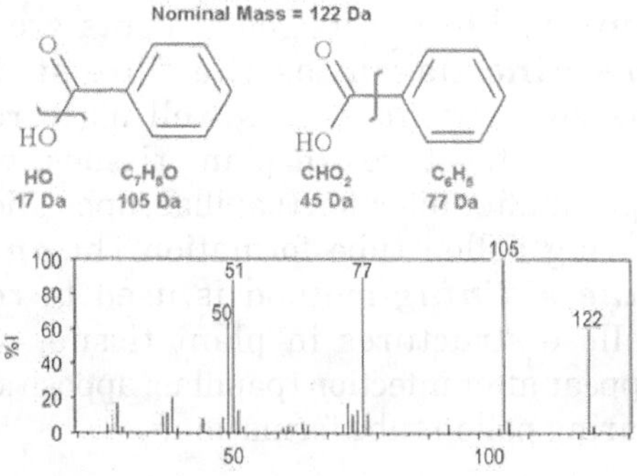

The mass spectrum of benzoic acid will generate the fragment as a base peak (100%, relative abundance) of *m*/*z* (mass to charge ratio) at 77.

20. **The standard** Gibbs **free energy** of formation of a compound is the change of Gibbs **free energy** that accompanies the formation of 1 mole of that substance from its component elements, at their **standard** states (the most stable form of the element at 25 degrees Celsius and 100 kilopascals). Its symbol is $\Delta_f G°$

(i) Citrate ↔ Citrate Acetate + Oxaloacetate;

Where $\Delta G_1° = -670$ cal/mole

(ii) Acetyl-CoA + Oxaloacetate + H_2O ↔ Citrate + CoA

Where $\Delta G_2° = -8192$ cal/mole

Therefore standard Gibbs **free energy** ($\Delta_f G°$) of acetyl-CoA hydrolysis will be

= (–670) + (–8192) = – 8862 **cal/mole**

BOTANY

1. ***Xanthium*** **(cocklebur)** is a genus of flowering plants in the sunflower tribe within the daisy family, native to the Americas and eastern Asia. Xanthium italicum (Asteraceae) is an annual species bearing dimorphic seeds. Each of its capitulum produces only one upper seed and one lower seed. It is productive, adaptable, and harmful to crops and environment.

2. Similar to protein-coding genes, most microRNA (miRNA) genes are transcribed by RNA polymerase II (Pol II), resulting in 5′ capped and poly(A)-tailed transcripts, named primary miRNAs (pri-miRNAs) [1, 2]. In plants, processing pri-miRNAs into precursor miRNAs (pre-miRNAs), then into ~ 21-nt miRNA/miRNA* duplexes is mediated by two sequential cleavages of Dicer-like 1 (DCL1).

3. A **transposable element (TE** or **transposon)** is a DNA sequence that can change its position within a genome, sometimes creating or reversing mutations and altering the cell's genetic identity and genome size. Transposition often results in duplication of the same genetic material.

Transposition can be classified as either "autonomous" or "non-autonomous" in both

Class I and Class II TEs. Autonomous TEs can move by themselves, whereas non-autonomous TEs require the presence of another TE to move. This is often because dependent TEs lack transposase (for Class II) or reverse transcriptase (for Class I).Activator element (*Ac*) is an example of an autonomous TE, and dissociation elements (*Ds*) is an example of a non-autonomous TE. Without *Ac, Ds* is not able to transpose.

Therefore"Only *Ac* is autonomous because it encodes its own transposase" is **TRUE** statement for transposable elements *Ac* and *Ds*.

4. A variety of experimental approaches resulted in identification of the S-ribonuclease (S-RNase) as the style-recognition component of gametophytic SI, acting together with both the previously elusive "pollen-S" gene and a number of other genes that play critical, supporting, or yet unclear roles in this response.

   The Solanaceae, Rosaceae, and Scrophulariaceae families all possess an RNase-mediated self-incompatibility mechanism through which their pistils can recognize and reject self-pollen to prevent inbreeding. The highly polymorphic S-locus controls the self-incompatibility interaction, and the S-locus of the Solanaceae has been shown to be a multi-gene complex in excess of 1.3 Mb

5. **An ecotone** is a transition area between **two** biomes. It is where **two** communities meet and integrate. It may be narrow or wide, and it may be local (the **zone** between a field and forest) or regional (the transition between forest and grassland **ecosystems**).

6. Normal, clean **rain** has a **pH** value of between 5.0 and 5.5, which is slightly **acidic**. However, when **rain**combines with sulfur dioxide or nitrogen oxides—produced from power plants and automobiles—the **rain**becomes much **more acidic**. Typical **acid rain** has a **pH**value of **4.0**.

   The pH scale is logarithmic rather than linear, and so there is a tenfold increase in acidity with each pH unit, such that rainfall with pH 5 is ten times more acidic than pH 6, rainfall with pH 4 is 100 times more acidic than pH 6 and rainfall with pH 3 is 1000 times more acidic than pH 6.

   The pH scale ranges from 0, which is strongly acid, to 14 which is strongly alkaline, the scale point 7 being neutral, invented by a Danish scientist called Sorenson in 1909. Examples of solutions with differing pH values include car battery acid (pH 1), lemon juice (pH 2), beer (pH 4), natural rain (pH 5-6), milk (pH 6), washing-up liquid (pH 7), seawater (pH 8), milk of magnesia (pH 10) and ammonia (pH 12).

7. Cananga odorata, known as the cananga tree, is a tropical tree that originates in Indonesia, which in the early 19th century spread to Malaysia and the Philippines. Ylangylang (Canangaodorata) essential oil comes from flower petals of the large, tropical ylangylang tree. Ylangylang actually means "flower of flowers" and was given this name because of its sweet, floral scent. In fact, ***ylangylang oil*** is one of the key ingredients used in the legendary perfume.

8. In plants, auxin is a key regulator of development and is unique among plant hormones in that its function requires polarized transport between neighboring cells to form concentration gradients across various plant tissues. AUX1 resides at the apical plasma membrane of protophloem cells and at highly dynamic subpopulations of Golgi apparatus and endosomes in all cell types. AUX1 action in the lateral root cap and/or epidermal cells influences lateral root initiation and positioning. Shoot supplied ammonium targets AUX1 and inhibits lateral root emergence.

   The Arabidopsis AUX1 gene encodes a transmembrane protein that shares homology with transporters of plant amino acid permeases, and appears to play a role in auxin influx.

9. **Aniline blue** or its constituents are used to **stain**collagen, as the fibre **stain** in Masson's trichrome, as well as to reveal callose structures in plant tissues, which appear after infection (papillae, apposition) or during pollen tube formation.The ***aniline blue staining*** method is used to reveal callose structures in plant tissue, which appear after infection (papillae, apposition) or during pollen tube formation.

10. AN ORF of 783 bp will code for a peptide with 783 / 3 amino acids i.e. 261.
Average MW of an amino acid is 110 daltons. Therefore MW of a peptide with 261 amino acids will be 261 × 110 = 28710 daltons or 28.710 Kda.

11. Statement "Mitosis occurs exclusively in diploid mother cell" is false however statement "Mitosis occurs both in diploid and haploid mother cells" is true. Statement "Meiosis occurs exclusively in diploid mother cell" is true however statement "Meiosis occurs both in diploid and haploid mother cells" is false.

12. A genetic construct for high-level expression of a gene encoding the therapeutic protein 18 (TP18) via plastid transformation. The **correct** set of genetic elements for this construct is as :

rbcL promoter → TP18 coding sequence → rbcL transcription terminator

13. The correctcombination of the statements are:

(Q) The cyclic electron transport chain involving PSI results in net production of ATP

(S) Rubisco enzyme usually converts RuBP and O2 into 2-phosphoglycolate and 3-phosphoglycerate

14. Correct match of the fruit characters with their families and representative plant species is as follows:

Fruit character	Family	Plant species
P. Syconus	1. Moraceae	iii. Ficus religiosa
Q. Capsule, opening by apical pores or valves	3. Papaveraceae	iv. Papaver somniferum
R. Legume	2. Fabaceae	i. Canavalia ensiformis
S. An etaerio of drupe	4. Annonaceae	ii. Artabotrys odoratissimus

15. The **correct** combination of the disease, affected plant and the causal organism is as:

Disease	Affected Plant	Causal organism
P. Black rot	4. Apple	iii. Botrysophaeria obtusa
Q. Loose smut	1. Corn	iv. Ustilago maydis
R. Panama wilt	2. Banana	i. Fusarium oxysporum f.sp. cubense
S. Bacterial fruit blotch	3. Watermelon	ii. Acidovorax avenae subsp. citrulli

16. The **correct**combination by matching **Group-I** with **Group-II is :**

Group-I	Group-II
P. Photorespiration	4. Glycine ? Serine
Q. Respiration	3. 2-Oxglutarate ? Succinyl-CoA
R. Amino acid degradation	1. Glutamate → 2-Oxglutarate
S. Fatty acid synthesis	2. Acetyl-CoA → Malonyl-CoA

17. The correct match of the plant alkaloids with their uses and source species are as follows:

Alkaloid	Use	Source species
P. Codeine	2. Analgesic	iv. Papaver somniferum
Q. Caffeine	1. Stimulant	iii. Cola nitida
R. Scopolamine	4. Anticholinergic	i. Hyoscyamus niger
S. Vinblastine	3. Antineoplastic	ii. Catharanthus roseus

18. The **correct** combination of statements with respect to chemical defense in plants is as follows:

(Q) *Phaseolus vulgaris* produces Phaseolus agglutinin I, which is toxic to the cowpea weevil

(S) Avenacin, a triterpenoid saponin from oat prevents infection by *Gaeumannomycesgraminis*, a major pathogen of cereal roots

19. Total recombinants

= Tall plants with terminal flowers
+ Dwarf plants with a axial flowers

Hence Total recombinants = 79 + 83 = 162

Now % of recombinants

= (Total recombinants / Total progeny) × 100

Then % of recombinants

= (162 / 320 + 318 + 79 + 83) × 100 or

% of recombinants = (162/800) x100

= 20.25 cM

20. Let A be the event for pink, B be the event for red and C be the event for white.

PhenotypicRatio = 1 : 2 : 1 (Red : pink : white)

Therefore, P (A) = 2/4 = 1/2; P(B) = 1/4; and P(C) = ¼

Let us consider any one order (e.g. :1 white, 2pink and 2 red flowers plants) will be = BBAAC

Since the individual's characteristic for all the 5 plants are independent events.

Then

$P(B) \cap B) \cap A) \cap A) \cap C)$

$= P(B) \times P(B) \times P(A) \times P(A) \times P(C)$

$= 1/4 \times 1/4 \times 1/2 \times 1/2 \times 1/4$

$= 1/256$

But the total order will be = $5! / [(2)! \times (2)! \times 1!]$

However each order will have same probability. Therefore total probability will be

$= (1/256 + 1/256 + 1/256.........30$ times)

$= 30/256 = 15/128$

Or % probability = $(15/128) \times 100 = 11.7\%$.

Hence the probability that out of the five plants picked up randomly, two would be with pink flowers, two with white flowers and one with red flowers is 11.7%.

MICROBIOLOGY

1. The **Baltimore classification**, developed by David Baltimore, is a virus classification system that groups viruses into families, depending on their type of genome (DNA, RNA, single-stranded (ss), double-stranded (ds), etc..) and their method of replication

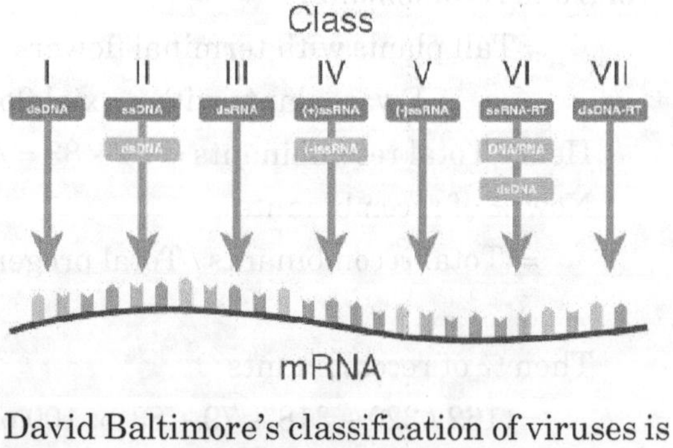

David Baltimore's classification of viruses is based on **differences in** the pathways required to synthesize virus mRNA.

2. An **opsonin** is any molecule that enhances phagocytosis by marking an antigen for an immune response or marking dead cells for recycling (i.e., causes the phagocyte to "relish" the marked cell).

Different opsonins perform different functions. Opsonin molecules include: Antibodies (IgM), Complement proteins (C3b, C4b, and C1q) and **Circulating proteins** (Pentraxins, collectins, and ficolins).

- Antibodies are part of the adaptive immune response and are generated by B cells in response to antigen exposure. The Fab region of the antibody binds to the antigen, whereas the Fc region of the antibody binds to an Fc receptor on the phagocyte, facilitating phagocytosis.
- The **T-cell receptor**, or TCR, is a molecule found on the surface of **T cells**, or **T lymphocytes**, that is responsible for recognizing fragments of antigen as peptides bound to major histocompatibility complex (MHC) molecules.
- **Histamine** is an organic nitrogenous compound involved in local immune responses, as well as regulating physiological function in the gut and acting as a neurotransmitter for the brain, spinal cord, and uterus.Histamine is involved in the inflammatory response and has a central role as a mediator of itching.
- **Interferons** (**IFN**s) are a group of signalling proteins made and released by host cells in response to the presence of several pathogens, such as viruses, bacteria, parasites, and also tumour cells. In a typical scenario, a virus-infected cell will release interferons causing nearby cells to heighten their anti-viral defences.

3. Oral poliovirus vaccines (OPV) have been the mainstay in the fight against polio. There are different types of oral poliovirus vaccine, which may contain one (mOPV), a combination of two (bOPV), or all the three (tOPV) serotypes of attenuated poliovirus.

4. **Autophagy** is a normal physiological process in the body that deals with destruction of cells in the body. It maintains homeostasis or normal functioning by protein degradation and turnover of the destroyed cell organelles for new cell formation

A **lysosome** is a membrane-bound organelle found in nearly all animal cells. They are spherical vesicles that contain hydrolytic enzymes that can break down many kinds of biomolecules.

The lysosomes also act as the waste disposal system of the cell by digesting unwanted materials in the cytoplasm, both from outside the cell and obsolete components inside the cell. Material from outside the cell is taken-up through endocytosis, while material from the inside of the cell is digested through autophagy.

5. Nuclear and mitochondrial DNA are thought to be of separate evolutionary origin, with the mtDNA being derived from the circular genomes of the bacteria that were engulfed by the early ancestors of today's eukaryotic cells. This theory is called the endosymbiotic theory. Each mitochondrion is estimated to contain 2–10 mtDNA copies. In the cells of extant organisms, the vast majority of the proteins present in the mitochondria (numbering approximately 1500 different types in mammals) are coded for by nuclear DNA, but the genes for some, if not most, of them are thought to have originally been of bacterial origin, having since been transferred to the eukaryotic nucleus during evolution.

6. Viruses are mainly classified by phenotypic characteristics, such as morphology, nucleic acid type, mode of replication, host organisms, and the type of diseases they cause. Currently, two main schemes are used for the classification of viruses: the International Committee on Taxonomy of Viruses (ICTV) system and Baltimore classification system, which places viruses into one of seven groups. Therefore, Binomial nomenclature has NOT yet been adopted forviruses classification. However Binomial nomenclature ("two name naming system") is a formal system of naming species of living things by giving each a name composed of two parts, both of which use Latin grammatical forms, although they can be based on words from other languages.

7. Some of the methods used to achieve sterilization are:
   - Autoclaves: Highly effective and inexpensive. Unsuitable for heat sensitive objects.
   - Hot air ovens: Inefficient compared to autoclaves.
   - Ethylene oxide: Suitable for heat sensitive items but leaves toxic residue on sterilized items.
   - Low-temperature steam and formaldehyde: Effective for instruments with cavities or tubular openings.
   - Sporicidal chemicals: Often used as disinfectants but can also sterilize instruments if used for prolonged periods.
   - Irradiation: Gamma rays and accelerated electrons are excellent at sterilization.
   - Gas plasma.

   However UV is also effective for sterilization, but its use is affected for some factors, especially concerning:
   - When the object produces "shades" on its own surface, where UV cannot reach, its global effect is lower.
   - If working with water, and its turbidity is considerable, UV's is not much effective, and you should use complementary treatments.
   - Its application time depends on many factors. In general, to affect DNA of microorganisms in water, it takes at least 20-30 minutes, depending on the lamp capacity, turbidity, water flow, etc.
   - UV applied directly in humans is not advisable, generally.

8. **Nitrogen fixation**, any natural or industrial process that causes free nitrogen (N_2), which is a relatively inert gas plentiful in air, to combine chemically with other elements to form more-reactive nitrogen compounds such as ammonia, nitrates, or nitrites.

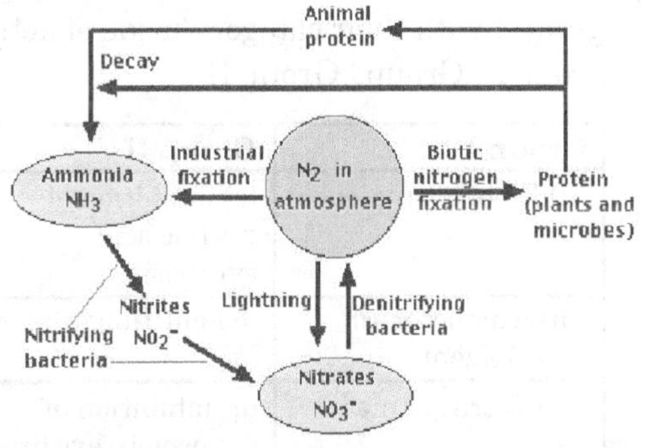

9. The natural ecology of malaria involves malaria parasites infecting successively two types of hosts: humans and female *Anopheles* mosquitoes. In humans,

the parasites grow and multiply first in the liver cells and then in the red cells of the blood. In the blood, successive broods of parasites grow inside the red cells and destroy them, releasing daughter parasites ("merozoites") that continue the cycle by invading other red cells.

The blood stage parasites are those that cause the symptoms of malaria. When certain forms of blood stage parasites ("gametocytes") are picked up by a female *Anopheles* mosquito during a blood meal, they start another, different cycle of growth and multiplication in the mosquito.

10. Given: 50 mg/mL stock solution of arginine.To prepare 1 litre of growth medium for an arginine auxotroph requires 70 μg/mL of arginine, the volume of this stock solution that should be added, would be calculated as:

$70/1000 = 50 \times vol. /1000$ {70 microgm = $70 \times 10^{-6}g = 70 \times 10^{-3}mg$}

Hence, volume of the stock solution that should be added = 1.4 ml

11. The **Three Domain System of Classification** by **Carl Woese** (1977) based on variations in 16S rRNA sequence, divided the entire living organism in the biosphere into three major groups called Domains namely (1). **Archaea**, (2). **Eubacteria** (Bacteria) and (3). **Eukarya** or Eukaryota. Properties shared between eukaryotes and archaea are:

(i) Protein biogenesis

(ii) Ribosomal subunit structures

12. Correct matchof the antimicrobial agents in group I with their category/mode of action in group II. Group I Group II

Group I	Group II
(i) Fluoroquinolones	(r) inhibition of nucleic acid synthesis
(ii) Amphotericin B agent	(s) antifungal agent
(iii) Tetracycline	(q) inhibition of protein synthesis
(iv) Amoxicillin	(p) beta lactam antimicrobial

13. Correct match of the microorganisms to their predominant modes of transmission

Microorganism	Mode of Transmission
Bordetella pertussis	(r) Droplet infection
Dengue virus	(p) Vector-borne
Entamoeba histolytica	(s) Contaminated food
Hepatitis B virus	(q) Blood-borne

Pertussis, a respiratory illness commonly known as whooping cough, is a very contagious disease caused by a type of bacteria called Bordetella pertussis.

Dengue virus (DENV) is the cause of dengue fever. It is a mosquito-borne single positive-stranded RNA virus of the family Flaviviridae. Vertical transmission from mosquito to mosquito has also been observed in some vector species.

E. histolytica: Transmission of E. histolytica from man to man occurs through its encysted stage and infection is effected through the ingestion of these cysts in food or drinks. It is to be noted that mature quadrinucleate cysts are the infective forms of this parasite.

Hepatitis B virus (HBV) is a bloodborne virus. HBV is transmitted when blood, semen, or other body fluid infected with Hepatitis B virus enters the body of a person not infected. Once inside the host, HBV is transported in the blood to the liver, where it infects liver cells. The incubation period of acute HBV infection is usually about 75 days, but can range from 45 to 200 days. The virus spreads in the liver and causes a spectrum of disease, ranging from acute hepatitis to chronic liver disease and liver tumours.

14. Correct match of the precursors/ intermediates with the corresponding metabolic pathways:

Precursor/ Intermediates	Metabolic pathway
(i) Inosine monophosphate	(r) Purine biosynthesis
(ii) Ornithine	(s) L-arginine biosynthesis
(iii) Chorismate	(q) L-tryptophan biosynthesis
(iv) Homocysteine	(p) L-methionine biosynthesis

Inosinic acid or inosine monophosphate (IMP) is a nucleoside monophosphate. Widely used as a flavor enhancer, it is typically obtained from chicken byproducts or other meat industry waste. Inosinic acid is important in metabolism. It is the ribonucleotide of hypoxanthine and the first nucleotide formed during the synthesis of purine. It is formed by the deamination of adenosine monophosphate, and is hydrolysed to inosine. IMP is an intermediate ribonucleoside monophosphate in purine metabolism.

Ornithine is a non-proteinogenic amino acid that plays a role in the urea cycle. Ornithine is abnormally accumulated in the body in ornithine transcarbamylase deficiency. The radical is **ornithyl**. L-Ornithine is one of the products of the action of the enzyme arginase on L-arginine, creating urea. Therefore, ornithine is a central part of the urea cycle, which allows for the disposal of excess nitrogen. Ornithine is recycled and, in a manner, is a catalyst. First, ammonia is converted into carbamoyl phosphate.

Chorismic acid, more commonly known as its anionic form **chorismate**, is an important biochemical intermediate in plants and microorganisms. It is a precursor for:

- The aromatic amino acids phenylalanine, tryptophan, and tyrosine
- Indole, indole derivatives and tryptophan
- The biosynthesis of Vitamin K and folate in plants and microorganisms.

15. Correct match the scientists to their area of major contribution

Scientists	Area of major contribution
(i) Antonie van Leeuwenhoek	(s) Microscopy
(ii) Carl Linnaeu	(p) Taxonomy
(iii) Sir Alexander Fleming	(q) Antimicrobial agents
(iv) Louis Pasteur	(r) Vaccination

Antonie Philips van Leeuwenhoek. He is commonly known as "the Father of Microbiology". Van Leeuwenhoek is best known for his pioneering work in **microscopy**.

Carl Linnaeus formalised **the modern system of naming organisms called binomial nomenclature**. He is known by the epithet "**father of modern taxonomy**". Many of his writings were in Latin and his name is rendered in Latin as **Carolus Linnæus.**

Sir Alexander Fleming discovered world's **first antibiotic** substance **benzylpenicillin** (Penicillin G) from the mould Penicilliumnotatum in 1928, for which he shared the Nobel Prize in Physiology or Medicine in 1945 with Howard Florey and Ernst Boris Chain.

Louis Pasteur renowned for his discoveries of the principles of vaccination, microbial fermentation and pasteurization. He is remembered for his remarkable breakthroughs in the causes and prevention of diseases. He reduced mortality from puerperal fever, and created the first vaccines for rabies and anthrax.

16. Combinations which improve the resolution of a microscope are:

(i) Increasing the half aperture angle of the objective lens

(ii) Decreasing the wavelength of the illumination source

The resolution of a microscope is intrinsically linked to the numerical aperture (NA) of the optical components as well as the wavelength of light which is used to examine a specimen. **Abbe's equation** in order to calculate approximate resolving power:

resolving power = wavelength of light used/2 (numerical aperture of objective)

17.

$$C_o = 0.005 \text{ M}$$
$$C_i = 0.5 \text{ M}$$
$$T = 298 \text{ K}$$
$$R = 1.98 \text{ cal/mol.K}$$

Amount of energy required for transport

$$\Delta G^\circ = -RT \ln K$$

$$K = \frac{C_o}{C_i}$$

$$\therefore \quad \Delta G^\circ = -(1.98)(298) \ln \frac{0.005}{0.5}$$

$$= 2717 \text{ cal/mol}$$

$$= 2.717 \text{ K col/mol.}$$

18. $S_F = 10$ g/L, $Y_{x/s} = 0.5$

$F = 5$ ml/min = 0.3 litre

$V = 3$ litre

$$D = \frac{F}{V} = \frac{0.3}{3} = 0.1\ h^{-1}$$

$$\mu = \frac{0.3\ S}{1+S} h^{-1}$$

Now, at steady state

$$D = \mu$$

$$0.1 = \frac{0.3\ S}{1+S}$$

$$\therefore \quad 0.1 + 0.13 = 0.35$$

$$\Rightarrow \quad 0.25 = 0.1$$

$$\therefore \quad S = \frac{1}{2} = 0.5\ g/litre$$

19. $N_o = 1.0 \times 10^6$ cells/ ml

$N_t = 1.0 \times 10^8$ cells/ml

$\mu = 0.1\ h^{-1}$

$t = ?$

$$\mu = \frac{1}{N}\frac{dN}{dT}$$

$$\therefore \quad \int_0^t dt = \frac{1}{\mu}\int_{N_o}^{N_t}\frac{dN}{N}$$

$$\therefore \quad t = \frac{1}{\mu}\ln\left(\frac{N_t}{N_o}\right)$$

$$= \frac{1}{0.1}\ln\left(\frac{10^8}{10^6}\right)$$

$$= 46.05 \text{ hours}$$

20. Glucose + 2Pi + 2ADP → 2Lactate + 2ATP $+2H_2O$

The 1 mole of glucose will hydrolyse 2 mole of ATP.

The total free energy of the conversion.

i.e. input energy = –47000 cal/mol

= – 47 kcal/mol

Total amount of energy available

= 2 × (–7.3 kcal/mol)

= – 14.6 kcal.

∴ Efficiency of energy transfer

$$= \frac{\text{Output energy}}{\text{Input energy}} \times 100$$

$$= \frac{14.6}{47} \times 100$$

$$= 31.06\%$$

ZOOLOGY

1. **Deuterostomia**, (Greek: "second mouth"), group of animals—including those of the phyla Echinodermata (*e.g.*, starfish, sea urchins), Chordata (*e.g.*, sea squirts, lancelets, and vertebrates), Chaetognatha (*e.g.*, arrowworms) and Brachiopoda (*e.g.*, lamp shells)—classified together on the basis of embryological development and by molecular criteria. During development the mouth of deuterostomes develops from an opening into the embryonic gut other than the blastopore, which develops into the anus. The coelom (a fluid-filled body cavity lined with mesoderm) develops from buds off the embryonic gut. A number of deuterostomes have distinctive larval forms. The Deuterostomia constitute one of two divisions of the coelomates (animals having a coelom).

2. **Polymerase chain reaction (PCR)** is a technique used in molecular biology to amplify a single copy or a few copies of a segment of DNAacross several orders of magnitude, generating thousands to millions of copies of a particular DNA sequence. Developed in 1983 by Kary Mullis. PCR is based on using the ability of DNA polymerase to synthesize new strand of DNA complementary to the offered template strand. Because DNA polymerase can add a nucleotide only onto a preexisting 3'-OH group, it needs a primer to which it can add the first nucleotide. This requirement makes it possible to delineate a specific region of template sequence that the researcher wants to amplify. At the end of the PCR reaction, the specific sequence will be accumulated in billions of copies (amplicons).

3. In a chemical reaction where the substrate and product are in equilibrium in solution. If an enzyme is added then the equilibrium of the reaction will not change.

4. **Tay-Sachs** is an autosomal recessive **disease** caused by mutations in both alleles of a gene (HEXA) on chromosome 15. HEXA codes for the

alpha subunit of the enzyme β-hexosaminidase A. This enzyme is found in lysosomes, **organelles** that break down large molecules for recycling by the **cell**.

5. Directional selection occurs when individuals with traits on one side of the mean in their population survive better or reproduce more than those on the other. It has been demonstrated many times in natural populations, using both observational and experimental approaches. Directional selection is the process that comes most easily to mind when thinking about natural selection, and it is the form of selection that has taken place in the best-known examples of evolution (e.g., the peppered moth, antibiotic resistance, finch beaks).

6. Cancer is occurs when mitosis has gone wrong! Genes control mitosis and if these are disrupted in some way, the cell division can go out of control. Meiosis do not cause cancer. The cells produced in meiosis are not a permanent part of the body. I mean they are used or given out of the body. Cancer is unchecked cell growth. Mutations in genes can cause cancer by accelerating cell division rates or inhibiting normal controls on the system, such as cell cycle arrest or programmed cell death. As a mass of cancerous cells grows, it can develop into a tumor. Cancer cells can also invade neighboring tissues and sometimes even break off and travel to other parts of the body, leading to the formation of new tumors at those sites.

7. The mesoderm is one of the three(the other two being the ectoderm and endoderm) germinal layers that appears in the third week of embryonic development. It is formed through a process called gastrulation. Some of the mesoderm derivatives include the muscle (smooth, cardiac and skeletal), the muscles of the tongue (occipital somites), the pharyngeal arches muscle (muscles of mastication, muscles of facial expressions), connective tissue, dermis and subcutaneous layer of the skin, bone and cartilage, dura mater, endothelium of blood vessels, red blood cells, white blood cells, and microglia, the kidneys and the adrenal cortex.

   Ectoderm: One of the three primary germ cell layers that make up the very early embryo. The ectoderm is the outermost of the three layers. It differentiates to give rise to many important tissues and structures including the outer layer of the skin and its appendages (the sweat glands, hair, and nails), the teeth, the lens of the eye, parts of the inner ear, the nerves, brain, and spinal cord.

8. The definition of **LATENT LEARNING** is and happens when an animal (or human) stores information in its long-term memory and then uses this knowledge when needed at a later date.

   A form of learning in which there is apparently no immediate reward for the animal, and what is learnt remains 'latent'. The prime example is an animal exploring its surroundings. Learning about the geography of its home area may bring an animal no immediate benefits, but can prove vital in the future when fleeing a predator or searching for food. Many insects learn the details of landmarks near their nest by making orientation flights. This process enables them to locate the nest when returning from distant sites.

9.
   - The kidneys are the primary functional organ of the renal system. The renal cortex, renal medulla, and renal pelvis are the three main internal regions found in a kidney.
   - Nephrons, masses of tiny tubules, are largely located in the medulla and receive fluid from the blood vessels in the renal cortex.
   - The renal cortex produces erythropotein.
   - The kidneys are made up by three external layers, which include the renal fascia (the outermost layer), the perirenal fat capsule, and lastly, the innermost layer,

the renal capsule, which then surround the space of the renal cortex.

- The Bowman's or renal capsule, located at one end of each nephron in the cortex of the kidney, is the blood-filtering region of the nephron.
- The renal pelvis contains a hilium the concave site in which the renal artery and vein and nerves enter the kidney and the ureter leaves the kidney.

10. Lung surfactants are made from animal lung extract. Lung surfactant is a complex with a unique phospholipid and protein composition. Its specific function is to reduce surface tension at the pulmonary air-liquid interface. Natural surfactants are produced by the alveolar cells in the lungs and line mainly the alveoli and small bronchioles, and prevent the alveoli from collapsing. Lung surfactant makes it easier for oxygen to penetrate the lung surface lining and move into the blood. Without the lung surfactant it would be extremely hard to breathe, and transfer of oxygen through the surface that lines the lungs would be very difficult.

11. Disorders/diseases listed in Column I to their respective causative agents in Column II.

S.No.	Column I	Column II
1	African tick bite fever	*Rickettsia sp.*
2	Yellow fever	Flavivirus
3	Microcephaly	Zika virus
4	Sleeping sickness	*Trypanosoma gambiense*

12. Glucose monomers are joined together by glycosidic linkages to form a cellulose polymer. During this process, changes in the free energy, total energy, and entropy respectively are represented correctly by + ΔG, + ΔH, –ΔS.

13. Mutations of the Ubx gene will lead to transformation of dorsal and ventral appendages of the third thoracic segment(T3), which includes the haltere and third leg, into the counterparts on the second thoracic segment(T2). If Ubx is present in T3, it will prevent the original fate of the T2 segment. Such mutations can produce a second set of wings.

In Drosophila, the Hox gene Ultrabithorax (Ubx) controls the differential development between wing and haltere. Ubx is expressed throughout haltere development but not in the developing wing. Reduced Ubx function in imaginal discs or in Ubx mutant clones results in transformation of haltere tissue into wing tissue. Total loss of Ubx function in the developing halteres results in the complete transformation of halteres to wings, giving rise to a four-winged fly. Conversely, mutations that cause ectopic expression of Ubx in the developing wing disc [e.g., Contrabithorax (Cbx)] transform wing into haltere tissue. Although these spectacular Ubx mutant phenotypes have been known for decades, no Ubx-regulated genes in the haltere have been identified.

14. Respiratory acidosis is a condition that occurs when the lungs can't remove enough of the carbon dioxide (CO_2) produced by the body. Elevated partial pressure of carbon dioxide ($P_a\ CO_2$) above the normal range (>44 mm Hg) causes the pH of blood and other bodily fluids to decrease, making them too acidic. Normally, the body is able to balance the ions that control acidity. This balance is measured on a pH scale from 0 to 14. Acidosis occurs when the pH of the blood falls below 7.35 (normal blood pH is between 7.35 and 7.45). Acute respiratory acidosis can be life-threatening when a sudden and sharp increase in $P_a\ CO_2$ is associated with severe hypoxemia and acidemia. In contrast, chronic respiratory acidosis (>24 h) is characterized by a gradual and sustained increase in $P_a\ CO_2$.

15. Proteins / molecules listed in column I with the cellular location mentioned in the column II.

S.No.	Column I	Column II
1	Galactosyl transferase	Golgi complex
2	Cytochrome oxidase	Mitochondria
3	Clathrin	Vesicles
4	Tubulin	Cytosol

16. In an experiment, nucleus from a Drosophila oocyte was transplanted into the anterior part of another oocyte, at a region opposite to the existing nucleus. "A dorsalized egg with four dorsal appendages" phenotypes will be the developing egg show.

17. The organisms listed in Column I with the features listed in Column II

S.No.	Column I	Column II
1	Tapeworm	Microvilli on the body surface
2	Jellyfish	Bioluminescence
3	Trichinella	Viviparous
4	Earthworm	Lateral heart

18. A trait which is constantly used will get inherited by next generation is NOT part of the classical Darwinian theory of evolution by natural selection.

19. Berth Rate means number of births per thousand of animals. Similarly mortality rate means mortality per thousand of animals.

Therefore, A population of rabbits have a birth rate of 200 means

= 200 rabbits /1000 of rabbits per year

After one year rabbit population will be

= 4000 + (800 birth – 200 mortality) = 4600

After 2nd year rabbit population will be

= 4600 + (920 birth – 230 mortality)

= 4600 + 690 = 5290 rabbits

20. The frequency of occurrence of a disorder caused by recessive allele (q) is 1 in 1100 i.e.

$q^2 = 1/1100 = 0.000909$ or $q = 0.030151$

As we know $p + q = 1$, then $p = 1.0 – 030151 = 0.969849$

Then the frequency of heterozygotes in the population will be = 2pq

Therefore, $2\ pq = 2 \times 0.969849 \times 0.030151$

$= 2 \times 0.029241 = 0.058482$

■■

GATE-2017

XL : LIFE SCIENCES

Time : 3 Hours | *Maximum Marks : 100*

CHEMISTRY

1. CO reacts readily with
   (a) Fe (b) Fe^{2+}
   (c) Fe^{4+} (d) Fe^{3+}

2. Molecules that are NOT isoelectronic to NO_2^+ ion are
   (a) CO_2 and N_3^-
   (b) NCO^- and H_3BCN^-
   (c) BO_2^- and $H_3CC \equiv CH$
   (d) OF_2 and O_3^-

3. The extensive quantity among the following is
   (a) Pressure
   (b) Temperature
   (c) Chemical potential
   (d) Volume

4. The compound that gives characteristic foul smell upon heating with potassium hydroxide and chloroform is

   (a) 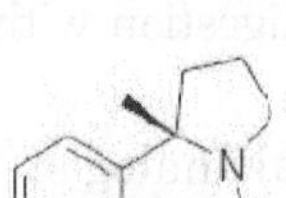
   Nicotine

   (b) 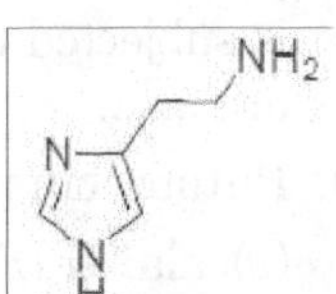
   Histamine

   (c) 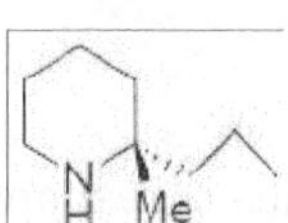
   Coniine

   (d) 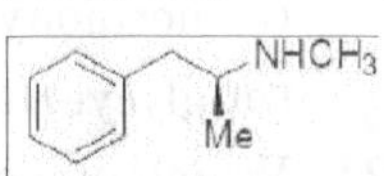
   Methamphetamine

5. The correct order of stability in water is

   (a) 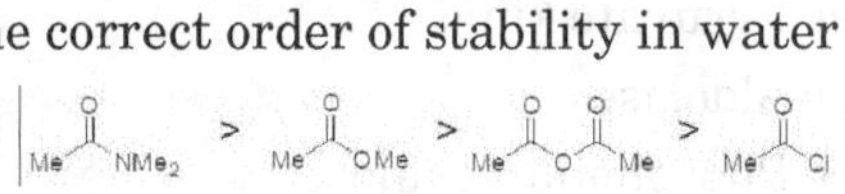

   (b) 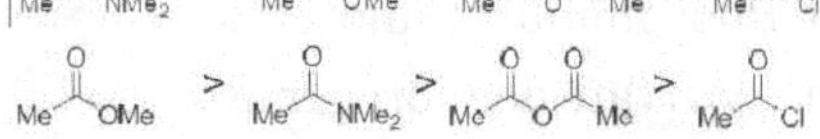

   (c) 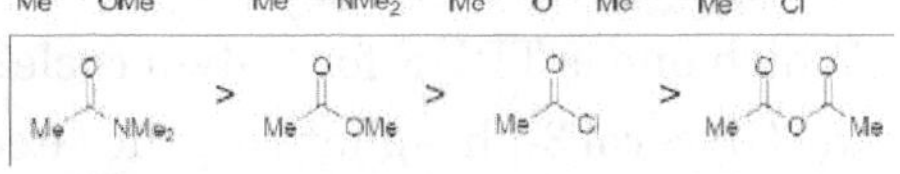

   (d) 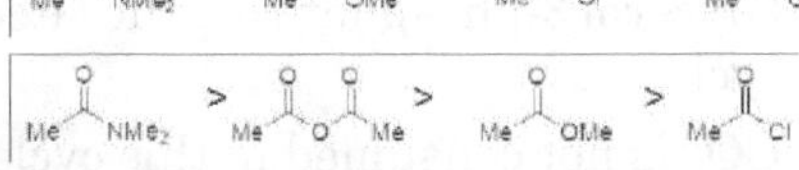

6. The pair of molecules having non-linear structures is
   (a) ICl_2^- and BeH_2 (b) CS_2 and I_3^-
   (c) SCl and ClO_2^- (d) XeF_2 and CN_2^{2-}

7. The decreasing order of bond lengths for O_2, B_2, N_2 and C_2 is
   (a) $B_2 > C_2 > N_2 > O_2$
   (b) $B_2 > C_2 > O_2 > N_2$
   (c) $N_2 > C_2 > O_2 > B_2$
   (d) $B_2 > O_2 > N_2 > C_2$

8. The octahedral metal oxide with the highest CFSE value is
   (a) ZnO (b) MnO
   (c) VO (d) TiO

9. Assuming independent non-interacting electrons, the first ionization energy of Helium atom is
   (a) 13.6 eV (b) 27.2 eV
   (c) 54.4 eV (d) 108.8 eV

10. For a reaction A + B $\longrightarrow$ products, the following data was obtained.

$[A]_0$ (M)	$[B]_0$ (M)	Initial rate
0.1	0.1	r
0.2	0.1	4r
0.1	0.2	2r

   A_0 and B_0 are initial concentrations of A and B, respectively. The overall order of the reaction is
   (a) 2 (b) 3
   (c) 4 (d) 6

11. The EMF for the following cell at 298.15 K is
   $Ag(s)|Ag^+$ (aq.. 0.01 M)||Ag^+(aq., 1.0 M)|Ag(s)
   (Standard reduction potential for $Ag^+ + e^- \longrightarrow Ag$ is – 0.80 V)
   (a) 0.12 V (b) 0.68 V
   (c) 0.80 V (d) 0.92 V

12. One gram of a protein is dissolved in one liter of water. The resulting solution exerts an osmotic pressure of 1.4 Torr at 298 K. Assuming that the protein does not ionize in solution, the molecular weight of the protein is ________ g mol^{-1}.
   (R = 0.082 L atm mol^{-1} K^{-1})

13. The type of nucleophilic substitution and the possible products for each of the reactions P and Q are

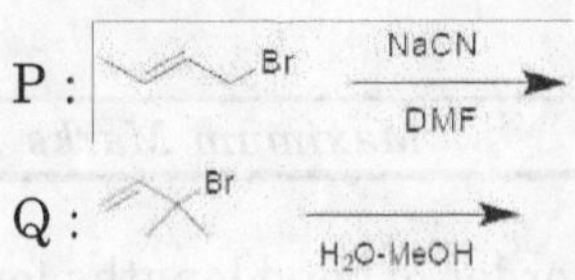

(a) 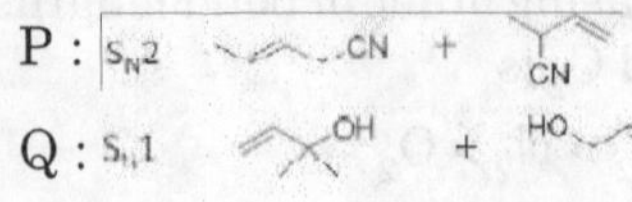

(b) 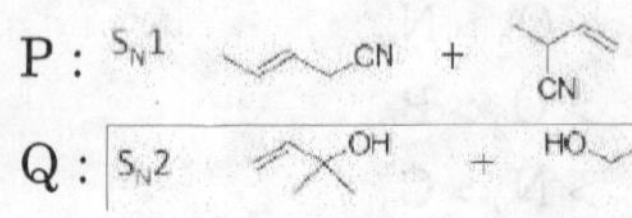

(c) 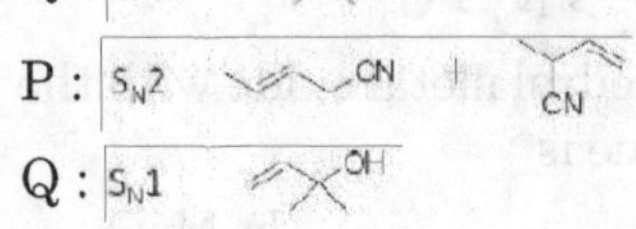

(d) 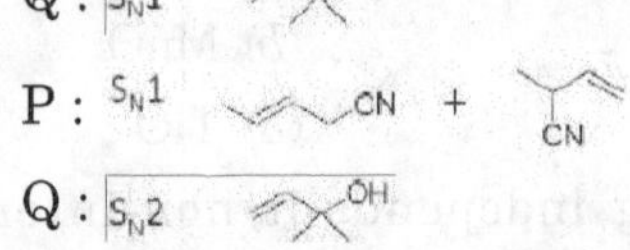

14. If mono-chlorination occurs at every carbon in the following reaction, the number of isomers (stereo isomers + constitutional isomers) that one can have is

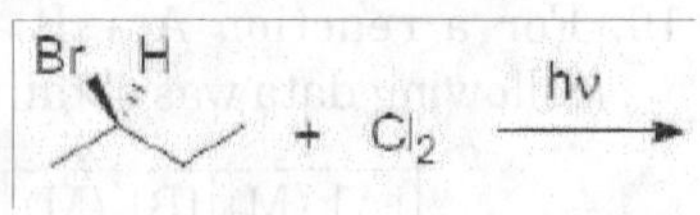

(a) 4
(b) 5
(c) 6
(d) 8

15. The major product in the following reactions is

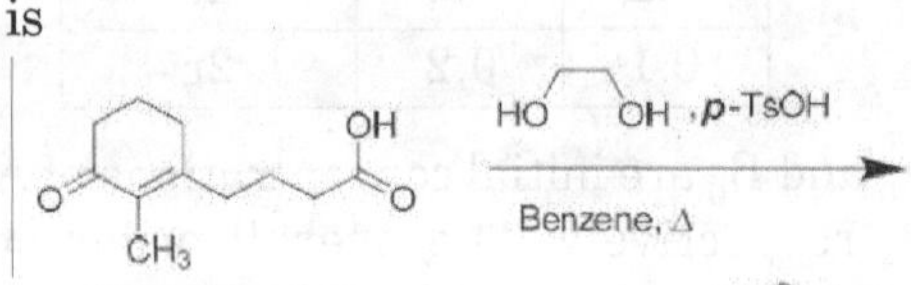

(a) 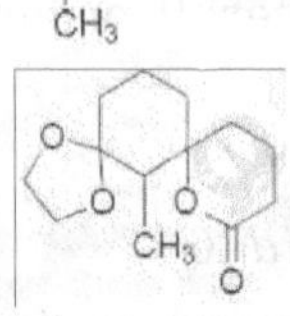

(b) 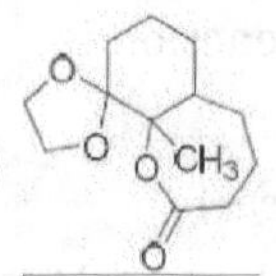

(c) 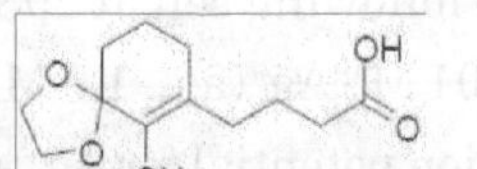

(d) 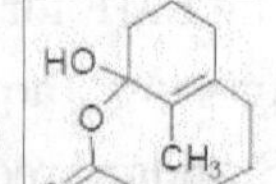

BIOCHEMISTRY

16. The molecular weight of a protein as determined by native PAGE is 400 kDa. This protein when run on a lion-reducing SDS-PAGE gave a band of 200 kDa. and on a reducing SDS-PAGE. gave a band of 100 kDa. The protein has
   (a) four subunits of which two sets are linked by two disulfide bridges
   (b) four subunits which are linked by four disulfide bridges
   (c) two subunits only and none are linked by disulfide bridges
   (d) two subunits which are linked by disulfide bridges

17. Which one of the following techniques CANNOT be used to determine the sequence of a novel protein?
   (a) De novo sequencing by ESI-MS/MS
   (b) Edman degradation
   (c) Sanger sequencing
   (d) Peptide mass fingerprinting

18. Which type of polyacrylamide gel can be used tor analyzing the four different proteins listed below?
   Protein P: 60 kDa, pi 4
   Protein Q: 45 kDa, pi 8
   Protein R: 60 kDa, pi 6
   Protein S: 45 kDa, pi 7.5
   (a) 20% gel, pH 4-7
   (b) 20% gel, pH 3-10
   (c) 12% gel, pH 3-10
   (d) 12% gel, pH 4-7

19. The number of fragments generated when the peptide 'ANDCQEGKFMLKPDTWRYVSFMRPA' is subjected to complete digestion with trypsin are ....

20. Putomycin is a structural analog of
   (a) alanyl-tRNA
   (b) tyrosyl-tRNA
   (c) methionyl-tRNA
   (d) glycyl-tRNA

21. Which one of the enzymes is responsible for arsenic toxicity?
   (a) Pyruvate kinase
   (b) Aldolase
   (c) Phosphofiuctokinase
   (d) Pyruvate dehydrogenase

22. Which one is TRUE for Calvin cycle?
   (a) Glycerol 3-phosphate is generated in this cycle
   (b) CO_2 is not consumed in this cycle
   (c) This is a reductive pentose phosphate cycle
   (d) Ribose 5-phosphate is a carboxylation substrate in this cycle

23. Administration of primaquine causes severe hemolytic anemia because it

(*a*) increases the demand for NADPH to a level that cells can't meet

(*b*) decreases the demand for NADPH

(*c*) inactivates glutathione peroxidase of erythrocytes

(*d*) increases reduced glutathione level of erythrocytes

24. Which one of the following will NOT form lipid bilayer?

(*a*) Cholesterol

(*b*) Phosphatidyl ethanolamine

(*c*) Triacylglycerol

(*d*) Phosphatidyl serine

25. Which one of the following features is NOT appropriate for Fab fragment of IgG?

(*a*) Contains antigen binding site

(*b*) Contains an intact L chain

(*c*) Two fragments are formed from one IgG molecule

(*d*) Mediates complement fixation in the intact IgG molecule

26. The duration of DNA synthesis (S phase) in plant cells is 11 h and the DNA is replicated at a rate of 100 bp/s/fork. A plant species has about 3.0×10^{10} bp DNA/genome. The number of bidirectional forks per genome required for replication will be.................

27. In a PCR reaction, with one double stranded DNA of 600 bp, nano gram of DNA produced after 40 cycles of amplification will be ....

28. A solution containing GTP has molar extinction coefficient of 1.55×10^4 mol^{-1} $dm^3 cm^{-1}$ at a given wavelength. The concentration of GTP solution is 1.290×10^{-5} mol din^{-3}. The absorbance of GTP solution in 1 cm cuvette at the same wavelength will be ....

29. Which one of the following is NOT TRUE for class I MHC protein?

(*a*) MHC class I protein are polymorphic

(*b*) T-cell receptors recognizes MHC class I protein

(*c*) MHC class I protein are displayed on the surfaces of nucleated vertebrate cells

(*d*) β_2-microglobulin is covalently associated with MHC class I protein

30. In an enzyme catalyzed reaction, the initial reaction velocity is only one fourth of its maximum velocity. If the substrate concentration is 3.0×10^{-3} mM. the value of K_m hi micro molar (μM) will be ....

31. Match the following enzymes in column I with their cofactors in column II

Column - I

(P) Pyruvate decarboxylase

(Q) Glyceraldehyde 3-phosphate dehydrogenase

(R) Pyruvate carboxylase

(S) Glucose-6-phosphate dehydrogenase

Column - II

i. Biocytin

ii. $NADP^+$

iii. NAD^+

iv. Thiamine pyrophosphate

(*a*) P-ii, Q-i, R-iv, S-iii

(*b*) P-iv, Q-iii, R-i, S-ii

(*c*) P-i, Q-ii, R-iii, S-iv

(*d*) P-iii, Q-i, R-iv, S-ii

32. Match the molecule in column I with its function in column II

Column - I

(P) Cholera toxin

(Q) Pertussis toxin

(R) IP3

(S) Caffeine

Column -II

i. modifies $G_{\alpha i}$

ii. inhibits c- AMP phosphodiesterase

iii. modifies $G_{\alpha s}$

iv. increases intracellular Ca^{2+} level

(*a*) P-iii, Q-i, R-iv, S-ii

(*b*) P-iv, Q-i, R-iii, S-ii

(*c*) P-ii, Q-iv, R-i, S-iii

(*d*) P-iii, Q-i, R-ii, S-iv

33. In an *in vitro* dehydrogenation reaction of succinate catalyzed by succinate dehydrogenase, malonate is added. Which one of the following curves represents the effect of malonate on the catalysis of succinate dehydrogenase?

(a) 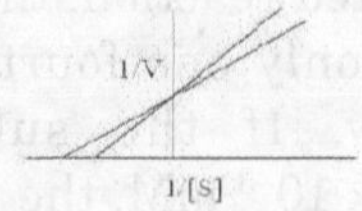

(b) 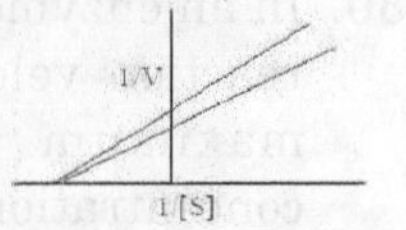

(c) 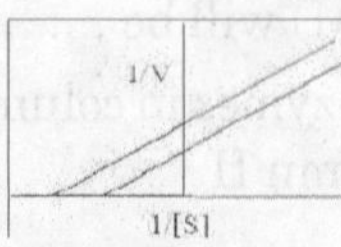

(d) 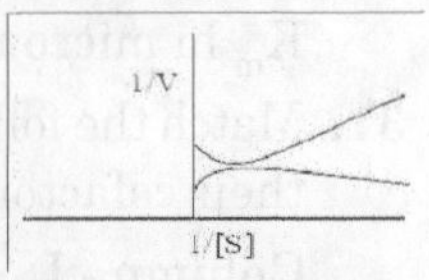

34. Cardiotonic steroids have ability to strengthen heart muscle contraction due to the fact that these steroids

(a) inhibit K^+-dependent dephosphory-lation of Na^+-K^+ ATPase

(b) activate Na^+-K^+ ATPase

(c) increase uptake of Na^+ by activation of Na^+-Ca^{2+} exchanger

(d) increase uptake of Ca^{2+} by activation of Na^+-Ca^{2+} exchanger

35. A newly isolated circular plasmid gave two bands of 3.2 and 3 kb on digestion with EcoRI and two bands of 5.0 kb and 1.2 kb on digestion with BamHI. Double digestion with EcoRI and BamHI, yielded four bands of 2.6 kb, 2.4 kb, 0.8 kb and 0.4 kb. Digestion with SalI led to disruption of ampicillin resistance gene cassette. The correct restriction map is

(a) 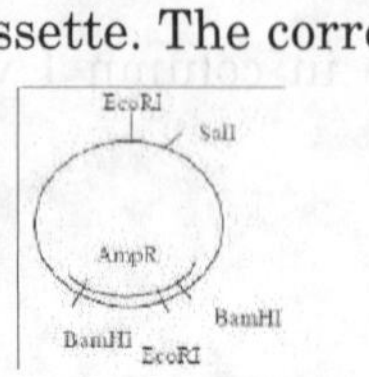

(b) 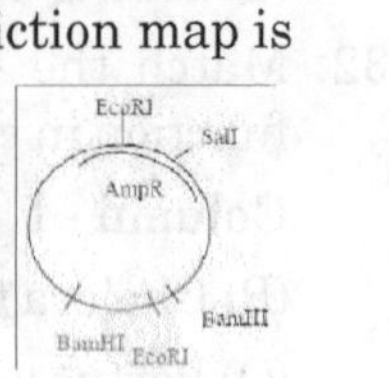

(c) 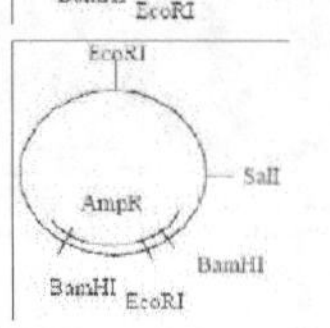

(d) 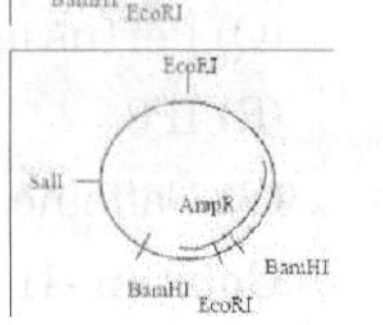

BOTANY

36. As per the Angiosperm Phylogeny Group (APG II. 2003) classification, which of the following plant families comprises of only single genus with single species?

(a) Lauraceae (b) Aristolochiaceae

(c) Amborellaceae (d) Typhaceae

37. A cavity, lysigenous in origin and possessing volatile oil is found in the pericarp of one of the following plants. Identify the CORRECT answer.

(a) Litchi

(b) Citrus

(c) Mango

(d) Coconut

38. Among the following, which genetic material is naturally inherited through maternal inheritance in higher plants?

(a) Nuclear DNA

(b) Plasmid DNA

(c) Chloroplast DNA

(d) T-DNA

39. A typical floral meristem differs from shoot apical meristem on the basis of

(a) Determinate growth

(b) Presence of auxin

(c) Presence of stem cells

(d) Negative geotropism

40. Which of the following plant hormones is a carotenoid-cleavage product?

(a) Phytosulfokine

(b) Brassinosteroid

(c) Methyl jasmonate

(d) Strigolactone

41. Two of the *vir* operons of Ti plasmid in *Agrobacterium tumefaciens* are constitutively expressed. Identify the CORRECT pair.

(a) vir A and virG (b) virF and virH

(c) virC and virD (d) virB and virE

42. Which of the following fungi is an example of obligate biotrophic plant pathogen?

(a) Alternaria brassicicola

(b) Botrytis cinerea

(c) Puccinia triticina

(d) Sclerotina sclerotiorum

43. The phenomenon where an organism lives at the expense of another organism by harming it but not killing, is called

(a) Commensalism

(b) Predation

(c) Symbiosis

(d) Parasitism

44. Which of the following is TRUE for K-strategist species?

(a) Produce relatively large number of offspring

(b) Population often grow exponentially

(c) Provide relatively little or no parental care to offspring

(d) Occur in stable and predictable habitats

45. Identity the INCORRECT statement with relation to plant secondary metabolites.

(*a*) Atropine is a member of indole alkaloids

(*b*) Limonene is a cyclic terpene found in citrus plants

(*c*) Green tea is rich in polyphenols

(*d*) Cyanidin contributes to the red color in rose petals

46. Choose the CORRECT set of matches between group I and group II in relation to nitrogen fixation and assimilation

GROUP I	GROUP II
P. Nitrobacter	1. $NO_3^- \rightarrow NO_2^-$
Q. Nitrite reductase	2. $N_2 \rightarrow 2NH_3$
R. Nitrogenase	3. $NO_2^- \rightarrow NH_4^+$
S. Nitrate reductase	4. $NO_2^- \rightarrow NO_3^-$

(*a*) P-4, Q-3, R-2, S-1 (*b*) P-4, Q-3, R-1, S-2

(*c*) P-1, Q-2, R-4, S-3 (*d*) P-3, Q-4, R-2, S-1

47. Two plant cells M and N are lying side by side making direct contact. "M" has osmotic potential (Ψs) of-10 bar and pressure potential (Ψp) of 4 bar. On the other hand, "N" has osmotic potential (Ψs) of-12 bar and pressure potential (Ψp) of 5 bar.

Based on these data, what would be the direction of movement of water between M and N?

(*a*) M to N

(*b*) N to M

(*c*) There will be no movement

(*d*) In both directions

48. Two independent non-segregating recessive mutants (m1 and m2) display similar defects in petal formation. When they were crossed with each other (m1 x m2), all the F1 plants developed normal petals. In view of this observation, which of the following conclusions is CORRECT?

(*a*) Mutations in both ml and m2 are in the same gene

(*b*) Mutations in both ml and m2 are in two separate genes

(*c*) Inheritance is non-Mendelian

(*d*) None of the above

49. In a hypothetical trihybrid cross of three loci (*viz.* A. B. C). all were inherited in a complete dominant manner over their recessive alleles a, b, c, respectively. When a test cross between F1 and parent 'aabbcc' was performed, following genotypes of eight phenotypically distinct classes were observed with respective numbers

Class	Genotype	Number
1	ABC	412
2	abc	406
3	Abc	85
4	aBC	80
s	ABc	08
6	abC	07
7	AbC	01
8	aBc	01

The genetic distance (up to one decimal) between A and C loci will be________cM.

50. In a typical sexually reproducing angiospermic plant, if an endosperm cell contains 4.8×10^8 nucleotide pairs of DNA. then a microsporocyte of this plant will have________ $\times 10^8$ nucleotide pairs of DNA

51. Identify the CORRECT matching between group I and group II in relation to ecology

Group-I

P. The physical environment of an organism

Q. The totality of the needs of a population for survival and its resource utilization

R. The position of a species in a food chain

S. Basic functional unit comprising living community and its physical environment

Group-II

1. Trophic level
2. Habitat
3. Ecosystem
4. Niche
5. Ecological pyramid

(*a*) P-2, Q-5, R-4, S-1 (*b*) P-2, Q-4, R-1, S-3

(*c*) P-5, Q-2, R-3, S-1 (*d*) P-1, Q-3, R-4, S-2

52. Choose the CORRECT set of matches between group I and group II in relation to plant genetic transformation methods.

GROUP-I	GROUP-II
P. Helium	1. *Agrobacterium tumefaciens*
Q. Acetosyringone	2. Microinjection
R. Polyethylene glycol	3. Particle bombardment
S. Agarose embedding	4. Protoplast

(*a*) P-4, Q-3, R-2, S-I
(B) P-2, Q-1, R-4, S-3
(C) P-3, Q-4, R-1, S-2
(D) P-3, Q-1, R-4, S-2

53. Match the pathogen, disease caused and the affected plant in the CORRECT combination.

Pathogen
P. Blumeri a graminis
Q. Magnaporthe grisea
R. Venturia inaequalis
S. Cercosodra personata

Disease
i. Blast disease
ii. Powdery mildew
iii. Tikka disease
iv. Scab disease

Plant
1. Groundnut 2. Apple
3. Barley 4. Rice

(*a*) P-i-1, Q-ii-2, R-iii-3, S-iv-4
(*b*) P-i-2, Q-ii-1, R-iii-4, S-iv-3
(*c*) P-ii-3, Q-i-4, R-iv-2, S-iii-1
(*d*) P-ii-3, Q-i-4, R-iii-2, S-iv-1

54. Choose the plant part, its use and the source species in CORRECT combination.

Plant Part	Use
P. Bark	i. Insecticide
Q. Leaf	ii. Food colorant
R. Capsule	iii. Flavoring agent
S. Stigma	iv. Analgesic

Species
1. Crocus sativus
2. Papaver somniferum
3. Azadirachta indica
4. Cinnamomum zeylanicum

(*a*) P-i-1, Q-ii-2, R-iii-3, S-iv-4
(*b*) P-iii-4, Q-ii-1, R-iv-2, S-i-3
(*c*) P-ii-1, Q-i-3, R-iv-2, S-iii-4
(*d*) P-iii-4, Q-i-3, R-iv-2, S-ii-1

55. Which TWO of the following reactions are INCORRECT in relation to C_2 oxidative photosynthetic carbon cycle in land plants?

P. 2 (Ribulose-1, 5-biphosphate) + $2(CO_2)$ $\rightarrow$ 2 (phosphoglycolate) + 2 (3-phosphoglycerate) + $4H^+$
Q. Serine + α-ketoglutarate $\rightarrow$ hydroxypyruvate + glutamine
R. 2 (Phosphoglycolate) + $2(H_2O)$ $\rightarrow$ 2 (glycolate) + 2Pi
S. Hydroxypyruvate + NADH + H^+ $\rightarrow$ glycerate + NAD^+

(*a*) P and Q (*b*) Q and R
(*c*) R and S (*d*) S and P

MICROBIOLOGY

56. Which one of the following is the end product of dissimilatory sulfate reduction by sulfate reducing bacteria?
(*a*) Hydrogen sulfide
(*b*) Sulfur dioxide
(*c*) Sulfur
(*d*) Thiosulfate

57. Which one of the following is the terminal electron acceptor in the given metabolic reaction catalyzed by methanogens?

$$4H_2 + CO_2 \longrightarrow CH_4 + 2H_2O$$

(*a*) H_2 (*b*) CO_2
(*c*) CH_4 (*d*) H_2O

58. Microbes that have their optimal growth rate near 15 °C but can still grow at 0 °C to 20 °C are known as
(*a*) mesophiles (*b*) psychrotrophs
(*c*) psychrotolerant (*d*) psychrophiles

59. Which one of the following is NOT a contribution by Robert Koch?
(*a*) Identification of causative agent of anthrax.
(*b*) Discovery of causative agent of tuberculosis.
(*c*) Discovery of causative agent of leprosy.
(*d*) Identification of causative agent of cholera.

60. Unicellular eukaryotic organisms belong to which one of the following kingdoms of classification?
(*a*) Monera (*b*) Plantae
(*c*) Protista (*d*) Animalia

61. Which one of the following is a contagious disease?
(*a*) Chickenpox (*b*) Tetanus
(*c*) Malaria (*d*) Filariasis

62. The inner mitochondrial membrane comprises of a series of folds known as
(*a*) cristae (*b*) thylakoids
(*c*) cisterns (*d*) cilia

63. Which one of the following antibiotics is NOT produced by Streptomyces sp.?
(*a*) Amphotericin B (*b*) Neomycin
(*c*) Vancomycin (*d*) Gentamicin

64. Which one of the following statements is TRUE about MacConkey (MAC) agar medium?
(*a*) MAC agar medium is a selective and differential medium for Gram-positive bacteria.
(*b*) MAC agar medium is a selective and differential medium for Gram-negative bacteria.
(*c*) MAC agar medium is an enriched medium for Gram-positive bacteria.
(*d*) MAC agar medium is a synthetic medium for Gram-positive and Gram-negative bacteria.

65. As an antiseptic, alcohol is effective against
(*a*) bacteria and non-enveloped viruses
(*b*) bacterial endospores and fungi
(*c*) bacteria and fungi
(*d*) fungi and non-enveloped viruses

66. An antigen X was injected into a rabbit for the first time at time P. Then the rabbit was given a booster dose of X at time Q. Which one of the following figures accurately depicts the adaptive immune response by the rabbit against X?

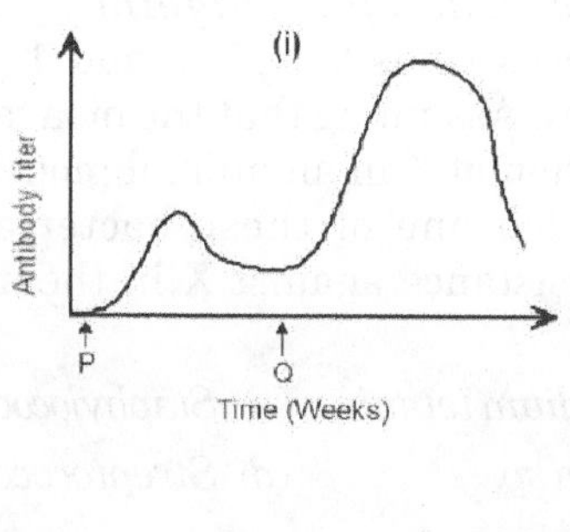

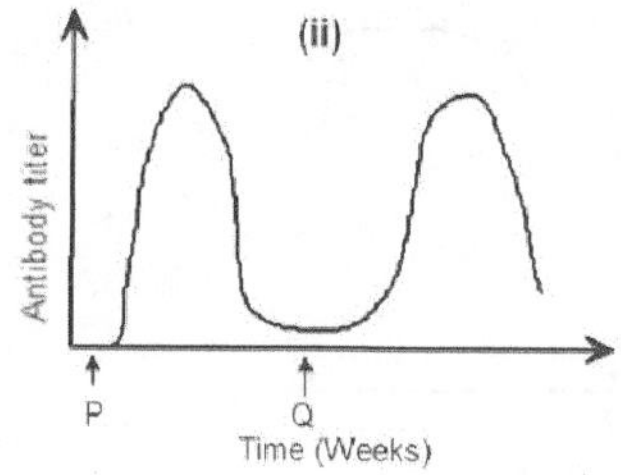

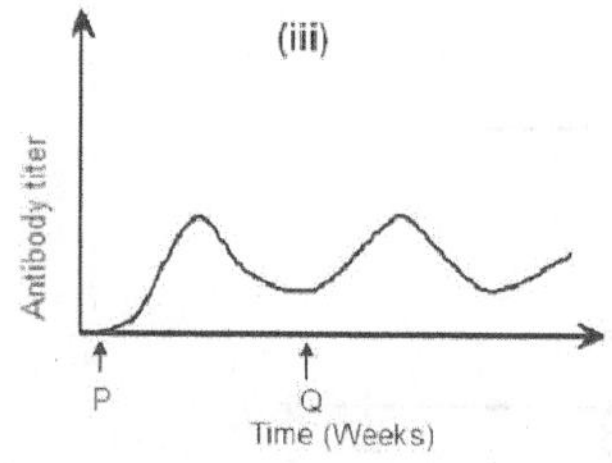

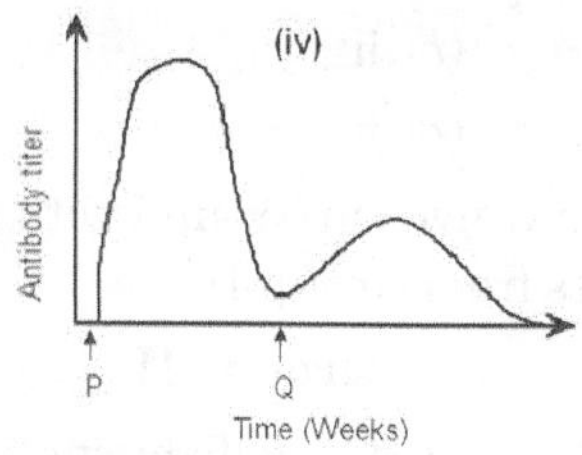

(*a*) i (*b*) ii
(*c*) iii (*d*) iv

67. A bactericidal agent X is added after 3 hours of growth of a bacterial culture. Following the addition of X. the bacterial growth was measured using the standard plate count method till 24 hours. Which one of the following figures is the most accurate representation of the action of X?

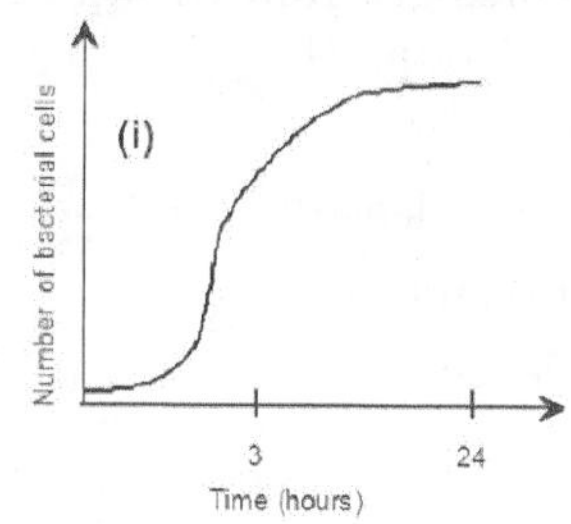

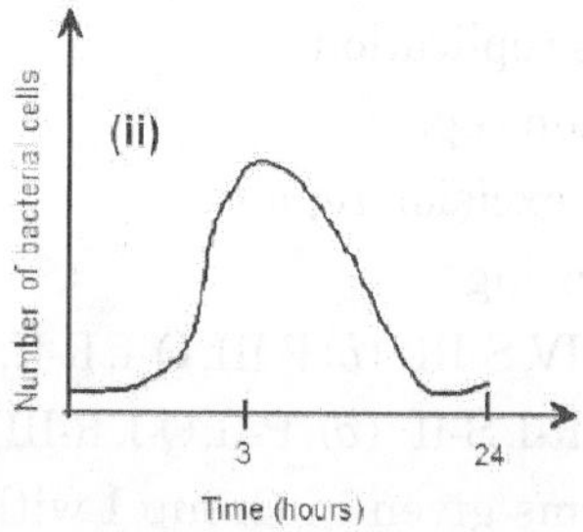

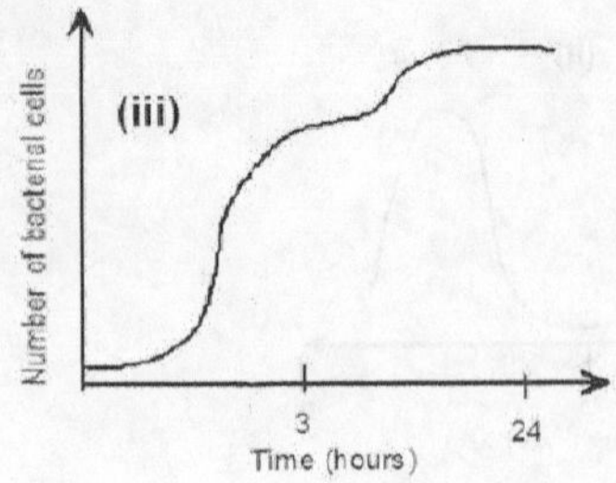

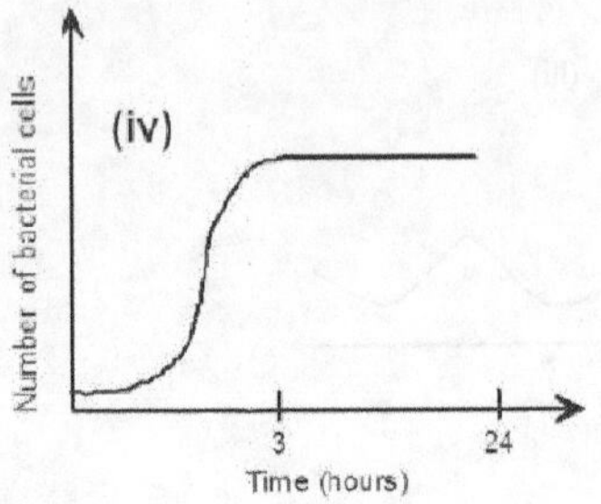

(*a*) i (*b*) ii
(*c*) iii (*d*) iv

68. Match the diseases given in Group-I with their causative agents from Group-II.

Group - I	Group - II
(P) Plague	(I) Coxiella burnetii
(Q) Rabies	(II) Plasmodium spp.
(R) Q fever	(III) Yersinia pestis
(S) Malaria	(IV) Lyssavirus

(*a*) P-III, Q-IV, R-I, S-II
(*b*) P-III, Q-I, R-II, S-IV
(*c*) P-IV, Q-III, R-I, S-II
(*d*) P-III, Q-I, R-IV, S-II

69. Match the enzymes given in Group - I with the events from Group - II.

Group - I
(P) UvrABC endonuclease
(Q) Reverse transcriptase
(R) AP endonuclease
(S) ATP sulfurylase

Group - II
(I) Retro virus replication
(II) Base excision repair
(III) Nucleotide excision repair
(IV) Pyrosequencing

(*a*) P-II, Q-I, R-IV, S-III (*b*) P-III, Q-I, R-II, S-IV
(*c*) P-IV, Q-III, R-I, S-II (*d*) P-II, Q-I, R-III, S-IV

70. Match the terms given in Group I with the descriptions from Group II.

Group - I
(P) Photoautotrophs
(Q) Chemoautotrophs
(R) Photoheterotrophs
(S) Chemoheterotrophs

Group - II
(I) Use inorganic chemical reactions for energy production
(II) Use organic compounds for energy production
(III) Use sunlight as energy source and carbon dioxide as carbon source
(IV) Use sunlight as energy sourcl and organic compounds as carbon source

(*a*) P-II, Q-I, R-IV, S-III (*b*) P-III, Q-I, R-IV, S-II
(*c*) P-IV, Q-III, R-I, S-II (*d*) P-II, Q-IV, R-III, S-I

71. One-nil sample of a bacterial culture was serially diluted to 10^5 times, and 46 colonies were obtained after plating this diluted sample on an agar medium. The number of cells present per ml in the undiluted original sample were ______.

72. The transformation efficiency of competent cells prepared in a laboratory is 10^4CFU/μg of plasmid DNA. If 0.01 μg of this plasmid is used to transform these competent cells, the number of transformed bacteria in CFU after plating will be ______

73. Assume that the average DNA content of a single microbial cell is 4 femtogram. A soil sample analyzed for its microbial community DNA is found to contain 0.32 μg DNA per gram of the soil. The number of microbial cells per milligrem of the soil are ______.

74. Assume that a bacterial culture has a mean generation time of 2 hours. If the number of bacteria present after 24 hours of culture are 4.1×10^7, the initial number of bacteria present were ______.

75. The minimal inhibitory concentration (MIC) of an antibiotic X against *Clostridium tetani*, *Staphylococcus sp.*, *Shigella sp.*, and *Streptococcus sp.* is 25. 15. 2 and 1 μg/ml. respectively. Assuming that the bioavailable concentration of X in an animal model is 20 μg/ml. which one of these bacteria may develop resistance against X in the animal model?

(*a*) *Clostridium tetani* (*b*) *Staphylococcus sp.*
(*c*) *Shigella sp.* (*d*) *Streptococcus sp.*

ZOOLOGY

76. The characteristic feature of deuterostomes is depicted by
   (*a*) coelom formed by the hollowing out of a previously solid cord of mesodermal cells
   (*b*) Spiral and determinate cleavage
   (*c*) formation of mouth from blastopore
   (*d*) formation of anus from blastopore

77. One of the most remarkable features of evolution is the formation of amnion and allantoin. This appeared for the "first time" in evolutionary time scale in
   (*a*) reptiles (*b*) birds
   (*c*) fishes (*d*) humans

78. A woman with blood group A gave birth to a baby with blood group AB. The blood group of the father would be
   (*a*) only AB (*b*) only B
   (*c*) either AB or B (*d*) blood group O

79. The enzyme amylase can break alpha glycosidic linkages between glucose monomers. Hence. amylase can digest which one of the following carbohydrates?
   (*a*) Cellulose (*b*) Starch
   (*c*) Chitin (*d*) Xylans

80. The metabolic pathway which is common to both fermentation and cellular respiration is
   (*a*) the TCA cycle
   (*b*) the election transport chain
   (*c*) glycolysis
   (*d*) synthesis of acetyl CoA from pyruvate

81. A female "Spotted sand piper" courts males repeatedly. This behavior can be explained by the term
   (*a*) polyandry
   (*b*) polygyny
   (*c*) monogamy
   (*d*) sexual cannibalism

82. Malaria is caused by *Plasmodium* species, which is a parasite having a complex life cycle. The fusion between male and female gametocytes of *Plasmodium* happens inside
   (*a*) human liver
   (*b*) human RBCs
   (*c*) mosquito midgut
   (*d*) mosquito salivary glands

83. Aromatase inhibitors are often prescribed for post-menopausal women to treat estrogen receptor positive breast cancer patients, because these class of drugs
   (*a*) reduce prostaglandin biosynthesis
   (*b*) reduce the level of estradiol biosynthesis
   (*c*) inhibit conversion of testosterone to dihydrotestosterone
   (*d*) are non-toxic in post-menopausal women

84. The covalent modification performed by kinases which regulate proteins in signaling pathways is
   (*a*) glycosylation (*b*) methylation
   (*c*) ubiquitination (*d*) phosphorylation

85. Which one of the following statements is NOT correct?
   (*a*) During metaphase, the 2 copies of chromosomal DNA are held together at the centromere
   (*b*) The short arm of chromosomes is referred to as p and the long arm is referred to as q
   (*c*) The terminal structures at the end of the chromatids are referred to as telomeres
   (*d*) The terms heterochromatin and euchromatin refer to the active and repressed regions of the chromosome respectively

86. A particular species is found to have $2n = 16$ chromosomes. The number of linkage groups in this species will be ___.

87. In the Meselson and Stahl experiment. *E. coli* was grown in a medium containing $^{15}NH_4Cl$. After 24 hours. *E. coli* were transferred to medium containing $^{14}NH_4Cl$. After the fourth generation in medium containing $^{14}NH_4Cl$. the ratio between hybrids ($^{15}N/^{14}N$) and light ($^{14}N/^{14}N$) labeled DNA will be 1: *n*, where the value of *n* is _______.

88. The population data present in an island is as follows

Genotype	Number
AA	300
Aa	500
aa	200
Total	1000

The allele frequency of A (upto two decimals) will be ________.

89. A cell in G1 phase has 16 chromosomes. The total number of chromatids that would be found per cell during Metaphase II of meiosis are ________

90. Upon activation of phospholipase C by ligand binding to G-protein coupled receptor, the Ca^{+2} concentration in cytosol will

(*a*) decrease due to blockage of $InsP_3$ gated channel on endoplasmic reticulum

(*b*) decrease due to blockage of $InsP_3$ gated channel on plasma membrane

(*c*) increase due to efflux of Ca^{+2} from $InsP_3$ gated channel on mitochondria

(*d*) increase due to efflux of Ca^{+2} from $InsP_3$ gated channel on endoplasmic reticulum as well as influx of Ca^{+2} from $InsP_3$ gated channel on plasma membrane

91. Match the following molecules in Group I with their function in Group II

Group I	Group II
P. Transferrin	(i) Uptake of glucose
Q. Insulin	(ii) Binds iron
R. α-macroglobulin	(iii) Substratum for cell attachment
S. Fibronectin	(iv) Proteinase inhibitor
	(v) Binds to oxygen in RBC

(*a*) P-ii, Q-i, R-iv, S-iii (*b*) P-ii, Q-i, R-v, S-iii

(*c*) P-ii, Q-i, R-iv, S-ii (*d*) P-i, Q-iii, R-ii, S-v

92. If a heavy chain of an antibody molecule weighs 65,000 Daltons (Da) and a light chain weighs 25,000 Da, the approximate calculated weight of an IgM antibody in Da will be

(*a*) 90,000 (*b*) 180,000

(*c*) 360,000 (*d*) 900,000

93. MATCH the signaling pathways in Group I with their functions in Group II, during the process of development

Group - I

P. Hedgehog signaling

Q. Hox proteins

R. Wnt signaling

S. Notch signaling

Group - II

(i) Involved in signaling at 4-cell embryo stage in *C. elegans* through *glp 1* expression

(ii) Involves frizzled receptor on target cell membrane and establish polarity in insects

(iii) Plays critical role in facial morphogenesis in vertebrates and its mutation causes cyclopia

(iv) Required for *T-bx* transcription factor expression for vertebrate limb development

(*a*) P-iii: Q-ii: R-iv: S-i

(*b*) P-iii: Q-iv; R-ii: S-i

(*c*) P-iv: Q-iii: R-ii: S-i

(*d*) P-iii: Q-iv: R-i: S-ii

94. In a population which is in Hardy-Weinberg equilibrium, the frequency of the recessive genotype of a certain trait is 0.09. The percentage of individuals with heterozygous genotype is ______%

95. An enzyme preparation has activity of 2 Units per 20 μl, and protein concentration 0.4 mg/ml. The specific activ ity (Units/mg) of this enzyme will be ________.

FOOD TECHNOLOGY

96. Indicate the correct group that contains a monosaccharide, a disaccharide and a trisaccharide.

(*a*) Glucose, sucrose, mannose

(*b*) Ribose, lactose, raffinose

(*c*) Mannose, maltose, lactose

(*d*) Raffionose, stachyose, glucose

97. In which of the following products. 'must' is used as the substrate for fermentation?

(*a*) Beer

(*b*) Wine

(*c*) Idli

(*d*) Tempeh

98. Identify the foodborne illness is not caused by bacteria.

(*a*) Botulism

(*b*) Listeriosis

(*c*) Vibriosis

(*d*) Cysticercosis

99. Nutrient composition of wheat flour changes with extent of extraction from whole wheat grain. Which of the following statements is true if the extraction rate increased from 50% to 90%?

(*a*) Starch increases, protein increases, fat increases, mineral increases

(*b*) Starch decreases, protein increases, fat increases, mineral increases

(*c*) Starch decreases, protein decreases, fat increases, mineral decreases

(*d*) Starch decreases, protein increases, fat decreases, mineral decreases

100. You have two samples of milk, one (X) with 3.8% fat and another (Y) with 0.5% fat. In order to produce a milk with 3.5% fat. 100 ml of Y should be mixed with _______ ml of X.

101. Match the items in column I with the items in column II in relation to food safety and standards.

	Column I		Column II
P.	HACCP	1.	International food standards
Q.	FSSAI	2.	Quality control protocol
R.	CIP	3.	Food plant sanitation and hygiene protocol
S.	CODEX	4.	Indian food standards

(*a*) P-2, Q-4, R-3, S-1 (*b*) P-4, Q-3, R-2, S-1

(*c*) P-1, Q-4, R-2, S-3 (*d*) P-4, Q-2, R-3, S-1

102. A 50% sucrose solution at 20°C is flowing at a rate of 3.5 m^3/h through a pipe with an inside diameter of 0.0475 m and length of 12 m. The viscosity and the density of the solution are 15.43 cp and 1232 kg/m^3, respectively. The Reynolds number of the follow is ________

103. In a pineapple juice, fibre particles having mean diameter of 160 μm and density of 1075 kg/m^3 are settling by gravity. If the density and viscosity of the juice are 1015 kg/m^3 and 0.98 cp, respectively, terminal velocity of the fibre particles is ______ mm/s.

104. Power consumption in liquid mixing is proportional to _______.

(*a*) Power number × liquid density × (rotational speed)^3 × (impeller diameter)^5

(*b*) Power number × liquid density × (rotational speed)^2 × (impeller diameter)^3

(*c*) Liquid density × viscosity of the liquid × (rotational speed)^2 × (impeller diameter)^3

(*d*) Acceleration due to gravity × liquid density × (rotational speed)^3 × (impeller diameter)^5

105. In dye-reduction test for estimation of viable microorganisms, the most commonly used dyes are methylene blue, triphenyltetrazolium-chloride and ______.

(*a*) Malachite green (*b*) Amaranth

(*c*) Tartrazine (*d*) Resazurin

106. Match the following items of group I with the items of group II in relation to the quality of fat.

	Group - I		Group - II
P.	Saponification number	1.	Unsaturation of fatty acid
Q.	Iodine number	2.	Volatile water soluble fattry acid
R.	Reichert Meissl number	3.	Hydroxy fatty acid
S.	Acetyl value	4.	Molecular weight of fatty acid

(*a*) P-1, Q-2, R-3, S-4 (*b*) P-1, Q-3, R-4, S-2

(*c*) P-4, Q-1, R-2, S-3 (*d*) P-2, Q-1, R-3, S-4

107. Match the following metabolic product (column I) that indicates the quality of food (Column II).

	Column I		Column II
P.	Ethanol	1.	Canned vegetable
Q.	Lactic acid	2.	Fish
R.	Trimethylamine	3.	Butter
S.	Volatile fatty acid	4.	Apple juice

(*a*) P-3, Q-2, R-4, S-1 (*b*) P-4, Q-1, R-2, S-3

(*c*) P-4, Q-3, R-2, S-1 (*d*) P-3, Q-4, R-2, S-1

108. Correlate the vitamins in column I with their role in promoting reaction/process in column II.

	Column I		Column II
P.	Riboflavin	1.	Visual cycle
Q.	Vitamin D	2.	Acyl group transfer
R.	Pantothenic acid	3.	Regulation of Ca^{2+} metabolism
S.	Vitamin A	4.	Oxidation-reduction reaction

(*a*) P-1, Q-2, R-4, S-3 (*b*) P-2, Q-1, R-3, S-4

(*c*) P-3, Q-4, R-1, S-2 (*d*) P-4, Q-3, R-2, S-1

109. A pure strain with generation time of 60 min is used in a fermentation process. Following inoculation (0 h), the strain takes 2 h for adaptation, 10 h to achieve maximum growth rate. If the inoculation load is 100 cells, the total population at the end of 10 h will be ______.

110. Refer to the shear stress – shear rate plot shown in the figure below. Match the lines (Column I) with appropriate rheological behavior (Column II).

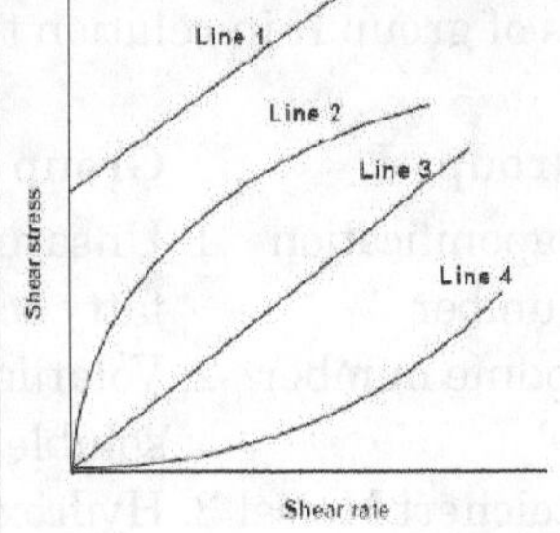

Column I	Column II
P. Line 1	1. Dilatant
Q. Line 2	2. Newtonian
R. Line 3	3. Pseudoplastic
S. Line 4	4. Bingham plastic

(*a*) P-2, Q-3, R-4, S-1
(*b*) P-1, Q-3, R-4, S-2
(*c*) P-2, Q-4, R-3, S-1
(*d*) P-4, Q-3, R-2, S-1

111. Water flowing at a rate of 1 kg/min is heated from 12 to 80°C with flue gas supplied at a rate of 3 kg/min. The temperature and specific heat of the flue gas are 180°C and 1.05 kJ/kg.K, respectively. If specific heat of water is 4.2 kJ/kg.K and the flow is parallel, then the logarithmic mean temperature difference will be ______ °C.

112. The Lineweaver-Burk plot of an enzymatic reaction shows V_{max} of 160 μmol/l.min and k_m of 60 μmol/l. For a substrate concentration of 40 μmol/l, the velocity of the reaction is estimated to be ______ μmol/l.min.

113. A suspension containing 2×10^4 spores of organism A having a $D_{121.1°C}$ value of 1.5 min and 8×10^5 spores of organism B having a $D_{121.1°C}$ value of 0.8 min is heated at a constant temperature of 121.1°C. The heating time needed to obtain a probability of spoilage '1 in 1000' is ______ min.

114. In an evaporation process, a compressor picks up 0.05 m^3 air in each revolution and compresses 500 kg of air per minute. If the specific volume of air is 0.9 m^3/kg, then the compressor speed is ______ rpm.

115. For a soybean oil extraction system, solvent:soy ratio is maintained at 0.5:1(w/w). Original seed contains 18% oil (w/w). If the meal (soy solid) after final desolventization has 0.01 kg oil per kg oil free meal, then the effectiveness of the solvent (kg oil/kg solvent) in the extraction process is ______.

GENERAL APTITUDE

116. The event would have been successful if you ______ able to come.

(*a*) are (*b*) had been
(*c*) have been (*d*) would have been

117. There was no doubt that their work was <u>thorough</u>.

Which of the words below is closest in meaning to the underlined word above?

(*a*) pretty (*b*) complete
(*c*) sloppy (*d*) haphazard

118. Four cards lie on a table. Each card has a number printed on one side and a colour on the other. The faces visible on the cards are 2, 3, red and blue.

Proposition: If a card has an even value on one side, then its opposite face is red.

The cards which MUST be turned over to verify the above proposition are

(A) 2, red (B) 2, 3, red
(C) 2, blue (D) 2, red, blue

119. What is the value of *x* when

$$81 \times \left(\frac{16}{25}\right)^{x+2} \div \left(\frac{3}{5}\right)^{2x+4} = 144?$$

(*a*) 1
(*b*) –1
(*c*) –2
(*d*) Cannot be determined

120. Two dice are thrown simultaneously. The probability that the product of the numbers appearing on the top faces of the dice is a perfect square is

(*a*) 1/9 (*b*) 2/9
(*c*) 1/3 (*d*) 4/9

121. Bhaichung w as observing the pattern of people entering and leaving a car service centre. There was a single window where customers were being served. He saw that people inevitably came out of the centre in the order that they went in. However, the time they spent inside seemed to vary a lot: some people came out in a matter of minutes while for others it took much longer.

From this, what can one conclude?

(*a*) The centr e operates on a first-come-first-served basis, but with variable service times, depending on specific customer needs.

(*b*) Customers were served in an arbitrary order, since they took varying amounts of time for service completion in the centre.

(*c*) Since some people came out within a few minutes of entering the centre, the system is likely to operate on a last-come-first-served basis.

(*d*) Entering the centre early ensured that one would have shorter service times and most people attempted to do this.

122. A map shows the elevations of Darjeeling. Gangtok. Kalimpong, Pelling. and Siliguri. Kalimpong is at a lower elevation than Gangtok. Pelling is at a lower elevation than Gangtok. Pelling is at a higher elev ation than Siliguri. Darjeeling is at a higher elevation than Gangtok.

Which of the following statements can be inferred from the paragraph above?

i. Pelling is at a higher elevation than Kalimpong

ii. Kalimpong is at a lower elevation than Darjeeling

iii. Kalimpong is at a higher elevation than Siliguri

iv. Siliguri is at a lower elevation than Gangtok

(*a*) Only ii

(*b*) Only ii and iii

(*c*) Only ii and iv

(*d*) Only iii and iv

123. P, Q, R, S, T and U are seated around a circular table. R is seated two places to the right of Q, P is seated three places to the left of R, S is seated opposite U. If P and U now switch seats, which of the following must necessarily be true?

(*a*) P is immediately to the right of R

(*b*) T is immediately to the left of P

(*c*) T is immediately to the left of P or P is immediately to theright of Q

(*d*) U is immediately to the right of R or P is immediately tothe left of T.

124. Budhan covers a distance of 19 km in 2 hours by cycling one fourth of the time and walking the rest. The next day he cycles (at the same speed as before) for half the time and walks the rest (at the same speed as before) and covers 26 km in 2 hours. The speed in km/h at which Budhan walks is

(*a*) 1

(*b*) 4

(*c*) 5

(*d*) 6

125. The points in the graph below represent the halts of a lift for durations of 1 minute, over a period of 1 hour.

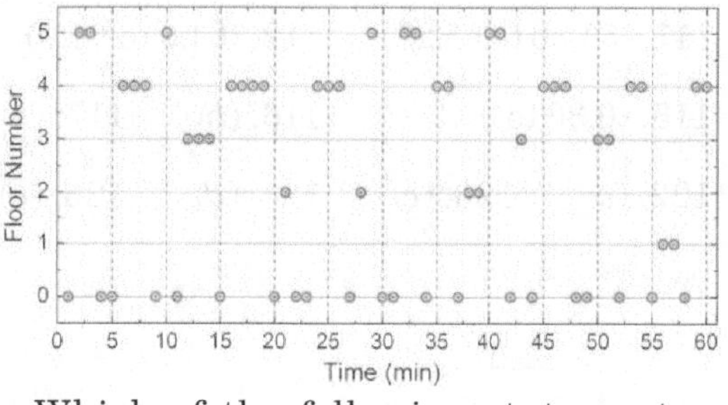

Which of the following statements are correct?

i. The elevator never moves directly from any non-ground floor to another non-ground floor over the one hour period

ii. The elevator stays on the fourth floor for the longest duration over the one hour period

(*a*) Only i (*b*) Only ii

(*c*) Both i and ii (*d*) Neither i nor ii

ANSWERS

1. (*a*) 2. (*d*) 3. (*d*) 4. (*b*) 5. (*a*) 6. (*c*) 7. (*b*) 8. (*c*) 9. (*c*)
10. (*b*) 11. (*a*) 12. (13260 to 13285) 13. (*a*) 14. (*c*) 15. (*a*) 16. (*a*) 17. (*d*)
18. (*c*) 19. (3.0 to 3.0) 20. (*b*) 21. (*d*) 22. (*c*) 23. (*a*) 24. (*c*) 25. (*d*)
26. (7575 to 7576) 27. (722 to 725) 28. (0.192 to 0.20) 29. (*d*) 30. (9.0 to 9.0)
31. (*b*) 32. (*a*) 33. (*a*) 34. (*a*) 35. (*b*) 36. (*c*) 36. (*c*) 37. (*b*) 38. (*c*)
39. (*a*) 40. (*d*) 41. (*a*) 42. (*c*) 43. (*d*) 44. (*d*) 45. (*a*) 46. (*a*) 47. (*a*)
48. (*b*) 49. (18.3 to 18.5) 50. (3.2 to 3.2) 51. (*b*) 52. (*d*) 53. (*c*) 54. (*d*)
55. (*a*) 56. (*a*) 57. (*b*) 58. (*d*) 59. (*c*) 60. (*c*) 61. (*a*) 62. (*a*) 63. (*d*)
64. (*b*) 65. (*c*) 66. (*a*) 67. (*b*) 68. (*a*) 69. (*b*) 70. (*b*)
71. (4550000 to 4650000) 72. (99 to 101) 73. (98000 to 82000)
74. (9990 to 10020) 75. (*a*) 76. (*d*) 77. (*a*) 78. (*c*) 79. (*b*) 80. (*c*) 81. (*a*)
82. (*c*) 83. (*b*) 84. (*d*) 85. (*d*) 86. (8.0 to 8.0) 87. (7.0 to 7.0)
88. (0.55 to 0.55) 89. (16 to 16) 90. (*d*) 91. (*a*) 92. (*b,d*) 93. (*b*)
94. (42.0 to 42.0) 95. (250 to 250) 96. (*b*) 97. (*b*) 98. (*d*) 99. (*b*)
100. (1000 to 1000) 101. (*a*) 102. (2078 to 2086) 103. (0.80 to 0.90) 104. (*a*)
105. (*d*) 106. (*c*) 107. (*b*) 108. (*d*) 109. (25550 to 25650) 110. (*d*)
111. (53.30 to 55.25) 112. (64.0 to 64.0) 113. (10.80 to 11.20) 114. (9000 to 9000)
115. (0.30 to 0.40) 116. (*b*) 117. (*b*) 118. (*c*) 119. (*b*) 120. (*b*) 121. (*a*)
122. (*c*) 123. (*c*) 124. (*d*) 125. (*d*)

EXPLANATIONS

1. The oxidation state of carbon in each CO is +2 so it readily reacts with Fe which has $3d^6$ $4S^2$ electronic configuration.
2. Isoelectronic refer to two atoms or molecules that have same electronic structure and same number of valence electron. In given question OF_2 and O_3^- have different valence electron i.e. 20 and 19 respectively. However other molecules given in option (A), (B) and (c) have 16 valence electron.
3. Physical properties of materials and systems can often be categorized as being either **intensive** or **extensive** quantities, according to how the property changes when the size (or extent) of the system changes. According to IUPAC, an intensive property is one whose magnitude is independent of the size of the system. An extensive property is one whose magnitude is additive for subsystems.

   Extensive property is additive for subsystems. This means the system could be divided into any number of subsystems, and the extensive property measured for each subsystem; the value of the property for the system would be the sum of the property for each subsystem. For example, both i.e. mass (*m*) and the volume (V) of a diamond are directly proportional to the amount that is left after cutting it from the raw mineral. Mass and volume are extensive properties, but hardness is intensive.
4. In the given reaction, the compound is heated with alcoholic potassium hydroxide and chloroform. If a primary amine is present in compound then isocyanides (carbylamines) is formed in which (NH_2) is foul smelling substance. Histamine contains the amine group among given compounds.
5. Structure (i) is soluble in water and having least reactivity with water. Structure (ii) 25 % soluble in water and having low reactivity with water. Structure (iii) React with OH ion and undergo hydration reaction. Structure (iv) readily react with water.
6. SCl_2 and ClO_2^- molecules having non-linear structures
7. The bond lengths for:

   O_2 = 148 Pm;

   B_2 = 159 Pm;

   N_2 = 145 Pm;

   C_2 = 154 Pm.
8. CFSE = $E_{ligand} - E_{isotropic\ field}$;

   Crystal field stabilization energies depend on the total d-electrons available on octahedral configuration. The stability of the given compound follows the following order as per Irving- Williams series.

   $Mn^{+2} < Ti^{+2} < Zn^{+2} < V^{+2}$.
9. He atom has $1S^2$ structure. The ground state energy is E = 79 eV; Energy required to remove 1 electron is E_1 = 24.6 eV.

   Therefore the first ionization energy of He atom = 79.00 – 24.6 = 54.4 eV.
10. We know that $r = k\,(A_0)^x\,(B_0)^y$

    Given, $r_1 = r$; $r_2 = 4r$; $r_3 = 2r$

    Therefore $r_1 = k\,(0.1)^x\,(0.1)^y$

    or $r = k\,(0.1)^x\,(0.1)^y$ ...(i)

    $r_2 = k\,(0.2)^x\,(0.1)^y$

    or $4r = k\,(0.2)^x\,(0.1)^y$ ...(ii)

    $r_3 = k\,(0.1)^x\,(0.2)^y$

    or $2r = k\,(0.1)^x\,(0.2)^y$ ...(iii)

    Now, Divide equation (iii) with equation (i)

    $2r/r = (0.2/0.1)^y$

    $2 = (2)^y$

    or $y = 1$;

    Now Divide equation (ii) with (i)

    $4r/r = (0.2/0.1)^x$

    $4 = (2)^x$

    or $x = 2$

    Therefore overall order of the reaction

    $= x + y = 3$
11. $$E_{cell} = E^{\circ}_{cell} - \frac{0.05916}{Z}\log Q$$

    and $$Q = \frac{[Ag^{+}0.01M]}{[Ag^{+}1M]}$$

$$= \frac{(0.01)}{(1)}$$

Where Z is no. of electron transfered = 1

$$\therefore \quad E^{\circ}_{cell} = \underset{Ag^+}{0.80} - \underset{Ag^+}{0.80} = 0$$

$$\therefore \quad E_{cell} = 0.0118 \approx 0.12$$

12. $\pi = mRT \Rightarrow M = \frac{\pi}{RT}$

$$= \frac{\frac{1.4}{760}}{0.082 \times 298}$$

$$= 7.5385 \times 10^{-5}\ M$$

$$\therefore \text{ Molar mass of protein} = \frac{1}{7.585 \times 10^{-5}}$$

$$= 13265.3\ g/mol.$$

13. P :

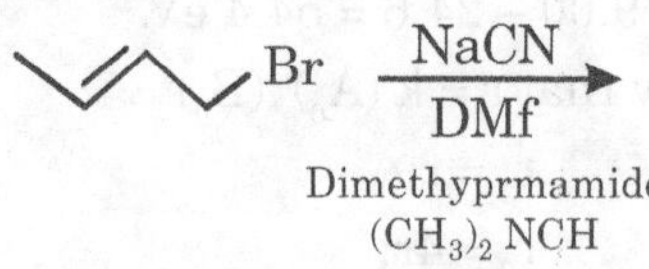

Q :

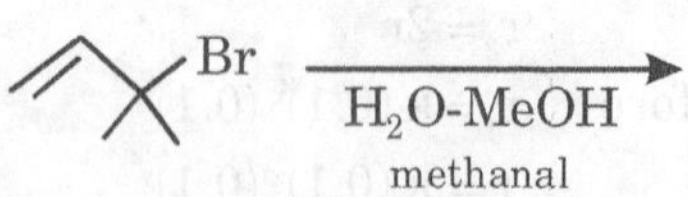

For P, SN_1 reaction of methyle helide (R – Br) is never happen, only SN_2 type reaction occured which is given by option (a) for Q main reaction is with strong bases such as OH^- from MeOH 4 and thus.

for tertiary (R_3C – Br). Compound only SN^1 reaction is possible which is given by option (*a*).

14.

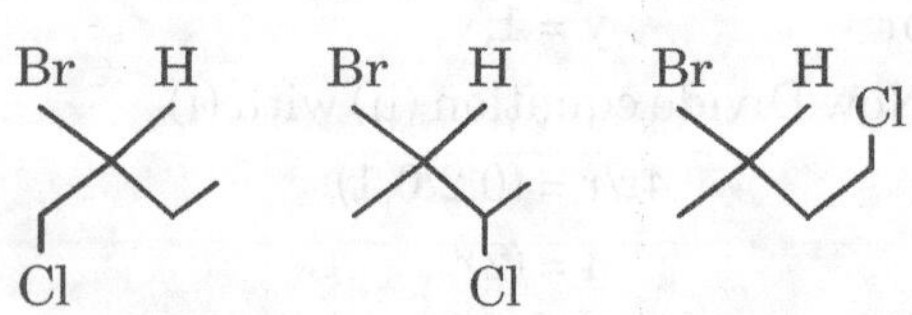

(1) (2) (3)

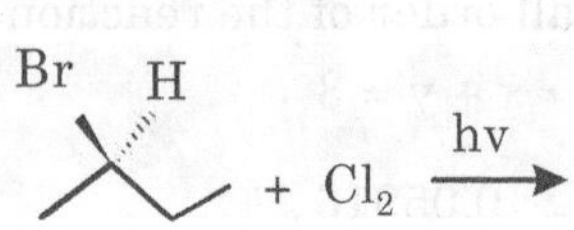

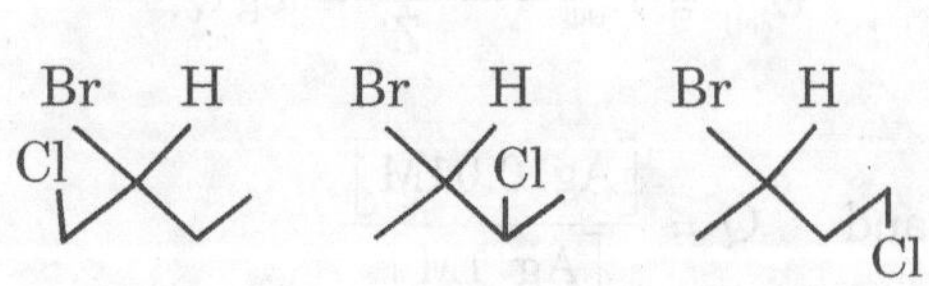

(4) (5) (6)

16. .Native-page: everything in-tact, separated by size and charge or shape.

SDS-page non-reducing: S-S are intact but protein is denatured

SDS-page reducing: S-S become reduced protein is still denatured.

In a native gel, you don't denature the protein at all. So the 3D shape becomes important in determining how the protein migrates. In a non-reducing SDS-PAGE, you still denature the protein - you just leave the disulfide bridges intact. So the protein will be mostly denatured and if it has disulfides, those will convey some 3D structure but very minimal compared to native gels.

If a protein has multiple subunits that are held together by disulfides, then those subunits will come apart under reducing SDS but not under non-reducing SDS. In other words, you'll see low-weight units under reducing conditions but heavier fragments under non-reducing SDS. If you ran a native gel on the same protein, you would see either apparently "lighter" or apparently "heavier" fragments than non-reducing SDS, depending on whether the protein is globular, predominantly beta-sheeted, etc. Keep in mind that disulfides can exist independently of subunits. So disulfides could be intra-unit and not function to hold multiple subunits together but rather to hold bits and pieces of one subunit together to convey local 3D topology.

17. **Edman degradation** is a method of sequencing amino acids in a peptide. In this method, the amino-terminal residue is labeled and cleaved from the peptide without disrupting the peptide bonds between other amino acid residues. **Sanger sequencing** is a method of DNA sequencing based on the selective incorporation of chain-terminating dideoxynucleotides by DNA polymerase during in vitro DNA replication. **Peptide mass fingerprinting (PMF)** is an analytical technique for *protein* identification in which the unknown protein of interest is first cleaved into smaller peptides, whose absolute masses can be accurately measured with a *mass spectrometer* such as **MALDI-TOF** or **ESI-TOF**. The peptide masses are compared to either a database containing known protein sequences or even the genome.The pattern of fragmentation of a peptide allows for direct determination of its sequence by **de novo sequencing**. This sequence may be used to match databases of protein sequences or to investigate post-translational or chemical modifications. It may provide additional evidence for protein identification.

18. Out of given 4 types of gel, the 12% gel, pH 3-10 type of polyacrylamide gel can be used for analysing the given four different proteins. The high percentage gel will not be able to resolve proteins of very narrow size range. Low % of gel is important for easy mobility of proteins. pH range should be picked in such a way that all pI (isoelectric point) of proteins must fall with in this range.

19. The aspartate residue (Asp 189) located in the catalytic pocket (S1) of trypsin is responsible for attracting and stabilizing positively charged lysine and/or arginine, and is, thus, responsible for the specificity of the enzyme. This means that trypsin predominantly cleaves proteins at the carboxyl side (or "C-terminal side") of the amino acids lysine and arginine except when either is bound to a C-terminal proline. Trypsin is considered an endopeptidase, i.e., the cleavage occurs within the polypeptide chain rather than at the terminal amino acids located at the ends of polypeptides. Therefore the number of fragments generated when the peptide ANDCQEGKFMLKPDTWRYVSFMRPA will be 3 i.e. (i) ANDCQEGK (ii) FMLKPDTWR (iii) YVSFMRPA

20. Puromycin (amino nucleoside antibiotic) is an analogue of the 3' end of a tyrosyl-tRNA with a part of its structure mimics a molecule of adenosine, and the other part mimics a molecule of tyrosine. Compared to the cleavable ester bond in a tyrosyl-tRNA, puromycin has anon-hydrolysable amide bond. As a result, puromycin interferes with translation, and causes premature release of translation products taking place in the ribosome.

21. **Arsenic poisoning** is a medical condition that occurs due to elevated levels of arsenic in the body. Arsenic interferes with cellular longevity by allosteric inhibition of an essential metabolic enzyme pyruvate dehydrogenase (PDH) complex, which catalyzes the oxidation of pyruvate to acetyl-CoA by NAD+. With the enzyme inhibited, the energy system of the cell is disrupted resulting in a cellular apoptosis.

22. The pentose phosphate pathway and the Calvin cycle have in common several enzymes and intermediates that attest to an evolutionary kinship. Like glycolysis and gluconeogenesis, these pathways are mirror images of one another: the Calvin cycle uses NADPH to reduce carbon dioxide to generate hexoses, whereas the pentose phosphate pathway breaks down glucose into carbon dioxide to generate NADPH. The Calvin cycle is sometimes referred to as the *reductive pentose phosphate pathway*.

Calvin cycle is part of the photosynthetic CO_2 fixation carried out in the chloroplasts, vegetable cell organelles. Chloroplasts are surrounded by a double outer membrane and contain in their interior membrane structures called thylakoids, which are piled up into stakes called grana. Grana bear chlorophyll and the enzymes responsible for the light reactions of photosynthesis leading to the synthesis of ATP and NADPH. The grana are immersed in the stroma, the gel-like matrix of the chloroplasts containing prokaryotic DNA, RNA, 70 S ribosomes, and soluble enzymes implicated in several biosynthetic processes such as fatty acids, isoprenoids, amino acids, nucleotides and conversion of CO_2 to carbohydrates, etc. This last conversion, carried out with the help of ATP and NADPH generated in the photosynthetic reactions, is called the Calvin cycle, reductive pentose phosphate pathway, or photosynthetic carbon reduction cycle. Three phases can be considered in the Calvin cycle: fixation of CO_2 into 3-phosphoglycerate (3PG), or the *carboxylation* phase; reduction of 3PG into glyceraldehyde-3-phosphate (GAP), or the *reduction*phase; and resynthesis of ribulose-1,5-bisphosphate, or the *regenerative* phase.

23. Primaquine is primarily used to prevent relapse of malaria due to Plasmodium vivax and Plasmodium ovale. It eliminates

hypnozoites, the dormant liver form of the parasite, after the plasmodia have been cleared from the bloodstream. Primaquine should not be administered to anyone with G6PD deficiency because a severe reaction can occur, resulting in hemolytic anemia. G6PD enzyme was demonstrated to play an active role in survival of erythrocytes for the production of NADPH and GSH. So it will increases the demand of NADPH level to cells.

24. In many naturally occurring bilayers, the compositions of the inner and outer membrane leaflets are different. In human red blood cells, the inner (cytoplasmic) leaflet is composed mostly of phosphatidylethanolamine, phosphatidylserine and phosphatidy-linositol and its phosphorylated derivatives. By contrast, the outer (extracellular) leaflet is based on phosphatidylcholine, sphingomyelin and a variety of glycolipids. In animal cell cholesterol, which helps strengthen the bilayer and decrease its permeability. Cholesterol also helps regulate the activity of certain integral membrane proteins.

25. Fab regions are used for the antigen-antibody binding studies without the interference from the non-antigen binding fragment (Fc region) and simplifies the characterization of MAb variants. IgG molecules have three protein domains. Two of the domains are identical and form the arms of the Y. Each arm contains a site that can bind to an antigen making IgG molecules bivalent. The third domain forms the base of the Y and this region is important in certain aspects of the immune response. The three domains may be separated from each other by cleavage with protease Papain. The two domains that carry the antigen binding sites are known as F(ab) fragments (named for the fragment having the antigen binding site) and the protein domain that is involved in immune regulation is termed as Fc fragment (for the fragment that crystallizes).

26. Replication rate

= 100 bp/second/fork (Given)

Total duration of DNA synthesis

= 11hrs

Plant species has

$= 3.0 \times 10^{10}$ DNA/genome

For 1 Fork;

100 bp replicated in = 1 second or

= 1/3600 hrs

Then, 1 bp will be replicated in

= (1/100) /3600 hrs

Then the given genome i.e. 3×10^{10} bpDNA will be replicated in = $3 \times 10^{10} \times (1/100)/3600$ hrs = 83,333 hrs

Because 1 Fork required 83,333 hrs to complete given genome replication

Hence No. of Fork required to complete given genome replication in 11 hrs = 83,333/11 = 7575.75 or the number of bidirectional forks per genome required for replication will be 7576.

27. The formula used is :

number of copies = (amount of DNA in Nano gram $\times 6.022 \times 10^{23}$)/(length $\times 1 \times 10^9 \times 650$)

$(2)^{40}$ = (amount $\times 6.022 \times 10^{23}$)/($600 \times 1 \times 10^9 \times 650$)

or Nano gram of DNA produced after 40 cycles of amplification will be = 722 Cordially yours

28. Given Data:

Molar extinction coefficient (ε)

$= 1.55 \times 10^4$ $mol^{-1}dm^3cm^{-1}$

Concentration (c) = 1.290×10^{-5} mol dm^{-3}

Path length (l) = 1 cm

Formula used: $A = \varepsilon cl$

$A = 1.55 \times 10^4 \times 1.290 \times 10^{-5} \times 1 = 0.1995$

The absorbance of GTP solution will be 0.1995 or 0.2000

29. MHC class I molecules are heterodimers that consist of two polypeptide chains, α and β2-microglobulin (b2m). The two chains are linked noncovalently via interaction of b2m and the α3 domain. Only α chain is polymorphic and encoded by a HLA gene, while the b2m subunit is not polymorphic and encoded by the Beta-2 microglobulin gene. The α3 domain is plasma membrane-spanning and interacts with the CD8 co-receptor of T-cells. The α3-CD8 interaction holds the MHC I molecule in place while the T cell receptor (TCR) on the surface of the cytotoxic T cell binds its α1-α2

heterodimer ligand, and checks the coupled peptide for antigenicity. The α1 and α2 domains fold to make up a groove for peptides to bind. MHC class I molecules bind peptides that are 8-10 amino acid in length

30. The Michaelis-Menten equation for this system is:

$$\nu = \frac{V_{max}[S]}{K_M + [S]}$$

Here, V_{max} represents the maximum velocity achieved by the system, at maximum (saturating) substrate concentrations. K_M (the Michaelis constant).

Then,

$\frac{1}{4} V_{max} = V_{max} (3.0 \times 10^{-3}) / (Km + 3.0 \times 10^{-3})$

i.e. $K_m = 4 \times (3.0 \times 10^{-3}) - (3.0 \times 10^{-3})$

$K_m = (3.0 \times 10^{-3})(4 - 1) = 9 \times 10^{-3}$mM.

Or $K_m = 9$ M

31. The pyruvate decarboxylase reaction provides our first encounter with thiamine pyrophosphate (TPP) by cleavage of bonds adjacent to a carbonyl group, such as the decarboxylation of α-keto acids, and in chemical rearrangements in which an activated acetaldehyde group is transferred from one carbon atom to another.

32. The CTA1 fragment of **cholera toxin** catalyses ADP-ribosylation of the Gs alpha subunit (Gαs) proteins using NAD that will cause loss of catalytic activity by inactivating GTP to GDP + Pi. Increased Gαs activation leads to increased adenylate cyclase activity, which increases the intracellular concentration of 3', 5'-cyclic AMP. The **pertussis toxin** (also an AB5 protein) produced by Bordetella pertussis acts in a similar manner with the exception that it ADP-ribosylates the Gαi subunit, rendering it inactive and unable to inhibit adenylyl cyclase production of cAMP.**Inositol trisphosphate** together with diacylglycerol (DAG), is a secondary messenger molecule used in signal transduction and lipid signaling in biological cells.The binding of IP3 ligand to InsP3R triggers the opening of the Ca2+ channel, and thus release of Ca2+ into the cytoplasm. **Caffeine** is a central nervous system (CNS) stimulant of the methylxanthine class. It is the world's most widely consumed psychoactive drug. At the cellular level, caffeine blocks the action of a chemical called phosphodiesterase (PDE).when caffeine stops the breakdown of cAMP, its effects are prolonged, and the response throughout the body is effectively amplified.These chemical messages lead to "fight or flight" behaviour.

33. Malonate is a competitive inhibitor of the reaction catalysed by succinate dehydrogenase. Malonate has two carboxyl groups, like succinate and can fill the succinate-binding site on the enzyme. The effect of competitive inhibitor depends on inhibitor concentration, the substrate concentration and the relative affinities of the substrate and inhibitor for the enzyme. Curve A represents the effect of malonate on the catalysis of succinate dehydrogenase.

34. Cardiotonic steroids (CTS) are a new class of hormones that circulate in the blood and are divided into two distinct groups, cardenolides, such as ouabain and digoxin, and bufadienolides, such as marinobufagenin, telocinobufagin and bufalin. They have the ability to bind and inhibit the ubiquitous transport enzyme sodium potassium pump, thus regulating intracellular Na^+concentration in every living cell. Although digoxin has been prescribed to heart failure patients for at least 200 years, the realization that CTS are endogenously produced has intensified research into their physiological and pathophysiological roles. Over the last two decades, substantial evidence has accumulated demonstrating the effects of endogenously synthesised CTS on the kidneys, vasculature and the heart. The Na,K-ATPase belongs to the P-type ATPase family of primary active cation pumps. It maintains the transmembrane gradients of Na(+) and K(+) across the cell membrane essential for cell homeostasis. The Na,K-ATPase is specifically inhibited by cardiotonic steroids like ouabain, which bind to the extracellular side of the enzyme and is of significant therapeutic value in the treatment of congestive heart failure.

35. If Sal I digestion is able to disrupt the ampicillin resistance function, the enzyme should be present with in the amp^r(AmpR) gene. Hence the correct restriction map is given in option (B). Rest of the information (about EcoRI and BamHI) is only to mislead/ distract the students.

36. Amborellaceae is a family of flowering plants native to New Caledonia. It consists of only one genus, Amborella, and one species, Amborella trichopoda. It is currently considered by plant systematists as the most basal lineage of angiosperms.

37. Lysigenous or schizolysigenous glands are present in the leaves and fruits of *Citrus* species. The glands occur for example in the outermost part of the pericarp of the orange and lemon peel. Schizolysigenous oil glands are also found in the floral parts of clove, *Eugenia caryophylata*, and are the source of clove oils.

38. The inherited characters can be transported from sires to progenies via 2 kinds of vehicles: nucleus (chromosomes) and cytoplasm (mitochondrial DNA or chloroplast DNA). Inheritance through the cytoplasm means that the locus of the determiners or representatives of a character is the cytoplasm, and since it is the egg alone which contains any significant amount of cytoplasm, this inheritance usually is refer to as maternal inheritance. Maternal inheritance of chloroplast DNA in higher plants is believed to be governed by methylation of specific DNA sites on maternal organelle, which protects it from degradation in the zygote.

39. In many cases the meristem is genetically programmed to stop producing new cells at a specific developmental stage. In these cases, the meristem is said to be determinate. A determinate meristem usually produces a part of the plant that has a predictable size and form, such as the flower, whereas an indeterminate meristem produces parts of the plant that can grow for variable periods of time, and vary in size and shape dependent on the local environment. Thus, the indeterminacy, or determinacy, of the meristem is directly related to the type of growth of an organ.

40. Strigolactones are terpenoid lactones and are derived from carotenoids. **Strigolactones** are plant hormones that stimulate the branching and growth of symbiotic arbuscular mycorrhizal fungi, increasing the probability of contact and establishment of a symbiotic association between the plant and fungus. Strigolactones also inhibit plant shoot branching, and trigger germination of parasitic plant seeds.

41. Genes in the virulence region are grouped into the operons *virABCDEFG*, which code for the enzymes responsible for mediating conjugative transfer of T-DNA to plant cells. *virG* activates vir-gene expression after binding to a consensus sequence,once it has been phosphorylated by *virA*.

42. **Wheat leaf rust** is a fungal disease that affects **wheat, barley** and **rye** stems, leaves and grains. In **temperate zones** it is destructive on **winter wheat** because the pathogen **overwinters**. Infections can lead up to 20% **yield** loss exacerbated by dying leaves which fertilize the fungus. The pathogen is **Puccinia rust fungus**. *Puccinia triticina* causes 'black rust', *P.recondita* causes 'brown rust' and *P.striiformis* causes 'Yellow rust'.

43. **Parasitism,** relationship between two **species** of **plants** or **animals** in which one benefits at the expense of the other, sometimes without killing the host organism. **Commensalism,** in biology a relationship between individuals of two **species** in which one species obtains **food** or other benefits from the other without either harming or benefiting the latter. **Predation,** in **animal behaviour**, the pursuit, capture, and killing of animals for food. Predatory animals may be solitary hunters, like the **leopard**, or they may be group hunters, like wolves. **Symbiosis,** any of several living arrangements between members of two different **species**, including **mutualism, commensalism**, and **parasitism**. Both positive (beneficial) and negative (unfavourable to harmful) associations are therefore included, and the members are called symbionts.

44. *K*-selected species possess relatively stable populations and tend to produce relatively low numbers of offspring; however, individual offspring tend to be quite large in comparison with *r*-selected species. *K*-selected species are characterized by long **gestation** periods lasting several months, slow maturation (and thus extended parental care), and long **life spans**. In addition, they tend to inhabit relatively stable **biological communities**, such as late-successional or climax **forests**.

45. **Atropine** is a type of secondary metabolite called a tropane alkaloid. **Alkaloids** contain nitrogens, frequently in a ring structure, and are derived from **amino acids**. Tropane is an organic compound containing nitrogen and it is from tropane that atropine is derived. Atropine is synthesized by a reaction between **tropine** and tropate, catalyzed by atropinase. **Atropine** is not a memberof indole alkaloids.

46. *Nitrobacter* uses energy from the oxidation of nitrite ions, NO_2^-, into nitrate ions, NO_3^-, to fulfill their energy needs. *Nitrobacter* fix carbon dioxide via the **Calvin cycle** for their carbon requirements. **Nitrite reductase** refers to any of several classes of **enzymes** that catalyze the reduction of **nitrite. Nitrogenases** are enzymes that are produced by certain bacteria, such as cyanobacteria (blue-green algae). These enzymes are responsible for the reduction of nitrogen (N_2) to ammonia (NH_3). **Nitrate reductases** are molybdoenzymes that **reduce nitrate** (NO_3^-) to **nitrite** (NO_2^-). This reaction is critical for the production of protein in most crop plants, as nitrate is the predominant source of nitrogen in fertilized soils.

47. Water potential (ψ) = pressure potential (P) + Osmotic potential (π);

    For M

    Water potential (ψ) = 4 + (–10) = –6

    For N

    Water potential (ψ) = 5 + (–12) = –7

    Because of water potential of M is more than N, therefore the direction of movement of water will be M to N.

48. Two independent non-segregating recessive mutants (m1 and m2) display defects in petal formation. When they were crossed with each other (m1 x m2), all the F1 plants developed normal petals. In view of this observation, mutations in both m1 and m2 are in two separate genes.

49. First we identify parental combination (ABC, abc) and double crossovers (AbC, aBc), then the distance between first two genes i.e. A and B loci was found to be = (85 + 80 + 01 + 01)/1000 = 0.167 (recombination frequency) or 16.7 cM. Now distance between B and C loci will be = (8 + 7 + 1 + 1) / 1000 = 0.017 (recombination frequency) or 1.7 cM. Therefore the distance between A and C loci will be = 16.7 + 1.7 = 18.4 cM.

50. As given, an endosperm cell contains = 4.8×10^8 nucleotide pairs of DNA. As we know endosperm cells have triploid nucleus i.e. 3N = 4.8×10^8, and microsporocytes have diploid nucleus (2N), hence microsporocytes of the given plant will have, (2N) = (4.8×10^8) $\times$ 3/2 = 3.2×10^8 nucleotide pairs of DNA.

51. A ***habitat*** is an ecological or environmental area that is inhabited by a particular species of animal, plant, or other type of organism. The term typically refers to the zone in which the organism lives and where it can find food, shelter, protection and mates for reproduction; The ecological ***niche*** describes how an organism or population responds to the distribution of resources and competitors (for example, by growing when resources are abundant, and when predators, parasites and pathogens are scarce) and how it in turn alters those same factors (for example, limiting access to resources by other organisms, acting as a food source for predators and a consumer of prey); The **trophic level** of an **organism** is the position it occupies in a **food chain.** Food chains start at trophic level 1 with **primary producers** such as plants, move to **herbivores** at level 2, **predators** at level 3 and typically finish with **carnivores** or **apex predators** at level 4 or 5; An ***ecosystem*** is a community of living organisms in conjunction with the nonliving components of their environment (things like air, water and mineral soil), interacting as a system. These biotic and abiotic components are regarded as linked together through nutrient cycles and energy flows.

52. (P) Plant transformation: a simple particle bombardment device based on flowing helium; (Q) *Agrobacterium tumefaciens* (updated scientific name *Rhizobium radiobacter*, synonym *Agrobacterium radiobacter*) is the causal agent of crown gall disease (the formation of **tumours**) in over 140 species of **eudicots.** Acetosyringone is a **phenolic natural product**, this substance has been best known for its involvement in plant-pathogen recognition, especially its role as a signal attracting and transforming unique, oncogenic bacteria in genus **Agrobacterium.** The *virA* gene on the **Ti plasmid** of **Agrobacterium tumefaciens** and the Ri plasmid of **Agrobacterium rhizogenes** is used by these soil bacteria to infect plants, via its encoding for a receptor for acetosyringone and other phenolic phytochemicals exuded by plant wounds; (R) Protoplasts may also be used for **plant breeding**, using a technique called **protoplast fusion.** Protoplasts from different species are induced to fuse by using an **electric field** or a solution of **polyethylene glycol.** This technique may be used to generate **somatic hybrids** in tissue culture; (S) Agarose plating is as anaid in the fixation of protoplasts for microinjection. The method for microinjection has been improved. An interesting method is the embedding of protoplasts in low melting point agarose.

53.

Pathogen	Disease	Plant
Blumeria graminis	Powdery mildew	Barley
Magnaporhe grisea	Blast disease	Rice
Ventturia inaequalis	Scab disease	Apple
Cercospora personata	Tikka disease	Groundnut

54.

Plant Part	Use	*Species*
Bark	Flavoring agent	*Cinmamomum zeylanicum*
Leaf	Insecticide	*Azadirachta indica*
Capsule	Analgesic	*Papaver somniferum*
Stigma	Food colorant	*Crocus sativus*

55. Ribulose-1, 5-bisphosphate + $2O_2 \rightarrow 2$ 2-phosphoglycolate + 2 3-Phophoglycerate; Serine+2-oxoglutarate → hydroxypyruvate + glutamate

56. **Sulfate-reducing bacteria** are those bacteria and archaea that can obtain energy by oxidizing organic compounds or molecular hydrogen (H_2) while reducing sulfate (SO_2^{-4}) to hydrogen sulfide (H_2S). In a sense, these organisms "breathe" sulfate rather than oxygen in a form of anaerobic respiration. Many bacteria reduce small amounts of sulfates in order to synthesize sulfur-containing cell components; this is known as assimilatory sulfate reduction. By contrast, the sulfate-reducing bacteria considered here reduce sulfate in large amounts to obtain energy and expel the resulting sulfide as waste; this is known as dissimilatory sulfate reduction. They use sulfate as the terminal electron acceptor of their electron transport chain. Most of them are anaerobes; however there are examples of sulfate-reducing bacteria that are tolerant of oxygen. Under oxygenated conditions these bacteria switch to aerobic respiration before reducing sulfate.

57. Methanogens use CO_2 taken up from their growth environment as the carbon substrate for growth. They use some CO_2 as the ultimate oxidizing agent of an electron transport chain which, by a chemiosmotic mechanism, maintains a transmembrane electrochemical ion gradient which powers ATP production.The equation shows the reduction of CO_2 by H_2 to produce methane. This redox reaction sustains anaerobic respiration which allows the production of ATP. CO_2 is the terminal electron acceptor in the given metabolic reaction.

$$CO_2 + 4H_2 \xrightarrow[\text{generation}]{\text{ATP}} CH_4 + 2H_2O$$

58. Psychrophiles are defined as organisms that can grow only in low temperatures up to a maximum of 20 °C. Many such organisms are bacteria, but psychrophiles also include eukaryotes such as lichens, snow algae, fungi, and wingless midges. Psychrotolerant organisms are like mesophiles (growing at 20–40 °C), but are able to tolerate lower temperatures albeit with slower growth rates.

59. **Robert Heinrich Hermann Koch** was a celebrated German physician and pioneering microbiologist. As the founder of modern bacteriology, he is known for his role in identifying the specific causative agents of tuberculosis, cholera, and anthrax and for giving experimental support for the concept of infectious disease. As a result of his groundbreaking research on tuberculosis, Koch received the Nobel Prize in Physiology or Medicine in 1905. He had not discovered the causative agent of leprosy. The **causative agent of leprosy**, Mycobacterium leprae, was **discovered** by G. H. Armauer Hansen in Norway in 1873, making it the first bacterium to be identified as **causing** disease in humans.

60. **A protist** is any eukaryotic organism that is not an animal, plant or fungus. The protists do not form a natural group, or clade, but are often grouped together for convenience, like

algae or invertebrates. In some systems of biological classification, such as the popular 5-kingdom scheme proposed by Robert Whittaker in 1969, the protists make up a kingdom called **Protista**, composed of "organisms which are unicellular or unicellular-colonial and which form no tissues. Protists can be heterotrophic, which means they obtain the energy they need to live by consuming other organisms. Or, they can be autotrophic, which means they obtain energy from the environment through photosynthesis, the process of capturing light energy and storing it in carbohydrates.

61. **Chickenpox**, also known as **varicella**, is a highly contagious disease caused by the initial infection with Varicella zoster virus (VZV).

62. A **crista** is a fold in the inner membrane of a mitochondrion. The name is from the Latin for crest or plume, and it gives the inner membrane its characteristic wrinkled shape, providing a large amount of surface area for chemical reactions to occur on. This aids aerobic cellular respiration, because the mitochondrion requires oxygen. Cristae are studded with proteins, including ATP synthase and a variety of cytochromes.

63. Gentamicin was discovered in 1963. It is made from the bacteria Micromonospora purpurea. Gentamicin is on the World Health Organization's List of Essential Medicines, the most effective and safe medicines needed in a health system. It is used to treat several types of bacterial infections. This may include bone infections, endocarditis, pelvic inflammatory disease, meningitis, pneumonia, urinary tract infections, and sepsis among others.

64. **MacConkey agar** is a selective and differential culture medium for bacteria designed to selectively isolate Gram-negative and enteric (normally found in the intestinal tract) bacilli and differentiate them based on lactose fermentation. The crystal violet and bile salts inhibit the growth of gram-positive organisms which allows for the selection and isolation of gram-negative bacteria. Enteric bacteria that have the ability to ferment lactose can be detected using the carbohydrate lactose, and the pH indicator neutral red.

65. **Antiseptic(s)** are antimicrobial substances that are applied to living tissue/skin to reduce the possibility of infection, sepsis, or putrefaction. Antiseptics are generally distinguished from antibiotics by the latter's ability to be transported through the lymphatic system to destroy bacteria within the body, and from disinfectants, which destroy microorganisms found on non-living objects. Although several alcohols have been shown to be effective antimicrobials, ethyl alcohol (ethanol, alcohol), isopropyl alcohol (isopropanol, propan-2-ol) and *n*-propanol (in particular in Europe) are the most widely used. Alcohols exhibit rapid broad-spectrum antimicrobial activity against vegetative bacteria (including mycobacteria), viruses, and fungi but are not sporicidal.

66. The function of adaptive immune responses is to destroy invading pathogens and any toxic molecules they produce. Because these responses are destructive, it is crucial that they be made only in response to molecules that are foreign to the host and not to the molecules of the host itself. Any substance capable of eliciting an adaptive immune response is referred to as an antigen (antibody generator). Adaptive immune responses are carried out by white blood cells called lymphocytes. There are two broad classes of such responses—antibody responses and cell-mediated immune responses, and they are carried out by different classes of lymphocytes, called B cells and T cells, respectively. Figure (i) accurately depicts the adaptive immune response by the rabbit against antigen X.

67. A **bactericide** or **bacteriocide**, sometimes abbreviated **Bcidal**, is a substance that kills bacteria. Bactericides are disinfectants, antiseptics, or antibiotics. Figure (ii) is the most accurate representation of the actionof bactericidal agent X.

68. The Gram-negative bacterium *Yersinia pestis* is the causative agent of the systemic invasive infectious disease classically referred

to as plague; The causative agent of rabies is ***rabies virus*** (RV), a negative-stranded RNA virus of the **rhabdovirus** family. **Lyssavirus** is a genus of RNA viruses in the family Rhabdoviridae, order Mononegavirales. Humans, mammals, and vertebrates serve as natural hosts. The genus Lyssavirus includes the rabies virus traditionally associated with that disease; Q fever is a disease caused by infection with ***Coxiella burnetii***, a **bacterium** that affects humans and other animals. This organism is uncommon, but may be found in cattle, sheep, goats, and other domestic mammals, including cats and dogs; ***Plasmodium malariae*** is a parasitic **protozoa** that causes malaria in humans. It is one of several species of **Plasmodium** parasites that infect humans including ***Plasmodium falciparum*** and ***Plasmodium vivax*** which are responsible for most malarial infection.

69. The process of nucleotide excision repair is controlled in Escherichia coli by the UvrABC endonuclease enzyme complex, which consists of four Uvr proteins: UvrA, UvrB, UvrC, and DNA helicase II (sometimes also known as UvrD in this complex); **Reverse transcriptase**, also called RNA-directed DNA polymerase, an enzyme encoded from the genetic material of retroviruses that catalyzes the transcription of retrovirus RNA into DNA. This catalyzed transcription is the reverse process of normal cellular transcription of DNA into RNA, hence the names reverse transcriptase and retrovirus; **Apurinic/apyrimidinic (AP)** endonuclease is an enzyme that is involved in the DNA base excision repair pathway (BER). Its main role in the repair of damaged or mismatched nucleotides in DNA is to create a nick in the phosphodiester backbone of the AP site created when DNA glycosylase removes the damaged base; **Pyrosequencing** is a method of DNA sequencing (determining the order of nucleotides in DNA) based on the "sequencing by synthesis" principle. It differs from Sanger sequencing, in that it relies on the detection of pyrophosphate release on nucleotide incorporation, rather than chain termination with dideoxynucleotides. The single-strand DNA (ssDNA) template is hybridized to a sequencing primer and incubated with the enzymes DNA polymerase, ATP sulfurylase, luciferase and apyrase, and with the substrates adenosine 5′ phosphosulfate (APS) and luciferin. ATP sulfurylase (ATPS) catalyzes a key reaction in the global sulfur cycle by reversibly converting inorganic sulfate (SO_4^{2-}) with ATP to adenosine 52 -phosphosulfate (APS) and pyrophosphate (PP_i).

70. An autotroph is an organism able to make its own food. **Photoautotrophs** are organisms that carry out photosynthesis. Using energy from sunlight, carbon dioxide and water are converted into organic materials to be used in cellular functions such as biosynthesis and respiration; **Photoheterotrophs** obtain their energy from sunlight and carbon from organic material and not carbon dioxide; **Chemoautotrophs** (or chemotrophic autotroph), in addition to deriving energy from chemical reactions, synthesize all necessary organic compounds from carbon dioxide. Chemoautotrophs use inorganic energy sources, such as hydrogen sulfide, elemental sulfur, ferrous iron, and also molecular hydrogen, and ammonia; **Chemoheterotrophs** are unable to fix carbon to form their own organic compounds. Chemoheterotrophs can be chemolithoheterotrophs, utilizing inorganic energy sources such as sulfur or chemoorganoheterotrophs, utilizing organic energy sources such as carbohydrates, lipids, and proteins.

71. Total Dilution Factor = 10^5

No. of colonies = 46

CFU/mL = (no. of colonies × dilution factor) / volume of culture plate

$= (46 \times 10^5)/1.0 = 46,00000.00$

Then the number of cells present per ml in the diluted original sample were = 46,00000.00

72. The transformation efficiency of component cells = 10^4 CFU/μg of plasmid DNA

Amount of plasmid used to transform the competent cells = 0.01 μg

CFU/ μg = (no. of colonies × dilution factor) / biomass of the culture plate

10^4 CFU/μg = (no. of colonies × 1) / 0.01 μg

no. transformed of bacteria in CFU after plating = $10^4 \times 0.01$ = 100.00

73. Femtogram = A unit of mass equal to 0.000 000 000 000 001 grams = 10^{-15} gm

Average DNA content of single microbial cell = 4×10^{-15} gm = 4×10^{-9} μg

DNA found in per gram soil sample contain = 0.32 μg

Then, DNA in per milligram soil sample contain = 0.32 μg/1000 = 0.00032 μg

Or DNA found in per milligram soil sample contain = 0.00032 μg = 32×10^{-5} μg

Then, No. of microbial cell per milligram of soil = $32 \times 10^{-5/4}$ X 10^{-9} = 8×10^4

i.e. No. of microbial cell per milligram of soil = 80,000

74. As we know,

$2.303(\log X_t - \log X_0)/t = 0.693/t_d$

Given,

$X_t = 4.1 \times 10^7$ numbers ;

t = 24 hrs ;

t_d = 2 hrs ;

X_0 = ?

Then,

$2.303(\log 4.1 \times 10^7 - \log X_0)/24 = 0.693/2$

Solving this we get, X_0 = 10005;

Hence the initial no. of bacteria present were = 10005;

The number of transformed bacteria in CFU after plating /mL = cfu/ml = (no. of colonies x dilution factor) / volume of culture plate

= $(46 \times 10^5)/1.0$ = 46,00000

Then the number of cells present per ml in the diluted original sample were = 46,00000

76. **Deuterostomia,** (Greek: "second mouth"), group of animals—including those of the phyla Echinodermata (*e.g.,* starfish, sea urchins), Chordata (*e.g.,* sea squirts, lancelets, and vertebrates), Chaetognatha (*e.g.,* arrowworms), and Brachiopoda (*e.g.,* lamp shells)—classified together on the basis of embryological development and by molecular criteria. During development the mouth of deuterostomes develops from an opening into the embryonic gut other than the blastopore, which develops into the anus. The defining characteristic of the deuterostome is the fact that the blastopore becomes the anus, whereas in protostomes the blastopore becomes the mouth.The coelom (a fluid-filled body cavity lined with mesoderm) develops from buds off the embryonic gut. A number of deuterostomes have distinctive larval forms. The Deuterostomia constitute one of two divisions of the coelomates (animals having a coelom).

77. Allantoin: Structure first evolved in reptiles and birds as a reservoir for nitrogenous waste, and also as a means for oxygenation of the embryo. Oxygen is absorbed by the allantois through the egg shell. The first amniotes, referred to as "basal amniotes", resembled small lizards and evolved from the amphibian reptiliomorphs about 312 million years ago,[3] in the Carboniferous geologic period. Their eggs could survive out of the water, allowing amniotes to branch out into drier environments. The eggs could also "breathe" and cope with wastes, allowing the eggs and the amniotes themselves to evolve into larger forms.

78. **ABO Blood Type Calculator**

		Father's Blood Type				
		A	B	AB	O	
Mother's Blood Type	A	A or O	A, B, AB, or O	A, B, or AB	A or O	Child's Blood type Must Be
	B	A, B, AB or O	B or O	A, B, or AB	B or O	
	AB	A, B, or AB	A, B, or AB	A, B, or AB	A or B	
	O	A or O	B or O	A or B	O	

		Child's Blood Type				
		A	B	AB	O	
Mother's Blood Type	A	A, B, AB or O	B or AB	B or AB	A, B, or O	Father's Blood Type Must Be
	B	A or AB	A, B, AB or O	A or AB	A, B, or O	
	AB	A, B, AB or O	A, B, AB or O	A, B, or AB		
	O	A or AB	B or AB		A, B, or O	

79. Amylase is a digestive enzyme that acts on starch in food, breaking it down into smaller carbohydrate molecules. The enzyme is made in two places. First, salivary glands in your mouth make salivary amylase, which begins the digestive process by breaking down starch when you chew your food, converting it into maltose, a smaller carbohydrate.

80. **Glycolysis** is the metabolic process that serves as the foundation for both aerobic and anaerobic cellular respiration. In **glycolysis**, glucose is converted into pyruvate.

81. Mating of a single female with several males is called polyandry. In sequential polyandry (the most typical form of this mating system), a female mates with a male, lays eggs, and then terminates the relationship with that male, leaving him to incubate the eggs while she goes off to repeat this sequence with another male. Spotted Sandpipers, Red-necked and Red Phalaropes are examples of sequentially polyandrous species that breed in North America.

82. The mosquito midgut and salivary glands are key entry and exit points for pathogens such as Plasmodium parasites and Dengue viruses. The malaria parasite Plasmodium has an absolute requirement for both a vertebrate and a mosquito host in order to complete its life cycle. The mosquito midgut represents one of the most challenging environments for the survival and development of Plasmodium, and is thus also one of the most attractive sites for novel targeted malaria control strategies.

83. Aromatase inhibitors and inactivators interfere with the body's ability to produce estrogen from androgens by suppressing aromatase enzyme activity. Before menopause, ovarian aromatase is responsible for the majority of circulating estrogen and is exquisitely sensitive to changes in luteinising hormone (LH). Following menopause, aromatase in fat and muscle may be responsible for much of the circulating estrogen. Aromatase in highly estrogen-sensitive tissues, such as the breast, uterus, vagina, bone, brain, heart and blood vessels, provides local estrogen in an autocrine fashion.

84. **Protein phosphorylation** is a post-translational modification of proteins in which an amino acid residue is phosphorylated by a protein kinase by the addition of a covalently bound phosphate group. Phosphorylation alters the structural conformation of a protein, causing it to become activated, deactivated, or modifying its function. The reverse reaction of phosphorylation is called dephosphorylation, and is catalyzed by protein phosphatases. Protein kinases and phosphatases work independently and in a balance to regulate the function of proteins. The amino acids most commonly phosphorylated are serine, threonine, and tyrosine in eukaryotes, and histidine in prokaryotes, which play important and well-characterized roles in signaling pathways and metabolism. One of the signal transduction pathways that are activated is called the mitogen-activated protein kinase (MAPK) pathway. The MAPK protein is an enzyme, a protein kinase that can attach phosphate to target proteins such as the transcription factor MYC and, thus, alter gene transcription and, ultimately, cell cycle progression.

85. Chromatin is found in two varieties: euchromatin and heterochromatin. Originally, the two forms were distinguished cytologically by how intensely they stained – the euchromatin is less intense, while heterochromatin stains intensely, indicating tighter packing. Heterochromatin is usually localized to the periphery of the nucleus. Despite this early dichotomy, recent evidence in both animals and plants has suggested that there are more than two distinct heterochromatin states, and it may in fact exist in four or five 'states', each marked by different combinations of epigenetic marks.

Heterochromatin mainly consists of genetically inactive satellite sequences, and many genes are repressed to various extents, although some cannot be expressed in euchromatin at all. Both centromeres and telomeres are heterochromatic, as is the Barr body of the second, inactivated X-chromosome in a female.

86. If you consider each chromosome as a linkage group (which would only be true if there were no recombination), there would be 8.0 linkage groups in a cell with 8 chromosomes (i.e. 2n = 16)

87. After 4 generations, there will be total 16 molecules i.e. 2 hybrid molecules and 14 14N molecules. Hence the ration between hybrid and light labeled DNA will be $(1 : n)$ = 2:14 or 1 : 7.

Then the value of n = 7.0.

88. **GENOTYPE FREQUENCIES:**

AA (p^2) = 300/1000 = 0.3

Aa (2pq) = 500/1000 = 0.5

aa (q^2) = 200/1000 = 0.2

ALLELE FREQUENCIES:

Frequency of $A = P = p^2 + 1/2\,(2pq)$

$= 0.3 + 1/2\,(0.5)$

$= 0.3 + 0.25 = 0.55$

Frequency of $a = Q = 1 - P$

$= 1 - 0.55 = 0.45$

89. After meiosis I, each cell will have 8 chromosomes. When at metaphase II, chromosomes will align at metaphoric plate, chromatids will separate hence each cell will have 16 chromatids as each chromosome has 2 chromatids.

90. **Phospholipase C (PLC)** is a class of membrane-associated enzymes that cleave phospholipids just before the phosphate group. Activators of each PLC vary, but typically include heterotrimeric G protein subunits, protein tyrosine kinases, small G proteins, Ca^{2+}, and phospholipids. Upon activation of phospholipase C by ligand binding toG-protein coupled receptor, the Ca^{+2} from $InsP_3$ gated channel on endoplasmic reticulum as well as influx of Ca^{+2} from $InsP_3$ gated channel on plasma membrane.

91. **Transferrins** are iron-binding blood plasma glycoproteins that control the level of free iron (Fe) in biological fluids. Human transferrin is encoded by the *TF* gene; **Insulin** is a peptide hormone produced by beta cells of the pancreatic islets. It regulates the metabolism of carbohydrates, fats and protein by promoting the absorption of, especially, glucose from the blood into fat, liver and skeletal muscle cells; **alpha-2-Macroglobulin** (**α2M**) is a large plasma protein found in the blood. It is mainly produced by the liver, and also locally synthesized by macrophages, fibroblasts, and adrenocortical cells. The alpha-macroglobulin (αM) family of proteins includes protease inhibitors, typified by the human tetrameric alpha-2-macroglobulin (α2M); they belong to the MEROPS proteinase inhibitor family I39, clan IL; **Fibronectin (FN)** mediates a wide variety of cellular interactions with the extracellular matrix (ECM) and plays important roles in cell adhesion, migration, growth and differentiation.

92. Immunoglobulin M (IgM), the largest pentameric immunoglobulin is used as a marker of recent primary infection for some diseases. The immunoglobulin **heavy chain** (IgH) is the large polypeptide subunit of an **antibody** (immunoglobulin). A typical **antibody** is composed of two immunoglobulin (Ig) **heavy chains** and two Ig light **chains**. Several different types of **heavy chain** exist that define the class or isotype of an **antibody**.

Therefore the approximate calculated weight of an IgM antibody

$= 5 \times (2 \times 65{,}000 + 2 \times 25{,}000)$

$= 5 \times (130{,}000 + 50{,}000)$

$= 900{,}000.$

93. The **Hedgehog signaling pathway** is a signaling pathway that transmits information to embryonic cells required for proper cell differentiation. The pathway is equally important during vertebrate embryonic development and is therefore of interest in evolutionary developmental biology. Disruption of hedgehog signaling during embryonic development, through either deleterious mutation or consumption of teratogens by the gestating mother, can lead to severe developmental abnormalities. Cyclopia, one of the most severe defects of holoprosencephaly, results if the pathway inhibitor cyclopamine is consumed by gestating mammals; **T-box** refers to a group of transcription factors involved in limb and heart development. The protein product of each Hox gene is a transcription factor. Each Hox gene contains a well-conserved DNA sequence known as the homeobox. Hox genes are thus a subset of the homeobox transcription factor genes. In many animals, the organization of the Hox genes in the chromosome is the same as the order of their expression along the anterior-posterior axis of the developing animal, and are thus said to display collinearity; The protein product of each Hox gene is a transcription factor. Each Hox gene contains a well-conserved DNA sequence known as the homeobox. Hox genes are thus a subset of the homeobox transcription factor genes. In many animals, the organization of the Hox genes in the chromosome is the same as the order of their expression along the anterior-posterior axis of the developing animal, and are thus said to display colinearity. Wnt signaling plays a critical role in embryonic development. It operates in both vertebrates and invertebrates, including humans, frogs,

zebrafish, *C. elegans*, *Drosophila* and others. It was first found in the segment polarity of Drosophila, where it helps to establish anterior and posterior polarities; he **Notch signaling pathway** is a highly conserved cell signaling system present in most multicellular organism. Notch signaling promotes proliferative signaling during neurogenesis, and its activity is inhibited by Numb to promote neural differentiation. It plays a major role in the regulation of embryonic development. The **Notch cascade** consists of Notch and Notch ligands, as well as intracellular proteins transmitting the notch signal to the cell's nucleus. The Notch/Lin-12/Glp-1 receptor family was found to be involved in the specification of cell fates during development in *Drosophila* and *C. elegans*.

116. The event would have been successful if you **had been** able to come.

117. From the given question the closest in meaning to the underlined word is **complete**.

118. According to given question, the cards which must be turned over to verify the above proposition are 2, blue.

119. Given,

$$81\times\left(\frac{16}{25}\right)^{x+2}\div\left(\frac{3}{5}\right)^{2x+4}=144$$

$$\Rightarrow (3)^4\times\left(\frac{16}{25}\right)^x\times\left(\frac{16}{25}\right)^2\div\left(\frac{3}{5}\right)^{2x}\times\left(\frac{3}{5}\right)^4=144$$

$$\frac{3^4\times\left(\frac{16}{25}\right)^x\times\left(\frac{16}{25}\right)^2}{\left(\frac{9}{25}\right)^x\times\left(\frac{9}{25}\right)^2}=144$$

$$3^4\times\left(\frac{\frac{16}{25}}{\frac{9}{25}}\right)^x\times\left(\frac{\frac{16}{25}}{\frac{9}{25}}\right)^2=144$$

$$\left(\frac{16}{9}\right)^x\times\left(\frac{16}{9}\right)^2=\frac{144}{81}$$

$$\left(\frac{16}{9}\right)^x\times\left(\frac{16}{9}\right)^2=\frac{16}{9}$$

$$\left(\frac{16}{9}\right)^x\times\frac{16}{9}=1$$

$$\left(\frac{16}{9}\right)^x=\frac{1}{\frac{16}{9}}$$

$$\left(\frac{16}{9}\right)^x=\left(\frac{16}{9}\right)^{-1}$$

$$\therefore\ x=-1$$

120. From given question when tow dices are thrown simutaneously, then

$n(S) = 6\times 6 = 36$

n(E) = (6, 6), (6, 5), (6, 4), (6, 3), (6, 2), (6, 1), (5, 6), (5, 5), (5, 4), (5, 3), (5, 2), (5, 1), (4, 6), (4, 5), (4, 4), (4, 3), (4, 2), (4, 1), (3, 6), (3, 5), (3, 4), (3, 3), (3, 2), (3, 1), (2, 6), (2, 5), (2, 4), (2, 3), (2, 2), (2, 1), (1, 6), (1, 5), (1, 4), (1, 3), (1, 2), (1, 1)

$$\therefore\ P(E)=\frac{n(E)}{n(S)}=\frac{8}{36}=\frac{2}{9}$$

121. From the given question, one can conclude the centre operates on a first-come-first-served (FCFS) basis, but with variable service times, depending on specific customer needs.

122. From the given paragraph, only statement (ii) and (iv) will be followed.

123. From the given question

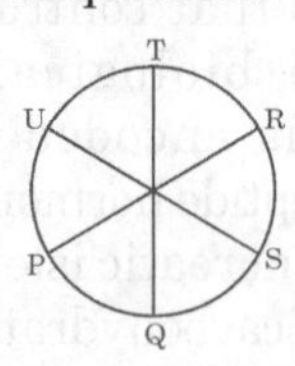

Now if P and U switch their seat, then the sitting arrangement is

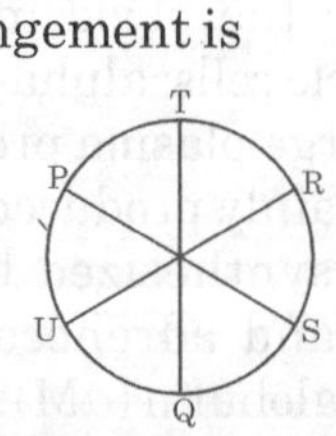

So, T is immediate to the left of P.

124. From the given question

$$\text{The speed (in km)}=\frac{19+26}{5\left(\frac{1}{2}+1\right)}$$

$$=\frac{45}{5\times\frac{3}{2}}=\frac{90}{15}$$

$$= 6\text{ km/hr}$$

125. From the given graph, neither (i) nor (ii) statements are correct.

GATE-2016

XL : LIFE SCIENCES

Time : 3 Hours | *Maximum Marks : 100*

GENERAL APTITUDE (GA)

(Q. 1 – 5) : Carry One Mark Each

1. The chairman requested the aggrieved shareholders to ______________ him.
   (*a*) bare with (*b*) bore with
   (*c*) bear with (*d*) bare

2. Identify the correct spelling out of the given options:
   (*a*) Managable
   (*b*) Manageable
   (*c*) Mangaeble
   (*d*) Managible

3. Pick the odd one out in the following:
   13, 23, 33, 43, 53
   (*a*) 23 (*b*) 33
   (*c*) 43 (*d*) 53

4. R2D2 is a robot. R2D2 can repair aeroplanes. No other robot can repair aeroplanes.
   Which of the following can be logically inferred from the above statements?
   (*a*) R2D2 is a robot which can only repair aeroplanes
   (*b*) R2D2 is the only robot which can repair aeroplanes
   (*c*) R2D2 is a robot which can repair only aeroplanes
   (*d*) Only R2D2 is a robot

5. If $|9y - 6| = 3$, then $y^2 - 4y/3$ is _______
   (*a*) 0 (*b*) + 1/3
   (*c*) – 1/3 (*d*) undefined

(Q. 6 – 10) : Carry Two Marks Each.

6. The following graph represents the installed capacity for cement production (in tonnes) and the actual production (in tonnes) of nine cement plants of a cement company. Capacity utilization of a plant is defined as ratio of actual production of cement to installed capacity. A plant with installed capacity of at least 200 tonnes is called a large plant and a plant with lesser capacity is called a small plant. The difference between total production of large plants and small plants, in tonnes is ____.

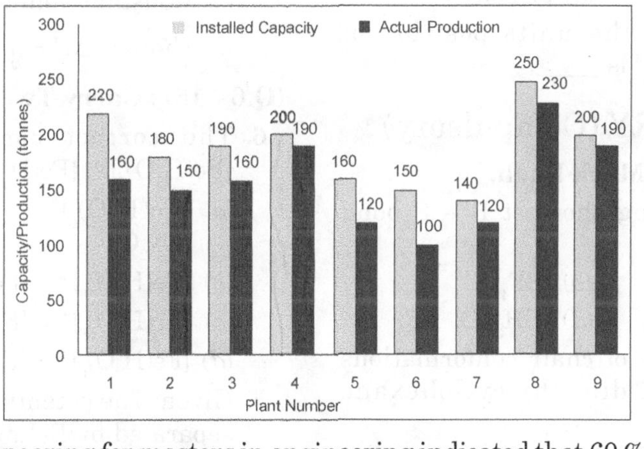

7. A poll of students appearing for masters in engineering indicated that 60 % of the students believed that mechanical engineering is a profession unsuitable for women. A research study on women with masters or higher degrees in mechanical engineering found that 99 % of such women were successful in their professions.
   Which of the following can be logically inferred from the above paragraph?
   (*a*) Many students have misconceptions regarding various engineering disciplines.
   (*b*) Men with advanced degrees in mechanical engineering believe women are well suited to be mechanical engineers.
   (*c*) Mechanical engineering is a profession well suited for women with masters or higher degrees in mechanical engineering.
   (*d*) The number of women pursuing higher degrees in mechanical engineering is small.

8. Sourya committee had proposed the establishment of Sourya Institutes of Technology (SITs) in line with Indian Institutes of Technology (IITs) to cater to the technological and industrial needs of a developing country.
Which of the following can be logically inferred from the above sentence?
Based on the proposal,
(i) In the initial years, SIT students will get degrees from IIT.
(ii) SITs will have a distinct national objective.
(iii) SIT like institutions can only be established in consultation with IIT.
(iv) SITs will serve technological needs of a developing country.
(*a*) (iii) and (iv) only
(*b*) (i) and (iv) only
(*c*) (ii) and (iv) only
(*d*) (ii) and (iii) only

9. Shaquille O' Neal is a 60% career free throw shooter, meaning that he successfully makes 60 free throws out of 100 attempts on average. What is the probability that he will successfully make exactly 6 free throws in 10 attempts?
(*a*) 0.2508 (*b*) 0.2816
(*c*) 0.2934 (*d*) 0.6000

10. The numeral in the units position of $211^{870} + 146^{127} \times 3^{424}$ is ____.

H : CHEMISTRY (Compulsory)

(Q. 1 – 5) : Carry One Mark Each.

1. The species having shortest B – F bond distance is
(*a*) BF_3 (*b*) $[BF_4]^-$
(*c*) $H_3N \cdot BF_3$ (*d*) $(CH_3)_2O \cdot BF_3$

2. The total number of chair conformations possible for 1, 2-dimethylcyclohexane is ____ .

3. 'A harmful substance persists in the environment for a very long period of time'. The UNACCEPTABLE statement for this fact is
(*a*) the substance degrades by second-order kinetics
(*b*) the substance degrades by first-order kinetics
(*c*) the substance is not biodegradable
(*d*) the substance has long half-life

4. For an enzyme catalyzed reaction, the plot that correctly represents the relationship between the rate and temperature is

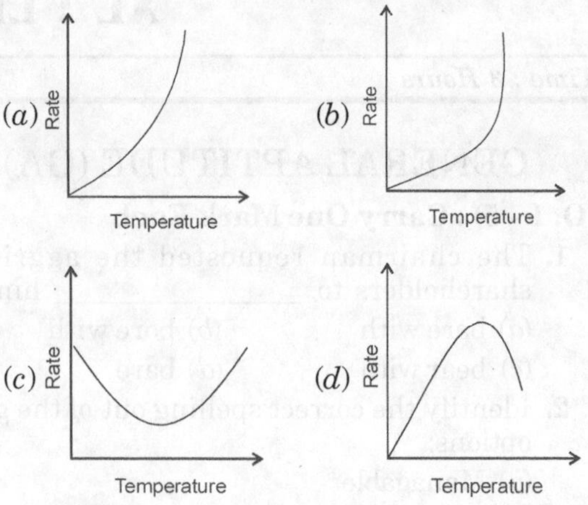

5. Combinations of a process and equation are given below. The INCORRECT combination is
(*a*) Constant pressure heating with no phase change; $w = -\int_1^2 P\,dV$
(*b*) Reversible adiabatic process in a perfect gas; $\Delta U = \int_1^2 C_p(T)\,dT$
(*c*) Reversible isothermal process in a perfect gas; $w_{rev} = -\int_1^2 P\,dV$
(*d*) Constant volume heating with no phase change; $\Delta U = \int_1^2 C_v\,dT$

(Q.6 – 15) : Carry Two Marks Each

6. The correct comparison of pK_a's of $[Fe(H_2O)_6]^{2+}$, $[Fe(H_2O)_6]^{3+}$, V_2O_5 and N_2O_5 is
(*a*) $[Fe(H_2O)_6]^{3+} < [Fe(H_2O)_6]^{2+}$ and $V_2O_5 < N_2O_5$
(*b*) $[Fe(H_2O)_6]^{3+} < [Fe(H_2O)_6]^{2+}$ and $V_2O_5 = N_2O_5$
(*c*) $[Fe(H_2O)_6]^{2+} = [Fe(H_2O)_6]^{3+}$ and $N_2O_5 < V_2O_5$
(*d*) $[Fe(H_2O)_6]^{3+} < [Fe(H_2O)_6]^{2+}$ and $N_2O_5 < V_2O_5$

7. Given: The potential energy of two electrons separated by Bohr radius is 27.211 eV. The first Bohr radius of hydrogen is 0.5292 Å. The electron makes an orbit of radius 0.5295Å around the nucleus in hydrogen.
The calculated ionization energy (eV) of hydrogen atom is ____.

8. The crystal field stabilization energy (excluding pairing energy, if any) of $[CoCl_4]^{2-}$ in Δ_o units is ____.

9. The correct statement is

(*a*) $TlBr_3$ is less soluble in water than TlBr

(*b*) Ag_2S is more soluble in water than Ag_2O

(*c*) LiF is less stable than CsF

(*d*) $[Co(NH_3)_5I]^{2+}$ is less stable than $[Co(NH_3)_5F]^{2+}$

10. Ferrous sulfate on reaction with potassium hexacyanochromate(III) produces a brick red complex. The number of unpaired electrons on Fe in the red complex is ________ .

11. The major product formed in the following reaction is (ignore product stereochemistry)

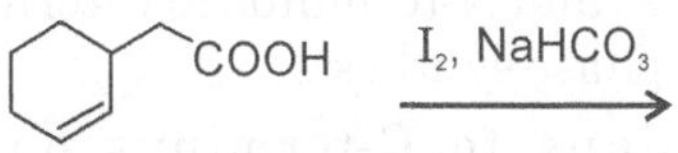

(*a*) 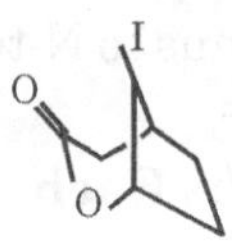
(*b*) 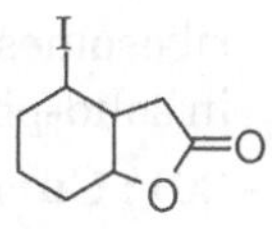

(*c*) 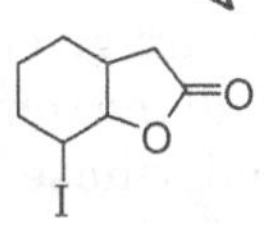
(*d*) 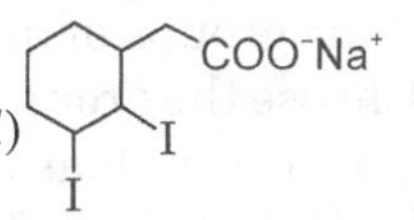

12. When 1.0 g of urea (Molecular Weight = 60) is dissolved in 200 g of solvent S, the freezing point of S is lowered by 0.25 °C. When 1.5 g of a non-electrolyte Y is dissolved in 125 g of S, the freezing point of S is lowered by 0.20 °C. The molecular weight of Y is ________.

13. The major product formed in the following reaction is

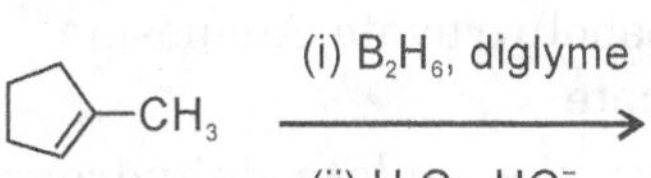

(*a*) 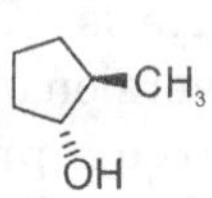
(*b*) 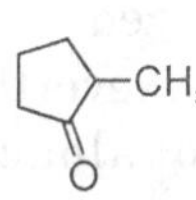

(*c*) 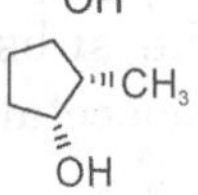
(*d*) 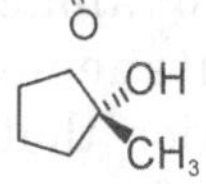

14. For a weak acid at 298 K the molar conductivities (in $ohm^{-1}\ m^2\ mol^{-1}$), at infinite dilution and 0.04 mol dm^{-3} are 4.3×10^{-3} and 1.0×10^{-3}, respectively. The degree of dissociation of the acid (0.04 mol dm^{-3}) at 298 K is ________ .

15. For propene at 298 K, the molar enthalpy of hydrogenation is – 124.27 kJ mol^{-1} and the standard enthalpy of formation is 20.42 kJ mol^{-1}. For propane at 298 K, the standard enthalpy of formation in kJ mol^{-1} is ____________ .

I : BIOCHEMISTRY

(Q. 1 – 10) : Carry One Mark Each

1. Heterologous expression of green fluorescent protein is possible because the genetic code is

(*a*) universal (*b*) triplet

(*c*) degenerate (*d*) non-overlapping

2. Phosphoglucose isomerase was incubated with 0.2 M of glucose 6-phosphate. On reaching equilibrium, 55% of glucose 6-phosphate was converted to fructose 6-phosphate. The equilibrium constant for this reaction is______.

3. Hydrolysis of a peptide involves cleavage of the bond between the atoms

(*a*) N and C_α (*b*) C and O

(*c*) C_α and C (*d*) N and C

4. Inter-conversion of UDP-glucose and UDP-galactose is catalyzed by

(*a*) an oxidase (*b*) a kinase

(*c*) an epimerase (*d*) a mutase

5. Gel filtration profile and corresponding activity data for a pure enzyme are shown in the figure below. The same enzyme sample on SDS-PAGE runs as a 30 kDa polypeptide.

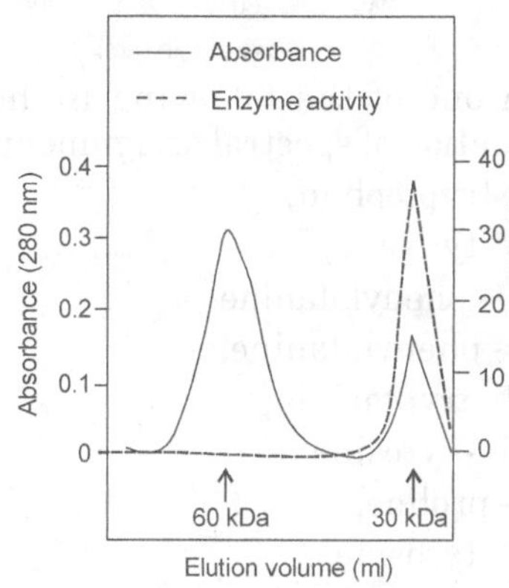

Which one of the following is the correct interpretation of the data?

(*a*) Both monomer and dimer are active

(*b*) Enzyme is active only as a monomer

(*c*) Protein does not form dimers

(*d*) Enzyme is active only as a dimer

6. Amino acid residues predominantly involved in protein-DNA interactions are

(*a*) alanines

(*b*) negatively charged

(*c*) prolines

(*d*) positively charged

7. Cellulose serves as a structural polymer whereas starch does not. This is because cellulose contains

(*a*) β1 → 4 linked glucose monomers and inter-chain hydrogen bonds

(*b*) β1 → 4 linked glucose monomers and intra-chain hydrogen bonds

(*c*) α1 → 4 linked glucose monomers and inter-chain hydrogen bonds

(*d*) α1 → 4 linked glucose monomers and intra-chain hydrogen bonds

8. Molar absorption spectra labeled (i), (ii) and (iii) for three different amino acids are shown below.

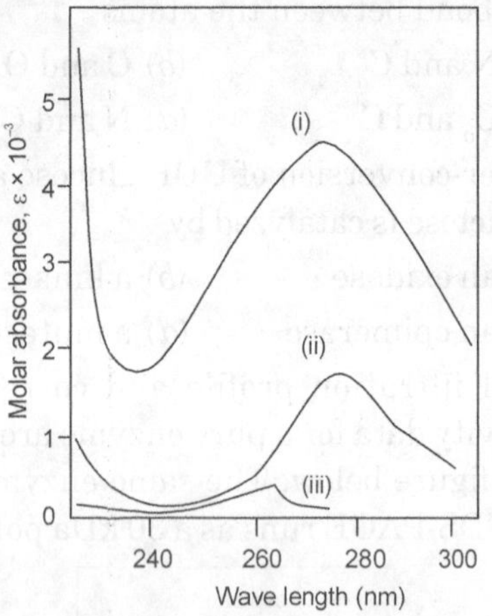

Which one of the following is the correct combination of spectral assignments?

(*a*) (i) - tryptophan,
(ii) - tyrosine,
(iii) - phenylalanine

(*b*) (i) - phenylalanine,
(ii) - tryptophan,
(iii) - tyrosine

(*c*) (i) - proline,
(ii) - tyrosine,
iii) - tryptophan

(*d*) (i) - tryptophan,
(ii) - proline,
(iii) - phenylalanine

9. The fluidity of a phospholipid membrane increases when the fatty acid

(*a*) chain length increases and degree of unsaturation decreases

(*b*) chain length decreases and degree of unsaturation increases

(*c*) chain length decreases and degree of unsaturation decreases

(*d*) chain length increases and degree of unsaturation increases

10. Polypeptides are biosynthesized on the ribosomes inside the cell. Chemical synthesis of polypeptides is also possible through Merrifield's solid-phase peptide synthesis. In both the cases the polypeptide chain is extended one amino acid at a time. The direction of polypeptide synthesis is from.

(*a*) C-terminus to N-terminus in both the cases

(*b*) N-terminus to C-terminus in both the cases

(*c*) C-terminus to N-terminus on the ribosomes and N-terminus to C-terminus in solid-phase synthesis

(*d*) N-terminus to C-terminus on the ribosomes and C-terminus to N-terminus in solid-phase synthesis

(Q. 11 – 20) : Carry Two Marks Each

11. Four groups of metabolites are given below. Choose the group in which all the compounds contain at least one bond whose $\Delta G'^{o}$ of hydrolysis is ≤ –7.0 kcal/mole.

(*a*) Glucose 1-phosphate, Adenosine triphosphate, Fructose 1,6-bisphosphate

(*b*) Creatine phosphate, Acetyl phosphate, Succinyl CoA

(*c*) Glycerol 3-phosphate, Acetyl CoA, 1, 3-Bisphosphoglycerate

(*d*) Glucose 6-phosphate, Phosphoenolpyruvate, Adenosine diphosphate

12. The $\Delta G'^{o}$ for the malate dehydrogenase catalyzed step of Krebs cycle is +7.1 kcal/mole. Nevertheless, the conversion of malate to oxaloacetate in vivo proceeds spontaneously because the subsequent reaction that consumes oxaloacetate has a $\Delta G'^{o}$ of

(*a*) – 3.0 kcal/mole (*b*) + 3.0 kcal/mole

(*c*) – 7.7 kcal/mole (*d*) + 7.7 kcal/mole

13. When freshly isolated intact mitochondria were incubated with ADP and inorganic phosphate neither the oxygen consumption nor the ATP synthesis could be detected. Addition of succinate resulted in increased oxygen consumption as well as ATP synthesis with time. Subsequent addition of cyanide to this system will result in which one of the following?

(*a*) Both oxygen consumption and ATP synthesis are inhibited
(*b*) Oxygen consumption continues but ATP synthesis is inhibited
(*c*) Oxygen consumption is inhibited but ATP synthesis continues
(*d*) Both oxygen consumption and ATP synthesis continue

14. Three micrograms of a circular plasmid of 4200 bp was digested with a restriction enzyme and subjected to agarose gel electrophoresis. Five DNA fragments of different sizes were observed and their sizes summed up to 4200 bp. The number of picomoles of DNA ends generated after complete digestion with the enzyme is______.
(Given: average molecular weight of each base pair is 660 Da)

15. An enzyme was purified using ion-exchange chromatography and the results are shown in the table below.

Step	Volume (ml)	Total protein (mg)	Total Activity (U)
Cell extract	8000	400	800
DEAE Sephacel	10	2	200

Which one of the following is the correct interpretation of these data?
(*a*) 50 fold purification was achieved with 25% yield of the enzyme
(*b*) 25 fold purification was achieved with 50% yield of the enzyme
(*c*) 50 fold purification was achieved with 4% yield of the enzyme
(*d*) 200 fold purification was achieved with 25% yield of the enzyme

16. Aspartate residues are found in the active sites of many enzymes. The pK_a for the β-carboxylate of aspartate is 3.86. At physiological pH this group can function as
(*a*) a nucleophile and a conjugate acid
(*b*) an electrophile and a conjugate acid
(*c*) a nucleophile and a conjugate base
(*d*) an electrophile and a conjugate base

17. Kinetic parameters for the enzyme fumarase with three different substrates are given below.

Substrate	K_M (μM)	k_{cat} (sec^{-1})
Fluorofumarate	27	2700
Fumarate	5	800
Chlorofumarate	111	20

The specificity of fumarase for the substrates decreases in the order
(*a*) Fluorofumarate > Fumarate > Chlorofumarate
(*b*) Chlorofumarate > Fluorofumarate > Fumarate
(*c*) Fumarate > Fluorofumarate > Chlorofumarate
(*d*) Fumarate > Chlorofumarate > Fluorofumarate

18. A polypeptide with the amino acid sequence 'AGKPDHEKAHL' was dissolved in a buffer of pH 1.8. The predominant form of the polypeptide will have a net charge of
(*a*) + 4 (*b*) + 5
(*c*) + 7 (*d*) + 11

19. An N-terminal His-tagged protein of molecular weight 40 kDa was purified using Ni-NTA column. This protein sample was subjected to SDS-PAGE. A western blot of the same using anti-His antibodies is shown below.

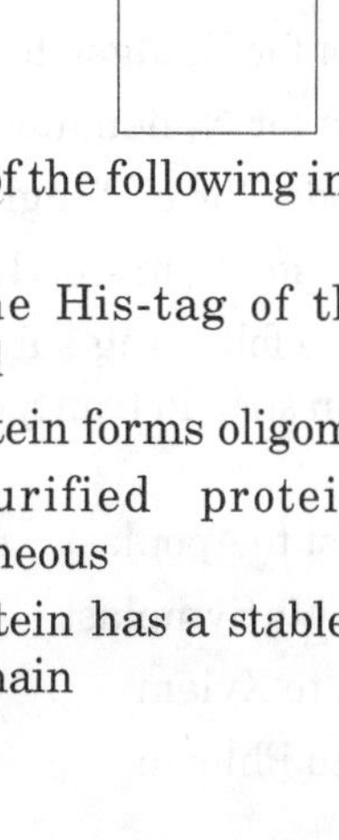

Which one of the following interpretations is correct?
(*a*) Only the His-tag of the protein got removed
(*b*) The protein forms oligomers
(*c*) The purified protein sample is homogeneous
(*d*) The protein has a stable N-terminal 20 kDa domain

20. The sequence of a polypeptide that forms a transmembrane helix is shown below.

```
1           11          21           31          41
|           |           |            |           |
TGERVQLAHH  FSEPEITLII  FGVMAGVIGT   ILLASYGIRR  LIKKSP
```

Which one of the following segments of the peptide is most likely to span the membrane?

(*a*) E3-G22 (*b*) V5-A25
(*c*) E15-A34 (*d*) F21-R40

J : BOTANY

(Q. 1– 10) : Carry One Mark Each.

1. Which of the following is most abundant in the aleurone layer of wheat seeds?

(*a*) Tannin (*b*) Starch
(*c*) Protein (*d*) Lipid

2. Which of the following does NOT use xylem to transport water?

(*a*) Miscanthus (*b*) Marchantia
(*c*) Selaginella (*d*) Magnolia

3. Which of the following is the closest ancestor of all land plants?

(*a*) Blue green algae (*b*) Red algae
(*c*) *Chara* (*d*) *Coleochaeteae*

4. 4',6 diamidino 2-phenylindole (DAPI) is a fluorescent dye used to stain the nucleus. Which of the following plant cells, when mature, cannot be stained by DAPI?

(*a*) Trichomes (*b*) Tracheids
(*c*) Collenchyma (*d*) Mesophyll

5. The uptake of nitrogen (N) and phosphorus (P) by plant roots often involves interaction between root and some symbiotic organisms. Which of the following associations is most commonly found for the uptake of these two nutrients?

(*a*) Bacteria for N, algae for P
(*b*) Bacteria for N, nematodes for P
(*c*) Nematodes for N, fungi for P
(*d*) Bacteria for N, mycorrhizae for P

6. Which of the following summarizes the role of Casparian strip in transport of water in the root?

(*a*) Symplast to Apoplast
(*b*) Apoplast to Symplast
(*c*) Phloem to Xylem
(*d*) Xylem to Phloem

7. Atropine is a drug used in the management of pesticide poisoning. Which of the following plants can serve as a commercial source of this anticholinergic drug?

(*a*) *Datura metel*
(*b*) *Medicago trancatula*
(*c*) *Mangifera indica*
(*d*) *Arachis hypogaea*

8. Which of the following is NOT involved in plant immune response?

(*a*) Antimicrobial proteins
(*b*) Hypersensitive response
(*c*) Pattern recognition receptors
(*d*) Interleukins

9. Which of the following is a neutral phenomenon?

(*a*) Natural selection
(*b*) Sexual selection
(*c*) Genetic drift
(*d*) Population bottleneck

10. When a plant is infected by a pathogen at one site, the distal parts of the plant and neighboring plants develop increased resistance to subsequent pathogen attack. Which of the following molecules mediates this long-distance signal?

(*a*) Nitric oxide
(*b*) Ethylene
(*c*) Jasmonic acid and its derivatives
(*d*) Salicylic acid and its derivatives

(Q. 11 – 20) : Carry Two Marks Each.

11. An inbred line of a plant with red flower and tall stem was crossed to another inbred line with white flower and short stem. The F_1 plants, which all had red flower and tall stem, were backcrossed to the line with white flower and short stem, and the following F_2 individuals were obtained: 103 red, tall; 89 white, short; 26 red, short; and 23 white, tall. What is the recombination percentage between the flower color locus and the stem height locus.

(*a*) 19-21% (*b*) 49-51%
(*c*) 79-81% (*d*) 0-2%

12. Consider the following pathway controlling time to flowering in wheat:

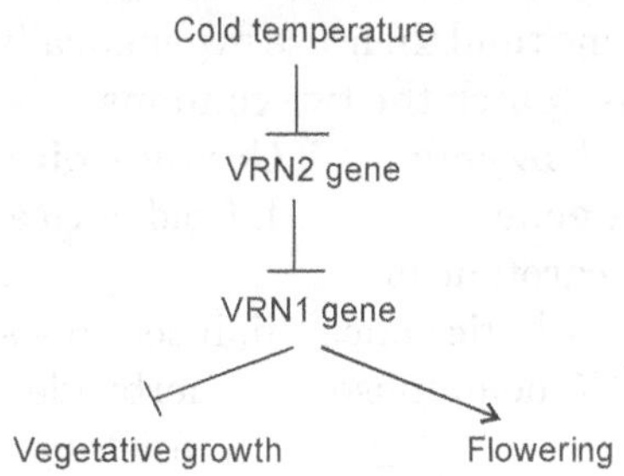

If batch P of wheat seed is vernalized before sowing and batch Q is not vernalized, then which of the following statements is most likely to be correct?

(*a*) P will have lower VRN2 transcript and will flower later than Q

(*b*) P will have lower VRN2 transcript and will flower earlier than Q

(*c*) P will have higher VRN2 transcript and will flower later than Q

(*d*) P and Q will have equal VRN2 transcript and will flower at the same time

13. The three plots P, Q and R (in different units) in the graph below represent the dependence of photosynthesis rate (PR), leaf expansion rate (LER) and translocation rate of assimilates (TR) in a plant on leaf water potential. Which of the following statements is correct in this regard?

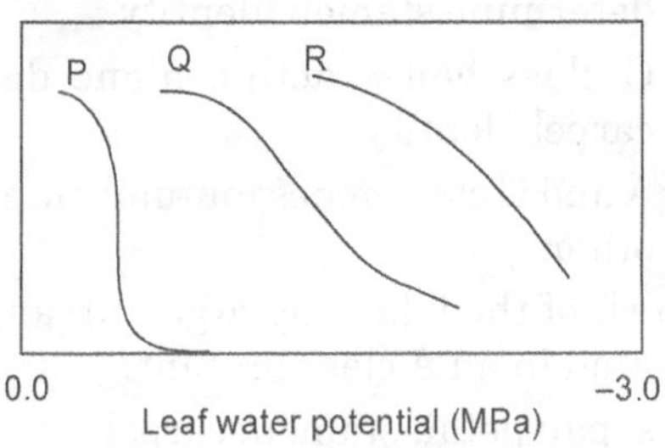

(*a*) P represents LER; Q represents TR; R represents PR

(*b*) P represents TR; Q represents PR; R represents LER.

(*c*) P represents PR; Q represents LER; R represents TR

(*d*) P represents LER; Q represents PR; R represents TR

14. PIN proteins are plasma membran e-localized carrier proteins required for polar auxin transport in plants. Four different carrier proteins are shown in the diagram below labeled P1-P4. Arrow indicates the direction of auxin flow. Which among these is most likely to be a PIN protein?

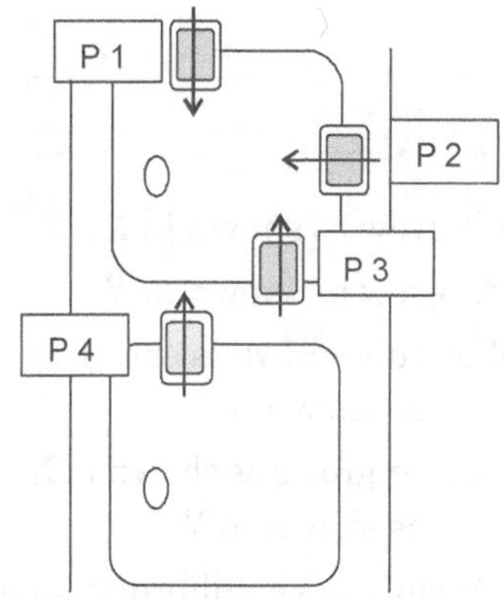

(*a*) P 1 (*b*) P 2

(*c*) P 3 (*d*) P 4

15. An RFLP marker shows sequence polymorphism in two ecotypes (X and Y) of a plant. In ecotype X, the marker contains one GAATTC site in its sequence, whereas in Y it has the sequence GAAATC at the same site. The rest of the sequence is identical in both ecotypes. In a genotyping experiment, the marker was PCR amplified from four different seedlings (P, Q, R, S), completely digested with *EcoRI* and the products were analyzed by electrophoresis. The diagram below shows the band patterns obtained. Based on the information provided, which of the following statements is correct?

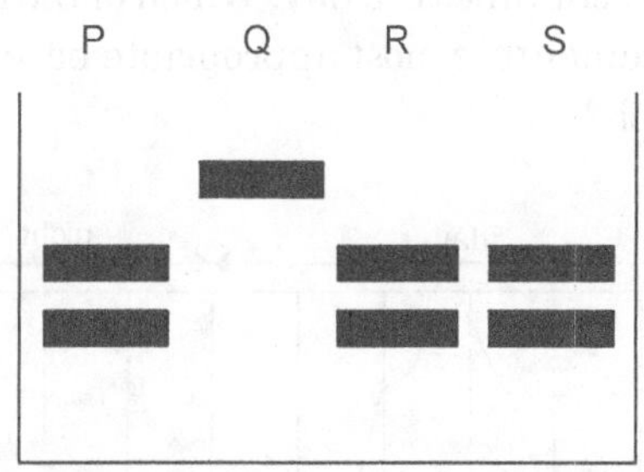

(*a*) Seedling Q belongs to ecotype Y

(*b*) Seedling Q belongs to ecotype X

(*c*) Seedling P belongs to ecotype Y

(*d*) Seedling R belongs to ecotype Y

16. The cell surface expands differently in different plant cells. Two common modes of expansion are shown below (X and Y). Each rectangular box represents a cell marked with dots on its surface. The spacing between the dots changes after the cell has undergone expansion as indicated by the arrow. Which of the following statements is correct with respect to the growth of root hair and pollen tube?

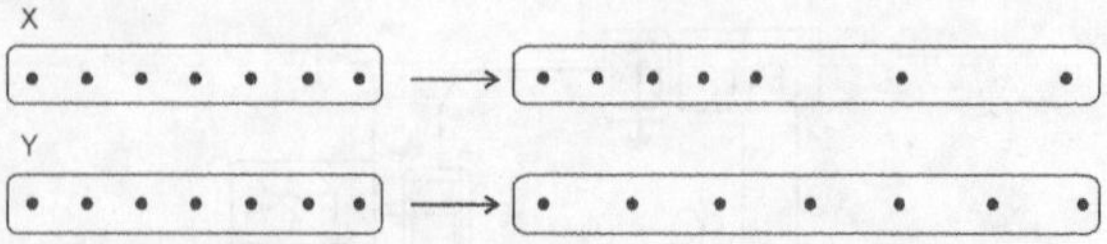

(*a*) Both grow as shown in X

(*b*) Both grow as shown in Y

(*c*) Pollen tube grows as shown in X, root hair grows as shown in Y

(*d*) Root hair grows as shown in X, pollen tube grows as shown in Y

17. Hardy Weinberg's equilibrium for a locus with two alleles p and q is mathematically defined as $P^2 + Q^2 + 2PQ = 1$. Which of the following equations represents the corresponding equilibrium for a locus with three alleles p, q and r? (P, Q and R represent the frequencies of p, q and r, respectively)

(*a*) $P^3 + Q^3 + R^3 + 3PQR = 1$

(*b*) $P^2 + Q^2 + R^2 + 2PQ + 2QR + 2PR = 1$

(*c*) $P^2Q + Q^2R + R^2P + 2PQ + 2QR + 2PR = 1$

(*d*) $P^2 + Q^2 + R^2 + 2P^2Q + 2Q^2R + 2P^2R = 1$

18. The continuous and dashed lines in the following graph represent the velocity of sap flow in two different parts of a plant at different times of a day. Which of the following statements is most appropriate based on this graph?

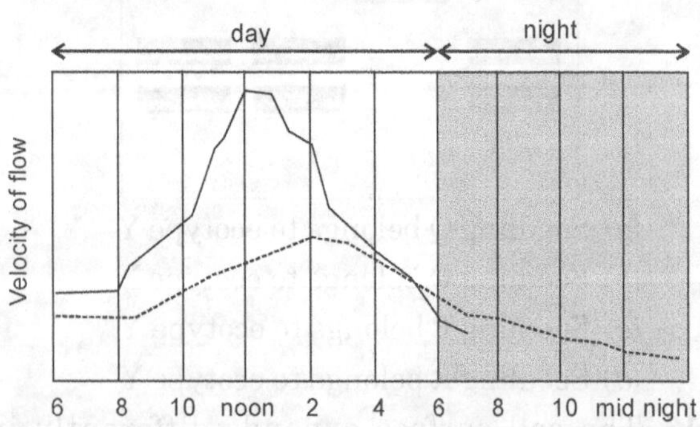

(*a*) The continuous line represents the trunk, and the dotted line a twig

(*b*) The continuous line represents a twig, and the dotted line the trunk

(*c*) The continuous line represents a root, and the dotted line a twig

(*d*) The continuous line represents a root, and the dotted line the trunk

19. Given below are the names of some genes/enzymes and their use in genetically modified crops. Match the two columns.

Gene/enzyme	**Commercial use**
P. Bt gene	i. Golden rice
Q. β-carotene bio synthetic genes	ii. insect resistance
R. ACC deaminase	iii. herbicide resistance
S. EPSP synthase	iv. fruit ripening

	P	**Q**	**S**	**R**
(*a*)	i	ii	iii	iv
(*b*)	ii	i	iv	iii
(*c*)	iii	i	ii	iv
(*d*)	ii	i	iii	iv

20. The basic tenets of the ABC model of Arabidopsis flower development are shown below along with a diagram.

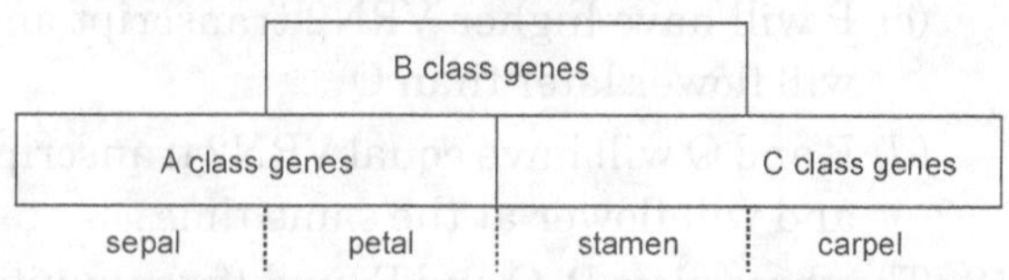

(i) A class genes acting alone determine sepal identity

(ii) A and B class genes acting together determine petal identity

(iii) B and C class genes acting together determine stamen identity

(iv) C class genes acting alone determine carpel identity

(v) A and C class genes mutually inhibit each other

Which of the following organ arrangements is found in an A class mutant?

(*a*) sepal; petal; stamen; carpel

(*b*) carpel; stamen; stamen; carpel

(*c*) petal; petal; stamen; carpel

(*d*) stamen; stamen; stamen; carpel

K : MICROBIOLOGY

(Q. 1 – 10) : Carry One Mark Each

1. Which one of the following is the most appropriate technique to determine the relatedness of two bacterial species?

(*a*) DNA hybridization

(*b*) Doubling time measurement

(*c*) Biochemical characterization

(*d*) Plasmid profiling

2. Which one of the following phages undergoes non-integrative lysogenic phase?
(*a*) λ (*b*) P1
(*c*) T7 (*d*) M13

3. Which one of the following is **NOT** a part of human microbiome?
(*a*) Propionibacterium acnes
(*b*) Lactobacillus casei
(*c*) Streptococcus suis
(*d*) Bacteroides fragilis

4. Resident macrophages of ________ are called Kupffer cells.
(*a*) brain (*b*) liver
(*c*) lung (*d*) kidney

5. The enzyme responsible for generation of hypochlorous ions during phagocytosis is
(*a*) NADPH oxidase
(*b*) catalase
(*c*) myeloperoxidase
(*d*) superoxide dismutase

6. Teichoic acid is composed of repetitive units of
(*a*) keto-deoxy octanoic acid
(*b*) glucose
(*c*) N-acetyl glucosamine
(*d*) glycerol

7. Biofilm produced by bacteria is detected by
(*a*) Saffranin (*b*) Malachite green
(*c*) Basic fuchsin (*d*) Congo red

8. The precursor for the synthesis of aromatic amino acids is
(*a*) phosphoenolpyruvate
(*b*) pyruvate
(*c*) oxaloacetate
(*d*) α-ketoglutarate

9. The net yield of NADH in the Embden-Meyerhof pathway in *E. coli* is _______.

10. *E. coli* ribonuclease contains 124 amino acids. The number of nucleotides present in the gene encoding the protein is ______________ .

(Q. 11 – 20) : Carry Two Marks Each

11. Which of the following infectious agents cross the blood-brain barrier?
(*a*) Streptococcus pneumoniae
(*b*) Coxsackie virus
(*c*) Rotavirus
(*d*) Streptococcus pyogenes

12. At OD_{540nm} = 0.5, which one of the following bacterial mono-dispersed cell suspensions will have
(i) maximum and
(ii) minimum number of cells?
(P) Mycoplasma pneumoniae
(Q) Micrococcus luteus
(R) Bacillus subtilis
(S) Escherichia coli
(*a*) P & Q (*b*) P & R
(*c*) Q & R (*d*) R & S

13. Which one of the following enzyme combinations allows some bacteria to utilize acetate through glyoxylate pathway?
(P) Isocitrate lyase
(Q) Isocitrate dehydrogenase
(R) Succinyl CoA synthetase
(S) Malate synthase
(*a*) P & S (*b*) P & R
(*c*) Q & S (*d*) Q & R

14. The decimal reduction time (D_{121}) for *Clostridium botulinum* spores is 0.2 min. The time required to reduce the spore count from 10^{12} to one spore at 121°C is_____minutes.

15. *E.coli* requires three genes, *galK* (kinase), *galT* (transacetylase) and *galE* (epimerase) to utilize galactose. If there is a mutation in any one of these genes, the mutant cannot utilize galactose. Which one of the following combinations of merodiploids will support the growth of mutants on galactose?
(P) $galK^+ galT^+ galE^-$ / $galK^- galT^+ galE^-$
(Q) $galK^- galT^+ galE^-$ / $galK^+ galT^- galE^+$
(R) $galK^+ galT^- galE^-$ / $galK^- galT^- galE^+$
(S) $galK^+ galT^+ galE^-$ / $galK^+ galT^- galE^+$
(*a*) P & Q (*b*) P & R
(*c*) R & S (*d*) Q & S

16. Nitrogenase reduces N_2 to NH_3. Metal co-factors required for this activity are_______.
(*a*) Fe & Cu
(*b*) Mo & Fe
(*c*) Mo & Mn
(*d*) Cu & Mn

17. If a bacterial cell contains 5,000 genes and if the average mutation frequency per gene is 2×10^{-4} per generation, the average number of new mutations per generation is ________.

18. The growth profile of *E. coli* on glucose plus lactose is shown below. The specific growth rate of the second exponential phase is____h^{-1}.

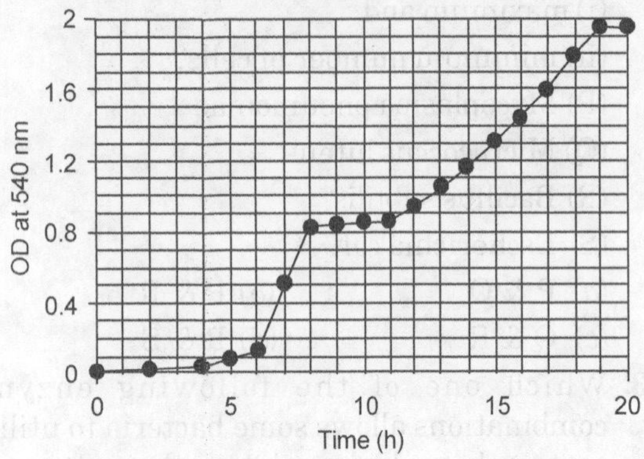

19. Match the cell structure components given in **Group I** with appropriate functions from **Group II.**

Group–I	Group–II
P. Cell membrane	I. Nutrient transport
Q. Purple membrane	II. Photosynthesis
R. Cisternae	III. Active transport
S. Outer membrane	IV. Protein glycosylation
	V. Light-driven proton transport

	P	Q	R	S
(*a*)	I	V	II	III
(*b*)	I	II	IV	III
(*c*)	III	II	V	I
(*d*)	III	V	IV	I

20. Match the antibiotics given in Group I with appropriate targets from Group II.

Group–I	Group–II
P. Nalidixic acid	I. RNA polymerase
Q. Tetracycline	II. DNA gyrase
R. Erythromycin	III. DNA polymerase
S. Rifampin	IV. 50S ribosomal subunit
	V. Aminoacyl tRNA

	P	Q	R	S
(*a*)	III	IV	V	I
(*b*)	V	I	IV	II
(*c*)	II	V	IV	I
(*d*)	II	V	I	IV

L : ZOOLOGY

(Q. 1 – 10) : Carry One Mark Each

1. Acorn worms (*Saccoglassus sp.*) belong to which ONE of the following Phyla?

(*a*) Platyhelminthes

(*b*) Achelminthes

(*c*) Hemichordata (Chordata)

(*d*) Annelida

2. A population of Bees develops resistance to pesticides and the trait gets fixed within a few generations. This is an example of

(*a*) macroevolution

(*b*) disruptive selection

(*c*) stabilizing selection

(*d*) microevolution

3. The nature of the polymorphic DNA fragment used for mapping is

(*a*) dominant (*b*) partial dominant

(*c*) co-dominant (*d*) recessive

4. The sex of a *Drosophila melanogaster*, which has 4 copies of X-chromosomes and 4 sets of autosomes will be

(*a*) female (*b*) male

(*c*) metafemale (*d*) metamale

5. Which of the following cations are found in higher concentration in extracellular fluid as compared to intracellular fluid in animals?

(*a*) Na^+ and Ca^{++} (*b*) K^+ and Ca^{++}

(*c*) K^+ and Mg^{++} (*d*) Na^+ and Mg^{++}

6. Detoxification of alcohol occurs in liver cells where peroxisomal enzymes remove hydrogen from it, which is

(*a*) combined with water molecules to generate hydrogen peroxide.

(*b*) used to break down hydrogen peroxide

(*c*) transferred to the mitochondria

(*d*) transferred to oxygen molecules to generate hydrogen peroxide.

7. When cells are treated with cyanide, which ONE of the following organelles will have the highest level of cyanide inside?

(*a*) Mitochondria

(*b*) Peroxisomes

(*c*) Lysosomes

(*d*) Endoplasmic reticulum

8. Toxoplasmosis in humans is caused by *Toxoplasma gondii*, an obligate intracellular parasite with two different life cycles, sexual and asexual. The sexual cycle occurs in which ONE of the following definitive hosts?

(*a*) Dog (*b*) Cat
(*c*) Rat (*d*) Human

9. Which ONE of the following is often a life-threatening systemic inflammatory response?

(*a*) Tuberculosis
(*b*) Lupus erythematosus
(*c*) Septic shock
(*d*) Hypertension

10. During the gastrulation stage of amphibian development, ectoderm formation takes place by the expansion of epithelial cell sheet over mesodermal cells. This type of cell movement is termed as

(*a*) ingression (*b*) epiboly
(*c*) involution (*d*) delamination

(Q. 11 – 20) : Carry Two Marks Each

11. In a population, 600 individuals have MM blood group, 300 have MN blood group and 100 have NN blood group. What will be the frequencies of M and N alleles in this population?

(*a*) M 0.75 and N 0.25
(*b*) M 0.65 and N 0.35
(*c*) M 0.85 and N 0.15
(*d*) M 0.55 and N 0.45

12. The molecules, hexanoic acid, lysine, histidine and glucose, each contain 6 carbon atoms, but have completely different properties due to the presence of different functional groups. Which ONE of these molecules has a high calorific value?

(*a*) Lysine
(*b*) Hexanoic acid
(*c*) Glucose
(*d*) Histidine

13. The primary function of polysaccharides attached to glycoproteins in the animal cell membrane is to

(*a*) facilitate diffusion of molecules down their concentration gradients
(*b*) maintain membrane fluidity at low temperatures
(*c*) maintain the integrity of a fluid mosaic membrane
(*d*) mediate cell-to-cell recognition

14. Which ONE of the following mechanisms is used to coordinate the expression of multiple, related genes in eukaryotic cells?

(*a*) Environmental signals enter the cell and bind directly to promoters
(*b*) Genes share a common intragenic sequence, and allow several activators to turn on their transcription, regardless of location
(*c*) Genes are organized into large operons, allowing them to be transcribed as a single unit
(*d*) Genes are organized into clusters, with local chromatin structures influencing the expression of all the clustered genes at once

15. In an experiment involving development of 64-cell stage sea urchin, an isolated animal hemisphere was combined with isolated micromeres. Which ONE of the following will be the resulting structure?

(*a*) A ball of ectomesodermal cells
(*b*) A ciliated ball of ectodermal cells
(*c*) A recognizable pluteus larva
(*d*) A ball of endodermal cells

16. Glycoprotein hormones, hCG and eCG, are synthesized in women and mares respectively, during pregnancy. Both of these chorionic gonadotropin hormones

(*a*) have only LH-like activity in their respective species
(*b*) have only FSH-like activity in other species
(*c*) are biologically inactive in other species
(*d*) are routinely employed to promote final stages of follicular maturation, ovulation and to treat infertility in women

17. *Entamoeba histolytica* is an intestinal parasite that causes dysentery in humans. This parasite resides in the isotonic environment of intestine and other tissues in the human body and does not possess contractile vacuoles. If this parasite is placed in fresh water, it will

(*a*) survive for long time, until they re-enter the host environment
(*b*) die due to hypoosmotic shock
(*c*) not survive in water as they require high salt content
(*d*) die due to hyperosmotic shock

18. In an experiment involving Drosophila development, a large amount of purified *bicoid* mRNA was injected into the posterior end of a wild-type embryo, the resulting developing embryo will have

(*a*) normal development with one each of head, thorax and abdomen
(*b*) head in the middle with two thoraces and two abdomens
(*c*) a head with two thoraces and an abdomen
(*d*) two heads and two thoraces with an abdomen segment in the middle

19. The migratory desert locust, *Schistocerca gregaria*, exists in two mutually exclusive forms: a short-winged, uniformly colored, solitary insect and a long-winged, brightly colored, gregarious morph. These phenotypes depend on crowding. Such phenotypic plasticity is called

(*a*) reaction norm
(*b*) polyphenism
(*c*) Batesian mimicry
(*d*) polymorphism

20. Given below is the list of animals and their respective characteristics.

Animals	**Characteristics**
I. Sea anemone	i. Three pairs of jointed legs
II. Bluefly	ii. Diploblastic acoelomate
III. Starfish	iii. Collar cells
IV. Sponge	iv. Tube feet

Which ONE of the following represents the correct match?

	I	II	III	IV
(*a*)	iv	i	ii	iii
(*b*)	iii	i	iv	ii
(*c*)	ii	i	iv	iii
(*d*)	ii	i	iii	iv

M : FOOD TECHNOLOGY

(Q. 1 – 10) : Carry One Mark Each.

1. Bread staling is caused by ______.

(*a*) Caramelisation
(*b*) Gelatinisation
(*c*) Retrogradation
(*d*) Aggregation

2. The grades of tea in the increasing order of their leaf size are ____, ____ and ____.

(*a*) Souchang, pekoe and orange pekoe
(*b*) Pekoe, souchang and orange pekoe
(*c*) Orange pekoe, souchang and pekoe
(*d*) Orange pekoe, pekoe and souchang

3. Fruit juice is being pasteurized in a tubular heat exchanger. The retention time in holding tube of 0.2 m^2 cross sectional area is 3 seconds. If the flow rate of juice is 0.4 m^3 s^{-1}, the length of the holding tube in m, is ____

4. The oil, which experiences flavor reversion even at the lower peroxide value is ____.

(*a*) Mustard
(*b*) Soybean
(*c*) Palm
(*d*) Sesame

5. 80 kg of wheat containing 10 kg of moisture has been dried to a moisture content of 8% wet basis in 3 hours under constant rate period of drying. The drying rate in kg h^{-1} is

6. The rate of cream separation in a disc bowl centrifuge can be increased by ____.

(*a*) Increasing the size of the bowl
(*b*) Lower viscosity of fluid
(*c*) Increasing RPM of the bowl
(*d*) All of these

7. Rigor mortis is caused due to ______.

(*a*) Unavailability of ATP which is necessary to break the link between actin and myosin
(*b*) Rupturing of tissue due to unavailability of oxygen
(*c*) Decrease in body temperature
(*d*) Breakage of rigid protein molecules in sarcoplasm

8. Oxygen is permeating through an EVOH film of thickness 't' and solubility coefficient 'S'. If diffusivity of oxygen through the film is 'D', then permeability of oxygen through the film will be ______.

(*a*) D/t
(*b*) D/S
(*c*) D × S
(*d*) S/D

9. Condensing steam is used to heat vegetable oil in a double pipe co-current heat exchanger. If the inlet and outlet temperature of steam are T_{hi} and T_{ho}, and for vegetable oil T_{ci} and T_{co} respectively, the log mean temperature difference (ΔT_{LM}) will be______.

(*a*) $\dfrac{T_{hi} - T_{co}}{\ln \dfrac{T_{hi} - T_{ci}}{T_{hi} - T_{co}}}$

(*b*) $\dfrac{(T_{ho} - T_{co}) - (T_{hi} - T_{co})}{\ln \dfrac{T_{ho} - T_{ci}}{T_{ho} - T_{co}}}$

(*c*) $\dfrac{(T_{hi} - T_{co}) - (T_{ho} - T_{ci})}{\ln \dfrac{T_{hi} - T_{ci}}{T_{ho} - T_{co}}}$

(*d*) $\dfrac{T_{co} - T_{ci}}{\ln \dfrac{T_{hi} - T_{ci}}{T_{hi} - T_{co}}}$

10. To produce Blue veined cheese, the curd is inoculated with strains of_______.

(*a*) Propioniobacterium shermanii
(*b*) Penicilium roqueforti
(*c*) Pencilium camemberti
(*d*) Brevibacterium linens

Q. 11 – Q. 20 Carry Two Marks Each.

11. Match the food spoilage organisms given in Column I with the associated foods given in Column II

Column –I	Column –II
P. Clostridium botulinum	1. Fish
Q. Salmonella spp.	2. Cooked starch foods
R. Vibrio parahaemolyticus	3. Meat, egg and poultry
S. Bacillus cereus	4. Canned foods

(*a*) P-4, Q-3, R-1, S-2 (*b*) P-3, Q-4, R-2, S-1
(*c*) P-2, Q-1, R-3, S-4 (*d*) P-4, Q-3, R-2, S-1

12. Fluid is flowing inside a pipe of radius 'R' in fully developed laminar flow. If the velocity of the fluid at the centre at a distance 'L' is 'v_{max}', velocity at radial distance of ¾ (R) will be __times v_{max}

(*a*) 9/16 (*b*) 7/16
(*c*) 16/9 (*d*) 16/7

13. The amount of sugar to be added (kg) to 40 kg of mango pulp to increase its total soluble solids from 20% wt. to 65% wt. is _______

14. (A) **Assertion :** Acidulates are added in soft drinks to provide a buffering action.

(R) **Reason :** Buffers tend to prevent changes in pH and prevent excessive tartness.

Choose the correct answer from the following

(*a*) Both (A) and (R) are true but (R) is not the correct reason
(*b*) Both (A) and (R) are true and (R) is the correct reason for (A)
(*c*) (A) is true but (R) is false
(*d*) Both (A) and (R) are false

15. The D_{121} and Z values for C. botulinum spores in canned food are 0.2 min and 10 °C, respectively. Total time required in min, to reduce the spores from 10^2 to 10^{-6} at 111 °C is ______ .

16. In a typical Psychrometric Chart shown below, the processes OP, OQ and OR related to air water vapor mixture are_____,_______ and _________.

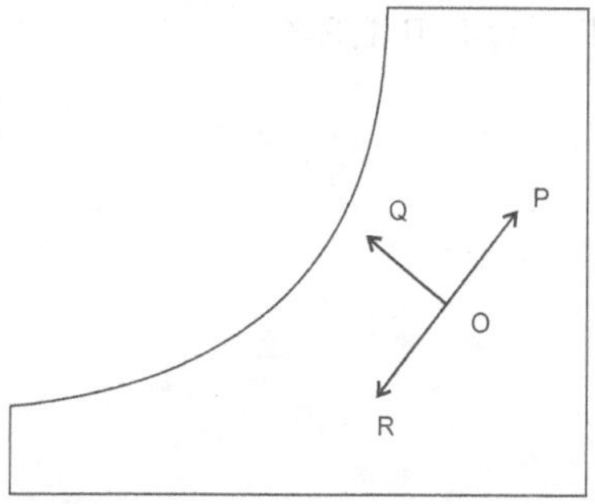

(*a*) Cooling & dehumidification, cooling & humidification, heating & humidification
(*b*) Cooling & dehumidification, heating & humidification, drying
(*c*) Heating & humidification, cooling & humidification, cooling & dehumidification
(*d*) Heating & humidification, cooling & dehumidification, drying

17. Match the enzymes in Column I with their functions in Column II

Column - I	Column - II
P. Amylase	1. Conversion of sucrose to glucose and fructose
Q. Invertase	2. Softening of dough
R. Phosphatase	3. Effectiveness of pasteurization
S. Protease	4. Conversion of starch to maltose

(*a*) P-1, Q-2, R-3, S-4 (*b*) P-4, Q-1, R-3, S-2
(*c*) P-1, Q-4, R-2, S-3 (*d*) P-2, Q-4, R-3, S-1

18. Match the terms in Column I with their most appropriate description in Column II

Column – I

P. Enrichment

Q. Fortification

R. Supplementation

S. Complementation

Column – II

1. Overcome the deficiency of nutrients by mixing of two plant sources
2. Overcome the deficiency of nutrients from a synthetic source
3. Restoration of nutrients which are lost during processing
4. Addition of nutrients which may or may not originally present

(*a*) P-3, Q-4, R-2, S-1

(*b*) P-4, Q-3, R-1, S-2

(*c*) P-1, Q-2, R-3, S-4

(*d*) P-2, Q-3, R-1, S-4

19. Match the products in Column I with their Original Phase in Column II

Column – I	Column – II
P. Milk	1. Colloidal
Q. Butter	2. Solution
R. Lactose	3. Water in oil emulsion
S. Casein	4. Oil in water emulsion

(*a*) P-3, Q-4, R-1, S-2

(*b*) P-3, Q-4, R-2, S-1

(*c*) P-4, Q-3, R-2, S-1

(*d*) P-4, Q-3, R-1, S-2

20. (A) **Assertion:** Presence of low sulphur containing amino acids makes casein in milk to boil, sterilize and concentrate without coagulation even at higher temperatures.

(R) **Reason :** This is due to the restricted formation of di-sulphide bonds resulting in increased stability.

Choose the correct answer from the following

(*a*) Both (A) and (R) are true and (R) is the correct reason for (A)

(*b*) Both (A) and (R) are true but (R) is not the correct reason for (A)

(*c*) Both (A) and (R) are false

(*d*) (A) is true but (R) is false

ANSWERS

GENERAL APTITUDE (GA)

1. (*c*) 2. (*b*) 3. (*b*) 4. (*b*) 5. (*c*) 6. (120 – 120) 7. (*c*) 8. (*c*) 9. (*a*) 10. (7.0 – 7.0)

H : CHEMISTRY

1. (*a*) 2. (4.0 – 4.0) 3. (*b*) 4. (*d*) 5. (*b*) 6. (*d*) 7. (13.55 – 13.64) 8. (0.52 – 0.54) 9. (*d*) 10. (4 – 4) 11. (*c*) 12. (180 – 182) 13. (*a*) 14. (0.22 – 0.24) 15. (–105 to –102)

I : BIOCHEMISTRY

1. (*a*) 2. (1.20 – 1.24) 3. (*d*) 4. (*c*) 5. (*b*) 6. (*d*) 7. (*a*) 8. (*a*) 9. (*b*) 10. (*d*) 11. (*b*) 12. (*c*) 13. (*a*) 14. (10 – 11) 15. (*a*) 16. (*c*) 17. (*c*) 18. (*b*) 19. (*d*) 20. (*c*)

J : BOTANY

1. (*c*) 2. (*b*) 3. (*c*) 4. (*b*) 5. (*d*) 6. (*b*) 7. (*a*) 8. (*d*) 9. (*c*) 10. (*d*) 11. (*a*) 12. (*b*) 13. (*d*) 14. (*d*) 15. (*a*) 16. (*a*) 17. (*b*) 18. (*b*) 19. (*b*) 20. (*b*)

K : MICROBIOLOGY

1. (*a*) 2. (*b*) 3. (*c*) 4. (*b*) 5. (*c*) 6. (*d*) 7. (*d*) 8. (*a*) 9. (2.0 – 2.0) 10. (375 – 375) 11. (*c*) 12. (*b*) 13. (*a*) 14. (2.4 – 2.4) 15. (*d*) 16. (*b*) 17. (1.0 – 1.0) 18. (0.10 – 0.11) 19. (*d*) 20. (*c*)

L : ZOOLOGY

1. (*c*) 2. (*d*) 3. (*c*) 4. (*a*) 5. (*a*) 6. (*d*) 7. (*a*) 8. (*b*) 9. (*c*) 10. (*b*) 11. (*a*) 12. (*b*) 13. (*d*) 14. (*d*) 15. (*c*) 16. (*a*) 17. (*b*) 18. (*d*) 19. (*b*) 20. (*c*)

M : FOOD TECHNOLOGY

1. (*c*) 2. (*a*) 3. (5.9 – 6.1) 4. (*b*) 5. (1.3 – 1.4) 6. (*d*) 7. (*a*) 8. (*c*) 9. (*d*) 10. (*b*) 11. (*a*) 12. (*b*) 13. (51 – 52) 14. (*b*) 15. (15 – 17) 16. (*c*) 17. (*b*) 18. (*a*) 19. (*c*) 20. (*a*)

EXPLANATIONS

GENERAL APTITUDE (GA)

3. All are prime numbers, except 33.

5. Given $|9y - 6| = 3$

It has two values,

i.e., $9y - 6 = 3$ ...(*i*)

and $-(9y - 6) = 3$ ...(*ii*)

From equation (*i*), we get

$$9y = 9$$

$$\therefore \quad y = 1$$

Also from equation (*ii*), we get

$$-(9y - 6) = 3$$

$$9y - 6 = 3$$

$$9y = 3$$

$$\therefore \quad y = \frac{1}{3}$$

So $y = 1, \frac{1}{3}$

Put $y = 1$, we get

$$y^2 - 4\frac{y}{3} = 1 - \frac{4.1}{3} = -\frac{1}{3}$$

and put $y = \frac{1}{3}$, we get

$$= \left(\frac{1}{3}\right)^2 - \frac{4}{3} \times \frac{1}{3}$$

$$= \frac{1}{9} - \frac{4}{9} = -\frac{3}{9} = -\frac{1}{3}$$

So, the required value is $-\frac{1}{3}$

6. From given graph,

Large plants = A plant with installed capacity of atleast 200 tonnes i.e the plant number is 1, 4, 8 and 9.

$\therefore$ Total production of large plants having plant number 1, 4, 8 and 9.

$= 160 + 190 + 230 + 190$

$= 770$ tonnes

Small plants = A plant with installed capacity is less then 200 tonnes i.e., plant number is 2, 3, 5, 6 and 7.

$\therefore$ Total production of small plants having plant numbers 2, 3, 5, 6 and 7

$= 150 + 160 + 120 + 100 + 120$

$= 650$ tonnes

Now the difference between total production of large plants and small plants

$= 770 - 650 = 120$ tonnes

10. Given $(211)^{870} + (146)^{127} \times (3)^{424}$

$= (211)^{4 \times 217} (211)^2 + (146)^{4 \times 31} \cdot (146)^3 \times (3)^{4 \times 106}$

$= 1 \cdot (211)^2 + 1 \cdot (146)^3 \times 1$

$= 1 + 1 \times 6 \times 1$

Unit digit $= 1 + 6 = 7$

So, the unit digit is 7.

H : CHEMISTRY

1.

Species	**B-F bond distance**
BF_3	130 PM
BF_4^-	143 PM
H_3NBF_3	170 PM
$(CH_3)_2OBF_3$	142 pm

So, BF_3 has shortest B-F bond distance

2. Following 4 confirmations possible for 1, 2– dimethylcyclo hexance

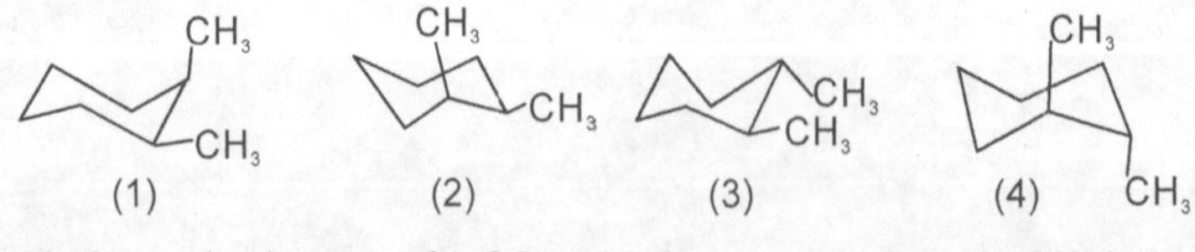

3. For substances which degrades by 1st order kinetics have very short half life i.e. they are removed/ degrade very fast from the any environment. Thus, the given statement contradict with this. So answer is B.

4.

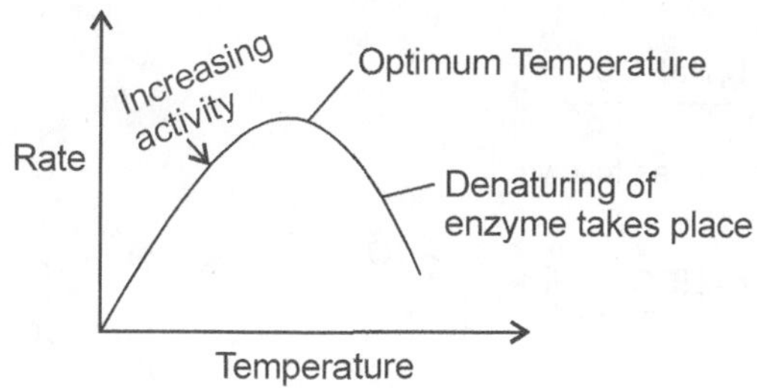

5. For reversible adiabatic process in a perfect gas $\Delta U = \int_1^2 C_V dT$

6. $K_c = \frac{[A^-][H^+]}{[H_A]}$, $Pk_a = -\log_{10} k_a$

Component	Pk_a
$[Fe(H_2O)_6]^{+2}$	11
$[Fe(H_2O)_6]^{+3}$	2.735
V_2O_5	10.25
N_2O_5	5.40

So, $[Fe(H_2O)_6]^{+2} > [Fe(H_2O)_6]^{+3}$

$V_2O_5 > N_2O_5$

7. Ionization energy (eV) = Potential energy + kinetic energy

Potential energy of two electron = 27.211 eV

So, PE of one electron = $\frac{27.211}{2}$ = 13.6055 eV

Now, the kinetic energy is given by $KE = -\frac{Ze^2}{2r}$

$Z = 1, e = 1, r = 0.5295 \text{ Å}$

Further 1eV = 96.485 KJ/ml.

$\therefore \quad K_E = -\frac{(1)(1)^2}{(2)(0.5295)(96.485)}$

$= -9.787 \times 10^{-3}$ eV

$\therefore$ Ionization energy

(eV) = $13.6055 - 9.787 \times 10^{-3}$

= 13.596 eV

8. $[CoCl_4]^{-2}$ has d^7 with high spin

$d^7 = e^4 t_2^3$.

Now, the CFSE (Crystal Field Stabilization Energy) = $[-0.4 t_2g + 0.6 eg]\Delta t$

Number of electrons in t_{2g} = 3

Number of electrons in e_g = 4.

$\therefore$ CFSE = $[-(0.4 \times 3) + (0.6)(4)]\Delta t = 1.2\, \Delta t$.

Now, $\Delta t = \frac{4}{9}\Delta_0$

$\therefore$ CFSE of $[CoCl_4]^{-2} = 1.2 \times \frac{4}{9}\Delta_0 = 0.533\, \Delta_0$.

11. 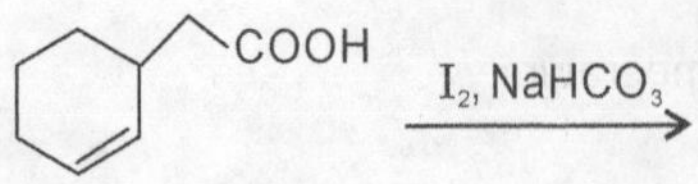

The reaction sequence is as follows:

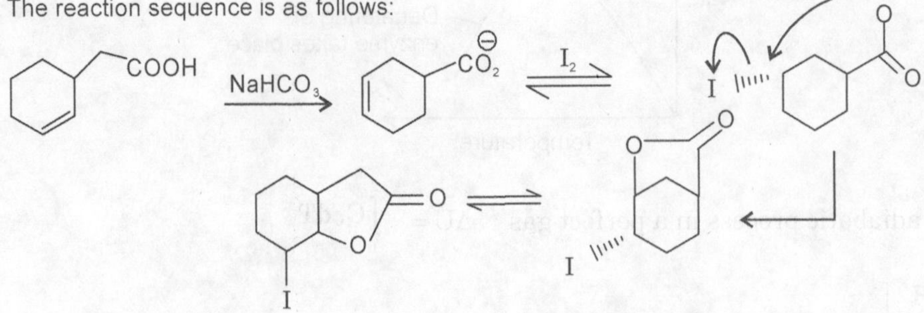

12. For urea in solvent: $\Delta T_{f_1} = k_f\, m_1$

ΔT_{f_1} = Freezing point decrease = 0.25 °C

K_f = constant °C/molal.

$$\therefore \quad m_1 = \text{molal} = \frac{1/60}{0.200} = 0.08333$$

$$K_f = \Delta T_{f1}/m_1 = \frac{0.25}{0.08333} = 3\ °\text{C/mol}$$

For non-electrolyte y.

$$\Delta T_{f_2} = K_f\, m_2$$

$$\therefore \quad m_2 = \frac{0.2}{3} = 0.06667$$

$$\therefore \quad 0.06667 = \frac{(1.5/\text{mol.wt of y})}{\text{Amount of S in kg}} = \frac{(1.5/\text{M.wt of y})}{0.125}$$

$$\therefore \quad M_{wy} = \frac{1.5}{0.06667 \times 0.125} = 180$$

13. 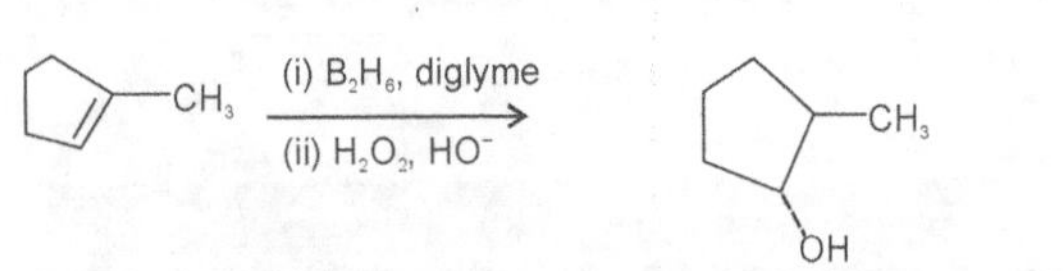

2-Methylcyclo pentanol
(86% yield of this product)
(i.e. major product.)

14. Degree of dissipation, $(\alpha) = \dfrac{\lambda_m c}{\lambda_m \infty}$

$$= \frac{\text{Molar conductivity at } 0.04\ \text{mol/dm}^3}{\text{Molar conductivity at infinite dilution}}$$

Given $\lambda_m^{\ c} = \dfrac{1.0 \times 10^{-3}}{4.3 \times 10^{-3}} = 0.233$

15. Propene is made by Hydrogenation of Propene as follows:

$C_3H_6 + H_2 \rightarrow C_3H_8; \Delta H_{hydro} = -124.27\ \text{KJ mol}^{-1}$

the standard enthalpy of formation is

$\Delta H°_{f\ propene} = 20.42\ \text{kJ mol}^{-1}$

So, net standard enthalpy of formation of Propene

$$\Delta H°_{f\ Propene} = \Delta H°_{f\ propene} + \Delta H_{Hydrogenation}$$
$$= 20.42 - 124.27$$
$$= -103.85\ \text{kJ mol}^{-1}$$

I : BIOCHEMISTRY

1. Heterologous expression of GFP is possible because the genetic code is universal. The technical revolution resulting from the discovery of GFP relates to a miraculous property of the chromophore that is responsible for its fluorescence. This chromophore is formed spontaneously from a tri-peptide motif in the primary structure of GFP, so that its fluorescence is "automatically" turned on in every organism where it is expressed. In other words, the maturation of the tri-peptide-based chromophore in GFP only requires oxygen and does not depend on the presence of enzymes or other auxiliary factors. GFP and its related variants thereby provide universal genetic tags that can be used to visualize a virtually unlimited number of spatio-temporal processes in virtually all living systems.
2. The molecular weight of glucose 6-phosphate = 260.13 and fructose 6-phosphate 259.81 i.e. approximately same. On reaching equilibrium, 55% of glucose 6-phosphate was converted to fructose 6-phosphate. The equilibrium constant for this reaction = 55/45 = 1.22.

3. Hydrolysis of peptide involves cleavage of N and C bond. A peptide bond can be broken by hydrolysis (the adding of water). In the presence of water they will break down and release 8 – 16 kilojoule/mol (2 – 4 kcal/mol) of free energy. This process is extremely slow. In living organisms, the process is catalyzed by enzymes. If the amine and carboxylic acid functional groups in amino acids join together to form amide bonds, a chain of amino acid units, called a peptide, is formed.

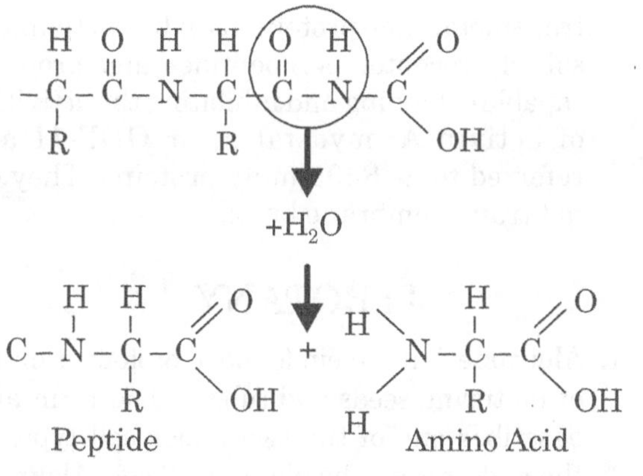

Hydrolysis of Peptide Bond

4. Inter-conversion of UDP glucose and UDP galactose is catalyzed by an epimerase. The enzyme UDP-glucose 4-epimerase, also known as UDP-galactose 4-epimerase or GALE, is a homodimeric epimerase found in bacterial, fungal, plant, and mammalian cells. This enzyme performs the final step in the Leloir pathway of galactose metabolism, catalyzing the reversible conversion of UDP-galactose to UDP-glucose. GALE tightly binds nicotinamide adenine dinucleotide (NAD^+), a co-factor required for catalytic activity.
5. According to the Gel filtration profile, there's no enzyme activity of 60kDa enzyme whereas the 30kDa protein has enzyme activity of >10U at a certain absorbance. Since SDS PAGE was performed the protein has been converted to its monomeric structure. Therefore the monomeric enzyme is active.
6. Amino acids involved in protein DNA interactions have to be positively charged because DNA is negatively charged due to phosphate groups present outside the double helix.
7. Cellulose serves as a structural polymer whereas starch does not because cellulose is a polysaccharide consisting of a linear chain of several hundred to many thousands of β (1 → 4) linked D-glucose units.
8. According to the graph, the molar absorbance of tryptophan will be highest followed by tyrosine and phenylalanine.
9. Fluidity of Phospholipid membrane increases when Fatty Acid chain length decreases and degree of unsaturation increases. The fluidity of membranes determines the extent to which molecules can be transported and signals can be transducted through the membrane. Membrane fluidity is a function of its fatty acid and cholesterol content. Fatty acid chains may be ordered and rigid or disordered and fluid which affects the fluidity of the membrane in which they are contained. Long fatty acid chains are able to form stronger intermolecular interactions which restrict fluidity. Bends and kinks in the fatty acid chains formed as a result of unsaturated *cis* and *trans* double bonds may interfere with intermolecular interactions which promotes fluidity. Membrane fluidity can therefore be controlled by varying the number of double bonds and the length of fatty acid chains. Meanwhile, the presence of bulky cholesterol molecules within the membrane restricts fluidity.
10. Chemical peptide synthesis starts at the C-terminal end of the peptide and ends at the N-terminus. This is the opposite of protein biosynthesis, which starts at the N-terminal end. Unlike ribosome protein synthesis, solid-phase peptide synthesis proceeds in a C-terminal to N-terminal fashion. The N-termini of amino acid monomers is protected by either of these two groups and added onto a deprotected amino acid chain.
11. Creatine Phosphate, Acetyl Phosphate and Succinyl CoA are the compounds those contain at least one bond whose ΔG of hydrolysis will be ≤ – 7.0 kcal/mol.
12. The ΔG for MDH catalyzed step of Krebs cycle is +7.1 kcal/mol. Nevertheless the conversion of malate to oxaloacetate in vivo proceeds spontaneously because the subsequent reaction that consumes oxaloacetate has a ΔG of –7.7 kcal/mol.
13. Both oxygen consumption and ATP synthesis are inhibited during addition of cyanide to the

system which blocks rotational catalysis of F0-F1 particle.

14. This formula converts micrograms of DNA and picomoles of DNA, according to the following formula where N is the length of the DNA:

$$\mu g\ DNA \times \frac{pmol}{660\ pg} \times \frac{10^6\ pg}{1\ \mu g} \times \frac{1}{N} = pmol\ DNA$$

$$\text{Then, } 3 \times \frac{pmol}{660\ pg} \times \frac{10^6\ pg}{1\ \mu g} \times \frac{1}{4200}$$

$$= 1.082\ pmol\ DNA$$

The number of picomoles of DNA ends generated after complete digestion with the enzyme is = 1.062 × 2 × 5 = 10.62 (Because 2 is the number of end in a linear DNA molecule and 5 is the no. of DNA fragments)

15. Through given table, the correct statement is 50 fold purification was achieved with 25% yield of the enzyme.

16. Aspartate residues found on active sites of many enzymes. The pKa value for ß-carboxylate of aspartate is 3.86. That is why at physiological pH, this group acts as a nucleophile and a conjugate base. Basicity is a subset of nucleophilicity. All nucleophiles are Lewis bases; they donate a lone pair of electrons. A "base" is just the name we give to a nucleophile when it's forming a bond to a proton (H+).

17. The Michaelis constant (Km) is a means of characterising an enzyme's affinity for a substrate. The Km in an enzymatic reaction is the substrate concentration at which the reaction rate is half its maximum speed. Thus, a low Km value means that the enzyme has a high affinity for the substrate (as a "little" substrate is enough to run the reaction at half its max speed). This is only true for reactions where substrate is limiting and the enzyme is NOT allosteric.

    As per above statement ant analyzing the given table the correct option is, Fumarate > Fluorofumarate > Chlorofumarate.

18. A polypeptide with the amino acid sequence 'AGKPDHEKAHL' was dissolved in a buffer of pH 1.8. The predominant form of the polypeptide will have a net charge = +5.

19. N terminal His tagged protein has molecular weight 40kDa. Its purified using Ni-NTA column. This is subjected to SDS PAGE. Therefore the tagged protein in halved so a 20 kDa fragment is produced. In western blotting anti His antibodies are used, which binds to the 20 kDa fragment forming the antigen(native protein) and antibody complex which is shown at 20kDa in the gel..

20. G22 is responsible for regulation of secretion of pancreatic spasmolytic polypeptide from porcine pancreas. A25: It is a protein involved in the lysis of bacterial cells during the phage life cycle. A 34: It can enhance the transcriptional activity of p53 on the promoters of Bax and PUMA; A34 can increase cell apoptosis and slow tumor growth in vitro and vivo therefore it is a transmembrane protein. R40: It is activin IIB soluble receptor polypeptides and proteins capable of binding and inhibiting the activities of activin A, myostatin, or GDF-11 are referred to as R40 family proteins. They do not transmembrane helix.

J : BOTANY

1. **Aleurone** is a protein found in protein granules of maturing seeds and tubers. The term also describes one of the two major cell types of the endosperm, the aleurone layer. Aleurone layer is the outer protein rich layer of living cells of the endosperm of wheat and other grain species.

2. Bryophytes are seedless plants without specialized water-conducting tissues. Bryophytes include mosses (phylum Bryophyta), liverworts (phylum Marchantiophyta Hepatophyta), and hornworts (phylum Anthocerophyta).

    There are several characteristic features of bryophytes. First, the green tissue that makes up most of the plant body is not vascularized; it does not have **xylem** and **phloem** cells. This absence of specialized tissues for transporting water and dissolved food throughout the organism limits terrestrial forms to being very short plants, since the only way to move substances through the plant body is by **osmosis** and diffusion from surface moisture.

3. Ancestors of green plants began to colonise the land about 500 million years ago and it is generally accepted that they evolved from streptophyte algae (a group of green, fresh water algae). But this group of algae is very diverse and currently ranges from simple, one

cell, flagellates to more complex, branching, algae such as stoneworts (Chara).

It was previously thought that land plants evolved from stonewort-like algae. However, new research published in BioMed Central's open access journal *BMC Evolutionary Biology* shows that the closest relatives to land plants are actually conjugating green algae such as Spirogyra.

4. Tracheids develop a thick lignified cell wall, and at maturity the protoplast has broken down and disappeared when there is no nucleus in tracheids at maturity how can they be stained by DAPI.

5. The uptake of nitrogen (N) and phosphorus (P) by plant roots often involves interaction between root and some symbiotic organisms. Bacteria for N, mycorrhizae for P associations are most commonly found for the uptake of these two nutrients. Through mycorrhization, the plant obtains phosphate and other minerals, such as zinc and copper, from the soil. The bacteria, rhizobia create ammonia from nitrogen in the air, which is used by the plant to create amino acids and nucleotides. The plant provides the bacteria with sugars.

6. At the root, the casparian strip is imbedded within the cell wall of endodermal cells in the non-growing region of the root behind the root tip. Here the casparian strip serves as a boundary layer separating the apoplast of cortex from the apoplast of the vascular tissue.This separation at the endodermis by the casparian strip obstrcuts water movement through the apoplastic pathway and forces water and solutes to pass through the plasma membrane via a symplastic route in order to cross the endodermis layer.

7. Hairy roots induced by Agrobacterium rhizogenes are distinguished by their high growth rate, genetic stability, and lateral branching. Datura metel is an important medicinal plant whose hairy roots are used for the production of atropine, a tropane alkaloid applied as an anticholinergic and parasympathetic agent. Atropine is a medication used to treat certain types of nerve agent and pesticide poisonings, some types of slow heart rate, and to decrease saliva production during surgery.

8. Plant disease resistance protects plants from pathogens in two ways: mechanisms and by infection-induced responses of the immune system.

Common mechanisms-Pre-formed structures and compounds: Plant cuticle/surface, Plant cell walls, Anti microbial chemicals (for example: glucosides, saponins), Antimicrobial proteins, Enzyme inhibitors, Detoxifying enzymes that break down pathogen-derived toxins, Receptors that perceive pathogen presence and activate inducible plant defences.

Inducible post-infection plant defenses: Cell wall reinforcement, Antimicrobial chemicals, including reactive oxygen species, **Anti-microbial proteins** such as defensins, thionins, or PR-1, Antimicrobial enzymes such as chitinases, beta-glucanases, or peroxidases, **Hyper-sensitive response** - a rapid host cell death response associated with defence mediated by "Resistance genes.

Endophyte assistance: Plant's roots release chemicals that attract beneficial bacteria to fight off infections.

The plant immune system consists of two interconnected tiers of receptors, one outside and one inside the cell. The first tier is primarily governed by pattern recognition receptors that are activated by recognition of evolutionarily conserved pathogen or microbial associated molecular patterns (PAMPs or MAMPs, here P/MAMP).

The second tier (again, primarily), effector-triggered immunity (ETI), consists of another set of receptors, the nucleotide-binding LRRs (NLRs). They operate within the cell, encoded by R genes.

9. **Genetic drift** (also known as ***allelic drift or the Sewall Wright effect*** after biologist Sewall Wright) is the change in the frequency of a gene variant (allele) in a population due to random sampling of organisms. Genetic drift may cause gene variants to disappear completely and thereby reduce genetic variation.

10. Salicylic acid (SA) is one of the key hormonal factors be involved in the plant defense-related actions against infection by various pathogens. Recently, intracellular SA receptors were finally identified after a long survey of SA-binding protein.

11. Given: Two types of plants:
Red flower (R) with tall stem (T) & white flower (W) with short stem (S). So, F_1 plant which all RT is back crossed with WS and F_2 has the following Proportion

Type	No.
RT	103
WS	89
RS	26
WT	23
Total	241

Now, we need to find re-combination % between RT & WS in terms of flower color locus & stem height i.e. the proportion of RS and WT Plants is i.e. RS + WT = 49

$\therefore$ % recombination = $\frac{49}{241} \times 100 = 20.33\%$

12. As, P seed is vernalized while Q seed is not vernalized. So, as per the chart, it is expressed that the seed which are vernalized has higher ability to flower faster.
So, from the given option (b) is correct, i.e. P will have lower VRN_2 transcript and will flower earlier than Q .

13. The three plots P, Q and R (in different units) in the graph represent the dependence of photosynthesis rate (PR), leaf expansion rate (LER) and translocation rate of assimilates (TR) in a plant on leaf water potential as P represents LER; Q represents PR; R represents TR.

14. Export of auxin from the cell requires an active component in plasma membrane, without these proteins, auxin can not leave the cell. The only carrier protein in the diagram which is exporting auxin is P4, rest of the proteins are importing.

15. In ecotype Y, the GAATTC site is missing hence *Eco*R1 will not be able to digest the PCR product of this ecotype. The undigested product appears in lane marked Q i.e. seeding Q belongs to ecotype Y.

16. In plants today, two types of tip-growing cells dominate; pollen tubes and root hairs. While pollen tubes provided for water-independent propagation of species, root hairs bestowed an increase in root surface area that could be used to increase nutrient uptake and better anchor plants in the soil. Root hairs and pollen tubes are filamentous cells that grow unidirectionally by depositing flexible cell wall material at one site of the cell and exploiting turgor pressure as the driving force for elongation; a process also referred to as tip growth.
Both root hairs and pollen tubes display a highly specialized growth form in which the cell elongates unidirectionally and only at the very tip. This extreme form of polarized growth, or tip-growth, sustains prodigious rates of elongation.

17. Hardy Weinberg's equilibrium for a locus with two alleles p and q is mathematically defined as $P^2 + Q^2 + 2PQ = 1$. The equation represents the corresponding equilibrium for a locus with three alleles p, q and r (P, Q and R represent the frequencies of p, q and r, respectively) will be, $(P+ Q +R)^2 =1$
i.e. $P^2 + Q^2 + R^2 + 2PQ + 2QR + 2PR = 1$

18. **Sapflow and Sap Velocity**
Sapflow is movement of water through the xylem of a plant, usually measured as litres of water perday. Measuring sapflow provides an estimation of transpiration. Sap velocity is the rate of sapflow, from which sap flow and sapflux density can be calculated. Sapflow, sap velocity and sapflux density are influenced by a number of environmental conditions such as soil moisture content, temperature, solar radiation and vapour pressure deficit.
The continuous and dashed lines in the graph represent the velocity of sap flow in two different parts of a plant at different times of a day: The most appropriate statement based on the graph is the continuous line represents a twig, and the dotted line the trunk .

19.

Gene/enzyme	Commercial use
P. Bt gene	ii. insect resistance
Q. β-carotene biosynthetic genes	i. Golden rice
R. ACC deaminase	iv. fruit ripening
S. EPSP synthase	iii. herbicide resistance

20. As A class genes are matured, C class gene will express in the sepal whorl. In the pettle whorl B class genes will act together with C class, giving rise to stamen. The two inner most whorls are controlled by B and C genes and hence will appear normally. Therefore moving from outside to inside the whorls will be carpel; stamen; stamen; carpel.

K : MICROBIOLOGY

1. DNA-DNA hybridization has been established as an important technology in bacterial species taxonomy and phylogenetic analysis. The genomic DNA from one species hybridizes to the genomic DNA of another species (DNA-DNA hybridization) in microarray analysis relates to the similarity between two genomes. Between closely related strains, significant numbers of highly divergent genes (<55% identity) and/or the accumulation of mismatches between conserved genes lowered the DNA-DNA hybridization signal, and this reduced the hybridization signals to below 70% for even bacterial strains with over 97% 16S rRNA gene identity. In addition, our results also suggest that a DNA-DNA hybridization signal intensity of over 40% indicates that two genomes at least shared 30% conserved genes (>60% gene identity).
2. p1 undergoes non integrative lysogenic phase.
3. Streptococcus suis is not a part of human microbiome.
4. Macrophages of Liver is called Kupffer cells.
5. Myeloperoxidase (MPO) is a peroxidase enzyme that in humans is encoded by the MPO gene on chromosome 17.MPO is most abundantly expressed in neutrophil granulocytes and produces hypohalous acids to carry out their antimicrobial activity. It is a lysosomal protein stored in azurophilic granules of the neutrophil and released into the extracellular space during degranulation.
6. Teichoic acids are bacterial copolymers of glycerol phosphate or ribitol phosphate and carbohydrates linked via phos-phodiester bonds.
7. Biofilm produced my bacteria is detected by Congo Red dye.
8. Phenylalanine, tyrosine, and tryptophan are known as the aromatic amino acids. The synthesis of all three share a common beginning to their pathways; the formation of chorismate from phosphoenolpyruvate (PEP) and erythrose 4- phosphate (E4P). The first step, condensation of 3-deoxy-D-arabino-heptulosonic acid 7-phosphate (DAHP) from PEP/E4P, uses three isoenzymes AroF, AroG, and AroH. Each one of these has its synthesis regulated from tyrosine, phenylalanine, and tryptophan, respectively. These isoenzymes all have the ability to help regulate synthesis of DAHP by the method of feedback inhibition. This acts in the cell by monitoring the concentrations of each of the three aromatic amino acids.
9. The net yield of NADH in the Embden-Meyerhof pathway in *E. coli* = 2.
10. 3 nucleotide code for one specific amino acid and last codon (3 nucleotide) will be the stop codon hence the number of nucleotides present in the gene encoding the 124 amino acids (ribonuclease protein) will be $(124 \times 3) + 3 = 372 + 3 = 375$.
11. *S. pneumoniae* and Rotavirus can cross blood brain barrier.
12. The use of optical-density (OD) readings after a 6-h incubation period, as a suitable method to quantify the bacterial contamination on hatching eggs, was established by the use of pure cultures of five bacterial isolates found to be the most prevalent on the hatching eggs examined. These isolates were identified as Micrococcus luteus, Staphylococcus gallinarum, Streptococcus epidermidis, Pseudomonas cepacei and Bacillus cereus. A direct relationship was established between the OD reading (at 540 nm) after 6 h and the log of the bacterial concentration at the start of incubation. The OD reading after 6 h of incubation is a repeatable, rapid and simple method to quantify the bacterial concentration at the start of the incubation period.
13. Many bacteria and plants are able to subsist on acetate or other compounds that yield acetyl CoA. They make use of a metabolic pathway absent in most other organisms that converts two-carbon acetyl units into four-carbon units (succinate) for energy production and biosyntheses. This reaction sequence, called the glyoxylate cycle, bypasses the two decarboxylation steps of the citric acid cycle. Another key difference is that two molecules of acetyl CoA enter per turn of the glyoxylate cycle, compared with one in the citric acid cycle.The glyoxylate cycle like the citric acid cycle, begins with the condensation of acetyl CoA and oxaloacetate to form citrate, which is then isomerized to isocitrate. Instead of being

decarboxylated, isocitrate is cleaved by isocitrate lyase into succinate and glyoxylate. The subsequent steps regenerate oxaloacetate from glyoxylate. Acetyl CoA condenses with glyoxylate to form malate in a reaction catalyzed by malate synthase, which resembles citrate synthase. Finally, malate is oxidized to oxaloacetate, as in the citric acid cycle.

14. Given Dr = 0.2 min,

$N_o = 10^{12}$ & $N_t = 1$

$$\Rightarrow Dr = \frac{2.303}{K_d} \text{ or } K_d = \frac{2.303}{0.2}$$

$$\therefore \quad \ln\left(\frac{N_o}{N_t}\right) = K_d t$$

$$\text{then} \quad \ln\left(\frac{10^{12}}{1}\right) = \frac{2.303}{0.2} \times t$$

$$\text{or } t = \frac{2.303 \times 12 \log 10 \times 0.2}{2.303}$$

$$t = 2.4 \text{ min}$$

15. *E.coli* requires three genes, *galK* (kinase), *galT* (transacetylase) and *galE* (epimerase) to utilize galactose. If there is a mutation in any one of these genes, the mutant cannot utilize galactose.

(Q) *galK-galT+galE-/ galK+galT-galE+ and*
(S) *galK+galT+galE-/galK+galT-galE+*,
combinations of merodiploids will support the growth of mutants on galactose.

16. Nitrogenase reduces N2 to NH3. Metal co-factors required for this activity are Mo and Fe.

17. Given, Total genes = 5,000

Average mutation frequency per gene

$= 2 \times 10^{-4}$ per generation

The average number of new mutations per

$$\text{generation} = \frac{1}{5000 \times 2 \times 10^{-4}} = \frac{104}{104} = 1$$

18. From the graph, the two points of second exponential phase are at time 15 hr and 17 hr.

$$\mu = \frac{\ln X_2 - \ln X_1}{t_2 - t_1}$$

$$\mu = \frac{\ln 1.6 - \ln 1.3}{17 - 15}$$

By solving this equation

Specific growth rate (μ) = 0.1038 hr^{-1}

19. Cell membrane : Active transport;

Purple membrane: Light driven proton transport;

Cisternae: Protein Glycosylation;

Outer membrane: Nutrient transport.

20. Nalidixic acid, Tetracycline, Erythro-mycin, Rifampin inhibits the action of DNA gyrase, Aminoacyl tRNA, 50S ribosomal subunit; RNA polymerase respectively.

L : ZOOLOGY

1. The acorn worms or Enteropneusta are a hemichordate class of invertebrates consisting of one order of the same name. They are closely related to the echinoderms. There are about 90 species of acorn worm in the world, the main species for research being *Saccoglossus kowalevskii*.

2. Micro evolution is simply a change in gene frequency (allele frequencies) within a population. Evolution at this scale can be observed over short periods of time — for example, between one generation and the next, the frequency of a gene for pesticide resistance in a population of crop pests increases. This change is due to four different processes: mutation, selection (natural and artificial), gene flow, and genetic drift. This change happens over a relatively short (in evolutionary terms) amount of time compared to the changes termed 'macroevolution' which is where greater differences in the population occur.

3. Properties desirable for ideal DNA markers : Highly polymorphic nature
   - Codominant inheritance (deter-mination of homozygous and heterozygous states of diploid organisms)
   - Frequent occurrence in genome
   - Selective neutral behaviour (the DNA sequences of any organism are neutral to environmental conditions or management practices)
   - Easy access (availability)
   - Easy and fast assay
   - High reproducibility
   - Easy exchange of data between lab

4. The individual *Drosophila* has four pairs of chromosomes. A female has two each of chromosomes 1 (more commonly called the

X chromosome), 2, 3, and 4. A male has one X chromosome, one Y chromosome, and two each of chromosomes 2, 3, and 4. The Y chromo-some and chromosome 4 are both very small, and carry few genes. The majority of the fly's genes are carried on chromosomes X, 2, and 3. The X and Y chromosomes are involved in sex determination, and are thus called the sex chromosomes. Chromosomes 2, 3, and 4 are called the autosomes. In the fruit fly, sex is determined by the relative number of X chromosomes and autosomes. If a fly has two X chromo-somes, and two of each autosome (an X:autosome ratio of 1:1), it will develop as a female. If a fly has only one X chromosome, and two of each autosome (an X:autosome ratio of 1:2), it will develop as a male. In *Drosophila*, the Y chromosome does not determine maleness! (This is in contrast to the case in mammals, in which the presence of the Y chromosome determines male-ness.). In fact, a fly that has two X chromosomes and a Y chromosome will develop as a female.

5. Extracellular fluid (ECF) or extracellular fluid volume (ECFV) usually denotes all body fluid outside the cells. The remainder is called intracellular fluid (ICF). The ECF and ICF are the two major fluid compartments. In some animals, including mammals, the ECF can be divided into two major sub-compartments, interstitialfluid and blood plasma, which make up at least 97%. The volume of ECF is typically 15 L, of which 12 L is interstitial fluid and 3 L is plasma. Interstitial fluid makes up 16% of human body weight, and blood plasma, 4%. It is poorer in proteins, as compared to intracellular fluid.

   Extracellular fluid (ECF) Constituents:
   Main cations:
   Sodium (Na^+ = 136 – 145 Eq/L),
   Potassium (K^+ = 3.5 – 5.5 mEq/L),
   Calcium (Ca^{2+} = 2.2 – 2.6 mEq/L),
   Main anions:
   Chloride (Cl^- = 99 –109 mEq/L),
   Hydrogen Carbonate (HCO_3^- 22–26 mM),
   Ionic Composition: Na^+ 150 (mM),
   K^+ 5 (mM), Cl^- 110 (mM).

6. **Detoxify Alcohol**: Alcohol is a common toxin that can be ingested in large quantities. The liver must detoxify the alcohol that is transported through the blood flow via the hepatic artery from the intestines in order to protect the build-up of alcohol toxins. The peroxisomes in the hepatocytes carry out this function by transferring hydrogen from the ethanol or alcohol molecules to oxygen. Peroxisomes use the enzyme catalyst peroxidase to facilitate this reaction.

   Certain enzymes within the peroxisome, by using molecular oxygen, remove hydrogen atoms from specific organic substrates (labeled as R), in an oxidative reaction, producing hydrogen peroxide (H_2O_2, itself toxic):

   $$RH_2 + O_2 \rightarrow R + H_2O_2$$

7. Cyanide binds to at least one molecule involved in producing ATP. If a cell is exposed to cyanide, most of the cyanide will be found within the mitochondria.

8. *Toxoplasma gondii* is an obligate intracellular, parasitic protozoan that causes the disease toxoplasmosis. Found worldwide, *T. gondii* is capable of infecting virtually all warm-blooded animals, but felids such as domestic cats are the only known definitive hosts in which the parasite can undergo sexual reproduction.

9. Septic shock is often a life-threatening systemic inflammatory response. Septic shock is a serious medical condition that occurs when sepsis, which is organ injury or damage in response to infection, leads to dangerously low blood pressure and abnormalities in cellular metabolism. The primary infection is most commonly by bacteria, but can also be by fungi, viruses, or parasites, and can be located in any part of the body, but most commonly in the lungs, brain, urinary tract, skin, or abdominal organs. It can cause multiple organ dysfunction syndrome and death.

10. Epiboly process that occurs during gastrulation in vertebrates, in which cells on one side of the blastula grow over and surround theremaining cells and yolk and eventually form the ectoderm. During the gastrulation stage of amphibian development, ectoderm formation takes place by the expansion of epithelial cell sheet over mesodermal cells. This type of cell movement is termed as epiboly.

11. Given MM = 600
    MN = 300
    NN = 100

Now given type frequencies of

$$MM\,(p^2) = \frac{600}{1000} = 0.60$$

$$MN(2pa) = \frac{300}{1000} = 0.30$$

$$NN(q^2) = \frac{100}{1000} = 0.1$$

Now, Allele frequencies

$$\text{Frequency of M} = p = p^2 + \frac{1}{2}(2pq)$$

$$= 0.6 + \frac{1}{2}(0.30) = 0.75$$

$$\text{Frequency of N} = q = 1-p$$

$$= 1-0.75 = 0.25$$

or $$N = q^2 + \frac{1}{2}(2pq)$$

$$= 0.1 + \frac{1}{2}(0.30) = 0.25$$

∴ Answers M 0.75 and N 0.25

12. All given molecules has 6 carbon. But the most stable structure is of $C_6H_{12}O_2$ i.e. hexanoic acid. So, the more the calorific value. So, hexanoic and has a high calorific value.

13. Many proteins, especially those destined for secretion or insertion into membranes, are post-translationally modified by attachment of carbohydrates. They are usually attached through either Asn or Ser side chains. Carbohydrate modifications on the protein appear to be involved in recognition of other binding molecules, prevention of aggregation during protein folding, protection from proteolysis, and increased half-life of the proteins. In contrast to a protein sequence which is determined by a DNA template, sugars are attached to proteins by enzymes which recognize appropriate sites on proteins and attach the sugars. Since there are many sugars which contain many functional groups that can serve as potential attachment sites. Thus polysaccharides attached to glycoproteins has primary function to mediate cell-to-cell recognition.

14. Mechanisms which is used to coordinate the expression of multiple, related genes in eukaryotic cells is as: Genes are organized into clusters, with local chromatin structures influencing the expression of all the clustered genes at once.

15. Ability of the micromeres to induce presumptive ectodermal cells to acquire other fates as: (A) Normal development of the 64-cell sea urchin embryo, showing the fates of the different layers. (B) An isolated animal hemisphere becomes a ciliated ball of ectodermal cells. (C) When an isolated animal hemisphere is combined with isolated micromeres, a recognizable pluteus larva is formed, with all the endoderm derived from the animal hemisphere.

16. Human gonadotropin is human chorionic gonadotropin (hCG), produced by the placenta during pregnancy. The human chorionic gonadotropin (hCG) are the primary target organs for LH and FSH.

Equine chorionic gonadotropin (acronym given as eCG) is a gonadotropic hormone produced in the chorion of pregnant mares. Most commonly called pregnant mare's serum gonadotropin (PMSG). In mares PMSG has only LH like activity, but in other species it has activity like both follicle-stimulating hormone (FSH) and luteinizing hormone (LH).

So, for Both hCG and eCG have LH like activity is common.

17. *Entamoeba histolytica* is an intestinal parasite that causes dysentery in humans. This parasite resides in the isotonic environment of intestine and other tissues in the human body and does not possess contractile vacuoles. If this parasite is placed in fresh water, it will die due to hypoosmotic shock. Osmotic shock or osmotic stress is a sudden change in the solute concentration around a cell, causing a rapid change in the movement of water across its cell membrane. Under conditions of high concentrations of either salts, substrates or any solute in the supernatant, water is drawn out of the cells through osmosis. This also inhibits the transport of substrates and cofactors into the cell thus "shocking" the cell. Alternatively, at low concentrations of solutes, water enters the cell in large amounts, causing it to swell and either burst or undergo apoptosis.

18. In an experiment involving Drosophila development, a large amount of purified *bicoid* mRNA was injected into the posterior end of a wild-type embryo, the resulting developing embryo will have two heads and two thoraces with an abdomen segment in the middle.

19. A polyphenism is a biological mechanism that causes a trait to be polyphenic. For example, crocodiles possess a sex-determining polyphenism, and therefore their gender is a polyphenic trait. A polyphenic trait is a trait for which multiple, discrete phenotypes can arise from a single genotype as a result of differing environmental conditions. It is therefore a special case of phenotypic plasticity. The migratory desert locust, *Schistocerca gregaria*, exists in two mutually exclusive forms: a short-winged, uniformly colored, solitary insect and a long-winged, brightly colored, gregarious morph. These phenotypes depend on crowding. Such phenotypic plasticity is called polyphenism.

20. The correct match in the list of animals and their respective characteristics.are

Animals	*Characteristics*
I. Sea anemone	ii. Diploblastic acoelomate
II. Bluefly	i. Three pairs of jointed legs
III. Starfish	iv. Tube feet
IV. Sponge	iii. Collar cells

■■

GATE-2015

XL : LIFE SCIENCES

Time : 3 Hours *Maximum Marks : 100*

GENERAL APTITUDE

Q. (1–5) Carry One Mark Each

1. Choose the word most similar in meaning to the given word :

   Educe

   (*a*) Exert (*b*) Educate

   (*c*) Extract (*d*) Extend

2. If $\log_x\left(\frac{5}{7}\right) = -\frac{1}{3}$, then the value of x is

   (*a*) $\frac{343}{125}$ (*b*) $\frac{125}{343}$

   (*c*) $-\frac{25}{49}$ (*d*) $-\frac{49}{25}$

3. Operators $\square, \diamond$ and $\rightarrow$ are defined by

   $$a \square b = \frac{a-b}{a+b};\ a \diamond b = \frac{a+b}{a-b};\ a \rightarrow b = ab.$$

   Find the value of $(66 \square 6) \rightarrow (66 \diamond 6)$

   (*a*) – 2 (*b*) – 1

   (*c*) 1 (*d*) 2

4. Choose the most appropriate word from the options given below to complete the following sentence.

   The principal presented the chief guest with a ___________, as token of appreciation.

   (*a*) momento

   (*b*) memento

   (*c*) momentum

   (*d*) moment

5. Choose the appropriate word/phrase, out of the four options given below, to complete the following sentence :

   Frogs ________.

   (*a*) Croak

   (*b*) Roar

   (*c*) Hiss

   (*d*) Patter

(Q. 6–10) : Carry Two Marks Each

6. A cube of side 3 units is formed using a set of smaller cubes of side 1 unit. Find the proportion of the number of faces of the smaller cubes visible to those which are NOT visible.

   (*a*) 1 : 4

   (*b*) 1 : 3

   (*c*) 1 : 2

   (*d*) 2 : 3

7. Fill in the missing value

   6 5 4

   7 4 7 2 1

   1 9 2 8 1 2 1

   4 1 5 2 3

   3 ? 3

8. Humpty Dumpty sits on a wall every day while having lunch. The wall sometimes breaks. A person sitting on the wall falls if the wall breaks.

   Which one of the statements below is logically valid and can be inferred from the above sentences?

   (*a*) Humpty Dumpty always falls while having lunch

   (*b*) Humpty Dumpty does not fall sometimes while having lunch

   (*c*) Humpty Dumpty never falls during dinner

   (*d*) When Humpty Dumpty does not sit on the wall, the wall does not break

9. The following question presents a sentence, part of which is underlined. Beneath the sentence you find four ways of phrasing the underline part. Following the requirements of the standard written English, select the answer that produces the most effective sentence.

Tuberculosis, together with its effects, <u>ranks one of the leading causes of death</u> in India.

(*a*) ranks as one of the leading causes of death

(*b*) rank as one of the leading causes of death

(*c*) has the rank of one of the leading causes of death

(*d*) are one of the leading causes of death

10. Read the following paragraph and choose the correct statement.

Climate change has reduced human security and threatened human well being. An ignored reality of human progress is that human security largely depends upon environmental security. But on the contrary, human progress seems contradictory to environmental security. To keep up both at the required level is a challenge to be addressed by one and all. One of the ways to curb the climate change may be suitable scientific innovations, while the other may be the Gandhian perspective on small scale progress with focus on sustainability.

(*a*) Human progress and security are positively associated with environmental security.

(*b*) Human progress is contradictory to environmental security.

(*c*) Human security is contradictory to environmental security.

(*d*) Human progress depends upon environmental security.

H : CHEMISTRY

Q. (1–10) Carry One Mark Each

1. For the electrochemical reaction, $Cu^{2+}(aq) + Zn(s) \rightleftharpoons Cu(s) + Zn^{2+}(aq)$ the equilibrium constant at 20°C is 1.7×10^{37}. The change in standard Gibbs free energy (ΔG°) for this reaction at that temperature will be _______ kJ mol^{-1} (up to one decimal place).
(Given : R = 8.314 JK^{-1} mol^{-1})

2. The Diels-Alder adduct from the reaction between cyclopentadiene and benzyne is

(*a*) 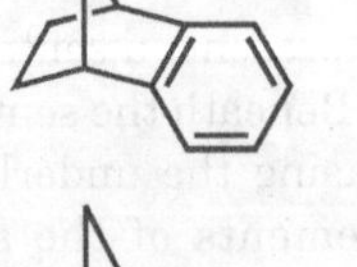 (*b*) 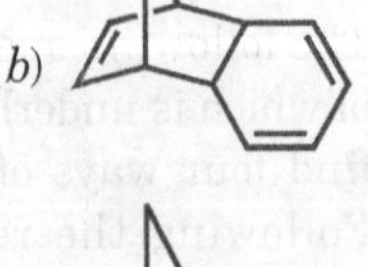

(*c*) 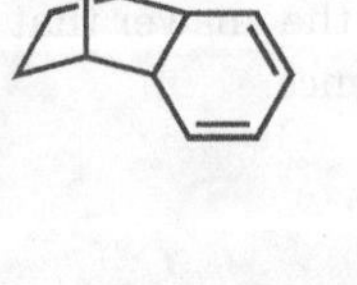 (*d*) 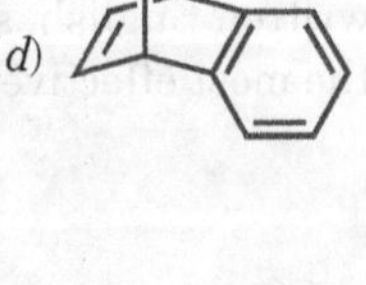

3. Among the following diagrams, the one that correctly describes a zero order reaction
(X → product) is
(Given : $[X]_0$ = initial concentration of reactant X; [X] = concentration of reactant X at time *t* and $t_{1/2}$ = half-life period of reactant X)

(*a*) 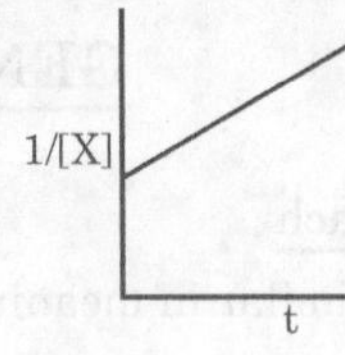

(*b*) 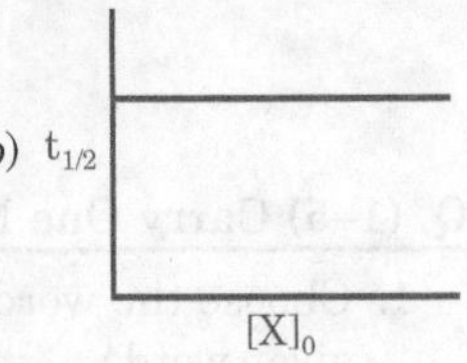

(*c*) 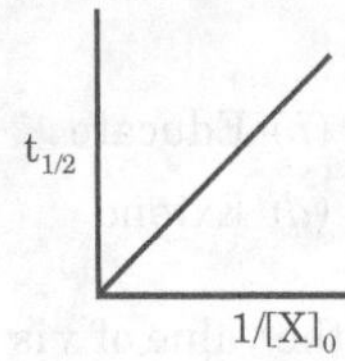

(*d*) 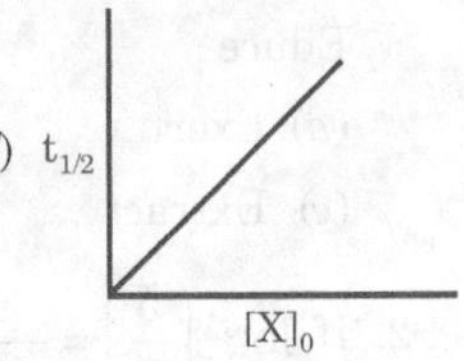

4. The number of possible enantiomeric pair(s) in HOOC-CH(OH)–CH(OH)–COOH is _______.

5. The molecule having net 'non-zero dipole moment' is

(*a*) CCl_4 (*b*) NF_3

(*c*) CO_2 (*d*) BCl_3

6. The molar enthalpy of vaporization for a liquid (normal boiling point = 78.3 °C) is kJ mol^{-1}. If the liquid has to boil at 25°C, the pressure must be reduced to _______ Torr (up to one decimal place).
(Given : R = 8.314 JK^{-1} mol^{-1}; 1 atm = 760 Torr)

7. If the radius of first Bohr orbit is 0.53 Å, then the radius of the third Bohr orbit is

(*a*) 2.12 Å (*b*) 4.77 Å

(*c*) 1.59 Å (*d*) 3.18 Å

8. The order of resonance energy for the following molecules is

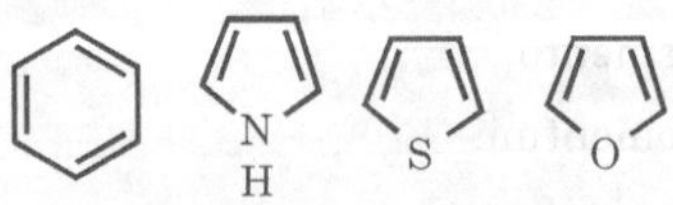

(1) (2) (3) (4)

(*a*) (1) > (3) > (2) > (4) (*b*) (1) > (3) > (4) > (2)

(*c*) (1) > (4) > (2) > (3) (*d*) (1) > (4) > (3) > (2)

9. In compounds $K_4[Fe(CH)_6]$(P) and $Fe(CO)_5$ (Q), the iron metal centre is bonded to

(*a*) C of CN^- in P and C of CO in Q

(*b*) N of CN^- in P and C of CO in Q

(*c*) C of CN^- in P and O of CO in Q

(*d*) N of CN^- in P and O of CO in Q

10. Among the following pairs, the paramagnetic and diamagnetic species, respectively, are

(*a*) CO and O_2^-

(*b*) NO and CO

(*c*) O_2^{2-} and CO

(*d*) NO^+ and O_2^-

11. Stability of $[CrCl_6]^{3-}$ (X), $[MnCl_6]^{3-}$ (Y) and $[FeCl_6]^{3-}$ (Z) follows the order

(Given : Atomic numbers of Cr = 24, Mn = 25 and Fe = 26)

(*a*) X > Y > Z (*b*) X < Y < Z

(*c*) Y < X < Z (*d*) X < Y = Z

12. Among the following reactions, the one that produces achiral alcohol (after hydrolysis) is

(*a*) 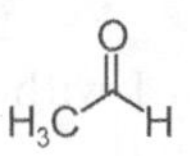 + $CH_3CH_2MgBr \longrightarrow$

(*b*) 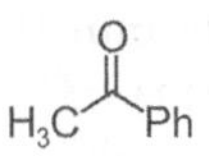 + $CH_3CH_2MgBr \longrightarrow$

(*c*) 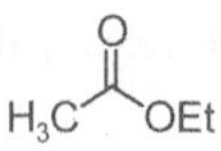 + $CH_3CH_2MgBr \longrightarrow$

(*d*) 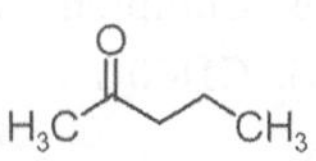 + $CH_3CH_2MgBr \longrightarrow$

13. If 50 mL of 0.02 M HCl is added to 950 mL of H_2O, then the pH of the final solution will be _____

14. The major product from the following reaction is

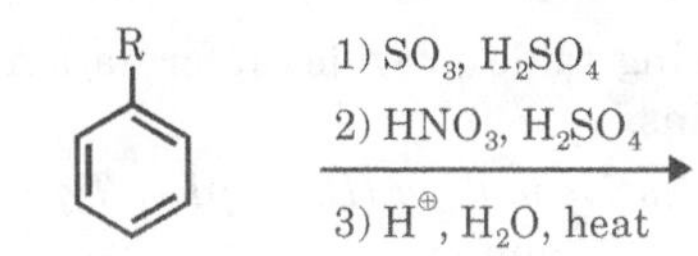

R = tert-Butyl

(*a*) 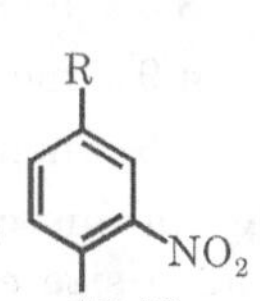 (*b*) 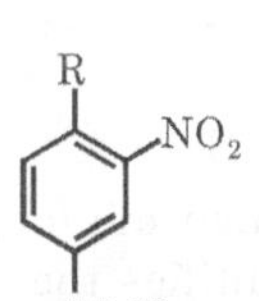

(*c*) 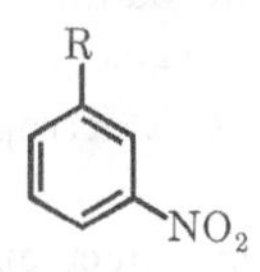 (*d*) 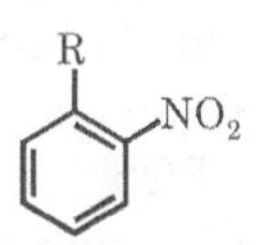

15. For the process, $H_2O(l) \rightleftharpoons H_2O(s)$ at 0°C and 1 atm, the correct statement is

(*a*) $\Delta S_{system} = 0$ (*b*) $\Delta S_{total} > 0$

(*c*) $\Delta S_{total} = 0$ (*d*) $\Delta S_{total} < 0$

I : BIOCHEMISTRY

1. Which one of the following amino acid substitutions is likely to cause the largest change in protein conformation?

(*a*) Phe → Ile (*b*) Ser → Thr

(*c*) Gln → Tyr (*d*) Glu → Val

2. Ribulose-5-phosphate epimerase is involved in which one of the following processes?

(*a*) Glycolysis

(*b*) TCA cycle

(*c*) Glycosylation

(*d*) Pentose phosphate pathway

3. The formation of a carbocation, also called an oxonium ion, occurs during the reaction catalyzed by

(*a*) aldolase (*b*) lysozyme

(*c*) ribonuclease A (*d*) carboxypeptidase

4. A closed circular B-DNA of 4000 base pairs is negatively supercoiled by introduction of 4 writhes. The super helical density of the resultant DNA molecule will be ________.

5. Which one of the following is NOT a receptor tyrosine kinase?

(*a*) Platelet derived growth factor receptor

(*b*) Insulin like growth factor -1 receptor

(*c*) Macrophage colony stimulating factor receptor

(*d*) Transforming growth factor β receptor

6. Which one of the following does NOT constitute the lipid moiety in lipid-linked membrane proteins?

(*a*) Palmitic acid (*b*) stearic acid

(*c*) Farnesyl groups (*d*) Myristic acid

7. Proteolytic enzymes are usually biosynthesized as large, inactive precursors known as

(*a*) holoenzymes (*b*) ribozyme

(*c*) zymogens (*d*) apoenzymes

8. Which one of the following small molecules is a prerequisite for fatty acid oxidation?

(*a*) Inositol (*b*) Choline

(*c*) Carnitine (*d*) Glycerol

9. Oxidation of one molecule of glucose via the glycerol-phosphate shuttle produces

(*a*) 32 molecules of ATP

(*b*) 32 molecules of NADPH

(*c*) 30 molecules of ATP

(*d*) 30 molecules of NADPH

10. Which one of the following bases is NOT found in the T-arm of an aminoacyl *t*-RNA?

(*a*) Dihydrouridine

(*b*) Pseudouridine

(*c*) Uracil

(*d*) Guanine

11. Match the entries of Column-I with those in Column-II

Column-I	Column-II
P. Vitamin B1	1. Thiamine pyrophosphate
Q. Carboxypeptidase	2. Aconitase
R. TCA cycle	3. Sucrose
S. Reducing sugar	4. Zn^{2+}
	5. Riboflavin
	6. Lactose

	P	Q	R	S
(*a*)	1	4	2	6
(*b*)	5	1	2	3
(*c*)	1	4	5	6
(*d*)	5	2	1	6

12. A cell suspension was subjected to membrane disruption followed by differential centrifugation to fractionate the cellular components. Match the centrifugal conditions in Column I to the appropriate subcellular components in Column II.

Column-I	Column-II
P. 1000 g, 10 min	1. Microsomes and small resicles
Q. 20000 g, 30 min	2. Ribosomes
R. 80000 g, 1 hour	3. Nuclei
S. 150000 g, 3 hours	4. Lysosomes and peroxisomes

	P	Q	R	S
(*a*)	3	4	1	2
(*b*)	1	4	3	2
(*c*)	3	4	2	1
(*d*)	2	1	4	3

13. The predicted molar extinction coefficient at 280 nm for the peptide GEEFHISFLLIMFGAWSTHMYRTYWFIHEMISTRY is ________ $M^{-1} cm^{-1}$.

[Molar extinction coefficients for phenylalanine, tryptophan and tyrosine at 280 nm are 200, 5600 and 1400 $M^{-1} cm^{-1}$, respectively]

14.

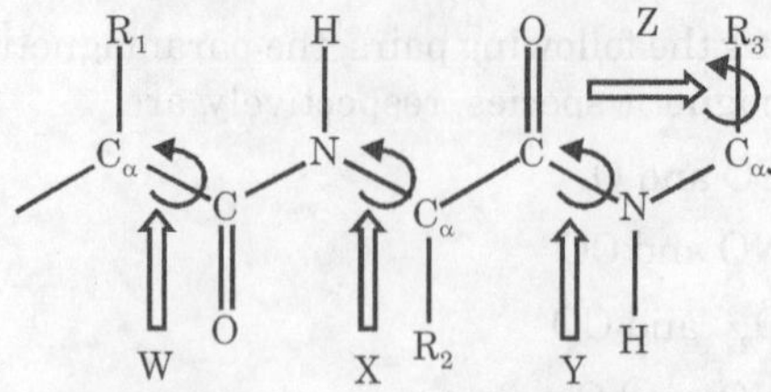

Column-I	Column-II
W	1. ψ
X	2. χ
Y	3. ϕ
Z	4. ω

	W	X	Y	Z
(*a*)	3	1	4	2
(*b*)	1	3	4	2
(*c*)	1	3	2	4
(*d*)	3	1	2	4

15. Match the contents of Column I with the most appropriate options in Coloumn II

Column-I	Column-II
P. Complement C1q	1. CD34
Q. L-Selectin	2. Complement C5b
R. Membrane Attack Complex	3. FC region of antibody
S. T-Helper cells	4. Complement C5a
	5. CD40L

	P	Q	R	S
(*a*)	3	5	4	1
(*b*)	1	2	4	5
(*c*)	3	1	2	5
(*d*)	4	5	2	1

16. The following table provides information about four proteins.

Protein	*Native mol. wt.(Da)*	*pI*	*Type*
P	32000	6.4	monomer
Q	40000	8.5	homodimer
R	25000	4.9	monomer
S	45000	8.5	homotrimer

Which one of the following options correctly identifies the order of elution in size exclusion chromatography and the increasing order of mobility in SDS polyacrylamide gel?

(*a*) Chromatrography : SQPR; Electrophoresis: RPQS

(*b*) Chromatrography : RPQS; Electrophoresis: SQPR

(*c*) Chromatrography : PRQS; Electrophoresis: PRQS

(*d*) Chromatrography : SQPR; Electrophoresis: PRQS

17. The value of ΔG at 37°C for the movement of Ca^{2+} ions from the endoplasmic reticulum where $[Ca^{2+}]$ is 1 mM to the cytosol where $[Ca^{2+}]$ is 0.1 μM at – 50 mV membrane potential is ______ kJ mol^{-1}.

[R = 8.314 JK^{-1} mol^{-1} and 1 Faraday = 96500 Coulombs]

18.

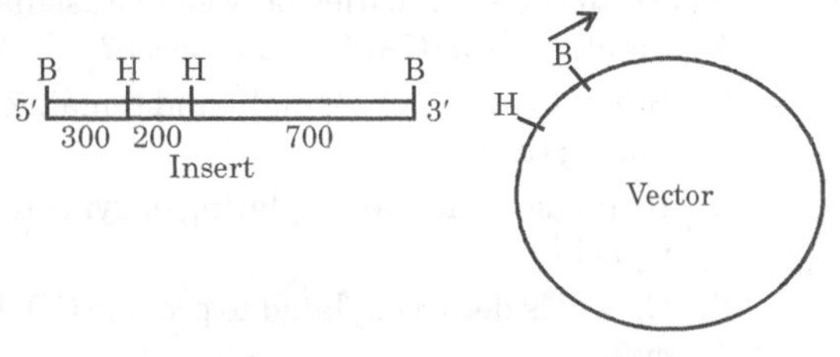

The insert is cloned into the vector at the *Bam*HI site and the desired orientation is shown by the arrow. After cloning, the orientation of the insert in the recombinant plasmid is tested by complete HindIII digestion followed by agarose gel electrophoresis. Which one of the following band patterns reveals the correct orientation of the insert in the construct?

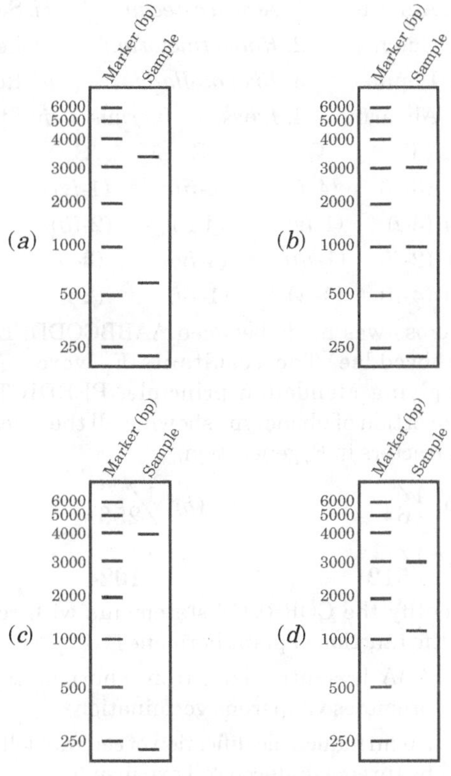

19. A 1.2 kb DNA fragment was used as template for PCR amplification using primers P1, P2, P3 and P4 as shown in the scheme below. The annealing positions of primers on the template are indicated by numbers. Primers P2 and P3 contain single base mismatches as indicated by filled triangles.

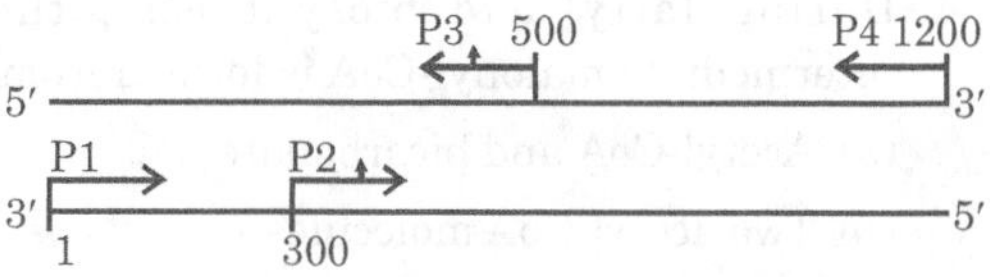

PCR was performed using primer pair P1 and P3 in one vial and P2 and P4 in another vial. The purified PCR products from the two vials were mixed and subjected to another round of PCR with primers P1 and P4. The final PCR product will correspond to a

(*a*) 1.2 kb wild type DNA

(*b*) 1.2 kB DNA with two point mutations

(*c*) 0.9 kb DNA with one point mutation

(*d*) 0.5 kb DNA with one point mutation

20. Which of the following statements is/are INCORRECT about hemoglobin (Hb)?

I. Hb demonstrates higher oxygen carrying capacity compared to myoglobin

II. There is covalent bonding between the four subunits of Hb

III. During deoxygenation the loss of the first oxygen molecule from oxygenated Hb promotes the dissociation of oxygen from the other subunits

(*a*) II (*b*) II and III

(*c*) I and III (*d*) III

J : BOTANY

1. A tube like membrane structure that forms the connection between the endoplasmic reticulum of neighboring cells through plasmodesmata is

(*a*) Desmotubule

(*b*) Desmosome

(*c*) Dictyosome

(*d*) Microtubule

2. An organized and differentiated cell having cytoplasm but no nucleus is found in

(*a*) Companion cell

(*b*) Xylem parenchyma

(*c*) Sieve tube element

(*d*) Phloem parenchyma

3. Which one of the followings is NOT a cryoprotectant for plant tissue?

(*a*) Dimethyl sulfoxide

(*b*) Glycerol

(*c*) Ethylene glycol

(*d*) Liquid nitrogen

4. During fatty acid biosynthesis, the first intermediate malonyl-CoA is formed from
(a) Acetyl-CoA and bicarbonate
(b) Two acetyl-CoA molecules
(c) Acetyl-CoA and biotin
(d) Palmitoyl CoA and acyl-carrier protein (ACP)

5. Identify the CORRECT family possessing the following characters : presence of glucosinolates, tetradynamous stamens, superior ovary with parietal placentation and siliqua type fruit
(a) Brassicaceae
(b) Capparidaceae
(c) Fumariaceae
(d) Papavaraceae

6. Two similar holotypes are called
(a) Monotype (b) Neotype
(c) Isotype (d) Syntype

7. Nuclear membrane is absent in
(a) *Chlamydomonas* (b) *Nostoc*
(c) *Volvox* (d) *Chlorella*

8. Double haploids in plants can be induced by
(a) Mitomycin-C (b) Mirin
(c) Colchicine (d) 5-Azacytidine

9. Which of the following reduces the transpiration rate when applied to aerial parts of plants?
(a) Phosphon-D
(b) Paraquat
(c) Phenyl mercuric acetate
(d) Valinomycin

10. Which of the following techniques in NOT applicable for evaluating the expression of a transgene?
(a) Northern blot (b) RT-PCR
(c) Western blot (d) Southern blot

11. Match the name of the diseases with their causal organisms.

Disease	Causal Organism
P. Loose smut of wheat	1. *Cercospora personata*
Q. Wart disease of potato	2. *Alternaria solani*
R. Panama disease of banana	3. *Synchytrium endobioticum*
S. Tikka disease of groundnut	4. *Ustilago tritici*
	5. *Fusarium oxysporum*
	6. *Erwinia amylovora*

	P	Q	R	S
(a)	6	4	3	2
(b)	4	6	1	3
(c)	4	3	5	1
(d)	2	3	2	6

12. Which of the following statements are TRUE with regard to the similarities between Crassulacean Acid Metabolism (CAM) and C_4 cycle?
P. Stomata open during night and remain closed during the day
Q. PEP case is the carboxylating enzyme to form C_4 acid
R. C_4 acid is decarboxylated to provide CO_2 for C_3 cycle
S. Kranz anatomy is predominant in both CAM and C_4 plants
(a) P, S (b) Q, R
(c) P, Q (d) R, S

13. Match the plant products with their sources and the plant parts from which they are obtained.

Product	Source	Plant Part
P. Annatto	1. *Acacia catechu*	*i.* Seed
Q. Cutch	2. *Rubia tinctorum*	*ii.* Leaf
R. Henna	3. *Bixa orellana*	*iii.* Root
S. Alizarin	4. *Lawsonia inermis*	*iv.* Stem

	P	Q	R	S
(a)	(3-*ii*)	(4-*i*)	(2-*iii*)	(1-*iv*)
(b)	(3-*i*)	(1-*iv*)	(4-*ii*)	(2-*iii*)
(c)	(2-*ii*)	(1-*iii*)	(4-*iv*)	(3-*i*)
(d)	(4-*ii*)	(3-*iv*)	(1-*iii*)	(2-*i*)

14. A cross was made between AABBCCDDEE and aabbccddee. The resultants F_1 were selfed. Applying Mendelian principle, PREDICT the proportion of phenotype showing all the recessive characters in F_2 generation.
(a) $1/64$ (b) $1/256$
(c) $1/512$ (d) $1/1024$

15. Identify the CORRECT statements with regard to the function of plant hormones
P. ABA is synthesized from chorismate and promotes viviparous germination
Q. Auxin induces acidification of cell wall followed by turgour-induced cell expansion
R. Gibberellin-reponsive genes become activated by the repression of DELLA protein
S. Cytokinin regulates the G_2 to M transition in the cell cycle
(a) P, Q (b) Q, R
(c) Q, S (d) P, R

16. Identify the CORRECT statements with respect to functioning of ecosystem.

P. A food chain is a series of organisms, each one feeding on the organism succeeding it

Q. Food web presents a complete picture of the feeding relationships in any given ecosystem

R. In ecosystem, energy flows in unidirectional way, whereas nutrients flow in cyclic fashion

S. In biogeochemical cycles, nutrients do not alternate between organisms and environment

(*a*) P, Q (*b*) P, R

(*c*) R, S (*d*) Q, R

17. With respect to germination of seeds, the CORRECT sequence of events is

P. Seed imbibes water

Q. Mobilization of starch reserve to embryo

R. Diffusion of gibberellin from embryo to aleurone layer

S. Synthesis of α-amylase in the aleurone layer

(*a*) P, Q, S, R (*b*) P, R, S, Q

(*c*) R, P, Q, S (*d*) R, Q, P S

18. Identify the INCORRECT statements with respect to plastid transformation.

P. Antibiotic used for selection of transplastomic plant is spectinomycin

Q. Chances of gene escape from transplastomic plants are high

R. Microprojectile bombardment is the method of DNA delivery

S. Levels of transgene expression are low

(*a*) P, R (*b*) P, Q

(*c*) Q, S (*d*) R, S

19. Match the floral structures with the families and representative plant species.

Floral structure

P. Gynostegium

Q. Gynostemium

R. Gynobasic style

S. Gynophore

Family

1. Orchidaceae
2. Lamiaceae
3. Capparidaceae
4. Asclepiadaceae

Plant

i. *Ocimum sanctum*

ii. *Cleome gynandra*

iii. *Calotropis procera*

iv. *Vanilla planifolia*

	P	Q	R	S
(*a*)	(2-*i*)	(3-*iii*)	(4-*ii*)	(1-*iv*)
(*b*)	(3-*ii*)	(4-*i*)	(2-*iii*)	(1-*iv*)
(*c*)	(4-*iii*)	(1-*iv*)	(2-*i*)	(3-*ii*)
(*d*)	(4-*ii*)	(2-*iii*)	(1-*iv*)	(3-*i*)

20. Statements given below are either TRUE (T) or FALSE (F). Find the correct combination.

P. Somatic embryo is unipolar in nature

Q. Heterokaryon can be selected using a fluorescence-activated cell sorter (FACS)

R. The term somaclonal variation is coined by Larkin and Scowcroft

S. Differentiation of shoot buds during *in vitro* culture isknown as somatic embryogenesis

(*a*) P-T, Q-F, R-T, S-F

(*b*) P-F, Q-T, R-F, S-T

(*c*) P-T, Q-F, R-F, S-T

(*d*) P-F, Q-T, R-T, S-F

K : MICROBIOLOGY

1. Of the following, the most effective method to kill bacterial endospores is

(*a*) moist heat sterilization

(*b*) UV irradiation

(*c*) filtration

(*d*) pasteurization

2. The classical way of representing taxonomic hierarchy of living organisms in ASCENDING ORDER is

(*a*) genus, species, class, order, family

(*b*) species, genus, order, family, class

(*c*) species, genus, family, order, class

(*d*) genus, species, order, class, family

3. The class of enzymes, which catalyze addition of groups to double bonds and non-hydrolytic removal of chemical groups, is

(*a*) oxidoreductase

(*b*) transferase

(*c*) hydrolase

(*d*) lyase

4. Lophotrichous bacteria have

(*a*) one flagellum

(*b*) a cluster of flagella at one or both ends

(*c*) flagella that are spread evenly over the whole surface

(*d*) a single flagellum at each pole

5. In aerobic respiration, the final electron acceptor is
   (*a*) hydrogen
   (*b*) nitrogen
   (*c*) sulfur
   (*d*) oxygen
6. Match scientists in Group I with terms related to their major scientific contributions in Group II

Group-I	Group-II
P. Sanger	1. DNA double helix structure
Q. Watson and Crick	2. DNA sequencing
R. Waksman	3. Complement
S. Bordet	4. Streptomycin
	5. Immune tolerance

	P	Q	R	S
(*a*)	3	4	2	1
(*b*)	2	3	4	5
(*c*)	4	1	2	5
(*d*)	2	1	4	3

7. Anammox organisms carry out
   (*a*) anaerobic reduction of NO_3^-
   (*b*) anaerobic oxidation NH_4^+
   (*c*) aerobic oxidation of NH_4^+
   (*d*) aerobic oxidation of NO_2^-
8. Limulus Amoebocyte Lysate (LAL) assay is used to identify the presence of
   (*a*) endotoxin
   (*b*) exotoxin
   (*c*) anthrax toxin
   (*d*) tetanus toxin
9. A process in which fatty acids are shortened by two carbons at a time resulting in release of acetyl-CoA is known as
   (*a*) photophosphorylation
   (*b*) carboxylation
   (*c*) β-oxidation
   (*d*) oxidative phosphorylation
10. Base-pair substitutions caused by the chemical mutagen ethyl methane sulfonate are a result of
    (*a*) hydroxylation
    (*b*) alkylation
    (*c*) deamination
    (*d*) intercalation
11. The volume (in ml) of a 1.0 mg/ml stock solution of ampicillin to be added to 0.1 liter of growth medium for achieving a final ampicillin concentration of 50 μg/ml is ________.
12. A bacterial culture is grown using 2.0 mg/ml fructose as the sole source of carbon and energy. The bacterial biomass concentrations immediately after inoculation and at the end of the growth phase are 0.1 mg/ml and 0.9 mg/ml, respectively. Assuming complete utilization of the substrate, the bacterial growth yield (Y) on fructose is ________.
13. Which combination of profiles in the following figure accurately represents the transport rate of glycerol and oxygen into E. *coli* cells as a function of their extracellular concentration?

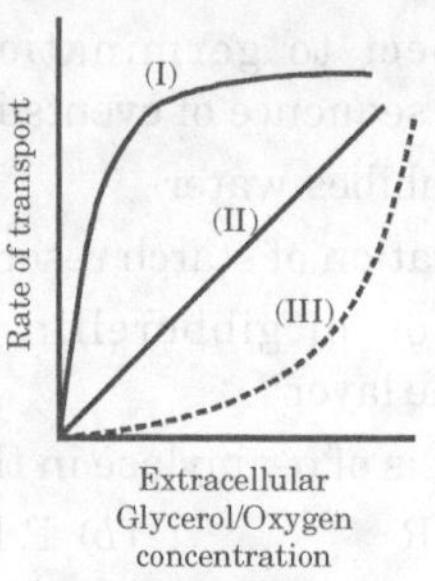

    (*a*) glycerol-(*ii*) and oxygen-(*iii*)
    (*b*) glycerol-(*ii*) and oxygen-(*i*)
    (*c*) glycerol-(*iii*) and oxygen-(*i*)
    (*d*) glycerol-(*i*) and oxygen-(*ii*)
14. The doubling time (in minutes) of a bacterium with a specific growth rate of 2.3 h^{-1} in 500 ml of growth medium is ________.
15. An *E. coli* strain is grown initially on glucose as the sole carbon source. Upon complete consumption of glucose following 12 h of growth, lactose is added as the sole carbon source and the strain is further grown for 12 h. Assuming that the *E. coli* strain has a functional wild type *lac* operon, which one of the following profiles is the most ACCURATE representation of β-galactosidase (*β-gal*) expression (in arbitrary units)?

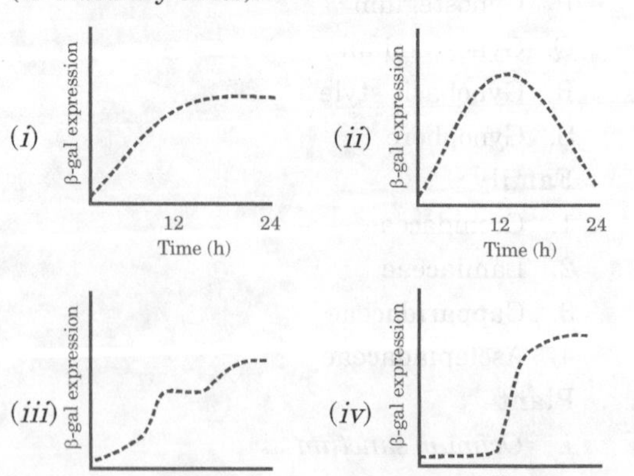

    (*a*) (*i*)
    (*b*) (*iii*)
    (*c*) (*ii*)
    (*d*) (*iv*)

16. The working volume (in liter) of a chemostat with 0.1 h^{-1} dilution rate and 100 hl/h feed flow rate is ________.

17. If the decimal reduction time for spores of a certain bacterium at 121°C is 12 seconds, the time required (in minutes) to reduce 10^{10} spores to one spore by heating at 121°C is ________.

18. Which combination of the following statements about specialized transduction is TRUE?

P. Specialized transducing phages can transport only certain genes between bacteria

Q. Specialized transducing phages can transport any gene between bacteria

R. Phage P22 is a specialized transducing phage

S. Phage lambda (λ) is a specialized transducing phage

(*a*) P and S only (*b*) Q and R only

(*c*) P and R only (*d*) Q and S only

19. Which one of the following about the standard free energy change ($\Delta G^{\circ\prime}$) and the equilibrium constant (K_{eq}) of an exergonic reaction, at pH 7.0, is TRUE?

(*a*) $\Delta G^{\circ\prime}$ is positive and K_{eq} is less than one

(*b*) $\Delta G^{\circ\prime}$ is negative and K_{eq} is less than one

(*c*) $\Delta G^{\circ\prime}$ is negative and K_{eq} is greater than one

(*d*) $\Delta G^{\circ\prime}$ is positive and K_{eq} is greater than one

20. An oil immersion objective of a light microscope has a numerical aperture of 1.25. Using the Abbe equation, the maximum theoretical resolving power (in nm) of the microscope with this objective and blue light (wavelength = 450 nm) is________.

L : ZOOLOGY

1. Which one of the following statements is FALSE with respect to phospholipids?

(*a*) Phospholipids have amphipathic character

(*b*) Phospholipids form the lipid bilayer of the cell membrane

(*c*) Phospholipids form micelles in living systems

(*d*) Some phospholipid molecules may contain a double bond in hydrophobic tails

2. Which one of the following life cycle stages of *Plasmodium falciparum* is infectious?

(*a*) Sporozoite (*b*) Cryptozoite

(*c*) Merozoite (*d*) Trophozoite

3. Which one of the following is a function of intermediate filaments?

(*a*) Chromosome movement during the cell division

(*b*) Cytoplasmic streaming

(*c*) Formation of tight junctions

(*d*) Anchorage of the nucleus

4. Which one of the following organs is INCORRECTLY paired with its function?

(*a*) Intestinal villi-absorption

(*b*) Epiglottis-closure of larynx

(*c*) Gall bladder-carbohydrate digestion

(*d*) Parietal cells-hydrochloric acid

5. Constitutive enzymes are

(*a*) Induced by effector molecules

(*b*) Repressed by repressors

(*c*) Encoded by sequences that occur as part of an operon

(*d*) Always produced in the cell

6. The term "paedomorphosis" refers to

(*a*) Accelerated reproductive development as compared to somatic development

(*b*) A transient stage in the developmental event

(*c*) Two independent structures resembling each other, yet performing different functions

(*d*) A form of mimicry

7. The behavior of young ducks following their mother is known as

(*a*) Imprinting

(*b*) Innate behavior

(*c*) Habituation

(*d*) Mimicry

8. Where do B lymphocytes acquire immune competence?

(*a*) Thymus

(*b*) Bone Marrow

(*c*) Lymph nodes

(*d*) Spleen

9. What is the role of the notochord during organogenesis in a vertebrate embryo?

(*a*) Signaling the development of placenta

(*b*) Induction of neural plate formation

(*c*) Stimulation of the umbilical chord formation

(*d*) Suppression of the development of extra-embryonic membranes

10. Which one of the following statements is TRUE when determining the age of a fossil using carbon dating?

(*a*) Carbon dating is based on carbon-13 to carbon-12 ratio in fossils

(*b*) Carbon dating is useful for determining the age of only fossils older than 100,000 years

(*c*) Older the fossil, lesser the carbon-14 to carbon-12 ratio

(*d*) Older the fossil, lesser the carbon-12 to carbon-14 ratio

11. Assuming equal frequency for all 4 nucleotides (G, A, T, C), how many EcoRI recognition sites (GAATTC) are possible in a bacterial artificial chromosome of 100,000 base pairs?

(*a*) 6 (*b*) 12

(*c*) 24 (*d*) 48

12. A population of spotted deer found in a national forest is in Hardy-Weinberg equilibrium. For a particular genetic locus in this deer species, only two alleles A and *a* are possible. If the frequency of the A allele in this population is 0.6, and the frequency of the *a* allele is 0.4, what will be the frequency of the genotype A*a*?

(*a*) 0.24 (*b*) 0.48

(*c*) 0.96 (*d*) 1.6

13. Choose the correct option that shows pairing of the organelle to its function

P. Smooth endoplasmic reticulum — 1. Internalization of receptors

Q. Peroxisome — 2. Protein secretion

R. Golgi apparatus — 3. Membrane biogenesis

S. Endosome — 4. Breakdown of fatty acids

	P	Q	R	S
(*a*)	1	2	3	4
(*b*)	1	3	2	4
(*c*)	3	4	2	1
(*d*)	2	3	4	1

14. Which one of the following statements DOES NOT explain altruism?

(*a*) Altruism reduces the fitness of the individual the displays this behavior

(*b*) Altruism increases the fitness of other individuals in the population

(*c*) Altruism reduces the fitness of the individual that displays this behavior and at the same time

(*d*) Altruistic behavior helps the individual escape from predators

15. In *Drosophila*, the gene for eye colour is present on the X chromosome. When a red-eyed female was mated with a white-eyed male, a total of 100 progeny were obtained – 50 females and 50 males. Of the 50 females, 25 were red-eyed, and 25 were white-eyed. How many of the male progeny were red-eyed?

(*a*) 0 (*b*) 10

(*c*) 20 (*d*) 25

16. The popular birth control pills for women have a combination of synthetic forms of estradiol and progesterone. Which one of the following statements is INCORRECT with regard to their function as contraceptive?

(*a*) The pills inhibit the release of GnRH leading to inhibition of gonadotropin-stimulated ovarian function

(*b*) They act directly on the pituitary gland to inhibit gonadotropin surges

(*c*) The low dose of estradiol in the pill inhibits the release of FSH, and thus blocks ovulation

(*d*) The synthetic forms of estradiol and progesterone bring about their effects by binding to their respective intracellular receptors

17. Which one of the following is consistent with the germplasm theory of August Weismann?

(*a*) Regulative development observed in frog embryos

(*b*) Mosaic development observed in tunicates

(*c*) Normal embryonic development of embryos formed by somatic nuclear transfer

(*d*) Ability of differentiated cells to form pluripotent stem cells under certain conditions

18. Choose the correct option based on your understanding of the circulatory system

P. Open circulatory system — 1. Fish

Q. Closed circulatory system — 2. Frog

R. Three chambered heart — 3. Earthworm

S. Two chambered heart — 4. Grasshopper

	P	Q	R	S
(*a*)	4	3	2	1
(*b*)	4	1	2	3
(*c*)	1	4	2	3
(*d*)	1	3	4	2

19. Match the species names with class names

P. *Calotes versicolor* — 1. Insecta

Q. *Periplaneta americana* — 2. Reptilia

R. *Glyphidrilus birmancus* — 3. Actinopterygii

S. *Clarias batracus* — 4. Clitellata

	P	Q	R	S
(*a*)	2	1	4	3
(*b*)	1	2	3	4
(*c*)	2	1	3	4
(*d*)	3	1	2	4

20. Defect in poly-A tail formation in eukaryotic mRNA leads to

(*a*) Increased translation of the resulting mRNA

(*b*) Decreased translation of the resulting mRNA

(*c*) Premature transcription termination

(*d*) Decreased mRNA stability

FOOD TECHNOLOGY

1. The enzyme that hydrolyzes starch to maltose is
(*a*) α-amylase
(*b*) β-amylase
(*c*) glucoamylase
(*d*) cyclodextrin glucanotransferase

2. What is the percent relative humidity at which both the dry bulb and wet bulb thermometers would record equal temperatures?
(*a*) 0 (*b*) 10
(*c*) 50 (*d*) 100

3. Among the following animal foods, the fat content is least in
(*a*) Beef
(*b*) Chicken meat
(*c*) Pork
(*d*) Lamb flesh

4. Which one of the following is NOT enriched in endosperm during parboiling of paddy?
(*a*) Thiamine (*b*) Niacin
(*c*) Iron (*d*) Fat

5. Standard pasteurization protocol for milk is adequate for destroying
(*a*) *Clostridium sporogenes*
(*b*) *Bacillus cereus*
(*c*) *Clostridium botulinum*
(*d*) *Listeria monocytogenes*

6. How many fold would the *g*-number of a centrifuge increase by doubling both the spinning speed and bowl diameter?
(*a*) 2 (*b*) 4
(*c*) 8 (*d*) 16

7. Which one of the following is NOT a component of an evaporator?
(*a*) Heat exchanger
(*b*) Vacuum separator
(*c*) Condenser
(*d*) Cyclone separator

8. The gradual decrease in viscosity of tomato paste during storage can be prevented by quickly heating it to 82°C, because
(*a*) water soluble pectin interacts with calcium
(*b*) hemicellulose prevents decrease in viscosity
(*c*) lignin prevents decrease in viscosity
(*d*) pectin methyl esterase is inactivated

9. Prolonged fermentation of cocoa seeds lead to "off-taste"due to the release of
(*a*) glucose
(*b*) short chain fatty acids
(*c*) carbon dioxide
(*d*) phospholipids

10. Heat-treated legume seed proteins are more digestible than those of untreated legume seed proteins due to
(*a*) reaction of reducing sugars with ε-amino group of lysine
(*b*) increased binding of lectins to intestinal mucosal cells
(*c*) thermolabile nature of lectins and Kunitz-type protease inhibitors
(*d*) thermolabile nature of Bowman-Birk type of inhibitor

11. Match the edible plant tissue in Group I with the type of carotenoid given in Group II

	Group-I	Group-II
P.	Corn	1. Lycopene
Q.	Red pepper	2. β-carotene
R.	Pumpkin	3. Capsanthin
S.	Tomato	4. Lutein

	P	Q	R	S
(*a*)	3	4	2	1
(*b*)	2	1	3	4
(*c*)	4	3	2	1
(*d*)	1	2	4	3

12. Granulated sugar, having an average particle size of 500 μm, is milled to produce icing sugar having an average particle size of 25 μm. The power requirement was 10 kW as obtained by Rittinger's law. If the same mill were to be used to produce fondant sugar having an average particle size of 20 μm at same capacity, the power requirement (kW) would be ________.

13. Green tea is considered to be a more healthy option than black tea because it
(*a*) has high content of polyphenols
(*b*) is richer in thearubigin
(*c*) does not require any sweetener during tea preparation
(*d*) has no microbial load

14. Match the enzyme is Group I with its corresponding application in Group II

Group-I	Group-II
P. Chymosin	1. Removal of cooked flavor from milk
Q. Sulfhydryl oxidase	2. Soybean milk coagulation
R. β-Galactosidase	3. For rennet puddings
S. Microbial proteases	4. Lactose removal

	P	Q	R	S
(*a*)	3	2	1	4
(*b*)	3	1	4	2
(*c*)	1	3	4	2
(*d*)	4	3	2	1

15. The order of succession of microbes in the spoilage of milk, involving (P) *Lactobacillus*, (Q) protein digesting bacteria, (R) *Lactococcus lactis*, (S) yeasts and molds, is

(*a*) S > R > Q > P

(*b*) S > Q > R > P

(*c*) R > P > S > Q

(*d*) Q > S > P > R

16. Whole milk (34,950 kg) containing 4% fat is to be separated in 6 h period into skim milk with 0.45% fat and cream with 45% fat. The flow rate of cream stream (kg/h) from the separator is ________.

17. One ton of soybean containing 18% oil, 35% protein, 27.1% carbohydrates, 9.4% of fibre and ash, and 10.5% moisture is crushed and pressed. The residual oil content in the pressed cake is 6%. Assuming that there is not loss of protein and water with oil, the amount of oil (kg) obtained from the crusher is ________.

18. A dilute pineapple juice is heated in a double pipe heat exchanger from 28 °C to 75 °C by heat exchanging with hot water flowing in shell in counter current direction. Hot water is entering the shell at 95 °C and leaving at 85 °C. The log mean temperature difference (°C) is ________.

19. Match the processing method in Group I with the operation carried out in Group II

Group-I	Group-II
P. Degumming	1. Crystallization of triacylgly-cerol by cooling to remove fat crystals
Q. Deacidifying	2. Passing heated oil over charcoal
R. Bleaching	3. Using alkaline solution to remove fatty acids
S. Winterizing	4. Wetting with water to remove lecithin

	P	Q	R	S
(*a*)	3	1	4	2
(*b*)	4	3	1	2
(*c*)	4	3	2	1
(*d*)	3	1	2	4

20. Milk is flowing at 0.12 m^3/min in a 2.5 cm diameter pipe. The temperature of the milk is 21 °C and the corresponding viscosity and density are 2.1×10^{-3} Pas and 1029 kg/m^3, respectively. If the flow is found to be turbulent under the given conditions, the Reynolds number is ________.

ANSWERS

GENERAL APTITUDE

1. (*c*)	2. (*a*)	3. (*c*)	4. (*b*)	5. (*a*)
6. (*c*)	7. (3)	8. (*b*)	9. (*a*)	10. (*a*)

H : CHEMISTRY

1. (–212.39 kJ/mol)	2. (*d*)	3. (*d*)	4. (1)	5. (*b*)
6. (69.76)	7. (*b*)	8. (*a*)	9. (*a*)	10. (*b*)
11. (*a*)	12. (*c*)	13. (6.86)	14. (*b*)	15. (*c*)

I : BIOCHEMISTRY

1. (*d*)	2. (*d*)	3. (*b*)	4. (– 0.0105)	5. (*d*)
6. (*b*)	7. (*c*)	8. (*c*)	9. (*c*)	10. (*a*)
11. (*a*)	12. (*a*)	13. (16200 $M^{-1}cm^{-1}$)		14. (*b*)
15. (*c*)	16. (*d*)	17. (–33.39 $kJmol^{-1}$)		18. (*a*)
19. (*b*)	20. (*a*)			

J : BOTANY

1. (*a*)	2. (*c*)	3. (*d*)	4. (*a*)	5. (*a*)
6. (*c*)	7. (*b*)	8. (*c*)	9. (*c*)	10. (*d*)
11. (*c*)	12. (*b*)	13. (*b*)	14. (*d*)	15. (*b*)
16. (*d*)	17. (*b*)	18. (*c*)	19. (*c*)	20. (*d*)

K : MICROBIOLOGY

1. (*a*)	2. (*c*)	3. (*d*)	4. (*b*)	5. (*d*)
6. (*d*)	7. (*b*)	8. (*a*)	9. (*c*)	10. (*b*)
11. (5)	12. (0.4)	13. (*d*)	14. (18.08)	15. (*d*)
16. (1 litre)	17. (2 min)	18. (*a*)	19. (*c*)	20. (180 nm)

L : ZOOLOGY

1. (*c*)	2. (*a*)	3. (*d*)	4. (*c*)	5. (*d*)
6. (*a*)	7. (*a*)	8. (*b*)	9. (*b*)	10. (*c*)
11. (*c*)	12. (*b*)	13. (*c*)	14. (*d*)	15. (*d*)
16. (*c*)	17. (*b*)	18. (*a*)	19. (*a*)	20. (*d*)

FOOD TECHNOLOGY

1. (*b*)	2. (*d*)	3. (*b*)	4. (*d*)	5. (*d*)
6. (*c*)	7. (*d*)	8. (*d*)	9. (*b*)	10. (*c*)
11. (*c*)	12. (12.63)	13. (*a*)	14. (*b*)	15. (*c*)
16. (464.17 Kg/hr)	17. (127 to 128 Kg)	18. (36)	19. (*c*)	20. (49906.5)

EXPLANATIONS

GENERAL APTITUDE

1. Educe → Extract

2. $$\frac{5}{7} = x^{-1/3}$$
$$\frac{7}{5} = x^{1/3}$$
$$\left(\frac{7}{5}\right)^3 = x$$
$$\frac{343}{125} = x$$

3. $$66\square 6 = \frac{66-6}{66+6} = \frac{60}{72} = \frac{5}{6}$$
$$66\diamond 6 = \frac{66+6}{66-6} = \frac{72}{60} = \frac{6}{5}$$
So, $(66\square 6)\rightarrow(66\diamond 6) = \frac{5}{6}\times\frac{6}{5} = 1$

4. The principal presented the chief guest with a <u>Memento</u> as token of appreciation.

5. Frogs croak.

6. Number of faces per cube = 6
Total number of cubes = 9 × 3 = 27
∴ Total number of faces = 27 × 6 = 162
∴ Total number of non-visible faces
= 162 – 54 = 108
$$\therefore \frac{\text{Number of visible faces}}{\text{Number of non-visible faces}} = \frac{54}{108} = \frac{1}{2}$$

7. Middle number is the average of the numbers on both sides :
Average of 6 and 4 is 5
Average of (7 + 4) and (2 + 1) is 7
Average of (1 + 9 + 2) and (1 + 2 + 1) is 8
Average of (4 + 1) and (2 + 3) is 5
Therefore, Average of (3) and (3) is 3

8. Humpty Dumpty does not fall sometimes while having lunch.

9. Ranks one of the leading causes of death → ranks as one of the leading causes of death

10. Human progress depends upon environmental security.

H : CHEMISTRY

1. $\Delta G^\circ = -\text{RT}\ln k$
$$K = -8.314\times 10^{-3}\times(273+25)\ln(1.7\times 10^{37})$$
$$= -212.39\ k\text{Jmol}^{-1}$$

2. Diels-Alder adduct is the product of cycloaddition in the sequence with another molecules without isolating the intermediates.

3. General equation for half life $t_{1/2} = \frac{2^{n-1}-1}{K(n-1)} C_{A_0}^{1-n}$

where n = order of reaction. The plot of ln $t_{1/2}$ vs ln$[x]_0$ gives the grap of option D.

4. HOOC–CH(OH)–CH(OH)–COOH
C_1 C_2 C_3 C_4

So, two assymetric carbon atoms C_2 & C_3. Hence $2^1 = 2$ enantiomeric i.e. (1pair) is possible.

5. The dipole moment of

$NF_3 = 0.24$ D
$CO_2 = 0$ D
$BCl_3 = 0$ D
$CCl_4 = 0$ D

also, apart from NF_3 all other molecules are symmetrical in their structures.

6. $\ln\left(\frac{P_1}{P_2}\right) = \frac{+\Delta H}{R}\left(\frac{1}{T_2} - \frac{1}{T_1}\right)$

$T_2 = 78.3°C = 351.3°K$
$T_1 = 25°C = 298°K$
$P_2 = 760$Torr
$P_1 = ?$
$\Delta H = 39.0$ kJ/mol = 39000 J/mol
$R = 8.314$ JK^{-1} mol^{-1}
$= 8.314 \times 10^{-3}$ KJ K^{-1}mol^{-1}

Putting all the values in equation and solving we get

$\therefore$ $P_1 = 69.76$ Torr

7. Ratio of radius of 1st Bohr orbit and 3rd. Bohr orbit is 1 : 9

$\therefore \frac{\text{radius 1}^{\text{st}}\text{ Bohr orbit}}{\text{radius 3}^{\text{rd}}\text{ Bohr orbit}} = \frac{1}{9}$

Bohr orbit is 1 : 9

$\Rightarrow$ radius of 3rd Bohr orbit
$= 9 \times 0.53 = 4.77$Å

8. The Resonance energy of four given molecules are as follows in Kcal/mol.

36 22 29 16

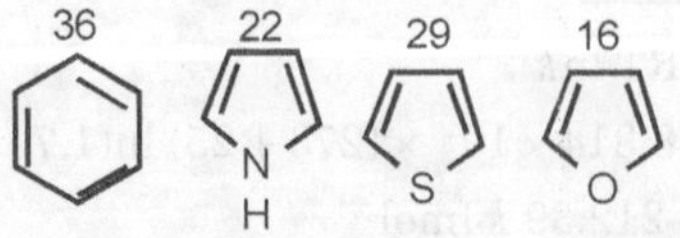

(1) (2) (3) (4)

so, 36 > 29 > 22 > 16
1 > 3 > 2 > 4

9.

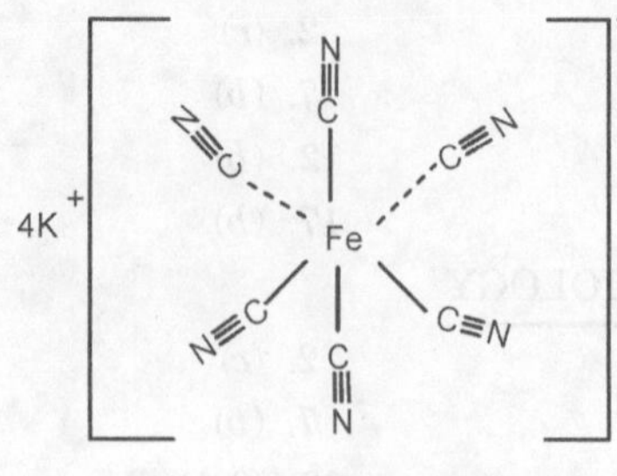

$K_4Fe(CN)_6$

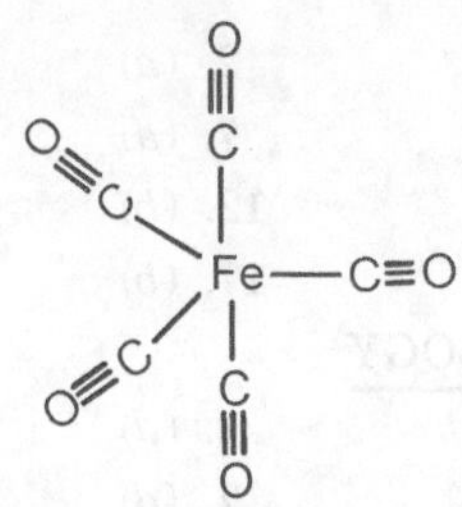

$Fe(CO)_5$

10. If species has unpaired electron then it is paramagnetic and if no unpaired electron then it is Diamagnetic.

NO has one unpaired electron so it is Paramagnetic
CO has no unpaired electron so it is Diamagnetic.

11. The CFS (crystal field splitting) energies are (Δ_0)

$[MnCl_6]^{-3} = 20000$ cm^{-1} = Y
$[CrCl_6]^{-3} = 13000$ cm^{-1} = X
$[FeCl_6]^{-3} = 41,000$ cm^{-1} = Z

so, higher the CFS energy and hence less stable molecules

so, X > Y > Z

12. 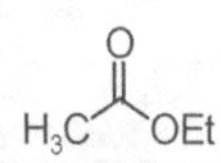 + $CH_3CH_2MgBr \longrightarrow$ 3–ethylpentan-3-ol

13. $N_1V_1 = N_2V_2$

$\Rightarrow N_2 = \frac{N_1V_1}{V_2}$

$= \frac{0.02 \times 50}{950} = 1.053 \times 10^{-3}$m

$\therefore$ pH = $-\log[1.053 \times 10^{-3}] = 6.86$

14. The Nitration of tert-butyl benzene never gives the meta-product and sulfonation of tert-butyl benzene gives para-product.

15. For, chemically equilibrium reaction the ΔS_{total} is zero. The given reaction is in equilibrium hence $\Delta S_{total} = 0$

I : BIOCHEMISTRY

1. **Glutamine to Valine** : It causes largest change in protein conformation. It causes sickle cell anemia thus it is the most significant substitution.
2. Ribulose-5- Phosphate epimerase is involved in pentose phosphate pathway it converts Ribulose-5- phosphate into xylulose-5-phosphate.
3. Lysozymes are glycoside hydrolases. The enzyme functions by attacking peptidoglycans and hydrolyzing the glycosidic bond that connects N-acetylmuramic acid with the fourth carbon atom of N-acetylglucosamine.

   The reaction catalyzed by lysozyme, the hydrolysis of a glycoside, is the conversion of an acetal into a hemiacetal Non-enzymatic, this is an acid-catalyzed reaction, involving the protonation of an oxygen atom, followed by cleavage of a O–C bond → transient formation of resonance stabilized carbocation = oxonium ion Enzymatic reaction should include an acid catalyst and a stabilization of the oxonium ion transition state.
4. Super helical density $(\sigma) = \frac{\Delta L_K}{L_{K_0}}$,

$$\Delta L_K = L_K - L_{K_0}$$

$$L_{K_0} = \frac{bp}{10.5} = \frac{4000}{10.5} = 380.95 \approx 380$$

$$L_K = T_w + W_r$$

$$T_w = \text{number of twist} = \frac{4000}{10.5} \approx 380$$

W_r = number of writhes = –4

(∴ DNA is negative supercoiled)

$$\therefore \quad L_K = 380 - 4 = 376$$

$$\therefore \quad \Delta L_K = 376 - 380 = -4$$

$$\therefore \quad \sigma = \frac{\Delta L_K}{L_{K_0}} = \frac{-4}{380} = -0.0105$$

5. Transforming growth factor β receptor is not a receptor tyrosine kinase.
6. Stearic acid does not constitute the lipid moiety in lipid linked membrane proteins.
7. Proteolytic enzymes are synthesised as inactive precursors or zymogens to prevent unwanted protein degradation and to enable spatial and temporal regulation of proteolytic activity. Upon sorting or appropriate compartmentalization, Zymogen conversion to active enzyme typically involves proteolysis and removal of active segment.
8. Carnitine molecule is a prerequisite for fatty acid oxidation.
9. As, FADH2 is produced in the glycerol phosphate pathway and each FAD worth only 2ATPs. In glycolysis, NADH is produced which then goes to shuttle and produces ATPs. If malate shuttle occurs, 6ATPs will be produced from 2NADH and in glycerol phosphate shuttle, 4ATPs will be produced from 2NADH. Now in the whole process of oxidation of one molecule of glucose:

   Glycolysis = 4ATP – 2ATP + 2NADH

   (resulting in 4ATPs in glycerol pathway) = 6ATPs

   Kreb's Cycle = 24ATPs

   Total = 6 + 24 = 30 ATPs
10. t-arm of an aminoacyl t-RNA contains a triplet sequence. It has G-U base pairing and a modified base pseudouridine whereas dihydrouridine is present in the D-arm of t-RNA.
11.
    - **Metabolics Vitamin B1** is in the form of **Thiamine Pyrophosphate**.
    - **Carboxypeptidase** is also known as **Zinc Carboxypeptidase** as the zinc ligands have been determined as two histidines and a glutamate, and the catalytic residue has been identified as a C-terminal glutamate
    - **Aconitase** is an enzyme that catalyses the stereospecific isomerization of citrate to isocitrate via cis-aconitate in the tricarbo xylic acid cycle
    - A **reducing sugar** is any sugar that either has an aldehyde group or is capable of forming one in solution through isomerism. Lactose is a reducing sugar.
12.
    - Nuclei is centrifuged with 1000g for 10 mins.
    - Lysosomes and peroxisomes are centrifuged with 20000g for 30 mins.
    - Microsomes and small vesicles are centrifuged with 80000g for 1 hour.
    - Ribosomes are centrifuged with 150000g fractionate for 3 hours.
13. (*i*) The molar extinction coefficient of given peptide is found using molar extinction coefficient of pheny-lalanine (E_{Phe}), tryptophan (E_{Trp}) and tyrosine (E_{Tyr}) by following equation

    $$E_{peptide} = a\,E_{phe} + b\,E_{Trp} + c\,E_{Tyr}$$

    a, b, c are number of residue of Phe , Trp + Tyr in peptide.

    (*ii*) So in a given Peptide

    a = number of Phe (F) = 4

    b = number of Trp (W) = 2

    c = number of Tyr (Y) = 3

Now, given

$$E_{Phe} = 200\ M^{-1}\ cm^{-1}$$
$$E_{Trp} = 5600\ M^{-1}cm^{-1}$$
$$E_{Tyr} = 1400\ M^{-1}cm^{-1}$$
$$\therefore\quad E_{peptide} = (4{\times}200)+(2{\times}5600) + 3(1400)$$
$$= (800 + 11200 + 4200)$$
$$= 16{,}200\ M^{-1}cm^{-1}$$

14. The angle around $C_\alpha - C$ bond is Psi angle (ψ) *i.e.* W

The angle around $N - C_\alpha$ bond is Phi angle (ϕ) *i.e.* X

The angle around $C - N$ bond is omega angle (ω) *i.e.* Y

The angle around $C_\alpha - R$ bond is Chi angle (χ) *i.e.* Z

$\therefore$ W – *i*, X – *iii*, Y – *iv* and Z – *ii*

15. 1. Complement C1q → Fe region of antibody
2. L-selection → CD34
3. Membrane Attack complex → complement C5b
4. T– Helper cells – CD40L

16. Size Exclusion Chromatography (SEC) is the separation technique based on the molecular size of the components. A sample of proteins passing through a gel filtration column will separate based on molecular size: the big ones will elute first and the smallest ones will elute last (and "middle" sized proteins will elute in the middle).

Polyacrylamide gels restrain larger molecules from migrating as fast as smaller molecules. Because the charge-to-mass ratio is nearly the same among SDS-denatured polypeptides, the final separation of proteins is dependent almost entirely on the differences in relative molecular mass of polypeptides. In a gel of uniform density the relative migration distance of a protein is negatively proportional to the log of its mass.

17. $$\Delta G = \Delta G^\circ + RT\ \ln \frac{\left[Ca^{+2}\right]_{in}}{\left[Ca^{+2}\right]_{out}}$$

$$\left[Ca^{+2}\right]_{in} = 0.1\mu m$$

$$\left[Ca^{+1}\right]_{out} = 1mm$$

$R = 8.314 \times 10^{-3}\ kJ\ K^{-1}\ mol^{-1}$

$T = (273 + 37) = 310^\circ\ K$

n = number of electrons transported = 2

F = 96500 coulombs

$$E_{cell} = -50mV$$
$$= -50 \times 10^{-3}\ V$$
$$\Delta G^\circ = +\,nFE_{cell}$$
$$\therefore\quad \Delta G^\circ = +\,2 \times 96500 \times (-50 \times 10^{-3})$$
$$= -\,9650\ J/mol = -\,9.650\ kJ/mol$$
$$\Delta G = -\,9.650 + (18.314 \times 10^{-3}) \times (310)\ \ln \frac{\left(0.1 \times 10^{-3}\right)}{(1)}$$
$$\Delta G = -9.650 - 23.74$$
$$= -\,33.39\ kJmol^{-1}$$

18. 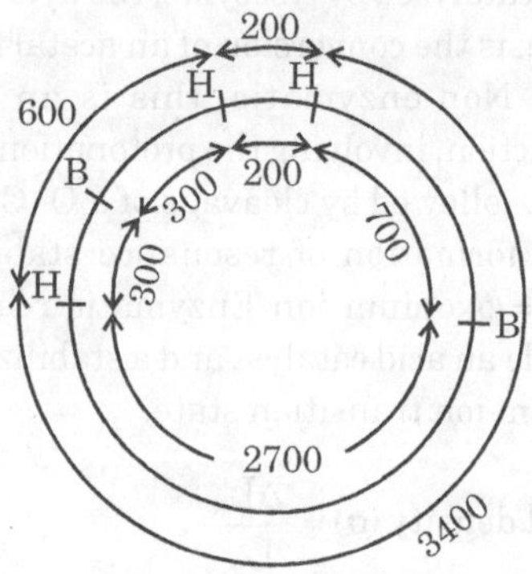

The correct orientation of the bands pattern inserted in the construct are

1. 200 bp,
2. 600 bp and
3. 3400 bp

19. 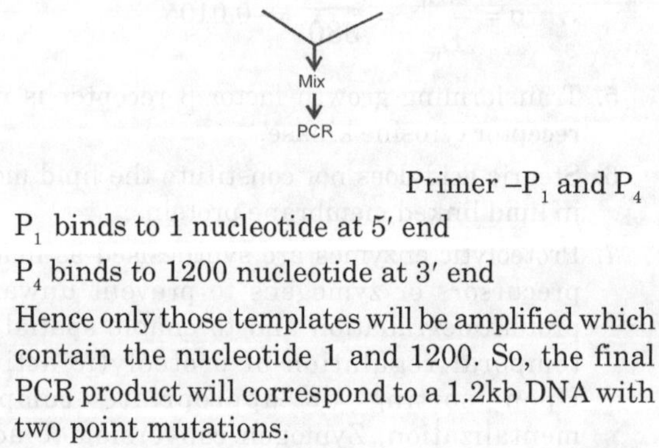

Primer – P_1 and P_4

P_1 binds to 1 nucleotide at 5′ end

P_4 binds to 1200 nucleotide at 3′ end

Hence only those templates will be amplified which contain the nucleotide 1 and 1200. So, the final PCR product will correspond to a 1.2kb DNA with two point mutations.

20. (*i*) Myoglobin binds to one molecule of O_2 whereas Hemoglobin binds to 4 molecules of O_2. Hence oxygen carrying capacity of Hb is more than that of myoglobin.

(*ii*) The 4 subunits of Hb are bound by non-covalent bonding.

(*iii*) During deoxygenation, the loss of first molecule of O_2 results due to cooperativity. This facilatates release of second oxygen molecule and so on.

J : BOTANY

1. Desmotubule : Cylindrical membrane-lined channel through a plasmodesma, linking the cisternae of endoplasmic reticulum in the two cells.
2. In plant anatomy, sieve tube elements, also called sieve tube members, are a specialised type of elongated cell in the phloem tissue of flowering plants. The ends of these cells are connected with other sieve tube members, and together they constitute the sieve tube. The main function of the sieve tube is transport of carbohydrates, primarily sucrose, in the plant (e.g., from the leaves to the fruits and roots). Unlike the water-conducting xylem vessel elements that are dead when mature, sieve elements are living cells. They are unique in lacking a nucleus at maturity.
3. A cryoprotectant is a substance used to protect biological tissue from freezing damage. Liquid nitrogen is used for cell lysis. Liquid nitrogen is not a cryo-protectant for plant tissue.
   Common cryoprotectants are :
   1. DMSO
   2. Ethylene glycol
   3. Glycerol
   4. 2-Methyl-2, 4-pentanediol (MPD)
   5. Propylene glycol
   6. Sucrose
4. Acetyl-CoA Carboxylase catalyzes the 2-step reaction by which acetyl-CoA is carboxylated to form malonyl-CoA :

$$HCO_3^- + ATP + acetyl-CoA \rightarrow ADP + P_i + malonyl-CoA$$

5. Brassicaceae posses the following charecters : presence of glucosinolates, tetradynamous stamens, superior ovary with partial placentation and siliqua type fruit.
6. A holotype is a single physical example (or illustration) of an organism, known to have been used when the species (or lower-ranked taxon) was formally described. It is either the single such physical example (or illustration) or one of several such, but explicitly designated as the holotype. Under the ICZN, a holotype is one of several kinds of name-bearing types. An isotype is a duplicate of the holotype.
7. *Nostoc* is a genus of cyanobacteria found in a variety of environmental niches that forms colonies composed of filaments of moniliform cells in a gelatinous sheath. Cells have no nucleus nor internal membrane system.
8. Colchicine, an alkaloid derived from *Colchicum autumnal* can be used to double the number of chromosomes of the cell. Colchicine prevents cellular mitosis by affecting the functionality of tubulin, the protein of microtubules. As a result, the chromosomes cells are duplicated but not divided.
9. Phenylmercuric acetate is an organo-mercury compound. This compound was formerly used as a preservative in paints, and as a disinfectant. When applied to the leaves of plants, it is an antitranspirant.
10. A Southern blot is a method used in molecular biology for detection of a specific DNA sequence in DNA samples, but not for gene expression. Southern blotting combines transfer of electro-phoresis-separated DNA fragments to a filter membrane and subsequent fragment detection by probe hybridization.
11. 1. Loose smut of wheat is caused by *Ustilago tritici*.
    2. *Synchytrium endobioticum* is a chytrid fungus that causes the potato wart disease or *black scab*.
    3. Panama disease is a plant disease of the roots of banana plants. It is caused by the fungal pathogen *Fusarium oxysporum*.
    4. Groundnut is subjected to various airborne fungal diseases like Tikka leaf spot caused by *Cercosporidium personatum, Cerocospora arachidicola*.
12. PE Pease is the carboxylating enzyme to form C_4 acid. C_4 acid is decarboxylated to provide CO_2 for C_3 cycle.
13. Annatto, sometimes called *roucou* or *achiote*, is derived from the seeds of the achiotetree. The seeds are sourced to produce a carotenoid-based yellow to orange food coloring and flavor. Its scent is described as "slightly peppery with a hint of nutmeg" and flavor as "slightly nutty, sweet and peppery".In commercial processing, annatto coloring is extracted from the reddish pericarp which surrounds the seed of the achiote (*Bixa orellana* L.).

    Catechu is an extract of Acacia used variously as a food additive, astringent, tannin, and dye. It is extracted from several species of *Acacia*, but especially *Acacia catechu*, by boiling the wood in water and evaporating the resulting brew. Henna (*Lawsonia inermis*,) is a flowering plant and the sole species of the *Lawsonia* genus. The name *henna* also refers to the dye prepared from the plant and the art of temporary tattooing based on those dyes (see also mehndi). Alizarin is a product from roots of *Rubia tinctorum*. *Rubia tinctorum,* the common madder or dyer's madder, is a plant species in the genus *Rubia*. The plant's roots contain several polyphenolic compounds, such as 1,3-Dihydroxyanthraquinone (purpuroxanthin), 1,4–Dihydroxyanthra-quinone (quinizarin), 1,2,4-Trihydroxyan-thraquinone (purpurin) and 1,2-dihy-droxyanthraquinone (alizarin).

14. In Gametogenesis 2^n gametes will be produced where n is the no. of heterozygotes i.e. $2^5 = 32$ Gametes. After fusion of all 32 types of gametes, $32 \times 32 = 1024$ characters will appear. Out of 32 gametes, one gamete has only abcde genotype that produces only one recessive character in F_2 generation. Genotype of that character will be aabbccddee. Hence the proportion of phenotype showing all the recessive character in F_2 generation will be 1/1024.

15. Function of plant hormones-

Q. Auxin induces acidification of cell wall followed by turgour-induced cell expansion

R. Gibberellin-reponsive genes become activated by the repression of DELLA protein

16. Food web presents a complete picture of feeding relationship in any given ecosystem. In ecosystem, energy flows in unidirectional way, whereas nutrients flow in cyclic fashion.

17. With respect to germination of seeds, the correct sequence of events are:

1. Seed imbibes water
2. Diffusion of gibberellins from embryo to aleurone layer
3. Synthesis of α – amylase in the aleurone layer
4. Mobilization of starch reserve to embryo

18. Statements with respect to plastid transformation are as follows:

Antibiotic used for selection of transplastomic plant is spectinomycin----Correct

Chances of gene escape from transplastomic plants are high---------- Incorrect

Microprojectile bombardment is the method of DNA delivery-------- Correct

Levels of transgene expression are low--------- Incorrect

19. *Vanilla planifolia* is a species of vanilla orchid, Family - Orchidaceae. *Calotropis procera* is a species of flowering plant in the family of Asclepiadaceae. *Ocimum tenuiflorum*, also known as Ocimum sanctum, holy basil, or *tulasi*, is an aromatic plant in the family of Lamiaceae. *Cleome gynandra* , is a species of *Cleome* known by the common name Shona cabbage in the family of Cleomaceae. The Cleomaceae are a small family of flowering plants in the order Brassicales, comprising about 300 species in 10 genera, or about 150 species in 17 genera. These genera were previously included in the family Capparaceae.

20. Somatic embryo is unipolar in nature ---- False, Shoots and roots are monopolar while somatic embryos are bipolar, allowing them to form a whole plant without culturing on multiple media types. Heterokaryon can be selected using a fluorescence-activated cell sorter (FACS) -------- True.

The term somaclonal variation is coined by Larkin and Scowcroft ----True. Differentiation of shoot buds during in vitro culture is known as somatic embryogenesis ------ False.

K : MICROBIOLOGY

1. Bacterial endospores can be destroyed by burning or by autoclaving at a temper-ature exceeding the boiling point of water, 100°C. Moist heat sterilization is the most effective method to kill Bacterial endospores .

2. The classical way of representing taxonomic hierarchy of living organism : species, genus, family, order, class.

3. lyase is an enzyme that catalyzes the breaking (an "elimination" reaction) of various chemical bonds by means other than hydrolysis (a"substitution" reaction) and oxidation, often forming a new double bond or a new ring structure.

4. Lophotrichous bacteria have multiple flagella located at the same spot on the bacteria's surfaces which act in concert to drive the bacteria in a single direction. Tuft of flagella at one or both ends e.g. Spirilla

5. In aerobic respiration the final electron acceptor is oxygen, whereas in anaerobic respiration the final electron acceptor is a molecule other than oxygen

6. Selman A. Waksman has discovered streptomycin, the first antibiotic effective against tuberculosis. Jules Bordet received his Nobel Prize for his discoveries relating to immunity. Sanger sequencing is a method of DNA sequencing based on the selective incorporation of chain-terminating dideoxynucleotides by DNA polymerase during in vitro DNA replication. Watson and Crick produced their double helix model of DNA.

7. Anammox, an abbreviation for **AN**aerobic **AMM**onium **OX**idation, is a globally important microbial process of the nitrogen cycle. In this biological process, nitrite and ammonium are converted directly into dinitrogen gas.

Globally, this process may be responsible for 30-50% of the dinitrogen gas produced in the oceans.

The overall catabolic reaction is:

$$NH_4^+ + NO_2^- \rightarrow N_2 + 2H_2O$$

8. Limulus amebocyte lysate (LAL) is an aqueous extract of blood cells (amoebocytes) from the horseshoe crab, *Limulus polyphemus.* LAL reacts with bacterialendotoxin or lipopolysaccharide (LPS), which is a membrane component of Gram negative bacteria. This reaction is the basis of the **LAL test**, which is the used for the detection and quantification of bacterial endotoxins.
9. Beta-oxidation is the catabolic process by which fatty acid molecules are broken down in the mitochondria to generate acetyl-CoA, which enters the citric acid cycle, and NADH and FADH2, which are co-enzymes used in the electron transport chain.
10. Ethyl methanesulfonate (EMS) is a mutagenic, teratogenic, and possibly carcinogenic organic compound with formula $CH_3SO_3C_2H_5$. It produces random mutations in genetic material by nucleotide substitution; particularly by guaninealkylation.
11. $N_1 V_1 = N_2V_2$,

    Where N_1 = 1 Mg/ml,

    N_2 = 50 g/ml = 50×10^{-3} mg/ml,

    V_2 = 100ml, V_1 = ?

    Then $V_1 = N_2V_2 / N_1$

    $= 50 \times 10^{-3} \times 100 / 1 = 5$ ml
12. $$Y_{X/S} = \frac{\Delta X}{\Delta S} = \frac{(0.9 - 0.1)}{(2-0)} = \frac{0.8}{2} = 0.4$$
13. Glycerol-(i) and Oxygen-(ii)
14. Given; = 2.3 h^{-1}

    But $t_d = 0.693/\mu$

    then $t_d = \frac{0.693}{2.3} = 0.301$ hr

    Or $t_d = 0.301 \times 60$ min. = 18.08 min.
15. The *lac* operon consists of **three genes** each involved in processing the sugar lactose. One of them is the gene for the enzyme **β-galactosidase**. This enzyme hydrolyses lactose into glucose and galactose. *E. coli* can use either glucose, which is a monosaccharide, or lactose, which is a disaccharide. However, lactose needs to be hydrolysed (digested) first. So the bacterium prefers to use glucose when it can.

    Four situations are possible.

    1. When glucose is present and lactose is absent the *E. coli* does not produce β-galactosidase.
    2. When glucose is present and lactose is present the E. coli does not produce β-galactosidase.
    3. When glucose is absent and lactose is absent the E.coli does not produce β-galactosidase.
    4. When glucose is absent and lactose is present the E. coli does produce β-galactosidase.
16. $D = \frac{F}{V}$ or $V = \frac{F}{D} = \frac{100}{0.1} = 1000$ ml = 1 lit
17. F = n D, Time required to kill the spores,

    n = number of log cycles between start and finish,

    D = Decimal reduction time

    Then F = 10 × 12 = 120 sec = 2 Minutes
18. *Specialized transduction* is the process by which a restricted set of bacterial genes is transferred to another bacterium. The genes that get transferred (donor genes) depend on where the phage genome is located on the chromosome. Example of specialized transduction is λ phages in *Escherichia coli* discovered by Esther Lederberg
19. An **exergonic reaction** is a chemical reaction where the change in the free energy is negative (there is a net release of free energy), indicating a spontaneous reaction. For processes that take place under constant pressure and temperature conditions, the Gibbs free energy is used whereas the Helmholtz energy is used for processes that take place under constant volume and temperature conditions. Symbolically, the release of free energy, G, in an exergonic reaction (at constant pressure and temperature) is denoted as:

    $$\Delta G = G_{products} - G_{reactants} < 0$$

    The standard Gibbs Free Energy change for a reaction can be related to the reaction's equilibrium constant (K_{eq}) by a simple equation:

    $$\Delta G^\circ = - RT \ln K_{eq}$$

    where:

    $$K_{eq} = \frac{[product]}{[reactant]} \text{ at equilibrium,}$$

    $R = 8.314\ J \times K^{-1} \times mol^{-1}$

    or $1.987\ cal \times K^{-1} \times mol^{-1}$,

    T = temperature in Kelvin (K)

    Negative value for ΔG°_{mx} (an exergonic reaction) corresponds to K_{eq} being greater than 1, an equilibrium constant which favors product formation.
20. $D = \frac{\lambda}{2NA} = \frac{450}{2} \times 1.25 = 180nm$

L : ZOOLOGY

1. Phospholipid structure prevents the formation of micelles because the two fatty acids, one of which is usually unsaturated, prevent aggregation into a tight sphere. Instead, phospholipids form liposomes, in which phospholipid molecules form a double layer, or bilayer, in a much larger sphere.

2. Sporozoite stages of *Plasmodium falciparum is infectious.*
3. Anchorage of the nucleus is a function of intermediate filaments.
4. Gall bladder stores bile which is necessary for emulsification of fats aiding in fat digestion.
5. Constitutive enzymes are produced constitutively by the cell under all physiological conditions. They are not controlled by induction or repression.
6. The term "paedomorphosis" refers to accelerated reproductive development as compared to somatic development.
7. In imprinting young animals acquires several of its behavioral characteristics from its mother or parents.
8. Produce in Bone Marrow but mature in spleen.
9. **Neural plate** : A thick, flat bundle of ectoderm formed in vertebrate embryos after induction by the notochord.
10. ^{14}C decay as the age of fossil increases *i.e.* the concentration of ^{14}C in the atmosphere decreases. Thus reduces the ratio of ^{14}C to ^{12}C.
11. There are 4 different bases, so the probability of finding a particular base at one location on a DNA strand = ¼. So, the probability of finding the required base at each of *n* locations = (¼) to the power of *n* where *n* can be 4, 6, or 8, thus frequency of sites = 4 to the power of *n*.
If DNA strand length >> 1/ frequency, then: number of cuts is almost equal to bp × frequency.
Therefore, Frequency of sites
$$= \left(\frac{1}{4}\right)^6 = \frac{1}{4096} = 0.0000244$$
Here frequency of sites < <100000
Therefore recognition sites
$$= 0.0000244 \times 1000000 = 24.4$$
12. The amount of genetic variation in a population will remain constant from one generation to the next in the absence of disturbing factors.
An equation of hardy Weinberg of two alleles : (AA) + (2Aa) + (aa) = 1
Then, $(0.4 \times 0.4) + 2Aa + (0.6 \times 0.6) = 1$
Solving the equation, we get
$$2Aa = 0.48$$
Note : In question the frequency of the genotype Aa has been asked but the frequency of the genotype is represented by 2Aa.
13. Major function of **Golgi apparatus**- modifying, sorting and packaging of proteins for secretion .
Peroxisome - Breakdown of long chain fatty acids through β-oxidation.
Smooth endoplasmic reticulum - Helps in membrane phospholipid synthesis.
14. An organism is said to behave altruistically when its behaviour benefits other organisms, at cost to itself. Altruism makes organism more prone to attacks or predators, for e.g:- vervet monkeys give alarm calls to warn fellow monkeys of presence of predators, even though in doing so they attract attention to themselves, increasing their personal chance of being attacked.
15.

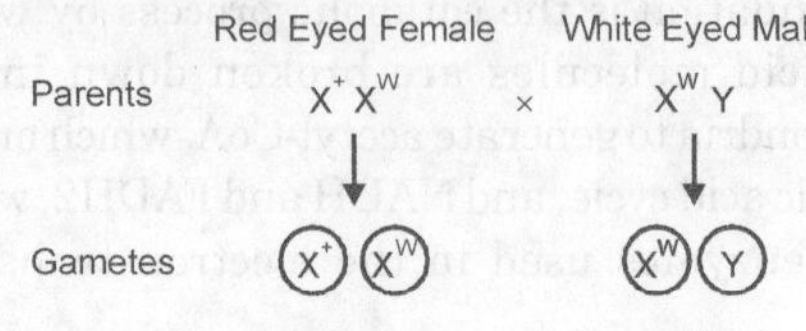

	X^+	X^W
X^W	X^+X^W 25 Red Female	X^WX^W 25 White Female
Y	X^+Y 25 Red male	X^WY 25 White Male

16. Estradiol and progesterone inhibit the GnRH hence inhibiting the ovarian function. The pill contains estradiol which will act on pitutary gland (negative feed- back) to inhibit gonadotropin surge. The hormones have the specific receptors on which they bind to bring about the effects.
17. The germplasm theory of August Weismann says mosaic development observed in tunicates.
18. Open circulatory system is present in grasshopper. Grasshopper has a direct oxygen delivery system through air tubes called trachae that are found throughout the body. Open circulatory system is an efficient way to allow wing muscles to get enough oxygen. Earthworms have closed circulatory system that consists of heart that pumps blood through blood vessels, distributing nutrients and oxygen and retrieving waste products discarded from tissues.
Fish has a two-chambered heart
Frog has a three-chambered heart.
19. **Calotes Versicolor**
Kingdom : Animalia
Family : Agamidae
Class : Reptilia
Periplaneta Americana
Kingdom : Animalia
Family : Blattidae
Class : Insecta
Glyphidrilus Birmancus
Kingdom : Animalia
Family : Almidae
Class : Clitella

Clarias batracus
Kingdom : Animalia
Family : Clariidae
Class : Actinopterygii

20. Poly A tail formation is addition of poly A tail to a messenger RNA.

In Eukaryotes it is a part of process that produces mature mRNA for translation. Poly A tail is important for nuclear export, translation and stability of mRNA. It protects the mRNA molecule from enzymatic degradation in cytoplasm and aids in transcription termination, export of mRNA from nucleus and translation. If there is a defect in Poly A tail formation, then stability of mRNA will be disturbed.

FOOD TECHNOLOGY

1. Beta-amylase is an enzyme with system name 4-alpha-D-glucan maltohydrolase. β-Amylase is an exoenzyme that releases successive maltose units from the nonreducing end of a polysaccharide chain by hydrolysis of *a*-1, 4-glucan linkages. The shortest normal saccharide attacked is maltotetraose.
2. At 100% relative humidity the water cannot evaporated and both dry bulb and wet bulb temperature are same.
3. The fat content of different food are as follows :

Beef – 15g/100gm
Chicken meat – 1.5g/100gm
Pork – 15g/100gm
Lamb flesh – 10-15g/100gm

4. Parboiling drives nutrients, especially thiamin, from the bran to the endosperm. Parboiling reduced the breakages, fat, protein and amylose content of the rice while the water uptake and thiamine contents were increased.
5. *Listeria monocytogenes* can be a pathogen for humans causing miscarriages or severe meningitis. This aerobic bacteria can develop at low temperatures of even 5°C and is destroyed through pasteurisation. *Listeria monocytogenes* is the bacterium that causes the infection listeriosis. It is a facultative anaerobic bacterium, capable of surviving in the presence or absence of oxygen. It has long been known that the pasteurization process effectively kills many pathogenic organisms, including the bacteria Listeria monocytogenes, which should make pasteurized milk and other products safe for human consumption.
6. $RCF = \frac{rw^2}{g}$

As, *r* and *w* both double then RCF increases by 8 fold

$$\text{New RCF} = 2\frac{r\times(2w)^2}{g} = 8\frac{rw^2}{g}$$

7. Heat exchanger is provide heat for evaporation. Evaporated material is collected by Vacuum separator and remaining material collected in condenser to utilize heat of hot material.
8. The gradual decrease in viscosity of tomato paste during storage can be prevented by quickly heating it to 82°C, because pectin methyl esterase is inactivated. Heating (blanching) during the hot break process deactivates pectin methyl esterase before it has a chance to hydrolyse the pectin; therefore hot break processing yield high viscosity tomato products.
9. Prolonged fermentation of cocoa seeds release the fatty acids which are responsible for off-taste.
10. These inhibitors have significant anti-nutritive effects, affecting digestion by hindering protein hydrolysis and activation of other enzymes in gut.
11. Corn – Lutein found in leafy vegetables.

Red pepper – Capsanthin found in Red pepper
Pumpkin – β-Carotene abundant in Pumpkin
Tomato – Lycopene found in red vegetables

12. According to Rittinger's law

$$\frac{P}{\dot{m}} = k_r\left(\frac{1}{D_{S_b}} - \frac{1}{D_{S_a}}\right)$$

D_{S_a} = average particle size of feed = 500μm

D_{S_b} = average particle size of 1st product = 25μm

If D_{S_c} = 20 μm

P_1 = 10kW

P_2 = ?

$$\therefore \frac{\frac{P_1}{\dot{m}} = k_r\left(\frac{1}{D_{S_b}} - \frac{1}{D_{S_a}}\right)}{\frac{P_2}{\dot{m}} = k_r\left(\frac{1}{D_{S_c}} - \frac{1}{D_{S_a}}\right)} \Rightarrow \frac{P_1}{P_2} = \frac{\left(\frac{1}{D_{S_b}} - \frac{1}{D_{S_a}}\right)}{\left(\frac{1}{D_{S_c}} - \frac{1}{D_{Sa}}\right)}$$

$$\Rightarrow \frac{10}{P_2} = \frac{\left(\frac{1}{25} - \frac{1}{500}\right)}{\left(\frac{1}{20} - \frac{1}{500}\right)} \Rightarrow P_2 = 12.63\text{kW}$$

13. Because the oxidation is arrested in green tea, so it preserve more polyphenols.
14. P. Chymosin – For rennet puddings

Q. Sulfhydryl oxidase – Removal of cooked flavour from milk

R. β- Galactosidase – Lactose removal

S. Microbial proteases – Soybean milk coagulation.

15. (R) Lactococcus generer microbes have most dominant population in milk.

16.

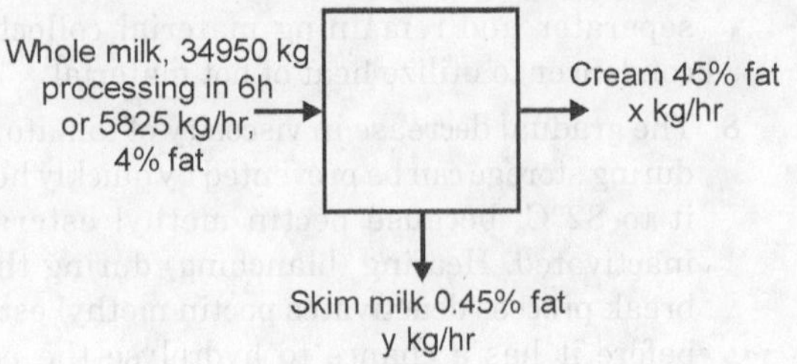

$$x + y = 5825 \quad ...(i)$$

Fat balance gives :-

$$(0.04)(5825) = x(0.45) + y(0.0045)$$

Substitude the value of $y = 5825 - x$ and solve

So, $x = 464.17$ kg/hr

17. Let the amount of oil obtained form crusker = y kg

% of oil in the product = 94% = 0.94 y kg

residual oil conten = 0.06 × 1000 = 60 kg

Taking material (oil) balence

oil input = oil in product + residual oil

$$1000 \times (0.18) = 0.94\,y + 60$$

$$\therefore \quad y = \frac{180 - 60}{0.94} = 127.66 \text{ kg}$$

18.

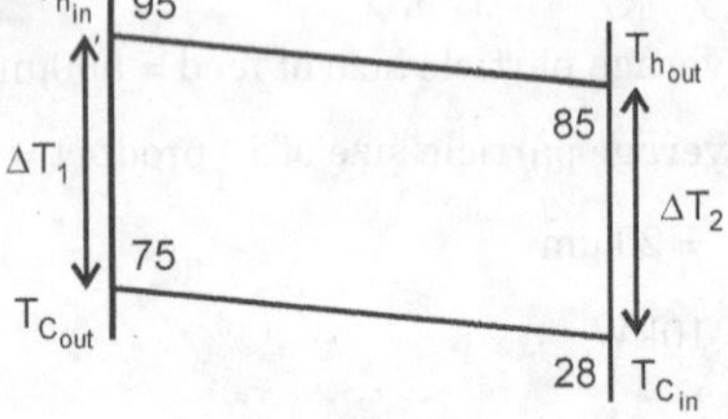

$$\Delta T_2 = (85 - 28) = 57$$

$$\Delta T_1 = (95 - 75) = 20$$

$$\Delta T_{LMTD} = \frac{\Delta T_1 - \Delta T_2}{\ln\left(\frac{\Delta T_1}{\Delta T_2}\right)} = 36°C$$

19. P. Degumming – Wetting with water to remove lecithin

Q. Deacidifying – Using alkaline solution to remove fatty acids

R. Bleaching – Passing heated oil over charcoal

S. Winterizing – Crystallization of triacylglycerol by cooling to remove fat crystals

20. $N_{Re} = \frac{DV\rho}{\mu}$, $\quad D = 0.025$ mt

$\rho = 1029$ kg/m^3

$\mu = 2.1 \times 10^{-3}$ Pas

$Q = 0.12$ m^3/min

$Q = uA$, $\quad A = \frac{\pi}{4} D^2 = 4.91 \times 10^{-4}$

$$\therefore \quad u = \frac{Q}{A} = \frac{0.12}{4.91 \times 10^{-4}}$$

$= 244.46$ m^3/min

$= 4.074$ m^3/sec.

$$N_{Re} = \frac{0.025 \times 4.074 \times 1029}{2.1 \times 10^{-3}}$$

$= 49906.5$

■■

GATE-2014

XL : LIFE SCIENCES

Time : 3 Hours *Maximum Marks : 100*

GENERAL APTITUDE

(Q. 1 - 5) Carry One Mark Each.

1. Choose the most appropriate word from the options given below to complete the following sentence.

A person suffering from Alzheimer's disease ____ short-term memory loss.

(*a*) experienced (*b*) has experienced

(*c*) is experiencing (*d*) experiences

2. Choose the most appropriate word from the options given below to complete the following sentence.

______ is the key to their happiness; they are satisfied with what they have.

(*a*) Contentment (*b*) Ambition

(*c*) Perseverance (*d*) Hunger

3. Which of the following options is the closest in meaning to the sentence below?

"As a woman, I have no country."

(*a*) Women have no country

(*b*) Women are not citizens of any country

(*c*) Women's solidarity knows no national boundaries

(*d*) Women of all countries have equal legal rights

4. In any given year, the probability of an earthquake greater than Magnitude 6 occurring in the Garhwal Himalayas is 0.04. The average time between successive occurrences of such earthquakes is ____ years.

5. The population of a new city is 5 million and is growing at 20% annually. How many years would it take to double at this growth rate?

(*a*) 3-4 years (*b*) 4-5 years

(*c*) 5-6 years (*d*) 6-7 years

(Q. 6-10) Carry Two Marks Each.

6. In a group of four children, Som is younger to Riaz. Shiv is elder to Ansu. Ansu is youngest in the group. Which of the following statements is/are required to find the eldest child in the group?

Statements

1. Shiv is younger to Riaz.
2. Shiv is elder to Som.

(*a*) Statement 1 by itself determines the eldest child

(*b*) Statement 2 by itself determines the eldest child

(*c*) Statements 1 and 2 are both required to determine the eldest child

(*d*) Statements 1 and 2 are not sufficient to determine the eldest child

7. Moving into a world of big data will require us to change our thinking about the merits of exactitude. To apply the conventional mindset of measurement to the digital, connected world of the twenty-first century is to miss a crucial point. As mentioned earlier, the obsession with exactness is an artefact of the information-deprived analog era. When data was sparse, every data point was critical, and thus great care was taken to avoid letting any point bias the analysis. From "BIG DATA" *Viktor Mayer- Schonberger and Kenneth Cukier*

The main point of the paragraph is:

(*a*) The twenty-first century is a digital world

(*b*) Big data is obsessed with exactness

(*c*) Exactitude is not critical in dealing with big data

(*d*) Sparse data leads to a bias in the analysis

8. The total exports and revenues from the exports of a country are given in the two pie charts below. The pie chart for exports shows the quantity of each item as a percentage of the total quantity of exports. The pie chart for the revenues shows the percentage of the total revenue generated through export of each item. The total quantity of exports of all the items is 5 lakh tonnes and the total revenues are 250 crore rupees. What is the ratio of the revenue generated through export of Item 1 per kilogram to the revenue generated through export of Item 4 per kilogram?

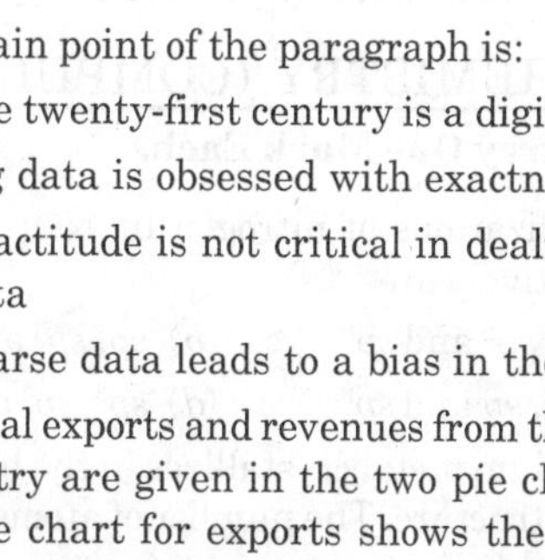

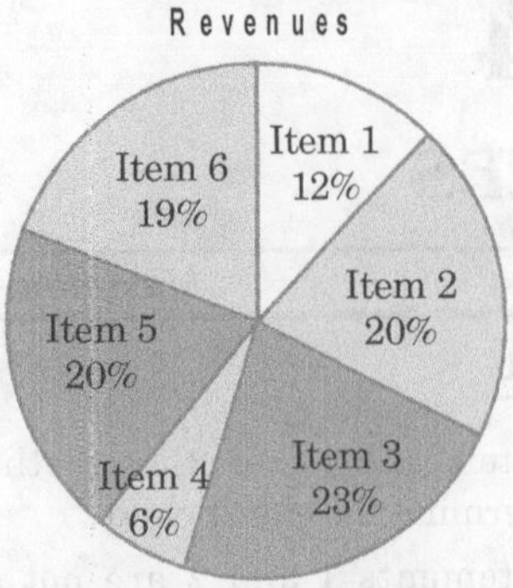

(*a*) 1 : 2 (*b*) 2 : 1 (*c*) 1 : 4 (*d*) 4 : 1

9. X is 1 km northeast of Y. Y is 1 km southeast of Z. W is 1 km west of Z. P is 1 km south of W. Q is 1 km east of P. What is the distance between X and Q in km?

(*a*) 1 (*b*) $\sqrt{2}$ (*c*) $\sqrt{3}$ (*d*) 2

10. 10% of the population in a town is HIV^+. A new diagnostic kit for HIV detection is available; this kit correctly identifies HIV^+ individuals 95% of the time, and HIV^- individuals 89% of the time. A particular patient is tested using this kit and is found to be positive. The probability that the individual is actually positive is ______

H : CHEMISTRY (COMPULSORY)

(Q. 1-5) Carry One Mark Each.

1. Hybridizations of nitrogen in NO_2^+, NO_3^-, NH_4^+ respectively are

(*a*) *sp*, *sp*^{2} and *sp*^{3} (*b*) *sp*, *sp*^{3} and *sp*^{2}
(*c*) *sp*^{2}, *sp* and *sp*^{3} (*d*) *sp*^{3}, *sp*^{2} and *sp*

2. Potassium metal crystallizes in the body-centered cubic structure. The number of atoms per unit cell is equal to

(*a*) one (*b*) two (*c*) three (*d*) four

3. Assuming ideal condition, the solution that has the highest freezing point is

(*a*) 0.002 M aqueous solution of copper nitrate
(*b*) 0.001 M aqueous solution of potassium dichromate
(*c*) 0.001 M aqueous solution of sodium chloride
(*d*) 0.002 M aqueous solution of magnesium chloride

4. The major product formed in the following reaction is

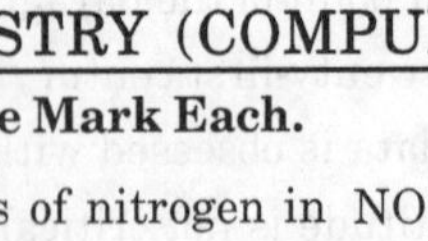

(*a*)
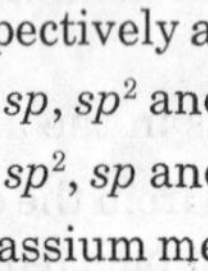

(*b*)
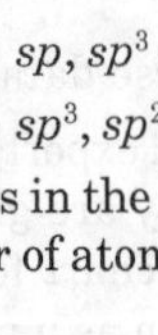

(*c*)
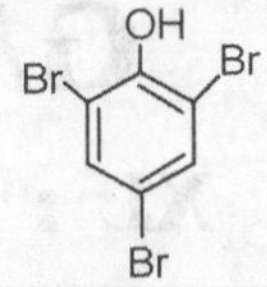

(*d*)
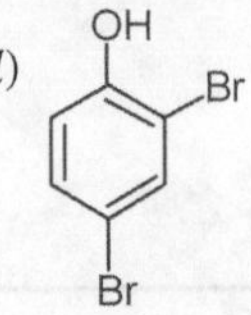

5. The acid that undergoes decarboxylation most readily upon heating is

(*a*)
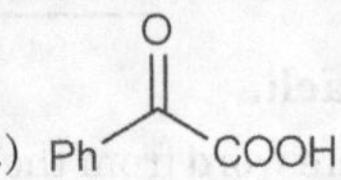

(*b*)
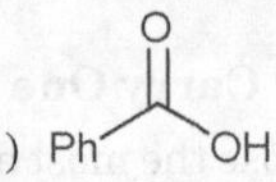

(*c*)
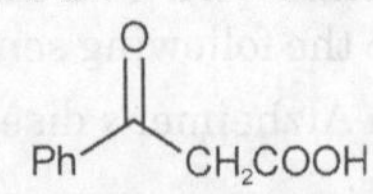

(*d*)
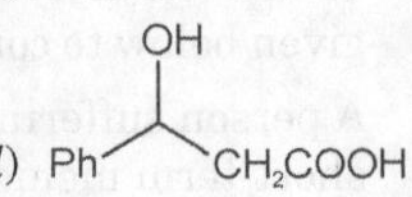

(Q. 6-15) Carry Two Marks Each.

6. A ball of mass 330 g is moving with a constant speed, and its associated de Broglie wavelength is 1×10^{-33} m. The speed of the ball is ______ m s^{-1}. ($h = 6.6 \times 10^{-34}$ J s)

7. Diphosphonic acid ($H_4P_2O_5$) has no P – P bond. This acid is

(*a*) tetrabasic (*b*) tribasic
(*c*) dibasic (*d*) monobasic

8. The magnetic moment of an octahedral Co(II) complex is approximately 4.0 μB (atomic number of Co is 27). The CFSE for this complex, in Δ_o units, is ___ .

9. The complex ion $[Cr(H_2O)_6]^{3+}$ (atomic number of Cr is 24) exhibits

(*a*) slightly distorted octahedral geometry
(*b*) tetragonally elongated octahedral geometry
(*c*) tetragonally compressed octahedral geometry
(*d*) perfect octahedral geometry

10. Assuming ideal behavior, the density of fluorine gas at 20 °C and 0.3 atm is __ gL^{-1}.
(Molecular weight of F_2 = 38 g mol^{-1}, R = 0.082 L atm mol^{-1} K^{-1})

11. For a first order reaction, the time required for 50% completion is 20 minutes. The time required for 99.9% completion of the reaction is ___ minutes.

12. At 298 K, the bond dissociation energies of C–H, C–C and C=C are 415, 344 and 615 kJ mol^{-1}, respectively. The enthalpy of atomization of carbon is 717 kJ mol^{-1} and that of hydrogen is 218 k Jmol^{-1}. The heat of formation of naphthalene at 298 K is ___ kJ mol^{-1}.

13. The Fisher projection that represents (2R,3S)-2,3-dihydroxybutanoic acid is

(*a*)
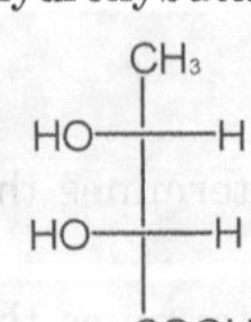

(*b*)
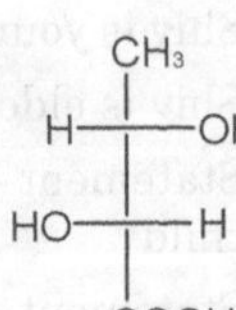

(c) 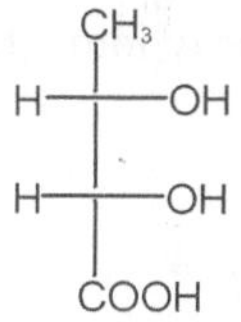

(d) 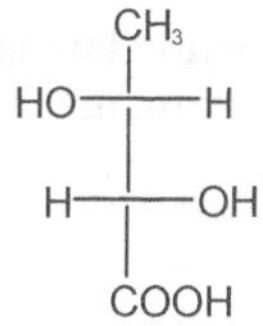

14. A hydrocarbon that undergoes ozonolysis (reaction with ozone followed by reduction with Me_2S) to form formaldehyde and glyoxal is

(a) 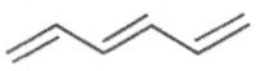 (b) 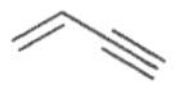

(c) 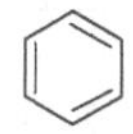 (d) 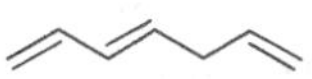

15. The order of acidity of the following acids is

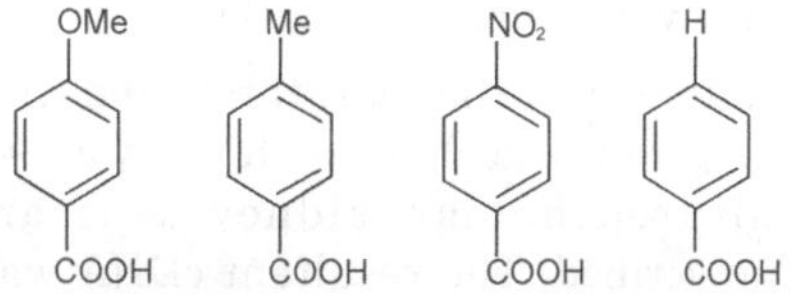

(a) 3 > 2 > 1 > 4 (b) 1 > 4 > 3 > 2

(c) 4 > 3 > 2 > 1 (d) 3 > 4 > 2 > 1

I : BIOCHEMISTRY

(Q. 1-10) Carry One Mark Each.

1. During an enzyme catalyzed reaction, the equilibrium constant

(a) increases

(b) decreases

(c) remains unchanged

(d) can increase or decrease, depending on the enzyme

2. A mixture of Arginine, Phenylalanine and Histidine was fractionated using cation exchange chromatography at neutral pH. The amino acids were eluted with an increasing salt gradient. Identify the correct order of elution.

(a) Arginine, Histidine, Phenylalanine

(b) Phenylalanine, Histidine, Arginine

(c) Histidine, Phenylalanine, Arginine

(d) Arginine, Phenylalanine, Histidine

3. Which one of the following proteases does **NOT** cleave on the carboxyl side of any Arginine residue in a protein?

(a) Trypsin (b) Proteinase K

(c) Thrombin (d) Chymotrypsin

4. The receptor for epinephrine is a

(a) Tyrosine kinase receptor

(b) Serine-threonine kinase receptor

(c) G-protein-coupled receptor

(d) Ligand activated transcription factor

5. Choose the option with two reducing sugars.

(a) Lactose and Maltose

(b) Trehalose and Sucrose

(c) Maltose and Trehalose

(d) Lactose and Sucrose

6. The affinity of an antibody can be determined quantitatively by

(a) MALDI-TOF MS (b) isoelectric focusing

(c) SDS-PAGE (d) equilibrium dialysis

7. Which one of the following molecules is an allosteric activator of phosphofruct-okinase-1?

(a) Fructose 1,6-bisphosphate

(b) Fructose 2,6-bisphosphate

(c) Glucose 6-phosphate

(d) Citrate

8. For a single substrate enzyme, a reaction is carried out at a substrate concentration four times the value of K_m. The observed initial velocity will be ________ % of V_{max}.

9. Consider the following biochemical reaction:

Fructose 6-phosphate + ATP → Fructose 1, 6-bisphosphate + ADP

The equilibrium constant under biochemical standard conditions (K'_{eq}) for the above reaction is 254. The standard free energy change ($\Delta G'^{\circ}$) for the conversion of fructose 6-phosphate is ________ kJ/mol.

10. Given below is the hydropathy plot of a monomeric transmembrane protein.

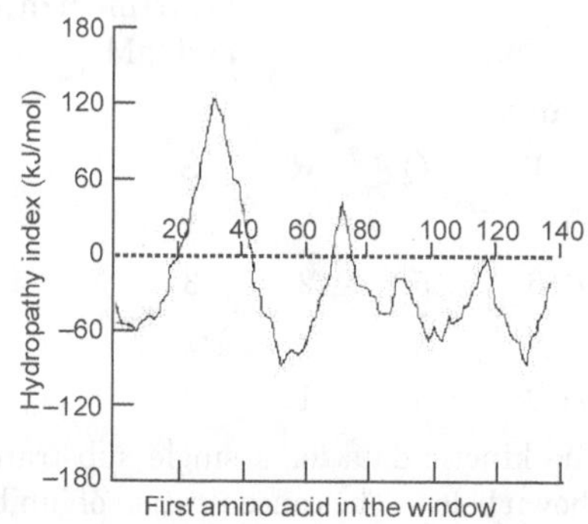

How many transmembrane α-helices are present in the protein?

(a) 1 (b) 2 (c) 4 (d) 5

(Q. 11-20) Carry Two Marks Each.

11. An aqueous solution contains two compounds X and Y. This solution gave absorbance values of 1.0 and 0.4 at 220 and 280 nm, respectively, in a 1 cm path length cell. Molar absorption coefficients (ε) of the compounds X and Y are as shown in the table below.

	ε_{220} ($M^{-1}cm^{-1}$)	ε_{280} ($M^{-1}cm^{-1}$)
Compound X	1000	200
Compound Y	800	400

The concentration of Y in the solution is _____ mM.

12. A purified oligomeric protein was analyzed by SDS-PAGE under reducing and non-reducing conditions. A one litre solution of 1 mg/ml concentration has 4.01×10^{18} molecules of the oligomeric protein. Based on the data shown below, deduce the total number of polypeptide chains that constitute this protein.

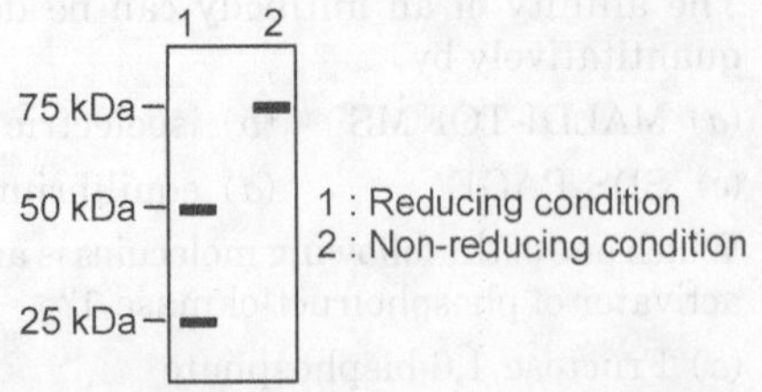

(*a*) 2 (*b*) 4 (*c*) 6 (*d*) 12

13. The concentration of Mg^{2+} ions outside a cell is twice the concentration inside. If the transmembrane potential of the cell is – 60 mV (inside negative), the free energy change of transporting Mg^{2+} ions across the membrane against the concentration gradient at 37 °C is ______ kJ/mol.

Faraday constant: 96.5 kJ/V mol

14. Match the entries in Group I with those in Group II

Group I	Group II
P. J chain	1. VDJ recombinase complex
Q. Serpin	2. Component of MHC class I
R. β2-microglobulin	3. B cell co-receptor complex
S. Artemis	4. C1 complement inhibitor
	5. Component of MHC class II
	6. Multimerization of IgA and IgM

Codes :

	P	Q	R	S
(*a*)	3	4	5	1
(*b*)	6	5	2	3
(*c*)	6	4	2	1
(*d*)	3	4	1	6

15. The kinetic data for a single substrate enzyme is shown below. The concentration of inhibitor [I] used in the reaction was equal to the K_i of the inhibitor. The K_m value of an uninhibited reaction is 2×10^{-5} M. In the presence of the inhibitor, the observed K_m value is ___ $\times 10^{-5}$ M.

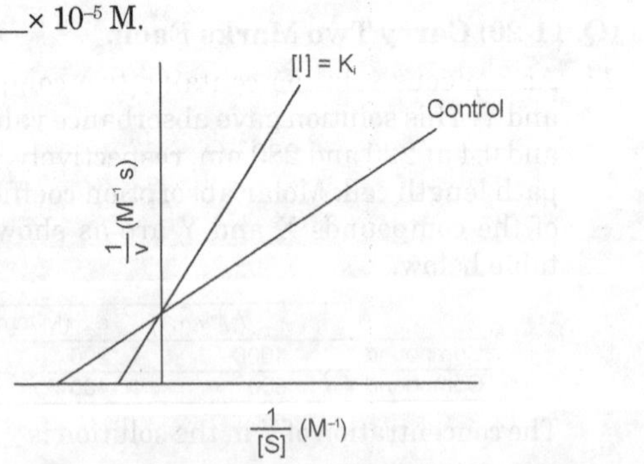

16. One litre of phosphate buffer was prepared by adding 208 grams of Na_2HPO_4 (Mol. wt. 142) and 71 grams of NaH_2PO_4 (Mol. wt. 120) in water. If the pK_a for the dissociation of $H_2PO_4^-$ into HPO_4^{2-} and H^+ is 6.86, the pH of the buffer will be ______.

17. Shown below is an electrospray ionization mass spectrum of a protein:

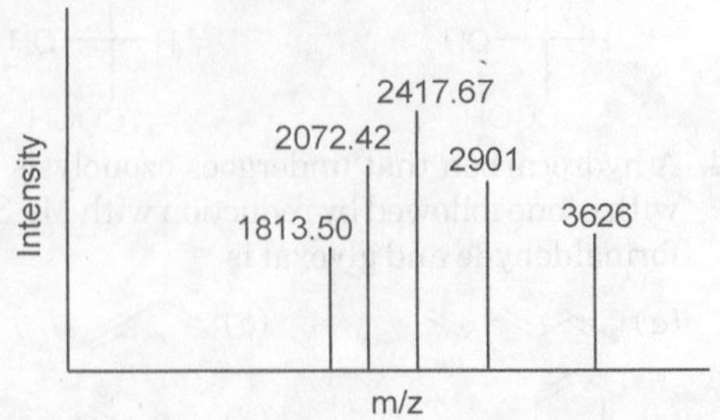

The numbers written on top of the peaks are the m/z values. The mass of the protein deduced from the given data is _____ kDa.

18. A human gene has only three exons (I, II and III in the given order). Total RNA was isolated from cultured human kidney cells and reverse transcribed. The resultant cDNA was used as a template in a PCR reaction containing a forward primer specific to Exon I and a reverse primer specific to Exon III. When the PCR product was analyzed by gel electrophoresis, two bands were observed of sizes 2.5 kb and 1 kb. However, when Northern blotting was performed with the same total RNA using a radiolabeled probe specific to Exon II, only one band was observed. Based on these observations, which one of the following statements is **FALSE** ?

(*a*) Northern blotting with a probe specific to Exon III will show two bands

(*b*) The gene codes for two mRNA splice variants

(*c*) If the forward primer were specific to Exon II, two bands will be observed

(*d*) The Exon II is 1.5 kb in size

19. Using the Sanger's dideoxy chain termination method, a particular exonic region of a protein coding gene was sequenced for two individuals referred to as Subject 1 and Subject 2. The figure below shows a segment of the autoradiogram corresponding to a small window of the DNA sequence.

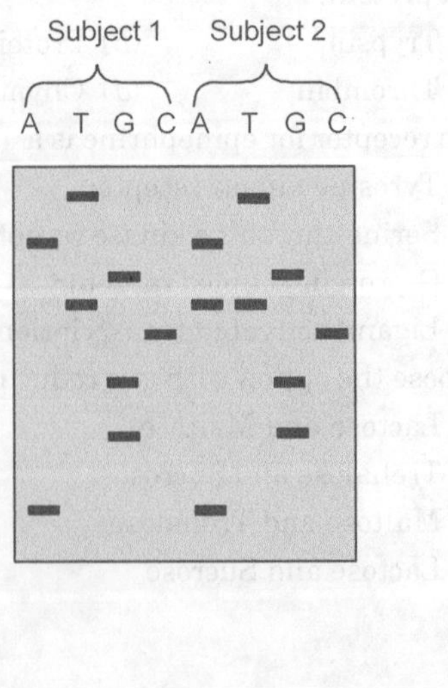

Which one of the following interpretations is correct for the sequenced DNA fragments?

(*a*) Subject 2 has two allelic variants

(*b*) Subject 1 has the sequence 5'- TAGTCGGA -3'.

(*c*) Subject 2 has the sequence 5'- AGGCTAGAT -3'.

(*d*) Subject 1 has a single nucleotide deletion in the gene

20. A 7 kb DNA molecule of a specific sequence has two E*co*RI and one P*vu*II restriction endonuclease sites. The restriction sites are shown below. The DNA was completely digested with both EcoRI and P*vu*II. The digestion product was purified and added to an appropriately buffered reaction mixture at 37 °C, which contained the Klenow fragment of DNA polymerase I and α-^{32}P dNTPs. After one hour, the DNA in the reaction product was purified and analyzed by electrophoresis. The bands were visualized by both ethidium bromide (EtBr) staining and autoradiography. The result is shown below.

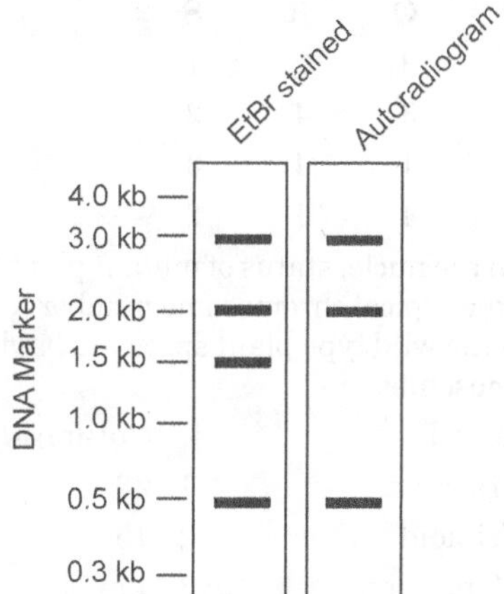

E*co*RI : GAATTC
CTTAAG

P*vu*II: CAGCTG
GTCGAC

Which one of the following restriction maps is in agreement with the above result?

(*a*)

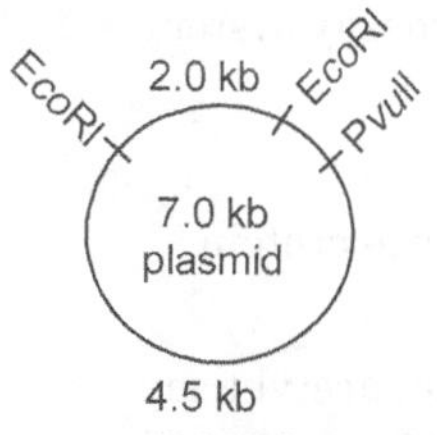

(*b*)

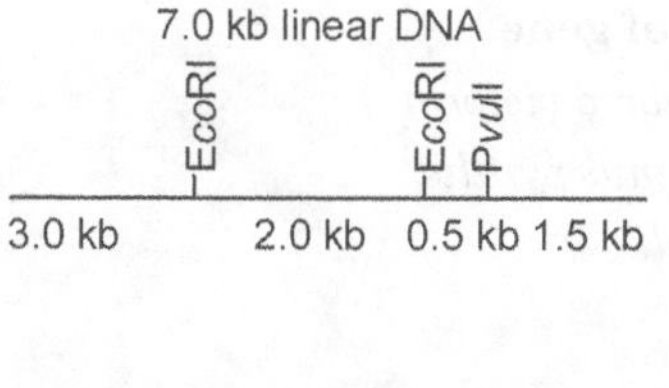

(*c*)

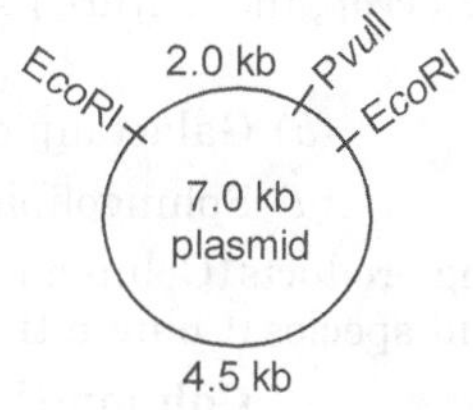

(*d*)

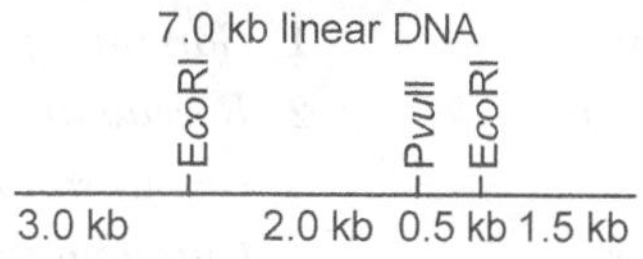

J : BOTANY

(Q. 1-10) Carry One Mark Each.

1. Plant which grows attached to another plant species but is not a parasitic is known as

(*a*) Endophyte (*b*) Halophyte

(*c*) Epiphyte (*d*) Lithophyte

2. An ideal cybrid should have

(*a*) both nuclear genome and cytoplasmic genome equally from both the parents

(*b*) nuclear genome from one of the parents and cytoplasmic genome from other parent

(*c*) nuclear genome predominantly/exclusively from one of the parents and cytoplasmic genome equally from both the parents

(*d*) nuclear genome equally from both the parents and cytoplasmic genome predominantly/ exclusively from one of the parents

3. Transmission Electron Micrograph of fungal cell can usually be distinguished from plant cell due to lack of P and having less abundant Q. Find the correct combination of P and Q.

(*a*) P- Plastid; Q-Vacuoles

(*b*) P- Plastid; Q-Mitochondria

(*c*) P-Plastid; Q-Endoplasmic reticulum

(*d*) P- Mitochondria; Q-Plastid

4. Identify the CORRECT answer

RNA interference (RNAi)

P. is an event of post transcriptional gene silencing

Q. works through RNA induced silencing complex

(*a*) P only (*b*) Q only

(*c*) Both P and Q (*d*) Neither P nor Q

5. Find the odd one out.

(*a*) Petal (*b*) Sepal

(*c*) Petiole (*d*) Tepal

6. Plantibody is the

(*a*) Antibody expressed in transgenic plant

(*b*) Transgenic plant that expresses antibody

(*c*) Antibody against plant based antigen

(*d*) Transgenic plant that expresses antigen

7. In a typical oil-seed crop, the matured seeds are enriched with

(*a*) Phospholipid (*b*) Galactolipid
(*c*) Neutral lipid (*d*) Sphingolipid

8. Match the following products (Column I) with the corresponding plant species (Column II)

Column-I	**Column-II**
P. Saffron	1. *Garcinia sp*
Q. Gamboge	2. *Rocella tinctoria*
R. Litmus	3. *Crocus sativus*
S. Turmeric	4. *Curcuma sp*

Codes:

	P	Q	R	S
(*a*)	4	2	1	3
(*b*)	3	4	1	2
(*c*)	2	3	2	1
(*d*)	3	1	2	4

9. The semi-dwarf trait of corn, wheat and rice plants used in breeding program during 1960s resulted in green revolution. Later this 'green-revolution gene' has been identified to be involved in either signal transduction pathway or biosynthesis of

(*a*) Auxin (*b*) Gibberellin
(*c*) Cytokinin (*d*) Ethylene

10. In classical model to explain the plant-pathogen interaction, the host will not develop the disease upon the pathogen attack when

(*a*) The resistance gene (R) is non-functional
(*b*) The avirulence gene (Avr) is non-functional
(*c*) Both R and Avr are non-functional
(*d*) Both R and Avr are functional

(Q. 11-20) Carry Two Marks Each.

11. Select the **CORRECT** combination from the promoter (Column I), transcription machinery used (Column II) and target tissue type (Column III) to express a foreign gene in a plant system.

Column I	**Column II**	**Column III**
P. *Ubiquitin*	1. Chloroplast	i. Leaf
Q. *Napin*	2. Nucleus	ii. Seed
R. *RbcL*	3. Mitochondria	
S. *RbcS*		

(*a*) P-1-i, Q-3-ii, R-2-i, S-3-ii
(*b*) P-3-i, Q-1-i, R-2-ii, S-1-ii
(*c*) P-2-i, Q-2-ii, R-1-i, S-2-i
(*d*) P-1-ii, Q-3-ii, R-2-ii, S-3-ii

12. In a plant species, flower colour purple is dominant over white. One such purple-flowered plant upon selfing produced 35 viable plants, of which 9 were white-flowered and the rest were purple-flowered. What fraction of these purple-flowered progeny is expected to be pure purple-flowered line?

(*a*) 1/2 (*b*) 1/3 (*c*) 1/4 (*d*) 2/3

13. Following diagram represents the sequence of genes in a normal chromosome of a plant species:

GHIJ —o— KLMN

Match the **CORRECT** combination for chromosomal mutation using Column - I and Column - II.

Column–I

P. GHIKL —o— JMN
Q. GJ —o— KLHIMN
R. GHIJ —o— KLKLMN
S. GHJ —o— KLMN

Column–II

1. Tandem duplication
2. Deletion
3. Pericentric inversion
4. Non-reciprocal translocation

Codes:

	P	Q	R	S
(*a*)	4	3	2	1
(*b*)	1	3	4	2
(*c*)	2	1	4	3
(*d*)	3	4	1	2

14. Match the nuclei status of mutant plant (Column-I) with the typical chromosome number (Column- II), when the wild type plant species is having 2N = 46 chromosomes.

Column-I	**Column-II**
P. Trisomic	1. 23
Q. Triploid	2. 45
R. Monosomic	3. 47
S. Monoploid	4. 69

Codes:

	P	Q	R	S
(*a*)	1	2	3	4
(*b*)	2	3	4	1
(*c*)	3	4	2	1
(*d*)	4	3	1	2

15. Match the following reporter genes used in plant transformation experiments with the source of gene and detection/assay system

Reporter gene

P. β-glucuronidase
Q. Green fluorescence protein
R. Luciferase
S. Chloramphenicol acetyl transferase

Source of gene

1. *Aequorea victoria*
2. *Photinus pyralis*
3. *E. coli*

Detection/assay

i. Radioactive assay

ii. Fluorimetric

iii. Fluorescence

iv. Luminescence

(*a*) P-3-i, Q-1-ii, R-2-iii, S-3-iv

(*b*) P-3-ii, Q-1-iii, R-2-iv, S-3-i

(*c*) P-2-ii, Q-1-iii, R-3-iv, S-1-i

(*d*) P-1-ii, Q-2-iii, R-3-i, S-3-iv

16. Find the **CORRECT** statements in the context of Global warming effect on plant photosynthesis.

P. Decreasing aqueous solubility of dissolved CO_2 compared to dissolved O_2

Q. Decreasing oxygenase activity of Rubisco relative to carboxylation

R. Enhancing the ratio of CO_2 to O_2 in air equilibrated solution

S. Increasing photorespiration relative to photosynthesis

(*a*) P and Q (*b*) R and S

(*c*) P and R (*d*) P and S

17. Statements given below are either **TRUE** (T) or **FALSE** (F). Find the correct combination.

P. Regulation of cell cycle progression depends on cyclin dependent kinase (CDK) and protease activity.

Q. In photosynthesis, oxidation of water produces O_2 and releases electrons required by photosystem I (PSI).

R. Photorespiratory reaction occurring in oxidative photosynthetic carbon (C_2) pathway involves a cooperative interaction among three organelles: chloroplast, peroxisome and mitoch-ondria.

S. Ethylene acts as a promoter of senescence and cytokinins act as a senescence antagonist.

(*a*) P-T, Q-F, R-T, S-F (*b*) P-T, Q-T, R-T, S-F

(*c*) P-T, Q-F, R-F, S-T (*d*) P-T, Q-F, R-T, S-T

18. Match the following diagrams P, Q, R, and S with the inflorescence type (Column I) and the corresponding plant species (Column II).

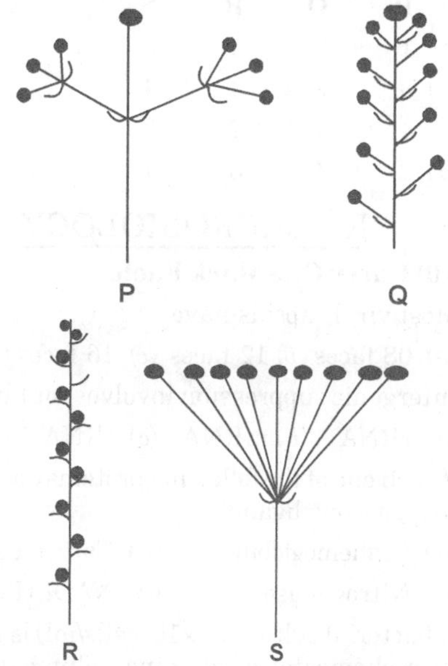

Column-I	Column-II
1. Umbel	i. *Pedicularis sp*
2. Raceme	ii. *Smilacina sp*
3. Compound determinate	iii. *Epilobium sp*
4. Spike	iv. *Pelargonium sp*

(*a*) P-2-i, Q-3-iv, R-4-ii, S-1-iii

(*b*) P-3-ii, Q-2-iii, R-4-i, S-1-iv

(*c*) P-1-iii, Q-3-ii, R-4-iv, S-2-i

(*d*) P-1-iv, Q-4-i, R-2-iii, S-3-ii

19. Find the right combination for P, Q, R and S with respect to gametophyte development in flowering plants.

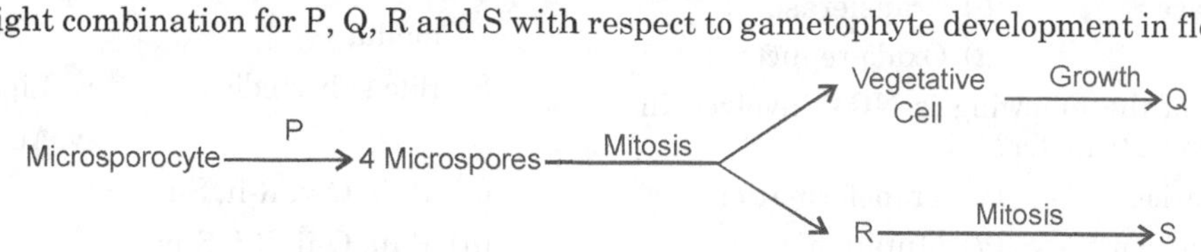

P. P-Meiosis, Q-Generative cell , R-Pollen Tube, S-2 Sperm Cells

Q. P-Meiosis, Q-Pollen Tube, R-Generative Cell, S-2 Sperm Cells

R. P-Mitosis, Q-Generative Cell, R-Pollen Tube, S-2 sperm Cells

S. P-Growth, Q-2 Sperm Cells, R-Pollen Tube, S-Generative Cell

20. Match the definition (Column I) with the type of plant community (Column II)

Column-I

P. The process of occupation of a particular area by different plant communities from their birth to maturity

Q. A major ecological unit of vegetation

R. A smaller unit of plant association

S. A subdivision of plant association which is related to minor differences in temperature and moisture relations

Column-II

1. Formation
2. Consociation
3. Faciation
4. Plant succession

Codes :

	P	Q	R	S
(*a*)	1	3	4	2
(*b*)	3	2	1	4
(*c*)	4	1	2	3
(*d*)	2	4	3	1

K : MICROBIOLOGY

(Q. 1-10) Carry One Mark Each.

1. Most viral capsids have

(*a*) 08 faces (*b*) 12 faces (*c*) 16 faces (*d*) 20 faces

2. Intergenic suppression involves mutation in

(*a*) rRNA (*b*) mRNA (*c*) tRNA (*d*) cDNA

3. Which one of the following proteins does **NOT** bind to a gaseous ligand?

(*a*) Leghemoglobin (*b*) Carbonic anhydrase

(*c*) Nitrogenase (*d*) NADPH oxidase

4. A bacterial culture (5×10^8 cells/ml) is maintained in a chemostat of working volume 10 L. If the doubling time of the bacteria is 50 min, the required rate of flow of nutrients (in ml/min) is ________.

5. Rheumatic fever is an example of

(*a*) autoimmune disease

(*b*) type IV hypersensitive reaction

(*c*) immunodeficiency disease

(*d*) neurodegenerative disorder

6. Oxygenases that catalyse the initial step in the degradation of polycyclic aromatic hydrocarbons by using molecular oxygen belong to which enzyme class?

(*a*) Hydrolase (*b*) Transferase

(*c*) Lyase (*d*) Oxido-reductase

7. Which one of the following is **NOT** involved in horizontal gene transfer?

(*a*) Conjugation (*b*) Transformation

(*c*) Transduction (*d*) Mutation

8. The principle of immunization was first explained by

(*a*) Edward Jenner (*b*) Elie Metchnikoff

(*c*) Louis Pasteur (*d*) Robert Koch

9. Lysozyme catalyzes the breakdown of

(*a*) NAG-NAM (*b*) lipopolysaccharide

(*c*) teichoic acid (*d*) lipoprotein A

10. Which one of the following microscopic techniques can be used to study the contour of proteins?

(*a*) SEM (*b*) TEM

(*c*) AFM (*d*) Confocal microscopy

(Q. 11-20) Carry Two Marks Each.

11. Match compounds in **Group I** with inhibitory activities in **Group II.**

Group I	**Group II**
P. Vancomycin	i. Folate metabolism
Q. Rifampin	ii. DNA synthesis
R. Puromycin	iii. Protein synthesis
S. Ciprofloxacin	iv. RNA synthesis
	v. Cell wall synthesis

(*a*) P-v, Q-iv, R-iii, S-ii (*b*) P-iv, Q-iii, R-i, S-ii

(*c*) P-iv, Q-i, R-iii, S-ii (*d*) P-v, Q-iii, R-ii, S-iv

12. Match the organisms with the appropriate growth curves.

P. Bacteria

Q. Extracellular virus

R. Intracellular virus

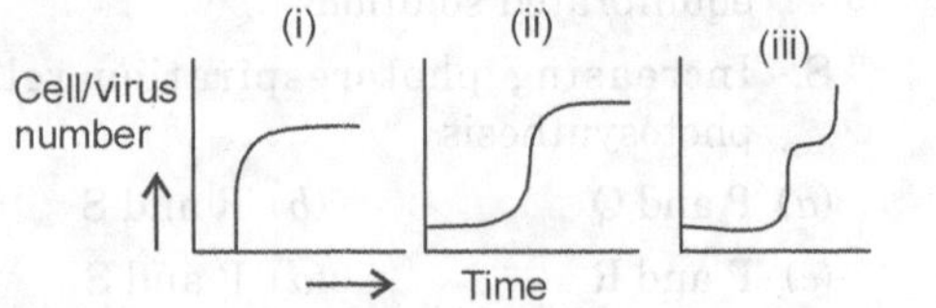

(*a*) P-iii, Q-i, R-ii (*b*) P-ii, Q-i, R-iii

(*c*) P-ii, Q-iii, R-i (*d*) P-i, Q-ii, R-iii

13. The length of a coding region in an mRNA is 897 bases. How many amino acids will be there in the polypeptide synthesized using this mRNA?

(*a*) 297 (*b*) 298

(*c*) 299 (*d*) 897

14. Match the media in **Group I** for screening microbial isolates in **Group II.**

Group-I	**Group-II**
P. Blood agar media	i. Coliforms
Q. Minimal media	ii. Protease producers
R. Skimmed milk agar media	iii. Hemolytic microbes
S. Bile salt media	iv. Lipase producers
	v. Autotrophs

(*a*) P-iii, Q-v, R-ii, S-i

(*b*) P-iii, Q-ii, R-i, S-iv

(*c*) P-i, Q-iii, R-ii, S-iv

(*d*) P-ii, Q-i, R-iv, S-v

15. During a bacterial growth experiment, the total viable cell count at 2 *h* and 6 *h* was 1×10^4 cells/ml and 1×10^9 cells/ml, respectively. The specific growth rate (in h^{-1}) of the culture is ________.

16. The concentration of sodium chloride in the cytoplasm of a *Halobacterium sp.* was found to be 250 ng/nl. The molarity (in M) of sodium chloride is ________.

17. Match organisms in **Group I** with shapes in **Group II** and flagellar arrangements in **Group III**.

Group-I	**Group-II**
P. *Salmonella typhi*	i. helical
Q. *Saccharomyces cerevisiae*	ii. rod
R. *Aquaspirillum serpens*	iii. curved rod
S. *Vibrio cholerae*	iv. ovoid

Group-III

1. non-motile
2. amphitrichous
3. peritrichous
4. polar

(*a*) P-ii-3, Q-iv-1, R-i-2, S-iii-4
(*b*) P-iii-1, Q-iv-2, R-ii-4, S-i-3
(*c*) P-i-2, Q-ii-4, R-iii-2, S-iv-3
(*d*) P-ii-2, Q-iii-1, R-i-3, S-iv-4

18. Lethal dose curves of different microorganisms (1, 2, 3 and 4) are shown below. Which of these microorganisms are the most lethal?

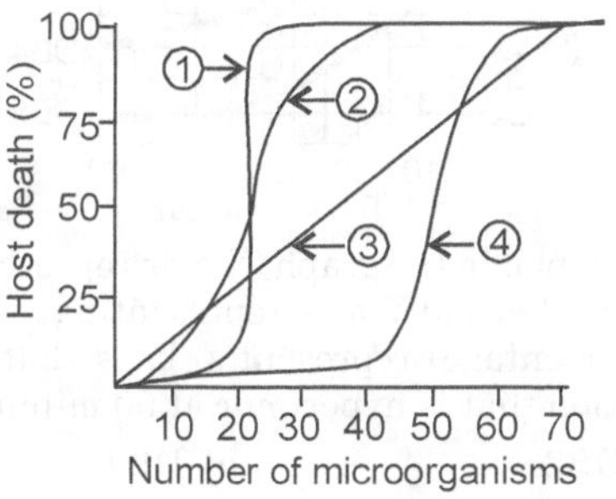

(*a*) 1 and 3 only (*b*) 1 and 2 only
(*c*) 3 and 4 only (*d*) 2 and 3 only

19. Match items in **Group I** with sterilization methods in **Group II**.

Group I

P. Ampicillin
Q. 1% glucose in phosphate buffer
R. Plastic syringe
S. Luria broth

Group-II

i. 70 % alcohol treatment
ii. Autoclaving at 15 psi for 15 min
iii. Autoclaving at 10 psi for 20 min
iv. Membrane filtration
v. γ-ray irradiation

(*a*) P-iv, Q-iii, R-v, S-ii (*b*) P-iii, Q-iv, R-ii, S-v
(*c*) P-i, Q-ii, R-v, S-iii (*d*) P-v, Q-ii, R-iii, S-i

20. Which of the following statements are **TRUE** regarding *recA* mutants of *E. coli*?

P. Exhibit much reduced recombination
Q. Do not survive UV irradiation
R. Show no effect on doubling time
S. Exhibit pleiotropy

(*a*) P, Q & R only (*b*) P, Q & S only
(*c*) P, R & S only (*d*) Q, R & S only

L : ZOOLOGY

(Q. 1-10) Carry One Mark Each.

1. Small geographic areas with high concentrations of endemic species and a large number of endangered and threatened species are known as

(*a*) endemic sinks
(*b*) critical communities
(*c*) biodiversity hot spots
(*d*) endemic metapopulations

2. Which one of the following animals has "Osculum" as an excretory structure?

(*a*) Hydra (*b*) Sponge
(*c*) Jelly Fish (*d*) Sea pen

3. During development of which one of the following organisms, bilateral meroblastic cleavage is found?

(*a*) Mollusc (*b*) Fish
(*c*) Bird (*d*) Amphibian

4. The mitochondrion is one considered a part of the endomembrane system on account of which one of the following reasons?

(*a*) It does not undergo structural changes
(*b*) It is not derived from the ER or Golgi
(*c*) It does not synthesize proteins
(*d*) It is not attached to the outer nuclear envelope

5. The end products of glycolysis include ATP,

(*a*) CO_2 and H_2O
(*b*) H_2O and pyruvate
(*c*) NADH and pyruvate
(*d*) CO_2 and NADH

6. The TATA box is found in the vicinity of the transcription start site. The role of this box is to

(*a*) serve as a ribosome recruitment site
(*b*) serve as RNA polymerase binding site
(*c*) provide 3-D structural integrity to a DNA molecule
(*d*) act as a terminator sequence

7. Which ONE of the following processes does NOT occur in prokaryotic gene expression, but occurs in eukaryotic gene expression?

(*a*) Transcription of mRNA, tRNA, and rRNA
(*b*) Binding of RNA polymerase to the promoter
(*c*) Addition of a poly-A tail to the 3′ end and the 5′ capping of an mRNA
(*d*) Translation begins as soon as transcription is initiated

8. In Graves' disease, the presence of auto antibodies against which one of the following molecules is the direct cause of hyperthyroidism?

(*a*) Thyroperoxidase
(*b*) Thyroxine
(*c*) Thyroid stimulating hormone
(*d*) Thyroid stimulating hormone receptor

9. In mammals, the two important organs associated with the production and elimination of urea are

(*a*) gastrointestinal tract and lungs
(*b*) gastrointestinal tract and liver
(*c*) kidneys and lungs
(*d*) liver and kidneys

10. Some endocrine glands produce hormones that stimulate functions of other endocrine glands. Which one of the following hormones specifically acts to increase secretion of other hormones?

(*a*) Thyroxine (*b*) Prolactin
(*c*) ACTH (*d*) ADH

(Q. 11-20) Carry Two Marks Each.

11. If the recombination frequency between X - Y loci is 12, X - Z loci is 4, and Y - Z loci is 8, then the order of the loci on the chromosome is

(*a*) X-Y-Z (*b*) Y-X-Z (*c*) X-Z-Y (*d*) Z-Y-X

12. A cross is made between a white eyed-miniature winged female with a red eyed-normal winged male of *Drosophila melanogaster*. Further crossing of F1 female offspring from this cross with a white eyed-miniature winged male fly gave 95 white eyed-normal winged, 102 red eyed-miniature winged, 226 red eyed-normal winged and 202 white eyed-miniature winged offspring in F2 generation. What is the percent frequency of recombination between the two genes?

(*a*) 20.11 (*b*) 31.52 (*c*) 49.10 (*d*) 34.12

13. A green fluorescent protein (GFP) encoding gene is fused to a gene encoding specific protein for expression in cells. What is the advantage of using GFP over staining cells with fluorescently labeled antibodies that bind to the target protein?

(*a*) It bleaches less compared to fluorescent probes
(*b*) It allows imaging at higher resolution than fluorescent probes
(*c*) It provides more precise location of the protein than fluorescent probes
(*d*) Its fusion allows tracking the location of the protein in living cells, while staining usually requires fixation of cells

14. A newborn was accidentally given a drug that destroyed the thymus. Which one of the following would be the most likely outcome?

(*a*) Lack of class I MHC molecules
(*b*) Inability to rearrange antigen receptors
(*c*) Inability to differentiate to mature T cells
(*d*) Reduction in T-independent number of B cells

15. One individual has a parasitic worm infection and another is responding to an allergen such as pollen. Which one of the following features is common to both of them?

(*a*) Increase in cytotoxic T cell population
(*b*) Risk of developing an autoimmune disease
(*c*) Reduced innate immune response
(*d*) Increased levels of IgE

16. Five dialysis bags (DB1-DB5), impermeable to sucrose, were filled with various concentrations of sucrose. The bags were placed in separate beakers containing 0.6 M sucrose solution. Every 10 minutes, the bags were weighed and the percent change in mass of each bag was plotted as a function of time.

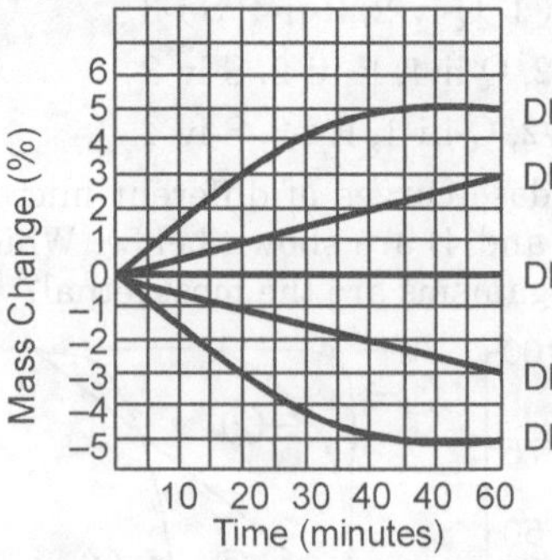

Which plot in the graph (X-axis representing time in minutes and Y-axis representing mass change in percentage) represent(s) bags that contain a solution that is hypertonic at 50 minutes?

(*a*) DB2 (*b*) DB4
(*c*) DB3 (*d*) DB4 and DB5

17. Which ONE of the following combinations of products will result, when 3 molecules of acetyl CoA is fed into TCA cycle?

(*a*) 1 ATP, 2 CO_2, 3 NADH, and 1 $FADH_2$
(*b*) 3 ATP, 6 CO_2, 9 NADH, and 3 $FADH_2$
(*c*) 3 ATP, 3 CO_2, 3 NADH, and 3 $FADH_2$
(*d*) 38 ATP, 6 CO_2, 3 NADH, and 12 $FADH_2$

18. A DNA fragment shown below has restriction sites I and II, which create fragments X, Y, and Z. Which one of the following agarose gel electrophoresis patterns represents the separation of these fragments?

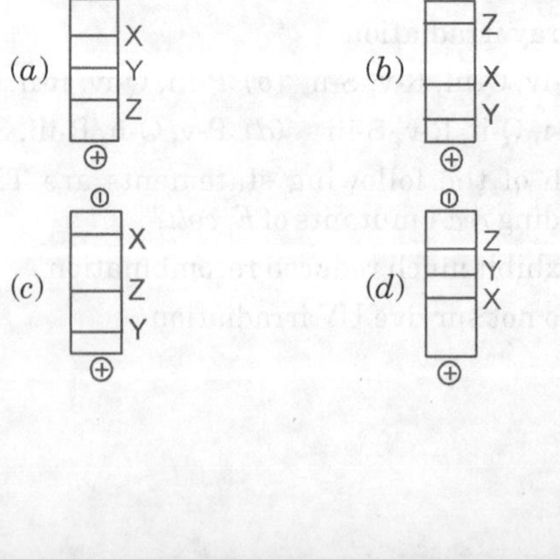

19. Theoretically, it is possible to resurrect the extinct woolly mammoth by which one of the following methods?

(*a*) Transferring cell nuclei from the frozen tissue into enucleated unfertilized eggs of a suitable mammal

(*b*) Introducing sequenced mammoth genome into donor eggs of a suitable mammal

(*c*) Transferring mammoth nuclear material into stem cells

(*d*) Collection of oocytes from ovaries of the frozen mammoth for *in vitro* fertilization and transfer of fertilized eggs into animals such as elephants

20. Regions of higher abundance of cholesterol molecules on the plasma membrane will

(*a*) be more fluid

(*b*) result in clogged arteries as it can detach from the plasma membrane

(*c*) be more rigid than the surrounding membrane

(*d*) have higher rates of lateral movement of proteins into and out of plasma membrane

M : FOOD TECHNOLOGY

(Q. 1-10) Carry One Mark Each.

1. Which one of the following is not a source of caffeine?

(*a*) Coffee (*b*) Cocoa beans

(*c*) Corn syrup (*d*) Tea leaves

2. Yoghurt is prepared using a pair of microorganisms. Choose the correct pair from the following:

(*a*) *Lactobacillus bulgaricus, Streptococcus thermophilus*

(*b*) *Lactobacillus lactis, Streptococcus thermophilus*

(*c*) *Lactobacillus bulgaricus, Streptococcus lactis*

(*d*) *Lactobacillus lactis, Streptococcus lactis*

3. Choose the target organism for milk pasteurization from the following:

(*a*) *Mycobacterium tuberculosis*

(*b*) *Coxiella burnetii*

(*c*) *Clostridium botulinum*

(*d*) *Bacillus cereus*

4. Hypobaric storage is also known as ____

(*a*) Modified atmospheric storage

(*b*) Controlled atmospheric storage

(*c*) Low pressure storage

(*d*) Modified aseptic package

5. In a solution of vegetable oil (molecular mass = 292 kg $kmol^{-1}$) and ethanol (molecular mass = 46 kg $kmol^{-1}$), the concentration of vegetable oil in the solution is measured to be 60% (total mass basis). Therefore, mole fraction of ethanol in the solution is _______.

6. An experiment started with 4 numbers of bacterial cells. After n^{th} generation, number of cells becomes 128. Therefore, value of 'n' is _______.

7. One ton of refrigeration means one of the following options:

(*a*) Cooling provided by one kg of ice in one hour

(*b*) Cooling provided by one ton of ice in one hour

(*c*) Energy extracted to freeze one ton of water in one day

(*d*) Coefficient of performance is unity

8. Fruit juice is flowing in a circular pipe (inner diameter 2 cm) at a mass flow rate of 2 kg s^{-1} and at a temperature of 25°C. The density and viscosity of the juice at 25°C are 1045 kg m^{-3} and 0.5 Pa s, respectively. Take $\pi = 22/7$. The Reynolds number for this flow will be _________.

9. Shear stress (τ, Pa) and shear rate (γ, s^{-1}) relationship of a pseudoplastic fluid follows the Power law equation given by, $\tau = k\gamma^n = 2.6\,\gamma^{0.45}$, where 'n' and 'k' are flow behavior index and consistency index respectively. The apparent viscosity (μ_a) of the fluid at a shear rate of 5 s^{-1} is _______ Pa s.

10. In a sterilization process, $D_{121.1}$ value of the target organism is 0.22 minute. Time required for 99.999% inactivation of the target organism at 121.1°C will be ____ minutes.

(Q. 11-20) Carry Two Marks Each.

11. A centrifuge having diameter of 10 cm is rotating at 10000 rpm. Take π = 22/7 and g = 9.81 m s^{-2}. The ratio of centrifugal force to gravitational force will be _______.

12. Match the items under **Group I** with items under **Group II**

Group-I	**Group-II**
P. Threonine	1. Fatty acid
Q. Pyridoxine phosphate	2. Sugar
R. Xylose	3. Amino acid
S. Oleic acid	4. Co-enzyme

Codes :

	P	**Q**	**R**	**S**
(*a*)	4	3	1	2
(*b*)	3	4	2	1
(*c*)	1	2	3	4
(*d*)	2	1	4	3

13. Match the items under **Group I** with items under **Group II**

Group-I	**Group-II**
P. Iron	1. Osteoporosis
Q. Calcium	2. Anemia
R. Zinc	3. Goiter
S. Iodine	4. Dwarfism

Codes :

	P	Q	R	S
(*a*)	2	1	4	3
(*b*)	1	2	3	4
(*c*)	3	4	1	2
(*d*)	4	3	2	1

14. In a counter-current double pipe heat-exchanger, milk is cooled from 110 to 40°C using chilled water as coolant. Water enters at 5°C and leaves at 60°C. Heat flux for the system with overall heat transfer coefficient of 950 W m^{-2} K^{-1} will be ______ W m^{-2}.

15. Saturated steam at 100°C is injected at 0.2 kg s^{-1} into air stream flowing at 3 kg s^{-1} and 25°C. Air contains 0.012 kg moisture per kg dry air. If the atmospheric pressure is 101.1 kPa, absolute humidity of air will be ______ kg kg^{-1}.

16. In an evaporator, milk is concentrated from 9.8% TSS to 52% TSS. Assume the solutes in the milk are non-volatile. The amount of vapour produced for 100 kg feed will be ______ kg.

17. Water enters a cylindrical tank at a steady uniform rate of 0.1 m^3 s^{-1}; simultaneously water is discharged from the tank through an orifice (area 0.05 m^2) located at the bottom of the tank. Initial level of water in the tank from the bottom is 5 m. If the acceleration due to gravity = 9.81 m s^{-2} and coefficient of discharge = 0.30, the final value of the steady-state height of water level from the bottom of tank is ______ m.

18. Match the following between **Group I and Group II** in relation to pretreatments.

Group-I

P. Ascorbic acid dip

Q. Heat blanching

R. Deaeration

S. Rendering

Group-II

1. Sogginess in fruits
2. Minimizes fruit oxidation
3. Melting of fat in meat
4. Removal of odours
5. Minimizes destruction of vitamin C

Codes :

	P	Q	R	S
(*a*)	1	2	3	4
(*b*)	2	1	5	3
(*c*)	1	3	4	5
(*d*)	3	4	5	2

19. A chocolate mix at 100°C is flowing through a 2 cm diameter and 4 m long stainless steel tube at 13.2 kg per minute. The density of the mix is 1750 kg m^{-3} and its viscosity at 100°C is 2 Pa s. Take $\pi = 22/7$. The pressure drop for this flow will be ______ Pa.

20. In a tray dryer, 100 kg of a vegetable material in a suitably reduced form is dried to yield a final product of 75 kg. The dried sample of 5 g, when kept in an oven at 105°C for 24 hours results in 3.56 g of dry matter. The moisture content of the vegetable, before drying, in dry basis is______%.

ANSWERS

GA : GENERAL APTITUDE

1. (*d*)	2. (*a*)	3. (*c*)	4. (25 to 25)	5. (*a*)
6. (*a*)	7. (*c*)	8. (*d*)	9. (*c*)	10. (0.48 to 0.49)

H : CHEMISTRY (Compulsory)

1. (*a*)	2. (*b*)	3. (*c*)	4. (*b*)	5. (*c*)
6. (1.9 to 2.1)	7. (*c*)	8. (–0.8 to –0.8)	9. (*d*)	10. (0.40 to 0.55)
11. (190 to 240)	12. (440 to 470)	13. (*b*)	14. (*a*)	15. (*d*)

I : BIOCHEMISTRY

1. (*c*)	2. (*b*)	3. (*d*)	4. (*c*)	5. (*a*)
6. (*d*)	7. (*b*)	8. (80 to 80)	9. (13.6 to 13.8)	10. (*a*)
11. (0.82 to 0.84)	12. (*b*)	13. (13.3 to 13.4)	14. (*c*)	15. (4 to 4)
16. (7.2 to 7.3)	17. (14.4 to 14.6)	18. (*c*)	19. (*a*)	20. (*b*)

J : BOTANY

1. (*c*)	2. (*c*)	3. (*a*)	4. (*c*)	5. (*c*)
6. (*a*)	7. (*c*)	8. (*d*)	9. (*b*)	10. (*d*)
11. (*c*)	12. (*b*)	13. (*d*)	14. (*c*)	15. (*b*)
16. (*d*)	17. (*d*)	18. (*b*)	19. (*b*)	20. (*c*)

K : MICROBIOLOGY

1. (*d*)	2. (*c*)	3. (*d*)	4. (200 to 200)	5. (*a*)
6. (*d*)	7. (*d*)	8. (*c*)	9. (*a*)	10. (*c*)
11. (*a*)	12. (*c*)	13. (*b*)	14. (*a*)	15. (2.8 to 2.9)
16. (4.2 to 4.4)	17. (*a*)	18. (*b*)	19. (*a*)	20. (*b*)

L : ZOOLOGY

1. (*c*)	2. (*b*)	3. (*a*)	4. (*b*)	5. (*c*)
6. (*b*)	7. (*c*)	8. (*d*)	9. (*d*)	10. (*c*)
11. (*c*)	12. (*b*)	13. (*d*)	14. (*c*)	15. (*d*)
16. (*a*)	17. (*b*)	18. (*b*)	19. (*a*)	20. (*c*)

M : FOOD TECHNOLOGY

1. (*c*)	2. (*a*)	3. (*b*)	4. (*c*)	5. (0.80 to 0.82)
6. (5 to 5)	7. (*c*)	8. (254 to 255)	9. (1.05 to 1.08)	10. (1.0 to 1.2)
11. (5590 to 5600)	12. (*b*)	13. (*a*)	14. (39900 to 40000)	15. (0.078 to 0.080)
16. (81 to 82)	17. (0.55 to 0.58)	18. (*b*)	19. (256000 to 256000)	20. (87.0 to 87.5)

EXPLANATIONS

GA : GENERAL APTITUDE

1. The correct word to fill in the blank is experiences. This is because the sentence is in present tense and the sense is in present indefinite.
2. Contentment is the right word which is appropriate to the meaning of the sentence. Contentment is the sign of true happiness as it gives a sense of fulfillment.
3. The sentence "As a woman, I have no country" implies that a woman's endeavour and reach transcends all boundaries. So, the correct sentence would be Woman's solidarity knows no national boundaries.
4. Given, in one year, probability of an earthquake > 6 magnitude = 0.04

   So, average time between successive earthquakes = 1/0.04 = 25 years

5. $$A = P\left[1+\frac{r}{100}\right]^t$$

   10 million = 5 million $\left[1+\frac{20}{100}\right]^t$

   $$2 = \left[1+\frac{1}{5}\right]^t$$

   $$2 = \left(\frac{6}{5}\right)^t$$

   $$= \log 2 = t \log\left(\frac{6}{5}\right)$$

   $$0.301 = t\ 0.0791$$

   $$t = \frac{0.301}{0.0791} = 3.8 \text{ years}$$

   ∴ Hence around 3–4 years would it take to double the growth rate

6. Riaz > Som ...(*i*)

   Shiv > Ansu ...(*ii*)

   Ansu is youngest in the group

   ∴ From equations (*i*) and (*ii*)

   ∴ Riaz > Som > Shiv > Ansu

   ∴ Statement I itself determines the eldest child

   which statement 2 is incorrect as Ansu is youngest in the group is not satisfied by statement 2

   Hence option (*a*) is correct

7. The main point of the paragraph is

   "Exactitude is not critical in dealing with big data"

8. Total quantity of exports = 5 lakh tonnes

$$= 5 \times 10^8 \text{ kg.}$$

And, total revenue = ₹ 25×10^8

Now for item 1,

Item 1 is 11% of total exports

i.e., $\frac{11}{100} \times 5 \times 10^8 \text{ kg} = 55 \times 10^6 \text{kg}$

And revenue for item 1

= 12% of total revenue

$$= \frac{12}{100} \times 25 \times 10^8$$

$$= 25 \times 12 \times 10^6$$

$$= ₹\, 3 \times 10^8$$

$\therefore$ 55 × 10^6 kg of item 1 generates revenue of ₹ 3×10^8

$\therefore$ 1kg of item 1 generates revenue

$$= \frac{3 \times 10^8}{55 \times 10^6} = ₹\frac{60}{11}$$

Similarly, for item 4,

Item 4 is 22% of total exports

i.e., $\frac{22}{100} \times 5 \times 10^8$ kg

$$= 22 \times 5 \times 10^6 \text{ kg}$$

$$= 110 \times 10^6 \text{ kg}$$

$$= 11 \times 10^7 \text{ kg}$$

And revenue for item 4

= 6% of total revenue

$$= ₹\left(\frac{6}{100} \times 25 \times 10^8\right)$$

$$= ₹\left(\frac{6 \times 10^8}{4}\right)$$

$$= ₹\left(\frac{3}{2} \times 10^8\right)$$

$$= ₹(15 \times 10^7)$$

$\therefore$ 11×10^7 kg of item 4 generates revenue of ₹ (15×10^7)

$\therefore$ 1 kg of item 4 generates revenue

$$= ₹\frac{15}{11}$$

$\therefore$ Ratio of revenue generated through export of item 1 per kilogram to the revenue generated through export of item 4 per kilogram

$$= \frac{\frac{60}{11}}{\frac{15}{11}} = 60 : 15 = 4 : 1$$

9.

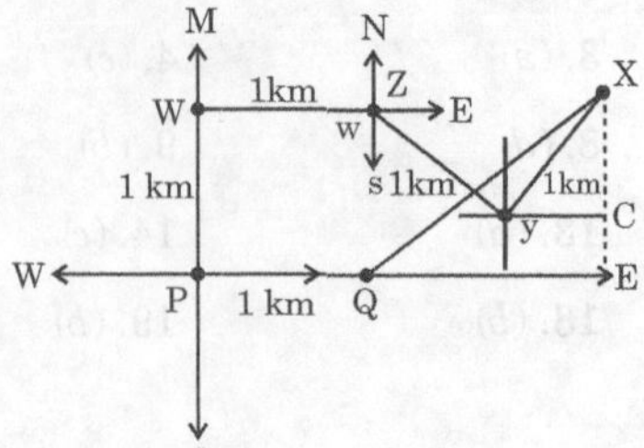

Here XE = 1km

$$QE = \frac{2}{\sqrt{2}} = \sqrt{2}$$

$\therefore$ using Pythagoras theorem,

$$XQ = \sqrt{(QE)^2 + (XE)^2}$$

$$= \sqrt{2+1}$$

$$= \sqrt{3} \text{ km}$$

10. Given, 10% of the population is HIV^+, so probability = 0.1 for HIV^+ and 0.9 for HIV^-

The diagnostic kit identifies → 0.95 HIV^+ and 0.89 HIV^- correctly

So, the required probability that the person is actually HIV^+ = 0.95/2 = 0.475

H : CHEMISTRY

1. In case of NO_2^+, nitrogen has *sp* hybridization according to VSEPR theory as only one *p*-orbital electron of nitrogen participates in bonding. In NO_3^-, the three lone pair electrons bond to three oxygen electrons but there is an additional pair of electrons which makes the hybridization sp^2. And in case of NH_4^+, it has sp^3 hybridization according to VSEPR and valence bond theory.

2. The body-centered cubic unit cell is a cube (all sides of the same length and all face perpendicular to each other) with an atom at each corner of the unit cell and an atom in the center of the unit cell. In determining the number of atoms inside the unit cell, one must count only that portion of an atom that actually lies within the unit cell. So, there are two atoms per unit cell in a *bcc* structure for Potassium.

3. Since the conditions are ideal, so the solution which has the least number of moles present in it and which has the lowest molecular weight for the compound will have the highest freezing point. In this case, 0.001M of $NaCl_2$ has the least molecular weight amongst all the four and has equivalent number of moles as that of potassium dichromate. So, it has the highest freezing point.

4. Phenols are potentially very reactive towards electrophilic aromatic substitution. This is because the hydroxyl group, -OH, is a strongly activating, ortho-/para-directing substituent. Substitution typically occurs para to the hydroxyl group unless the para position is blocked, then ortho substitution occurs. The strong activation often means that milder reaction conditions than those used for benzene itself can be used. Phenols are so activated that poly-substitution can be a problem.

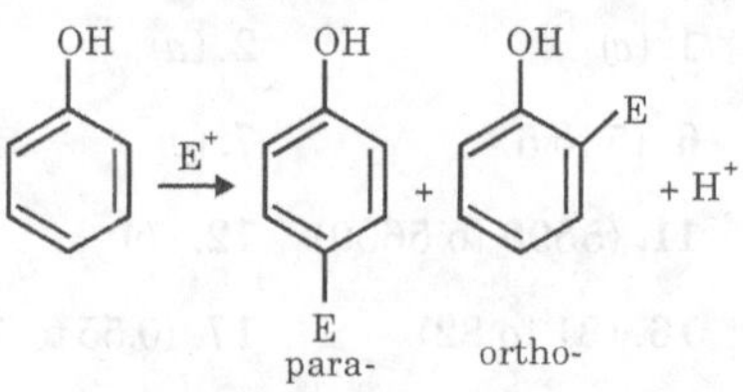

In the given reaction, the product formed will be *p*-Bromo phenol.

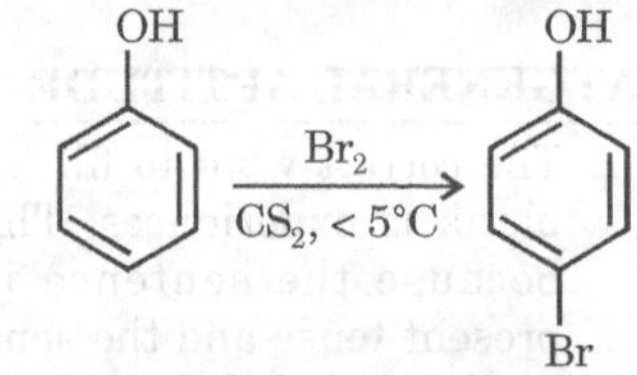

5. The elimination of CO_2 from the carboxyl group of carboxylic acids RCOOH leads to decarboxylation. Heating such an acid with soda lime yields the hydrocarbon RH and CO_2. Aromatic acids undergo decarboxylation when heated in quinoline in the presence of copper powder. Amino acids are decarboxylated by decarboxy-lases, whose coenzyme is primarily phosphopyridoxal. So, Ph-O-CH_2COOH being an aromatic compound and a longer chain of carboxylic acid group, undergoes decarboxylation as the CH_2- group destabilizes it.

6. We know, according to Wave particle duality and de Broglie hypothesis,

$\lambda = h/mv$

Given, $\lambda = 10^{-33}$ m, h = 6.6 × 10^{-34} Js and m = 330g = 0.33 kg

So, the velocity of the particle is,

$v = h/m\lambda = 6.6 \times 10^{-34}/\ 10^{-33} \times 0.33 = 2ms^{-1}$

7. Diphosphonic acids ($H_4P_2O_5$) do not have any kind of p-p bond in their chemical structure. So, these acids are dibasic in nature.

8. Given, an octahedral complex of cobalt Co (II),

Magnetic moment = 4 μ_B, Atomic number of Co = 27

So, the atomic configuration of Co in the octahedral complex = Ar $4s^1 3d^6$, so there are four unpaired *d*-orbital electrons.

Crystal field splitting energy of the octahedral complex

= ½ × Magnetic moment × –0.4 Δ_0

= ½ × 4 × (–0.4) Δ_0 = – 0.8 Δ_0.

9. Given, complex ion $[Cr(H_2O)_6]^{3+}$

Here the electronic configuration of Cr is Ar $4s^1 3d^2$

So, this gives the compound a perfect octahedral geometry

10. We have Density, ρ = mass (m) / volume (V)

And for ideal behaviour of a gas,

PV = nRT (Ideal gas equation)

Therefore, P m/ρ = nRT

Given, Temperature, T = 20°C = 293K; R = 0.082 L atm $mol^{-1}K^{-1}$; Molecular weight of F_2 = 38 $gmol^{-1}$; P = 0.3 atm

So, density of fluorine gas,

ρ = P × m/nRT

= 0.3 × 38/(1 × 0.082 × 293)

= 0.4068 g/L

11. Given, for a 1st order reaction,

$t_{1/2}$ = 20 minutes

We have, $\lambda = 0.693/t_{1/2}$

= 0.03465 min^{-1}

Now, rate of decay of substrate in the reaction is given by,

Log (N_0/N) = 2.303 λt

⇒ t = log (100/100 – 99.9)/ (2.303 × 0.03465)

= 37.598 minutes

The required time is approximately 38 minutes

12. 440 to 470

The molecular formula for naphthalene is $C_{10}H_8$ and the structure is

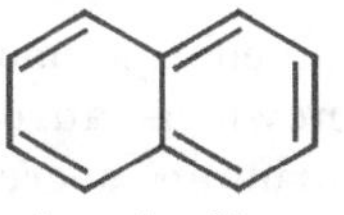

Given, bond dissociation energies of

C – H = 415 kJ/mol,

C – C = 344 kJ/mol

and C = C is 615 kJ/mol

Enthalpy of atomization of

C = 717 kJ/mol

and H = 218 kJ/mol

Number of C – H bonds = 8,

Number of C – C bonds = 6

and C = C bonds = 5

Now, heat of formation of naphthalene is given by:

Enthalpy of products – Enthalpy of reactants

$= 8 \times \Delta_{C-H} + 6 \times \Delta_{C-C} + 5 \times \Delta_{C=C} - (10 \times \Delta_C + 8 \times \Delta_H)$

= 8 × 415 + 6 × 344 + 5 × 615 – (10 × 717 + 8 × 218)

= 3320 + 2064 + 3075 – (7170 + 1744) kJ/mol

= 8459 – 8914 kJ/mol

= – 455 kJ/mol

13. (2R, 3S) –2, 3 Dihydroxybutanoic acid has a molecular weight of 120.10392 g/mol and molecular formula is $C_4H_8O_4$. Its structure is as follows:

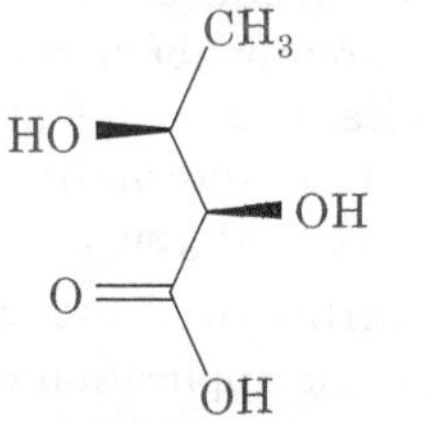

The Fisher projection of the compound is:

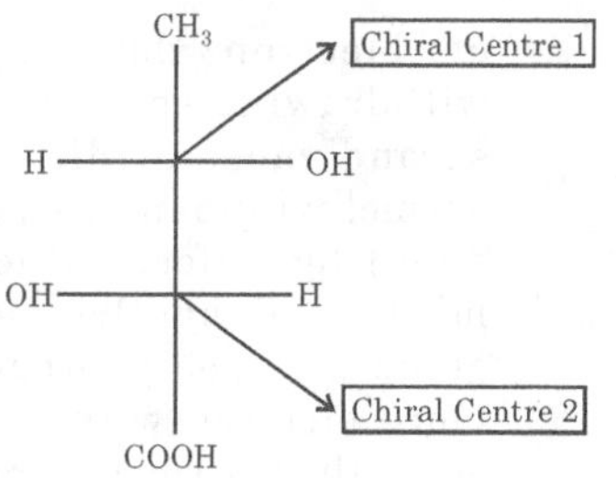

Fisher Representation

14. Ozonolysis is the process by which ozone (O_3) reacts with alkenes (olefins) to break the double bond and form two carbonyl groups. If the double bond of the alkene is substituted with hydrogen or carbon atoms, the carbonyl groups that are formed are either aldehydes or ketones. Acyclic alkenes form two carbonyl compounds while cyclic alkenes produce a single compound containing two carbonyl groups. Thus, the generic, stereoisomeric alkenes 1 and 2 give rise to the same pair of carbonyl compounds.

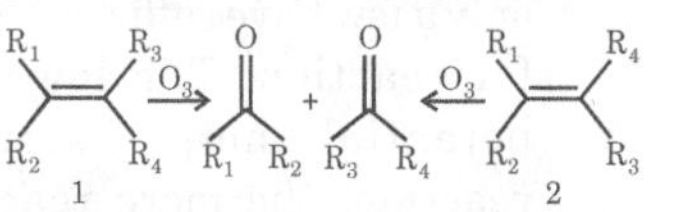

Here, the alkene that forms formaldehyde and glyoxal after ozonolysis is Hex-1, 3, 5- ene which is given by:

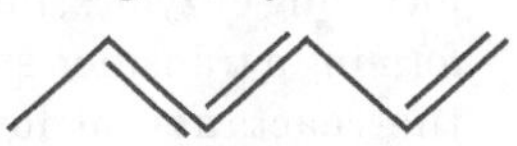

15. The electron donating groups amongst the following electronic species is NO_2. While the electron withdrawing or electrophiles amongst the following species are OMe and Me. Acidity of aromatic carboxylic groups depends on the position and the nature of the other electronic species present in the benzene ring. Here, all the species are present in the ortho position to the carboxylic group. So, electron donating species NO_2 makes the aromatic ring rich in electrons and so it can easily lose its hydrogen atom thereby making it the most acidic compound. Normal benzoic acid with absence of any kind of electron donating or withdrawing species is the second most acidic. Now, oxymethyl group has partial donating effect which is minimized by the methyl group. So, methyl group has more electron withdrawing effect than oxymethyl and so the order is as follows:

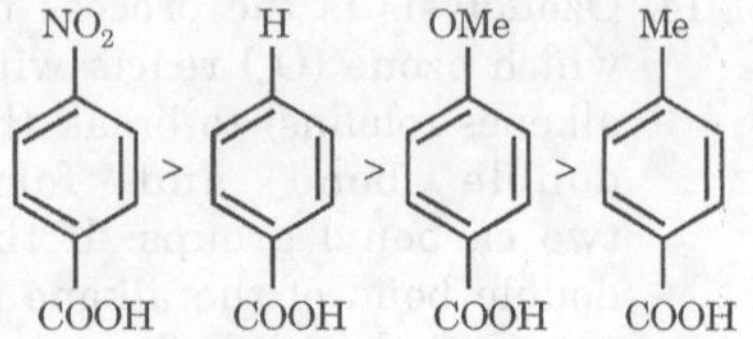

I : BIOCHEMISTRY

1. In order for a reaction to occur, reactant molecules must contain sufficient energy to cross a potential energy barrier, the activation energy. All molecules possess varying amounts of energy depending, for example, on their recent collision history but, generally, only a few have sufficient energy for reaction. The lower the potential energy barrier to reaction, the more reactants have sufficient energy and, hence, the faster the reaction will occur. All catalysts, including enzymes, function by forming a transition state, with the reactants, of lower free energy than would be found in the un-catalyzed reaction. During the catalysis of a reaction by an enzyme, the equilibrium constant of the reaction does not change.

2. In a cation-exchange resin of neutral pH, proteins are eluted out on the basis of their ability to produce anionic biproducts. So, the correct order is: Phenylalannine followed by histidine and arginine.

3. Chymotrypsin is a digestive enzyme that can perform proteolysis. Chymotrypsin preferentially cleaves peptide amide bonds where the carboxyl side of the amide bond (the P1 position) is a tyrosine, tryptophan, or phenylalanine. The main substrates of chymotrypsin include tryptophan, tyrosine, phenylalanine, leucine, and methionine, which are cleaved at the carboxyl terminal. So, chymotrypsin does not cleave any Arginine residue in a protein at the carboxyl side.

4. Epinephrine, more commonly known as adrenaline, is a hormone secreted by the medulla of the adrenal glands. Epinephrine is formed in the body from Tyrosine through a four-step process. Relaxation and contraction of smooth muscle cells (i.e. heart, arteries, and veins) are controlled through epinephrine receptors. Epinephrine will bind to the receptor on the outside of a liver cell allowing a conform-ational change to occur. This receptor shape change allows G protein to bind, and become active. The activation G protein causes a conformational change on the molecule causing adenylate cyclase to bind. Cyclic AMP activates protein kinase, which activates phosphorylase catalyzing the breakdown of glycogen to glucose.

5. A reducing sugar is a carbohydrate that is oxidized by a weak oxidizing agent (an oxidizing agent capable of oxidizing aldehydes but not alcohols, such as the Tollen's reagent) in basic aqueous solution. The characteristic property of reducing sugars is that, in aqueous medium, they generate one or more compounds containing an aldehyde group. Lactose and maltose are the two reducing sugars.

6. Equilibrium dialysis is a specific application of dialysis that is important for the study of the binding of small molecules and ions by proteins. It is one of several methods available for this purpose, and its attractive feature continues to be its physical simplicity. Another attractive feature of equilibrium dialysis is the ability to perform interaction studies without the use of fluorescent or radiolabeled tags. So, it can be used for quantitative determination of the affinity of an antibody.

7. In biochemistry, allosteric regulation is the regulation of an enzyme or other protein by binding an effector molecule at the protein's allosteric site (that is, a site other than the protein's active site). Effectors that enhance the protein's activity are referred to as allosteric activators, whereas those that decrease the protein's activity are called allosteric inhibitors. In case of pyruvate synthesis in glycolysis pathway, fructose-2, 6–bisphosphate is the allosteric activator of phosphofructoki-nase-1 as it enhances the synthesis of pyruvate in the process.

8. We know, from Michaelis-Menten equation for the rate of a reaction,

$$V = (V_{max}\,[S])/(K_M + [S])$$

Where, V_{max} = maximum velocity for the reaction of enzyme with the substrate,

[S] = substrate concentration and

K_M = Michaelis-Menten constant

Given, $[S] = 4\,K_M$

Therefore, $V = V_{max}\,4K_M/(K_M + 4\,K_M)$

$\Rightarrow \quad V = 4/5\,V_{max}\,K_M/K_M$

$\Rightarrow \quad V = 0.8\,V_{max}$

So, the initial velocity for the reaction of the enzyme with the substrate is 80% of V_{max}

9. Given, under standard biochemical conditions, equilibrium constant for the reaction:

Fructose 6-phosphate + ATP
→ Fructose 1, 6 – bisphosphate + ADP

$K'_{eq} = 254$

We have, standard free energy change for a reaction,

$\Delta G'^0 = -RT\, lnK$

$= -8.314 \times 298 \times ln(254)$

$= 2477.572 \times 5.537$

$= 13,719.1443$ J/mol

$= 13.7191$ kJ/mol

10. Hydropathy is a numeric representation of the tendency of each amino acid residue to enter a non-polar environment. A sequence is scanned in linearly and a moving average of hydropathy values is computed. The hydropathy plot is based on a moving average H(n) spanning a "window" of (2n + 1) amino acids. The orientation of a side chain is predictable based on standard geometries of the alpha-helix and beta-sheet. So, in the given monomeric protein, the hydropathy index with the largest window shows only one peak of high intensity. So, number of transmembrane α-helices in the protein is 1.

11. Given, in an aqueous solution there are two compounds X and Y.

We know, from Beer-Lambert's law, Absorbance of an aqueous solution,

$$A = \varepsilon C L$$

Where, ε = molar absorption coefficient,

C = concentration of the solution and

L = path length of light to pass through the solution

Here, absorbance was taken at 220 nm and 280 nm.

So, for a mixture, we have $A = \varepsilon_1 C_1 (l) + \varepsilon_2 C_2 (l)$ at a particular wavelength

Here, at 220 nm,

$\varepsilon_1 = 1000\ M^{-1}cm^{-1}$

and $\varepsilon_2 = 800\ M^{-1}cm^{-1}$

Concentration of the mixture,

$C_1 = [X]\ M$

and $C_2 = [Y]\ M$

Given, path length = 1 cm

Therefore, at 220 nm, A = 1

$\Rightarrow 1 = 1000\ [X] + 800\ [Y]$ ...(i)

Again, at 280 nm, we have

$\varepsilon'_1 = 200\ M^{-1}cm^{-1}$,

$\varepsilon'_2 = 400\ M^{-1}cm^{-1}$

So, $A = 0.4$

$\Rightarrow 0.4 = 200\ [X] + 400\ [Y]$ ...(ii)

$(0.2) \times (i) \Rightarrow 0.2 = 200\ [X] + 160\ [Y]$

$1 \times (ii) \Rightarrow 0.4 = 200\ [X] + 400\ [Y]$

$(ii) - (i) \Rightarrow 0.2 = 240\ [Y]$

$[Y] = 8.33333 \times 10^{-4}$ M

$= 0.83333 \times 10^{-3}$ M

$= 0.8333$mM

So, the concentration of the compound Y is 0.83333mM

12. From the data obtained from the SDS-PAGE run of the oligomeric protein, we have:

Under reducing conditions, the protein separates into two fragments of 50kDa and 25kDa peptides. But under non-reducing conditions, the protein separates on the gel as a single polypeptide of 75kDa size. So, the size of the oligomeric protein is 75kDa.

Now, number of molecules in 1litre of the solution = 4.01×10^{18} in 1 gram solution (Since concentration is 1mg/mL; so weight of the protein in 1L solution is 1 g)

We know,

$1kDa = 1.66 \times 10^{-24}$ kg

$= 1.6605 \times 10^{-21}$ grams

so $75kDa = 124.5375 \times 10^{-21}$ grams

$= 1.245375 \times 10^{-19}$ grams

In 1 gram solution of the oligomeric protein, number of molecules

$= 4.01 \times 10^{18}$

Therefore, number of molecules in 1.245375×10^{-19}gram of the protein

$= 4.01 \times 10^{18} \times 1.245375 \times 10^{-19}$

$= 4.99939 \times 10^{-1}$

$= 0.4999939$

Hence, number of polypeptide chains that constitute the oligomeric protein

$= 4.9999$

$= 5$ (approx.)

13. We know, Free energy change,

$\Delta G = -nFE^0$

Where, n = number of moles in the reaction which are exchanged,

F = Faraday's constant and

E = potential of a cell

Given, number of Mg^{2+} = twice the concentration in the outside, so n = 2

F = 96.5 kJ/V mol

and E = – 60 mV

$= -60 \times 10^{-3}$ V

Therefore, free energy change across the membrane against a concentration gradient is

$\Delta G = -2 \times 96.5 \times (-60 \times 10^{-3})$ kJ/mol

$= 11.58$ kJ/mol

14. IgM and IgA are usually synthesized as multimers in association with an additional polypeptide chain, the J chain. Genes in the SERPIN gene super family provide instructions for making proteins called serine peptidase inhibitors or serpins. Most serpins help control certain chemical reactions by blocking (inhibiting) the function of proteins, specifically enzymes called serine proteases. Serpin inhibits C1 complement proteins. β-2-microglobulin (β-2-M) is a small membrane protein (11,800 Dalton) associated with the heavy chains of class I major histocompatibility complex proteins and is, therefore, on the surface of all nucleated cells. V(D)J recombination represents one of the three mechanisms that contribute to the diversity of the immune repertoire of B lymphocytes and T lymphocytes. The V(D)J recombination process insures the somatic diversification of immunoglobulin and antigen T cell receptor encoding genes. Artemis, whose mutations cause human RS-SCID is a novel protein involved in V(D)J recombination/DNA repair. Artemis belongs to the metallo-β-lactamase super family.

15. In case of competitive inhibition, the Michaelis-Menten equation becomes:

Initial rate of the reaction,

$$V_0 = V_{max} [S]/\{K_M^{observed} + [S]\}$$

Where, $K_M^{observed}$ = apparent value of Michaelis-Menten constant which is determined by the inhibitor as:

$$K_M^{observed} = K_M(1 + [I]/K_i],$$

where is [I] is the concentration of the inhibitor and K_i is the dissociation constant of the inhibitor.

Given, K_i = [I] and K_M of uninhibited reaction = 2×10^{-5}M

So, $K_M^{observed} = 2 \times 10^{-5}(1 + 1)$

$= 4 \times 10^{-5}$ M.

16. We have, pH of a buffer solution is given by:

$$pH = pK_a + \log [Salt]/[Base]$$

Here, [Salt] = $[Na_2HPO_4]$

$= w/M \times 1000/V$

$= 208/142 \times 1000/V$

And [Base] = $[NaH_2PO_4]$

$= 71/120 \times 1000/V$

Given, pK_a for dissociation of

$H_2PO_4^- = 6.86$

Therefore, pH = 6.86 + log

$[Na_2HPO_4]/[NaH_2PO_4]$

$= [208/142]/[71/120]$

$= 6.86 + 0.3937$

$= 7.2537$

17. In order to form a multiple-charge ion, an analyte molecule must have more than one site which can be ionized. With very large numbers of charges we do not observe a single multiple-charge species in the mass spectrum (i.e., a single value for z), but rather a heterogeneity of charge. We can read the m/z of the peak in the spectrum and if we solve for m we can determine the molecular mass of the protein represented by this spectrum. Starting with a molecule of mass M we can adduct z protons to create a multiple charge ion. The mass-to-charge ratio of that ion can be defined as follows, where H is the mass of a proton:

$$m/z = (M + zH)/z \text{ (Eq.1)},$$

where m is the mass of the ion, i.e., the molecular mass of the protein plus the mass of all adducted protons.

$$m = (M + zH) \text{ (Eq. 2)}$$

$$m - zH = M \text{ (Eq. 3)}$$

$$M = z\,(m/z - H) \text{ (Eq. 4)}$$

We know, m/z values of two adjacent peaks are m_1/z_1 and m_2/z_2 where $z_1 = z_2 + 1$. Using equations 1 and 4, we have:

$$z_2 = ((m_1/z_1) - H) / ((m_2/z_2) - (m_1/z_1)) \text{ (Eq. 5)}$$

Let us pick any two peaks of m/z values 2072.42 and 2417.67

So, here $z_2 = z_{2417.67}$

and $z_1 = z_{2072.42}$

So, from equation 5 we have,

$Z_{2417.42} = (2072.42 - 1)/(2417.67 - 2072.42)$

$= 2071.42/345.25$

$= 5.99977$

Now, Mass of the protein, from equation 4,

$M = z_{2417.67}\,(m_{2417.67}/z_{2417.67} - H)$

$= 5.99977\,(2417.67 - 1)$

$= 14,\ 499.46$Da

Therefore, the required mass of protein is 14.49946kDa.

18. The three exons I, II and III of human gene obtained from kidney cells showed two different fragments of PCR products when amplified using a forward primer specific to exon 1 and a reverse primer specific to exon III. The two fragments were of size 2.5kb and 1kb. On northern blotting the same total RNA which was reverse transcribed to obtain cDNA, a single band was observed on gel when a probe specific to exon II was used. So, it is clear that exon I and II amplify to give rise to single cDNA transcript while the exon III coded region gives rise to an mRNA splice variant. So, northern blotting of the exon III region with specific radioactive probes will certainly result in the formation of two bands. Since, on amplification, size of the 1st band came to be 2.5kb and the second to be 1kb, so size of the exon II encoded region is 2.5 – 1 = 1.5kb. Also, it is clear that variations in the spliced mRNAs comes from the exon III region and a forward primer directed at exon I or exon II will not result in two bands formation.

19. The DNA sequences of two individuals, subject 1 and subject 2 were determined using Sanger's dideoxy method of chain termination. A partial portion of the autoradiogram shows sequences as follows:

Subject 1 → 5' – AGGCTGAT-3' and

subject 2 → 5' – AGGC (A ⇔T) GAT-3'

It is seen from the autoradiogram of subject two that there occurs allelic inversion at one position with A and T being the two nucleotides. So, subject two has 2 allelic variants present in it.

20. After double digestion of the 7kb DNA molecule with EcoRI and PvuII restriction endonucleases, they were synthesized into whole DNA fragments by sealing of the sticky ends using radioactive α-^{32}P d-NTPs using Klenow fragment of DNA polymerase I. When stained with EtBr, four fragments were noticed on gel electrophoresis. In case of autoradiography, the autoradiogram showed 3 fragments. So, it is clear that

EcoRI first cuts the DNA into fragments of 3kb and 4kb respectively. The 4kb fragment is then cut into two 2kb fragments. Now, PvuII with a relatively smaller restriction site than EcoRI, cuts the other 2kb fragment into fragments of 0.5kb and 1.5kb. In case of EtBr staining, all the four fragments generated could be seen because of intercalation of EtBr into stacked DNA bases. In case of autoradiography, the fragments which took up radioactive dNTPs could be seen while the 1.5kb fragment with no sticky ends which did not take up any dNTPs did not display any reading on the autoradiogram. So, the correct restriction map would be→

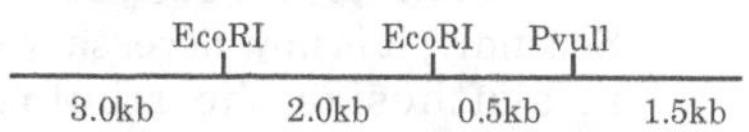

7.0 kb Linear DNA

J : BOTANY

1. An epiphyte is a plant that normally grows on another plant for support. It is not parasitic, but uses the host plant for support only. Epiphytes can be found in many different environments all over the world, but many of the most beautiful come from the tropic rain forests.

2. A cybrid is an artificial hybrid cell produced by introducing nuclear material from one organism into a cell (of the same or different species) from which the nucleus has been removed. It contains a nuclear genome from one source and a mitochondrial genome from another. Thus an ideal cybrid has nuclear genome exclusively from one of the parents and cytoplasmic genome from both the parents.

3. A plant cell consists of plastids and vacuoles. Thus a Transmission Electron Micrograph (TEM) of a fungal cell can be distinguished from plant cell due to lack of plastid and having less abundant vacuoles.

4. RNA interference (RNAi) is an endogenous post-transcriptional gene regulatory mechanism mediated by non-coding RNA molecules known as microRNAs. This mechanism can be utilized for targeted gene silencing by introduction of nucleic acid based tools that are specially designed to trigger the RNAi mechanism. These molecules are taken up by the RNA induced silencing complex (RISC) to target specific mRNAs for degradation or to modulate endogenous microRNAs.

5. Petals are modified leaves that surround the reproductive parts of flowers. Sepals are one of the four basic parts of a flower. They are found below the petals. Tepals are elements of the perianth, or outer part of a flower, which includes the petals or sepals. Petiole is the stalk attaching the leaf blade to the stem. Thus petiole is the odd one out.

6. A plantibody is an antibody that is produced by plants that have been genetically engineered with animal DNA. Plantibodies are engineered in plants via insertion of recombinant DNA gene transfer.

7. A neutral lipid is a term that is used to refer to any of lipids that are soluble only in solvents of very low polarity. Neutral lipids are basically a triglyceride made of 3 fatty acids linked to a glycerol and have no polar group as phospholipids do. So although they have a hydrophobic tail they do not have a hydrophilic (charged) head. Oleaginous seeds store lipids in specialized structures called oil bodies (OBs). These organelles consist of a core of neutral lipids bound by proteins embedded in a phospholipid monolayer. Thus in a typical oil- seed crop, the matured seeds are enriched with neutral lipids.

8. *Crocus sativus*, commonly known as saffron crocus, is a species of flowering plant of the *Crocus* genus in the Iridaceae family.

   Garcinia is a plant genus of the family Clusiaceae. Most species in Garcinia are known for their gum resin, brownish-yellow from xanthonoids such as mangostin, and used as purgative or cathartic, but most frequently – at least in former times – as a pigment. The colour term gamboge refers to this pigment. Gamboge is partially transparent deep saffron to mustard yellow pigment.

   Roccella tinctoria is a species of fungus in the genus Roccella. It is used to make litmus, a mixture of several organic compounds.

   Curcuma is a genus of about 80 accepted species in the plant family Zingiberaceae that contains such species as turmeric and Siam Tulip.

9. The 'green revolution gene' has been identified to be involved in either single transduction pathway or biosynthesis of Gibberellins. There are many genes associated with a semi-dwarf growth habit in wheat. They are known as Reduced height (Rht) genes and many of them are dominant or semi-dominant, indicating that they actively inhibit growth through a so-called gain-of-function mutation. The identity and function of most of these genes are not known, but some have been found to prevent the action of gibberellins.

10. Plants, in nature, are generally resistant to most pathogens. The ability of a pathogen to cause disease in a host plant is usually the exception, not the rule. The inheritance of both resistances in the host and parasite ability to cause disease is controlled by pairs of matching genes. One is a plant gene called the resistance (R) gene. The other is a parasite gene called the avirulence (Avr) gene. Plants producing a specific R gene product are resistant towards a pathogen that produces the corresponding Avr gene product.

11. The ubiquitin-proteasome system is active in distinct nuclear domains and plays a major role controlling the initial steps of gene expression, DNA repair and nuclear quality-control mechanisms. The target tissue type is leaf.

Napin is a seed storage protein from Brassica napus (rape) that is encoded by a gene family. The transcription machinery used is nucleus and target tissue type is seed.

Ribulose-bisphosphate carboxylase gene (rbcL) catalyzes the carboxylation of ribulose-1,5-bisphosphate. The large-chain gene (rbcL) is part of the chloroplast DNA molecule in plants. Its transcription machinery is chloroplast and target tissue type is seed.

The small subunit of ribulose 1, 5- bisphosphate carboxylase is encoded by a multigene family of RbcS genes in the nucleus. The target tissue type is seed.

12. The fraction of purple- flowered progeny expected to be pure purple- flowered line is 1/3.

13. The sequence of genes in a normal chromosome of a plant species is given as:

GHIJ o KLMN

An inversion is when there's a breakage of the chromosome and the genetic material is flipped over before it reconnects to the rest of the chromosome again. A pericentric inversion does include the centromere, meaning that the break points are on different arms. It can be represented as: GHIKL o JMN.

Non-reciprocal translocation involves the transfer of genes from one chromosome to another, non-homologous chromosome. It can be represented as :

GJ o KLHIMN

If the duplicated sections are adjacent to the original, the process is known as tandem duplication. It can be represented as: GHIJ o KLKLMN

Deletion is the absence of a section of genetic material from a gene. It can be represented as: GHJ o KLMN.

14. Trisomy X is a sex chromosome anomaly with a variable phenotype caused by the presence of an extra X chromosome in females (47,XXX instead of 46,XX).

Triploid syndrome is an extremely rare chromosomal disorder. Individuals with triploid syndrome have three of every chromosome for a total of 69 rather than the normal 46 chromosomes.

In a monosomic, the homologous chromosome(s) is represented only once in a cell or all cells of an individual. The gametes of diploids are monosomic for all chromosomes. A monosomic individual of an allopolyploid has 2n – 1 chromosomes i.e. 45 chromosomes.

Monoploid refers to the number of chromosomes of the cell, meaning that the cell has only one chromosome from every one of the "n" pairs (n = 23 for the human cells).

15. Escherichia coli produce the enzyme beta-D-glucuronidase. Beta-D-glucuronidase is an enzyme which hydrolyzes the beta-D-glucopyranosid-uronic derivatives to aglycons and D-glucuronic acid. The detection system is fluorimetric.

Green Fluorescent Protein (GFP) is a protein produced by a jellyfish Aequorea victoria; which produces glowing points of light around the margin of its umbrella. The detection system used is fluorescence.

Luciferase is a generic term for the class of oxidative enzymes used in bioluminescence. Luciferases are enzymes that emit light. One example is the firefly luciferase from the firefly Photinus pyralis. The detection system used is luminescence.

Chloramphenicol acetyltrans-ferase (or CAT) is a bacterial enzyme that detoxifies the antibiotic chloramphenicol and is responsible for chloramphen-icol resistance in bacteria (*E. coli*).

16. Climate change affects plants in many different ways. Increasing CO_2 concen-tration can increase photosynthetic rates. Photosynthesis can help in reducing the global warming by taking in carbon dioxide. But global warming has led to an increase in the photorespiration relative to photosynthesis. Photorespiration reduces the efficiency of photosynthesis for a couple of reasons. First, oxygen is added to carbon. In other words, the carbon is oxidized, which is the reverse of photosynthesis—the reduction of carbon to carbohydrate. Secondly, it is now necessary to re-synthesize the ribulose bisphosphate and to reduce the phosphoglycolate. Thus the aqueous solubility of dissolved CO_2 is decreased as compared to dissolved O_2.

17. Regulation of a cell cycle progression depends on cyclin dependent kinase (CDK) and protease activity.

The oxidation of water is catalyzed in photosystem II by a redox-active structure that contains four manganese ions; this oxygen-evolving complex binds two water molecules and stores the four oxidizing equivalents that are required to drive the water-oxidizing reaction. Photosystem II is the only known biological enzyme that carries out this oxidation of water.

Photorespiratory reaction occurring in oxidative photosynthetic carbon (C_2) pathway involves a cooperative interaction among three organelles: chloroplast, peroxisome and mitochondria.

Ethylene acts as a promoter of senescence and cytokinins act as a senescence antagonist.

18. The inflorescence type of Smilacina sp. is compound determinate.

Epilobium is a species of flowering plant in the evening primrose family known by the common names Talus Willowherb and Clavatefruit Willowherb. The inflorescence is an erect raceme of flowers, each with four small pink petals.

Pedicularis is a genus of perennial green root parasite plants currently placed in the broomrape family Orobanchaceae. The inflorescence is spike.

Pelargonium is a genus of flowering plants which includes about 200 species of perennials, succulents, and shrubs, commonly known as geraniums. The inflorescence of Pelargonium comprises an umbel of three to seven flowers on a long peduncle that bends down as the flowers wither.

19. P-Microsporocyte undergoes meiosis and gives rise to four haploid microspores.

R-A microspore undergoes mitosis and cytokinesis in order to produce two separate cells, the generative cell and the tube cell. A generative cell is a cell of the male gametophyte or pollen grain in seed plants that divides to give rise directly or indirectly to sperm.

Q-Pollen itself is not the male gamete. Each pollen grain contains vegetative (non-reproductive) cells (only a single cell in most flowering plants but several in other seed plants) and a generative (reproductive) cell. In flowering plants the vegetative tube cell produces the pollen tube, R-and the generative cell divides to form the two sperm cells.

20. Plant succession can be defined as the process of gradual replacement of one plant community by another plant community which is of stable type. It occurs over a period of time. The first plant community which develops in a bare area is known as pioneer community and the last invading community is called the climax community. The plant comm-unities that develop during the succession are called the seral communities.

Formation is a major ecological unit of vegetation. Formation Class is a vegetation classification unit of high rank (1st level) defined by a characteristic combination of dominant growth forms adapted to a very basic set of moisture / temperature regimes.

Consociation can be defined as a small climax community of plants having a characteristic dominant species.

Faciation refers to a part of a climax association which lacks some of the dominants of the normal association due to slight differences in environmental fundamentals. It is related to minor differences in temperature and moisture relations.

K : MICROBIOLOGY

1. A capsid is the protein shell of a virus. The icosahedral shape has 20 equilateral triangular faces, approximates a sphere, while the helical shape is cylindrical.

2. Intergenic mutation is a mutation that alters the anticodon in a tRNA so that it is complementary to a termination codon, thus suppressing termination of the amino acid chain.

3. The NADPH oxidase (nicotinamide adenine dinucleotide phosphate-oxidase) is a membrane-bound enzyme complex. It can be found in the plasma membrane as well as in the membranes of phagosomes used by neutrophil white blood cells to engulf microorganisms. Thus NADPH oxidase does not bind to a gaseous ligand.

4. Given, Working volume = 10L

or 10,000ml (As 1L = 1000ml)

Doubling time = 50min

Rate of flow of nutrients

= volume/doubling time

= 10000/50 = 200ml/min

5. Rheumatic fever is an autoimmune disease in which the body's own antibodies to strep attack different parts of a person's body such as the heart valves, the brain's basal ganglia, and the joints. It is an inflammatory disease that occurs following a Streptococcus pyogenes infection, such as streptococcal pharyngitis.

6. Oxidoreductases are a class of enzymes that catalyze oxidoreduction reactions. Oxidorecuctases can be oxidases or dehydrogenases. Oxidases are enzymes involved when molecular oxygen acts as an acceptor of hydrogen or electrons. Oxygenases incorporate oxygen from molecular oxygen into organic substrates. Thus oxygenases that catalyze the initial step in the degradation polycyclic aromatic hydrocarbons by using molecular oxygen belong to oxido-reductase class of enzyme.

7. Horizontal Gene Transfer Horizontal gene transfer (HGT) is the introduction of genetic material from one species to another species by mechanisms other than the vertical transmission from parent(s) to offspring. Horizontal gene transfer may occur via three main mechanisms: transformation, transduction or conjugation.

Transformation involves uptake of short fragments of naked DNA by naturally transformable bacteria. Transduction involves transfer of DNA from one bacterium into another via bacteriophages. Conjugation involves transfer of DNA via sexual pilus and requires cell –to-cell contact.

Thus mutation is not involved in horizontal gene transfer.

8. Louis Pasteur was a French chemist and microbiologist renowned for his discoveries of the principles of vaccination, microbial fermentation and pasteurization. The principle of vaccination or immunisation is based on the property of 'memory' of the immune system. A vaccine is always given before the occurrence of the disease.

9. Lysozyme is an enzyme used to break down bacterial cell walls to improve protein or nucleic acid extraction efficiency. The enzyme acts by catalyzing the hydrolysis of 1,4-beta-linkages between N-acetylmuramic acid (NAM) and N-acetyl-D-glucosamine (NAG) residues in peptidoglycans and between the N-acetyl-D-glucosamine residues in chitodextrins.

10. Atomic force microscopy (AFM) is a technique for analyzing the surface of a rigid material all the way down to the level of the atom. AFM uses a mechanical probe to magnify surface features up to 100,000,000 times, and it produces 3-D images of the surface. Thus it can be used to study the contour of proteins.

11. Vancomycin is used to treat colitis (inflammation of the intestine caused by certain bacteria) that may occur after antibiotic treatment. Vancomycin acts by inhibiting proper cell wall synthesis in Gram-positive bacteria. Due to the different mechanism by which Gram-negative bacteria produce their cell walls and the various factors related to entering the outer membrane of Gram-negative organisms, vancomycin is not active against Gram-negative bacteria.

Rifampicin inhibits bacterial DNA-dependent RNA synthesis by inhibiting bacterial DNA-dependent RNA polymerase.

Puromycin is an aminonucleoside antibiotic produced by the bacterium Streptomyces alboniger. It inhibits protein synthesis by disrupting peptide transfer on ribosomes causing premature chain termination during translation.

Ciprofloxacin is a broad-spectrum antibiotic active against both Gram-positive and Gram-negative bacteria. It functions by inhibiting DNA gyrase, a type II topoisomerase, and topoisomerase IV, enzymes necessary to separate bacterial DNA, thereby inhibiting cell division.

12. A growth curve is an empirical model of the evolution of a quantity over time.

Growth curve of bacteria can be represented as:

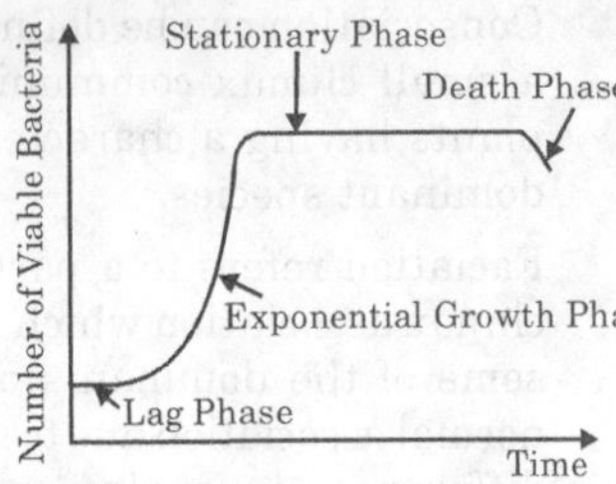

Growth curve of extracellular virus can be represented as:

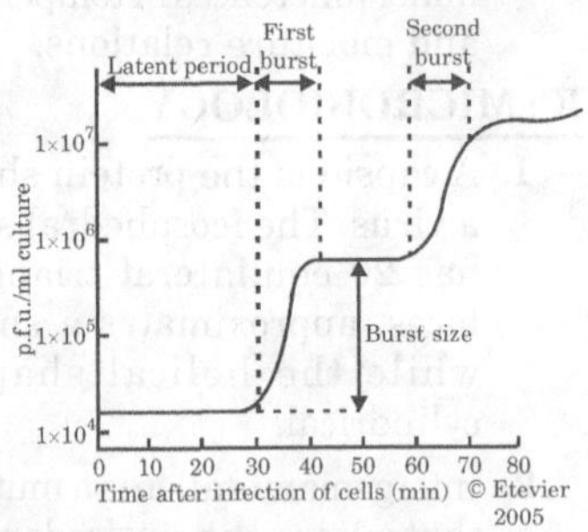

Growth curve of intracellular virus can be represented as:

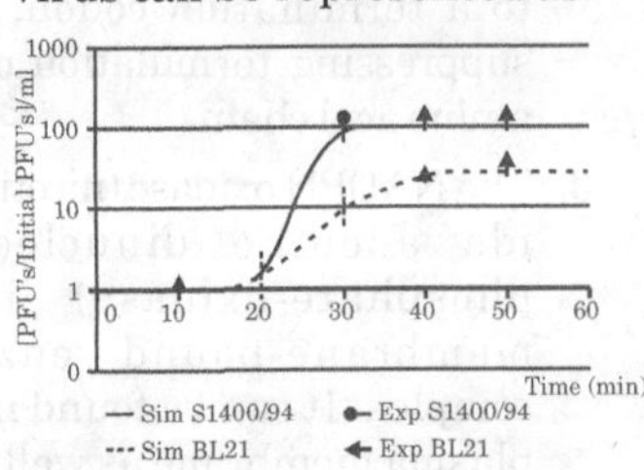

13. The length of a coding region in an amino acid is 897 bases. There will be 298 amino acids in the polypeptide synthesized using this mRNA.

14. Hemolytic microbes are grown in blood agar media. The ability of bacterial colonies to induce hemolysis when grown on blood agar is used to classify certain microorganisms.

Autotrophs are those organisms that are able to make energy-containing organic molecules from inorganic raw material by using basic energy sources such as sunlight. Thus they can be grown in a minimal media. Minimal Media contains the essentials for bacterial species to grow.

Skim Milk Agar is used for the demonstration of coagulation and proteolysis of casein. Proteolytic bacteria hydrolyze casein to form soluble nitrogenous compounds indicated as clear zone surrounding the colonies. More clear zones are seen on milk agar if, the bacteria produce acid from fermentable carbohydrates in the medium.

There is a wide range of media available that use different substrates for the detection of *E. coli* and coliforms. The media are also supplemented with agents like bile salts, brilliant green, sodium lauryl sulphate and other substances to enhance their selectivity.

15. At time 2hrs, total viable cell count

$= 1 \times 10^4$ cells/ml.

At time 6hrs, total viable cell count

$= 1 \times 10^9$ cells/ml.

Specific growth rate (k) = ?

We know,

$\log 10N_2 - \log 10N_1 = k(t_2 - t_1)/2.303$

Thus, $k = (9 - 4)2.303/6-2$

$k = 5 \times 2.303/4$

Therefore, Specific growth rate (k)

$= 2.87\ h^{-1}$

16. Molecular weight of Sodium Chloride

= 58.44ng/mol

Concentration of Sodium chloride in cytoplasm = 250ng/nl

Thus, Molarity of Sodium Chloride

= 250/58.44

= 4.277M

17. Salmonella is a genus of rod-shaped, Gram-negative bacteria. Salmonella are non-spore-forming, predominantly motile enterobacteria with diameters around 0.7 to 1.5 µm, lengths from 2 to 5 µm, and peritrichous flagella (flagella that are all around the cell body).

Saccharomyces cerevisiae is a species of yeast. S. cerevisiae cells are round to ovoid, 5–10 micrometres in diameter and they are non-motile.

Aquaspirillum serpens is a harmless, saprophytic, aerobic bacterium, obtainable from the culture collections, easy to grow in simple broth. It has a helical shape and its flagellar arrangement is amphitrichious.

Vibrio cholerae is a "comma" (curved rod) shaped Gram-negative bacteria with a single, polar flagellum for movement.

18. LD_{50} is the lethal dose required to kill half the members of a tested population after specified test duration.

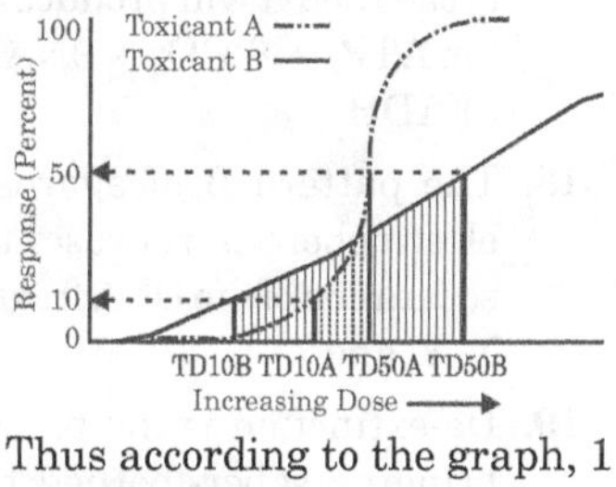

Thus according to the graph, 1 and 2 microorganisms are the most lethal.

19. Ampicillin belongs to the penicillin group of beta-lactam antibiotics. It is sterilized by filtering through a sterile membrane filter with a porosity of 0.22 micron or less.

1% glucose in phosphate buffer can be sterilized by autoclaving at 10psi for 20 min.

Gamma rays are also used to sterilize hospital equipment, especially plastic syringes that would be damaged if heated.

Luria broth can be sterilized by heating the mixture to boiling to dissolve agar and sterilizing by autoclaving at 15 psi, from 121-124°C for 15 minutes.

20. The recA and recB mutants decrease the ability of the cells to survive UV and to undergo genetic recombination thus they exhibit reduced recombination. RecA and recB mutants also show pleiotropic effects.

L : ZOOLOGY

1. A biodiversity hotspot is a biogeographic region that is both a significant reservoir of biodiversity and is threatened with destruction. They are areas that support natural ecosystems that are largely intact and where native species and communities associated with these ecosystems are well represented. They are also areas with a high diversity of locally endemic species, which are species that are not found or are rarely found outside the hotspot.

2. The osculum is an excretory structure in the living sponge, a large opening to the outside through which the current of water exits after passing through the spongocoel. Wastes diffuse into the water and the water exits through the osculum at a velocity of nearly 8.4 cm/second, carrying away with it the sponge's wastes. The size of the osculum is regulated by the myocyte. Its size, in turn, determines the amount of water flowing through the sponge.

3. Cleavage is a unique embryological process which transforms the single fertilized egg cell into a sphere of closely aggregated multitude of cells. Bilateral cleavage results in bisection of the zygote into left and right halves. This type of cleavage is found in Molluscs which are an important phylum of invertebrate animals.

4. Mitochondriais is not considered to be a part of Endomembrane system. The endomembrane system consists of the endoplasmic reticulum and the Golgi apparatus - i.e. things that are formed within the cell. The mitochondria were originally formed from a captured bacterial cell- as it has its own DNA and its own ribosomes. It is a separate organelle on its own, although it has connections with the endomembrane system, but it is not considered a part of it.

5. The end products of glycolysis are two molecules of pyruvic acid (or pyruvate) with the formation of a small amount of ATP. This is produced from a molecule of glucose. Also two molecules of NAD^+ capture and are reduced to 2 molecules of $NADH + H^+$.

6. A TATA box is a DNA sequence that indicates the point at which a genetic sequence can be read and decoded. The TATA box assists in directing RNA polymerase II to the initiation site downstream on DNA. RNA polymerases bind to regions of DNA known as promoters.

7. The eukaryotic pre-mRNA undergoes extensive processing before it is ready to be translated. The additional steps involved in eukaryotic mRNA maturation create a molecule with a much longer half-life than a prokaryotic mRNA. Eukaryotic mRNAs last for several hours, whereas the typical *E. coli* mRNA lasts no more than five seconds. Thus the Eukaryotic pre-mRNA receives a 5' cap and a 3' poly-A tail before introns are removed and the mRNA is considered ready for translation. The 5' cap protects the mRNA from degradation by RNase, and enzyme that degrades unprotected mRNA. 3' poly A tail offers protection from exonucleases (enzymes that degrade nucleotide sequences) and assists the mRNA strand in leaving the nucleus.

8. Hyperthyroidism, often referred to as an overactive thyroid, is a condition in which the thyroid gland produces and secretes excessive amounts of the free thyroid hormones triiodothyronine (T3) and thyroxine (T4). Graves' disease is the most common cause of hyperthyroidism. There are several causes of hyperthyroidism. Most often, the entire gland is overproducing thyroid hormone. Hypersecretion of thyroid stimulating hormone (TSH), which in turn is almost always caused by a pituitary adenoma, accounts for much less than 1 percent of hyperthyroidism cases. Measuring the level of thyroid-stimulating hormone (TSH), produced by the pituitary gland in the blood is typically the initial test for suspected hyperthyroidism. Measuring specific antibodies, such as anti-TSH-receptor antibodies in Graves' disease which is a common cause of hypothyroidism — may also contribute to the diagnosis.

9. Urea is the waste created when the body metabolizes protein. Urea is produced in the Liver. It is produced when the liver breaks down the protein and ammonia. The urea is then transferred to the urine from the blood via kidneys. The kidney filters it from the blood before it enters the bladder to be excreted.

10. Adrenocorticotropic hormone (ACTH), also known as corticotropin, is a polypeptide tropic hormone produced and secreted by the anterior pituitary gland. It acts to increase the secretion of other hormones. ACTH stimulates secretion of glucocorticoid steroid hormones from adrenal cortex cells. Within the pituitary gland, ACTH is produced in a process that also generates several other hormones.

11. In genetics, a locus (plural loci) is the specific location of a gene or DNA sequence or position on a chromosome. Recombination data is used to find the loci on a chromosome. The recombination frequency between X-Y is 12, between X-Z is 4 and between Y-Z is 8. Thus the order of loci on the chromosome would start from the smallest frequency between two loci i.e. 4 between X-Z. Then comes the frequency between Z-Y or Y-Z i.e. 8. Thus the order of loci on the chromosome would be X-Y-Z as the frequency between X and Z loci in X-Y-Z would be (4 + 8 = 12).

12. Given,

95-White eyed-normal winged

102-Red eyed-miniature winged

226-Red eyed-normal winged

202-White eyed-miniature winged offspring.

The percentage frequency of recombination between the two genes would be 31.52%.

13. An advantage of Green Fluorescent Protein (GFP) over antibody staining often emerges if a protein is highly localized within a cell. GFP expression analysis can help suggest where the gene of interest may act. It allows easy identification of the nature of the living cell. Thus the fusion of GFP allows tracking the location of the protein in living cells, while staining usually requires fixation of cells.

14. If a newborn was accidently given a drug that would destroy the thymus then his T cells would mature and differentiate appropriately as thymus is the site for T cell maturation and when it is destroyed then the T cells would not be able to mature properly.

15. IgE's main function is immunity to parasites such as parasitic worms. IgE also plays an essential role in type I hypersensitivity, which manifests various allergic diseases, such as allergic asthma, most types of sinusitis, allergic rhinitis, food allergy, and some types of chronic urticaria and atopic dermatitis. Thus if an individual has parasitic worm infection and another is responding to an allergen such as pollen, then they both will have an increased levels of IgE. As high IgE levels indicate a parasitic infection.

16. All the dialysis bags are impermeable to sucrose and are filled with different concentrations of sucrose. The bags are placed in different beakers containing 0.6M sucrose solution. Thus according to the graph, the Dialysis Bag 2 (DB2) represents the bags that contain solutions that are hypertonic at 50 minutes.

17. Acetyl CoA is the fuel for the citric acid cycle. The tricaboxylic acid (TCA) cycle produces 2 moles of CO_2, 3 moles of NADH, 1 molecule of GTP (or ATP) and 1 mole of $FADH_2$ for each mole of acetyl-CoA that enters the cycle. Thus when 3 molecules of Acetyl CoA are fed into the TCA cycle, then it will produce 3GTP (or ATP) + 6 CO_2 + 9NADH + 3$FADH_2$.

18. The pattern B of agarose gel electrophoresis represents the separation of the DNA fragments X, Y, and Z.

19. De-extinction is the process of bringing saber-toothed tigers, woolly mammoths and other extinct animals back into the world. It is possible to resurrect the extinct woolly mammoth by transferring cell nuclei from the frozen tissue into the enucleated unfertilized eggs of a suitable mammal.

20. Regions of higher abundance of cholesterol molecules on plasma membrane will be more rigid than the surrounding membrane as cholesterols reduce the membrane fluidity by reducing phospholipid movement thus making it more rigid.

M : FOOD TECHNOLOGY

1. Corn syrup is a food syrup, which is made from the starch of maize and contains varying amounts of maltose and higher oligosaccharides, depending on the grade. Thus it is not a source of caffeine. Whereas, coffee, cocoa beans and tea leaves are all a source of caffeine.

2. Yoghurt is a fermented milk product produced by bacterial fermentation of milk. The bacteria used to make yogurt are known as "yogurt cultures". Fermentation of lactose by these bacteria produces lactic acid, which acts on milk protein to give yogurt its texture and its characteristic tang. It is produced using a culture of *Lactobacillus delbrueckii subsp. bulgaricus* and *Streptococcus* salivarius subsp. thermophilus bacteria.

3. *Coxiella burnetti* is an obligate intracellular Gram-negative *coccobacillus* bacterium that is known to be the main pathogen that causes Q fever in mammals and humans. *Coxiella burnetti* been known to possibly be found in milk. Milk pasteurization aims to kill all harmful bacteria through extensive heat treatment.

4. Hypobaric storage is also known as low pressure storage. Hypobaric storage involves the cold storage of fruit under partial vacuum. Typical conditions include pressures as low as 80 and 40 millimeters of mercury and temperatures of 5° C (40° F). Hypobaric conditions reduce ethylene production and respiration rates; the result is an extraordinarily high-quality fruit even after months of storage.

5. In a solution of vegetable oil (molecular mass = 292 kg $kmol^{-1}$) and ethanol (molecular mass 46 kg $kmol^{-1}$), the concentration of vegetable oil in the solution is measured to be 60% (total mass basis). Therefore, mole fraction of ethanol in the solution is 0.809.

Given,

Molecular mass of vegetable oil
$= 292 \text{ kg kmol}^{-1}$

Molecular mass of ethanol
$= 46 \text{ kg kmol}^{-1}$

Concentration of vegetable oil in the solution = 60%.

Let the mass of the solution be 100 kg.

Thus, mass of vegetable oil
= 60 kg

Mass of ethanol = 100 – 60
= 40 kg

Moles of vegetable oil = mass/ molar mass
= 60/292
= 0.205 mol

Moles of ethanol = 40/46
= 0.869 mol

Total number of moles in the solution
= 0.205 + 0.869
= 1.074

Thus mole fraction of ethanol
= 0.869/1.074
= 0.809

6. An experiment started with 4 numbers of bacterial cells. After n^{th} generation, number of cells becomes 128. Therefore the value of n is 5.

$2^{\text{number of generations}}$ × initial number of bacterial cells
= total number of bacterial cells.

$$2^n * 4 = 128$$
$$2^n = 32$$
$$2^n = (2)^5$$
$$n = 5.$$

7. One ton of refrigeration means energy extracted to freeze one of water in one day. It can be defined as the amount of Refrigeration Effect produced by uniform melting of 1 ton of ice from and at 0°C in 24 hrs.

8. Fruit juice is flowing in a circular pipe (inner diameter 2cm) at a mass flow rate of 2 kg s^{-1} and at a temperature of 25°C. The density and viscosity of the juice at 25°C are 1045 kg m^{-3} and 0.5 Pa s, respectively.

Take $\pi = 22/7$.

The Reynolds number for this flow will be 255.

Reynolds number (Re)
$= \rho Dv/\mu$

D = 2cm = 0.002 m

$\rho = 1045 \text{ kg m}^{-3}$

$\mu = 0.5$ Pa s

9. Shear stress (τ, Pa) and shear rate (γ, s^{-1}) relationship of a pseudoplastic fluid follows the power law equation given by, $\tau = k\gamma^n = 2.6\,\gamma^{0.45}$, where 'n' and 'k' are flow behavior index and consistency index respectively. The apparent viscosity (μ_a) of the fluid at a shear rate $5s^{-1}$ is 1.05 to 1.08 Pa s.

Apparent viscosity (μ_a)
$= k\,|du/dy|^{n-1}$. Du/dy

Where du/dy = τ (shear rate)

10. In a sterilization process, $D_{121.1}$ value of the target organism is 0.22 minute; time required for 99.999% sterilization of the target organism at 121°C will be 1.0 to 1.2 minutes.

11. A centrifuge having diameter of 10 cm is rotating at 10000 rpm.

Take $\pi = 22/7$

and $g = 9.81 \text{ m s}^{-2}$.

The ratio of centrifugal force to gravitational force will be 5590 to 5600.

Ratio = Centrifugal force /Gravitational force
$= mv^2/r/Gm1m2/r^2$

12. Threonine is an α-amino acid. This essential amino acid is classified as polar.

Pyridoxine 5'-phosphate, vitamin B-6, is an essential coenzyme in various transamination, decarboxylation, glycogen hydrolysis, and synthesis pathways involving carbohydrate, sphingolipid, amino acid, heme, and neurotransmitter metabolism.

Xylose is a sugar which is classified as a monosaccharide of the aldopentose type, which means that it contains five carbon atoms and includes a formyl functional group.

Oleic acid is a monounsaturated fatty acid found naturally in many plant and animal products.

13. Iron-deficiency anemia is a common anemia caused by insufficient dietary intake and absorption of iron, and/or iron loss from bleeding which can originate from a range of sources such as the intestinal, uterine or urinary tract.

Osteoporosis is a disease of the bones. Vitamin D and calcium are essential for bone health. Thus insufficient dietary intake of calcium causes osteoporosis.

Chronic Zinc deficiency in humans can cause retarded growth also called as dwarfism.

Goiter is a swelling of the neck or larynx resulting from enlargement of the thyroid gland, associated with a thyroid gland that is functioning properly or not. One of the most common causes of goiter formation worldwide is iodine deficiency.

14. In a counter-current double pipe heat- exchanger, milk is cooled from 110 to 40°C using chilled water as coolant. Water enters at 5°C and leaves at 60°C. Heat flux for the system, with overall heat transfer coefficient of 950 $Wm^{-2}K^{-1}$ will be 39900 to 40000W m^{-2}.

15. Saturated steam at 100°C is injected at 0.2 kg^{-1} into air stream flowing at 3 kg s^{-1} and 25°C. Air contains 0.012 kg moisture per kg dry air. If the atmosphere pressure is 101.1 kPa, absolute humidity of air will be 0.078 to 0.080 kg.

16. In an evaporator, milk is concentrated from 9.8% TSS to 52% TSS. Assume the solutes in the milk are non-volatile. The amount of vapour produced for 100 kg feed will be 81 to 82 kg.

17. Water enters a cylindrical tank at a steady uniform rate of 0.1m^3 s^{-1}; simultaneously water is discharged from the tank through an orifice (area 0.05 m^2) located at the bottom of the tank. Initial level of water n the tank from the bottom is 5m. If the acceleration due to gravity = 9.81 m s^{-2} and coefficient of discharge = 0.30, the final volume of the steady-state height water level from the bottom of tank is 0.55 to 0.58 m.

18. Ascorbic acid dip minimizes the fruit oxidation. The fruit pieces are pretreated by dipping in ascorbic acid. Ascorbic acid (vitamin C) is an antioxidant that keeps fruit from darkening and enhances destruction of bacteria during drying.

Fruits generally are not heat-blanched because the heat causes loss of turgor, resulting in sogginess and juice drainage after thawing.

Deaeration means mechanical removal of dissolved and free gasses from a fluid (by vacuum). Deaeration is a processing step applied immediately before pasteuri-zation to remove air, in particular oxygen, incorporated into orange juice during extraction or mixing. Vitamin C is believed to be the compound the most affected (oxidized) by dissolved oxygen (DO) in orange juice. Thus it minimizes destruction of vitamin C.

Rendering is a process that converts waste animal tissue into stable, value-added materials. Rendering can refer to any processing of animal products into more useful materials, or more narrowly to the rendering of whole animal fatty tissue into purified fats like lard or tallow. Thus rendering causes melting of fat in meat.

19. A chocolate mix at 100°C is flowing through a 2 cm diameter and 4 m long stainless steel tube at 13.2 kg/min. The density of the mix is 1750 kg m^{-3} and its viscosity at 100°C is 2 pa s.

Take $\pi = 22/7$.

The pressure drop for this flow will be 256000 Pa.

20. In a tray dryer, 100 kg of a vegetable material in a suitably reduced form is dried to yield a final product of 75 kg. The dried sample of 5 g, when kept in an oven at 105°C for 24 hours results in 3.56 g of dry matter, the moisture content of the vegetable before drying, in dry basis is 87 to 87.5%.

■■

GATE-2013

XL : LIFE SCIENCES

Time : 3 Hours | *Maximum Marks : 100*

GA : GENERAL APTITUDE

Q. 1 – Q. 5 carry one mark each.

1. If $3 \le X \le 5$ and $8 \le Y \le 11$ then which of the following options is TRUE?

   (*a*) $\frac{3}{5} \le \frac{X}{Y} \le \frac{8}{5}$ (*b*) $\frac{3}{11} \le \frac{X}{Y} \le \frac{5}{8}$

   (*c*) $\frac{3}{11} \le \frac{X}{Y} \le \frac{8}{5}$ (*d*) $\frac{3}{5} \le \frac{X}{Y} \le \frac{8}{11}$

2. The Headmaster _____ to speak to you.

   Which of the following options is incorrect to complete the above sentence?

   (*a*) is wanting (*b*) wants

   (*c*) want (*d*) was wanting

3. Mahatama Gandhi was known for his humility as

   (*a*) he played an important role in humiliating exit of British from India.

   (*b*) he worked for humanitarian causes.

   (*c*) he displayed modesty in his interactions.

   (*d*) he was a fine human being.

4. All engineering students (I) should learn mechanics, (II) mathematics and (III) how to do computation. (IV)

   Which of the above underlined parts of the sentence is not appropriate?

   (*a*) I (*b*) II (*c*) III (*d*) IV

5. Select the pair that best expresses a relationship similar to that expressed in the pair:

   water: pipe::

   (*a*) cart: road (*b*) electricity: wire

   (*c*) sea: beach (*d*) music: instrument

Q. 6 to Q. 10 carry two marks each.

6. Velocity of an object fired directly in upward direction is given by $V = 80 - 32t$, where t (time) is in seconds. When will the velocity be between 32 m/sec and 64 m/sec?

   (*a*) (1, 3/2) (*b*) (1/2, 1) (*c*) (1/2, 3/2) (*d*) (1, 3)

7. In a factory, two machines M1 and M2 manufacture 60% and 40% of the autocomponents respectively. Out of the total production, 2% of M1 and 3% of M2 are found to be defective. If a randomly drawn autocomponent from the combined lot is found defective, what is the probability that it was manufactured by M2?

   (*a*) 0.35 (*b*) 0.45 (*c*) 0.5 (*d*) 0.4

8. Following table gives data on tourists from different countries visiting India in the year 2011.

Country	Number of Tourists
USA	2000
England	3500
Germany	1200
Italy	1100
Japan	2400
Australia	2300
France	1000

   Which two countries contributed to the one third of the total number of tourists who visited India in 2011?

   (*a*) USA and Japan (*b*) USA and Australia

   (*c*) England and France (*d*) Japan and Australia

9. If $|-2X + 9| = 3$ then the possible value of $|-X| - X^2$ would be:

   (*a*) 30 (*b*) – 30 (*c*) – 42 (*d*) 42

10. All professors are researchers

    Some scientists are professors

    Which of the given conclusions is logically valid and is inferred from the above arguments:

    (*a*) All scientists are researchers

    (*b*) All professors are scientists

    (*c*) Some researchers are scientists

    (*d*) No conclusion follows

H : CHEMISTRY (COMPULSORY)

Q. 1 – Q. 5 carry one mark each.

1. $N(CH_3)_3$ and $N(SiH_3)_3$ are congeners, but around N-atom the former has pyramidal geometry whereas the latter is nearly planar. The bonding responsible for planarity of $N(SiH_3)_3$ is

   (*a*) pπ-pπ (*b*) pπ-dπ

   (*c*) dπ-dπ (*d*) δ

2. The type of electronic transition responsible for the yellow colour of K_2CrO_4 is

   (*a*) metal to ligand charge transfer

   (*b*) ligand to metal charge transfer

   (*c*) intra-ligand charge transfer

   (*d*) d-d transition

3. The given equation

$$\left(\frac{d(\Delta H)}{dT}\right)_p = \Delta C_p$$

where H, T and C_p are the enthalpy, temperature and heat capacity at constant pressure, respectively, is called

(*a*) Clausius-Clapeyron equation
(*b*) Hess's law
(*c*) Kirchhoff's equation
(*d*) Trouton's rule

Q.4 - 5 are questions with numerical answer.

4. The number of 2-center–2-electron bonds in anhydrous $AlCl_3$ is __________

5. When dissolved in water, the number of H^+ ions released from a molecule of H_3BO_3 is __________

Q. 6 - Q. 15 carry two marks each.

6. In NaCl crystal, the arrangement and coordination number of the ions are

(*a*) fcc and 6 (*b*) fcc and 4
(*c*) hcp and 6 (*d*) hcp and 4

7. The solubility product (K_{sp}) of $Ca_3(PO_4)_2$ is 1.3×10^{-32}. In a 0.02 M solution of $Ca(NO_3)_2$, the solubility of $Ca_3(PO_4)_2$ (in units of M) is

(*a*) 6.5×10^{-31} (*b*) 1.6×10^{-26}
(*c*) 8.0×10^{-16} (*d*) 4.0×10^{-14}

8. Identify the **CORRECT** product in the following reaction:

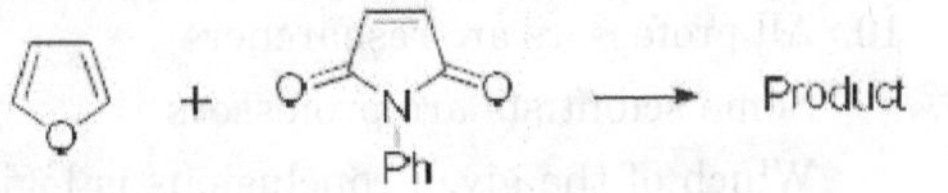

(*a*)
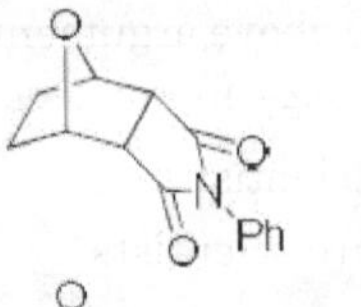
(*b*)
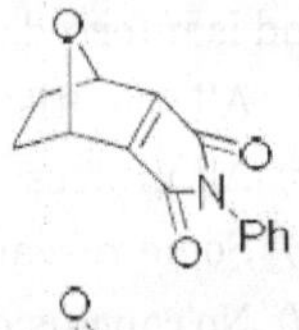
(*c*)
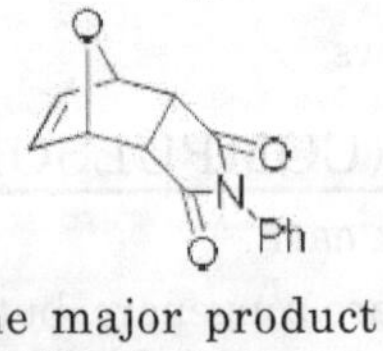
(*d*)
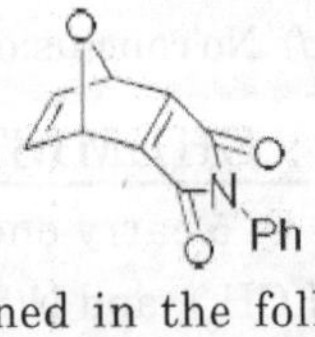

9. The major product obtained in the following reaction is

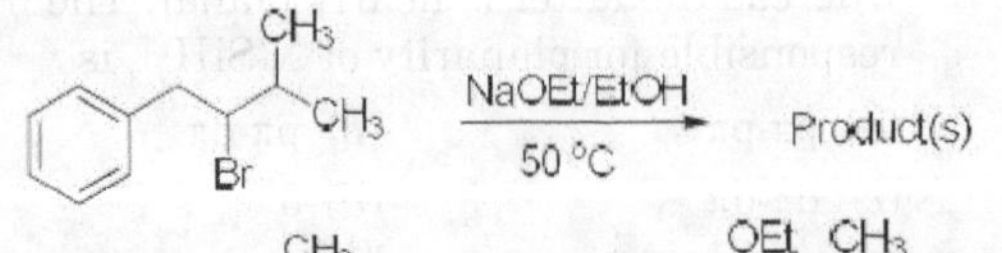

(*a*)
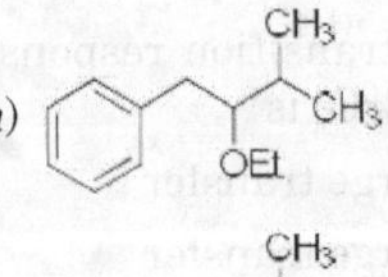
(*b*)
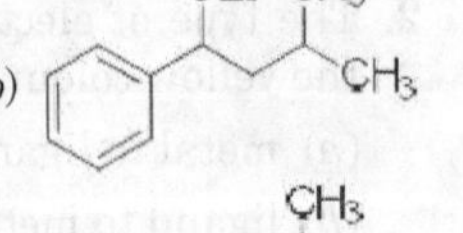
(*c*)
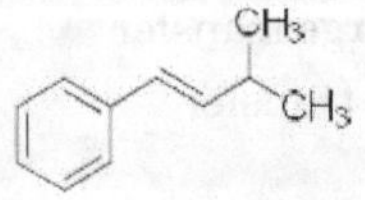
(*d*)
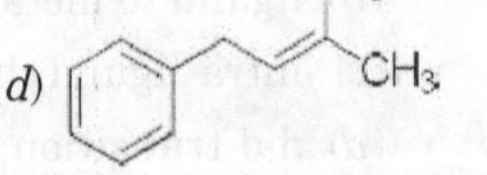

Q.10 - 11 are questions with numerical answer.

10. Iodine forms an anionic species Q in aqueous solution of iodide (I^-). The number of lone pair(s) of electrons on the central atom of Q is __________

11. The rate of a chemical reaction is tripled when the temperature of the reaction is increased from 298 K to 308 K. The activation energy (in kcal $mol^{-1} K^{-1}$, up to one decimal place) for the reaction is (Given R = 1.987cal $mol^{-1} K^{-1}$) __________

Common Data Questions

Common Data for Questions 12 and 13:

Consider the following S_N2 reaction of optically pure 1-chloro-3-ethylcyclopentane (**X**).

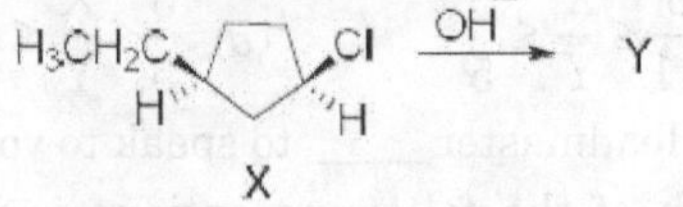

X

12. The structure of Y in the above reaction is

(*a*)
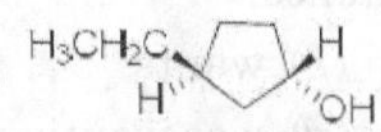
(*b*)
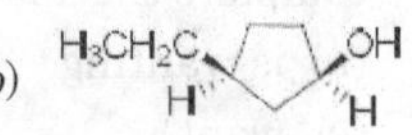
(*c*)
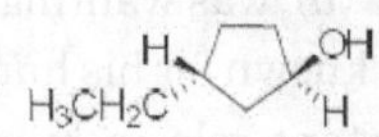
(*d*)
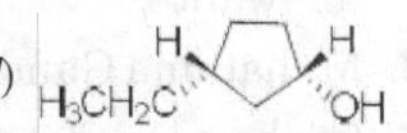

13. The absolute configuration of1-chloro-3-ethylcyclopentane (X) shown above is

(*a*) (1S,3R) (*b*) (1S,3S) (*c*) (1R,3R) (*d*) (1R,3S)

Linked Answer Questions

Statement for Linked Answer Questions 14 and 15:

The molar conductance at infinite dilution of sodium acetate, sodium sulfate and sulfuric acid solutions are 91.0×10^{-4}, 259.8×10^{-4} and 859.3×10^{-4} S m^2 mol^{-1}, respectively.

14. The molar conductance at infinite dilution (in S m^2 mol^{-1})of acetic acid is

(*a*) 1028×10^{-4} (*b*) 820.4×10^{-4}
(*c*) 690.5×10^{-4} (*d*) 390.8×10^{-4}

15. If the molar conductance of an acetic acid solution is 15.2×10^{-4} Sm^2 mol^{-1},then the percentage (%) dissociation of acetic acid in the solution will be

(*a*) 3.89 (*b*) 2.20
(*c*) 1.85 (*d*) 1.48

I : BIOCHEMISTRY

Q. 1 – Q. 10 carry one mark each.

1. Which one of the following statements is **TRUE** when a cell is kept in a hypotonic solution?

(*a*) Water moves out of the cell
(*b*) Size of the cell remains same
(*c*) No movement of water takes place
(*d*) Size of the cell increases

2. Which one of the following amino acids has a higher propensity for *cis* peptide bond formation?

(*a*) Histidine (*b*) Cysteine
(*c*) Glycine (*d*) Proline

3. The length of an α-helix composed of 36 amino acid residues is
(*a*) 10 Å (*b*) 54 Å (*c*) 27 Å (*d*) 360 Å

4. The order *n* for a given substrate concen-tration in an enzyme catalyzed reaction following Michaelis-Menten kinetics, is
(*a*) $n = 1$ (*b*) $n = 0$
(*c*) *n* is not defined (*d*) $0 \leq n \leq 1$

5. Which one of the following amino acid residues is specifically recognised by chymotrypsin during peptide bond cleavage?
(*a*) Phe (*b*) Leu (*c*) Val (*d*) Asp

6. The terminal electron acceptor during mitochondrial respiration is
(*a*) O_2 (*b*) FAD^+ (*c*) NAD^+ (*d*) ATP

7. During the biosynthesis of urea in the urea cycle, the two nitrogen atoms are derived from
(*a*) Two free ammonium groups
(*b*) Free ammonium group and aspartate
(*c*) Both nitrogen atoms are derived from arginine
(*d*) One nitrogen atom is derived from citrulline and one from glutamate.

8. An enzyme has two binding sites for an inhibitor molecule. When the inhibitor binds to the first site, the dissociation constant of the inhibitor for the second site increases, leading to negative co-operativity. The Hill coefficient for such an inhibitor is
(*a*) equal to one (*b*) greater than one
(*c*) less than one (*d*) less than zero

9. An oligonucleotide was sequenced by the dideoxy method of Sanger and the following autoradiogram was obtained

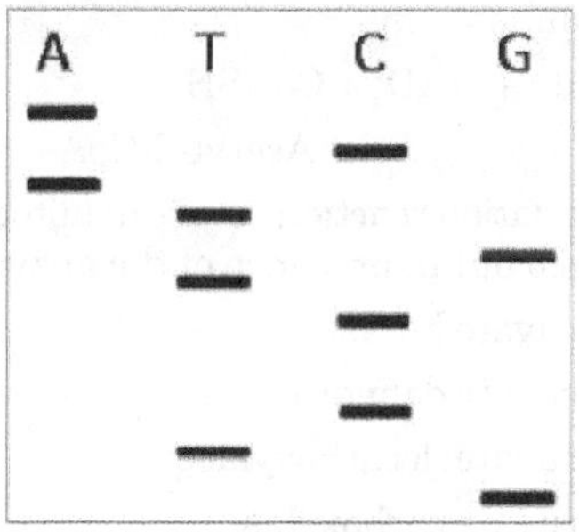

The sequence of the oligonucleotide is
(*a*) 3'-GTCCTGTACA-5' (*b*) 5'-GTCCTGTACA-3'
(*c*) 5'-ACATGTCCTG-3' (*d*) 3'-AATTTCCCGG-5'

10. In different types of tissue transplantations, the rate of graft rejection in decreasing order is
(*a*) Isograft > Xenograft > Allograft
(*b*) Allograft > Isograft > Xenograft
(*c*) Xenograft > Autograft > Allograft
(*d*) Xenograft > Allograft > Isograft

Q. 11 - Q. 20 carry two marks each.

11. You have prepared 1.0 liter of 0.5 M acetate buffer (pH = 5.0). The dissociation constant of acetic acid is 1.7×10^{-5} M. What would be the acetate ion concentration in the buffer?
(*a*) 0.1 M (*b*) 0.25 M (*c*) 0.315 M (*d*) 0.415 M

12. The following figures show the plot of reaction rate versus substrate concentration (mM) for an enzyme catalyzed reaction in the presence and absence of an inhibitor. Match the possible reaction types with the plots.
(P) Competitive inhibition
(Q) Substrate inhibition
(R) Michaelis-Menten
(S) Non-competitive inhibition

(i)

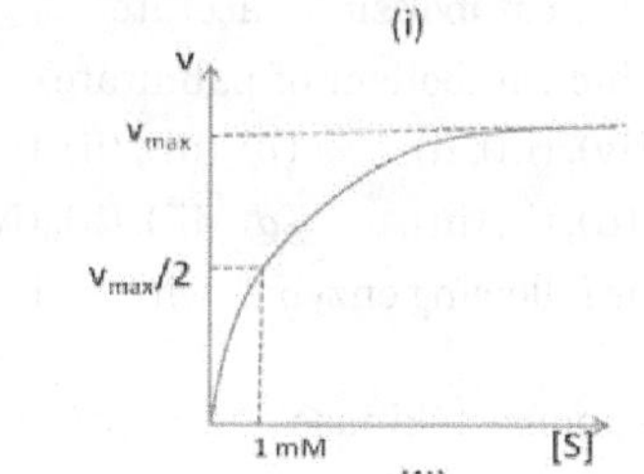

(ii)

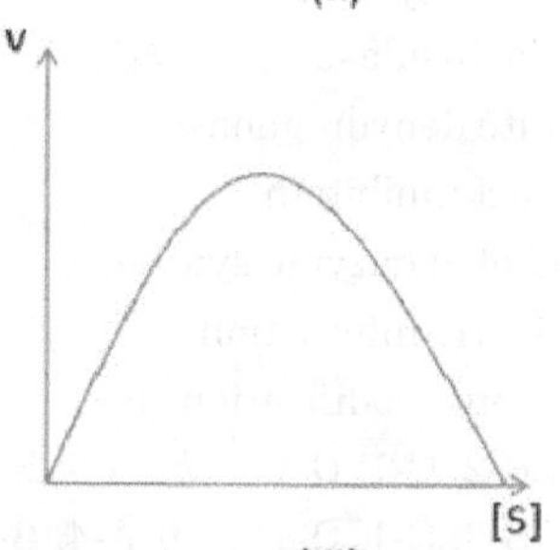

(iii)

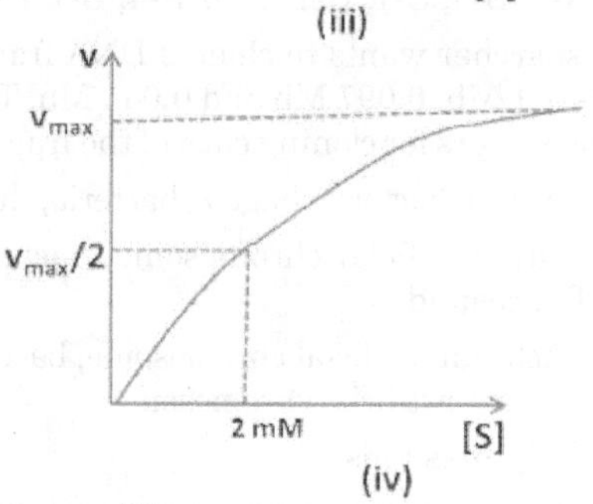

(iv)

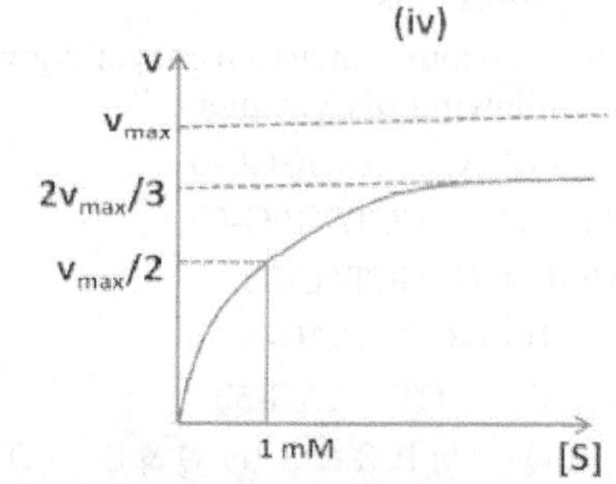

(*a*) P – i, Q – iii, R – ii, S – iv
(*b*) P – iii, Q – ii, R – i, S – iv
(*c*) P – iii, Q – iv, R – i, S – ii
(*d*) P – iv, Q – ii, R – i, S – iii

13. Arrange the following in the decreasing order of their permeability coefficients across a lipid bilayer membrane.

(i) Urea (ii) Glucose
(iii) H2O (iv) Na+
(v) Tryptophan

(*a*) (i), (iii), (v), (ii), (iv) (*b*) (iii), (v), (ii), (iv), (i)
(*c*) (iii), (i), (v), (ii), (iv) (*d*) (i), (iii), (iv), (v), (ii)

14. Arrange the following in the increasing order of amount of ATP generated by metabolism of one molecule of the following compounds.

(i) Anaerobic catabolism of starch with 300 glucose units
(ii) Aerobic catabolism of glucose
(iii) Aerobic catabolism of acetate
(iv) Aerobic catabolism of palmitate

(*a*) (ii), (iv), (iii), (i) (*b*) (iii), (ii), (i), (iv)
(*c*) (iv), (ii), (i), (iii) (*d*) (iii), (ii), (iv), (i)

15. Match the following enzymes with their regulatory mechanism

A. Phosphofructokinase
B. Glycogen synthase
C. β-galactosidase
D. Lactate dehydrogenase
1. Product inhibition
2. Control of enzyme synthesis
3. Allosteric interaction
4. Covalent modification

(*a*) A-3, B-2, C-1, D-4 (*b*) A-3, B-4, C-2, D-1
(*c*) A-4, B-3, C-1, D-4 (*d*) A-4, B-1, C-2, D-3

16. A researcher wants to clone 3 DNA fragments of sizes 1.1 Mb, 0.097 Mb and 0.045 Mb. The choice of the vectors for cloning each of the fragments are

(*a*) Cosmid, bacteriophage λ, bacteriop-hage P1
(*b*) Yeast artificial chromosome, bacteriop-hage P1, cosmid
(*c*) Bacterial artificial chromosome, bacteriophage λ, yeast artificial chromosome
(*d*) Only plasmids

17. Which of the four restriction enzymes given below cut the following DNA sequence?

5'-CCGATATCTCGAGGGC-3'

(P) BamH1 (3'-CCTAG^G-5')
(Q) XhoI (3'-GAGCT^C-5')
(R) EcoRI (3'-CTTAA^G-5')
(S) EcoRV (3'-CTA^TAG-5')

(*a*) P & Q (*b*) P, R & S (*c*) Q & S (*d*) P & R

18. You have expressed the following protein that has an isoelectric point of 6.0. The best order of protein purification methodologies to obtain a pure protein is?

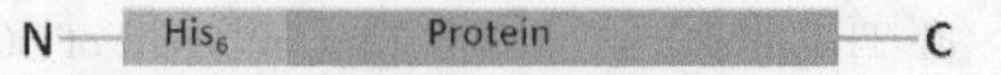

(*a*) Gel filtration chromatography, Anion exchange chromatography at pH = 4.0, Ammonium sulphate precipitation
(*b*) Cation exchange chromatography at pH = 9.0, Ni-affinity chromatography, Gel filtration chromatography
(*c*) Anion exchange chromatography at pH = 8.0, Ni-affinity chromatography, Gel filtration chromatography
(*d*) Ammonium sulphate precipitation, Anion exchange chromatography at pH = 4.0, Niaffinity chromatography

19. An enzyme of 40 kDa is added to a substrate solution in a molar ratio of 1:3. The concentration of the enzyme in the mixture is 12 mg/ml. What would be the corresponding substrate concentration?

(*a*) 0.4 mM (*b*) 0.12 mM
(*c*) 0.9 mM (*d*) 0.3 mM

20. A patient suffering from pneumonia and tuberculosis was found to have very low CD4$^+$ T cells. In all probability the **PRIMARY** causative infectious agent belongs to

(*a*) Klebsiella family (*b*) Mycobacterium family
(*c*) Retrovirus family (*d*) Streptococcus family

J : BOTANY

Q. 1 – Q. 10 carry one mark each.

1. Bast fibres are present in

(*a*) Xylem (*b*) Phloem
(*c*) Collenchyma (*d*) Parenchyma

2. During cellular respiratory process, pyruvate must be oxidized to acetyl CoA and CO_2 before it enters the citric acid cycle. The corresponding simplified equation is

Pyruvate + NAD$^+$ + CoASH
$\longrightarrow$ Acetyl-S-CoA+ NADH + CO_2

This oxidation reaction occurs in mitochondria and is carried out in presence of the enzyme

(*a*) Pyruvate kinase
(*b*) Pyruvate dehydrogenase
(*c*) Pyruvate decarboxylase
(*d*) Pyruvate carboxylase

3. Which one of the following statements having the terms - gene, chromosome and genome is **CORRECT**?

(*a*) The rice gene contains about 50,000 genomes located on 12 different chromosomes
(*b*) The rice genome contains about 50,000 genes located on 12 different chromosomes
(*c*) The rice chromosome contains about 50,000 genes located on 12 different genomes
(*d*) The rice genome contains about 50,000 chromosomes located on 12 different genes

4. The aflatoxin found in post-harvested grains is injurious to health due to
   (*a*) *Aspergillus* (*b*) *Alternaria*
   (*c*) *Fusarium* (*d*) *Phytopthora*
5. Identify the event that exclusively occurs in meiotic cell division
   (*a*) Chromatid formation
   (*b*) Spindle formation
   (*c*) Synapsis
   (*d*) Chromosome movement to pole
6. In the symbiotic nitrogen fixation process, Leghemoglobin present in the nodule helps in fixing nitrogen in presence of the enzyme
   (*a*) Nitrate synthetase
   (*b*) Nitrate synthase
   (*c*) Glutathione synthetase
   (*d*) Nitrogenase
7. Considering environment and ecosystem, identify the **INCORRECT** statement
   (*a*) In detrital food chain, it is very difficult to measure the energy flow although the use of radioactive tracers give some idea about the energy flow
   (*b*) The change in species composition, community structure and function over time is ecological succession
   (*c*) The slower rise of environmental temperature may be attributed to the increase in pollution in environment which reflects enough solar energy back to other spacer to slow down global warming
   (*d*) Photoperiodism has no relation with the environment and ecosystem, rather it is a biological event taking place in every plant
8. The two enzymes commonly used for isolation of protoplasts from plants are
   (*a*) Cellulase and Lipase
   (*b*) Cellulase and Amylase
   (*c*) Pectinase and Cellulase
   (*d*) Pectinase and Lipase
9. For successful transfer of a foreign gene from the engineered Ti-plasmid to the plant genome, few *cis*-acting DNA elements and *trans*-acting protein factors are very much essential. Select the **CORRECT** combination from the following
   (*a*) Opine catabolism genes, Left border sequence, Right border sequence
   (*b*) Opine catabolism genes, Left border sequence, Virulence genes
   (*c*) Hormone biosynthetic genes, Right border sequence, Virulence genes
   (*d*) Left border sequence, Right border sequence, Virulence genes
10. In naturally occurring cytoplasmic male sterility, the molecular determinant is located in
   (*a*) Chloroplast
   (*b*) Endoplasmic reticulum
   (*c*) Golgi complex
   (*d*) Mitochondria

Q. 11 - Q. 20 carry two marks each.

11. Identify the floral formula with the family and the corresponding plant species

General Floral Formula

P. $\oplus$ ⚥ $P_{0\text{ or }2\text{-}3}, A_{3\text{ or }3+3}, \underline{G_{1\text{ or }(3)}}$

Q. $\oplus$ ♂ $P_{3+3}, A_{3+3\text{ or }3}$ / $\oplus$ $P_{3+3}, \underline{G_{(3)}}$

R. $\oplus$ ⚥ $P_{3+3}, A_{3+3}, \underline{G_{(3)}}$

S. $\cdot|\cdot$ ⚥ $P_{3+3}, A_{6\text{ or }5}, G_{(3)}$

Family	**Plant**
1. Liliaceae	i. *Cocos nucifera*
2. Cannaceae	ii. *Musa paradisiaca*
3. Graminae (Poaceae)	iii. *Maranta bicolor*
4. Palmae (Arecaceae)	iv. *Canna indica*
5. Musaceae	v. *Allium cepa*
6. Marantaceae	vi. *Oryza sativa*

   (*a*) P-1-iv, Q-2-iii, R-6-i, S-4-ii
   (*b*) P-2-v, Q-4-vi, R-3-iii, S-5-iv
   (*c*) P-3-v, Q-6-iii, R-5-i, S-2-ii
   (*d*) P-3-vi, Q-4-i, R-1-v, S-5-ii
12. A plant of genotype *GGHH* is crossed with another plant of the genotype *gghh*. If the F_1 is test crossed, what percentage (%) of the test cross progeny will have the genotype *gghh* when the two genes are - (P) unlinked, (Q) completely linked with no crossing over, (R) 10 m.u. (genetic map unit) apart, (S) 24 m.u. apart?
   (*a*) P-25, Q-25, R-25, S-25
   (*b*) P-25, Q-50, R-45, S-38
   (*c*) P-50, Q-50, R-90, S-76
   (*d*) P-25, Q-50, R-10, S-24
13. Which two of the following are the **CORRECT** statements ?
   P. Nondisjunction in the parental meiosis is not essential to produce diploid organisms
   Q. Nondisjunction in the parental meiosis is essential to produce aneuploid organisms
   R. Nondisjunction in the parental meiosis is essential to produce hexaploid organisms
   S. Nondisjunction in the parental meiosis is essential to produce tetraploid organisms
   (*a*) P,Q (*b*) Q,R
   (*c*) R,S (*d*) P,S

14. Identify the correct matching by taking one item from each column

Column -I	Column -II
P. Morphine	1. Cinchona officinalis
Q. Nicotine	2. Hyoscyamus niger
R. Atropine	3. Papaver somniferum
S. Vinblastine	4. Nicotiana tabacum
	5. Coffea arabica
	6. Catharanthus roseus

Column -III

i. Antineoplastic
ii. Respiratory paralysis
iii. Antibacterial
iv. Narcotic analgesic
v. Anticholinergic
vi. Antifungal

(*a*) P-1-*i*, Q-2-*ii*, R-3-*iii*, S-4-*iv*
(*b*) P-2-*iii*, Q-3-*i*, R-1-*iv*, S-5-*v*
(*c*) P-3-*iv*, Q-4-*ii*, R-2-*v*, S-6-*i*
(*d*) P-4-*iii*, Q-1-*v*, R-5-*i*, S-2-*vi*

15. Which two of the following are the **INCORRECT** statements ?

P. All plants fix CO_2 by the action of ribulose biphosphate carboxylase. The reaction occurs in the bundle sheath of C_4 plants

Q. All plants fix CO_2 by the action of ribulose biphosphate carboxylase. The reaction occurs in the mesophyll cells of C_4 plants

R. Phosphoenol pyruvate + $CO_2 \rightarrow$ Oxaloacetate + Pi, catalyzed by the enzyme phosphoenol pyruvate carbxylase occurs in the mesophyll cells of C_4 plants

S. Phosphoenol pyruvate + $CO_2 \rightarrow$ Oxaloacetate + Pi, catalyzed by the enzyme phosphoenol pyruvate dehydrogenase occurs in the mesophyll cells of C_4 plants

(*a*) P,Q (*b*) Q,R (*c*) Q,S (*d*) P,R

16. Select the **CORRECT** set comprising only the synthetic analogues of auxin and cytokinin

(*a*) IAA and Kinetin (*b*) 2, 4-D and Zeatin
(*c*) IAA and Zeatin (*d*) 2, 4-D and Kinetin

17. Which two of the following are the **INCORRECT** statements ?

P. In monocotyledonous stems with closed vascular bundle, secondary growth takes place without any cambium

Q. In dicotyledonous stems hypodermis is collenchymatous

R. Mobilization of storage reserves takes place during post-germination of embryo

S. Osborne's classification of seed storage proteins is based upon solubility in *n*-hexane

(*a*) P,R (*b*) Q,S (*c*) Q,R (*d*) P,S

18. Identify two **CORRECT** characteristic features of (P) Autogamy and (Q) Allogamy from the following statements

1. Plant species usually does not depend on external agents
2. Plant species usually depends on external agents
3. Plant species normally produces progeny that are healthier and better adapted in nature
4. Plant species normally produces weaker progeny in several generations

(*a*) P-1,3; Q-2,4 (*b*) P-2,4; Q-1,3
(*c*) P-1,4; Q-2,3 (*d*) P-2,3; Q-1,4

19. Identify the correct matching by taking one item from each column

Column-I

P. Coenzyme
Q. Holoenzyme
R. Prosthetic group
S. Apoenzyme

Column-II

1. Holoenzyme + Apoenzyme
2. Non-protein part in anactive enzyme
3. Only the proteinpart in an active enzyme
4. Cofactor in an enzymatic reaction
5. Apoenzyme + Prosthetic group
6. Holoenzyme + inorganic phosphate

(*a*) P-4 Q-5 R-2 S-3
(*b*) P-4 Q-3 R-1 S-2
(*c*) P-4 Q-3 R-5 S-6
(*d*) P-4 Q-1 R-3 S-5

20. Identify two **CORRECT** statements from the following which are related to the ion transportation in the root system of plant

P. The proton pumps and H^+-pyrophospha-tase appear to work in anti-parallel with the vacuolar ATPase to create a proton gradient across the tonoplast

Q. Calcium is one of the important ion whose concentration is strongly regulated by the concentration of apoplastic spaces in the millimolar level

R. Solute move through both apoplast and symplast, and xylem parenchyma cells participate in xylem loading

S. The limitation of Nerst equation for relating the membrane potential to the distribution of ion at equilibrium is that it cannot distinguish between active and passive transport

(*a*) P,S (*b*) Q,R (*c*) R,S (*d*) Q,S

K : MICROBIOLOGY

Q. 1 – Q. 10 carry one mark each.

1. In 1976, Tonegawa's experiment gave clue about gene rearrangement during differentiation of B-cells. The two different types of cells used in this experiment were
   (*a*) HeLa cells and fibrosarcoma cells
   (*b*) embryonic cells and fibroblasts
   (*c*) adult myeloma cells and HeLa cells
   (*d*) embryonic cells and adult myeloma cells
2. To which one of the following groups, the antibiotics kanamycin, streptomycin and gentamicin belong
   (*a*) cephalosporins (*b*) macrolides
   (*c*) aminoglycosides (*d*) quinolones
3. Shine Dalgarno's sequence present in mRNA binds to
   (*a*) 3′ end of rRNA (*b*) 5′ end of rRNA
   (*c*) 5′ end of tRNA (*d*) 3′ end of tRNA
4. Which one of the following transport mechanism is **NOT** employed by prokaryotes?
   (*a*) Passive diffusion (*b*) Group translocation
   (*c*) Endocytosis (*d*) Active transport
5. The most common indicator organism of faecal pollution in water is
   (*a*) *Clostridium botulinum*
   (*b*) *Bacillus subtilis*
   (*c*) *Escherichia coli*
   (*d*) *Clostridium tetani*
6. The theoretical maximum number of ATP molecules produced from aerobic oxidation of glucose by eukaryotic cells is
   (*a*) 38 (*b*) 24 (*c*) 12 (*d*) 8
7. Which one of the following **DO NOT** use water as an electron source during photosynthesis?
   (*a*) Sulfate reducing bacteria
   (*b*) Methanogenic bacteria
   (*c*) Green and purple bacteria
   (*d*) Nitrifying bacteria
8. If the radius of a spherical coccus is 0.8 μm, the value of $\frac{surface\ area}{volume}$ in μm^{-1} will be
   (*a*) 7.45 (*b*) 4.05 (*c*) 3.75 (*d*) 0.85
9. The enzyme that catalyzes the reduction of nitrogen to ammonia is
   (*a*) nitrogenase (*b*) nitrate reductase
   (*c*) nitrite reductase (*d*) deaminase
10. Chemostat is a continuous culture system in which sterile medium is fed into the culture vessel at the same rate as the spent medium is removed. If in a chemostat culture, the flow rate is 30 ml h^{-1} and volume of the medium inside the vessel is 100 ml, the dilution rate in h^{-1} is
   (*a*) 3.33 (*b*) 1.50 (*c*) 0.75 (*d*) 0.30

Q. 11 - Q. 20 carry two marks each.

11. In an experiment the structural genes *lacZYA*of *lac* operon were found to be constitutively expressed. The following explanations were given for the constitutive expression
   (P) absence of a functional repressor due to mutation in the repressor gene *lacI*
   (Q) mutation in the operator that can no longer bind the repressor
   (R) mutation in the *lacA*gene
   Which of the following is **CORRECT**
   (*a*) Only P (*b*) Only Q
   (*c*) Both P & Q (*d*) Only R
12. Which one of the following is **TRUE** about siderophores in bacteria?
   (*a*) Siderophores are secreted only when soluble iron is available in the medium
   (*b*) Siderophores form complex with ferrous ions in the medium
   (*c*) Siderophores are the only route of iron uptake
   (*d*) Siderophores form complex with ferric ions in the medium
13. In a population containing fast and slow growing bacteria, the slow growing bacteria can be enriched by supplementing the medium with
   (*a*) chloramphenicol
   (*b*) penicillin
   (*c*) penicillin & chloramphenicol
   (*d*) rifampin
14. When the supply of tryptophan is plentiful, the tryptophan operon is repressed because the
   (*a*) repressor protein-corepressor complex is bound at the operator
   (*b*) repressor protein is synthesized in large quantity
   (*c*) repressor-corepressor complex is not formed
   (*d*) repressor becomes inactive and therefore has reduced specificity for the operator
15. Match the scientists in **Group I** with their contributions in microbiology in **Group II**
   Group I
   P. Robert Hooke
   Q. Paul Ehrlich
   R. Antony van Leeuwenhoek
   S. Sergei Winogradsky
   Group II
   I. Proved that microbes can cause diseases
   II. First to observe cells
   III. First to observe bacteria
   IV. Used the first synthetic chemothera-peutic agent
   V. Linked specific bacteria to biogeoche-mical transformations
   (*a*) P-I, Q-II, R-III, S-V (*b*) P-II, Q-IV, R-III, S-V
   (*c*) P-II, Q-I, R-III, S-IV (*d*) P-V, Q-III, R-IV, S-II

16. Match the infectious agents in **Group I** with the associated diseases in **Group II**

Group I	**Group II**
P. *Bordetellapertusis*	I. Mumps
Q. *Mycobacterium leprae*	II. Meningitis
R. *Haemophilusinfluenzae*	III. Tuberculosis
S. *Rubella*	IV. Whooping cough
	V. Hansen's disease

(*a*) P-IV, Q-V, R-II, S-I (*b*) P-V, Q-III, R-I, S-IV
(*c*) P-I, Q-III, R-V, S-IV (*d*) P-III, Q-II, R-V, S-I

17. Match the microscopes in **Group I** with their working principles in **Group II**

Group I
P. Phase contrast
Q. Dark field
R. Bright field
S. Electron microscopy

Group II
I. Light reaches the specimen only from the sides
II. Uses fluorescent dyes
III. Difference in the refractive index of cells from their surrounding medium
IV. Difference in contrast between specimen and its surrounding medium
V. Uses electrons instead of photons as energy source

(*a*) P-V, Q-II, R-III, S-V (*b*) P-III, Q-I, R-IV, S-V
(*c*) P-III, Q-II, R-V, S-I (*d*) P-II, Q-I, R-III, S-V

18. In a phenol coefficient test for determining the efficacy of a disinfectant **X**, the maximum effective dilution for **X** and phenol was found to be 1/450 and 1/90, respectively. Calculate the phenol coefficient for **X**.
(*a*) 10.0 (*b*) 5.0 (*c*) 1.0 (*d*) 0.2

19. How many electrons are accepted when sulfate acts as the terminal electron acceptor in bacteria such as *Desulfovibrio*?
(*a*) 8 (*b*) 6 (*c*) 4 (*d*) 2

20. A bacterial population increases from 10^3 cells to 10^9 cells in 10 h. Calculate the number of generations per hour.
(*a*) 20 (*b*) 10 (*c*) 4 (*d*) 2

L : ZOOLOGY

Q. 1 – Q. 10 carry one mark each.

1. Which one of the following provides the strongest support for the theory of "descent with modification"?
(*a*) Early embryonic forms of diverse organisms (examples: fishes, birds and mammals) appear similar
(*b*) Ability of fishes and whales to swim
(*c*) Variation in flower colour in a given species
(*d*) Skin colour variation among individuals in a human population

2. Which one of the following is an example of sympatric speciation?
(*a*) Origin of new species among wasps that pollinate figs
(*b*) Emergence of a new species among finches that migrated to an island and thus isolated from their ancestors
(*c*) Evolution of birds' and bats' wings
(*d*) Speciation of squirrels separated by a wide river

3. The primary difference between glycogen and cellulose is in the
(*a*) types of constituent monosaccharides
(*b*) number of monomers per molecule
(*c*) configuration of the monomers
(*d*) susceptibility to acid hydrolysis

4. Control mechanisms operate at any of the several steps involved in gene expression. Which one of the following is the key mode of regulation during the cell cycle?
(*a*) Transcription
(*b*) mRNA processing
(*c*) Activation of protein function resulting from protein-protein interaction
(*d*) mRNA export

5. Testicular feminization syndrome is a genetic condition wherein an individual with a XY genotype will have an external female-like phenotype. This is caused by
(*a*) Functional loss of androgen receptor
(*b*) Increased production of estrogen and its receptor
(*c*) Functional loss of Mullerian inhibiting hormone
(*d*) Functional loss of androgen receptor and Mullerian inhibiting hormone

6. Which one of the following defects do you expect to see if you were able to specifically block apoptosis in the developing limb bud of a frog embryo?
(*a*) The digits will remain connected through a web-like extension
(*b*) The bones will not form, and the limb would look like a paddle
(*c*) The limb would look normal but would be larger in size
(*d*) The anterior-posterior polarity of the limb will be lost

7. The formation of antigen-antibody complex helps in disposing antigen through the following pathways EXCEPT:
(*a*) Neutralizing the antigen by blocking its activity
(*b*) By directly hydrolyzing the antigen
(*c*) By promoting the precipitation of antigen
(*d*) By activating cell lysis pathway

8. The term "ecological succession" refers to:
   (*a*) A process wherein newer species populate a region that was devoid of flora and fauna
   (*b*) A transition phase wherein one particular set of species is replaced by another set of species
   (*c*) Changes in the community due to a disturbance in the habitat
   (*d*) All the above
9. Which one of the following options provide example for the term "habituation" in behavioral ecology?
   (*a*) A fish transferred to a fish tank startles initially for a hand clap, but not later
   (*b*) Migratory birds from the temperate zone migrating towards the tropical part during the winters
   (*c*) Adult kingfisher birds are more successful in catching fishes than their younger siblings
   (*d*) Female lizard getting used to a new male lizard during the courtship period
10. Among the following cell structure-function pairs, identify the correctly paired one
   (*a*) Microvilli – engulfment of foreign bodies
   (*b*) Cytoskeleton – cell migration
   (*c*) Peroxisomes – cellular respiration
   (*d*) Nucleolus – mRNA transcription

Q. 11 - Q. 20 carry two marks each.

11. Which of the following most accurately states the goal of systematics?
   (*a*) Classification scheme should reflect phylogenetic relationship
   (*b*) All animals should be classified based on the relatedness at the early embryonic stage
   (*c*) All animals should be grouped based on DNA sequence data
   (*d*) Classification of animals should be based on morphological characters
12. Among the following options, choose the one that is probably a cause of rapid diversification of animal groups during the Cambrian explosion.
   (*a*) Adaptation of organisms to live in the salty environment of ocean
   (*b*) Emergence of coelom
   (*c*) The movement of animals to land
   (*d*) The accumulation of sufficient atmosp-heric oxygen to support the metabolism of actively moving animals
13. A newly discovered, recessively-inherited disease-susceptibility trait (DS) is observed only in cotton plants with white flowers, although the flower colour (R) and DS are independently inherited. In a breeding programme, one variety that is homozygous for the absence of DS, but heterozygous for R was mated to another having white flowers but heterozygous for DS. What is the probability that a given plant among the cross progeny will be susceptible to the disease?
   (*a*) 25 % (*b*) 12.5 % (*c*) 75 % (*d*) 0 %
14. In a new species of moth, the genes for body colour (black, *B*, is dominant over grey, *b*), wing size (normal wing, *W*, is dominant over vestigial, *w*) and eye colour (red, *R*, is dominant over white, *r*) are linked. In this species, only one cross-over event has been observed between any two homologous chromosomes during meiosis. In a cross between *BB; ww* and *bb; WW*, 5 % of the progeny were black with normal wings. In a separate cross between *RR; WW* and *rr; ww*, 15 % of the progeny were red-eyed with vestigial wings. In a third cross between *BB; rr* and *bb; RR*, 10 % of the progeny were black-coloured with red eyes. Which among the following is the correct order of these three genetic loci?
   (*a*) Body colour – Eye colour – Wing size
   (*b*) Eye colour – wing size – Body colour
   (*c*) Wing size – Body colour – Eye colour
   (*d*) Eye colour – Body colour – Wing size
15. In vertebrates, the variations in the structure and function of nephrons are directly linked to the osmoregulatory requirements of the organisms depending on the habitats they live in. From the options given below, identify the correct combination that truly represents the adaptation seen in desert mammals:
   i. Long loops of Henle
   ii. Short loop of Henle
   iii. Hyperosmotic urine
   iv. Large volume of urine
   v. Removal of nitrogen as uric acid
   (*a*) Options *i* and *iii* (*b*) Options *ii* and *iii*
   (*c*) Options *i* and *iv* (*d*) Options *i* and *v*
16. In *Drosophila*, mutations in homeotic genes result in which one of the following developmental defects?
   (*a*) The anterior portion of the embryo will not develop
   (*b*) Several segments in the anterior region of the embryo will be lost
   (*c*) Segmentation will be lost, and the embryo will have only one segment
   (*d*) Segment-specific identities will be lost
17. Retroviruses, like the influenza virus, escape the detection of pre-existing antibodies in the host by generating surface antigen variants. They do so:
   (*a*) By editing the surface antigen post-translationally
   (*b*) Because RNA polymerase of these viruses display high mutation rate during RNA synthesis
   (*c*) Because the surface antigens are attacked by the proteases present in the host cell
   (*d*) Because DNA polymerase of the host mutates the viral genome in the infected cell

18. The relative number of individuals in each age group is an important demographic factor for the study of future growth trends, and this is normally depicted in the form of an age-structure pyramid. Based on your understanding on population dynamics, match the following distribution properties of age structure (Group 1) with the individual forecast given (Group 2):

Group 1

I. Uniform age distribution in the pyramid
II. Distribution skewed towards younger age groups
III. Distribution skewed towards older age groups
IV. Reduction in the number of males in the middle age group

Group 2

i. Emigration in the recent past and the possible increase in the older age groups in the near future.
ii. Likely to be a stable population
iii. Possible unemployment in the near future
iv. Increased government expenditure on medical needs and social security related issues in the near future

(*a*) I – *iii*; II – *ii*; III– *i*; IV – *iv*
(*b*) I – *ii*; II – *iii*; III – *iv*; IV – *i*
(*c*) I – *ii*; II – *i*; III – *iii*; IV – *iv*
(*d*) I – *i*; II – *iii*; III – *ii*; IV – *iv*

19. Like any other trait, animal behavior also evolves by natural selection. Which one of the following examples is NOT true with regard to the evolution of behavior by natural selection?
(*a*) The behavioral trait is determined only by genes
(*b*) The behavioral trait varies within the population of that species
(*c*) The reproductive success partly dependent upon the behavioral trait
(*d*) The behavioral trait is influenced by the genotype

20. Among the following molecular process-biological effect pairs, identify the mismatched pair.
(*a*) Histone deacetylation – activation of gene expression
(*b*) Protein phosphorylation – signal transduction
(*c*) DNA methylation – sex-specific control of gene expression
(*d*) Proteolytic cleavage – activation of signaling by peptide hormones

M: FOOD TECHNOLOGY

Q. 1 – Q. 10 carry one mark each.

1. Kawashiorkor disease is caused due to the deficiency of
(*a*) lysine
(*b*) unsaturated fatty acids
(*c*) vitamin K
(*d*) protein

2. Which of the following statements is TRUE in case of oxidative rancidity of vegetable oils and fats?
(*a*) It is caused by the reaction of saturated fatty acids and oxygen
(*b*) It involves polymerization of fatty acids
(*c*) It is caused by the reaction of unsaturated fatty acids with oxygen
(*d*) It is caused by oxidative enzymes

3. The food borne disease, Q fever is caused by the organism
(*a*) *Clostridium perfringens*
(*b*) *Coxiella burnetti*
(*c*) *Bacillus cereus*
(*d*) *Staphylococcus aureus*

4. The primary bacterial spoilage of poultry meat at low temperature, with characteristic sliminess at outer surface, is caused by
(*a*) *Pseudomonas spp.* (*b*) *Aspergillus spp.*
(*c*) *Bacillus spp.* (*d*) *Candida spp.*

5. The weight gain (in gram) per gram protein consumed is called
(*a*) Net Protein Ratio (NPR)
(*b*) Biological Value (BV)
(*c*) Protein Efficiency Ratio (PER)
(*d*) Chemical Score (CS)

6. Which of the following carbohydrates is NOT classified as dietary fibre?
(*a*) Agar (*b*) Pectin
(*c*) Sodium alginate (*d*) Tapioca starch

7. In the extruder barrel, the compression is achieved by back pressure created by the die and by
(*a*) increasing pitch and decreasing diameter of the screw
(*b*) using the tapered barrel with constant pitch
(*c*) increase in the clearance between barrel surface and screw
(*d*) opening of the die

8. The brown colour of bread crust during baking is due to Maillard reaction between
(*a*) aldehyde groups of sugars and amino groups of proteins
(*b*) aldehyde groups of sugars and vitamins
(*c*) aldehyde groups of sugars and salt
(*d*) starch and yeast

9. Blanching influences vegetable tissues in terms of
(*a*) enzymes production
(*b*) alteration of cytoplasmic membrane
(*c*) stabilization of cytoplasmic proteins
(*d*) stabilization of nuclear proteins

10. When garlic is cut or processed, the crushed garlic odour is due to the formation of

(*a*) diacetyl (*b*) diallyl disulfide
(*c*) ethyl butyrate (*d*) benzaldehyde

Q. 11 - Q. 20 carry two marks each.

11. Match the toxicants of plant foods in **Group I** with their main plant source given in **Group II.**

Group I

P. Gossypol
Q. Vicine
R. Glucosinolates
S. BOAA (beta-N- Oxalyl Amino L-Alanine)

Group II

1. Khesari Dahl (*Lathyrus sativus*)
2. Cotton seeds
3. Fava beans
4. Rapeseeds

(*a*) P-2, Q-3, R-4, S-1 (*b*) P-2, Q-4, R-3, S-1
(*c*) P-3, Q-1, R-2, S-4 (*d*) P-4, Q-3, R-1, S-2

12. Match the products in **Group I** with the enzymes used for their preparation given in **Group II.**

Group I

P. Aspartame
Q. Cocoa butter substitute
R. High fructose corn syrup
S. Lactose free milk

Group II

1. Lipase
2. Glucose isomerase
3. Thermolysin
4. Invertase
5. Beta galactosidase

(*a*) P-2, Q-1, R-4, S-3 (*b*) P-3, Q-1, R-2, S-5
(*c*) P-1, Q-3, R-2, S-4 (*d*) P-1, Q-2, R-4, S-5

13. Match the food items in **Group I** with the type of colloidal dispersion given in **Group II.**

Group I	**Group II**
P. Mayonnaise	1. Sol
Q. Tomato ketchup	2. Emulsion
R. Cake	3. Gel
S. Curd	4. Solid foam

(*a*) P-4, Q-1, R-2, S-3 (*b*) P-3, Q-1, R-2, S-5
(*c*) P-2, Q-3, R-4, S-5 (*d*) P-2, Q-1, R-4, S-3

14. ***Assertion (A)***: In the presence of sucrose, the temperature and time for gelatini-zation of starch increases.

Reason (R): Sucrose, due to its hygros-copic nature, competes with starch for water needed for gelatinization.

(*a*) Both [A] and [R] are true and [R] is the correct reason for [A]
(*b*) Both [A] and [R] are true but [R] is not the correct reason for [A]
(*c*) Both [A] and [R] are false
(*d*) [A] is true but [R] is false

15. Thermal death of viable spores of *Bacillus subtilis* in a food sample follows a first order kinetics with a specific death rate constant of 0.23 min^{-1} at 100°C. The time (in minutes) required to kill 99% of spores in the food sample at 100°C will be

(*a*) 10 (*b*) 20 (*c*) 23 (*d*) 60

16. How much skim milk (in kg) containing 0.1% fat should be added to 500 kg of cream containing 50% fat to produce standardized cream containing 36% fat?

(*a*) 140 (*b*) 165 (*c*) 195 (*d*) 210

17. Which of the following statements is NOT CORRECT in relation to muscle proteins ?

(*a*) Actin and myosin interact to form actomyosin which is responsible for muscle contraction
(*b*) Collagen contributes to the toughness of muscles due to its abundant presence
(*c*) Elastin, a constituent of ligaments, is tougher than collagen
(*d*) Actomyosin is not the main state of actin and myosin in post-mortem muscles

18. A cold storage plant is used for storing 50 tonnes of apples in perforated plastic crates. During the storage, apples are cooled down from 28°C to storage temperature of 2°C. (Specific heat of the apple = 0.874 kCal kg^{-1} $°C^{-1}$). If the required cooling is attained in 16 hours, the refrigeration plant capacity (in Tons) is

(*a*) 19 (*b*) 24 (*c*) 29 (*d*) 32

19. An actively growing culture of *Acetobacter aceti* is added to the vigorously aerated fermented fruit juice medium containing 10 g l^{-1} ethanol to produce vinegar. After some time, the ethanol concentration in the medium is 0.8 g l^{-1} and acetic acid produced is 8.4 g l^{-1}. What is the conversion efficiency of the process with respect to theoretical yield?

(*a*) 30 (*b*) 50 (*c*) 70 (*d*) 90

20. An enzyme catalyzed reaction (following Michaelis-Menten kinetics) exhibits maximum reaction velocity (V_m) of 75 nmol l^{-1} min^{-1}. The enzyme at a substrate concentration of 1.0×10^{-4} M shows the initial reaction velocity of 60 nmol l^{-1} min^{-1}. The K_m value of the enzyme in molar concentration (M) is

(*a*) 2.5×10^{-5} (*b*) 5.0×10^{-5}
(*c*) 2.5×10^{-4} (*d*) 5.0×10^{-4}

ANSWERS

GA : GENERAL APTITUDE

1. (*b*)	2. (*c*)	3. (*c*)	4. (*d*)	5. (*b*)	6. (*c*)	7. (*c*)	8. (*c*)	9. (*b*)	10. (*c*)

H : CHEMISTRY (Compulsory)

1. (*b*)	2. (*b*)	3. (*c*)	4. 8	5. 1	6. (*a*)	7. (*d*)	8. (*c*)	9. (*c*)	10. 3
11. 19.8 to 20.2	12. (*a*)	13. (*d*)	14. (*d*)	15. (*a*)					

I : BIOCHEMISTRY

1. (*d*)	2. (*d*)	3. (*b*)	4. (*d*)	5. (*a*)	6. (*a*)	7. (*b*)	8. (*c*)	9. (*b*)	10. (*d*)
11. (*c*)	12. (*b*)	13. (*c*)	14. (*d*)	15. (*b*)	16. (*b*)	17. (*c*)	18. (*c*)	19. (*c*)	20. (*c*)

J : BOTANY

1. (*b*)	2. (*b*)	3. (*b*)	4. (*a*)	5. (*c*)	6. (*d*)	7. (*d*)	8. (*c*)	9. (*d*)	10. (*d*)
11. (*d*)	12. (*b*)	13. (*a*)	14. (*c*)	15. (*c*)	16. (*d*)	17. (*d*)	18. (*c*)	19. (*a*)	20. (*b*)

K : MICROBIOLOGY

1. (*d*)	2. (*c*)	3. (*a*)	4. (*c*)	5. (*c*)	6. (*a*)	7. (*c*)	8. (*c*)	9. (*a*)	10. (*d*)
11. (*c*)	12. (*d*)	13. (*b*)	14. (*a*)	15. (*b*)	16. (*)	17. (*b*)	18. (*b*)	19. (*a*)	20. (*d*)

L : ZOOLOGY

1. (*a*)	2. (*)	3. (*c*)	4. (*c*)	5. (*a*)	6. (*a*)	7. (*b*)	8. (*d*)	9. (*a*)	10. (*b*)
11. (*a*)	12. (*d*)	13. (*d*)	14. (*)	15. (*a*)	16. (*d*)	17. (*b*)	18. (*b*)	19. (*a*)	20. (*a*)

M: FOOD TECHNOLOGY

1. (*d*)	2. (*)	3. (*b*)	4. (*a*)	5. (*c*)	6. (*d*)	7. (*b*)	8. (*a*)	9. (*b*)	10. (*b*)
11. (*a*)	12. (*b*)	13. (*)	14. (*a*)	15. (*b*)	16. (*c*)	17. (*d*)	18. (*b*)	19. (*c*)	20. (*a*)

Note (*) : None of the option is correct.

EXPLANATIONS

H: CHEMISTRY

1. If there is bonding between two atoms where one atom is having one vacant orbital and another is having one lone pair of electrons, then if this electron pair is donated to that respective vacant orbital then the bonding is called pπ- pπ or pπ- dπ depending on the orbital to which the electron pair is donated and from which the electron pair is donated. If both the orbitals are d orbitals, then bonding is called dπ – dπ bonding. In case of $N(SiCH_3)_3$, the planarity is caused by pπ – dπ bonding.

2. Potassium chromate (K_2CrO_4) is a yellow chemical indicator used for identifying concentrations of chloride ions in a salt solution with silver nitrate ($AgNO_3$). The type of electronic transition that occurs in K_2CrO_4 is metal to ligand charge transfer which results in the yellow colour of the coordinate compound.

3. Given equation, $\left(\dfrac{d(\Delta H)}{dT}\right)_p = \Delta C_p$.

Kirchhoff's Law describes the enthalpy of a reaction's variation with temperature changes. In general, enthalpy of any substance increases with temperature, which means both the products and the reactants' enthalpies increase. The overall enthalpy of the reaction will change if the increase in the enthalpy of products and reactants is different.

4. Given, Compound is anhydrous $AlCl_3$

A dipolar bond, also known as a dative covalent bond or coordinate bond is a kind of 2-center, 2-electron covalent bond in which the two electrons are derived from the same atom. Typically, a dipolar bond is formed when a Lewis base donates a pair of electrons to a Lewis acid.

In $AlCl_3$, the number of dipolar bonds is 8

5. Structure of Orthoboric acid, H_3BO_3:

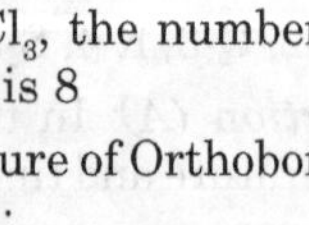

Boric acid does not dissociate in aqueous solution as a Brønsted acid, but is a Lewis acid which interacts with water molecules to form the tetrahydroxyborate ion, as confirmed by Raman spectroscopy:

$$B(OH)_3 + H_2O \rightarrow B(OH)_4^- + H^+$$

So, one H^+ molecule is released in the aqueous solution.

6. The NaCl crystal is face centered cubic (fcc) unit cell with the counter ion filling the octahedral holes in the structure. The sodium ions, which are smaller than the chloride ions, are inserted into octahedral holes and push the chloride ions apart so that no two chloride ions are in contact with each other. The resulting structure has (6, 6)-coordination.

7. In the given question, Solubility product for $Ca_3(PO_4)_2$,

$$K_{sp} = 1.3 \times 10^{-32}$$

Now, $K_{sp} = [Ca^{2+}]^3 \times [PO_4^{2-}]^2$

Given, Solubility of a $Ca(NO_3)_2$ solution

$= 0.02$ M

Therefore, Solubility of Ca in this solution

$= 0.02$ M

Let x M be the solubility of $Ca_3(PO_4)_2$

Again for $Ca(NO_3)_2$ solution, we have solubility of $Ca_3(PO_4)_2$ as

$$K_{sp} = [3x + 0.02]^3[2x]^2$$

$$\Rightarrow K_{sp} = [27x^3 + 8 \times 10^{-6} + 0.06x^2 + 0.0012x] \times [4x^2]$$

$$\Rightarrow K_{sp} = [108x^5 + 32x^2 \times 10^{-6} + 0.24\,x^4 + 0.0048x^3]$$

{The higher power terms are negligible}

$$\Rightarrow K_{sp} = [32\,x^2 \times 10^{-6}]$$

$$\Rightarrow x^2 = \frac{K_{sp}}{(32 \times 10^{-6})}$$

$$\Rightarrow x^2 = \frac{(1.3 \times 10^{-32})}{(32 \times 10^{-6})}$$

$$\Rightarrow x^2 = 4.0625 \times 10^{-28}$$

$$\Rightarrow x = 2.0155 \times 10^{-14}$$

The required solubility in the $Ca(NO_3)_2$ solution $= 2x = 4.031 \times 10^{-14}$ M

8. 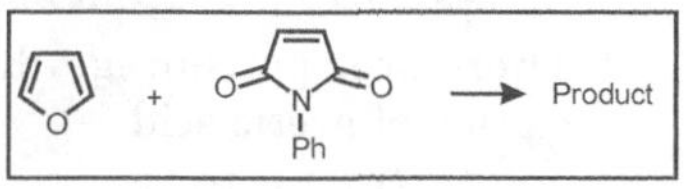

In the given reaction, the required product that is formed is:

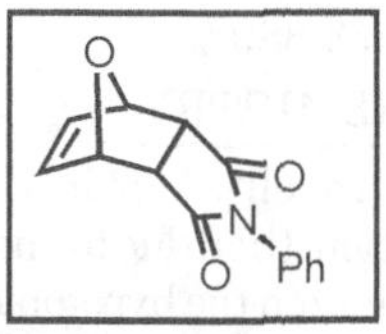

which is a half chair or boat conformational product.

9. Given, a reaction undergone is by Sodium ethoxide in presence of alcohol at a temperature of 50°C.

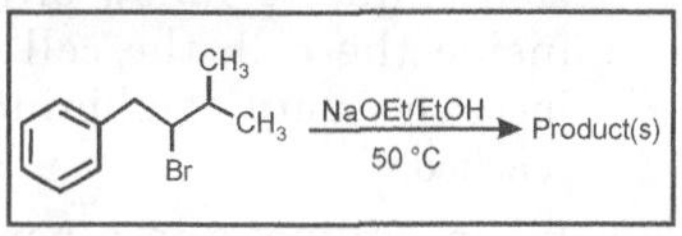

In the given reaction, Sodium ethoxide in presence of OH^- triggers the debromination from the alky side chain of the benzene ring. The resultant product that is formed is a double bond in the 3rd and 4th carbon position. The required product is:

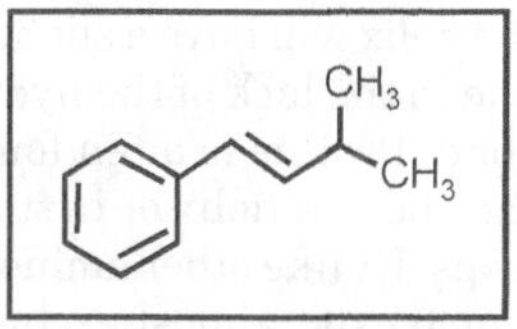

10. Iodine having valence electrons in the 4th energy level will also have access to the 4d sublevel, thus allowing for more than 8 electrons. I^{3-} is dsp3 hybridized and contains 3 lone pairs and 2 bonding pairs of valence electrons around the Iodine. The VSEPR predicts the linear shape. The outer iodine atoms have an octet. The middle iodine has 7 of its own electrons, plus 2 shared by the other iodine atoms, plus the one extra electron from somewhere else.

11. **19.8 to 20.2**

Activation energy is the amount of energy required to initiate a chemical reaction. The activation energy can be determined from reaction rate constants at different temperatures by the equation

$$\ln\left(\frac{k_2}{k_1}\right) = \frac{E_a}{R} \times \left(\frac{1}{T_1} - \frac{1}{T_2}\right)$$

Where, E_a is the activation energy of the reaction in cal mol^{-1} K^{-1}

R is the ideal gas constant

$= 1.987$ cal mol^{-1} K^{-1}

T_1 and T_2 are absolute temperatures

k_1 and k_2 are the reaction rate constants at T_1 and T_2

Given, $k_2 = 3k_1$, $T_1 = 298$ K and $T_2 = 308$ K

$$\Rightarrow E_a = \frac{\left\{\ln\left(\frac{k_2}{k_1}\right) \times R\right\}}{\left(\frac{1}{T_1} - \frac{1}{T_2}\right)}$$

$$\Rightarrow E_a = \frac{\{\ln(3) \times 1.987\}}{\left(\frac{10}{91784}\right)}$$

$$\Rightarrow E_a = \frac{(1.0986 \times 1.987)}{(1.089 \times 10^{-4})}$$

$$\Rightarrow E_a = 2.004 \times 10^4$$

The required activation energy is given by

2.004×10^4 cal mol^{-1} K^{-1}

$= 20.004 \times 10^3$ cal $mol^{-1}K^{-1}$

$= 20.004$ Kcal $mol^{-1}K^{-1}$

12. In the given nucleophilic substitution reaction of the compound X which is 1-chloro-3-ethyl cyclopentane:

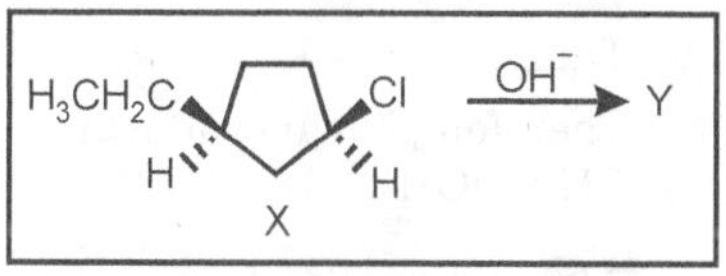

The hydroxyl substitution would occur at the 2-carbon position because of the deficit or the electrophilic nature of the 2-C atom due to the electron withdrawing capacity of the 1-chloro atom.

Hence, the product formed after substitution will be:-

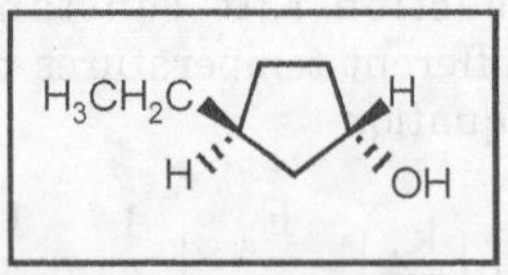

This is the product Y

13. The spatial arrangement of the atoms of a chiral molecular entity (or group) and its stereochemical description is known as absolute configuration. To name the enantiomers of a compound unambiguously, their names must include the "handedness" of the molecule. The method that has been developed to do this is formally known as R, S nomenclature. The absolute configuration of 1-chloro-3-ethylcyclopentane (X) is (1 R, 1 S).

14. At infinite dilution,

Molar conductance of $(CH_3COO)Na$

$= 91 \times 10^{-4}$ Sm^{2}mol^{-1}

Molar conductance of Na_2SO_4

$= 259.8 \times 10^{-4}$ Sm^{2}mol^{-1}

Molar conductance of H_2SO_4

$= 859.3 \times 10^{-4}$ Sm^{2}mol^{-1}

At infinite dilution, when dissociation is complete, each ion makes a definite contribution towards equivalent conductance of the electrolyte irrespective of the nature of the ion with which it is associated and the value of equivalent conductance at infinite dilution for any electrolyte is the sum of contribution of its constituent ions, i.e., anions and cations.

Thus, $\wedge_\infty = \lambda_a + \lambda_c$

Therefore, molar conductance of CH_3COOH

$$= \lambda_{(CH_3COO)Na} + \tfrac{1}{2}\lambda_{H_2SO_4} - \tfrac{1}{2}\lambda_{Na_2SO_4}$$

$$= \left(\frac{91 + 859.3}{2} - \frac{259.8}{2}\right) \times 10^{-4} \text{ Sm}^2\text{mol}^{-1}$$

$= 390.75 \times 10^{-4}$ Sm^{2}mol^{-1}

15. Given, Molar conductance of acetic acid on dissociation

$= 15.2 \times 10^{-4}$ Sm^{2}mol^{-1}

Molar conductance of acetic acid on infinite dilution

$= 390.75 \times 10^{-4}$ Sm^{2}mol^{-1}

Therefore, percentage dissociation of acetic acid

$$= \frac{(15.2 \times 10^{-4})}{(390.75 \times 10^{-4})} \times 100$$

$= 3.889$ %

I: BIOCHEMISTRY

1. When a cell is kept in a hypotonic solution, then due to endosmosis, water from the hypotonic solution flows into the cell through the cell membrane (which acts as the semi-permeable barrier) and dilutes the hypertonic concentration present in the cell. Hence, due to inflow of fluid inside the cell, the cell size increases until equilibrium is reached.

2. When proline is in a peptide bond, it does not have a hydrogen on α amino group, so it cannot donate a hydrogen bond to stabilize an α helix or a β sheet. It is often said, inaccurately, that proline cannot exist in α helix. When proline is found in an α helix, the helix will have a slight bend due to the lack of the hydrogen bond. Proline is often found at the end of α helix or in turns or loops. Unlike other amino acids which exist almost exclusively in the trans- form in polypeptides, proline can exist in the cis-configuration in peptides. The configuration of the peptide bond is central to the sort of secondary structure the protein backbone can adopt. It is easy to understand by imagining a normal helix and converting a trans peptide bond into its cis form.

3. An alpha-helix is formed from a connected stretch of amino acids. Its main characteristics are: The R groups of the amino acids all extend to the outside. The helix makes a complete turn every 3.6 amino acids. It rises 1.5 Å per residue. An alpha-helix is a right-handed helix. It twists in a clockwise direction. The carbonyl (-C=O) group of each peptide bond extends parallel to the axis of the helix and points directly at the -N-H group of the peptide bond 4 amino acids below it in the helix. Hydrogen bonds occur between the -C=O of residues and the -N-H of residues n+4.

Here,

No. of amino acids given = 36

Per residue rise of the helix

= 1.5 Å

Therefore, length of the helix

= 36 × 1.5 Å = 54 Å

4. In an enzyme catalyzed reaction where the kinetics are governed by Michaelis-Menten equation, the order of reaction for the substrate should always remain $0 \leq n \leq 1$ where n is the order of the substrate concentration. This is because for higher order substrate concentration, the Michaelis-Menten equation is not defined and the graph of the double reciprocal plot follows irregular kinetics.

5. Chymotrypsin is a digestive enzyme belonging to a super family of enzymes called serine proteases. It uses an active serine residue to perform hydrolysis on the C-terminal of the aromatic amino acids of other proteins. Chymotrypsin is a protease enzyme that cleaves on the C-terminus phenylalanine (F), tryptophan (W), and tyrosine (Y) on peptide chains. It has specificity for aromatic amino acids because of its hydrophobic pocket.

6. A final electron acceptor is a molecule that accepts an electron at the final stage of an electron transport chain. In cells, energy is obtained by oxidation reactions. Oxidation involves a loss of electrons from the substance being oxidized, and these electrons are passed to carriers. In mitochondria, the compounds of the electron transport chain are embedded in the inner membrane. The final acceptor of the electrons is oxygen, which is reduced to water: $2\ H^+ + 1/2\ O_2 \rightarrow H_2O$.

7. Urea is the major end product of nitrogen metabolism in humans and mammals. Ammonia, the product of oxidative deamination reactions, is toxic in even small amounts and must be removed from the body. The urea cycle or the ornithine cycle describes the conversion reactions of ammonia into urea. Since these reactions occur in the liver, the urea is then transported to the kidneys where it is excreted. The overall urea formation reaction is:

   2 Ammonia + carbon dioxide + 3ATP $\rightarrow$ urea + water + 3 ADP.

   One amine group comes from oxidative deamination of glutamic acid while the other amine group comes from aspartic acid. Aspartic acid is regenerated from fumaric acid produced by the urea cycle. The fumaric acid first undergoes reactions through a portion of the citric acid cycle to produce oxaloacetic acid which is then changed by transamination into aspartic acid.

8. A frequently used measure for the extent of cooperativity in ligand binding by an allosteric protein is the Hill coefficient, obtained by fitting data of initial reaction velocity (or fractional binding saturation) as a function of substrate concentration to the Hill equation. In practice, however, by fitting experimental binding data with the Hill equation, a value between 1 and the total number of binding sites (n) is frequently observed for nH. nH, therefore, is an index of cooperativity in ligand binding. Whereas nH = n reflects cooperative and concerted ligand binding to the enzyme, nH = 1 reflects non-cooperative (independent) sequential binding. In the given problem, because of negative cooperativity, the Hill coefficient for the inhibitor will always be less than 1.

9. From the given autoradiogram, it is fairly clear that the oligonucleotides sequence was analysed using the dideoxy method of Sanger sequencing. In the dideoxy method, the autoradiogram is read from the bottom or the far most end of the wells and eventually progress closer to the wells. So the read from the autoradiogram is: 5′-GTCCTGTACA-3′

10. Organ transplantation is the surgical replacement of diseased organs with healthy organs (grafts) from live or cadaver donors. An isograft is an organ transplanted from a donor who is genetically identical to the recipient (i.e., identical twins). Isografts are also called isogeneic and syngeneic grafts. An allograft is an organ transplanted from a donor to a recipient of the same species who is not genetically identical. Allografts are also called allogeneic grafts and homografts. Although isografts would be preferable to allografts, for obvious reasons the majority of organs transplanted are allografts. A xenograft is an organ transplanted from a donor to a recipient of a different species (eg, baboon to human). So, the decreasing order of graft rejection is:

    Xenograft > Allograft > Isograft.

11. We know, from Henderson-Hasselbach equation,

$$pH = pK_a + \log\left\{\frac{[Salt]}{[Acid]}\right\}$$

Given, pH = 5, $K_a = 1.7\times10^{-5}$ M

$\Rightarrow \quad pK_a = 4.769$

[Salt] = [acetate buffer]

= 0.5 M

Therefore, $5 = 4.769 + \log\left\{\frac{[0.5]}{[\text{acetate ion}]}\right\}$

$\Rightarrow \quad 0.231 = \log 0.5 - \log[\text{acetate ion}]$

$\Rightarrow \quad \log[\text{acetate ion}] = 0.231 - \log 0.5$

$\Rightarrow \quad \log[\text{acetate ion}] = 0.532$

$\Rightarrow \quad [\text{acetate ion}] = 0.3154$

The required concentration of the acetate ion is 0.3154 M

12. The study of the rate at which an enzyme works is called enzyme kinetics. K_m is (roughly) an inverse measure of the affinity or strength of binding between the enzyme and its substrate. In the presence of a competitive inhibitor, it takes a higher substrate concentration to achieve the same velocities that were reached in its absence. So while V_{max} can still be reached if sufficient substrate is available, one-half V_{max} requires a higher [S] than before and thus K_m is larger. With non-competitive inhibition, enzyme molecules that have been bound by the inhibitor are taken out of the game so enzyme rate (velocity) is reduced for all values of [S], including V_{max} and one-half V_{max} but K_m remains unchanged because the active site of those enzyme molecules that have not been inhibited is unchanged. Many enzymes are inhibited by their own substrates, leading to velocity curves that rise to a maximum and then descend as the substrate concentration increases.

13. H_2O is the most permeable substance across a cell membrane. This is because of the ability of water to form hydrogen bonds while permeating through the lipid bilayer whose hydrophilic heads are exposed to the flowing polar water. Urea is an organic compound with a simple structure. So it can easily permeate through the membrane. The amino acid tryptophan also percolates through the lipid bilayer because of its organic nature and its hydrophobic character. Glucose, being a water soluble organic molecule can pass through the lipid bilayer if and only if there

is an imbalance of glucose level inside and outside the cell. Na^+ cannot enter the membrane through simple physical processes like other molecules and can only enter when there is the action of the active Na-K pump through active transport. So the order is:

H_2O > Urea > Tryptophan > Glucose > Na^+

14. Anaerobic catabolism of starch having one glucose unit would have produced approximately 2 moles of ATP. Since there are 300 glucose units in the starch molecule, the number of ATPs generated will be 600. Aerobic catabolism of glucose generates 4 ATP molecules which is then transported to mitochondria to perform the electron transport to generate 36 moles of ATP. Aerobic catabolism of acetate will generate roughly 1 mole of ATP only. Aerobic catabolism of palmitate (a fatty acid) generates large amount of reserved energy which can amount to 37-65 moles of ATP.

15. Phosphofructokinase-1 (PFK-1) is a glycolytic enzyme that catalyzes the transfer of a phosphoryl group from ATP to fructose-6-phosphate (F6P) to yield ADP and fructose-1, 6-bisphosphate (FBP). It is an allosteric enzyme that is described using the symmetry model of allosterism whereby there is a concerted transition from its high-activity R state to its low-activity T state. Glycogen Synthase catalyzes elongation of glycogen chains. Glycogen Synthase catalyzes transfer of the glucose moiety of UDP-glucose to the hydroxyl at C4 of the terminal residue of a glycogen chain to form α (1, 4) glycosidic linkage. This is a covalent modification. β-galactosidase, also called beta-gal or β-gal, is a hydrolase enzyme that catalyzes the hydrolysis of β-galactosides into monosaccharides. It controls enzyme synthesis by the use of galactosides. Lactate dehydrogenase is an enzyme that catalyzes the conversion of lactate to pyruvate. It is not tissue-specific, being found in a variety of tissues, including liver, heart and skeletal muscle. It is regulated by end product inhibition mechanism.

16. Yeast artificial chromosome (YAC) is a human-engineered DNA molecule used to clone DNA sequences in yeast cells. YACs are often used in connection with the mapping and sequencing of genomes. The development of a bacteriophage P1 cloning system capable of accepting DNA fragments as large as 100 kilobase pairs (kbp) is widely used. Cosmids are predominantly plasmids with a bacterial oriV, an antibiotic selection marker and a cloning site, but they carry one, or more recently two cos sites derived from bacteriophage lambda.

17. Given sequence: 5′-CCGATAT CTCGAGGGC-3′

From the given recognition sequences of the various restriction enzymes, the ones with recognition sites present in the given sequence are: XhoI (3′-GAGCT^C-5′) and EcoRV (3′-CTA^TAG-5′). So, Q and S cut the given DNA sequence.

18. Since the protein has a His tag at its N-terminal end and it has an isoelectric point of 6, so the first purification step would that be of Anion exchange chromatography with elution buffer of pH 8. Next Ni-NTA column of affinity chromatography can be used for further purification. Lastly, gel filtration chromatography can be used to isolate purified solution of proteins which can be crystallized later.

19. Given, concentration of the enzyme in the solution of the substrate = 12 mg/mL

Molecular weight of the enzyme = 40 kDa = 40 mg (approx.)

Therefore, molar concentration of the enzyme in the solution = 12/40 mM = 0.3 mM

Since the enzyme to substrate molar ratio = 1 : 3, therefore the concentration of the substrate is given by = 3 × 0.3 mM = 0.9 mM

20. A retrovirus is a virus whose genes are encoded in RNA instead of DNA. Although, like other viruses, retroviruses need to use the cellular machinery of the organisms they infect to make copies of themselves, infection by a retrovirus requires an additional step. The retrovirus genome needs to be reverse-transcribed into DNA by an enzyme called reverse-transcriptase before it can be copied in the usual way. The most well known retrovirus that infects humans is HIV. However, there are several other human retroviruses, including the human T-cell lymphotropic virus 1 (HTLV-1), which is associated with certain T-cell leukaemia and lymphomas. There are many additional retroviruses which have been identified as infecting other species. Since the patient is exhibiting very low level of $CD4^+$ T cells, hence the infection in all probability must be of a retrovirus family.

J: BOTANY

1. Bast fibres are soft, woody fibre obtained from stems of dicotyledonous plants (flowering plants with net-veined leaves) and used for textiles and cordage. Such fibres, usually characterized by fineness and flexibility, are also known as "soft" fibres, distinguishing them from the coarser, less flexible fibres of the leaf, or "hard," fibre group. They are present in phloem.

2. Pyruvate Dehydrogenase catalyzes oxidative decarboxylation of pyruvate, to form acetyl-CoA. Pyruvate Dehydrogenase is a large complex

containing many copies of each of three enzymes, E1, E2, and E3. The inner core of the mammalian Pyruvate Dehydrogenase complex is an icosahedral structure consisting of 60 copies of E2. The pyruvate dehydrogenase complex links glycolysis to the TCA cycle (also known as the Krebs cycle or the citric acid cycle). It is a large multi-enzyme complex composed of three enzymes involving five cofactors. The pyruvate dehyd-rogenase complex oxidizes pyruvate to generate acetyl-coA.

3. Rice is the first crop plant whose complete genetic sequence, or genome, has been compiled and placed in computer data banks around the world. The rice genome is well mapped and well characterized, and it is the smallest of the major cereal crop genomes at an estimated 400 to 430 Mb. The rice genome contains about 50,000 genes located on 12 different chromosomes.

4. Aflatoxin is a naturally occurring mycotoxin produced by two types of mould: *Aspergillus flavus* and *Aspergillus parasiticus*. *Aspergillus flavus* is common and widespread in nature and is most often found when certain grains are grown under stressful conditions such as drought. The mould occurs in soil, decaying vegetation, hay, and grains undergoing microbiological deterioration and invades all types of organic substrates whenever and wherever the conditions are favourable for its growth.

5. Meiosis is a special type of cell division that produces gametes with half as many chromosomes. The opposite process would be syngamy or fertilization, which is the union of the egg and sperm to restore the 2n number. This results in a zygote, the first cell formed by fertilization, a completely new and different organism with unique genetic information different from either parent. The zygote divides and grows to form an embryo which develops into a young organism, then an adult. The steps in meiosis are similar to mitosis and even have the same names. However, there is a significant difference in how the chromosomes line up initially. In mitosis, chromosomes line up individually, while in meiosis, the two chromosomes in each homologous pair line up next to each other. This pairing process is called synapsis, and the resulting homologous pair is called a bivalent in reference to the two chromosomes or a tetrad in reference to the four sister chromatids involved.

6. Leghaemoglobin is a haemoglobin-like red pigment in the root nodules of leguminous plants, as soybean, that is essential for nitrogen fixation. The enzyme nitrogenase is found in certain bacteria and blue-green algae, which can reduce N_2 to NH_3 (nitrogen fixation). Some of these bacteria are free-living while others are symbiotic (in the anaerobic environment of roots of legume plants). This bacterial reaction is the key step in the nitrogen cycle, which maintains a balance between two reservoirs of the nitrogen compounds: the Earth's atmosphere and the biosphere. The plants cannot extract nitrogen directly from the atmosphere. N_2 must be fixed by these bacteria (as NH_3) or converted by lightning to NOx and then NO^{3-} in the reaction with water. The fixed nitrogen is lost through leaching of the soil, harvesting of crops and the action of the denitrifying bacteria.

7. Photoperiodism is a biological response to a change in the proportions of light and dark in a 24-hour daily cycle. Plants use it to measure the seasons and to coordinate seasonal events such as flowering. Many angiosperms flower at about the same time every year. This occurs even though they may have started growing at different times. Their flowering is a response to the changing length of day and night as the season progresses. It helps promote cross pollination. Photoperiodic reactions can be reasonably predicted, but temperature, nutrition, and other environmental factors also modify an organism's response.

8. Protoplasts can be isolated from a range of plant tissues: leaves, stems, roots, flowers, anthers and even pollen. The isolation and culture media used vary with the species and with the tissue from which the protoplasts were isolated. Individual hydrolytic enzymes include cellulases, hemicellulase, pectinase, and pectolase which can also be used for isolation.

9. Ti (Tumour inducing) plasmids in *Agrobacterium tumefaciens* can transfer their T-DNA region into dicotyledonous plants, in which the expression of T-DNA genes causes plant tumours and the production of bacterial nutrients, e.g., opines such as nopaline. Naturally occurring Ti plasmids (pTi) are difficult to cure by conventional curing methods because of their high stability. Here, we developed a novel curing method based on plasmid incompatibility. This transformation method uses bacterial strains harbouring a modified tumour-inducing (Ti) plasmid that lacks the transfer DNA (T-DNA) region (disarmed Ti plasmid). It is desirable to develop strains that can broaden the host range. The transfer DNA (T-DNA) and virulence gene (vir) regions in the Ti plasmid are essential for tumorigenesis. The vir gene products nick the T-DNA region at its left border (LB) and right border (RB) and then transfer T-DNA into plant cells. T-DNA contains phytohormone

synthesis genes, whose expression causes infected plants to suffer from unregulated growth.

10. Cytoplasmic male sterility (CMS), a condition under which a plant is unable to produce functional pollen, is widespread among higher plants. CMS systems represent a valuable tool in the production of hybrid seed in self-pollinating crop species, including maize, rice, cotton, and a number of vegetable crops. Hybrids often exhibit heterosis, more commonly known as hybrid vigour, whereby hybrid progeny exhibit superior growth characteristics relative to either of the parental lines. CMS systems can be of considerable value in facilitating efficient hybrid seed production. CMS is a maternally inherited trait that is often associated with unusual open reading frames (ORFs) found in mitochondrial genomes. In many cases, it has been found that male fertility can be restored by nuclear-encoded fertility restorer (Rf) gene(s). CMS/Rf systems therefore are also of value in the study of interactions between nuclear and mitochondrial genomes.

11. *Oryza sativa*, commonly known as Asian rice, is the plant species most commonly referred to in English as rice. *Oryza sativa* is the cereal with the smallest genome, consisting of just 430Mb across 12 chromosomes. *Cocos nucifera* is a single stem palm that can grow to a height of 30m. The onion (*Allium cepa*), is also known as the bulb onion or common onion, is the most widely cultivated species of the genus Allium. *Musa paradisiaca* is about 30 feet high and produces green or greenish-yellow seedless fruits, so fruits develop parthenocarpically (in the absence of seed development). The name "plantain" refers to *Musa paradisiaca*, which requires cooking before it is eaten.

12. Given, P1 generation:

GGHH × gghh

F1 generation: GgHh

Test cross: GgGh × GgHh

⇒ GGHH, GgHh (1) ggHh, ggHH -(2)- Gghh, GGhh gghh (1)

In case of P, the normal phenotypic ratio of 1: 2: 1 is observed from the test cross which gives 25 % to gghh progeny.

In case of Q, when two genes G and H are linked, then they do not segregate and a single ratio of 1: 1 is observed. So gghh progeny is comprised of 50% of the total offsprings.

In case of R, when there is 10 m.u. distance between the two genes then the % of recombination of the two genes gghh

= 10m.u./2

= 5.

So the % of occurrence of gghh

= (50 – 5)%

= 45%

In case of S, when there is 24 m.u. distance between the two genes, then % recombination of the two genes in gghh

= 24 m.u./2

= 12.

So the % of occurrence of gghh

= (50 – 12)%

= 38%

13. Nondisjunction is the failure of two members of a homologous pair of chromosomes to separate during meiosis. It gives rise to gametes with a chromosomal content that is different from the norm. In normal meiosis, homologous chromosomes pair up and, by attachment to the spindle fibres, become aligned at the cell equator. Prior to the first meiotic division, the members of each homologous pair migrate to opposite poles of the cell by means of the pulling action of the spindle fibres. This ensures that, upon completion of meiosis, each gamete will contain one copy of every chromosome. Meiosis is a very tightly regulated process, and a whole series of control mechanisms (constituting a number of "checkpoints") exist to ensure that everything proceeds in the correct manner. If an error should occur during the process, it is usually corrected. Nondisjunction is the result of a mistake at the level of chromosome segregation, which involves the spindle fibres.

14. Morphine is a narcotic pain reliever used to treat moderate to severe pain. The milky latex sap of opium poppies contains isoquinoline alkaloids. This class of alkaloid contains a double carbon ring with one nitrogen atom (N). It is classified as a narcotic and is commonly found in certain members of the poppy family (Papaveraceae), such as the opium poppy (*Papaver somniferum*). Agrobacterium-mediated transformation of Nicotiana species, namely, *Nicotiana tobaccum* and *Nicotiana benthamiana*, using leaf disks as the target explant has provided the plant community with a valuable tool for rapid evaluation of transgenes in higher plants. Nicotine is an alkaloid found in the nightshade family of plants ("Solanaceae") which constitutes approximately 0.6–3.0% of dry weight of tobacco. As a nitrogenous base, nicotine forms salts with acids that are usually solid and water soluble. Atropine, a naturally occurring belladonna alkaloid, is a racemic mixture of equal parts of d- and l-hyocyamine, whose activity is due almost entirely to the levo isomer of the drug. Atropine is obtained from such solanaceous plants as *Atropa belladonaa* (deadly nightshade), *Hyoscyamus niger* (black henbane). Vinblastine is a vinca alkaloid antineoplastic agent. The vinca alkaloids have become clinically useful since the

discovery of their antitumour properties in 1959. Initially, extracts of the periwinkle plant (*Catharanthus roseus*) were investigated because of putative hypoglycemic properties, but were noted to cause marrow suppression in rats and antileukemic effects in vitro.

15. C4 plants are specially adapted to reduce photorespiration and promote photosynthesis in response to hot and dry conditions. These plants have unique cellular structures: tightly packed bundle sheath cells surrounding the leaf veins, and mesophyll cells surrounding the bundle sheath cells. The process of photosynthesis is split into two different types of cells. In the mesophyll cells, PEP carboxylase adds CO_2 to PEP. CO_2, in the form of malate, is moved from the mesophyll cells into the bundle sheath cells through plasmodesmata. In the bundle sheath cells, the CO_2 is released and enters the Calvin cycle. When CO_2 enters the stomata of a C4 plant, it diffuses directly into mesophyll cells, which lack the enzyme rubisco and, as a result, cannot carry out photorespiration. Instead, mesophyll cells contain the enzyme PEP carboxylase, which has a strong affinity for CO_2 and no affinity for O_2. PEP carboxylase adds a CO_2 to a 3-carbon compound called phosphoenolpyruvic acid (PEP). This produces the 4-carbon compound oxaloacetic acid (oxaloacetate). Oxaloacetic acid is then converted into malic acid or aspartic acid (both 4-carbon compounds).

16. 2, 4-D is a chlorophenoxy herbicide that is also sometimes used as a plant growth regulator. 2, 4-D has a number of chemical forms, including esters and salts. The different chemical forms of 2, 4-D affect organisms in different ways. It is a synthetic auxin. Kinetin (6-Furfuryladenine) is a kind of cytokinin, a class of plant hormone that promotes cell division. Kinetin is often used in plant tissue culture for inducing formation of callus (in conjunction with auxin) and to regenerate shoot tissues from callus.

17. Secondary growth is common in roots and shoots of all gymnosperms and many dicots, but is rare in monocots. Vascular cambium adds secondary xylem and secondary phloem tissue that improve vascular flow and mechanical support. Because this growth usually ruptures the epidermis of the stem or roots, plants with secondary growth usually also develop a cork cambium, which protects against water loss and pathogen invasion by producing a thick covering of wax impregnated cells. The analysis of plant proteins has a long and distinguished history, with work dating back over 250 years. Much of the work has focused on seed proteins, which are important in animal nutrition and food processing. Early studies classified plant proteins into groups based on solubility ('Osborne fractions') or protein function. More recently, families have been defined based on structural and evolutionary relationships.

18. Allogamy is a term used in the field of biological reproduction describing the fertilization of an ovum from one individual with the spermatazoa of another. Whereas, autogamy is the term used for self-fertilization as in the fertilisation of a flower by its own pollen. In plants, allogamy specifically mean the use of pollen from one plant to fertilize the flower of another plant termed as cross fertilization or cross pollination - pollen exchange between different plant strains or even different plant species (termed as hybridization).

19. Coenzyme is a nonproteinaceous organic substance that usually contains a vitamin or mineral and combines with a specific protein, the apoenzyme, to form an active enzyme system. Enzymes are proteins that catalyze (i.e., increase the rates of) chemical reactions, Coenzymes are small organic molecules that transport chemical group. Inhibitors are activators or molecules that increase or decrease enzyme activity. Apoenzyme is a protein component of an enzyme, to which the coenzyme attaches to form an active enzyme where as holoenzyme is an active, complex enzyme consisting of an apoenzyme and a coenzyme. Prosthetic group is a tightly bound, specific non-polypeptide unit required for the biological function of some proteins.

20. Transport in plants occurs on three levels: the uptake and release of water and solutes by individual cells, short-distance transport of substances from cell to cell,and long-distance transport of sap within the xylem and phloem. Water is transported by either apoplastic transportation or symplastic transportation. Apoplastic transport is when water is transported between cells up to the endodermis. Symplastic transport is when water is transported through the plasma membrane and cytoplasm. Water following this route may take longer to transport and require ATP. Symplastic transport can pass through the endodermis whereas apoplastic transport cannot. Material and water must be transported through the endodermis symplastically. Both of these pathways are needed to transport water and dissolved substances to the vascular bundle. To transport water and material across the endodermis, symplastic transport is needed (because the endodermis is relatively impermeable). Once transported across the endodermis and to the stele, materials must then move from the symplastic area to the apoplastic area (the xylem).

K: MICROBIOLOGY

1. Susumu Tonegawa was the one who finally answered the question how the gene material in B cells could suffice to create the structures of a seemingly endless number of different antibodies. In 1976 he could in a convincing and elegant manner show how different immunoglobulin genes which were far apart in the embryonic cell in the B lymphocyte had been moved in closer contact. Under development from the germ cells (the sperm and egg cell) to an antibody producing B lymphocyte the genes forming the immunoglobulins had accordingly been redistributed. In subsequent experiment Tonegawa could clarify how different pieces of the genome were moved around, recombined and even could be "lost" to finally give rise to the DNA which is found in the mature B lymphocyte.
2. Aminoglycosides are polar drugs and their distribution is mainly restricted to extracellular fluids. Protein binding of these antibiotics is less than 10%. Aminoglycosides distribute well in synovial, peritoneal, ascitic and pleural fluids. High concentrations of aminoglycosides are obtained in renal tissue especially in renal cortex. Penetration of these drugs is poor in eye and central nervous system. Concentrations of aminoglycosides in biliar and bronchial secretions are variable. Aminoglycosides are primarily excreted unchanged through the kidney by glomerular filtration. The 80-90% of the administered dose is excreted in the urine resulting in high urinary concentrations.
3. The Shine-Dalgarno sequence is a purine-rich tract of 3-10 nucleotides and precedes the start AUG codon by approximately 10 nucleotides upstream on the 5′ side. The Shine-Dalgarno sequence forms base pairing with a highly conserved, pyrimidine-rich region of the 16S rRNA which is part of the 30S ribosomal subunit. This base-pairing properly aligns the start AUG codon in the P site of the 30S ribosomal subunit.
4. In endocytosis, the cell engulfs some of its extracellular fluid (ECF) including material dissolved or suspended in it. A portion of the plasma membrane is invaginated and pinched off forming a membrane-bounded vesicle called an endosome. In endocytosis, the material to be internalized is surrounded by an area of plasma membrane, which then buds off inside the cell to form a vesicle containing the ingested material. Eukaryotic cells are also able to take up macromolecules and particles from the surrounding medium by a distinct process called endocytosis. The former of these activities is known as phagocytosis (cell eating) and the latter as pinocytosis (cell drinking).
5. Faecal pollution of water from a health point of view is the contamination of water with disease-causing organisms (pathogens) that may inhabit the gastrointestinal tract of mammals, but with particular attention to human faecal sources as the most relevant source of human illnesses globally. In recent years the WHO have strongly promoted the use of the faecal bacterium *Escherichia coli* (*E. coli*) as the principle faecal indicator for waters. Previously, a larger group of bacteria related to *E. coli* but not all specific to faeces (known as the total coliforms) had been promoted, but with the advent of more rapid and selective methods it is more reliable to directly measure *E. coli*, rather than either total or so-called faecal coliforms. The most commonly used indicators for surface waters are the faecal coliforms and E. coli, although another bacterial group, the entercocci are often used to better assess health risks associated with marine recreational waters.
6. The maximum number of ATP possibly produced is 38 but it is often not reached due to losses (leaky membranes) as well as the cost of moving pyruvate and ADP into the mitochondrial matrix. It is estimated that 29-30 ATP are produced per glucose. In eukaryotic cells, the theoretical maximum yield of ATP generated per glucose is 36 to 38, depending on how the 2 NADH generated in the cytoplasm during glycolysis enter the mitochondria and whether the resulting yield is 2 or 3 ATP per NADH.
7. The presently existing classification for the green and purple bacteria comprises physiological-ecological assemblages of phototrophic bacteria with anoxygenic photosynthesis. Since degrees of resemblance form the basis of the grouping, this classification cannot reflect the genetic or evolutionary relatedness of these bacteria, neither among themselves nor with other bacteria. The four existing families correspond to the four major recognized, ecophysiological groups, the Chlorobiaceae and Chloro-flexaceae among the green bacteria, and the Chromatiaceae and Rhodospirillaceae among the purple bacteria. Amino acid sequence studies of cytochromes c from Rhodospirillaceae, other bacteria and eukaryotic organisms have led to the recognition of four different groups of cytochrome c molecules (long, medium and two groups of short protein chains). The subdivision of the Rhodospirillaceae into three species groups, each possessing one of the three types of cytochrome c, proved to be in total agreement with the results of oligonucleotide cataloging of the 16 S ribosomal RNA of these bacteria.

8. Given, radius (r) of the spherical coccus

$= 0.8$ m

Therefore, area of the spherical coccus

$= 4\Pi r^2$

Volume of the spherical coccus

$= 4/3\ \Pi r^3$

Now, Surface area/Volume of the coccus

$= 4\Pi r^2 / (4/3\ \Pi r^3)$

$= 3/r = 3/0.8 = 3.75$ m

9. The enzyme nitrogenase is found in certain bacteria and blue-green algae, which can reduce N_2 to NH_3 (nitrogen fixation). Some of these bacteria are free-living while others are symbiotic (in the anaerobic environment of roots of legume plants). This bacterial reaction is the key step in the nitrogen cycle, which maintains a balance between two reservoirs of the nitrogen compounds: the Earth's atmosphere and the biosphere.

10. In a chemostat culture, flow rate (F)

$= 30$ mL/*hr*

Volume of the culture vessel (V) $= 100$mL

Therefore, Dilution rate of the continuous culture system,

$D = F/V = 30/100\ hr^{-1} = 0.3\ h^{-1}$.

11. The lac operon encodes a set of genes that are involved in the metabolism of a simple sugar, lactose. Lactose is a disaccharide composed of two sugars (galactose and glucose) with a β-linkage between carbon 1 of galactose and carbon 4 of glucose. The lac operon encodes three proteins: β-galactosidase (the product of the lacZ gene), lactose permease (the product of the lacY gene), and lactose transacetylase (the product of the lacA gene). The function of lacA is not known, but a mutation in either lacZ or lacY means that the cell can't grow by using lactose as a sole carbon source. All three structural genes are transcribed from a common promoter site, in the direction Z-Y-A. The lac transcript is termed polycistronic because it contains more than one coding sequence. The unregulated, "always on" expression caused by a $lacI^-$ mutation is called constitutive expression. This behavior is characteristic of a negative control element. LacO is also a negative element. Deletion of lacO leads to constitutive expression of the lac genes. The difference between the two types of constitutive mutation is seen when the genes are put into an artificial situation where two copies of the relevant control genes exist.

12. Siderophores are biosynthetically produced and secreted by many bacteria, yeasts, fungi and plants, to scavenge for ferric iron (Fe(3+)). They are selective iron-chelators that have an extremely high affinity for binding this trivalent metal ion. The ferric ion is poorly soluble but it is the form of iron that is predominantly found in oxygenated environments. Of the various siderophore systems present in *E. coli*, the enterobactin and aerobactin genes, encoded on the chromosome and pColV respectively, have been the most intensively studied to date as regards their molecular genetics.

13. Penicillin is an antibiotic and is used to treat and prevent a variety of bacterial infections. It works by stopping the growth of bacteria. In media containing slow growing bacteria, penicillin enriches their growth by removal of the fast growing bacteria from the culture and making the nutrient media available for the slow growing bacteria to feed upon.

14. The trp operon of *E. coli* controls the biosynthesis of tryptophan in the cell from the initial precursor chorismic acid. This operon contains genes for the production of five proteins which are used to produce three enzymes. The trp operon is a repressible system. The primary difference between repressible and inducible systems is the result that occurs when the effector molecule binds to the repressor. With inducible systems, the binding of the effector molecule to the repressor greatly reduces the affinity of the repressor for the operator, the repressor is released and transcription proceeds. The lac operon is an example of an inducible system. With repressible systems, the binding of the effector molecule to the repressor greatly increases the affinity of repressor for the operator and the repressor binds and stops transcription. Thus, for the trp operon, the addition of tryptophan (the effector molecule) to the *E. coli* environment shuts off the system because the repressors bind at the operator.

15. In 1663 an English scientist, Robert Hooke, discovered cells in a piece of cork, which he examined under his primitive microscope. Actually, Hooke only observed cell walls because cork cells are dead and without cytoplasmic contents. In 1906 Paul Ehrlich discovered the structural formula of atoxyl, a chemical compound that had been shown to be able to treat sleeping sickness (Silesia). Anton Van Leeuwenhoek was the first to see and describe bacteria (1674), yeast plants, the teeming life in a drop of water, and the circulation of blood corpuscles in capillaries. Sergei Winogradsky was the first to develop the concept of chemolithotrophy and to thereby reveal the essential role played by microorganisms in geochemical processes.

16. *Bordetella pertussis* is a Gram-negative, aerobic coccobacillus capsulate of the genus *Bordetella*, and the causative agent of pertussis or whooping cough.

Mycobacterium leprae is responsible for leprosy or Hansen's disease. It is a strongly acid-fast rod-shaped organism with parallel sides and rounded ends. In size and shape it closely resembles the tubercle bacillus. *Haemophilus influenzae* type b (Hib) disease is a serious disease caused by bacteria. It usually strikes children under 5 years of age. Rubella — commonly known as German measles or 3-day measles — is an infection that primarily affects the skin and lymph nodes. It is caused by the rubella virus, which is usually transmitted by droplets from the nose or throat that others breathe in.

17. In phase contrast microscopy, highly refractive structures bend light to a much greater angle than do structures of low refractive index. The same properties that cause the light to bend also delay the passage of light by a quarter of a wavelength or so. In dark field microscopy, the light coming from the source of light of the microscope is led past the object to be examined. Only light which is strewn through the preparations in the path of rays - the Tyndall – effect - arrives in the objective and produces a picture with bright structures on a dark underground. Bright field microscopy is the simplest of a range of techniques used for illumination of samples in light microscopes and its simplicity makes it a popular technique. The typical appearance of a bright field microscopy image is a dark sample on a bright background. The conventional electron microscope requires that the electron beam be in a vacuum, because electrons cannot ordinarily travel an appreciable distance in air at atmospheric pressure. The column of the electron microscope is evacuated by pumps, and the specimens and any other necessary apparatus are introduced into the vacuum by means of air locks.

18. Given, Maximum effective dilution for the disinfectant

$$X = \frac{1}{450}$$

Maximum effective dilution for phenol $= \frac{1}{90}$

Now, the phenol coefficient for X

$$= \frac{\left(\frac{1}{90}\right)}{\left(\frac{1}{450}\right)}$$

$$= \frac{450}{90}$$

$$= 5$$

19. *Desulfovibrio* is known as a sulphate reducing bacterium, which has put it to the forefront of biological research. Because of its metal corroding ability, which has consequently led to numerous health and safety concerns in industry, a means to neutralize and better understand *Desulfovibrio* species is the goal of research on *Desulfovibrio.* In a sulphate reducing bacteria, the terminal acceptor sulphate accepts 8 electrons.

20. Original number of cells in bacterial population

$$= 10^3$$

After 10 hours, the number of bacterial cells

$$= 10^9$$

After 1st generation, number of bacterial cells would be

$$= 10^{3\times 2} = 10^6$$

After 2nd generation, number of bacterial cells would be

$$= 10^{6\times 2} = 10^{12}$$

So, the number of generations/hour = 2

L: ZOOLOGY

1. Descent with modification is the term Darwin used for evolution. It explains both the unity of life and the diversity of life. The unity of life comes from descent; offspring resemble their parents, even over many generations. But organisms are not identical to their parents, they are also modified in the process; and this - over long periods of time - explains the diversity of life. "The framework of bones being the same in the hand of a man, wing of a bat, fin of the porpoise, and leg of the horse, – the same number of vertebrae forming the neck of the giraffe and of the elephant, - and innumerable other such facts, at once explain themselves on the theory of descent with modification with slow and slight successive modifications."
2. Sympatric speciation occurs when there are no physical barriers preventing any members of a species from mating with another, and all members are in close proximity to one another. A new species, perhaps based on a different food source or characteristic, seems to develop spontaneously. The theory is that some individuals become dependent on certain aspects of an environment—such as shelter or food sources—while others do not. A possible example of sympatric speciation is the apple maggot, an insect that lays its eggs inside the fruit of an apple, causing it to rot. As the apple falls from the tree, the maggots dig in the ground before emerging as flies several months later. The apple maggot originally laid its eggs in the fruit of a relative of the apple—a fruit called a hawthorn.
3. The main structural difference comes from the difference in the sequence of bonds in glycogen

and cellulose and starch where the three of them composed mainly of glucose and its derivatives. Starch, glycogen and cellulose are all polymers of glucose. They differ in the type of glucose present and the bonds which link the glucose monomers together. Glycogen is similar in structure to amylopectin, but branches more frequently. Cellulose is an un-branched polymer composed of beta glucose molecules. Beta glucose is an isomer of glucose in which the hydroxyl group attached to carbon 1 is above the plane of the ring. The glucose monomers are linked by 1, 4 glycosidic bonds.

4. By switching genes off when they are not needed, cells can prevent resources from being wasted. There should be natural selection favouring the ability to switch genes on and off. Complex multicellular organisms are produced by cells that switch genes on and off during development. A typical human cell normally expresses about 3% to 5% of its genes at any given time. Gene expression in eukaryotes is controlled by a variety of mechanisms that range from those that prevent transcription to those that prevent expression after the protein has been produced. Some proteins are not active when they are first formed. They must undergo modification such as folding, enzymatic cleavage, or bond formation. Many proteins are activated by adding phosphate groups. They can be inactivated by removing phosphate groups. These are the post-translational modifications.

5. Testicular feminization syndrome is a genetic disorder that makes XY foetuses insensitive (unresponsive) to androgens (male hormones). Instead, they are born looking externally like normal girls. Internally, there is a short blind-pouch vagina and no uterus, fallopian tubes or ovaries. There are testes in the abdomen or the inguinal canal. These defects make the body unable to respond to the hormones that produce a male appearance. The complete androgen insensitivity syndrome is usually detected at puberty when a girl should but does not begin to menstruate. Many of the girls with the syndrome have no pubic or axillary (armpit) hair. They have luxuriant scalp hair without temporal (male-pattern) balding. They are sterile and cannot bear children. They are at high risk for osteoporosis and so should take oestrogen replacement therapy.

6. If the apoptosis in the developing limb bud of the frog embryo was specifically blocked, it would result in the non-disjunction of the digits. As such the digits will remain connected and joined to each other. This would give the appearance of a web-like extensive feature.

7. When an antigen enters the body, the immune system produces antibodies against it. Antibodies are always Y-shaped. It is like a battle with the army (antibody) fighting off the invader (antigen). A type of white blood cell called a lymphocyte recognizes the antigen as being foreign and produces antibodies that are specific to that antigen. Each antibody has a unique binding site shape which locks onto the specific shape of the antigen. The antibodies destroy the antigen (pathogen) which is then engulfed and digested by macrophages. When an antigen enters the body, the immune system produces antibodies against it. Antibodies are always Y-shaped. The complex formed by the binding of an antibody to an antigen is known as antigen-antibody complex. Antigen-antibody complexes initiate immune responses.

8. Ecological Succession is an orderly sequence of different communities over a period of time in a particular area. Two different types of succession—primary and secondary—have been distinguished. Primary succession occurs in essentially lifeless areas—regions in which the soil is incapable of sustaining life as a result of such factors as lava flows, newly formed sand dunes, or rocks left from a retreating glacier. Secondary succession occurs in areas where a community that previously existed has been removed; it is typified by smaller-scale disturbances that do not eliminate all life and nutrients from the environment. In some environments, succession reaches a climax, which produces a stable community dominated by a small number of prominent species. This state of equilibrium, called the climax community, is thought to result when the web of biotic interactions becomes so intricate that no other species can be admitted.

9. Habituation involves a loss of responsiveness to unimportant stimuli or stimuli that do not provide appropriate feedback. For example, some animals stop responding to warning signals if signals are not followed by a predator attack (the "cry wolf" effect). In terms of ultimate causation, habituation may increase fitness by allowing an animal's nervous system to focus on meaningful stimuli, rather than wasting time on irrelevant stimuli. In the same way, the

given example of a fish after being habituated with the clap of hands do not startle through a certain passage of time and behavioural modification.

10. The cytoskeleton provides an important structural framework. For cells without cell walls, the cytoskeleton determines the shape of the cell. This is one of the functions of the intermediate filaments. The dynamic collection of micro-filaments and microtubules can be continually in the process of assembly and disassembly, resulting in forces that move the cell. There can also be sliding motions of these structures. Microtubules and microfilaments can help move organelles from place to place in the cell. In the case of endocytosis when a vesicle is formed to engulf some particle from outside the cell, microfilaments attach to the vesicle and pull it into the cell.

11. Systematics is the study of biological diversity and its evolution. Taxonomy, a subdivision of systematics, is the science of biological classification. Classification systems help to clarify relationships among organisms; they help us remember organisms and their traits; they enable us to communicate clearly the identity of organisms being studied; they improve our predictive powers; and they provide stable names. Systematics is the study of biological diversity and its origins. It focuses on understanding evolutionary relationships among organisms, species, higher taxa, or other biological entities, such as genes, and the evolution of the properties of taxa including intrinsic traits, ecological interactions, and geographic distributions. An important part of systematics is the development of methods for various aspects of phylogenetic inference and biological nomenclature/classification.

12. The rapid diversification of multi-cellular animal life around the beginning of the Cambrian Period, resulting in the appearance of almost all modern animal phyla is the Cambrian Explosion. The theory of the Cambrian Explosion holds that, beginning some 545 million years ago, an explosion of diversity led to the appearance over a relatively short period of 5 million to 10 million years of a huge number of complex, multi-celled organisms. Natural selection is generally believed to have favoured larger size, and consequently the need for hard skeletons to provide structural support - hence, the Cambrian gave rise to the first shelled animals and animals with exoskeletons.

13. Given, a recessive disease susceptibility trait is present in cotton plants with white flowers. Now, when a heterozygous coloured cotton plant having homozygous allele for the absence of the disease susceptibility trait is crossed with a white plant which has heterozygous trait for the presence of the disease susceptibility, the overall offsprings formed after the cross would be either homozygous or heterozygous for the absence of the trait because the recessive nature of the disease susceptibility trait. Hence, the probability of disease susceptibility in the offsprings will be 0.

14. The body colour Black (BB) against grey (bb), the eye colour Red (RR) against white (rr) and the wing type normal (WW) against vestigial (ww) are given to linked to each other. When homologous recombination takes place through crossing over, these linked genes will segregate together in the next generation of alleles.

15. Many desert animals live in underground burrows and emerge to feed at night, when conditions are cooler. Mammals such as the kangaroo rat have very efficient kidneys to cope with this problem: the nephrons contain long loops of Henle, to promote high water re-absorption, and dry nasal passages, to reduce water loss. The kidneys of reptiles, having only cortical nephrons, produce urine that is, at best, isosmotic to body fluids. Among mammals, those able to excrete the most hyperosmotic urine, such as kangaroo rats and other mammals adapted to the desert, have exceptionally long loops of Henle that maintain steep osmotic gradients in the kidney.

16. The homeotic gene Antennapedia (Antp) controls determination of many different cell types in the thorax and abdomen of *Drosophila melanogaster*. Mutations in homeotic genes do not eliminate elements of the pattern but rather cause these elements to develop with inappropriate identities. One of the best studied examples of these is the gene Antennapedia(Antp), which as the name suggests causes the transformation of antennal structures to the corresponding (homologous) leg structures. The dominant phenotype of Antp mutants is a result of inappropriate expression of the normal Antp gene product. Antp is normally required in PS4 which corresponds to the posterior part of the first thoracic segment (T1p) and the anterior part of the second thoracic segment. If ANTP is expressed in the antenna (far anterior to PS4) transformation of antennal structures to leg

structures occurs. This can result from a mutation that brings normal coding sequences under inappropriate control or by regulated mis-expression of a cDNA encoding the protein under heat shock control.

17. Retroviral DNA synthesis is absolutely dependent on the two distinct enzymatic activities of RT: a DNA polymerase that can use either RNA or DNA as a template, and a nuclease, termed ribonuclease H (RNase H), that is specific for the RNA strand of RNA:DNA duplexes. First, retroviruses can become integrated into germ line DNA as endogenous viruses, leading to permanent genetic consequences for the descendants of the original host, a property they share with a variety of nonviral, but related, reverse-transcriptase-containing elements. Second, the special replication properties of retroviruses permit development of vectors for modifying the genetic composition of the host. Third, retroviruses display a remarkable variety of pathogenic interactions with their host.

18. Every organism in an ecosystem divides its energy among three competing goals: growing, surviving, and reproducing. Ecologists refer to an organism's allocation of energy among these three ends throughout its lifetime as its life history strategy. There are tradeoffs between these functions: for example, an organism that spends much of its energy on reproduction early in life will have lower growth and survival rates, and thus a lower reproductive level later in life. An optimal life history strategy maximizes the organism's contribution to population growth. In a growing population, survival and reproduction rates will not stay constant over time. Eventually resource limitations will reduce one or both of these variables. Populations grow fastest when they are near zero and the species is uncrowded. A simple mathematical model of population growth implies that the maximum population growth rate occurs when the population size (N) is at one-half of the environment's carrying capacity, K (i.e., at N = K/2). In theory, if a population is harvested at exactly its natural rate of growth, the population will not change in size, and the harvest (yield) can be sustained at that level. In practice, however, it can be very hard to estimate population sizes and growth rates in the wild accurately enough to achieve this maximum sustainable yield.

19. Behavioural nature is not only determined by the constitutive regulation of the genes but also it depends on the behavioural modification and natural adaptation of the genes that are quoting a particular function. Natural selection is one of the basic mechanisms of evolution, along with mutation, migration, and genetic drift. In natural selection, those variations in the genotype that increase an organism's chances of survival and procreation are preserved and multiplied from generation to generation at the expense of less advantageous ones. Evolution often occurs as a consequence of this process. Natural selection may arise from differences in survival, in fertility, in rate of development, in mating success, or in any other aspect of the life cycle. All such differences result in natural selection to the extent that they affect the number of progeny an organism leaves.

20. It has been a long-term puzzle whether chromatin can be further divided into distinct gene expression domains. Because histone deacetylation affects chromatin structure, that in turn may affect the expression of nearby genes, histone deacetylation sites may act to partition chromatin into different gene expression domains. Histone deacetylation is also related to aberrant gene expressions in human cancer. It is well known that there is correlation between histone acetylation level and gene expression. But the detailed relationship between histone acetylation patterns and gene expression domains is less clear.

M: FOOD TECHNOLOGY

1. Kwashiorkor is a form of severe malnutrition that affects children living in poverty in tropical and subtropical parts of the world. It is caused by a lack of protein in the diet. Kwashiorkor stunts growth and causes children to have bloated bellies and thin arms and legs.

2. Rancidity is a term generally used to denote unpleasant odours and flavours in foods resulting from deterioration in the fat or oil portion of a food. Three different mechanisms of rancidity may occur. These are oxidative, hydrolytic, and ketonic. Oxidative rancidity arises from the decomposition of peroxides. Peroxides are the result of the oxidation of unsaturated fats. The products resulting from the decomposition of peroxides include aldehydes, ketones, and hydrocarbons. These help to produce the flavours and odours associated with oxidative rancidity.

3. Q fever is a bacterial infection that can affect the lungs, liver, heart, and other parts of the body. Q fever is found around the world and is caused by the bacteria *Coxiella burnetii.* The bacteria infect sheep, goats, cattle, dogs, cats, birds, rodents, and ticks, as well as some other animals.

4. Several genera of moulds grow on the surface of meat and can cause spoilage, but cannot grow on meat stored below 5°C. Usually, fresh cut meats in the refrigerator at high humidity undergo bacterial spoilage by: Gram negative aerobes like *Pseudomonas*, *Acinetobacter* and *Moraxella spp.* The intrinsic and extrinsic parameters of ground beef favour these bacteria so strongly that they are almost exclusive spoilage agents.

5. Proteins are essential to human health. To better assess the quality of protein in various foods, analysts often use the protein efficiency ratio, or PER, a measure of a specific protein's ability to promote growth. The way that protein in a food or supplement is usually measured is by using the Protein Efficiency Ratio (PER). The protein efficiency ratio for a food is determined in a lab by dividing the weight gain of a test subject who had been given certain types of foods or, more specifically, proteins, by the intake of that particular protein during the test period.

6. Dietary fibre comes from the portion of plants that is not digested by enzymes in the intestinal tract. Part of it, however, may be metabolized by bacteria in the lower gut. Different types of plants vary in their amount and kind of fibre. Fibre includes pectin, gum, mucilage, cellulose, hemicellulose and lignin. Pectin and gum are water-soluble fibres found inside plant cells. They slow the passage of food through the intestines but do nothing to increase faecal bulk. Insoluble fibres also decrease cholesterol and can help lower blood glucose. Beans, oat bran, fruit and vegetables contain water-soluble fibre.

7. The extruder barrel is the holding chamber of an extrusion or injection moulding machine. The barrel holds the resin as the screw melts and mixes it. In the extrusion of plastics, raw thermoplastic material in the form of nurdles (small beads, often called resin in the industry) is gravity fed from a top mounted hopper into the barrel of the extruder. Additives such as colorants and UV inhibitors (in either liquid or pellet form) are often used and can be mixed into the resin prior to arriving at the hopper. The process has much in common with plastic injection moulding from the point of the extruder technology though it differs in that it is usually a continuous process.

8. The Maillard reaction is occurring for most of cooking: such as caramel, or roasting. The Maillard reaction occurs when the denatured proteins on the surface of the meat recombine with the sugars present. The combination creates the "meaty" flavour and changes the colour. For this reason, it is also called the browning reaction. The Maillard reaction occurs most readily at around 300° F to 500° F. When meat is cooked, the outside reaches a higher temperature than the inside, triggering the Maillard reaction and creating the strongest flavours on the surface.

9. Blanching is a term that usually refers to the very brief cooking of a fresh vegetable prior to freezing. Blanching typically involves vegetables rather than other types of food (like fruit or meat) because vegetables are particularly susceptible to enzyme-triggered changes that can result in lost flavour, lost colour, and lost texture during freezing. The prevention of unwanted changes in flavour, colour, and texture is not the only purpose of blanching, however. Other purposes include: Thoroughly cleansing of the vegetable surface, and increasing the safety of frozen vegetables in terms of potentially unwanted microorganisms.

10. Crushing or chopping garlic releases an enzyme called allinase that catalyzes the formation of allicin. Allicin rapidly breaks down to form a variety of organosulfur compounds. Allicin breaks down *in vitro* to form a variety of fat-soluble organo-sulphur compounds, including diallyl trisulfide (DATS), diallyl disulfide (DADS), and diallyl sulfide (DAS), or in the presence of oil or organic solvents, ajoene and vinyldithiins. Crushing garlic does not change its gamma-glutamylcysteine content. Water-soluble organo-sulphur compounds, such as S-allylcysteine, are formed from gamma-glutamylcysteines during long-term incubation of crushed garlic in aqueous solutions, as in the manufacture of aged garlic extracts.

11. Gossypol is a natural phenol derived from the cotton plant. Gossypol is a phenolic aldehyde that permeates cells and acts as an inhibitor for several dehydrogenase enzymes. Vicine

is an alkaloid glycoside found in fava beans. Vicine is toxic, causing the disease favism, in individuals who have a hereditary loss of the enzyme glucose-6-phosphate dehydrogenase. Glucosinolates are thioethers. They generally consist of a sugar entity, β-D-thioglucose, with an ester bond to an organic aglycone that is an alkyl group yielding isothiocyanate, nitrile, thiocyanate or a similar compound upon hydrolysis. Rapeseed meal contains several glucosinolates and produces not only oxazolidine-2-thiones but also isothiocyanates, nitriles and thiocyanates. β-N-Oxalylamino-L-alanine (BOAA) is a dicarboxylic diamino acid present in *Lathyrus sativus* (chickling pea). Excessive oral intake of this legume in remote areas of the world causes humans and animals to develop a type of spastic paraparesis known as lathyrism.

12. Aspartame is a methyl ester of the dipeptide of the natural amino acids L-aspartic acid and L-phenylalanine. Under strongly acidic or alkaline conditions, aspartame may generate methanol by hydrolysis. Thermolysin is involved in its preparation. Cocoa butter equivalents, healthy oil containing medium-chain fatty acids, phosphatidyl serine, and phenol lipids from enzyme technology have been reported for commercial operation. As the demand for better quality functional lipids is increasing, the production of structured lipids becomes an interesting area. Lipases act as biocatalysts for the synthesis of structured lipids. Glucose isomerase (GI) (D-xylose ketol-isomerase) catalyzes the reversible isomerization of D-glucose and D-xylose to D-fructose and D-xylulose, respectively. The enzyme has the largest market in the food industry because of its application in the production of high-fructose corn syrup (HFCS). The enzyme β-galactosidase most commonly known as lactase, which hydrolyses lactose into its monomers that is glucose and galactose has potential applications in food processing industry. Because of low levels of the enzyme in intestine, large fraction of the population shows lactose intolerance and they have difficulty in consuming milk and dairy products.

13. Mayonnaise is a thick, creamy sauce often used as a condiment. The oil and the water in yolks form a base of the emulsion, while lecithin and protein from the yolks are the emulsifiers that stabilize it. Ketchup is a sweet and tangy sauce, typically made from tomatoes, vinegar, a sweetener, and assorted seasonings and spices. The sweetener is most commonly sugar or high-fructose corn syrup. Cake is a form of bread or bread-like food. Curds are a dairy product obtained by curdling (coagulating) milk with rennet or an edible acidic substance such as lemon juice or vinegar, and then draining off the liquid portion.

14. Starch is a non homogeneous polymer (i.e., a complex of simpler bits), a "polysaccharide" of thousands of simple sugars in a similar way that fats are polymers of aliphatic acids, proteins of amino acids and tannins of simple phenols. The gel/sol interaction is reversible, with increasing water and temperature and enzymatic activity favouring the sol. The gel is a COLLOIDAL structure that is it has inter-particle bonds (usually hydrogen bonds) of lower potential energy than starch in true SOLUTION. Thus enzymatically unconverted mash starch extracted by lauter will form a gel haze by complexing when the boiled wort is cooled and the lower thermodynamic condition is favoured. This is called "starch haze". Starch is insoluble in cold water but in warm water it swells until "gelatinisation temperature" when it begins to lose structure and leach out compounds.

15. From Thermal death kinetics, we have

$$\log_e(N/N_0) = -\int_0^t Kdt$$

where,

N = no. of microorganisms at time t,

N_0 = initial no. Of micro-organisms

K = thermal death constant

Therefore, $\log_e(N/N_0) = -Kt$

Given, $K = 0.23\ min^{-1}$,

$N/N_0 = 0.01$

Thus, $-0.23 \times t = \log_e(0.01)$

$\Rightarrow t = 20.022$

The required time of death is 20 minutes

16. Let x kg be the weight of skim milk to be added

We have,

50% of fat present in 500 kg cream

= 250 kg of fat present

Now,

$250 - 0.1\% x = (500 + x) \times 36\%$

$\Rightarrow 250 - 0.001 x = 180 + 0.36 x$

$\Rightarrow 250 - 180 = 0.36 x + 0.001 x$

$\Rightarrow$ 0.361 x = 70

$\Rightarrow$ x = 193.90

The required weight of the skim milk is 194 kg (approx.)

17. Myosins are a class of molecular motors responsible for many motile processes in eukaryotic organisms. Myosins produce force and displacement through their interaction with actin. Actin, a major constituent of the cytoskeleton, can form filaments which act as "tracks" for myosin-driven motility. The system of actin and myosin working together is referred to as actomyosin.

18. Given, storage weight of the apples

= 50 tonnes

Temperature drop for cooling

$= (28 - 2)^0C$

Time required for cooling

= 16 hours

Specific heat of apple

$= 0.874 \text{ Kcal kg}^{-1}\ {}^0C^{-1}$

The required weight of the storage capacity

= 24 tonnes

19. Theoretical yield of the reaction of conversion of ethanol to acetic acid,

$CH_3CH_2OH + O_2$

$\rightarrow CH_3COOH + H_2O$

So 1 mole of ethanol gives rise to 1 mole of acetic acid

Molar mass of acetic acid

= 60 g/mol

Molar mass of ethanol

= 46 g/mol

Therefore, theoretical yield

$= 46/60 \times 100\ \%$

$= 76.67\ \%$

Actual yield in the process

$= \frac{(8.4 \text{ g/L})}{(10 - 0.8)\text{g/L}}$

$= \frac{8.4}{9.2}$

= 0.9130 x 100%

= 91.30 %

Conversion efficiency in terms of theoretical yield

= 76.67% of 91.30

= 70.003 %

20. We know, From Michaelis-Menten equation,

$V = (V_{max}[S])/(K_m + [S])$

Given, $V = 60 \text{ nmol l}^{-1} \text{ min}^{-1}$,

$V_{max} = 75 \text{ nmol l}^{-1} \text{ min}^{-1}$,

$[S] = 1 \times 10^{-4}$ M

Therefore, $60 = \frac{75 \times 10^{-4}}{(K_m + 10^{-4})}$

$\Rightarrow K_m + 10^{-4} = 1.25 \times 10^{-4}$

$\Rightarrow K_m = 0.25 \times 10^{-4}$

$\Rightarrow K_m = 2.5 \times 10^{-5}$

The K_m value is 2.5×10^{-5} M

GATE-2012

XL : LIFE SCIENCES

Time : 3 Hours | *Maximum Marks : 100*

GA : GENERAL APTITUDE (*Compulsory*)

Q. 1 – 5 carry one mark each.

1. If $(1.001)^{1259} = 3.52$ and $(1.001)^{2062} = 7.85$, then $(1.001)^{3321} =$

   (*a*) 2.23 (*b*) 4.33 (*c*) 11.37 (*d*) 27.64

2. One of the parts (A, B, C, D) in the sentence given below contains an ERROR.

   Which one of the following is **INCORRECT?**

   I requested that he should be given the driving test today instead of tomorrow.

   (*a*) requested that (*b*) should be given
   (*c*) the driving test (*d*) instead of tomorrow

3. Which one of the following options is the closest in meaning to the word given below?

   Latitude

   (*a*) Eligibility (*b*) Freedom
   (*c*) Coercion (*d*) Meticulousness

4. Choose the most appropriate word from the options given below to complete the following sentence:

   Given the seriousness of the situation that he had to face, his _____ was impressive.

   (*a*) beggary (*b*) nomenclature
   (*c*) jealousy (*d*) nonchalance

5. Choose the most appropriate alternative from the options given below to complete the following sentence:

   If the tired soldier wanted to lie down, he ___ the mattress out on the balcony.

   (*a*) should take (*b*) shall take
   (*c*) should have taken (*d*) will have taken

Q. 6 – 10 carry two marks each.

6. **One of the legacies of the Roman legions was discipline. In the legions, military law prevailed and discipline was brutal. Discipline on the battlefield kept units obedient, intact and fighting, even when the odds and conditions were against them.**

   Which one of the following statements best sums up the meaning of the above passage?

   (*a*) Thorough regimentation was the main reason for the efficiency of the Roman legions even in adverse circumstances.

   (*b*) The legions were treated inhumanly as if the men were animals.

   (*c*) Discipline was the armies' inheritance from their seniors.

   (*d*) The harsh discipline to which the legions were subjected to led to the odds and conditions being against them.

7. A and B are friends. They decide to meet between 1 PM and 2 PM on a given day. There is a condition that whoever arrives first will not wait for the other for more than 15 minutes. The probability that they will meet on that day is

   (*a*) 1/4 (*b*) 1/16 (*c*) 7/16 (*d*) 9/16

8. The data given in the following table summarizes the monthly budget of an average household.

Category	Amount (Rs.)
Food	4000
Clothing	1200
Rent	2000
Savings	1500
Other expenses	1800

   The approximate percentage of the monthly budget NOT spent on savings is

   (*a*) 10% (*b*) 14% (*c*) 81% (*d*) 86%

9. There are eight bags of rice looking alike, seven of which have equal weight and one is slightly heavier. The weighing balance is of unlimited capacity. Using this balance, the minimum number of weighings required to identify the heavier bag is

   (*a*) 2 (*b*) 3 (*c*) 4 (*d*) 8

10. Raju has 14 currency notes in his pocket consisting of only ₹ 20 notes and ₹ 10 notes. The total money value of the notes is ₹ 230. The number of ₹ 10 notes that Raju has is

    (*a*) 5 (*b*) 6 (*c*) 9 (*d*) 10

H : CHEMISTRY (*Compulsory*)

Q. 1 – 5 carry one mark each.

1. Among the following, the most reactive diene in the Diels-Alder reaction is

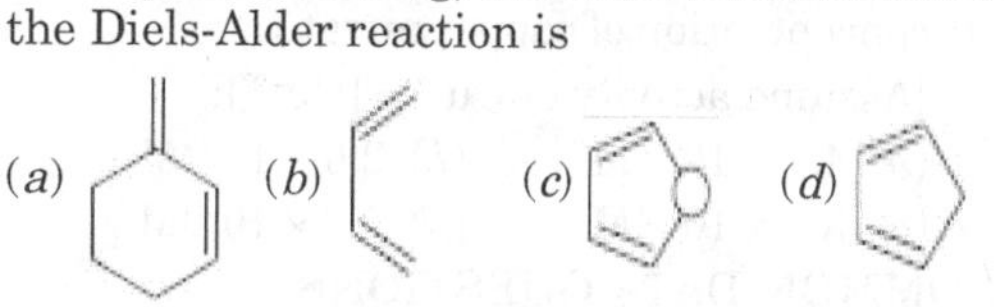

2. The molecule that does **NOT** absorb the microwave radiation is

   (*a*) CO_2 (*b*) H_2O (*c*) CO (*d*) NO

3. The hybridization of atomic orbitals of sulphur in SF_4 is

   (*a*) dsp^2 (*b*) sp^3d^2 (*c*) sp^3d (*d*) sp^3

4. The ionic size of Na^+, F^-, Mg^{2+} and Al^{3+} varies as

   (*a*) $Al^{3+} > Mg^{2+} > Na^+ > F^-$ (*b*) $F^- > Na^+ > Mg^{2+} > Al^{3+}$
   (*c*) $Al^{3+} > Mg^{2+} > F > Na$ (*d*) $Na > F > Mg > Al$

5. The non-aromatic compound/ion is

(*a*) 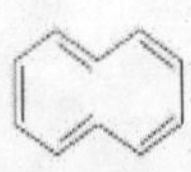 (*b*) 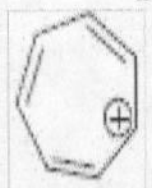 (*c*) 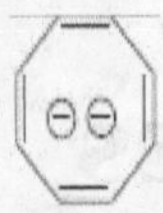 (*d*) 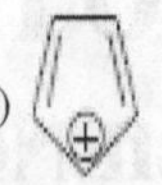

Q. 6 – 15 carry two marks each.

6. As predicted by MO theory, the bond order and magnetic nature of NO^+ are
(*a*) three and paramagnetic
(*b*) two and diamagnetic
(*c*) two and paramagnetic
(*d*) three and diamagnetic

7. The value of ionic product of water changes with temperature. It is 1×10^{-14} at 25°C and 1×10^{-13} at 60°C. The **CORRECT** statement with respect to ΔH and ΔS is
(*a*) ΔH is negative and ΔS is negative
(*b*) ΔH is positive and ΔS is zero
(*c*) ΔH is positive and ΔS is negative
(*d*) ΔH is negative and ΔS is positive

8. 10 micrograms of the enzyme carbonic anhydrase (molecular weight = 30,000 g/mole) removes 300 milligrams of carbon dioxide per minute from the cells. The turnover number of the enzyme is
(*a*) 20 min^{-1} (*b*) 2×10^7 min^{-1}
(*c*) 2×10^{10} min^{-1} (*d*) 7.2×10^{10} min^{-1}

9. The iodide which reacts most slowly with cyanide ion as a nucleophile in a SN^2 reaction is
(*a*) CH_3 $CH_2CH_2CH_2I$ (*b*) 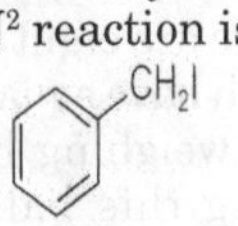
(*c*) 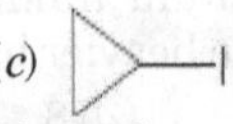 (*d*) (CH_3) CH-I

10. The value of K_a of acetic acid is 1.7×10^{-5} mol/dm^3. The pH of a buffer solution prepared by mixing 100 ml of 0.1 M acetic acid with a solution of 100 ml of 0.2 M sodium acetate is
(*a*) 4.1 (*b*) 4.5 (*c*) 5.1 (*d*) 5.5

11. The value of standard half cell potential of Cu^{+2}, Cu couple ($E^0_{Cu(+2), Cu}$) is 0.34 V. A wire of pure copper is immersed into a solution of copper nitrate. If the measured cell potential against standard hydrogen electrode at 298 K is 0.24 V, the molar concentration of copper nitrate is
{Assume activity of Cu^{+2} = $[Cu^{+2}]$}.
(*a*) 4.1×10^{-4} M (*b*) 2.0×10^{-2}M
(*c*) 3.4×10^{-2} M (*d*) 1.8×10^{-1}M

COMMON DATA QUESTIONS

Common Data for Questions 12 and 13:
$[FeCl_4]^{2-}$(I), $[CoCl_4]^{2-}$ (II) and $[NiCl_4]^{2-}$ (III) are paramagnetic tetrahedral complexes.

12. The order of values of crystal field stabilization energy is
(*a*) I > III > II (*b*) III > I > II
(*c*) I > II > III (*d*) II > III > I

13. The order of values of spin only magnetic moment is
(*a*) III > II > I (*b*) III > I > II
(*c*) II > I > III (*d*) I > II > III

Linked Answer Questions

Statement for Linked Answer Questions 14 and 15:
Bromine water is decolourised upon reaction with (E)-3-hexene.

14. It is due to
(*a*) electrophilic addition of bromine to C = C
(*b*) nucleophilic addition of bromine to C = C
(*c*) electrophilic allylic bromination
(*d*) nucleophilic allylic bromination

15. The structure of the product obtained is
(*a*) 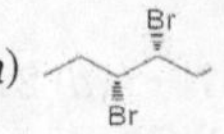 (*b*) 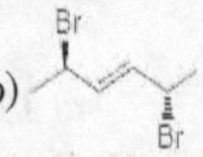 (*c*) 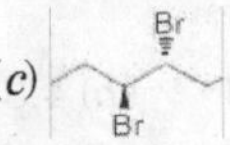 (*d*) 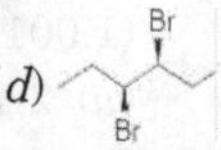

I : BIOCHEMISTRY

Q. 1 – 10 carry one mark each.

1. Four proteins (P1, P2, P3 and P4) have 17, 10, 21 and 14 percent hydrophobic amino-acids respectively. The order of precipitation of these proteins using ammonium sulphate will be
(*a*) P3, P1, P4, P2 (*b*) P3, P1, P2, P4
(*c*) P2, P4, P3, P1 (*d*) P2, P4, P1, P3

2. Which one of the following pairs of amino-acids in the protein has high propensity to take up the α-helix conformation?
(*a*) Gly-Asp (*b*) Pro-His (*c*) Gly-Pro (*d*) Ala-Arg

3. Which one of the following closely defines 'Molten Globule' state of a protein?
(*a*) State with high degree of secondary structure and loss of tertiary structure
(*b*) State with complete loss of secondary structure
(*c*) Completely unfolded state
(*d*) Loss of quaternary structure

4. Which one of the following amino-acids has highest fluorescence quantum yield (Φ) in aqueous solution?
(*a*) Tyrosine (*b*) Tryptophan
(*c*) Phenylalanine (*d*) Histidine

5. Which one of the following compounds does **NOT** block electron transport?
(*a*) Cyanide (*b*) Rotenone
(*c*) Oligomycin (*d*) Antimycin A

6. The pair of amino-acids which does **NOT** undergo post-translational modification is
(*a*) Asn-His (*b*) Tyr-Ser (*c*) Asn-Ser (*d*) Ala-Gly

7. Match the hormones in **Group I** with their metabolic precursor in **Group II**

Group I	Group II
P. 17-β estradiol	1. Arachidonic
Q. Thromboxane A2	2. Tyrosine
R. Epinephrine	3. β-carotene
S. Retinoic acid	4. Cholesterol

Codes:

	P	Q	R	S
(*a*)	4	2	3	1
(*b*)	1	3	2	4
(*c*)	4	1	2	3
(*d*)	1	2	4	3

8. Upon stimulation of a eukaryotic cell, the intracellular calcium (Ca^{2+}) is released from
   (*a*) Endoplasmic reticulum
   (*b*) Nucleus
   (*c*) Peroxisome
   (*d*) Mitochondria
9. Leguminous plants maintain a very low concentration of free oxygen in their root nodules because
   (*a*) the nitrogen fixing bacteria living in the root nodules are anaerobic
   (*b*) of binding of oxygen to leghemoglobin
   (*c*) reductase enzyme of the nitrogenase complex helps in removal of O_2
   (*d*) nitrogenase enzyme of the nitrogenase complex helps in removal of O_2
10. The membrane of mature B cells have
   (*a*) both IgG and IgM (*b*) both IgG and IgD
   (*c*) both IgM and IgE (*d*) both IgM and IgD

Q. 11 – 20 carry two marks each.

11. An amino-acid has one proton donating group in the side chain (R). The pK_{COOH}, pK_{NH2} and pK_R values for this amino-acid are 2.19, 9.67 and 4.25, respectively. Which one of the following statements about this amino-acid is **CORRECT**?
   (*a*) Majority of the molecules will have a net charge of –1 at pH of 7.0
   (*b*) Majority of the molecules will have a net charge of 0 at pH of 4.25
   (*c*) All the molecules will have a deprotonated R group at pH of 3.22
   (*d*) During titration with a strong base, deprotonation will start with the R group
12. Which one of the following bacterial toxins does **NOT** have ADP-ribosyl transferase activity?
   (*a*) Pertussis toxin
   (*b*) Diphtheria toxin
   (*c*) Pseudomonas Exotoxin A
   (*d*) *S. aureus* α-toxin
13. The **CORRECT** pair of amino-acid sequence and the corresponding target organelle is
   (*a*) KDEL -Golgi
   (*b*) K-K/R-X-K/R -Lysosome
   (*c*) SKL -Peroxisome
   (*d*) NPVY -Endoplasmic reticulum
14. β-oxidation of a 16 carbon fatty acid and a 17 carbon fatty acid leads to formation of
   (*a*) (8 Acetyl CoA) and (8 Acetyl CoA + CO_2), respectively
   (*b*) (5 Propionyl CoA +1CO_2) and (5 Propionyl CoA +1 Acetyl CoA), respectively
   (*c*) (5 Propionyl CoA + 1CO_2) and (5 Propionyl CoA + 2 CO_2), respectively
   (*d*) (8 Acetyl CoA) and (7 Acetyl CoA + 1 Propionyl CoA), respectively
15. Pick the correctly matched pairs.
   P. Immature B cells — Terminal deoxynucleotidyl transferase
   Q. Activated B cells — Class switching
   R. Pre B cells — Surrogate light chain
   S. Mature B cells – Recombination activating gene 1
   (*a*) P and R (*b*) Q and R (*c*) Q and S (*d*) Q and P
16. The actual free energy change of a given biochemical reaction carried out under standard conditions with 1 M initial concentration of each of the reactants and products will be
   (*a*) equal to zero
   (*b*) equal to standard free energy change for the reaction
   (*c*) less than the standard free energy change for the reaction
   (*d*) greater than the standard free energy change for the reaction
17. Match the enzymes in Group I with their corresponding activity in Group II

Group I

P. Flippase Q. Floppase
R. Lipase S. Scramblase

Group II

1. Catalyzes the movement of any phospholipid across the lipid bilayer down its concentration gradient
2. Catalyzes the translocation of amino-phospholipids from the extracellular to the inner leaflet
3. Catalyzes the translocation of membrane phospholipids from cytosolic to the extracellular leaflet
4. Degradation of phospholipids from the lipid bilayer including the inner and outer leaflets

Codes:

	P	Q	R	S
(*a*)	2	3	4	1
(*b*)	1	2	3	4
(*c*)	4	1	2	3
(*d*)	3	2	4	1

18. Match the antibiotics in Group I with their mechanism of action in Group II

Group I

P. Tetracyclines Q. Chloramphenicol
R. Cycloheximide S. Streptomycin

Group II

1. Inhibits bacterial protein synthesis by blocking peptidyl transfer
2. Inhibits bacterial protein synthesis by blocking the A-site on the ribosome
3. Misreads the genetic code and inhibits initiation of protein synthesis
4. Inhibits protein synthesis by blocking peptidyl transferase on 80S ribosome

Codes:

	P	Q	R	S
(*a*)	2	1	3	4
(*b*)	2	1	4	3
(*c*)	4	3	1	2
(*d*)	3	4	2	1

19. The kinetics of an enzyme in the presence (+I) or absence (–I) of a reversible inhibitor is described in the following graph.

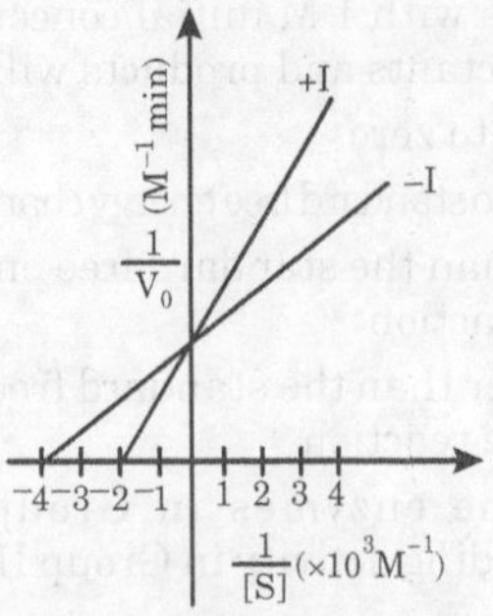

If concentration of the reversible inhibitor in + I experiment was equal to 3.0×10^{-3} M, then the dissociation constant for the enzyme-inhibitor complex is

(*a*) 1×10^{-3}M (*b*) 2×10^{-3}M
(*c*) 3×10^{-3}M (*d*) 4×10^{-3}M

20. The figure below is a schematic of a linear double stranded DNA containing the indicated restriction sites. The DNA was completely digested with *Pvu*II and *Eco*RI. The products were purified and added to an appropriately buffered reaction mixture containing dNTP mix, $\alpha-^{32}P$ dATP, and Klenow fragment of *E. coli* DNA polymerase I. The Klenow reaction products were analyzed by gel electrophoresis and autoradiography. Which of the following products depicts the expected result?

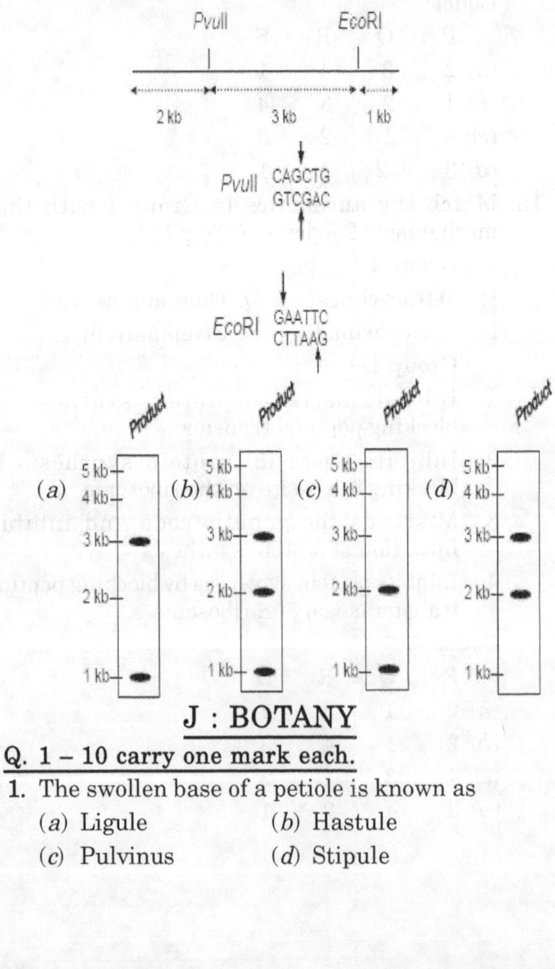

J : BOTANY

Q. 1 – 10 carry one mark each.

1. The swollen base of a petiole is known as

(*a*) Ligule (*b*) Hastule
(*c*) Pulvinus (*d*) Stipule

2. An estimate of phylogenetic relationships among the taxa is commonly represented in the form of a

(*a*) Cladogram (*b*) Idiogram
(*c*) Phenogram (*d*) Dendrogram

3. Parenchyma cells associated with sieve tube members are called

(*a*) Albuminous cells
(*b*) Companion cells
(*c*) Bulliform cells
(*d*) Subsidiary cells

4. Cytoplasmic male sterility via the chloroplast genome can be induced by the expression of *Pha A* gene encoding

(*a*) β-Ketothiolase
(*b*) Acetoacetyl CoA carboxylase
(*c*) Acetoacetyl CoA reductase
(*d*) PHB synthase

5. The number of nucleosomes present in a 30 nm solenoid structure of a chromatin is

(*a*) 2 (*b*) 4 (*c*) 6 (*d*) 8

6. Which one of the following performs normal C_3 photosynthesis when water is available, but switches to crassulacean acid metabolism (CAM) during salt or drought stress?

(*a*) *Mesembryanthemum crystallinum*
(*b*) *Cynodon dactylon*
(*c*) *Eleucine coracana*
(*d*) *Hordeum vulgare*

7. Which one of the following is a free-living photosynthetic nitrogen fixer?

(*a*) *Frankia* (*b*) *Clostridium*
(*c*) *Rhodospirillum* (*d*) *Rhizobium*

8. Carbon dioxide and other 'greenhouse gases' act by

(*a*) destroying ozone in the stratosphere
(*b*) trapping heat in the earth's atmosphere
(*c*) allowing more visible light to reach the earth's surface
(*d*) reducing the amount of radiant energy which reaches the surface of the earth

9. Which of the following best represents the flow of energy through an ecosystem?

(*a*) Producers → Primary consumers → Secondary consumers
(*b*) Sun → Producers → Secondary consumers → Primary consumers
(*c*) Sun → Producers → Primary consumers → Secondary consumers
(*d*) Secondary consumers → Primary consumers → Producers → Sun

10. Which one of the following drugs is obtained from the capsule of *Papaver somniferum*?

(*a*) Papain (*b*) Codeine
(*c*) Digoxin (*d*) Bromelain

Q. 11 – 20 carry two marks each.

11. Which of the following statements are TRUE for plant growth regulators?
    P. The release of cellulase and polygalacturonase into the cell wall is promoted by abscissic acid
    Q. The early biosynthetic steps of gibberellic acid, up to the formation of ent-kaurene take place in the plastid
    R. The naturally occurring zeatin belongs to the aromatic group of cytokinins
    S. Induction of protease inhibitors as a result of wounding and pathogen attack is activated by jasmonic acid
    (*a*) P, R (*b*) Q, S (*c*) Q, R (*d*) P, Q

12. Which of the following statements are TRUE for the transposable elements?
    P. Barbara McClintock discovered the autonomous and non-autonomous transposable elements in Maize
    Q. Variations in flower pigmentation in *Antirhinum* are due to the presence of transposable elements Ac and Ds
    R. The Ac transposable element is 4563 bp long and has an 11 bp inverted repeats
    S. Ds produces the transposase and mobilize the Ac elements
    (*a*) Q, S (*b*) P, Q (*c*) P, R (*d*) R, S

13. Match the recombinant proteins produced through molecular farming with their applications.

Recombinant proteins	**Applications**
P. Hirudine	1. HIV therapy
Q. Trichosanthin	2. Anticoagulant
R. Somatotrophin	3. Growth hormone
S. β-Interferon	4. Hypertension
	5. Cystic fibrosis
	6. Treatment for hepatitis-B

Codes:

	P	Q	R	S
(*a*)	2	3	4	1
(*b*)	4	1	5	2
(*c*)	1	5	3	2
(*d*)	2	1	3	6

14. Which of the following statements are CORRECT for somatic cell hybridization?
    P. For fusion of protoplast, dimethy-lsulfoxide (DMSO) is used as a fusogen
    Q. The enzyme 'Cellulase Onozuka' used for protoplast isolation is sourced from *Trichoderma viride*
    R. The first report of somatic hybrid plants resulted from the fusion of protoplasts of *Nicotiana glauca* and *N. tabacum*
    S. Viability of isolated protoplasts can be determined by Evan's blue staining
    (*a*) P, Q (*b*) Q, S (*c*) R, S (*d*) Q, R

15. Which of the following statements are TRUE on transgene approach?
    P. T-DNA integration occurs mainly through non-homologous recombination
    Q. The Gateway cloning depends on recombination technology as opposed to standard uses of restriction enzymes and DNA ligase
    R. The localization of β-glucuronidase (GUS) activity as a result of expression of GUS reporter gene can be visualized in a histochemical assay using the X-gal
    S. The green fluorescent protein gene (GFP) is isolated from the bacterium *Photinus pyralis*
    (*a*) P, Q (*b*) Q, R (*c*) P, S (*d*) R, S

16. Identify the free radicals (marked as '?') in sequence from the inter-conversion of reactive oxygen species as shown below.

$$O_2 \rightarrow ? \rightarrow H_2O_2 \rightarrow ? \rightarrow H_2O$$

    P. $O_2^{\bullet -}$ Q. OH^-
    R. HO_2^- S. $^1O_2$
    (*a*) P, Q (*b*) R, Q (*c*) P, R (*d*) Q, S

17. With respect to adhesion and cohesion of stamens, identify the INCORRECT statements.
    P. Adnation of stamens to petals is described as epiphyllous stamens
    Q. In *Calotropis*, stamens and carpels are united to form gynostegium
    R. In syngenesious stamens, filaments are united to form a bundle while the anthers are free
    S. Synandrous stamens found in *Cucurbita* represent the union of filaments as well as anthers
    (*a*) P, Q (*b*) P, R (*c*) Q, S (*d*) Q, R

18. Identify the CORRECT statements in plant secondary metabolism.
    P. Tropane alkaloids in *Atropa belladonna* are synthesized from tyrosine
    Q. Antioxidative food ingredient rosmarinic acid is obtained from cell suspension cultures of *Coleus blumei*
    R. Thiophenes are produced from hairy root cultures of *Tagetes patula*
    S. Cyanidin, the principal antho-cyanin responsible for red color in *Rosa hybrida* is produced from cinnamaldehyde
    (*a*) P, S (*b*) R, S (*c*) P, Q (*d*) Q, R

19. Which of the following statements are TRUE for respiration?
    P. The conversion of one molecule of pyruvate to three molecules of CO_2 generates four molecules of NADH
    Q. Fructose 6-phospate is the principal substrate for glycolysis
    R. The oxidation of glucose 6-phosphate to 6-phosphogluconate is the first step in the oxidative pentose phosphate pathway

S. The mitochondrial 'alternative oxidase' provides an alternative pathway for transfer of electrons from ubiquinone to oxygen utilizing proton pumping complex of the respiratory chain

(*a*) P, R (*b*) P, S (*c*) Q, R (*d*) Q, S

20. 'Match the name of the disease with the causal organism.

Disease	Causal organism
P. Black rot of sugarcane	1. *Cercospora personata*
Q. Stem rot of jute	2. *Macrophomina phaseolina*
R. Tikka disease of groundnut	3. *Ceratocystis adiposa*
S. Crown gall of grapes	4. *Synchytrium endobioticum*
	5. *Agrobacterium tumefaciens*
	6. *Colletotrichum corchorum*

Codes:

	P	Q	R	S
(*a*)	1	3	6	5
(*b*)	2	3	1	5
(*c*)	3	2	1	5
(*d*)	2	6	3	4

K : MICROBIOLOGY

Q. 1 – 10 carry one mark each.

1. Which ONE of the following components is NOT an electron acceptor during anaerobic respiration?
(*a*) Lactate (*b*) Carbonate (*c*) Nitrate (*d*) Sulphate

2. Bergey's Manual of Systematic Bacteriology groups bacteria into species according to their
(*a*) nutritional requirement
(*b*) phylogenetic relationships
(*c*) pathogenic properties
(*d*) morphology

3. An auxotrophic mutant arises spontaneously in a wild type *E.coli* culture growing in a rich medium. Which ONE of the following techniques will ensure the isolation of the auxotrophic mutant?
(*a*) Replica plating
(*b*) Streaking for single colonies
(*c*) Pour plating method
(*d*) Direct microscopic observation

4. Which ONE of the following mutants is used to carry out genetic analysis to determine the function of an essential gene?
(*a*) Knock out mutant
(*b*) Deletion mutant
(*c*) Insertion mutant
(*d*) Temperature sensitive mutant

5. An *E.coli* mutant constitutive for the *lac* operon was mated with a wild type strain. The merodiploid thus obtained was inducible by lactose. This observation indicates that the original mutation is
(*a*) dominant (*b*) trans-dominant
(*c*) recessive (*d*) cis-dominant

6. A rich medium is inoculated with a bacterium that divides every 30 minutes. The number of bacteria at the end of 50 hours is
(*a*) 2×10^{10} (*b*) 2×10^{20} (*c*) 1×10^{50} (*d*) 1×2^{100}

7. Which ONE of the following statements about *E.coli* is NOT true ?
(*a*) *E.coli* was the first disease-causing bacterium identified by Robert Koch
(*b*) *E.coli* is part of the normal microbiota of humans
(*c*) Certain *E.coli* strains can cause bloody diarrohea
(*d*) *E.coli* is beneficial to human

8. Antibody coated pathogens are recognized by effector cells through
(*a*) CD4 receptor (*b*) F_C receptor
(*c*) CD8 receptor (*d*) IFN gamma receptor

9. Match the disease in Group I with their corresponding organism in Group II

Group I	Group II
P. African sleeping sickness	I. Rubulavirus
Q. Rocky mountain spotted fever	II. Trypanosoma brucei
R. Mumps	III. Wuchereria bancrofti
S. Filariasis	IV. Rickettsia rickettsii
	V. Leishmania donovani

Codes:

	P	Q	R	S
(*a*)	III	V	II	I
(*b*)	II	I	III	IV
(*c*)	II	IV	I	III
(*d*)	I	V	II	IV

10. Select the technique most appropriate to demonstrate that lactose induces the synthesis of β-galactosidase enzyme.
(*a*) Northern Blot (*b*) Western Blot
(*c*) Quantitative PCR (*d*) Southern Blot

Q. 11 – 20 carry two marks each.

11. Frederick Griffith used smooth (S) and rough (R) strains of *Streptococcus pneumoniae* in his classical experiment that showed DNA might be the genetic element. Which ONE of the following observations gave the clue for this discovery?
(*a*) R strain became S strain when mixed with heat killed S strain
(*b*) R strain remained R strain when mixed with heat killed S strain
(*c*) S strain became R strain when mixed with heat killed R strain
(*d*) R strain became S strain when mixed with live S strain

12. Entry of λ phage lysogen to lytic phase is triggered by
(*a*) mutation in the λ genome
(*b*) loss of co-operativity in binding of λ repressor
(*c*) increase in the λ repressor concentration
(*d*) decrease in *rec*A function

13. Match the Phylum in **Group I** with their characteristic motility appendage listed in **Group II**

Group I	Group II
P. Archaezoa	I. Flagella
Q. Amoebozoa	II. Fimbriae
R. Ciliophora	III. Pseudopods
S. Apicomplexa	IV. Cilia
	V. Pili

Codes:

	P	Q	R	S
(*a*)	V	II	IV	IV
(*b*)	II	I	IV	III
(*c*)	I	III	IV	I
(*d*)	III	II	IV	V

14. Ten bacteria were inoculated into a rich medium. If at the end of ten hours the total number of cells is 10^4, then the number of elapsed generations and the generation time respectively is

(*a*) 10, 120 minutes (*b*) 10, 60 minutes
(*c*) 20, 30 minutes (*d*) 40, 15 minutes

15. The first step in the replication of a virus with the reverse transcriptase deals with the synthesis of

(*a*) complementary strand of RNA
(*b*) double stranded RNA
(*c*) complementary strand of DNA
(*d*) double stranded DNA

16. An *E.coli* mutant defective for an enzyme is unable to grow on acetate but grows on glycerol as the sole carbon source. Which ONE of the following enzymes is likely to be defective in this mutant?

(*a*) Isocitrate dehydrogenase
(*b*) Glyceraldehyde 3-phospahte dehydrogenase
(*c*) Pyruvate dehydrogenase
(*d*) Isocitrate lyase

17. Which one of the following pairs of bacterial species fixes atmospheric Nitrogen?

(*a*) *Clostridia* and *Rhizobia*
(*b*) *Clostridia* and *Lactobacillus*
(*c*) *Rhizobia* and *Enterococcus*
(*d*) *Actinomycetes* and *Mycoplasma*

18. Nalidixic acid inhibits gyrase activity. Resistance to this antibiotic arises mainly due to

(*a*) nonsense mutation in the gyrase gene
(*b*) deletion mutation in the gyrase gene
(*c*) missense mutation in the gyrase gene
(*d*) degradation of the gyrase gene product

19. Transformation of normal cyanobacterial cells into heterocysts involves

(*a*) synthesis of nitrogenase and retention of photosystem I
(*b*) synthesis of nitrogenase and loss of photosystem I
(*c*) loss of nitrogenase but retention of photosystem I
(*d*) loss of both nitrogenase and photosystem I

20. Methane belched (eructation) out by cattle arises from the carbon dioxide produced

(*a*) during normal respiration
(*b*) oxidation of food stuff occurring in mitochondria
(*c*) lactic acid fermentation occurring in muscles
(*d*) bacterial fermentation occurring in the gut

L : ZOOLOGY

Q. 1 – 10 carry one mark each.

1. Trees in the equatorial region of earth supply oxygen into the atmosphere that sustains species living in distant polar regions. This relationship is called as

(*a*) mutualism (*b*) symbiosis
(*c*) commensalism (*d*) parasitism

2. A swimmer is preparing to swim 'non-stop' across the English channel (a distance of 34 kilometers). Consumption of which of the following category of food/s should the swimmer increase to accomplish this feat?

(*a*) Proteins
(*b*) Fats
(*c*) Proteins and Carbohydrates
(*d*) Carbohydrates

3. Some species of beetles and fishes can survive at sub freezing temperature. They accomplish this by maintaining cellular integrity using one of the following mechanisms.

(*a*) Expressing anti-freeze proteins
(*b*) Accumulating fats
(*c*) Increasing accumulation of complex polyols
(*d*) Reducing the availability of total water in the body

4. Zygotic genes required for the formation of a group of adjacent segment in the developing Drosophila embryo is called

(*a*) Maternal gene (*b*) Pair rule gene
(*c*) Homeotic gene (*d*) Gap gene

5. A typical receptor senses extracellular stimuli by virtue of its localization on plasma membrane. The receptor to which of the following ligands is an exception to this rule?

(*a*) γ-amino butyric acid (*b*) Acetylcholine
(*c*) Estrogen (*d*) Luteinizing hormone

6. The relationship between genes and enzymes was first suggested by the discovery of

(*a*) in-born errors of metabolism in human
(*b*) sexual phenotype in insects
(*c*) metabolic pathways in fungi
(*d*) gene regulation in bacteria

7. The blind spot in the retina is blind because of which of the following reasons?

(*a*) It is the region where the optical nerve leaves the retina.
(*b*) The opsin is not expressed in this region.
(*c*) It lies in the shadow of pupil.
(*d*) It is the junction between rods and cones.

8. Lamprey, a jawless fish, belongs to which one of the following 'Classes'?
(*a*) Myxini (*b*) Cephalaspilomorphi
(*c*) Conodonta (*d*) Anaspida

9. Chorionic gonadotropin plays an important role in the establishment and maintenance of pregnancy and is synthesized in the placenta of
(*a*) Cattle (*b*) Pigs (*c*) Mice (*d*) Human

10. Glucose and hexanoic acid, each having six carbon atoms can undergo complete biological oxidation. In terms of net ATP generation, which of the following statements is CORRECT?
(*a*) Glucose produces more ATP than hexanoic acid
(*b*) Only glucose can generate ATP
(*c*) Both glucose and hexanoic acid produce same amount of ATP
(*d*) Hexanoic acid produces more ATP than glucose

Q. 11 – 20 carry two marks each.

11. Match the following evolutionary biologists with their respective theory
(I) August Weisman
(II) Jean-Baptiste Lamark
(III) Amotz Zahavi
(IV) Motoo Kimura
(i) Neutral theory of molecular evolution
(ii) Handicap principle
(iii) Germ plasm theory
(iv) Inheritance of acquired characteristics
(*a*) I-ii, II-iv, III-i, IV-iii (*b*) I-iii, II-iv, III-ii, IV-i
(*c*) I-iii, II-iv, III-i, IV-ii (*d*) I-iii, II-i, III-iv, IV-ii

12. A female cat with a mutant phenotype was bred with a wild-type male cat. All progeny (4 males and 4 females) show the mutant phenotype. On the other hand, all progeny (4 males and 4 females) from the reciprocal cross between a mutant male and a wild-type female show the wild-type phenotype. Which of the following explain the inheritance pattern of the mutation?
(*a*) Recessive
(*b*) Linked inheritance
(*c*) Mitochondrial inheritance
(*d*) Autosomal inheritance

13. If all the nucleotides have equal probability of occurrence in a 4 Mbp long DNA sequence, then how many times will the site of *Eco*RI, restriction endonuclease occur?
(*a*) 976 (*b*) 4^6 (*c*) 6^4 (*d*) 1000

14. Seasonally breeding animals and birds measure the day length, i.e. photoperiod and use these measurements as predictive information to prepare themselves for breeding. Besides melatonin, which of the following hormones is involved in this biological process?
(*a*) Gonadotropin releasing hormone
(*b*) Growth hormone
(*c*) Thyroxine
(*d*) Adrenocorticotropic hormone

15. Red-Green color blindness is an X-linked recessive disorder. In a population which is in the Hardy-Weinberg equilibrium, the incidence of occurrence of this in males is 1 : 1000. What will be the expected incidence of affected homozygous females?
(*a*) 1 in 1002000 (*b*) 1 in 2000000
(*c*) 1 in 1001000 (*d*) 1 in 1000000

16. Golgi apparatus is also termed as cellular post office, since it packages and transports cellular proteins across various organelles and outside the cell. In general, the Golgi is perinuclear in location and is closely associated with the endoplasmic reticulum. A chemical compound, Monensin inhibits all trafficking from Golgi. If Golgi is visualized by immunofluorescence microscopy after treatment with this compound, the Golgi will be
(*a*) absent (*b*) normal (*c*) swollen (*d*) fragmented

17. In an individual, three distinct proteins bind oxygen depending on the location and development stage. While hemoglobin is the major oxygen binding protein in adults, myoglobin is present in skeletal muscles and fetal hemoglobin is present in fetal stage only. The following graph shows the oxygen binding capacity of these proteins. The A, B and C plots represent oxygen binding capacity of

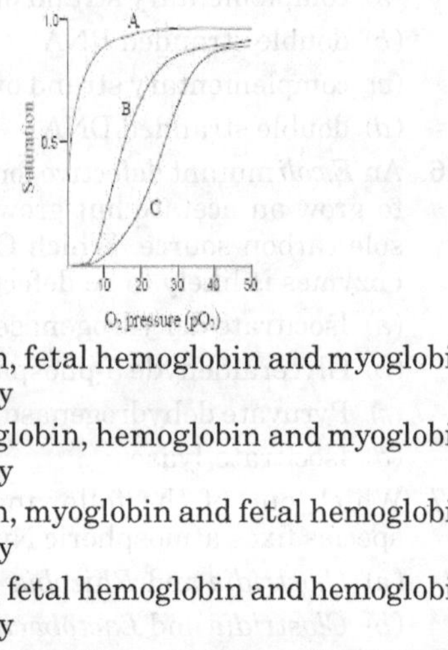

(*a*) hemoglobin, fetal hemoglobin and myoglobin, respectively
(*b*) fetal hemoglobin, hemoglobin and myoglobin, respectively
(*c*) hemoglobin, myoglobin and fetal hemoglobin, respectively
(*d*) myoglobin, fetal hemoglobin and hemoglobin, respectively

18. A patient comes with symptoms of autonomic hemolysis. The diagnostic tests reveal that he has auto-antibodies to red blood cells (RBCs). Which one of the following mechanisms is the cause of this condition?
(*a*) Neutrophils release granzymes which lyse RBCs
(*b*) Complement is activated and membrane attack complex lyse RBCs
(*c*) Cytotoxic T-cells lyse RBCs
(*d*) Interleukin-2 binds to the receptor on RBCs

19. The nerve impulse at the neuromuscular junction results in discharge of acetylcholine (Ach) from its vesicles into the synaptic cleft. Ach gets degraded by acetylcholine esterase and is present in which one of the following locations?
(*a*) Post synaptic membrane
(*b*) Both pre and post – synaptic clefts
(*c*) Presynaptic membrane
(*d*) Synaptic cleft

20. Increasing estradiol (E2) hormone from ovarian follicles prior to ovulation has been hypothesized to play a critical role for induction of pheromones. These pheromones render females sexually receptive to males to facilitate mating. An investigator performs experiments in sheep in which females are gonadectomized, then treated with E2 or vehicle alone and allowed to breed. Which one of the findings listed below will validate the hypothesis that pheromones are induced by E2?
(*a*) Sexual receptivity is regained only in vehicle treated females.
(*b*) Sexual receptivity is regained only in E2 treated females
(*c*) Sexual receptivity was regained irrespective of E2 treatment
(*d*) Sexual receptivity is not regained by any treatment

M : FOOD TECHNOLOGY

Q. 1 – 10 carry one mark each.

1. Among the following fatty acids, which group is known as essential fatty acids?
(*a*) 9,11-Octadecadienoic & 9,11, 13-Octadecatrienoic
(*b*) 9,12-Octadecadienoic & 9,12, 15-Octadecatrienoic
(*c*) 9-Octadecenoic and 9,11-Octadec-adienoic
(*d*) 9,11-Octadecadienoic and 9-Eicosenoic

2. Cellulose, the structural polysaccharide of plant, is a polymer of
(*a*) β-D-Glucose (*b*) α-D-Glucose
(*c*) β-D-Galactose (*d*) α-D-Galcturonic acid

3. The important role of carotenoids in the human diet is their ability to serve as precursors of
(*a*) Vitamin C (*b*) Vitamin D
(*c*) Vitamin A (*d*) Vitamin K

4. Which one of the following microorganisms is used in the preparation of bread?
(*a*) *Candida utilis*
(*b*) *Saccharomyces cerevisiae*
(*c*) *Saccharomyces cevarum*
(*d*) *Aspergilus niger*

5. Which one of the microorganisms given below is NOT RESPONSIBLE for ropy or stringyfermentation of milk?
(*a*) *Alcaligenes viscolactis*
(*b*) *Enterobacter aerogenes*
(*c*) *Streptococcus cremoris*
(*d*) *Streptococcus lactis*

6. A mild heat treatment of foods that destroys pathogens and extends its shelf life is called
(*a*) Baking (*b*) Blanching
(*c*) Sterilization (*d*) Pasteurization

7. The most common and least expensive plastic film used for packaging of solid food materials is
(*a*) Polyethylene (*b*) Polystyrene
(*c*) Polypropylene (*d*) Polyvinylchloride

8. Reassociation of amylose and formation of crystalline structure upon cooling of cooked starch solution is termed as
(*a*) Synersis (*b*) Gelatinization
(*c*) Retrogradation (*d*) Denaturation

9. Thermal destruction of microorganisms follows a kinetics of
(*a*) Zero order (*b*) First order
(*c*) Second order (*d*) Fractional order

10. 100 kg tomato juice containing 5% Total Solids (w/w) is concentrated to 25% Total Solids (w/w). The total amount of water removed from tomato juice in kg is
(*a*) 65 (*b*) 70 (*c*) 75 (*d*) 80

Q.11 – 20 carry two marks each.

11. Which one of the following is NOT A CORRECT statement?
(*a*) Meatiness is the taste produced by compounds such as glutamate in products like cheese, soy sauce.
(*b*) Astringency is a dry mouth feel in the oral cavity that is most associated with phenolic compounds.
(*c*) Saltiness is a taste that is mainly produced by chloride ions.
(*d*) Sourness is related to acidity and is sensed by hydrogen ion channels in the human tongue.

12. The following plot represents the *Lineweaver-Burk* equation of an enzymatic reaction both in the presence and the absence of inhibitor. Here, V is the velocity of reaction and S is the substrate concentration.

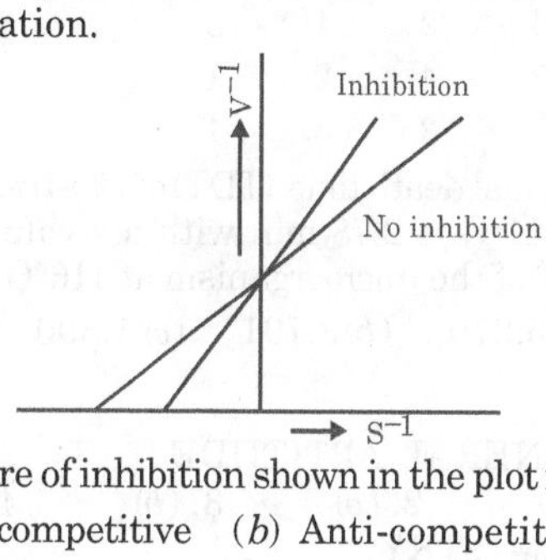

The nature of inhibition shown in the plot is
(*a*) Non-competitive (*b*) Anti-competitive
(*c*) Competitive (*d*) Mixed type

13. Make the correct match of the food constituents in Group I with their nature given in Group II.

Group I	Group II
(P) Ascorbic Acid	(1) Sugar
(Q) Phenyl alanine	(2) Chelate
(R) Dextrose	(3) Amino Acid
(S) Haemoglobin	(4) Antioxidant

Codes:

	P	Q	R	S
(*a*)	4	3	1	2
(*b*)	4	1	3	2
(*c*)	3	4	2	1
(*d*)	4	2	1	3

14. Make the correct match of the fermented food products in **Group I** with the microorganisms in **Group II.**

Group I	Group II
P. Yoghurt	1. *Lactobacillus acidophilus and Lactobacillus delbrueckii*
Q. Cheese	2. *Leuconostoc mesenteroides and Lactobacillus plantarum*
R. Sauerkraut	3. *Lactobacillus delbrueckii and Streptococcus thermophillus*
S. Kefir	4. *Lactobacillus casei and Streptococcus thermophillus*

Codes:

	P	Q	R	S
(*a*)	1	4	2	3
(*b*)	4	3	1	2
(*c*)	3	4	2	1
(*d*)	3	2	4	1

15. Match the following between organelle or cellular components of a bacterium cell in Group I with the constituents and functionalities in Group II.

Group I	Group II
(P) Cytoplasmic membrane	(1) Protein synthesis
(Q) Flagellum	(2) Peptidoglycan
(R) Cell wall	(3) Phospholipid bilayer
(S) Ribosome	(4) Motility of cell

Codes:

	P	Q	R	S
(*a*)	3	2	4	1
(*b*)	4	2	1	3
(*c*)	3	4	2	1
(*d*)	2	3	4	1

16. Thermal death time (TDT) of *Clostridium botulinum* at 121°C is 2.78 min with a z-value of 10°C. The TDT of the microorganism at 116°C (in min) is

(*a*) 5.270 (*b*) 8.791 (*c*) 1.390 (*d*) 0.712

17. Make the correct match between specific food processing operations in **Group I** with their mechanism of action in **Group II.**

Group I	Group II
P. Ball Mill	1. Compression & shear
Q. Roller Mill	2. Pressure bursting
R. Flash Peeling	3. Friction and shear
S. Abrasive Peeling	4. Impact and shear

Codes:

	P	Q	R	S
(*a*)	4	2	1	3
(*b*)	4	1	2	3
(*c*)	4	3	2	1
(*d*)	3	1	4	2

18. 650 g of a wet food containing 405 g water is dried in a tray dryer to a final moisture content of 6.8 % (dry basis). It is observed that the drying process occurs under constant rate period and it takes 8 h. The rate of drying (in kg/h) is

(*a*) 128.79 (*b*) 126.35 (*c*) 77.81 (*d*) 0.0485

19. Air at 1 atmospheric pressure (101.325 kPa) and 30°C with absolute humidity of 0.0218 kg/kg of dry air is flowing in a drying chamber. The saturated vapor pressure of water (p^0_w, in kPa) is related to temperature (T, in °C) as given below

$$\ln p^0_w = 18.6556 - \frac{5217.635}{T + 273}$$

The relative humidity of air (in percentage) is

(*a*) 62.82 (*b*) 68.22 (*c*) 86.62 (*d*) 81.80

20. The total solids content in a milk sample is 18 %. It is desired to produce 1000 kg of sweetened condensed milk (SCM) having 40 % sugar, 25 % moisture and rest milk solids. What is the 'Sugar Ratio' (in percentage) in the SCM in terms of sugar and water content in the final product?

(*a*) 48.19 (*b*) 61.54 (*c*) 54.16 (*d*) 56.14

ANSWERS

GA : GENERAL APTITUDE

1. (*d*) 2. (*b*) 3. (*b*) 4. (*d*) 5. (*a*) 6. (*a*) 7. (*c*) 8. (*d*) 9. (*a*) 10. (*a*)

H : CHEMISTRY

1. (*d*) 2. (*a*) 3. (*c*) 4. (*b*) 5. (*a*) 6. (*d*) 7. (*d*) 8. (*b*) 9. (*c*) 10. (*c*)
11. (*a*) 12. (*d*) 13. (*d*) 14. (*a*) 15. (*c*)

I : BIOCHEMISTRY

1. (*a*) 2. (*d*) 3. (*a*) 4. (*b*) 5. (*c*) 6. (*d*) 7. (*c*) 8. (*a*) 9. (*b*) 10. (*d*)
11. (*a*) 12. (*d*) 13. (*c*) 14. (*d*) 15. (*b*) 16. (*b*) 17. (*a*) 18. (*b*) 19. (*c*) 20. (*a*)

J : BOTANY

1. (*c*) 2. (*a*) 3. (*b*) 4. (*a*) 5. (*c*) 6. (*a*) 7. (*c*) 8. (*b*) 9. (*c*) 10. (*b*)
11. (*b*) 12. (*c*) 13. (*d*) 14. (*) 15. (*a*) 16. (*a*) 17. (*b*) 18. (*d*) 19. (*a*) 20. (*c*)

K : MICROBIOLOGY

1. (*a*) 2. (*b*) 3. (*a*) 4. (*d*) 5. (*c*) 6. (*d*) 7. (*a*) 8. (*b*) 9. (*c*) 10. (*b*)
11. (*a*) 12. (*b*) 13. (*c*) 14. (*b*) 15. (*c*) 16. (*d*) 17. (*a*) 18. (*c*) 19. (*a*) 20. (*d*)

L : ZOOLOGY

1. (*c*) 2. (*b*) 3. (*a*) 4. (*d*) 5. (*c*) 6. (*a*) 7. (*a*) 8. (*b*) 9. (*d*) 10. (*d*)
11. (*b*) 12. (*c*) 13. (*a*) 14. (*c*) 15. (*d*) 16. (*c*) 17. (*d*) 18. (*b*) 19. (*a*) 20. (*b*)

M : FOOD TECHNOLOGY

1. (*b*) 2. (*a*) 3. (*c*) 4. (*b*) 5. (*d*) 6. (*d*) 7. (*a*) 8. (*c*) 9. (*b*) 10. (*d*)
11. (*c*) 12. (*c*) 13. (*a*) 14. (*c*) 15. (*c*) 16. (*b*) 17. (*b*) 18. (*d*) 19. (*d*) 20. (*b*)

Note (*) : Marks to all

EXPLANATIONS

H : CHEMISTRY

1. The Diels-Alder reaction is a conjugate addition reaction of a conjugated diene to an alkene (the dienophile) to produce a cyclohexene. Since the reaction forms a cyclic product, via a cyclic transition state, it can also be described as a "cyclo-addition". Due to the high degree of regio- and stereoselectivity (due to the concerted mechanism), the Diels-Alder reaction is a very powerful reaction and is widely used in synthetic organic chemistry. The reaction is usually thermodynamically favourable due to the conversion of 2 π-bonds into 2 new stronger σ-bonds.

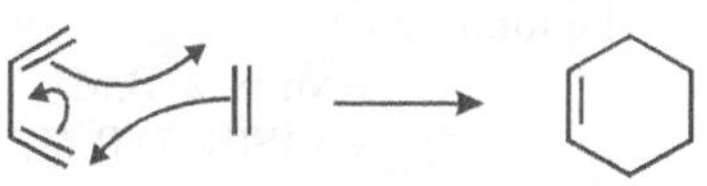

The two reactions shown above require harsh reaction conditions, but the normal Diels-Alder reaction is favoured by electron withdrawing groups on the electrophilic dienophile and by electron donating groups on the nucleophilic diene.

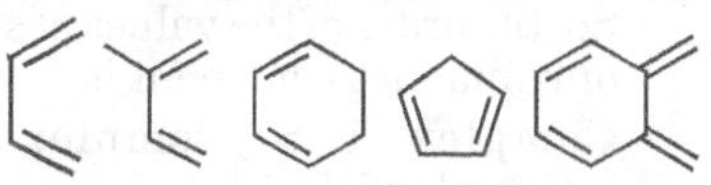

These are some of the common component dienes involved in Diels-Alder reaction.

2. Microwaves are electromagnetic rays with a frequency range of 0.3 GHz to 300 Ghz. They are found between the radio waves and the infrared waves in the electromagnetic spectrum. Microwave radiation is the radiating wave movement in which microwave energy travels. Microwaves are of a non-ionizing character, which means that they do not have the energy to cause chemical changes in substances as would happen in the case of radioactivity. CO_2 does not absorb microwave radiation as molecules of carbon dioxide (CO_2) absorb energy from infrared (IR) radiation which maintains the temperature on the earth's atmosphere.

3. In the molecule SF_4, there are five electron pairs which should lead to trigonal bi pyramidal structure. However, out of the five electron pairs, one is a lone pair. This lone pair could occupy an axial position or an equatorial position. When the lone pair is in axial position, then there will be three Lone pair - Bond pair repulsion but when lone pair is in equatorial position, then there will be two Lone pair - Bond pair repulsion.

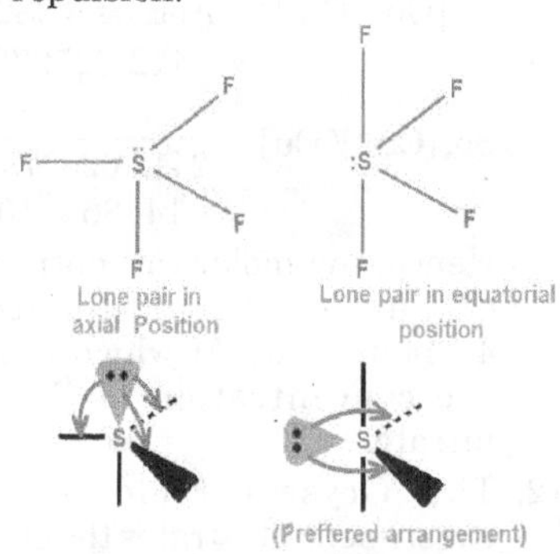

S atom in SF_4 is sp^3d hybridized. The fifth sp^3d orbital accommodates a lone pair of electrons. Hence SF_4 is not square planar. The most stable arrangement of SF_4 is when a lone pair is in axial position it would be 90° from the three closest other pairs and 180° from the other axial pair.

4. The size of an ion is governed by its electronic structure, but also by its charge. The size of the atom is relative to the atom that it was formed from. The size of the ion involved has influence on both the chemical and physical properties of ionic compounds. This shows a strong correlation between ionic size and the melting point of the ionic compound. So, an atom which has lost its valence shell electrons has reduced size compared to an atom which has gained electrons in its outermost shell. So, the ionic size of the electronic species varies as: $F^- > Na^+ > Mg^{2+} > Al^{3+}$ since they belong to the same series in the periodic table and have the same number of total electrons so size varies based on the number of valence shell electrons and the number of electrons lost or gained.

5. Aromaticity of a cyclic compound depends on Huckel's rule. In order to be aromatic, a molecule must have a certain number of π electrons (electrons with π bonds or lone pairs) within a closed loop of parallel, adjacent p orbitals. The π electron count is defined by the series 4n + 2 where n = zero or a positive integer (0, 1, 2, etc.). Amongst the given compounds, the one that does not have a closed loop for parallel π electrons though it has (4n + 2) = 10 where $n = 2$, is:

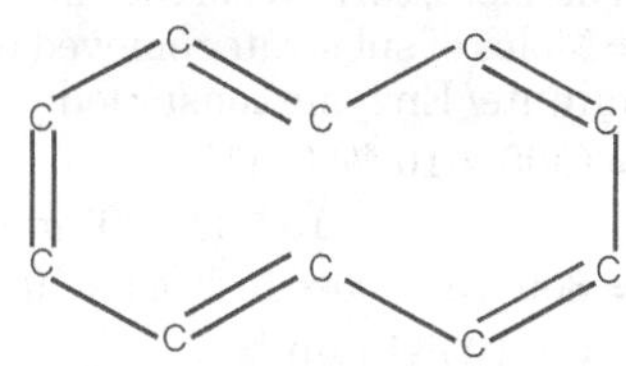

6. In molecular orbital (MO) theory, we calculate bond orders by assuming that two electrons in a bonding molecular orbital contribute one net bond and that two electrons in an anti-bonding molecular orbital cancel the effect of one bond. Atoms or molecules in which the electrons are paired are diamagnetic and repelled by both poles of a magnetic field. Those that have one or more unpaired electrons are paramagnetic and attracted to a magnetic field. So, according to MO theory, NO^+ has 10 electrons, a triple bond between N and O and two pairs, one on each atom. This means that both N and O follow the octet rule. Bond order is 3. Since there is one unpaired electron present in NO^+, so it is diamagnetic in nature.

7. The Ionic Product of Water, K_W, is the equilibrium constant for the reaction in which water undergoes an acid-base reaction with itself. That is, water is behaving simultaneously as both an acid and a base.

$$H_2O\,(l) + H_2O\,(l) \Rightarrow H_3O^+\,(aq) + OH^-\,(aq)$$

Since at different temperatures the value of ionic product for water changes, it means that with increase in temperature from 25^0C to 60^0C the entropy of water increases as the ionic product increases. So ΔS of the system will be positive as there is increase in entropy. However, since entropy is positive, so enthalpy will be negative to balance the system.

8. Number of moles of enzyme carbonic anhydrase in 10 g of enzyme

$= 10 \times 10^{-6}/30{,}000$ moles

Moles of CO_2 removed per minute by the enzyme

$= 300 \times 10^{-3}/44$ moles/min.

Therefore, turnover of the enzyme = Moles of substrate removed per minute/ Enzyme consumed

$= (300 \times 10^{-3}/44)/ (10 \times 10^{-6}/30{,}000)\ min^{-1}$

$= 300 \times 30{,}000 \times 10^{-3}/ (44 \times 10^{-5})$

$= 9 \times 10^8/44\ min^{-1}$

$= 0.204545 \times 10^8\ min^{-1}$

$= 2.045454 \times 10^7\ min^{-1}$

9. In the given iodides, 1-iodo-cyclopropane reacts slowly with cyanide ion than with the rest through S_N2 substitution reaction. This is because in cyclopropane, the cyclic ring destabilizes the iodide ion and it is very slow to be substituted as a nucleophile.

10. We know, from Henderson-Hasselbach's equation:

$pH = pK_a + \log[Salt]/ [Acid]$

Here K_a of acetic acid

$= 1.7 \times 10^{-5}\ mol/dm^3$

Therefore,

$pK_a = -\log (1.7 \times 10^{-5})$

$= 5 - 0.230449$

$= 4.76955$

[Salt] = [Sodium acetate]

= 0.2M

[Acid] = [Acetic acid] = 0.1M

Therefore,

$pH = 4.76955 + \log[0.2/0.1]$

$= 4.76955 + 0.3010299$

$= 5.0706 = 5.1$ (approx.)

11. Given,

$E^0_{Cu(+2), Cu} = 0.34 V$,

Temperature = 298K

We know, F = 96,500 C,

R = 8.314 J/K/mole

$E_{Cell} = 0.24$ V

We have, from Nernst equation:

$E_{cell} = E^0 - RT/nF * \ln (a_{red}/a_{ox})$

$0.24 = 0.34 - 8.314 \times 298/ (2 \times 96{,}500) * 2.303 \log_{10} (a_{red}/a_{ox})$

[Since, $Cu^{2+} \rightarrow Cu$, so n = 2 e^-]

$-0.1 = -0.029564 \log_{10} (a_{red}/a_{ox})$

Since activity of $Cu^{2+} = [Cu^{2+}]$

Therefore,

$\log_{10} (a_{red}/a_{ox}) = \log_{10} ([Red]/[Ox])$

$$\log_{10}([Red]/[Ox]) = \frac{0.1}{0.029564} = 3.38249$$

Therefore,

$[Cu]/[Cu^{2+}] = \text{Antilog}\{3.38249\}$

$= 2412.62597919$

$$\text{So, } [Cu^{2+}]/[Cu] = \frac{1}{2412.62597919} = 4.14486 \times 10^{-4}$$

Hence, the molar concentration of Cu^{2+} in Copper nitrate = 4.14486×10^{-4} M which is also the concentration of Copper nitrate.

12. The Crystal Field Theory experiment illustrates the effects on metal d orbital energies of moving a set of negative point charges close to a metal ion. A consequence of Crystal Field Theory is that the distribution of electrons in the d orbitals can lead to stabilization for some electron configurations. Each geometry of point charges (linear, square planar, tetrahedral, or octahedral) produces a characteristic splitting pattern for the five d orbitals (xy, xz, yz, x^2-y^2, and z^2).

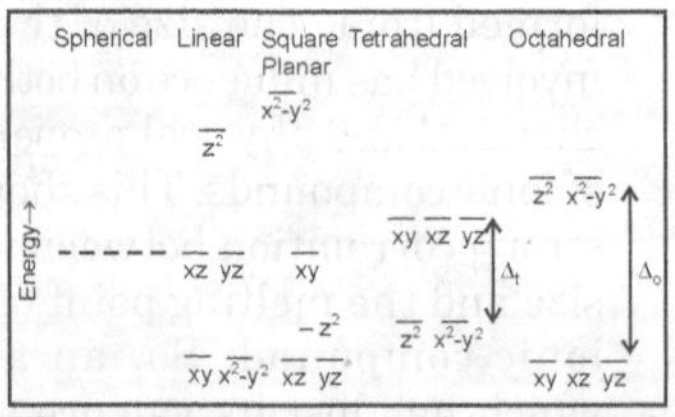

The splitting crystals and field stabilization energies vary according to the elements present in the d-series of the periodic table. Since all the tetrahedral complexes given are paramagnetic in nature and are positioned in the periodic table as Ni→Fe→Co, so the order of values of the energy of stabilization would be Complex II > Complex III > Complex I.

13. Magnetic moments are often used in conjunction with electronic spectra to gain information about the oxidation number and stereochemistry of the central metal ion in coordination complexes. Tetrahedral complexes are all high spin since the difference between the 2 subsets of energies of the orbitals is much smaller than is found in octahedral complexes. The formula used to calculate the spin-only magnetic moment can be written in two forms; the first based on the number of unpaired electrons, n, and the second based on the electron spin quantum number, S. Since for each unpaired electron, n=1 and S=1/2 then the two formulae are clearly related and the answer obtained must be identical.

$\mu_{so} = \sqrt{n(n+2)}$ B.M.

and $\mu_{so} = \sqrt{4S(S+1)}$ B.M.

Comparison of calculated spin-only magnetic moments with experimental data for some tetahedral complexes:

Ion	Configuration	μ_{so}/B.M.	μ_{obs}/B.M.
Fe(II)	$d^6 (e^3 t_2^3)$	$\sqrt{24} = 4.90$	5.3-5.5
Co(II)	$d^7 (e^4 t_2^3)$	$\sqrt{15} = 3.88$	4.2-4.8
Ni(II)	$d^8 (e^4 t_2^4)$	$\sqrt{8} = 2.83$	3.7-4.0

So, the order of the values of spin only magnetic moment is:

Complex I > Complex II > Complex III

14. The reaction (electrophilic addition) of an alkene (which has a C=C bond) with 'bromine water' will produce at least two products: a small amount of a dibromo-compound as well as a bromo-alcohol (bromohydrin) as the main product. In this main product one of the carbons originally joined by the double bond will end up attached to a bromine atom and the other carbon that was joined by the double bond will end up with an -OH group attached. This is the main product because after the initial attack by bromine the intermediate carbonium ion (carbocation) will be attacked by water. The solution becomes colourless as alkenes decolourise bromine water. So (E)-3- hexane decolourizes bromine water through electrophilic addition of bromine to C=C.

15. The reaction between hexene, bromine, and water is an addition reaction resulting in the formation of a bromohydrin. The reaction is as follows:

3-hexene + bromine —H_2O
→ 3, 4-dibromo-hexane

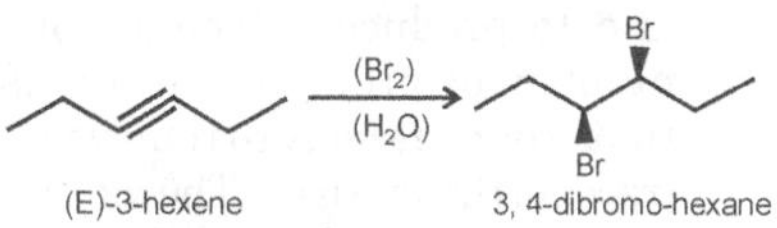

I : BIOCHEMISTRY

1. Given, there are four proteins P1, P2, P3 and P4. The amounts of hydrophobic amino acids in them are:

P1 = 17%, P2 = 10%, P3 = 21% and P4 = 14%.

Ammonium sulphate precipitation is dependent on the ionic charge on the amino acids present in the protein. This salt precipitation is given by Cohn equation, $\log S/S_0 = \beta - kI$, where S = solubility of the amino acid at any time, S_0 = initial solubility of the amino acids, β = constant dependent on temperature and pressure but is independent of the salt, k = salt specific constant and I = ionic strength. The ionic strength and the ionic charge resulting in precipitation of the amino acids are given by the Hoffmeister series. The rate of precipitation of a protein is inversely proportional to the amount of non-covalent interactions (hydrogen bonds, Vander Waal's interactions, hydrophobic bonds) present in the protein. Thus, more the hydrophobic bonds or amino acids present in the protein, lesser will be the time required for precipitation. Hence, the orders of precipitating proteins are: P3 (21% hydrophobicity), P1 (17%), P4 (14%) and P1 (10%).

2. The amino acids in an α helix are arranged in a right-handed helical structure where each amino acid residue corresponds to a 100° turn in the helix (i.e., the helix has 3.6 residues per turn), and a translation of 1.5 Å (0.15 nm) along the helical axis. The N-H group of an amino acid forms a hydrogen bond with the C = O group of the amino acid four residues earlier. This repeated i + 4 → i hydrogen bonding is the most prominent characteristic of an α-helix. Helices observed in proteins can range from four to over forty residues long, but a typical helix contains about ten amino acids (about three turns). Different amino-acid sequences have different propensities for forming α-helical structure. Methionine, alanine, leucine, uncharged glutamate, and lysine all have especially high helix-forming propensities, whereas proline and glycine have poor helix-forming propensities. Thus, alanine-arginine will form a high propensity α helix conformation.

3. Molten globules are compact, partially folded conformations of proteins that have near-native compactness, substantial secondary structure, little detectable tertiary structure and increased solvent-exposed hydrophobic surface area relative to the native state. These compact intermediates are characterised by certain properties including the presence of secondary structure and considerable conformational mobility compared to the native, functional state. Those intermediates that are thermodynamically stable under mild denaturing conditions have many features in common with the transient intermediates that accumulate significantly during the process of folding. The cooperative nature of folding results in only minute amounts of these intermediates at equilibrium. There is some evidence that these intermediates, termed "molten globules," also occur along the kinetic pathway.

4. When a fluorophore absorbs a photon of light, an energetically excited state is formed. The fate of this species is varied, depending upon the exact nature of the fluorophore and its surroundings, but the end result is deactivation (loss of energy) and return to the ground state. The fluorescence quantum yield is the ratio of photons absorbed to photons emitted through fluorescence. In other words the quantum yield gives the probability of the excited state being deactivated by fluorescence rather than by another, non-radiative mechanism. Proteins contain three aromatic amino acid residues (tryptophan, tyrosine, and phenylalanine) which may contribute to their intrinsic fluorescence. Cofactors such as FMN, FAD, NAD and porphyrins also exhibit fluorescence. Tryptophan has much stronger fluorescence and higher quantum yield than the other two aromatic amino acids. The intensity, quantum yield, and wavelength of maximum fluorescence emission of tryptophane are very solvent dependent. Tyrosine, like tryptophan, has strong absorption bands at 280 nm, and when excited by light at this wavelength, has characteristic emission profile. Phenylalanine with only a benzene ring and a methylene group is weakly fluorescent.

5. The electron transport system (ETS) accepts energy from carriers in the matrix and stores it to a form that can be used to phosphorylate ADP. The inhibitors of the Electron Transport Chain are substances that bind to some of the components of the ETC blocking its ability to change in a reversible form from an oxidized state to a reduced state. Amytal, a barbiturate, and Rotenone, a plant product are used as insecticide and pesticide, block the ETC between NADH dehydrogenase (Complex I) and CoQ. Antymicin A interferes with electron flow from cytochrome bH in Complex III (Q-cytochrome c oxidoreductase). Cyanide affects practically all metalloenzymes, but its principal toxicity derives from the binding to the Fe^{3+} in the Hem groups in cytochrome Oxidase, inhibiting the functioning of the Electron Transport Chain. Oligomycin inhibits the H^+- ATP-synthase by binding to the Oligomycin sensitivity-conferring protein (OSCP) at the F(0) subunits 6 and 9 which are found in the stalk of the F_1F_0-ATPase complex. This binding blocks the proton conductance and inhibits the synthesis of mitochondrial ATP.

6. Post-translational modifications of proteins control many biological processes, and examining their diversity is critical for understanding mechanisms of cell regulation. Polypeptides encoded by genes are primarily made up of the 20 common amino acids that are directly translated using the genetic code. However, many of these amino acids can be further modified post-translationally to yield a set of additional amino acids that contribute to the function of the mature protein. Together the 20 primary amino acids and these "secondary" amino acids which are found in proteins comprise the set of proteinogenous amino acids. Of the 20 common amino acids, alanine, glycine, isoleucine, leucine, and valine, which lack side chain functional groups, have not been implicated in post-translational modifications.

7. Estradiol-17-beta is the most potent form of mammalian estrogenic steroids whose metabolic precursor is cholesterol. Thromboxane A2 is a positive feedback lipid mediator produced following platelet activation. Upon exposure to activating agonists (e.g. thrombin, ADP, and collagen), platelets liberate arachidonic acid stored as phospholipid in the platelet plasma membrane that is converted into thromboxane A2 by sequential oxygenation of arachidonic acid by cycloxygenase and thromboxane A2 synthase. Epinephrine, more commonly known as adrenaline, is a hormone secreted by the medulla of the adrenal glands. It is produced in some neurons of the central nervous system, and in the chromaffin cells of the adrenal medulla from the amino acids phenylalanine and tyrosine. Retinoic acid (RA) is a vitamin A-derived, non-peptidic, small lipophilic molecule that acts as ligand for nuclear RA receptors (RARs), converting them from transcriptional repressors to activators. It acts through Hox genes, which ultimately control anterior/posterior patterning in early developmental stages having β-carotene as the precursor.

8. Calcium regulates a wide range of vital cell functions including enzyme activities, attachment, motility, morphology, metabolic processes, cell-cycle progression, signal-transduction, replication, gene expression and electrochemical responses. Calcium is stored in the endoplasmic reticulum (ER). Proteins that bind calcium within the ER lumen include protein disulfide isomerase, calreticulin, endoplasmin and reticulocalbin. Calcium acts as a diffusible second messenger when it is released from the endoplasmic reticulum by inositol-3-phosphate (IP3), a metabolite of the cleavage of phosphatidylinositol 4, 5 bisphosphate (PIP2) by members of the PI-phospholipase C family of enzymes. Signaling is activated by temporary increases in intracellular calcium concentration through the opening of calcium channels in the plasma membrane or the endoplasmic reticulum (ER). Prolonged elevation of intracellular calcium levels can lead to apoptosis.

9. Leguminous plants belong to the family Fabaceae (or Leguminosae). This ability in them is due a mutualistic symbiotic relationship with bacteria (*Rhizobium*) found in root nodules of these plants. These plants are used in a crop rotation to replenish soil nitrogen. These plants need root nodules because the bacteria in these nodules covert nitrogen into nitrates and give it to the plant. The plant uses this nitrogen to make proteins and other substances. In return the plants use to provide shelter and carbohydrates to the bacteria. In plants infected with *Rhizobium*, (such as alfalfa or soybeans), the presence of oxygen in the root nodules would reduce the activity of the oxygen-sensitive nitrogenase - an enzyme responsible for the fixation of atmospheric nitrogen. Leghemoglobin buffers the concentration of free oxygen in the cytoplasm of infected plant cells to ensure the proper function of root nodules. This allows an oxygen concentration that is low enough to allow nitrogenase to function but high enough so that it can provide the bacteria with oxygen for respiration.

10. B cells and antibodies together provide one of the most important functions of immunity, which is to recognize an invading antigen and to produce a tremendous number of protective proteins that scour the body to remove all traces of that antigen. The mature membranes of B cell after differentiation consist of IgM and IgD antibodies while IgG remains in the blood and IgA in mucous lining of the tissues.

11. Given, $pK_{COOH} = 2.19$, $pK_{NH2} = 9.67$ and $pK_R = 4.25$. Here, the R-side chain of the amino acid has a proton donating group. From the data it can be inferred that the amino acid is acidic in nature. That means at neutral pH (pH =7), the overall charge on the amino acid will be negative with most of the molecules carrying a charge of -1.

12. *Corynebacterium diphtheriae* cells lysogenized with the b-phage produce a diphtheria toxin which is a bipartite molecule, composed of a B subunit which mediates binding to a specific human cell surface receptor and an A subunit which possesses enzymatic (ADP-ribosyl transferase) activity. The substrate of the reaction is human elongation factor 2 (EF2), an essential part of the protein synthetic machinery. *Pseudomonas aeruginosa* exotoxin A works in the same manner as diphtheria toxin, i.e., it catalyzes the ADP-ribosylation of EF-2. During an episode of whooping cough, the *Bordetella pertussis* toxin cell produces an exotoxin composed of an A portion and 4 B portions. The A subunit is an ADP-ribosyl transferase which elevates cAMP but in a way different from cholera toxin. Alpha-toxin, the major cytotoxic agent elaborated by *Staphylococcus aureus*, was the first bacterial exotoxin to be identified as a pore former.

13. Peroxisomal and glyoxysomal matrix proteins are synthesized on free ribosome and then translocated through the peroxisomal membrane. The

carboxyl-terminal amino acid sequence serine-lysine-leucine (SKL) is the consensus peroxisomal targeting sequence 1 (PTS1) and is sufficient to direct a polypeptide to peroxisomes *in vivo* in plants, animals, and yeasts. Many mature peroxisomal proteins have the carboxylterminal amino acid sequence SKL or a similar sequence and this motif have been designated PTSl. Additionally, a second peroxisomal-targeting sequence (PTS2) with the consensus sequence of RLXXXXXHL has been identified near the amino terminus of some peroxisomal proteins.

14. Fatty acid β-oxidation is a multi step process by which fatty acids are broken down by various tissues to produce energy. Fatty acids primarily enter a cell via fatty acid protein transporters on the cell surface. Once inside, FACS adds a CoA group to the fatty acid. CPT1 then converts the long chain acyl-CoA to long chain acylcarnitine. The fatty acid moiety is transported by CAT across the inner mitochondrial membrane. CPT2 then converts the long chain acylcarnitine back to long chain acyl-CoA. The long chain acyl-CoA can then enter the fatty acid β-oxidation pathway, resulting in the production of one acetyl-CoA from each cycle of β-oxidation. This acetyl-CoA then enters the TCA cycle. The NADH and $FADH_2$ produced by both β-oxidation and the TCA cycle are used by the electron transport chain to produce ATP. Chains with an odd-number of carbons are oxidized in the same manner as even-numbered chains, but the final products are propionyl-CoA and acetyl-CoA. Thus, when a 16 carbon fatty acid is oxidised, it gives 8-acetyl CoA as product but when a 17 carbon fatty acid is oxidised, it gives 7-acetyl CoA and one propionyl CoA as the product.

15. A relatively high number of different subsets of B-cells are generated through the differentiation of early B-cell precursors into mature B-lymphocytes in the bone marrow (BM) and antigen-triggered maturation of germinal centre B-cells into memory B-lymphocytes and plasmablasts in lymphoid tissues. These B-cell subpopulations, which are produced in the BM and lymphoid tissues, recirculate through peripheral blood (PB), into different tissues including mucosa and the BM, where long-living plasma cells produce antibodies. These circulating PB B-cells can be classified according to their maturation stage into i) immature/transitional, ii) naïve, and iii) memory B-lymphocytes, and iv) plasmablasts/ plasma cells. Additionally, unique subsets of memory B-lymphocytes and plasmablasts/plasma cells can be identified based on their differential expression of unique Ig-heavy chain isotypes (e.g.: IgM, IgD, IgG, IgA). During early B cell genesis, productive Ig H chain gene rearrangement leads to assembly of the pre-B cell receptor (pre-BCR), which acts as an important checkpoint at the pro-B/pre-B transitional stage. After B-cell activation, class switching of antibodies occur for specific antigenic response.

16. The change in the Gibbs free energy is an indicator of the direction of spontaneous reaction for systems at constant pressure and temperature. Gibbs free energy change is given by $\Delta G_0 = \Delta H - T\Delta S$, where ΔH = enthalpy change in the system; T = absolute temperature and ΔS = entropy distribution or change in randomness of the system. We have, the actual free energy change for a system under specified conditions, including the concentrations of reactants and products is given by,

$$\Delta G = \Delta G_0 + RT \ln \frac{[\text{product}]}{[\text{reactant}]},$$

where R = universal gas constant. Now, under standard conditions of temperature and pressure, if initial concentration of both product and reactant are, [product] = [reactant] = 1 M, then actual free energy change ΔG = standard free energy change ΔG_0 for the reaction.

17. Flippase refer to lipid transporters that serve to equilibrate newly synthesized lipid across biogenic membranes such as the Endoplasmic reticulum (ER). Biogenic membrane flippases are energy-independent and belong to the class of transporters first envisioned by Bretscher. Phospholipid flippase mediates translocation of phosphilipids between the bilayer leaflets. Transporters hat transport lipids from the cytofacial surface to the opposite side of the membrane are called "floppases". The degree of substrate selectivity for lipids varies, but both classes of these transporters typically require an input of energy (usually in the form of ATP), allowing them to pump lipids against a concentration gradient. In contrast, "scramblases" transport lipids in both directions, are driven by a pre-existing trans-bilayer lipid gradient, and in the plasma membrane are Ca^{2+}-activated. Scramblases play an important role in the controlled randomization of lipid distribution that occurs during apoptosis or during cell activation. Lipases are water-soluble enzymes. Their job is to catalyze the hydrolysis of ester bonds found in lipid substrates. It helps the body absorb fat by breaking the fat down into fatty acids.

18. The tetracyclines are a family of antibiotics that inhibit protein synthesis by preventing the attachment of aminoacyl-tRNA to the ribosomal acceptor (A) site. Tetracyclines are broad-spectrum agents, exhibiting activity against a wide range of gram-positive and gram-negative bacteria. Chloramphenicol is lipid-soluble, allowing it to diffuse through the bacterial cell membrane. It then reversibly binds to the L16 protein of the 50S subunit of bacterial ribosomes, where transfer of amino acids to growing peptide chains is prevented, thus inhibiting peptide bond formation and subsequent protein synthesis. Cycloheximide blocks the elongation phase of eukaryotic translation. It binds the ribosome and inhibits eEF2-mediated translocation. Footprinting experiments revealed protection of a single cytidine nucleotide (C3993) in the E-site of the 60S ribosomal subunit (of 80S ribosome), defining a common binding pocket for both inhibitors in the ribosome. Aminoglycosides like Streptomycin "irreversibly" bind to specific 30S-subunit proteins and 16S rRNA. Specifically Streptomycin binds to four nucleotides of 16S rRNA and a single amino acid of protein S12. This interferes with decoding site in the vicinity of nucleotide 1400 in 16S rRNA of 30S subunit. This region interacts with the wobble base in the anticodon of tRNA. This leads to interference with the initiation complex, misreading of mRNA so incorrect amino acids are inserted into the polypeptide leading to non-functional or toxic peptides and the breakup of polysomes into non-functional monosomes.

19. For a reversible inhibitor, the kinetic schemes that could be possible are:

$$\begin{array}{ccccc} E & + S \Leftrightarrow & ES & \Leftrightarrow & E + P \\ + & & + & & \\ I \Leftrightarrow EI & & I \Leftrightarrow ESI & & \end{array}$$

The dissociation constant K_i for enzyme inhibitor complex is given by :

$$E + I \Leftrightarrow EI \text{ where, } K_i = \frac{\{[E][I]\}}{[EI]}.$$

Since the concentrations are very less, the enzyme-inhibitor complex would have a similar concentration to that of the enzyme. Therefore, the dissociation constant K_i is given by $K_i = [I] = 3 \times 10^{-3}$M.

20. From the full length DNA of 6 kb length, EcoRI restricted it to a 1kb and 5 kb fragment while PvuII restricted the 5 kb fragment into 3kb and 2kb fragments. The reaction mixture consists of dNTP mix, radiolabelled α-^{32}P dATP and Klenow fragment of *E.coli* DNA polymerase I. After the reaction is over, and the electrophoresed gel was analyzed through autoradiography, only those fragments would fluoresce extensively in the gel which is rich in adenine residues. From the restriction sites of EcoRI and PvuII, it can be clearly seen that EcoRI has more adenine and thymine residues in it than PvuII restriction site. So, when polymerization of the sites that are rich in thymine would take place, those sites complementary bonded with radiolabelled ^{32}P dATP would fluoresce. Hence, the 2 kb fragment against which PvuII makes cut through both ends would not fluoresce as much as the 3 kb and 1kb fragments consisting mainly of thymine residues. Thus, the product would show two fluorescing bands at 3kb and 1kb positions of the gel.

J : BOTANY

1. **Pulvinus** is a prominent swelling at the base of a petiole or pinna. It consists of cells (motor cells) that can rapidly move water into or out of their vacuoles. Such changes in turgor alter the position of the leaf or leaflet and are responsible for certain sleep movements and haptotropic movements. Pulvini are found in many members of the Leguminosae.
2. Cladogram is a diagram that depicts evolutionary relationships among groups. It is based on **PHYLOGENY**, which is the study of evolutionary relationships. Sometimes a cladogram is called a phylogenetic tree (though technically, there are minor differences between the two).
3. **Companian cells** are a number of specialised parenchymal cells adjacent to a sieve tube in the phloem of flowering plants, believed to regulate the flow of nutrients through the tube.
4. Cytoplasmic male sterility, as the name indicates, is under extranuclear genetic control (under control of the mitochondrial or plastid genomes). It shows non-Mendelian inheritance, with male sterility inherited maternally. In general there are two types of cytoplasm: N (normal) and aberrant S (sterile) cytoplasms.
   β-Ketothiolase is a protein coded by expression of Pha A gene.
5. The **solenoid** defines the packing of DNA as a 30 nm fiber of chromatin and results from the helical winding of at least five or six nucleosome strands.
6. *Mesembryantheum crystallinum* (the common ice plant, Aizoaceae, Caryophyllales), a halophyte with a developmentally programmed switch from C3 photosynthesis to Crassulacean acid metabolism (CAM) which is accelerated by salinity and drought. Since there has been controversy regarding the interplay between genes and environmental stimuli during the development of *M. Crystallinum.*
7. It is a facultative anaerobe; it can therefore use alcoholic fermentation under low oxygen conditions or use aerobic respiration in aerobic conditions. Under aerobic growth photosynthesis is genetically suppressed and *R. rubrum* is then colorless. After the exhaustion of oxygen, *R. rubrum* immediately starts the production of photosynthesis apparatus including membrane proteins, bacteriochlorophylls and carotenoids, i.e. the bacterium becomes photosynthesis active. *R. rubrum* is also a nitrogen fixing bacterium, i.e., it can express and regulate nitrogenase, a protein complex that can catalyse the conversion of atmospheric dinitrogen into ammonia.
8. Solar radiation at the frequencies of visible light largely passes through the atmosphere to warm the planetary surface, which then emits this energy at the lower frequencies of infrared thermal radiation. Infrared radiation is absorbed by greenhouse gases, which in turn re-radiate much of the energy to the surface and lower atmosphere.
9. Solar energy is fixed by the photoautotrophs, called primary producers, like green plants. Primary consumers absorb most of the stored energy in the plant through digestion, and transform it into the form of energy they need, such as

adenosine triphosphate (ATP), through respiration. Secondary consumers, carnivores, then consume the primary consumers, although omnivores also consume primary producers. Energy that had been used by the primary consumers for growth and storage is thus absorbed into the secondary consumers through the process of digestion. As with primary consumers, secondary consumers convert this energy into a more suitable form (ATP) during respiration.

10. **Opium poppy, *Papaver somniferum***, is the species of plant from which opium and poppy seeds are derived. Opium is the source of many narcotics, including morphine (and its derivative heroin), thebaine, codeine, papaverine, and noscapine.

11. The early biosynthetic steps of gibberellic acid, up to the formation of ent- kaurene take place in the plastid. The first true gibberellin is synthesized in plastids. Biosynthesis of gibberellins requires the action of plastid-localised terpene cyclases, membrane-bound cytochrome P450 monoxygenases and soluble 2-oxoglutarate-dependent dioxygenases.

    Jasmonic acid (JA) is derived from the fatty acid linolenic acid. It is a member of the jasmonate class of plant hormones. It has an important role in response to wounding of plants and systemic acquired resistance. When plants are attacked by insects, they respond by releasing JA, which activates the expression of protease inhibitors, among many other anti-herbivore defense compounds.

12. The first Transposable Elements were discovered in maize (Zea mays), by Barbara McClintock in 1948, for which she was awarded a Nobel prize in 1983. She noticed insertions, deletions, and translocations, caused by these elements. These changes in the genome could, for example, lead to a change in the color of corn kernels. About 85% of the genome of maize consists in TEs. The Ac/Ds system described by McClintock are class II TEs. Transposition of Ac in tobacco has been demonstrated by B. Baker. The Ac transposable element is 4563 bp long and has 11 bp inverted repeats.

13. Hirudin is a naturally occurring peptide in the salivary glands of medicinal leeches (such as Hirudo medicinalis) that has a blood anticoagulant property.

    Trichosanthin is a ribosome-inactivating protein. It has been studied as an anti-HIV therapy and has been shown to kill HIV-infected macrophages.

    Growth hormone (GH or HGH), also known as somatotropin or somatropin, is a peptide hormone that stimulates growth, cell reproduction and regeneration in humans and other animals.

    Interferons (IFN) have antiviral, antiproliferative, and immunomodulatory effects. IFN-alfa (IFNa) and IFN-beta have predominantly antiviral effects. Interferon- beta is used for the treatment of hepatitis B.

15. The Gateway T-DNA integration is the final step of the transformation process. During this step, the T-DNA, which traveled as a single-stranded DNA molecule from the bacterial cell through the host-cell cytoplasm into the nucleus, must covalently attach itself to the host cell's double-stranded genomic DNA. It occurs at random positions in the genome by a process of non-homologous recombinationCloning Technology is based on the site-specific recombination system used by phage l to integrate its DNA in the E. coli chromosome.

    For GUS expression there are actually different possible glucuronides that can be used as substrates for the beta-glucuronidase, depending on the type of detection needed (histochemical, spectrophotometrical, fluorimetrical). The most common substrate for GUS histochemical staining is 5-bromo-4-chloro-3-indolyl glucuronide (X-Gluc): the product of the reaction is in this case a clear blue color.

16. $O_2^- \rightarrow O_2^- \rightarrow H_2O_2 \rightarrow OH^- \rightarrow H_2O$.

17. Adnation of stamens to petals is described as epipetalous stamens. The stamens or lower part of filament may be fused to the petal.

    In syngenesious stamens, the filaments are free but anthers are fused e.g. sunflower while in Synandrous, stamens are fused throughout the length e.g., cocks-comb

18. Rosmarinic acid is an ester of caffeic acid and 3,4-dihydroxyphenyllactic acid. It has antioxidant and / or medicinal properties. Rosmarinic acid was first isolated and characterized in 1958 from rosemary (*Rosmarinus officinalis*). Suspension cultures of Coleus blumei accumulate very high amounts of rosmarinic acid in medium with elevated sucrose concentrations.

    Tagetes species (*Tagetes patula*) produce thiophenes, polyacetylenic compounds that possess strong biocidal activity, thus making Tagetes plants very useful for suppressing nematode populations in the soil and as sources of natural pesticides.

19. Glucose-6 phosphate is the principal molecule of glycolysis pathway not fructose-6 phosphate.

    The alternative oxidase provides an alternative route for electrons passing through the electron transport chain to reduce oxygen. However, as several proton-pumping steps are bypassed in this alternative pathway, activation of the oxidase reduces ATP generation. This enzyme was first identified as a distinct oxidase pathway from cytochrome c oxidase as the alternative oxidase is resistant to inhibition by the poison cyanide.

20.

DISEASE	CAUSAL ORGANISM
Black rot of sugarcane	Ceratocystis adipose
Stem rot of jute	Macrophomina phaseolina
Tikka disease of groundnut	Cercospora personata
Crown gall of grapes	Agrobacterium tumefaciens.

K : MICROBIOLOGY

1. Anaerobic respiration uses molecules other than oxygen as terminal electron acceptors; the most commonly used alternative electron acceptors are nitrate, sulfate, and CO_2 or carbonates. Thus lactate is not an electron acceptor during anaerobic respiration; instead lactate is an anaerobic electron donor.
2. Bergey's Manual of Systematic Bacteriology is the main resource for determining the identity of bacteria species, utilizing every characterizing aspect. Bergey's Manual of Systematic Bacteriology differs from Bergey's Manual of Determinative Bacteriology in that the former groups bacteria according to phylogenetic relationships.
3. Replica plating procedure can be used for the isolation of auxotrophic mutants. It is a method for the isolation of nutritional mutants in microorganisms. The colonies are grown from a microorganism suspension previously exposed to a mutagenic agent, on a complete medium in a petri dish. A velour surface is used to transfer the impression of all these colonies to a petri dish containing a minimal medium. The colonies that do not grow on the minimal medium are the auxotrophic mutants.
4. Temperature-sensitive (Ts) mutants of a gene are ones in which there is a marked drop in the level or activity of the gene product when the gene is expressed above a certain temperature (restrictive temperature). Temperature-sensitive mutants are a powerful tool with which to study gene function *in vivo*. These mutants provide a reversible mechanism to lower the level of a specific gene product at any stage in the growth of the organism simply by changing the temperature of growth. Ts mutants are typically generated by random mutagenesis followed by laborious screening procedures.
5. The observation that the merodiploid obtained was inducible by lactose indicates that the original mutation is recessive. A recessive mutation is one in which both alleles must be mutant in order for the mutant phenotype to be observed; that is, the individual must be homozygous for the mutant allele to show the mutant phenotype. Recessive mutations inactivate the affected gene and lead to a loss of function.

   Mutations can occur in the lac operon. Mutations can occur in the repressor genes such that the protein loses affinity for the operator, and causes the continual production of the inducible enzymes regardless of if lactose was present or not. Therefore, the lac operon becomes constitutive. The mutant bacterial cell could either be homozygous or heterozygous for this mutation whereby the mutant allele is recessive.
6. The equation is:

   Number of bacteria after x minutes = $1 * 2^{x/30}$

   Here, x = 50 hrs or 3000 mins

   Number of bacteria at the end of 50 hrs (or 3000mins)

   $$= 1 * 2^{3000/30}$$

   $$= 1 * 2^{100}$$
7. *E.coli* is the primary facultative anaerobe of the human gastrointestinal tract. Most *E. coli* are harmless and actually are an important part of a healthy human intestinal tract. However, some *E. coli* are pathogenic, meaning they can cause illness, either diarrhea or illness outside of the intestinal tract. The types of *E. coli* that can cause diarrhea can be transmitted through contaminated water or food, or through contact with animals or persons.

   Thus *E. coli* was not the first disease causing bacterium identified by Robert Koch. Instead Robert Koch identified specific causative agents of tuberculosis, cholera and anthrax.
8. Antibody coated pathogens are recognized by effector cells through F_C receptor. An F_C receptor is a protein found on the surface of certain cells that contribute to the protective functions of the immune system. F_C receptors bind to antibodies that are attached to infected cells or invading pathogens. All of the Fcγ receptors (FcγR) belong to the immunoglobulin super family and are the most important F_C receptors for inducing phagocytosis of opsonized (coated) microbes. The antibody-coated pathogens are more easily taken up by phagocytes that express F_C receptors which improves antigen presentation to T cells.

9. *Trypanosoma brucei* is a species of salivary trypanosome which causes African trypanosomiasis, known also as sleeping sickness in humans and nagana in animals.

Rickettsia rickettsii is a unicellular, Gram-negative coccobacillus. It belongs to the spotted fever group (SFG) of Rickettsia and is most commonly known as the causative agent of Rocky Mountain spotted fever (RMSF).

Rubulavirus is a genus of single stranded RNA viruses belonging to the subfamily *Paramyxovirinae*. The genus includes the mumps virus. Thus human diseases due to rubulaviruses include the mumps and respiratory tract diseases.

Wuchereria bancrofti is a human parasitic roundworm that is the major cause of lymphatic filariasis. It is one of the three parasitic worms, besides Brugia malayi and B. timori that infect lymphatic system to cause lymphatic filariasis.

10. Western blot is the technique that can be used to demonstrate that lactose induces the synthesis of β-galactosidase enzyme. Western Blotting (also called immunoblotting) is a technique used for analysis of individual proteins in a protein mixture. Antibodies are used to detect target proteins on the western blot (immunoblot). The antibodies are conjugated with fluorescent or radioactive labels or enzymes that give a subsequent reaction with an applied reagent, leading to a coloring or emission of light, enabling detection. In Western blot, beta-gal antibody can be used for detection of beta-gal.

11. Griffith's experiment, conducted in 1928 by Frederick Griffith, was one of the first experiments suggesting that bacteria are capable of transferring genetic information through a process known as transformation. Griffith used two strains of pneumococcus (*Streptococcus pneumoniae*) bacteria which infect mice – a type III-S (smooth) and type II-R (rough) strain. In this experiment, bacteria from the III-S strain were killed by heat, and their remains were added to II-R strain bacteria. While neither alone harmed the mice, the combination was able to kill its host. Griffith was also able to isolate both live II-R and live III-S strains of pneumococcus from the blood of these dead mice. Griffith concluded that the type II-R had been "transformed" into the lethal III-S strain by a "transforming principle" that was somehow part of the dead III-S strain bacteria.

12. The lambda repressor is a self assembling dimer also known as the cI protein. It binds DNA in the helix-turn-helix binding motif. It regulates the transcription of the cI protein and the Cro protein. The life cycle of lambda phages is controlled by cI and Cro proteins. The lambda phage will remain in the lysogenic state if cI proteins predominate, but will be transformed into the lytic cycle if cro proteins predominate. Thus the entry of lambda phage lysogen to lytic phase is triggered by the loss of co-operativity in binding of lambda repressor as cro dominates the repressor site.

13. Archezoa was a kingdom proposed for eukaryotes that diverged before the origin of mitochondria. Archaezoa lack mitochondria and have flagella.

The Amoebozoa are a major group of amoeboid protozoa, including the majority that moves by means of internal cytoplasmic flow. They contain amebas and other protozoans that move by using their mobile extensions of the cytoplasm called pseudopodia.

Ciliophora can be classified under Protista or Protozoa. The ciliates are a group of protozoans characterized by the presence of hair-like organelles called cilia, which are identical in structure to eukaryotic flagella, but typically shorter and present in much larger numbers with a different undulating pattern than flagella.

Apecomplexa are a large group of parasitic protists, most of which possess a unique organelle, a type of plastid called an apicoplast, and an apical complex structure involved in penetrating a host's cell. Motile structures such as flagella or pseudopods are present only in certain gamete stages.

14. Number of generations = log (cells at the beginning)- log (cells at the end)/ 0.301

Thus number of generations (n) = 10.

Generation time = t/n

= 10*60 / 10

= 600/10

= 60 minutes

15. The first step in the replication of a virus with the reverse transcriptase deals with the synthesis of complementary strand of DNA. Reverse transcriptase acts as DNA-dependent polymerase and transcribes the second DNA strand which is complementary to the 1st DNA strand.

16. The enzyme isocitrate lyase is likely to be defective in the *E. coli* mutant. It is an enzyme in the glyoxylate cycle that catalyzes the cleavage of isocitrate to succinate and glyoxylate. Together with malate synthase, it bypasses the two decarboxylation steps of the tricarboxylic acid cycle (TCA cycle) and is used by bacteria, fungi, and plants.

17. Nitrogen-fixing bacteria are microorganisms capable of transforming atmospheric nitrogen into fixed nitrogen, inorganic compounds usable by

plants. Two kinds of nitrogen fixers are recognized: free-living (non-symbiotic) bacteria, including the cyanobacteria (or blue-green algae) Anabaena and Nostoc and such genera as Azotobacter, Beijerinckia, and Clostridium; and mutualistic (symbiotic) bacteria such as Rhizobium, associated with leguminous plants, and Spirillum lipoferum, associated with cereal grasses.

18. Nalidixic acid is the first of the synthetic quinolone antibiotics. Nalidixic acid is effective against both gram-positive and gram-negative bacteria. Nalidixic acid and related antibiotics inhibit a subunit of DNA gyrase and topoisomerase IV and induce formation of cleavage complexes. It also inhibits the nicking-closing activity on the subunit of DNA gyrase that releases the positive binding stress on the supercoiled DNA. Thus naladixic acid resistant bacteria have mutant genes for DNA gyrase. The resistance to this antibiotic arises mainly due to missense mutation in the gyrase gene. In the missense mutation the codon is changed, so there is a different amino acid at that position.

19. Transformation of normal cyanobacterial cells into heterocysts involves synthesis of nitrogenase and retention of photosystem I. Heterocysts are specialized nitrogen-fixing cells formed during nitrogen starvation by some filamentous cyanobacteria. Heterocysts produce nitrogenase and other proteins involved in nitrogen fixation, degrade photosystem II, which produces oxygen and retain photosystem I.

20. Methane belching or eructation is the release of gas from the digestive tract (mainly esophagus and stomach) through the mouth. It is usually accom-panied with a typical sound and, at times, an odor. In the case of ruminants (cattle and other animals), the gas expelled is methane produced as a byproduct of the animal's digestive process. Thud the methane belched by cows arise from the CO_2 produced by the bacterial fermentation occurring in the gut.

L : ZOOLOGY

1. Commensalism is a relation between individuals of two species in which one species obtains food or other benefits from the other without either harming or benefiting the latter. The commensal (the species that benefits from the association) may obtain nutrients, shelter, support, or locomotion from the host species, which is substantially unaffected. The commensal relation is often between a larger host and a smaller commensal. Thus, the trees in the equatorial region of earth sustaining species living in distant polar regions through oxygen supply in the atmosphere is an example of commensalism.

2. For swimming across the English channel at one go without stopping which is a distance of 34 kilometres, a swimmer would require ample amount of reserved energy in the form of fats. This is because fats are the reservoir of energy which are stored in the body and are utilised when required. Thus, consumption of fats would be the best diet for the swimmer.

3. Natural freeze tolerance occurs in aquatic animals such as polar fishes and intertidal invertebrates, terrestrial amphibians and reptiles, and various polar and temperature insects. Since a few freeze tolerant insects produce antifreeze proteins (AFP's), it has been speculated that these proteins minimize the injury associated with re-crystallization of extracellular ice (AFP's are potent inhibitors of re-crystallization). In fact, many of the freeze tolerant species that produce AFP's contain them in too low a concentration to produce thermal hysteresis; they are concentrated enough to inhibit re-crystallization, however, since the thermodynamic driving force is much lower than for crystal growth in supercooled water. AFPs are thought to inhibit growth by an adsorption-inhibition mechanism.

4. The segmented body pattern along the longitudinal axis of the *Drosophila* embryo is established by a cascade of specific transcription factor activities. This cascade is initiated by maternal gene products that are localized at the polar regions of the egg. The initial long-range positional information of the maternal factors, which are transcription factors, is transferred through the activity of the zygotic segmentation genes. Expression of the gap genes occurs in discrete domains along the longitudinal axis of the pre-blastoderm and defines specific, overlapping sets of segment primordia. Their protein products, which are DNA-binding transcription factors mostly of the zinc finger type, form broad and overlapping concentration gradients which are controlled by maternal factors and by mutual interactions between the gap genes themselves. Once established, these overlapping gap protein gradients provide spatial cues which generate the repeated pattern of the subordinate pair-rule gene expression, thereby blue-printing the pattern of segmental units in the blastoderm embryo.

5. Given, a typical receptor is able to sense extracellular stimuli through its localization on the plasma membrane. Estrogens act on target tissues by binding to parts of cells called oestrogen receptors. An oestrogen receptor is a protein molecule found inside those cells that are targets for oestrogen action. Oestrogen receptors contain a specific site to which only estrogens (or closely related molecules) can bind. The target tissues affected by oestrogen molecules all contain oestrogen receptors. Thus, oestrogen is an exception to the rule. Therefore, when oestrogen molecules circulate in the bloodstream and move throughout the body, they exert effects only on cells that contain oestrogen receptors.

6. The first insight into the relationship between genes and enzymes came in 1909, when it was realized that the inherited human disease phenylketonuria results from a genetic defect in metabolism of the amino acid phenylalanine. This defect was hypothesized to result from a deficiency in the enzyme needed to catalyze the relevant metabolic reaction, leading to the general suggestion that genes specify the synthesis of enzymes. Clearer evidence linking genes with the synthesis of enzymes came from experiments of George Beadle and Edward Tatum, performed in 1941 with the fungus *Neurospora crassa.* Each mutation resulted in a deficiency in a specific metabolic pathway. Since such metabolic pathways were known to be governed by enzymes, the conclusion from these experiments was that each gene specified the structure of a single enzyme-the one gene-one enzyme hypothesis.

7. The human eye has a blind spot at the area of the retina where the optic nerve leads back into the brain. All the nerve impulses generated in the retina travel back to the brain by way of the axons in the optic nerve. At the point on the retina where the approximately 1 million axons converge on the optic nerve, there are no rods or cones. This spot, called the blind spot, is thus insensitive to light. The blind spots in each eye are aligned symmetrically so that most of the time, one eye's field of vision will compensate for the loss of vision in the other.

8. Lamprey eggs hatch into small larvae, known as ammocoetes, which are not predators at all; they lack the sucker mouths of the adults, and feed by producing strands of mucus and trapping food particles. Because they lack mineralized tissues such as bone, lampreys are rare as fossils, and their early evolutionary history is still poorly known. Some researchers have classified lampreys as the sole surviving representatives of the Linnean class Cephalaspi-domorphi. Cephalaspidomorpha is sometimes given as a subclass of the Cephalaspidomorphi.

9. Human chorionic Gonadotrophin (hCG) is a glycoprotein hormone which is produced in large amounts during pregnancy and also by certain types of tumour. The biological action of hCG is identical to that of luteinizing hormone, although the former has a much longer plasma half-life. Human chorionic Gonadotropin (hCG) is a protein secreted in large quantities by normal trophoblasts and the antibody detects cells and tumours of trophoblastic origin such as choriocarcinoma.

10. The formation of 1.5 moles of acetoacetate for each mole of hexanoate,2-A-hexenoate, or sorbate, which disappears in a liver enzyme system incapable of metabolizing either acetate or acetoacetate, is direct evidence for oxidation-recondensation mechanism for the oxidation of these 6-carbon acids. The net amount of ATP synthesis from oxidation of hexanoic acid is 44 ATP. While the oxidation of glucose through glycolysis results in the synthesis of net 2 ATP molecules. Thus, oxidation of hexanoic acid produces more ATP than glucose.

11. August Weismann is best known for his opposition to the doctrine of the inheritance of acquired traits and for his "germ plasm" theory, the forerunner of DNA theory. Amotz Zahavi is best known for his work on the handicap principle, which explains the evolution of characteristics, behaviours or structures that appear contrary to the principles of Darwinian evolution in that they appear to reduce fitness and endanger individual organisms. Motoo Kimura developed the neutral theory of molecular evolution in which genetic drift is the main force changing allele frequencies by combining theoretical population genetics with molecular evolution data. Jean-Baptiste Lamarck is a pioneer French biologist who is best known for his idea that acquired characters are inheritable, an idea known as Lamarckism, which is controverted by modern genetics and evolutionary theory.

12. When the female cat having a mutant phenotype was crossed with a wild-type male cat, all the progenies were depicting the mutant phenotype. At the same time, when the mutant male was crossed with a wild-type female cat, the progenies obtained were showing wild-type phenotype. This infers that the phenotype is not sex-linked and is inherited directly from the female cat. That means the inheritance of the mutant or the wild-type phenotype is due to the mitochondrial inheritance of the progenies from the mother.

13. Given, a DNA sequence of length
= 4 Mbp
= 4096 base pairs

Since all nucleotides have an equal probability of occurrence in the sequence, hence :

Number of A, G, C and

$T = \frac{4096}{4} = 1024$ base pairs per nucleotide.

Restriction site of EcoRI
= 5′-G′AATT′C-3′
3′-C′TTAA′G-5′

It consists of 1 G, 1 C, 2 A's and 2 T's.

14. Photoperiodism is a process whereby organisms are able to use both absolute measures of day length and the direction of day length change as a basis for regulating seasonal changes in physiology and behaviour. Two types of paradigms, designated as the external and internal coincidence models, have been proposed to account for photoperiodic time measurement by a circadian echanism. Both models postulate that the timing of light exposure, rather than the total amount of light, is critical to the organism's perception of day length. In mammals, a circadian oscillator(s) in the suprachiasmatic nucleus of the hypothalamus receives photic stimuli via the retino-hypothalamic tract. The circadian system regulates the rhythmic secretion of the pineal hormone, melatonin. Melatonin is secreted at night, and the duration of secretion varies in inverse relation to day length; thus, photoperiod information is "encoded" in the melatonin signal. Siberian hamsters exhibit a variety of seasonal responses when exposed to short days (SD), including decreases in body weight and fat, gonadal regression, and changes in several non-steroid serum hormone concentrations. One such SD-induced hormonal change is a modest decrease in serum thyroxine (T4) concentrations.

15. Hardy-Weinberg law is an algebraic equation that describes the genetic equilibrium within a population. In the simplest case of a single locus with two alleles: allele one is denoted A and allele two a and their frequencies are denoted by p and q; freq (A) = p; freq (a) = q; p + q = 1. If mating is random, then new individuals will have freq (AA) = p^2 for the AA homozygotes in the population, freq (aa) = q^2 for the aa homozygotes, and freq (Aa) = 2pq for the heterozygote. The formula is written as $(p^2) + (2pq) + (q^2) = 1$, representing the fact that probabilities must add up to one. Here, red-green colour blindness is an X-linked trait. Now, males are heterozygous for the trait. Therefore, we have p = 1 : 1000. Therefore, the homozygous female frequency of colour blindness would be $p^2 = 1^2 : 1000^2 = 1 : 1000000$.

16. Since the chemical Monensin inhibits the trafficking from Golgi apparatus, it would result in the blockage in the transport of cellular proteins to various organelles and also outside the cell. This would lead to the clustering of proteins in the vesicles of the golgi apparatus. As a result, the golgi apparatus would appear swollen if visualized using immuno fluorescence microscopy.

17. We know that haemoglobin is the major molecule in red blood corpuscles that bind oxygen and carry it to the tissues. From the graph, the plot of C shows the maximum partial pressure of oxygen with the least level of saturation. This plot C represents the haemoglobin protein binding oxygen. The plot B is intermediate with less oxygen partial pressure and relatively high saturation level. This is indicative of the foetal haemoglobin protein which binds and carries oxygen in case of foetus only and is absent in adults. The third plot A has the least partial pressure of oxygen and has the highest saturation level. That means these have the poorest binding capacity amongst the three proteins and are present in specific tissues only. Thus, the plot A represents the myoglobin present in muscles which transport oxygen into the tissues from the blood through the haemoglobin.

18. Hemolytic anemia is a condition in which red blood cells are destroyed and removed from the bloodstream before their normal lifespan is over. Autoimmune hemolytic anemia is a group of disorders characterized by a malfunction of the immune system that produces autoantibodies, which attack red blood cells as if they were substances foreign to the body. There are two main types of autoimmune hemolytic anemia: warm antibody hemolytic anemia and cold antibody hemolytic anemia. In the warm antibody type, the autoantibodies attach to and destroy red blood cells at temperatures equal to or in excess of normal body temperature. In the cold antibody type, the autoantibodies become most active and attack red blood cells only at temperatures well below normal body temperature. The lysis of the red blood cells occurs through the activation of complement against the RBCs leading to their destruction.

19. The mechanism of neuromuscular transmission is the liberation of acetyl choline which is synthesized in the terminal axoplasm from choline and acetyl coenzyme A under the influence of choline-O- acetyl

transferase. It is loaded into vesicles by a specific carrier mediated system. Eighty percent of acetyl choline is in these vesicles and 20% is dissolved in the axoplasm. These vesicles are synthesized in the cell bodies of lower motor neurons of the spinal cord or brain stem and transported to the nerve terminals with the help of micro-tubules. The neuromuscular junction is analogous to the synapse between two neurons. After the hydrolysis of acetyl choline to inactive choline and acetate catalysed by acetyl cholinesterase, these degraded fragments remain in the post synaptic membrane of the junction.

20. Pheromones are chemicals released by an organism into its environment enabling it to communicate with other members of its own species. The increased level of oestradiol from the ovarian follicles of a female has been inferred to induce production of pheromones. When an investigator gonadectomised female sheep, those female sheep which can sexually attract male sheep after treatment with oestradiol imply and indicate that oestradiol revives the sexual receptivity in those females. On the otherhand, vehicle treated females did not demonstrate any kind of sexual receptivity indicating the lack of pheromones due to no treatment of oestradiol.

M : FOOD TECHNOLOGY

1. Essential fatty acids (EFAs), linoleic acid (LA) (9, 12-Octadecadienoic acid), and alpha-linolenic acid (ALA) (9, 12, 15-Octadecatrienoic acid) are essential for humans, and are freely available in the diet. Hence, EFA deficiency is extremely rare in humans. To derive the full benefits of EFAs, they need to be metabolized to their respective long-chain metabolites, *i.e.*, dihomo-gamma-linolenic acid (DGLA), and arachidonic acid (AA) from LA; and eicosapentaenoic acid (EPA) and docosahexaenoic acid (DHA) from ALA. Some of these long-chain metabolites not only form precursors to respective prostaglandins (PGs), thromboxanes (TXs), and leukotrienes (LTs), but also give rise to lipoxins (LXs) and resolvins that have potent anti-inflammatory actions. Furthermore, EFAs and their metabolites may function as endogenous angiotensin-converting enzyme and 3-hdroxy-3-methylglutaryl coenzyme A reductase inhibitors, nitric oxide (NO) enhancers, anti-hypertensives, and anti-atherosclerotic molecules.

2. The major component in the rigid cell walls in plants is cellulose. Cellulose is a linear polysaccharide polymer with many glucose monosaccharide units. The acetal linkage is beta which makes it different from starch. The structure of cellulose consists of long polymer chains of glucose units connected by a beta acetal linkage. All of the monomer units are beta-D-glucose, and all the beta acetal links connect C-1 of glucose to C-4 of the next glucose.

3. Dietary carotenoids are thought to provide health benefits in decreasing the risk of disease, particularly certain cancers and eye disease. The carotenoids that have been most studied in this regard are β-carotene, lycopene, lutein, and zeaxanthin. In part, the beneficial effects of carotenoids are thought to be due to their role as antioxidants. β-Carotene may have added benefits due to its ability to be converted to vitamin A. Furthermore, lutein and zeaxanthin may be protective in eye disease because they absorb damaging blue light that enters the eye. Food sources of these compounds include a variety of fruits and vegetables, although the primary sources of lycopene are tomato and tomato products. Additionally, egg yolk is a highly bio-available source of lutein and zeaxanthin. These carotenoids are available in supplement form.

4. Preparation of bread is done using the fungi *Saccharomyces cerevisiae,* commonly known as Baker's Yeast. Yeast metabolises sugars for energy and produces carbon dioxide gas and alcohol as by-products just as in the fermentation of beer. Yeast spores are ubiquitous in air and on the surface of grain, and they readily infect a moist, nutritious grain paste. The reaction is:

$$C_6H_{12}O_6 \rightarrow 2C_2H_5OH + 2\ CO_2$$

In other words, one molecule of glucose sugar yields two of alcohol and two of carbon dioxide gas.

5. *Lactococcus lactis*, formerly named "streptococcus" are Gram-positive cocci that can, depending on growth conditions, appear ovoid and are typically 0.5 - 1.5 m in size. They do not form spores and they are not motile. *Lactococcus* species grow in pairs or in short chains and unlike many members of the Streptococcus genus, these organisms do not grow in long chains. *Lactococcus lactis* is one of the most important micro-organisms involved in the dairy industry. It is a non-pathogenic bacterium that is critical for manufacturing dairy products like buttermilk, yogurt and cheese. When *L. lactis ssp. lactis* is added to milk, the bacterium uses enzymes to produce energy molecules, called ATP, from lactose (milk sugar). The by-product of ATP energy production is lactic acid. The lactic acid produced by the bacterium curdles the milk that then separates to form curds, which are used to produce cheese and whey.

6. Pasteurization is partial sterilization of foods at a temperature that destroys harmful microorganisms without major changes in the chemistry of the food. It is the act or process of heating a beverage or other food, such as milk or beer, to a specific temperature for a specific period of time in order to kill microorganisms that could cause disease, spoilage, or undesired fermentation. It is the treatment of foods or beverages with mild heat, irradiation, or chemical agents to improve keeping quality or to inactivate disease-causing microorganisms.

7. Food packaging is an important step in food manufacturing operations. Food packaging ensures the shelf life of the food item protecting it from external barriers such as insect pests, microbes and also from light, moisture, oxygen etc. Polymers used for packaging include polyethylene, polypropylene, Polyvinyl chloride, Polyvinilydine chloride and Polyethylene terephthalate etc. PET and HDPE are recyclable. For respiring food items, packaging material with high barrier properties are not suitable as it leads to rotting due to moisture accumulation. Among them, polyethylene is the cheapest and the most widely used method.

8. Starch granules heated in excess water undergo an order-disorder phase transition called gelatinization over a temperature range characteristic of the starch source. This phase transition is a non-equilibrium process associated with the diffusion of water into the granule, hydration and swelling of the starch granules, uptake of heat, loss of crystallinity, and amylose leaching. On cooling, the starch chains (amylose and amylopectin) in the gelatinized paste associate, leading to the formation of a more ordered structure. These molecular interactions are termed collectively "retrogradation" and have important textural and dietary implications. This picture emphasizes the important roles played by the crystallization of the two starch polysaccharides (amylose and amylopectin).

9. Microorganisms, like all living things, are sensitive to heat, or thermal energy, and will not survive if subjected to sufficient quantities of heat at sufficient intensity. To kill the micro-organism, heat must be transferred to it in sufficient quantity to raise the temperature to a lethal level. Then the organism must be held at that level for sufficient time to ensure destruction of the life force, however that may be defined. The amount of heat delivered by a food process is dependent on both the way in which the product is heated and its physical nature. Process dependent factors can include: processing equipment design, type of heating media, container or food size and shape, product composition and viscosity. The thermal destruction kinetics of microorganisms or their ability to be killed within the food matrix is likewise dependent on a number of factors. These factors may include: pH of the product, levels and types of preservatives, water activity, the previous growth conditions of the micro-organisms of concern, product composition and competitive micro-organisms. Thermal destruction of microorganisms tends to follow first order rate reaction kinetics and have traditionally been described by the rate, at a specific temperature, required to reduce a population of organisms by 90%. This value is referred to as the D value, or decimal reduction time value. The change in D value with temperature also follows a first order relationship.

10. Given, Weight of tomato juice = 100 kg

Total solids present in the tomato juice

$$= 5\% \text{ (w/w)}$$

$$= \frac{(5 \times 100)}{100} = 5 \text{ kg}$$

When, total amount of solids in the juice is increased by concentrating the juice to 25% (w/w) solids, weight of solids

$$= \frac{(25 \times 100)}{100} = 25 \text{ kg}$$

Net increase in weight of the solids

$$= (25 - 5) \text{ kg} = 20 \text{ kg}$$

Therefore, remaining weight is of water

$$= (100 - 20) \text{ kg}$$

$$= 80 \text{ kg}$$

Thus, amount of water removed is 80 kg

11. Saltiness is the taste mainly due to the presence of sodium (Na^+) ions in water or food substances. Salty taste governs intake of Na^+ and other salts, essential for maintaining the body's water balance and blood's salt balance.

12. In competitive inhibition, a molecule similar to the substrate but unable to be acted on by the enzyme competes with the substrate for the active site. Because of the presence of the inhibitor, fewer active sites are available to act on the substrate. But since the enzyme's overall structure is unaffected by the inhibitor, it is still able to catalyze the reaction on substrate molecules that do bind to an active site. At the macroscopic level, the effect of competitive inhibition is to increase the substrate concentration required to achieve a given reaction velocity; in other words, to raise the K_m, the V_{max} is unchanged. If a reversible inhibitor can bind to the enzyme active site

in place of the substrate, it is described as a "competitive inhibitor." In pure competitive inhibition, the inhibitor is assumed to bind to the free enzyme but not to the enzyme-substrate (ES) complex. The given plot is that of competitive inhibition.

13. Vitamin C (Ascorbic acid) is a water-soluble vitamin. It acts as an antioxidant and can slow down the progression of atherosclerosis (hardening of the arteries). It helps prevent damage to LDL cholesterol, which then builds up as plaque in the arteries and can cause heart attack or stroke. Other studies suggest that vitamin C may help keep arteries flexible. Phenylalanine is an essential amino acid (a building block for proteins in the body), meaning the body needs it for health but cannot make it. Phenylalanine serves as the precursor to tyrosine, which in turn serves as the precursor to the catecholamines (dopamine, norepinephrine and epinephrine). Dextrose is a monosaccharide (d-glucose monohydrate). It is used chiefly as a fluid and nutrient replenisher, and also as a diuretic and for various other clinical purposes. Haemoglobin is composed of four polypeptide chains, which in adults consist of two alpha (α) globin chains and two beta (β) globin chains (i.e. $\alpha 2\beta 2$). Each polypeptide has a haeme prosthetic group attached, where each haeme can bind one oxygen molecule - so there are four haeme groups per haemoglobin molecule that together bind four oxygen molecules.

14. Yogurt is produced through the fermentation of milk by lactic acid bacteria, usually *Lactobacillus bulgarius* and *Streptococcus thermophilus*. After the milk has been heated to achieve evaporation, the bacteria are added, and the condensed milk is set aside at a warm temperature to produce the yogurt. Sauerkraut is produced by *Leuconostoc* and *Lactobacillus* species growing within shredded cabbage. Soft cheeses, such as Camembert, do not spoil rapidly. Camembert cheese is a product of the growth of the fungus *Penicillium camemberti*. Hard cheeses have less water and are ripened with bacteria or fungi. Swiss cheese is ripened by various bacteria, including species of *Propionibacterium*, which produces gas holes in the cheese. Bleu cheese is produced by *Penicillium roqueforti*, which produces veins within the cheese as it grows. Kefir is refreshing fermented milk with a slightly acidic taste. Kefir grains are clusters of microorganisms held together by a matrix of polysaccharides. The grains include primarily lactic acid bacteria (*Lactobacilli, Lactococci, Leuconnostoc*) and yeasts, and include acetic acid bacteria and possibly other microorganisms.

15. The bacterial cytoplasmic membrane is composed of a phospholipid bilayer and proteins and encloses the contents of the bacterial cell. Hydrophobic in nature, it acts as a barrier, preventing the leakage of the hydrophilic cytoplasmic constituents and protecting the inside of the cell from environmental insult. Flagellum is a hair-like structure that acts primarily as an organelle of locomotion in the cells of many living organisms. Flagellar motion causes water currents necessary for respiration and circulation in sponges and coelenterates. Most motile bacteria move by means of flagella. The bacterial cell wall consists of peptidoglycan (or murein), a polymer consisting of NAG and NAM and short chains of amino acids. Ribosomes are cell organelles that consist of RNA and proteins. They are responsible for assembling the proteins of the cell.

16. It has been found that if the logarithm of *t*, the thermal death time, is plotted against the temperature, a straight-line relationship is obtained, which is given by

$$\log t - \log F = m(121 - T)$$
$$= \log t/F,$$

where t is the thermal death time at temperature T, F is the thermal death time at temperature 121°C and m is the slope of the graph. Also, if we define the z value as the number of degrees below 121°C at which t increases by a factor of 10, that is by one cycle on a logarithmic graph,

$$t = 10F$$

when $T = (121 - z)$

so that, $\log 10F - \log F$

$$= \log\left(\frac{10F}{F}\right)$$
$$= 1 = m[121 - (121 - z)]$$

and so $z = \dfrac{1}{m}$.

Therefore,

$$\log\left(\frac{t}{F}\right) = \frac{(121 - T)}{z}$$

or $t = F \times 10^{(121-T)/z}$.

Now, given

$$F = 2.78 \text{ minutes},$$
$$z = 10^{0}C, T = 116^{0}C$$

Therefore, the thermal death time of *Clostridium botulinum* is:

$$t = 2.78 \times 10^{(121-116)/10}$$
$$= 2.78 \times 10^{5/10}$$
$$= 2.78 \times 10^{1/2}$$
$$= 8.7911$$

The required time is 8.7911 minutes

17. To reduce the ball mill energy consumption and improve productivity, the correlative working theories should be thoroughly understood and the reason why the energy efficiency is low should be dissected from various aspects, such as the crushing theory, the working principle and the design structure. The grinding is done with the force (mechanical force turned from the electrical force) produced by the crushing. The roller mill mainly applies the compression force and the shear force for the purpose of grinding. Flash peeling is carried out as a batch wise or continuous process. The raw materials are treated in a pressure vessel and subjected to high pressure steam. The peeling drum with protrusions on the inside surface rotates and detaches peel from raw materials by abrasion. The water spraying unit washes the raw materials and simultaneously peel is removed from the drum through the perforation along with the flow of water. Thus frictional shear is applied.

18. Given, Water content in the wet food = 405 g

After drying, water content left

= 6.8% of 405 g

= 27.54 g

Therefore, water removed by drying

= 405 – 27.54 g

= 377.46 g

= 0.37746 kg

Time taken for drying = 8 h

Therefore, rate of drying

= 0.37746/8 kgh^{-1}

= 0.04718 kgh^{-1}

19. The relation of saturated vapour pressure is given as:

$$Ln(p^0_w) = \frac{18.6556 - 5217.635}{(T + 273)},$$

given T = 30⁰C

$\Rightarrow$ $\ln(p^0_w)$ = 18.6556 – 17.2199

$\Rightarrow$ $\ln(p^0_w)$ = 1.4357

$\Rightarrow$ (p^0_w) = 4.20258

The relative humidity of air

$$= \frac{(101.325 \times 0.0218)}{4.20258} \times 100\%$$

= 81.80%

20. Total weight of the product = 1000kg

% of sugar in the Sweetened condensed milk

= 0% = 40% of 1000 kg

= 400kg

% of moisture in the sweetened condensed milk

= 25% = 25% of 1000kg

= 250 kg

Net weight of sugar + moisture = 650 kg

Now, Sugar Ratio in terms of sugar and water content

$$\frac{400}{650} \times 100\% = 61.538\%$$

■■

GATE-2011

XL : LIFE SCIENCES

Time : 3 Hours | ***Maximum Marks : 100***

GA : GENERAL APTITUDE

Q. (1–5) carry one mark each.

1. The question below consists of a pair of related words followed by four pairs of words. Select the pair that best expresses the relation in the original pair :
   Gladiator : Arena
   (*a*) dancer : stage (*b*) commuter : train
   (*c*) teacher : classroom (*d*) lawyer : courtroom
2. Choose the most appropriate word from the options given below to complete the following sentence:
   Under ethical guidelines recently adopted by the Indian Medical Association, human genes are to be manipulated only to correct diseases for which____treatments are unsatisfactory.
   (*a*) similar (*b*) most
   (*c*) uncommon (*d*) available
3. Choose the word from the options given below that is most nearly **opposite** in meaning to the given word :
   Frequency
   (*a*) periodicity (*b*) rarity
   (*c*) gradualness (*d*) persistency
4. Choose the most appropriate word from the options given below to complete the following sentence:
   It was her view that the country's problems had been___________by foreign technocrats, so that to invite them to come back would be counter-productive.
   (*a*) identified (*b*) ascertained
   (*c*) exacerbated (*d*) analysed
5. There are two candidates P and Q in an election. During the campaign, 40% of the voters promised to vote for P, and rest for Q. However, on the day of election 15% of the voters went back on their promise to vote for P and instead voted for Q. 25% of the voters went back on their promise to vote for Q and instead voted for P. Suppose, P lost by 2 votes, then what was the total number of voters?
   (*a*) 100 (*b*) 110 (*c*) 90 (*d*) 95

Q. (6 – 10) carry two marks each.

6. The horse has played a little known but very important role in the field of medicine. Horses were injected with toxins of diseases until their blood built up immunities. Then a serum was made from their blood. Serums to fight with diphtheria and tetanus were developed this way.
   It can be inferred from the passage, that horses were
   (*a*) given immunity of diseases
   (*b*) generally quite immune to diseases
   (*c*) given medicines to fight toxins
   (*d*) given diphtheria and tetanus serums
7. The sum of n terms of the series 4 + 44 + 444 + ... is
   (*a*) $(4/81)[10^{n+1} - 9n - 1]$ (*b*) $(4/81)[10^{n-1} - 9n - 1]$
   (*c*) $(4/81)[10^{n+1} - 9n - 10]$ (*d*) $(4/81)[10^{n} - 9n - 10]$
8. Given that $f(y) = |y|/y$, and q is any non-zero real number, the value of $|f(q) - f(-q)|$ is
   (*a*) 0 (*b*) –1 (*c*) 1 (*d*) 2
9. Three friends R, S and T shared toffee from a bowl. R took 1/3rd of the toffees, but returned four to the bowl. S took 1/4th of what was left but returned three toffees to the bowl. T took half of the remainder but returned two back into the bowl. If the bowl had 17 toffees left, how many toffees were originally there in the bowl?
   (*a*) 38 (*b*) 31 (*c*) 48 (*d*) 41
10. The fuel consumed by a motorcycle during a journey while traveling at various speeds is indicated in the graph below.

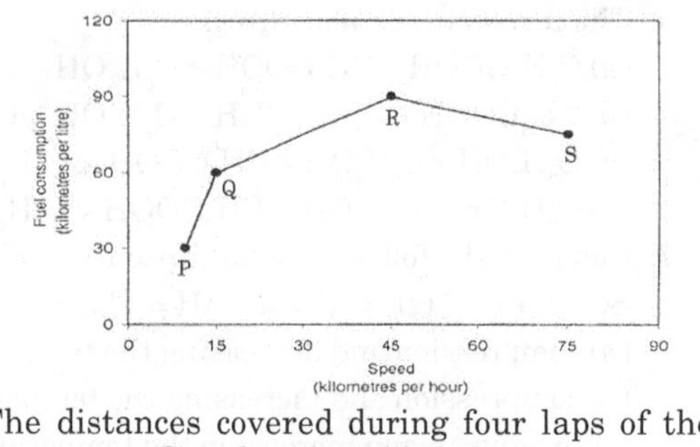

The distances covered during four laps of the journey are listed in the table below

Lap	Distance (kilometers)	Average speed (kilometers per hour)
P	15	15
Q	75	45
R	40	75
S	10	10

From the given data, we can conclude that the fuel consumed per kilometre was least during the lap
(*a*) P (*b*) Q (*c*) R (*d*) S

H : CHEMISTRY (*Compulsory*)

Q. (1 – 5) carry one mark each.

1. Electrophile among the following is
   (*a*) NH_3 (*b*) SO_3
   (*c*) NO_2 (*d*) $CH \equiv C^-$

2. The major product for the following reaction is

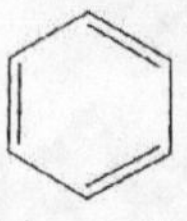 $+ (CH_3)_2\,CHCH_2Cl \xrightarrow{AlCl_3}$

(a) 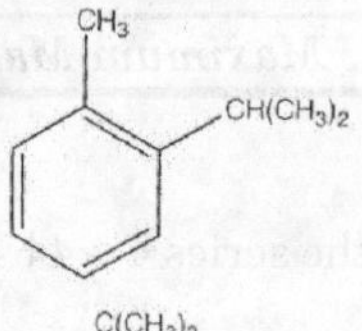 (b) 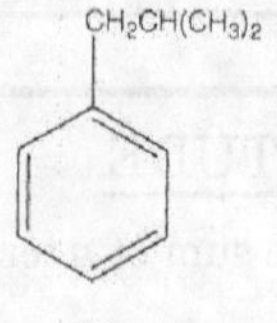

(c) 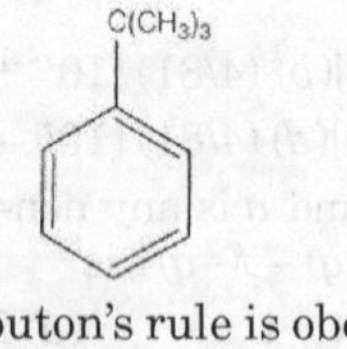 (d) 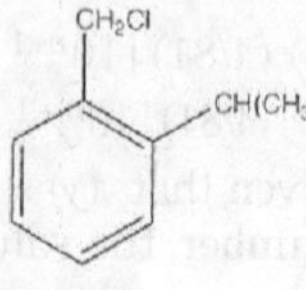

3. Trouton's rule is obeyed by
(a) hydrogen (b) methanol
(c) benzene (d) acetic acid

4. Which one of the following compounds is known as silanes?
(a) Silicon hydrides (b) Silicon halides
(c) Silicon hydroxides (d) Silicon oxides

5. The shape of PCl_5 is
(a) tetrahedral (b) square planar
(c) trigonal pyramidal (d) square pyramidal

Q. (6 – 15) carry two mark each.

6. The correct order of acidity is
(a) $C_6H_5COOH < CH_3COOH < C_6H_5OH < C_2H_5OH$
(b) $CH_3COOH < C_6H_5COOH < C_2H_5OH < C_6H_5OH$
(c) $C_2H_5OH < C_6H_5OH < CH_3COOH < C_6H_5COOH$
(d) $C_2H_5OH < C_6H_5OH < CH_3COOH < C_6H_5COOH$

7. Consider the following equilibrium
$SO_2(g) + ½O_2\,(g) \rightleftharpoons SO_3(g),\ \Delta H = -23.5\ \text{kCal mol}^{-1}$
(a) compression and decreasing the temperature
(b) compression and increasing the temperature
(c) expansion and increasing the temperature
(d) expansion and decreasing the temperature

8. A molecular electronic excited state has a life time of 10^{-9} s, the uncertainty in measuring the frequency (Hz) of the electronic transition is approximately
(a) $\frac{h}{4\pi} \times 10^9$ (b) $\frac{h}{4\pi} \times 10^{-9}$
(c) $\frac{1}{4\pi} \times 10^{-9}$ (d) $\frac{1}{4\pi} \times 10^9$

9. According to the molecular orbital theory, bond order for H_2^+ species is
(a) 0.5 (b) 1.0 (c) 1.5 (d) 2.0

10. According to crystal field theory, the electronic configuration of $[Ti(H_2O)_6]^{3+}$ in the ground state is
(a) $e^1t_2^0$ (b) $t_{2g}^{\,0}e_g^{\,1}$ (c) $e^0t_2^1$ (d) $t_{2g}^{\,1}e_g^{\,0}$

11. The ions with lowest and highest radii among O^{2-}, F^-, Na^+ and Mg^{2+} are respectively
(a) Mg^{2+} and O^{2-} (b) O^{2-} and F^-
(c) O^{2-} and Mg^{2+} (d) Na^+ and Mg^{2+}

Common Data Questions

Common Data for Questions (12 and 13):

The solubility products of FeS, ZnS, CuS and HgS are 1.0×10^{-19}, 4.5×10^{-24}, 4.0×10^{-38} and 3.0×10^{-53} respectively.

12. H_2S is passed through an aqueous solution containing all the four metal ions. The metal ion that precipitates first is
(a) Fe^{2+} (b) Zn^{2+} (c) Cu^{2+} (d) Hg^{2+}

13. The concentration of S^{2-}, at which FeS begins to precipitate from the mixture having 0.1 M Fe^{2+} is
(a) 1.0×10^{-17} M (b) 1.0×10^{-18} M
(c) 1.0×10^{-19} M (d) 1.0×10^{-20} M

Linked Answer Questions

Statement for Linked Answer Questions 14 and 15:

Consider the reaction

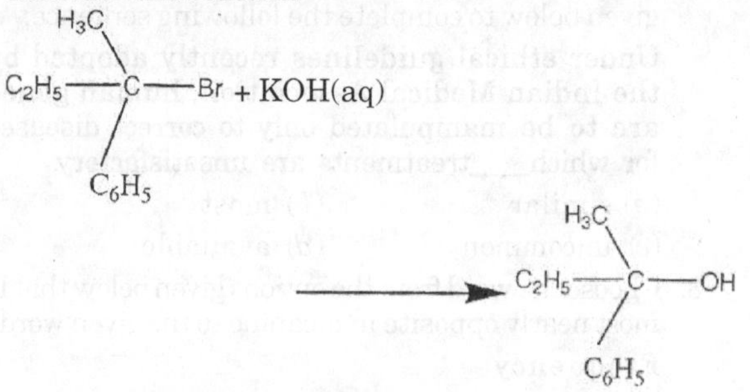

14. The above reaction is an example of
(a) addition reaction
(b) bimolecular elimination reaction (E2)
(c) unimolecular substitution reaction (SN_1)
(d) increased by four-times

15. If the concentration of KOH in the reaction mixture is doubled, the rate of the reaction will be
(a) decreased to one-half
(b) the same
(c) increased by two-times
(d) increased by four- times

I : BIOCHEMISTRY

Q. (1 - 10) carry one mark each.

1. Which one of the following DOES NOT inhibit protein biosynthesis?
(a) Puromycin (b) Chloramphenicol
(c) Cycloheximide (d) Oligomycin

2. The activation of the complement components occurs via three distinct pathways. Which of the following component(s) is specific to the 'Alternate Pathway'?
(a) Factor B and D (b) Mannose binding protein
(c) C1qr2s2 (d) C2

3. Which one of the following enzymes fixes CO_2 into organic form?
(a) Ribulose 5-phosphate kinase
(b) Ribulose 1, 5-bisphosphate carboxylase
(c) Pyruvate dehydrogenase
(d) Carbonic anhydrase

4. Cytochrome C is normally found in the inner mitochondrial membrane. It is released into the cytoplasm during
(*a*) Apoptosis (*b*) Necrosis
(*c*) Cell differentiation (*d*) Cell proliferation

5. Horseradish peroxidase and alkaline phosphatase are the two enzymes commonly utilized as reagents in ELISA, because these enzymes
(*a*) are colored proteins
(*b*) are very small
(*c*) have high turnover number
(*d*) bind to ELISA plates

6. The polarity of water molecule is due to
(*a*) its tetrahedral structure
(*b*) bonding electrons being attracted more to oxygen
(*c*) bonding electrons being attracted more to hydrogen
(*d*) its weak electrolytic property

7. Cyanide poisoning is due to its direct inhibition of
(*a*) Electron transport chain
(*b*) Fatty acid biosynthesis
(*c*) Fatty acid oxidation
(*d*) Nucleic acid biosynthesis

8. In humans, the largest energy reserve is
(*a*) liver glycogen
(*b*) muscle glycogen
(*c*) blood glucose
(*d*) adipose tissue triacylglycerol

9. A mixture of four proteins of pIs 11, 7, 5 and 3 are loaded on DEAE anion-exchange column equilibrated with low ionic strength buffer of pH 8. Which of the four proteins would be expected to be retained on the column?
(*a*) Protein with pI 11 but not the others
(*b*) Proteins with pIs 11 and 7 but not 5 and 3
(*c*) Proteins with pIs 7,5 and 3
(*d*) Protein with pI 7 but not the others

10. Valinomycin, a cyclic peptide antibiotic, facilitates the transport of which one of the following ions?
(*a*) K^+ (*b*) Ca^{2+} (*c*) Na^+ (*d*) H^+

Q. (11 - 20) carry two marks each.

11. Match P, Q, R and S with the appropriate numbers 1 to 6 on the right

P. Basophils	1. Perforin
Q. T cells	2. Phagocytosis
R. B cells	3. Albumin
S. Neutrophils	4. Macroglobulin
	5. Fc receptors for IgE
	6. Plasma cells

(*a*) P-5, Q-1, R-6, S-2
(*b*) P-1, Q-2, R-3, S-4
(*c*) P-3, Q-4, R-5, S-1
(*d*) P-2, Q-6, R-1, S-3

12. Two purified DNA samples A and B contain equal number of basepairs. Each of these DNA samples has one site each for *Eco*RI and *Bam*HI restriction enzymes. Complete digestion with both the enzymes yielded 3 DNA bands and 2 DNA bands respectively for A and B upon electrophoresis of the digestion products. Which one of the following explains the observation?
(*a*) A is circular DNA and B is linear
(*b*) B is circular DNA and A is linear
(*c*) A is circular DNA and B could be linear or circular
(*d*) B is circular DNA and A could be linear or circular

13. In the following enzyme catalyzed reaction which follows Michaelis-Menten kinetics

$$E + S \underset{k_{-1}}{\overset{k_1}{\rightleftharpoons}} ES \xrightarrow{k_2} E + P$$

K_m is equal to
(*a*) $k_{-1}/(k_1.k_2)$ (*b*) $(k_1.k_2)/k_{-1}$
(*c*) $k_1(k_2 + k_{-1})$ (*d*) $(k_2 + k_{-1})/k_1$

14. Match the items in **Group I** with those in **Group II**

Group I	**Group II**
P. Progesterone	1. Peptide
Q. Dopamine	2. Fatty acid
R. Vasopressin	3. Carbohydrate
S. Prostaglandin	4. Catecholamine
	5. Eicosanoid
	6. Steroid

	P	Q	R	S
(*a*)	3	4	1	2
(*b*)	6	4	1	4
(*c*)	3	5	4	1
(*d*)	6	5	1	4

15. Three samples of antibodies were electrophoresed under denaturing and reducing conditions on a 15% acrylamide gel, followed by staining with Coomassie blue dye. Samples 1, 2 and 3 showed two, three and four stainable bands respectively. Which one of the following conclusions can be made from these observations?
(*a*) Sample 1 is IgG, 2 is IgA and 3 is IgM
(*b*) Sample 1 is IgA, 2 is IgM and 3 is IgG
(*c*) Sample 1 is IgG, 2 is IgM and 3 is IgA
(*d*) Sample 1 is IgA, 2 is IgG and 3 is IgM

16. Four identical PCR reactions were carried out in tubes named I, II, III and IV. Besides the usual mix of dNTPs, each of the tubes respectively contained γ–^{32}P dATP, β–^{32}P dATP, α–^{32}P dATP and α–^{32} P rNTP. Which one of the tubes will have radiolabelled PCR product?
(*a*) Tube I
(*b*) Tube II
(*c*) Tube III
(*d*) Tube IV

17. Match the following:

Group I	Group II
P. Polynucleotide kinase	1. ATPase
Q. Fluoride	2. GTPase
R. Ras	3. Transketolase
S. *lac* operon	4. Enolase
	5. 5′ end of DNA
	6. 3′ end of DNA
	7. Only positive regulation
	8. Positive and negative regulation

	P	Q	R	S
(*a*)	5	4	2	8
(*b*)	6	3	1	7
(*c*)	4	2	1	6
(*d*)	1	7	5	3

18. Collagen, α-keratin and tropomyosin have common structural features. They are
P. disulfide bridges to neighboring proteins.
Q. repeating sequences of amino acids
R. a high β-sheet content
S. superhelical coiling
(*a*) P, Q (*b*) Q, R (*c*) Q, S (*d*) P, R

19. Match the following :

Group I
P. Tyrosine hydroxylation
Q. Tyrosine iodination
R. Tyrosine phosphorylation
S. Tyrosine oxidation

Group II

1. Thyroxine	2. T cell Receptor
3. DOPA	4. Estradiol receptor
5. Epinephrine	6. Melanin
7. Endorphin	8. Serotonin

	P	Q	R	S
(*a*)	1	6	5	4
(*b*)	5	7	4	8
(*c*)	2	5	3	4
(*d*)	3	1	2	6

20. Scatchard analysis of ligand-receptor interaction yielded the graph shown below. The affinity of the ligand-receptor interaction can be obtained from

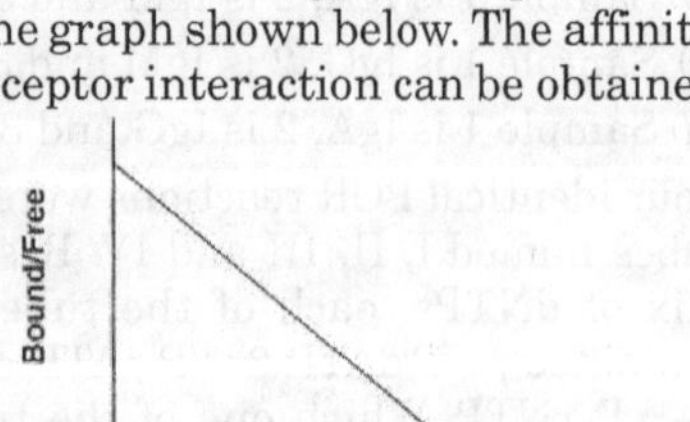

(*a*) Y intercept
(*b*) X intercept
(*c*) Slope of the line
(*d*) Product of X intercept and Y intercept

J : BOTANY

Q. (1 - 10) carry one mark each.

1. The stalk with which the ovule remains attached to the placenta is called
(*a*) Micropyle (*b*) Chalaza
(*c*) Funiculus (*d*) Hilum

2. The diploid chromosome number of an organism is $2n = 14$. What would be the expected chromosome numbers in a nullisomic?
(*a*) 12 (*b*) 13 (*c*) 15 (*d*) 16

3. The mutagen ethidium bromide acts as a
(*a*) Deaminating agent (*b*) Alkylating agent
(*c*) Intercalating agent (*d*) Base analogue

4. During photorespiration the reactive oxygen species, H_2O_2 is produced in
(*a*) Glyoxysome (*b*) Lysosome
(*c*) Peroxisome (*d*) Dictyosome

5. One of the defense mechanisms adopted by plants for detoxification of heavy metals is the synthesis of
(*a*) Phytochelatin (*b*) Calmodulin
(*c*) Tubulin (*d*) Systemin

6. In which one of the following phases of cell cycle the drug colchicine exerts its effect?
(*a*) G1 (*b*) G2 (*c*) S (*d*) M

7. The transition of water molecule from liquid to glassy state during cryopreservation is termed as
(*a*) Vitrification (*b*) Hyperhydricity
(*c*) Cryoprotectant (*d*) Habituation

8. The DNA content of a nucleus can be measured by
(*a*) ESR Spectroscopy (*b*) FTIR Spectroscopy
(*c*) Flow Cytometry (*d*) X-Ray Crystallography

9. Retrograde signaling involves communication of
(*a*) nucleus to the chloroplast
(*b*) endoplasmic reticulum to the nucleus
(*c*) nucleus to the mitochondria
(*d*) chloroplast to the nucleus

10. A photoautotrophic micropropagation system can be established by increasing the
(*a*) sucrose concentration in the culture medium
(*b*) CO_2 concentration in the culture medium
(*c*) agar concentration in the culture medium
(*d*) NH_4^+ concentration in the culture medium

Q.(11–20) carry two marks each.

11. Which of the following statements in photosynthesis are CORRECT?
P. The absorption maxima for photosystem I (PSI) and PS II are 680 nm and 700 nm, respectively
Q. Photosynthetic reactioncentre contains 300 chlorophyll molecules and the release of one molecule of oxygen requires a minimum of 8 photons
R. The non-photochemical quenching of excitation energy is enhanced by the presence of zeaxanthin
S. The photochemical splitting of water occurs in PS I
(*a*) P, Q (*b*) R, S
(*c*) P, S (*d*) Q, R

12. Which of the following statements are TRUE on DNA delivery methods during plant transformation?

P. Single stranded nicks are made in T-DNA border repeat by the VirD1, VirD2 ad VirD3 protein complex

Q. *vir*A gene products form the export apparatus on the membrane for the transfer of T-DNA

R. Gold/Tungsten particles are used as microprojectiles in biolistic method

S. Acceleration of DNA-coated micro-projectiles is carried out with compressed CO_2

(*a*) P, S (*b*) R, S (*c*) P, R (*d*) Q, S

13. Match the following plant secondary compounds with their uses and source plants

Compounds	**Uses**
P. Guggulusterol	1. Anti-Tumor
Q. Shikonin	2. Anti-rheumatic
R. Ajmalicine	3. Dye
S. Glycyrrhizin	4. Anti- Plaque
	5. Anti-Hypersensitive
	6. Sweetner

Plant species

i. Lithospermum erythrorhizon
ii. Catharanthus roseus
iii. Glycyrrhiza glabra
iv. Commiphora wightii
v. Swertia chirata
vi. Coptis japonica

(*a*) P-2-*iv*, Q-3-*i*, R-1-*ii*, S-4-*iii*
(*b*) P-3-*iv*, Q-1-*i*, R-5-*ii*, S-6-*iii*
(*c*) P-4-*iv*, Q-3-*i*, R-1-*v*, S-2-*vi*
(*d*) P-4-*iii*, Q-2-*ii*, R-5-*i*, S-6-*iv*

14. Match the gene of interest for various aspects of crop improvement

Gene insert

P. *bar* Q. *vip3A*
R. *b-lcy* S. *gsh-II*

Aspects of crop improvement

1. Tolerance to heavy metals
2. Nutritional improvement with increased vitamin A
3. Insect resistance
4. Herbicide resistance
5. Delayed ripening
6. Resistance to fungal infection

	P	Q	R	S
(*a*)	4	3	5	6
(*b*)	4	3	2	1
(*c*)	2	4	5	3
(*d*)	4	2	6	1

15. Match the plants with their seed storage proteins

Plant	**Protein**
P. Rape seed	1. Kafirin
Q. Pea	2. Vicillin
R. Sorghum	3. Gliadin
S. Wheat	4. Napin
	5. Zein
	6. Patatin

	P	Q	R	S
(*a*)	4	3	5	2
(*b*)	2	3	6	1
(*c*)	4	2	1	3
(*d*)	3	2	4	5

16. Match the name of the disease with the causal organism

Disease

P. False smut of rice
Q. Ring rot of potato
R. Red rot of sugarcane
S. Downy mildew of grape

Causal organism

1. *Plasmopara viticola*
2. *Colletotrichum falcatum*
3. *Corynebacterium sepidonicum*
4. *Ustilaginoidea virens*
5. *Erwinia amylovora*
6. *Synchytrium endobioticum*

	P	Q	R	S
(*a*)	1	5	2	4
(*b*)	4	3	2	1
(*c*)	6	2	4	1
(*d*)	5	3	2	4

17. Identify the CORRECT statements for phylogenetic systems of classification

P. The most popular phylogenetic systems of classification is that of George Bentham and Joseph Dalton Hooker and was published in 'Genera Plantarum'

Q. A true phylogenetic system of classification was proposed by Adlof Engler and was published in 'Die Naturlichen Pflanzenfamilien'

R. The phylogenetic system of classification proposed by John Hutchinson was appeared in 'The Families of Flowering Plants'

S. The origion of dicot from primitive monocot was proposed by Arthur Cronquist in his book 'Systema Naturae'

(*a*) Q, R (*b*) P, Q (*c*) R, S (*d*) P, S

18. Which of the following statements are TRUE for the plastid genomes?

P. Plastid genome is circular in nature with genome size of 120-160 kb

Q. The plastid ribosomes are with sedimentation coefficient of 80S

R. The gene for the small subunit of ribulose bisphospate carboxylase (Rubis CO) is located in the plastid

S. rRNAs in the plastid genome are arranged in one transcription unit

(*a*) P, R (*b*) Q, S (*c*) R, S (*d*) P, S

19. Identify the CORRECT statements.

P. Specialized parenchymatous cells with tannins and crystals of calcium oxalate are termed as sclereids

Q. The sieve elements of angiosperms are surrounded by companion cells and are essential component of phloem loading

R. The exudation of water by guttation occurs through trichomes

S. The bulliform cells control the unrolling and hygroscopic movement of grass leaves

(*a*) P, Q (*b*) P, R (*c*) Q, S (*d*) P, S

20. Which of the following statements are INCORRECT on ecological point of view?

P. Primary succession involving xerosere is initiated in a wet habitat

Q. Halones commonly found in electronic equipment are one of the active force destroying the protective ozone layer in the stratosphere

R. Sympatric speciation occurs when the new species evolves in geographic isolation from the parent species

S. α-Diversity is the diversity of species within a habitat or community

(*a*) P, Q (*b*) P, R (*c*) Q, R (*d*) Q, S

K : MICROBIOLOGY

Q. (1- 10) carry one mark each.

1. Quinolones inhibit bacterial growth by targeting

(*a*) DNA replication

(*b*) mRNA translation

(*c*) RNA polymerase

(*d*) active transport of nutrients into the cell

2. To select for spontaneously arising histidine auxotrophs in a population, you would use a medium containing

(*a*) Histidine and penicillin

(*b*) Penicillin but no histidine

(*c*) Histidine and lysozyme

(*d*) Lysozyme but no histidine

3. Which one of the following statements is NOT associated with contributions of Louis Pasteur?

(*a*) Anthrax is caused by anthrax bacillus

(*b*) Bacteria causing food spoilage come from air

(*c*) The disease causing organism must be isolated in pure culture

(*d*) Bacteria cause the wine disease

4. The active transport of solute in the cell is characterized by

(*a*) its uptake along the concentration gradient utilizing energy

(*b*) requirement of a carrier to support transport along the concentration gradient

(*c*) chemical modification of the solute during its uptake

(*d*) its uptake against the concentration gradient

5. Catabolite repression allows cells to save energy by

(*a*) inactivating catabolic enzymes

(*b*) inhibiting synthesis of total RNA

(*c*) regulating expression of genes required for utilization of less-efficient metabolites

(*d*) inhibiting translation of mRNAs encoding catabolic enzymes

6. A newly emerged variant of Influenza virus can be selectively propagated from the mixed population by addition of

(*a*) Gangcyclovir

(*b*) Tamiflu

(*c*) Interferon gamma

(*d*) Neutralizing antibody

7. The synthesis of an immunoglobulin in either a secretory or membrane bound form is governed by

(*a*) allelic exclusion

(*b*) class switching

(*c*) differential RNA processing

(*d*) affinity maturation

8. The *cis-trans* test can determine whether a gene codes for

(*a*) an activator or a repressor

(*b*) an RNA or a protein

(*c*) a protein with the same or different amino acids

(*d*) a diffusible or non-diffusible product

9. Which of the following are expected to be the abundant inhabitants of nitrate and sulfate rich soil naturally depleted for oxygen?

(*a*) *Pseudomonas* and *Azotobacter*

(*b*) *Pseudomonas* and *Desulfovibrio*

(*c*) *Azotobacter* and *Thiobacillus*

(*d*) *Nitrosomonas* and *Nitrobacter*

10. Which one of the following immersion oils would you use to get the best resolution in a light microscope (with 100 X objective)?

(*a*) an oil with refractive index of 1.6

(*b*) an oil with refractive index of 1.5

(*c*) an oil with refractive index of 1.4

(*d*) an oil with refractive index of 1.3

Q. (11 - 20) carry two marks each.

11. Four Hfr strains of *E.coli* were generated from the same F^+ strain. The Hfr strains donated markers in the following order:

Strain1 : DQWMT : Strain 2 : AXPTM; Strain 3: BNCAX; Strain 4: BDQWM

The order of the markers in the original F^+ strain is

(*a*) DQWMTPXACNB (*b*) AXPTMDQWBNC

(*c*) BNCAXPTMDQW (*d*) BDQWMNCAXPT

12. Which one of the following forms of the same DNA molecule would bind maximum ethidium bromide?
(*a*) Negatively supercoiled
(*b*) Covalently closed relaxed circle
(*c*) Linear
(*d*) Positively supercoiled

13. An actively growing culture of *E.coli* divides in about 20 min. Under laboratory conditions, time taken to replicate the entire genome of this bacterium would be about
(*a*) 20 min (*b*) 40 min
(*c*) 10 min (*d*) 18 min

14. Which of the statements about *Coryne bacterium diphtheriae* biology is NOT CORRECT?
(*a*) All strains of *C. diphtheriae* are producers of diphtheria toxin
(*b*) Diphtheria toxin production can be minimized by high concentration of iron in the medium
(*c*) Diphtheria toxin inhibits protein synthesis
(*d*) Diphtheria toxin is an A-B toxin secreted as a polypeptide of 62 kDa

15. Match the names of investigators in Group 1 with their contributions in Group 2

Group 1
P. Joseph Lister Q. John Needham
R. Elie Metchnikoff S. Lazaro Spallanzani

Group 2
1. Role of phagocytosis in infection
2. Disproved spontaneous generation
3. Proved spontaneous generation
4. Use of agar as solidifying agent
5. Use of carbolic acid as disinfectant

	P	Q	R	S
(*a*)	5	3	4	1
(*b*)	5	3	1	2
(*c*)	4	3	1	5
(*d*)	3	2	1	4

16. During replication of the *E. coli* chromosome, Okazaki fragments are produced from
(*a*) only one of the strands of the circular genome
(*b*) both the strands of the circular genome
(*c*) one of the strands in one generation and the other strand in the next generation
(*d*) both the strands of the circular genome provided that the heavy nitrogen (^{15}N) is present in the medium

17. A new isolate of a facultative anaerobe utilizes either oxygen or pyruvate as terminal electron acceptor. This bacterium was grown either anaerobically with glucose as sole carbon source; or aerobically with lactose as the sole carbon source. Net increase in ATP production (per mole of the carbon source) during the aerobic growth would be
(*a*) 2-fold (*b*) 4-fold (*c*) 19-fold (*d*) 38-fold

18. Based on their properties, match the "Genera" in Group 1 with those in Group 2

Group 1	Group 2
P. *Bacillus*	1. *Sarcina*
Q. *Neisseria*	2. *Azotobacter*
R. *Rhizobium*	3. *Hyphomicrobium*
S. *Caulobacter*	4. *Clostridium*

(*a*) P-4, Q-1, R-2, S-3 (*b*) P-4, Q-1, R-3, S-2
(*c*) P-2, Q-4, R-1, S-3 (*d*) P-1, Q-4, R-2, S-3

19. An actively growing culture (20 ml) of *E.coli* (1×10^5 per ml) was mixed with a total of 100 T4 phage particles, grown further for 40 min and mixed with a few drops of chloroform. Under the conditions used, the generation time of *E.coli* is 30 min, the infection cycle of phage T4 is 20 min, and the burst size is 100. Assuming that each infection was a successful one, many plaque forming units would you expect at the end of the experiment?
(*a*) 10^4 (*b*) 10^3 (*c*) 10^5 (*d*) 10^6

20. Match the pair of organisms in Group 1 with their characteristic interactions in Group 2.

Group 1
P. *Photoblepharon palpebratus* and *Vibrio fischeri*
Q. *Pseudomonas* and *Bdellovibrio*
R. *Aspergillus* and *Pseudomonas*
S. *Thiobacillus ferrooxidans* and *Beijerinckia lacticogenes*

Group 2
1. *Mutualism* 2. *Symbiosis*
3. *Antagonism* 4. *Parasitism*

	P	Q	R	S
(*a*)	2	4	3	1
(*b*)	1	3	4	1
(*c*)	4	2	3	1
(*d*)	2	4	1	3

L : ZOOLOGY

Q. (1 - 10) carry one mark each.

1. Which one of the following is an example of eumetazoans?
(*a*) Dictyostelium (*b*) Hydra
(*c*) Sponges (*d*) Volvox

2. Which one of the following is characteristic of deuterostomes?
(*a*) Radially symmetric body
(*b*) Bilaterally symmetric body
(*c*) Presence of well-defined digestive system
(*d*) Formation of anus from blastopore

3. Extraembryonic tissues are derived from which one of the following?
(*a*) Ectoderm (*b*) Endoderm
(*c*) Trophoectoderm (*d*) Mesoderm

4. Which one of the following type of immune cells is responsible for graft rejection?
(*a*) B cells (*b*) T cells
(*c*) Macrophages (*d*) Eosinophils

5. Which of the following is a main symptom of infection by *Wuchereria bancrofti*?
(*a*) Swelling of limbs (*b*) Skin rashes
(*c*) Blindness (*d*) Brain cyst

6. In insect's tracheal system, the transport of oxygen to the target tissue is done by
(*a*) fine branches of air tubes extending to almost every cell
(*b*) a liquid that fills the tracheal tube
(*c*) a specialized set of cells that produce myoglobin
(*d*) a specialized pigment

7. Which one of the following examples represents an adaptation or a physiological activity that DOES NOT minimize the loss of body temperature of animals?
(*a*) Feathers or fur
(*b*) Fat layers in the adipose tissue
(*c*) Snovering
(*d*) Vasodilation

8. Which one of the following hormones is **INCORRECTLY** paired with its function?
(*a*) Melatonin – biological rhythm
(*b*) Glucagon – increases blood glucose levels
(*c*) Prolactin – stimulates milk secretion
(*d*) Calcitonin – increases blood calcium level

9. The term *innate behavior* refers to an animal behavior
(*a*) that is triggered by an environmental change
(*b*) that is taught by the parent
(*c*) that is developmentally fixed
(*d*) that an organism learns on its own by "a hit-and trial" approach

10. Which of the following is **TRUE** about Kreb's cycle?
(*a*) Kreb's cycle generates NADPH
(*b*) The enzymes of Kreb's cycle reside in the inter-membrane space of a mitochondria
(*c*) It produces ATP, the energy currency of a cell
(*d*) None of these

Q. (11 - 20) carry two marks each.

11. A genetic experiment was performed to map the gene(s) for eye colour in a newly-discovered moth species. Sex determination in this moth species: XY – male and XX – female. When blue-eyed males were mated to green-eyed females, all of both male and female progeny had green eyes. When these progeny were mated among themselves, about half of the males of the resulting second generation had blue eyes; however, all females were green-eyed. Which one of the following is consistent with the above data?
(*a*) Multiple genes control eye colour in this moth species
(*b*) Gene(s) for eye colour is located on the X chromosome
(*c*) Gene(s) for eye colour is located on the Y chromosome
(*d*) Gene(s) for eye colour may not be sex linked

12. In a newly discovered organism, normal development was unaffected when a few blastomeres were removed from 100-cell stage embryo. However, removal of five cells at the 100-cell stage abolished the formation of kidney. Which one of the following options most accurately describes the type(s) of specification operating in the development of this organism?
(*a*) Conditional specification only
(*b*) Autonomous specification only
(*c*) Conditional and autonomous specifications
(*d*) Specification does not occur in this organism

13. In which one of the following organisms, it is easiest to distinguish mutations on adjacent base pairs of DNA through genetic recombination experiments?
(*a*) Bacteriophages (*b*) Yeast
(*c*) *Escherichia coli* (*d*) *Bacillus subtilis*

14. RNA is considered as the first genetic material to have evolved on the earth. Which one of the following properties of RNA is critical for its functioning as the genetic material in the absence of DNA and protein?
(*a*) The presence of uracil as a base in place of thymine
(*b*) The RNA is less stable than DNA; therefore RNA has higher probability to evolve as genetic material as compared to DNA
(*c*) The single stranded RNA has a genotype as well as phenotype
(*d*) RNA exists in 3 forms while DNA has only one form

15. The birth control pills contain hormonal formulations that may either arrest the ovulation or prevent the fertilization of egg. Some of the formulations do both. Which one of the following combinations represents a formulation that is likely to affect the process of ovulation and fertilization?
(*a*) Progesterone and estrogen
(*b*) Prostaglandin and estrogen
(*c*) Gonadotrophin and estradiol
(*d*) Prolactin and estradiol

16. Behavioral studies on animals have shown that there is relationship between mechanism of reproduction and male parental care (protecting eggs or the young ones). In aquatic invertebrates, fishes and amphibians for example, the species that practice internal fertilization rarely show male parental care while a majority of species that practice external fertilization tend to exhibit male parental care. This is likely due to
(*a*) the male sex in species that practice internal fertilization are unable to defend against the predators
(*b*) the male sex in species that practice internal fertilization live on female as parasite

(*c*) the fact that the females of species that practice external fertilization die soon after laying the eggs

(*d*) the certainty of paternity in species that practice external fertilization and this behavior is reinforced over generation by natural selection

17. The term *biological magnification* refers to the increased levels of a toxin seen in successive trophic levels in a food web. Which one of the following options correctly states the reason(s) for the increment of a toxin in the ecosystem?

(*a*) The toxin is highly toxic to primary producers, relatively less toxic to primary consumers, and non-toxic to secondary consumers. Thus, a higher level of toxin is seen in species representing higher trophic levels

(*b*) The toxin cannot be degraded by microorganism and consequently persist in the environment for years

(*c*) The toxin to begin with was not toxic or less toxic, but became more toxic by metabolism in the primary producers

(*d*) Both (*b*) and (*c*)

18. From the point of view of the enzymzatic reactions, which of the following **DOES NOT** belong here?

(*a*) Telomerase (*b*) Reverse transcriptase
(*c*) Taq polymerase (*d*) Primase

19. Which of the following statements is/are **TRUE** about JUXTACRINE signaling?

I. The ligand and the receptor engage in reciprocal signaling

II. Both the ligand and the receptor are membrane associated proteins

III. The ligand proteolytically cleaved after binding to the receptor

(*a*) I only (*b*) II only
(*c*) III only (*d*) I, II and III

20. Which of the following amino acid change (mutation) would **MOST** adversely affect the structure of an α-helix?

(*a*) A valine residue changed to an isleucine residue

(*b*) A methionine residue changed to a proline residue

(*c*) An aspartic acid residue changed to a glutamic acid residue

(*d*) A histidine residue changed to an arganine residue

M : FOOD TECHNOLOGY

Q. (1 - 10) carry one mark each.

1. The protein responsible for spongy structure in bread is

(*a*) Albumin (*b*) Zein (*c*) Gluten (*d*) Gliadin

2. The factor most responsible for making a good ice-cream is

(*a*) Water content (*b*) Homogenization
(*c*) Emulsifying agent (*d*) Mixing index

3. Listed below are some of the functions of fats in the human nutrition. Identify the INCORRECT function

(*a*) Concentrated source of energy

(*b*) Transport of oxygen to various organs

(*c*) Absorption of fat soluble vitamins

(*d*) Synthesis of cell membrane and hormones

4. During ripening of cheese by *Penicillium roqueforti* the characteristic aroma is because of

(*a*) Methyl ketones (*b*) Aceto acetic acid
(*c*) Diacetyl (*d*) Acetoin

5. Which of the following statements is NOT TRUE in case of oxidative rancidity of fatty foods?

(*a*) Peroxides and hydroperoxides are formed during auto-oxidation

(*b*) Auto-oxidation is a complex chain reaction

(*c*) The final breakdown products of auto-oxidation are aldehydes, ketones and alcohols

(*d*) The reaction is brought about by an enzyme, called lipase

6. Which of the following group of characteristics is **CORRECT** in respect of *Shigella* species found as pathogen?

(*a*) Gram positive, motile by gliding, spore forming cocci and transmitted by contaminated food

(*b*) Gram negative, motile by flagella, spore forming bacilli and transmitted by contaminated water

(*c*) Gram positive, non-motile, non-spore forming cocci and transmitted by contaminated air and water both

(*d*) Gram negative, non-motile, non-spore forming and transmitted by fecal-oral route

7. Relate the vitamins listed below Group I with the associated diseases Group II

Group I	**Group II**
P. Thiamin	1. Pellagra
Q. Nicotinic acid	2. Beriberi
R. Folic acid	3. Scurvy
S. Ascorbic acid	4. Anemia

	P	Q	R	S
(*a*)	1	2	3	4
(*b*)	4	3	2	1
(*c*)	2	1	4	3
(*d*)	3	4	1	2

8. Which of the following conditions for the heat resistance of microorganisms is CORRECT?

(*a*) Psychrophiles < Mesophiles < Thermophiles

(*b*) Psychrophiles > Mesophiles > Thermophiles

(*c*) Thermophiles > Psychrophiles > Mesophiles

(*d*) Mesophiles < Thermophiles < Psychrophiles

9. The solubility of sodium bicarbonate in water is 9.6g/100g at 20°C and 16.4g/100g at 60°C. If a saturated solution of sodium bicarbonate at 60°C is cooled to 20°C, the percentage of the dissolved salt crystallized out will be

(*a*) 20.5 (*b*) 25.4 (*c*) 41.5 (*d*) 45.2

10. Which one of the following statements is NOT TRUE in terms of nutritive evaluation of proteins?

(*a*) PER is defined as the live weight gain per unit weight of protein intake

(*b*) 'Metabolic nitrogen' is the amount of nitrogen present in the feces when a nitrogen free diet is fed to an animal

(*c*) Net protein utilization is a product of biological value and digestibility

(*d*) 'Chemical score' of a mixed protein diet can be calculated from the total amino acids present in the mixture

Q. (11 - 20) carry two marks each.

11. A sugar syrup (density = 1040 kg/m^3 and viscosity = 1600 × 10^{-6} Pa.s) is required to be pumped into a tank (1.5 m diameter and 3 m height) by a 3 cm inside diameter pipe. If the liquid is required to flow under laminar conditions the minimum time to fill the tank with the syrup will be

(*a*) 192.9 h (*b*) 19.3 h

(*c*) 38.6 h (*d*) 57.9 h

12. Match the following sauerkraut defects for their causative agents

P. Soft kraut Q. Slimy kraut

R. Rotted kraut S. Pink kraut

1. Due to growth of bacteria, mold and/or yeast
2. Due to surface growth of *Torula* yeast
3. Rapid growth of *Lactobacillus cucumens* and *L. plantarum* specially at elevated temperature

	P	Q	R	S
(*a*)	4	2	3	1
(*b*)	3	4	1	2
(*c*)	1	3	2	4
(*d*)	4	3	1	2

13. Match the following cabohydrates with their use in the food processing

P. High amylose starch

Q. Pectin

R. Starch phosphates

S. Glucose

1. White sauces in cook freeze operations
2. Edible film for wrapping candies
3. As humectant in confectionary
4. Setting agent in jams and jellies

	P	Q	R	S
(*a*)	1	2	4	3
(*b*)	2	4	1	3
(*c*)	3	1	2	4
(*d*)	4	3	1	2

14. Match the food items and their principal flavouring agents given in the two columns below

P. Butter 1. Menthol

Q. Orange 2. Limonene

R. Cloves 3. Eugenol

S. Mint 4. Diacetal

	P	Q	R	S
(*a*)	3	2	4	1
(*b*)	2	3	1	4
(*c*)	4	1	3	2
(*d*)	4	2	3	1

15. Match the food items on left hand side with their colloidal nature on right hand side

P. Curd 1. Foam

Q. Butter 2. Emulsion

R. Vegetable soup 3. Sol

S. Whipped egg white 4. Gel

(*a*) P-2, Q-1, R-3, S-4 (*b*) P-4, Q-3, R-2, S-1

(*c*) P-4, Q-2, R-3, S-1 (*d*) P-3, Q-4, R-1, S-2

16. In an actively growing (exponential phase) yeast culture, the cell concentration increased from 10^3 cells per ml to 10^7 cells per ml in 4 h. The doubling time of the year is

(*a*) 120 minutes (*b*) 30 minutes

(*c*) 18 minutes (*d*) 60 minutes

17. The steps followed in Gram's staining of microorganisms are

P. Washing with neutral organic solvent

Q. Counter staining with a contrast dye

R. Staining with basic dye

S. Fixing the colour with a suitable mordant

Identify the CORRECT sequence.

(*a*) Q→S→R→P (*b*) P→Q→R→S

(*c*) Q→P→S→R (*d*) R→S→P→Q

18. A continuous dryer was used to dry 12 kg/min of a blanched vegetable containing 50% moisture (wet weight basis) to give a product containing 10% moisture. As the dryer could handle feed material with moisture content not more than 25%, a part of dried material was recycled and mixed with the fresh feed. The evaporation rate in the dryer will be

(*a*) 2.08 kg/min (*b*) 5.33 kg/min

(*c*) 3.33 kg/min (*d*) 2.93 kg/min

19. An enzyme has a K_m of 4.7 × 10^{-5} M and V_m is 22 micro moles per litre per min. The enzyme reaction is carried out at a substrate concentration of 2 × 10^{-4} M. The initial reaction velocity for this enzyme catalyzed reaction will be

(*a*) 6.5 micro moles per litre per min

(*b*) 17.8 micro moles per litre per min

(*c*) 13.0 micro moles per litre per min

(*d*) 8.9 micro moles per litre per min

20. The F - value at 121.1°C, eqivalent to 99.9999 percent destruction of a strain of *Clostridium botulinum,* is 1.8 min. The D_0 value (decimal reduction time at reference temperature) of the organism will be

(*a*) 10.8 min (*b*) 0.3 min

(*c*) 6.0 min (*d*) 0.2 min

ANSWERS

GA : GENERAL APTITUDE

1. (*d*)	2. (*d*)	3. (*b*)	4. (*c*)	5. (*b*)	6. (*b*)	7. (*c*)	8. (*d*)	9. (*c*)	10. (*b*)

H : CHEMISTRY

1. (*b*)	2. (*b*)	3. (*c*)	4. (*a*)	5. (*c*)	6. (*d*)	7. (*a*)	8. (*d*)	9. (*a*)	10. (*d*)
11. (*a*)	12. (*d*)	13. (*b*)	14. (*c*)	15. (*b*)					

I : BIOCHEMISTRY

1. (*d*)	2. (*a*)	3. (*b*)	4. (*a*)	5. (*c*)	6. (*b*)	7. (*a*)	8. (*d*)	9. (*c*)	10. (*a*)
11. (*a*)	12. (*b*)	13. (*d*)	14. (*b*)	15. (*c*)	16. (*c*)	17. (*a*)	18. (*c*)	19. (*d*)	20. (*b*)

J : BOTANY

1. (*c*)	2. (*a*)	3. (*c*)	4. (*c*)	5. (*a*)	6. (*d*)	7. (*a*)	8. (*c*)	9. (*d*)	10. (*b*)
11. (*a*)	12. (*c*)	13. (*b*)	14. (*b*)	15. (*c*)	16. (*b*)	17. (*a*)	18. (*)	19. (*c*)	20. (*b*)

K : MICROBIOLOGY

1. (*a*)	2. (*a*)	3. (*c*)	4. (*d*)	5. (*c*)	6. (*b*)	7. (*c*)	8. (*c*)	9. (*b*)	10. (*b*)
11. (*a*)	12. (*c*)	13. (*b*)	14. (*a*)	15. (*b*)	16. (*a*)	17. (*c*)	18. (*a*)	19. (*d*)	20. (*a*)

L : ZOOLOGY

1. (*b*)	2. (*d*)	3. (*c*)	4. (*b*)	5. (*a*)	6. (*b*)	7. (*d*)	8. (*d*)	9. (*c*)	10. (*c*)
11. (*d*)	12. (*a*)	13. (*c*)	14. (*d*)	15. (*a*)	16. (*d*)	17. (*d*)	18. (*d*)	19. (*c*)	20. (*b*)

M : FOOD TECHNOLOGY

1. (*c*)	2. (*d*)	3. (*b*)	4. (*a*)	5. (*d*)	6. (*d*)	7. (*c*)	8. (*a*)	9. (*c*)	10. (*d*)
11. (*b*)	12. (*b*)	13. (*b*)	14. (*d*)	15. (*c*)	16. (*c*)	17. (*d*)	18. (*c*)	19. (*b*)	20. (*d*)

EXPLANATIONS

GA : GENERAL APTITUDE

1. Given relationship is worker: workplace.

   A gladiator is

   (*i*) a person, usually a professional combatant trained to entertain the public by engaging in mortal combat with another person or a wild.

   (*ii*) A person engaged in a controversy or debate, especially in public.

2. The context seeks to take a deviation only when the existing / present / current / alternative treatments are unsatisfactory. So the word for the blank should be a close synonym of existing / present/current/ alternative. Available is the closest of all.

3. The best antonym here is rarity which means shortage or scarcity.

4. Clues in the question are -- foreign technocrats did something negatively to the problems – so it is counter-productive to invite them. All other options are non-negative. The best choice is exacerbated which means aggravated or worsened.

5.

P	Q
40%	60%
–6%	+6%
+15%	–15%
49%	51%

since 2% = 2

∴ 100% = 100

6. From the passage it cannot be inferred that horses are given immunity as in (*a*), since the aim is to develop medicine and in turn immunize humans. (*b*) is correct since it is given that horses develop immunity after some time. Refer "until their blood built up immunities". Even (*c*) is invalid since medicine is not built till immunity is developed in the horses. (*d*) is incorrect since specific examples are cited to illustrate and this cannot capture the essence.

7. Let

$$S = 4\,(1 + 11 + 111 + ...)$$

$$= \frac{4}{9}(9 + 99 + 999 + ...)$$

$$= \frac{4}{9}\{(10 - 1) + (10^2 - 1) + (10^3 - 1) + ...\}$$

$$= \frac{4}{9}\{(10 + 10^2 + ... + 10^n) - n\}$$

$$= \frac{4}{9}\left\{10\frac{(10^n - 1)}{9} - n\right\}$$

$$= \frac{4}{81}\{10^{n+1} - 9n - 10\}$$

8. Given:

$$f(y) = \frac{|y|}{y}$$

$$\Rightarrow f(q) = \frac{|q|}{q};$$

$$f(-q) = \frac{|-q|}{-q} = \frac{-|q|}{q}$$

$$|f(q) - f(q)| = \frac{|q|}{q} + \frac{|q|}{q}$$

$$= \frac{2|q|}{q} = 2$$

9. Let total number of toffees in bowl be x

   R took $\frac{1}{3}$ of toffees and returned 4 to the bowl

   ∴ Number of toffees with

$$R = \frac{1}{3}x - 4$$

Remaining of toffees in bowl

$$= \frac{2}{3}x + 4$$

Number of toffees with

$$S = \frac{1}{4}\left(\frac{2}{3}x+4\right) - 3$$

Remaining toffees in bowl

$$= \frac{3}{4}\left(\frac{2}{3}x+4\right) + 3$$

Number of toffees with

$$T = \frac{1}{2}\left(\frac{3}{4}\left(\frac{2}{3}x+4\right)+3\right) - 2$$

Remaining toffees in bowl

$$= \frac{1}{2}\left[\frac{3}{4}\left(\frac{2}{3}x+4\right)+4\right] + 2$$

Given :

$$\frac{1}{2}\left[\frac{3}{4}\left(\frac{2}{3}x+4\right)+3\right] + 2 = 17$$

$$\Rightarrow \frac{3}{4}\left(\frac{2}{4}x+4\right) = 27$$

$$\Rightarrow x = 48$$

10. Fuel consumption Actual

	Fuel consumption	Actual
P	60 km/l	$\frac{15}{60} = \frac{1}{4} l$
Q	90 km/l	$\frac{75}{90} = \frac{5}{6} l$
R	75 km/l	$\frac{40}{75} = \frac{8}{15} l$
S	30 km/l	$\frac{10}{30} = \frac{1}{3} l$

H : CHEMISTRY

1. A molecule or ion that accepts a pair of electrons to make a new covalent bond is called an electrophile (from the Greek for "electron loving"). Any molecule, ion or atom that is electron deficient in some way can behave as an electrophile. Electron deficiency would include a formal positive charge (methyl carbocation), a partial positive charge (d+), usually in conjunction with a polar bond (such as H-Cl) or an open octet (borane). "E" or "E+" is common abbreviation for generic electrophiles. SO_3 has an atom which does not have an octet of electrons and so can accept a pair of electrons and is an electrophile.

2. Benzene undergoes Friedel Craft's reaction in presence of halogen carrier $AlCl_3$, conjugate molecule Benzene undergoes electromeric effect in presence of $(CH_3)_2$ $CHCH_2Cl$ and replaces H in Benzene

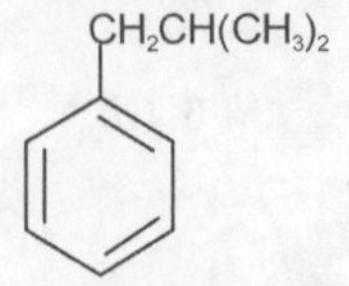

3. Trouton's rule states that for all liquids the entropy of vaporization is same i.e. 87–88 J K^{-1} mol^{-1}. Entropy of vaporization is the ratio of enthalpy of vaporization to the temperature. But this rule is not universal as there are many exceptions to this rule like water, ethanol do not meet the criteria of the law. But some follows it like benzene and chloroform.

4. Silanes serve, depending upon the type of the silane, as a radical H-donor or as a hydride donor. The range reaches from simple alkylsilanes (Et_3SiH) over different phenylsilanes (such as $PhSiH_3$) and halosilanes (such as trichlorosilane) up to tris (trimethylsilyl) silane, which is due to its structure an outstanding radical reducing agent. They are silicon hydrides. Silanes are often used as an alternative to toxic reducing agents, e.g. Bu_3SnH. But they offer their own chemistry due to the outstanding affinity from silicon to oxygen and fluorine.

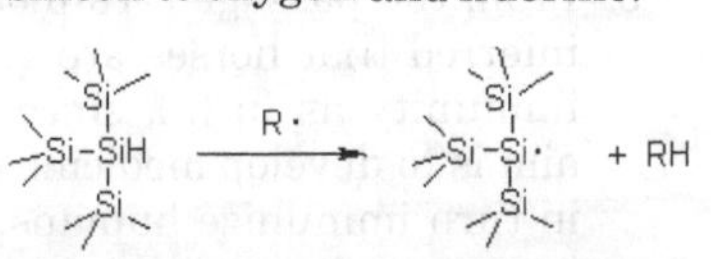

5. There are two P–Cl bonding environments in PCl_5 molecule. Each equatorial P Cl bond make two 90° and two 120° bond angles with the other bonds in the molecule. Each axial P–Cl bond makes three 90° and one 180° bond angles with the other bonds in the molecule. According to VSEPR theory, the shape of PCl_5 is trigonal bipyramidal.

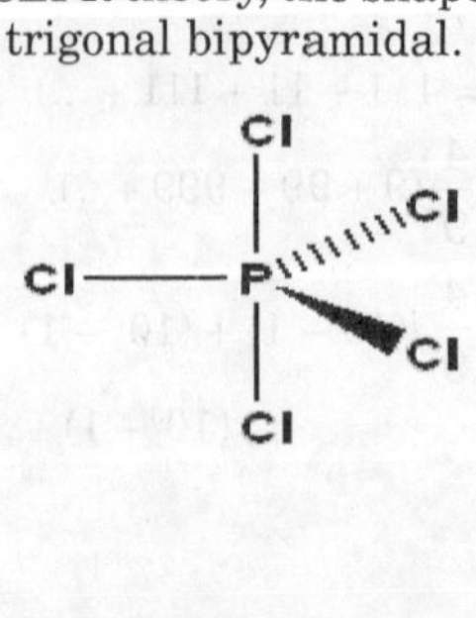

6. Carboxylic acids are the most acidic simple organic compounds (pKa ~ 5). But they are only weak acids compared to acids like HCl or H_2SO_4. Resonance stabilization of the carboxylate ion allows the negative charge to be delocalised between the two electronegative oxygen atoms. Adjacent electron withdrawing substituents increase the acidity by further stabilising the carboxylate. The polar nature of both the O-H and C=O bonds (due to the electronegativity difference of the atoms) results in the formation of strong hydrogen bonds with other carboxylic acid molecules or other H-bonding systems (e.g. water). The stability of the carboxylic acids is mainly due to the resonance stability present in the molecule. So, a carboxylic acid with a phenyl group is the most stable followed by alkyl carboxylic acid and then the alcohols which are rather basic in nature.

7. Given, a reaction for the formation of SO_3

$$SO_2(g) + \frac{1}{2}O_2(g) \Leftrightarrow SO_3(g)$$

And $\Delta H = -23.5$ Kcal/mol

Since ΔH is negative, means that the reaction is stable and spontaneous.

Also 1.5 moles of SO_2 and O_2 give rise to 1 mole of SO_3. So, the randomness or the entropy reduces to a slight extent. Now, for the reaction to be forward biased, that means to be favourable for the formation of SO_3, the reactants should be dealt with high pressure and by lowering the volume of the system through compression. Also, decreasing temperature directly affects the entropy ($-T\Delta S$) and so it favours the forward reaction.

8. Heisenberg's Uncertainty Principle is one of the fundamental concepts of Quantum Physics, and is the basis for the initial realization of fundamental uncertainties in the ability of an experimenter to measure more than one quantum

variable at a time. Heisenberg's Principle is typically written mathematically in either of two forms:

$\Delta E\ \Delta t \geq h/4\pi$ or $\Delta x\ \Delta p \geq h/4\pi$

The constant, h, is called Planck's Constant (where h/4p = 0.527 × 10-34 Joule-second).

Here, $\Delta E = h\upsilon$ where υ is the frequency.

Therefore, using it in the original equation, we have

$h\upsilon\ \Delta t \geq h/4\pi$

$\Rightarrow\ \upsilon > 1/(4\pi\Delta t)$; $\Delta t = 10^{-9}$ s

$\Rightarrow\ \upsilon > 1/4\pi \times 10^9$

The required frequency is

$1/4\pi \times 10^9$ Hz

9. There are two molecular orbitals for hydrogen; the lower energy orbital has its greater electron density between the two nuclei. This is the bonding molecular orbital - and is of lower energy than the two 1s atomic orbitals of hydrogen atoms making this orbital more stable than two separated atomic hydrogen orbitals. The upper molecular orbital has a node in the electronic wave function and the electron density is low between the two positively charged nuclei. The energy of the upper orbital is greater than that of the 1s atomic orbital and such an orbital is called an anti-bonding molecular orbital.

Normally, the two electrons in hydrogen occupy the bonding molecular orbital(σ), with anti-parallel spins. If molecular hydrogen is irradiated by ultra-violet (UV) light, the molecule may absorb the energy, and promote one electron into its anti-bonding orbital (σ^*), and the atoms will separate. According to molecular orbital theory, bond order for

$$H_2^+(1\ e^-) = \frac{(1-0)}{2} = 0.5$$

10. In the ionic Crystal Field Theory (CFT), it is assumed that the ions are simple point charges. For transition metal cations that contain varying numbers of d electrons in orbitals that are not spherically symmetric, however, the situation is quite different. The shape and occupation of these d-orbitals then becomes important in an accurate description of the bond energy and properties of the transition metal compound. To be able to understand and use CFT then, it is essential to have a clear picture of the shapes (angular dependence functions) of the d-orbitals. One of the important aspects of CFT is that not all ligands are identical when it comes to causing a separation of the energy of the d-orbitals. For transition metal compounds, there is clear evidence for this from the multitude of colours available for a given metal ion when the ligands or stereochemistry are varied. For octahedral complexes this is a reflection of the energy difference between the higher *dz2, dx2-y2* (e.g., subset) and the *dxy, dyz, dxz* (t2g subset). In the given complex $[Ti(H_2O)_6]^{3+}$, the Titanium atom exists as Ti^{3+} with electronic configuration as: [Ar] $3d^1$. So, the ground state electronic configuration of $[Ti(H_2O)_6]^{3+}$ is $t_{2g}^{\ 1}\ e_g^{\ 0}$.

11. Ionic radii are difficult to measure with any degree of certainty, and vary according to the environment of the ion. For example, it matters what the co-ordination of the ion is (how many oppositely charged ions are touching it), and what those ions are. There are several different measures of ionic radii in use, and these all differ from each other by varying amounts. In each case, the ions have exactly the same electronic structure - they are said to be isoelectronic. However, the number of protons in the nucleus of the ions is increasing. That will tend to pull the electrons more and more towards the centre of the ion - causing the ionic radii to fall. On the otherhand, in case of negative ions, the ionic radii rise. So, from the following ions, O^{2-} has the highest ionic radii and Mg^{2+} has the lowest radii.

12. In the question, the solubility products of four metal ion sulphates are given:

$FeS = 1 \times 10^{-19}$,

$ZnS = 4.5 \times 10^{-24}$,

$CuS = 4 \times 10^{-38}$,

$HgS = 3 \times 10^{-53}$

Now, on passing H_2S through an aqueous solution containing all the four metal ions, that metal ion will precipitate out at first which has the least solubility. That means the metal ion sulphate having the least solubility product will precipitate out first. Thus, HgS precipitates first because it has the least solubility product value.

13. Given, concentration of Fe^{2+} ion = 0.1 M

We know, for precipitation to occur, Ionic product > solubility product

So, the minimum concentration of S^{2-} ion required to precipitate Fe^{2+} as FeS is given by:

$$K_{sp} = [Fe^{2+}][S^{2-}]$$

$$\Rightarrow\ 1 \times 10^{-19} = 0.1\ [S^{2-}]$$

$$\Rightarrow\ [S^{2-}] = 1 \times 10^{-18}$$

The required concentration of $[S^{2-}]$ ion is 1×10^{-18} M

14. In the given reaction, the aqueous KOH substitutes the halide molecule (in this case Br) with the hydroxyl group –OH in a process of substitution. This is a single molecular substitution because only one set of molecules are being substituted in the compound. The Br^- is a nucleophile which is replaced by other nucleophile OH^- so that the reaction is that of a nucleophilic substitution type.

15. Aqueous KOH is the reagent in the reaction which provides the nucleophiles OH^- for substitution. But it does not affect the rate of the reaction. This is because the rate of the reaction is determined by the target molecule $CH_3(C_2H_5)C(C_6H_5)Br$ as rate is directly proportional to the molecule. The reaction follows first order kinetics. So, if the concentration of KOH is doubled, the rate of the reaction remains unchanged and same.

I : BIOCHEMISTRY

1. Puromycin inhibits protein synthesis at translation by prematurely terminating a peptide chain. It is a structural analog of the aminoacyl-adenylyl grouping characteristic of the 3'-end of aminoacyl tRNAs. Chloramphenicol inhibits prokaryotic systems and it binds to 50S subunit of ribosome and blocks peptidyl transferase activity. Cycloheximide mainly works in eukaryotic system by inhibiting the translocation of peptidyl-tRNA. Whereas, oligomycin is a natural antibiotic which is isolated from *Streptomyces diastatochromogenes* and it inhibits mitochondrial H^+-ATP synthase.
2. Components of the complement system that are unique to the alternative pathway are factor B, factor D, and properdin. The alternative pathway is capable of auto-activation because of a process termed "tickover" of C3. Once factor B associates with C3 (H_2O), factor B itself changes conformation and can then be cleaved by the constitutively active serum protease factor D, generating Ba and Bb. The Bb fragment remains associated with the complex and can then, through its own serine protease domain, cleave additional C3 molecules, generating a form designated C3b. Once C3b is generated, it associates with factor B to generate more C3-convertase. This overall series of successive proteolytic steps is enhanced by the serum protein properdin, which stabilizes protein-protein interactions during the process. The alternative pathway can also be initiated as an "amplification loop" when fixed C3b that is generated by classical or lectin pathway activation binds factor B, again resulting in conformational changes in factor B that allow factor D to cleave it similarly to the tickover process.
3. Carbon fixation is the process by which photosynthetic organisms such as plants turn inorganic carbon (usually carbon dioxide) into organic compounds such as carbohydrates. For the sugar glucose (one of the most abundant products of photosynthesis) the equation is : $6CO_2 + 12H_2O \rightarrow C_6H_{12}O_6 + 6H_2O + 6O_2$. CO_2 combines with the phosphorylated 5-carbon sugar ribulose bisphosphate which is catalyzed by the enzyme ribulose bisphosphate carboxylase oxygenase (RUBISCO). The resulting 6-carbon compound breaks down into two molecules of 3-phosphoglyceric acid (PGA). The PGA molecules are further phosphorylated (by ATP) and are reduced (by NADPH) to form phosphoglyceraldehyde (PGAL). Phosphoglyceraldehyde serves as the starting material for the synthesis of glucose and fructose. Glucose and fructose make the disaccharide sucrose, which travels in solution to other parts of the plant.
4. Cytochrome c is primarily known for its function in the mitochondria as a key participant in the life-supporting function of ATP synthesis. However, when a cell receives an apoptotic stimulus, cytochrome c is released into the cytosol and triggers programmed cell death through apoptosis. The release of cytochrome c and cytochrome-c-mediated apoptosis are controlled by multiple layers of regulation, the most prominent players being members of the B-cell lymphoma protein-2 (BCL2) family. As well as its role in canonical intrinsic apoptosis, cytochrome c amplifies signals that are generated by other apoptotic pathways and participates in certain non-apoptotic functions.
5. Enzymes have been used as detection probes for years and are still commonly used, even with the upsurge of fluorescent probes, because of their simplicity, sensitivity and broad-spectrum applications. Enzyme probes, including horseradish peroxidase (HRP) and alkaline phosphatase (AP), are used to detect target proteins through chromogenic, chemiluminescent or fluorescent outputs. HRP has a high turnover rate and produces abundant reaction products in a short amount of time at physiological pH (7.6). HRP-IgG conjugates are superior to alkaline phosphatase and β-galactosidase conjugates due to their higher specific enzyme activity (more HRP/mole of antibody) and immunological reactivity (less steric hindrance because of the size of HRP).
   Alkaline phosphatases (AP) are a widely distributed family of enzymes that hydrolyze phosphates from nucleotides and proteins. Optimal enzymatic activity occurs at pH 9.0-9.6. It has also a very good turn over number. This characteristic of both the enzymes is used in ELISA.
6. Water is polar because of the difference in electro negativity between hydrogen and oxygen. The highly electronegative oxygen atom attracts electrons or negative charge to it, making the region around the oxygen more negative than the areas around the two hydrogen atoms. However, the molecule would not be polar if H_2O was linear like, for example, carbon dioxide, CO_2. Each water molecule is bent so that the positive portions of the molecule (the hydrogen atoms) are flexed away from the two filled orbitals of the oxygen.
7. Cyanide causes intracellular hypoxia by reversibly binding to mitochondrial cytochrome oxidase a_3. Signs and symptoms of cyanide poisoning usually occur less than 1 minute after inhalation and within a few minutes after ingestion. Early manifestations include anxiety, headache, giddiness, inability to focus the eyes, and mydriasis. Cyanide has a high affinity for certain sulphur compounds (sulphanes, which contain two covalently bonded but unequally charged sulphur atoms) and for certain metallic complexes, particularly those containing cobalt and the trivalent form of iron (Fe^{3+}). The cyanide ion can rapidly combine with iron in cytochrome a_3 (a component of the cytochrome aa_3 or cytochrome oxidase complex in mitochrondria for electron transport system) to inhibit this

enzyme, thus preventing intracellular oxygen utilization. The cell then utilizes anaerobic metabolism, creating excess lactic acid and a metabolic acidosis.

8. Nearly all of the energy needed by the human body is provided by the oxidation of carbohydrates and lipids. Whereas carbohydrates provide a readily available source of energy, lipids function primarily as an energy reserve. Lipids ingested as food are digested in the small intestine where bile salts are used to emulsify them and pancreatic lipase hydrolyzes lipids into fatty acids, glycerol, soaps, or mono- and diglycerides. Since lipids are not soluble in blood, they are transported as lipoproteins after reaction with water-soluble proteins in the blood. Excess lipids in the blood are eventually converted into adipose tissue. If lipid levels in the blood become too low, the body synthesizes lipids from other foods, such as carbohydrates, or removes lipids from storage.

9. Given, four proteins of pIs = 11, 7, 5, 3

Amino acids having isoelectric point (pI) lower than 7 are basic amino acids and those having pIs greater than 7 are acidic amino acids. This basicity or acidity is induced whenever there is a buffer solution of pH either > 7 or pH < 7 respectively. Thus, when a pH of 8 for a low ionic strength buffer is utilised, the anion exchange column of DEAE would bind to the negatively charged ions released from the basic amino acids to neutralise the acidity (H^+ ions) of the solution. Thus, the proteins having pIs of 3, 5 and 7 will only bind to the anion-exchange matrix.

10. Valinomycin is a natural, lipid-soluble molecule (Mr = ~1,110) that binds potassium ions (K^+) and facilitates their transfer across lipid bilayers (i.e., it is an ionophore). It is a macrocyclic molecule formed from 12 alternating amino acids and esters, synthesized by specific *Streptomyces*. Valinomycin exhibits a 10,000-fold selectivity for K^+ over Na^+. Valinomycin is a potent antibiotic. It is commonly used as an agent to induce apoptosis and can also be used to calibrate potentiometric responses in membrane experiments involving potential-sensitive dyes.

11. Basophil, type of white blood cell, is characterized histologically by its ability to be stained by basic dyes and functionally by its role in mediating hypersensitivity reactions of the immune system. When antibodies of the immunoglobulin E (IgE) class bind to specialized receptor molecules on basophils, the cells release their stores of inflammatory chemicals, including histamine, serotonin, and leukotrienes. These chemicals have a number of effects, including constriction of the smooth muscles, which leads to breathing difficulty. Cytotoxic T lymphocytes (CTL) are lymphocytes that kill other ("target") cells. CTLs have cytoplasmic granules that contain the proteins perforin and granzymes. When the CTL binds to its target, the contents of the granules are discharged by exocytosis. CTLs express on their surface molecules of a transmembrane protein, the death activator designated Fas ligand (FasL). B cells regulate immune responses by producing antigen-specific antibodies. Many B cells mature into what are called plasma cells that produce antibodies (proteins) necessary to fight off infections while other B cells mature into memory B cells. Neutrophils provide the first line of defence of the innate immune system by phagocytosing, killing, and digesting bacteria and fungi.

12. Two purified samples of DNA, A and B have the same number of base pairs and one site each for restriction enzymes BamHI and EcoRI. The resulting product after digestion and electrophoresis yielded 3 bands for DNA A and 2 bands for DNA B. Now, if a DNA is circular, then digesting it with 2 restriction enzymes would yield 2 bands of DNA. On the otherhand, if a DNA is linear, digesting it with 1 restriction enzyme would yield 2 bands and using another enzyme will further fragment the bands into 3. Thus, DNA A is linear and DNA B is circular.

13. Enzymes are biological catalysts vital to life processes and have attracted century-long investigation. The classic Michaelis-Menten mechanism provides a highly satisfactory description of catalytic activities for large ensembles of enzyme molecules. The reactions are given below:

$E + S \Leftrightarrow ES \rightarrow E + P$; rate of forward reaction in formation of enzyme-substrate complex is k_1 and rate of backward reaction is k_{-1}. The rate of forward reaction for the formation of product is k_2. Now, the Michaelis-Menten equation is given as :

$$v = \frac{(v_{max}[S])}{(K_m + [S])}$$

and $$K_m = \frac{(k_2 + k_{-1})}{k_1}$$

14. Progesterone is one of the steroid hormones. It is secreted by the corpus luteum and by the placenta and is responsible for preparing the body for pregnancy and, if pregnancy occurs, maintaining it until birth. Dopamine is a neurotransmitter that helps control the brain's reward and pleasure centers. Dopamine (dopamine hydrochloride)HCl, anaturally occurring catecholamine, is an ionotropic vasopressor agent. Vasopressin, also called antidiuretic hormone, is a peptide hormone that plays a key role in maintaining osmolality and therefore helps in maintaining the volume of water in the extracellular fluid. Prostaglandins and related

compounds are collectively known as eicosanoids. Most are produced from arachidonic acid, a 20-carbon polyunsaturated fatty acid (5, 8, 11, 14-eicosatetraenoic acid). Examples of eicosanoids are prostaglandins, prostacyclins, thromboxanes, leukotrienes, and epoxyeicosatrienoic acids.

15. IgG, a monomer, is the predominant immunoglobulin (Ig) class present in human serum. Produced as part of the secondary immune response to an antigen, this class of immunoglobulin constitutes approximately 75% of total serum Ig. Serum IgM exists as a pentamer in mammals, predominates in primary immune responses to most antigens, is the most efficient complement fixing immunoglobulin and comprises approximately 10% of normal human serum Ig content. IgA exists in serum in both monomeric and dimeric forms, comprising approximately 15% of the total serum Ig. Since IgG is a monomer, it will denature to form the least number of bands, followed by IgA (dimer) and IgM (pentamer).

16. By including a radioactive triphosphate during polymerase chain reaction (PCR), probes of very high specific activity can be generated. The PCR technique can use protein-derived oligonucleotide sequences as primers to develop probes for screening recombinant libraries. The radioactive isotope α-^{32}P is labelled with any trinucleotide to form a triphosphate to trace the reaction and the product. Thus, out of the given four radiolabelled nucleotides, α-^{32}P dATP will have a radioactive product at the end of the PCR cycle.

17. T4 polynucleotide kinase (Pnk) exemplifies a family of bifunctional enzymes with 5′-kinase and 3′-phosphatase activities that play key roles in RNA and DNA repair. Enolase is a dimeric metal-activated metalloenzyme which uses two magnesium ions per subunit: the strongly bound conformational ion and the catalytic ion that binds to the enzyme-substrate complex inducing catalysis. One fluoride ion bridges the structural and catalytic magnesium ions while the other interacts with the structural magnesium ion and the ammonio groups of Lys 342 and Lys 393. The ras protein belongs to a large super-family of proteins known as "low-molecular weight G-proteins". These proteins are called "G-proteins" because they bind guanine nucleotides (GTP and GDP). Ras possesses a GTPase activity that converts GTP to GDP by hydrolyzing the gamma phosphate off the GTP. The lac operon is a positive and negative regulator of lactose in prokaryotes. In the absence of lactose, the repressor protein encoded by the I gene binds to the lac operator and prevents transcription. Binding of allolactose to the repressor causes it to leave the operator. This enables RNA polymerase to transcribe the three genes of the operon. The single mRNA molecule that results is then translated into the three proteins.

18. The triple-helical structure of collagen arises from an unusual abundance of three amino acids: glycine, proline, and hydroxyproline. These amino acids make up the characteristic repeating motif Gly-Pro-X, where X can be any amino acid. Keratin is a fibrous protein with numerous α-helices and β-pleated sheets and numerous sulfhydryl cross-bridges. Keratin is mechanically strong, and hydrophobic enough to create an effective moisture barrier. Tropomyosin is composed of two alpha-helical chains arranged as a coiled-coil. It is polymerized end to end along the two grooves of actin filaments and provides stability to the filaments. All these proteins have repetitive sequences of amino acids along with high level of super-coiling.

19. Tyrosine hydroxylase (TH) deficiency is associated with a broad phenotypic spectrum ranging from TH-deficient dopa-responsive dystonia (DRD) at the mild end to a levodopa-unresponsive infantile Parkinsonism or progressive infantile encephalopathy phenotype at the severe end. Iodide is rapidly bound as 3-iodotyrosine, 3,5-diiodotyrosine, and thyroxine during the chloroperoxidase-catalyzed iodination. Since iodination of thyroglobulin occurred very effectively in the presence of only a single crystalline enzyme, the results suggest that it may not be necessary to postulate the existence of a separate "tyrosine iodinase" in the thyroid. The reversible phosphorylation of tyrosine residues is an important mechanism for modulating biological processes such as cellular signalling, differentiation, and growth. Stimulation of the T cell antigen receptor (TCR) induces formation of a phosphorylation-dependent signalling network via multiprotein tyrosine complexes. Melanin synthesis begins in the liver where phenylalanine is converted to tyrosine by the action of phenylalanine hydroxylase. The oxidation of L-Tyrosine toL-DOPA is then catalysed by the action of tyrosinase enzymes within the melanocyte's melanosome.

20. The Scatchard plot is a graphical method of analyzing equilibrium ligand binding data. It is used to determine the number of ligand-binding sites on a receptor, whether these sites show cooperative interactions, whether more than one class of site exists, and the respective affinities of each site. The experimental parameters used for a Scatchard plot are the free ligand concentration [L] and the average number of ligand molecules bound to a receptor, n, at a particular ligand concentration at equilibrium. The intercept on the abscissa equals the total number of binding sites in the receptor, and the slope equals -K where Ka is the intrinsic equilibrium association constant. So, the affinity of the receptor-ligand interaction is obtained through the number of the binding sites present which is the abscissa or the X-intercept.

J : BOTANY

1. The stalk that attaches an ovule or seed to the wall of the ovary is called funicle or funiculus. It can also be defined as the part that joins the seed to the pod frame. The pod frame is called a replum. The crowning beak of the pod is termed a rostrum.
2. The diploid number of an organism is given as 14. We know nullisomy = $2n - 2$.

   Therefore, nullisomy

   $= 14 - 2 = 12.$

   Thus 12 chromosomes would be expected in its nullisomic.
3. Intercalating agents are usually associated with insertion mutations. The best known mutagen of this type is ethidium bromide, which fluoresces when exposed to UV radiation and so is used to reveal the positions of DNA bands after agarose gel electrophoresis. Ethidium bromide and other intercalating agents are flat molecules that can slip between base pairs in the double helix, slightly unwinding the helix and hence increasing the distance between adjacent base pairs.
4. Peroxisomes are small, membrane-enclosed organelles that contain enzymes involved in a variety of metabolic reactions, including several aspects of energy metabolism. Peroxisomes in leaves are involved in photorespiration, which serves to metabolize a side product formed during photosynthesis. Photorespiration involves a complex network of enzyme reactions that exchange metabolites between chloroplasts, leaf peroxisomes and mitochondria and it produces reactive oxygen species and H_2O_2.

   Glycolate + $O_2 \rightarrow$ glyoxylate + H_2O_2 (in the presence of oxidase)

   $2H_2O_2 \rightarrow 2H_2O + O_2$ (in the presence of catalase)
5. The defence mechanism adopted by plants for detoxification of heavy metals is the synthesis of phytochelatin. Phytochelatin synthase is the enzyme responsible for the synthesis of heavy-metal-binding peptides (phytochelatins) from glutathione and related thiols. Phytochelatins act as chelators, and are important for heavy metal detoxification.
6. The drug colchicine exerts its effect in the M phase of cell cycle. Colchicine is an alkaloid derived from the autumn crocus (Colchicum autumnale). It inhibits mitosis by inhibiting microtubule polymerization.
7. Vitrification is the transformation of a substance into a glass. Usually, it is achieved by rapidly cooling a liquid through the glass transition. Certain chemical reactions also result in glasses. An important application is the vitrification of an antifreeze-like liquid in cryopreservation.
8. Flow cytometry is a technique for counting and examining microscopic particles, such as cells and chromosomes, by suspending them in a stream of fluid and passing them by an electronic detection apparatus. Cellular DNA content can be measured by flow cytometry with the aim of revealing cell distribution within the major phases of the cell cycle, estimating the frequency of apoptotic cells with fractional DNA content, and/or disclosing the DNA-ploidy of the measured cell population.
9. Plant organelles emit signals that regulate the expression of nuclear genes, a process known as retrograde signaling. Retrograde signaling is a pathway of communication from chloroplast to the nucleus under normal and pathophysiological conditions.
10. Photoautotrophic micropropagation refers to micropropagation with no exogenous organic components (sugar, vitamins, etc.) added to the medium, and it has been developed along with the development of techniques of in vitro environmental control. CO_2 concentration, photosynthetic photon flux, relative humidity, and air speed in the vessel are some of the most important environmental factors affecting plantlet growth and development.
11. The chlorophyll molecules in the reaction center of photosystem II are P680 (sensitive to wavelengths up to about 680 nm), whereas those in photosystem I are P700, which can therefore respond to slighter longer wavelengths.

    For photosynthetic organisms, 200–300 chlorophyll molecules act as light-harvesting antennae for each reaction centre and release of one molecule of oxygen requires minimum of 8 photons.
12. The VirD1 and VirD2 proteins encoded by an inducible locus of the virulence (vir) region of the Agrobacterium tumefaciens Ti plasmid are required for site-specific nicking at T-DNA border sites along with VirD3 protein.

    A gene gun or a biolistic particle delivery system, originally designed for plant transformation, is a device for injecting cells with genetic information. The payload is an elemental particle of a heavy metal usually gold/tungsten coated with plasmid DNA.

13. Guggulsterone is a plant steroid found in the resin of the guggul plant, Commiphora mukul.

Shikonin and its derivatives are contained in the outer surface of the roots of Lithospermum erythrorhizori (Boraginaceae) and these purple-red compounds, with naphthazalin skeleton are present as low molecular weight fatty acid ester in the roots. Shikonin is a herbal medicine with anti-tumor activities in this root.

Ajmalicine, also known as δ-yohimbine or raubasine, is an antihypertensive drug used in the treatment of high blood pressure.

Glycyrrhizin is the main sweet-tasting compound from liquorice root.

14. A gene which confers resistance to the herbicide bialaphos (bar) is known as bar gene.

Vip3A protein possesses insecticidal activity against a wild spectrum of lepidopteran insect larvae.

Golden rice was created by transforming rice with three beta-carotene biosynthesis genes, one of which was beta lcy gene. It has a transit peptide sequence attached so it is targeted to the plastid, where geranylgeranyl diphosphate formation occurs. It is used for nutritional improvement with increase in vitamin A.

gshII genes are involved in the tolerance of heavy metals.

15. Napin is a basic, low molecular weight storage protein synthesized in rapeseed (Brassica napus) embryos during seed development.

Vicilin is the major protein in pea. It contains 7% lysine but no sulphur containing amino acids methionine and cysteine.

Grain sorghum and its proteins are safe for celiac patients and individuals with varying levels of gluten intolerances. However, the main sorghum protein i.e. kafirins, are resistant to digestion.

Gliadin is a class of proteins present in wheat and several other cereals within the grass genus Triticum.

16. *Ustilaginoidea virens*, perfect sexual stage Villosiclava virens, is a plant pathogen which causes the disease False Smut of rice which reduces both grain yield and grain quality.

The organism *Corynebacterium sepidonicium* causes ring rot of potato in many of the major potato-growing areas of the world.

Colletotrichum falcatum is an important pathogen of sugarcane causing red rot disease. The type specimen of this species could not be located in any herbaria.

Plasmopara viticola, the causal agent of grapevine downy mildew, is a heterothallic oomycete that overwinters as oospores in leaf litter and soil.

17. Adolf Engler was a German botanist. He is notable for his work on plant taxonomy and phytogeography, such as Die natürlichen Pflanzenfamilien (The Natural Plant Families).

John Hutchinson first proposed his classification of angiosperms in his book The Families of Flowering Plants, the first volume on Dicotyledons appearing in 1926 and the second on Monocotyledons in 1934.

18. The correct statements are A and C.

Plastid genomes typically range in size from 120 to 160 kilobase pairs (kb), and there is a relatively high degree of conservation in size, structure, gene content, and linear order of the genes in land plants.

The gene for the small subunit of ribulose carboxylase (Rubisco) is located in the plastid. One of the subunits of ribulose bisphosphate carboxylase (rubisco) is encoded by chloroplast DNA.

19. Sieve elements are an elongated, food-conducting cell in phloem in angiosperms. Sieve elements have living protoplasts when mature, but they lack a nucleus and are dependent upon companion cells for certain functions. The sieve-tube elements are aligned end to end and form continuous tubes, along which nutrients flow relatively unimpeded from cell to cell through the sieve plates.

Bulliform cells are large, bubble-shaped epidermal cells that occur in groups on the upper surface of the leaves of many grasses. They are thought to play a role in the unfolding of developing leaves and in the rolling and unrolling of mature leaves in response to alternating wet and dry periods.

20. The succession initiated in extremely dry situations such as bare rock, windblown sand, etc. is called xerach succession or primary succion in xerosere. It is a plant succession which is limited by water availability.

Sympatric speciation is the process through which new species evolve from a single ancestral species while inhabiting the same geographic region.

K : MICROBIOLOGY

1. Quinolones are antimicrobial agents effective in the treatment of selected community-acquired and nosocomial infections. Quinolones are bactericidal and exhibit concentration-dependent killing. The targets of quinolone activity are the bacterial DNA gyrase and topoisomerase IV, enzymes essential for DNA replication and transcription.

2. To select for spontaneously arising histidine auxotrophs in a population, the medium should contain histidine and penicillin. Auxotrophy is the inability of an organism to synthesize a

particular organic compound required for its growth. Thus the medium must contain histidine along with penicillin (antibiotic). The histidine auxotrophs cannot synthesize histidine and it must therefore be taken up from the environment.

3. Louis Pasteur was a French chemist and microbiologist, who began investigating anthrax in 1879. German physician Robert Koch announced the isolation of the anthrax bacillus, which Pasteur confirmed. Koch and Pasteur independently provided definitive experimental evidence that the anthrax bacillus was indeed responsible for the infection.

   In 1859, Louis Pasteur definitively showed that microorganisms were responsible for food spoilage for the first time. This discovery led to the coining of the term "pasteurization" to describe the process where liquids with the potential to spoil (milk in particular) are heated for preservation.

   In his early research Pasteur worked with the wine growers of France, helping with the fermentation process to develop a way to pasteurize and kill germs. Thus he confirmed that bacteria cause wine disease.

   Thus the statement "the disease causing organism must be isolated in pure culture" is not associated with Louis Pasteur's contributions.

4. Active transport involves expenditure of metabolic energy to move ions or other solutes across membranes against their electrochemical (concentration) gradient. Its importance to cells is readily demonstrated by inhibiting the production of ATP - in such cases, the concentration of ions inside the cell soon drifts toward that of extracellular fluid and the cell dies.

   Primary active transport involves a carrier protein that directly hydrolyzes ATP to drive the transport process.

   Secondary active transport utilizes energy stored in electrochemical gradients of ions to drive transport.

5. Carbon catabolite repression (CCR) is a regulatory mechanism by which the expression of genes required for the utilization of secondary sources of carbon is prevented by the presence of a preferred substrate. It inhibits the regulating expression of genes required for utilization of less-efficient metabolites, thus saves energy. The catabolite repression was first shown to be initiated by glucose and therefore sometimes referred to as the glucose effect.

6. Tamiflu (oseltamivir phosphate) is an oral anti-viral drug approved for the treatment of acute, uncomplicated influenza. This product is approved to treat Type A and B influenza.

7. Differential RNA processing governs the synthesis of an immunoglobulin in either a secretory or membrane bound form.

8. Cis- trans test is a test used to define the unit of genetic function, based on whether two mutations of the same character occur in a single chromosome (the cis position) or in different cistrons in each chromosome of a homologous pair (the trans position). Thus it can determine whether a gene codes for a protein with the same or different amino acids.

9. *Pseudomonas* and *Desulfovibrio* are expected to be the abundant inhabitants of a nitrate and sulphate rich soil naturally depleted for oxygen. *Desulfovibrio* are sulfate reducing bacteria and are gram negative, non-spore forming medium sized curved rod shaped cells that contain desulfoviridin and are motile. Members of the genus. This genus can grow easily on a sulfate-lactate medium in the absence of oxygen. *Pseudomonas* is also gram- negative sulphate and nitrate reducing bacteria.

10. In light microscopy, oil immersion is a technique used to increase the resolution of a microscope. This is achieved by immersing both the objective lens and the specimen in a transparent oil of high refractive index, thereby increasing the numerical aperture of the objective lens. Immersion oils are transparent oils that have specific optical and viscosity characteristics necessary for use in microscopy. Typical oils used have an index of refraction around 1.515.

11. Four Hfr strains of E. coli were generated from the same F^+ strain. The order of the markers in the original F^+ strain is DQWMTPXACNB as it satisfies the different possible results of Hfr * F^- strain conjugation.

12. Ethidium bromide is a common fluorescent stain used with double-stranded DNA. Ethidium intercalates between DNA bases. When EtBr binds to the linear DNA, it lengthens it by intercalating between the stacked bases. The intercalating agent doesn't bind to closed circular molecules because they can't be lengthened enough to allow insertion of the chemical between the bases. In case of close circular DNA the ends are constrained, thus it cannot bind to the extent that it does on linear DNA. This is because it reduces Twist of DNA, which in a plasmid causes increase in writhe (supercoils), which adds torsional stress on the helix and limits the amount of EtBr that can be bound.

13. E. coli (and certain other bacteria) is capable of very rapid growth in rich medium, with doubling times as short as 20 min. The replication time, however, remains long, with approximately 40-45 min required to replicate and segregate the chromosome. Thus replication time for entire genome of E coli is around 40-45 min while its double time is only

20 min. As overlapping rounds of DNA replication allow the bacteria to double in faster times than the time required to copy the genome.

14. C. diphtheriae is a Gram-positive, aerobic, nonmotile, toxin-producing, rod-shaped bacteria which causes diphtheria. Diphtheria toxin (DT) is an extracellular protein of Corynebacterium diphtheriae that inhibits protein synthesis and kills susceptible cells. Diphtheria toxin is a single polypeptide chain of 535 amino acids and of 62 kDa consisting of two subunits linked by disulfide bridges, known as an A-B toxin.

The tox gene which codes for the Diphtheria toxin is located on the right-handed end of an integrated corynephage. C. diptheriae contains the protein DtxR, an iron-dependent negative-regulatory protein which prevents the tox gene from being transcribed under high iron conditions, as well as the high-energy iron uptake system of the bacterium. Because a host often reacts to infection by lowering iron levels, the bacteria have developed a mechanism which couples Diphtheria toxin gene expression with low iron levels.

Thus the statement "all strains of C. diphtheria are producers of diphtheria toxin" is an incorrect statement".

15. Joseph Lister was a British Surgeon who is credited as being the 'father of antiseptic surgery'. He promoted the idea of sterile surgery by introducing carbolic acid to clean wounds and disinfect surgical instruments.

John Needham was an English microscopist who performed experiments on spontaneous generation in mutton broth and hay infusions. The experiments consisted of briefly boiling a broth mixture and then cooling the mixture in an open container to room temperature. Later, the flasks would be sealed, and microbes would grow a few days later. Those experiments seemed to show that there was a life force that produced spontaneous generation.

Elie Metchnikoff was a Russian scientist who was the first to discover phagocytosis, a cell-mediated immune response to foreign matter. He discovered that certain white blood cells, which he called phagocytes, engulf and digest bacteria. He called these cells the body's first line of defense against disease.

Lazzaro Spallanzani was one of the first to disprove spontaneous generation. He was an Italian scientist who proved microorganisms could be killed by boiling.

16. Okazaki fragments are short, newly synthesized DNA fragments without RNA primer at the 5′ terminus that are formed on the lagging template strand during DNA replication. Thus Okazaki fragments are produced from only one of the strands of the circular genome, i.e. the lagging strand.

17. Aerobic metabolism is 19 times more efficient than anaerobic metabolism (which yields 2 mol ATP per 1 mol glucose). Anaerobic respiration is less efficient at using the energy from glucose since 2 ATP are produced during anaerobic respiration per glucose, compared to the 38 ATP per glucose produced by aerobic respiration. Thus there is a 19- fold increase in the net ATP production.

18. Bacillus and Clostridium are both Gram positive, spore forming, bacilli (rods). Bacillus sp. are aerobic. Clostridium sp. are anaerobic.

Neisseria species are Gram-negative cocci, 0.6 to 1.0 μm in diameter. The organisms are usually seen in pairs with the adjacent sides flattened. Sarcina is a genus of Gram-positive cocci bacteria in the family Clostridiaceae.

Rhizobia are soil bacteria that fix nitrogen after becoming established inside root nodules of legumes. Rhizobia require a plant host; they cannot independently fix nitrogen. In general, they are Gram-negative, motile, non-sporulating rods. Azotobacter are usually motile, oval or spherical bacteria that form thick-walled cysts. They are aerobic, free-living soil microbes which play an important role in the nitrogen cycle in nature, binding atmospheric nitrogen, which is inaccessible to plants, and releasing it in the form of ammonium ions into the soil.

Caulobacter crescentus is a rod-shaped single-celled organism found in fresh water, soil and sea water. In Hyphomicrobium a hyphal filament (prostheca) grows out of one end of the cell, and the bud grows out of the tip of the prostheca, separated by a relatively long distance from the mother cell.

19. Given, T = 40 min = 0.66 hrs

Generation time,

$G = 30$ min $= 0.5$ hrs

$N_0 = 20 * 10^5$

$N = ?$

So, $G = t/3.3 (\log_{10}N - \log_{10}N_0)$

Therefore, on solving,

$N = 10^6$

Burst size = 100 (initial phage particles present)

Infection cycle of phage = 20 min

Therefore,

No. of phage particles produced + phage particles initially present = $(100 * 100)^2 = 10^8$

Thus, the no. of phage particles exceeds the no. of *E coli* cells.

Therefore, the plaque forming units = 10^6.

20. Vibrio fischeri is a marine species. It inhabits the light organ of the flashlight fish, Photoblepharon palpebratus, and so is usually found in the gut, skin and light organ of this

fish, but it is also abundant in free living form. It also has a symbiotic relationship with the squid, Euprymna scolopes. P. palpebratus is a tropical reef-associated fish which is especially notable for its symbiotic association with a luminous bacteria that lives in pouches or "light organs" under its eyes.

Bdellovibrio is a genus of small, highly mobile, vibrio shaped, monoflagellated, gram negative bacteria with the ability to parasitize and kill other gram negative bacteria. This includes many pathogens, a few of the genera being: Alcaligenes, Campylobacter, Erwinia, Escherichia, Helicobacter, Pseud-omonas, Salmonella, Legionella, and Shigella.

Antagonism is the procedure that enables one microorganism to injure, inhibit, or kill the growth of another microorganism. Aspergillus and Pseudomonas represent an antagonist relation-ship. They can cause infection, which antagonizes the immune system.

Thiobacillus ferrooxidans and Beijerinckia lacticogenes share a mutualistic relationship.

L : ZOOLOGY

1. Extraembryonic tissues have been long known for their implication in the formation of structures that support the growth of the embryo within the intrauterine environment. These are intrauterine tissues that support the embryo's placenta, umbilical cord, and amniotic sac. Vertebrate embryos have four extra-embryonic tissues: amnion, chorion, yolk sac and the allantois. In placental animals these tissues form the placenta. The outer layer of the blastocyst becomes the trophoblast, which forms the outer layer of the placenta. Trophoblasts are cells forming the outer layer of a blastocyst, which provide nutrients to the embryo and develop into a large part of the placenta. After gastrulation, this layer of trophoblasts is referred to as the trophoectoderm, as it is then contiguous with the ectoderm of the embryo. Thus, extraembryonic tissues originate from trophoectoderm during the gastrula stage of embryo development.

2. Animal evolution split into two major lineages approximately 600 million years ago: the deuterostomes and the protostomes. Both Protostomia and Deuterostomia belong to a larger group within the Animalia called the Bilateria. The defining characteristic of the deuterostome is the fact that the blastopore (the opening at the bottom of the forming gastrula) becomes the anus, whereas in protosomes the blastopore becomes the mouth. The deuterostome mouth develops at the opposite end of the embryo from the blastopore and a digestive tract develops in the middle connecting the two. The name deuterostome means "mouth second". In taxonomic classification, deuterostomes are the superphyla comprising of the phyla Chordata, Hemichordata, Echinodermata, Xenoturbellida, Vetulicolia.

3. Extraembryonic tissues have been long known for their implication in the formation of structures that support the growth of the embryo within the intrauterine environment. These are intrauterine tissues that support the embryo's placenta, umbilical cord, and amniotic sac. Vertebrate embryos have four extra-embryonic tissues: amnion, chorion, yolk sac and the allantois. In placental animals these tissues form the placenta. The outer layer of the blastocyst becomes the trophoblast, which forms the outer layer of the placenta. Trophoblasts are cells forming the outer layer of a blastocyst, which provide nutrients to the embryo and develop into a large part of the placenta. After gastrulation, this layer of trophoblasts is referred to as the trophoectoderm, as it is then contiguous with the ectoderm of the embryo. Thus, extraembryonic tissues originate from trophoectoderm during the gastrula stage of embryo development.

4. The immune system defends the body against disease. Lymphocytes are one type of white blood cell that helps the body resist infection by recognizing harmful foreign substances, such as bacteria, and eliminating them. The ability of the vertebrate immune system to distinguish self from nonself depends largely on a group of protein makers (antigens) known as the major histocompatibility complex (MHC). These receptor antigens are present on the surface of T-cell lymphocytes. These markers which are present on the surface of every cell are slightly different in different individuals. The genes that code for these proteins are found linked together on one chromosone (chromosome 6 in humans). In humans the MHC is called the HLA (human leukocyte antigen) group. HLA is determined by five different linked genes. These genes are all polymorphic - that is, within the population there are multiple alleles at each locus. Tissues from the same individual or from identical twins have the same HLA alleles and thus the same HLA antigens.

5. *Wuchereria bancrofti* is a common human parasite found in tropical regions worldwide. Lymphatic filariasis is a parasitic disease caused by thread-like worms called *Wuchereria bancrofti.* It is one of the three parasites that cause lymphatic filariasis, an infection of the lymphatic system by filarial worms. The life cycle of *Wuchereria bancrofti* starts, when a male and a female

mate inside lymphatic vessels of an infected human. The parasite is carried from person to person by mosquitoes. Repeated mosquito bites during several months are usually needed to develop lymphatic filariasis. *Wuchereria bancrofti* infection is usually asymptomatic. Some people can develop lymphedema, swelling, which is prevalent in the legs, but sometimes also in the arms, genitalia and breasts. The swelling and decreased flow of the lymph fluid will expose the body to skin and lymph system infections. Over time the disease causes thickening and hardening of the skin, a condition called elephantiasis which can be fatal.

6. Insects, being arthropods, have a relatively inefficient, open circulatory system with no vessels to carry oxygen to different parts of their body. The tracheal system is composed of chitin-ringed tubes called tracheae that connect directly to the air through openings in the body wall called spiracles. The tracheae are reinforced with rings of chitin, the same material that makes up the arthropod exoskeleton. The tracheae branch into smaller and smaller tubes, called tracheoles, which eventually terminate on the plasma membrane of every cell in the insect's body. The tips of the tracheoles are closed and contain fluid. Air enters the tracheae through the spiracles and travels through the tracheoles to the fluid-filled tips, where oxygen diffuses directly from the tracheoles into the cells, and CO_2 diffuses from the cells into the tracheoles.

7. Feathers are among the most complex integumentary appendages found in vertebrates and are formed in tiny follicles in the epidermis, or outer skin layer, that produce keratin proteins. Feathers insulate birds from water and cold temperatures. Fur is a synonym for hair, used in reference to non-human animals, usually mammals; particularly those with extensive body hair coverage (helps in insulation against heat loss from the body). Adipose tissue, or fat, is an anatomical term for loose connective tissue composed of adipocytes. Its main role is to store energy in the form of fat, although it also cushions and insulates the body. Shivering is a bodily function in response to early hypothermia in warm-blooded animals. When the core body temperature drops, the shivering reflex is triggered to maintain homeostasis. Vasodilation is the increase in the internal diameter of a blood vessel that results from relaxation of smooth muscle within the wall of the vessel. This causes an increase in blood flow, but a decrease in systemic vascular resistance and loss of energy in the form of heat.

8. Melatonin is a hormone secreted by the pineal gland in the brain. It helps regulate other hormones and maintains the body's circadian rhythm. Glucagon is a hormone produced in the pancreas. Glucagon is used to raise very low blood sugar. Glucagon is also used in diagnostic testing of the stomach and other digestive organs. Prolactin is a hormone released by the pituitary gland that stimulates breast development and milk production in women. There is no known normal function for prolactin in men. Calcitonin is a hormone found naturally in our bodies. It is made by the thyroid gland and controls the activity of the osteoclasts (bone-eroding cells). The most prominent factor controlling calcitonin secretion is the extracellular concentration of ionized calcium. Elevated blood calcium levels strongly stimulate calcitonin secretion, and secretion is suppressed when calcium concentration falls below normal. Thus, it reduces the concentration of calcium in blood to maintain homeostasis.

9. Innate behaviour is the behaviour determined by the "hard-wiring" of the nervous system. It is usually inflexible, a given stimulus triggering a given response. The simplest example of an innate behaviour is a fixed action pattern, in which a very short to medium length sequence of actions, without variation, is carried out in response to a clearly defined stimulus. Innate behaviour is genetically programmed. Individuals inherit a suite of behaviours (often called an ethogram) just as they inherit physical traits such as body colour and wing venation.

10. The tricarboxylic acid cycle (TCA) is a series of enzyme-catalyzed chemical reactions that form a key part of the aerobic respiration in cells. This cycle is also called the Kreb's cycle and the citric acid cycle. Within the Krebs cycle, energy in the form of ATP is usually derived from the breakdown of glucose, although fats and proteins can also be utilized as energy sources. The enzymes that cause each step of the process to occur are all located in the cell's "power plant"; in animals, this power plant is the mitochondrial matrix; in plants, it is the chloroplasts; and in microorganisms, it can be found in the cell membrane. Energy is generated in the form of ATP with the help of NADH generated in the process and through electron transport pathway. The NADH generated by the TCA cycle is fed into the oxidative phosphorylation pathway. The net result of these two closely linked pathways is the oxidation of nutrients to produce usable energy in the form of ATP.

11. As the given data is insufficient, it will be impossible to as certain whether the eye colour is a single gene or a multi-gene characteristic. Now, if the gene(s) for eye colour is located on the X-chromosome i.e., it is a X-limited

trait, then a cross between green-eyed females and blue-eyed males would result:-

Gametes--> XX^c x XY
(from the parents)
here c is the gene for green eye

F2 gene ration

--> XX^c XX XY X^cY

Here, though 50% of male have blue eyes and the rest have green eyes, but also 50% females have green eyes and nothing can be said about the rest 50%. So gene cannot be located on X-chromosome.

If the gene were located on the Y-chromosome, then all the men should have blue eyes (since Y^c will be present in both cases of the F2 generation). Thus, the gene(s) for eye colour is not sex dependent or linked. Hence, eye colour gene(s) may be sex-independent i.e., not sex-limited.

12. The development of specialized cell types is called differentiation. These overt changes in cellular biochemistry and function are preceded by a process involving the commitment of the cell to a certain fate. At this point, even though the cell or tissue does not appear phenotypically different from its uncommitted state, its developmental fate has become restricted. The first stage is a labile phase called specification. The second stage of commitment is determination. There are three general ways a cell can become specified for a particular fate - they are autonomous specification, conditional specification and syncytial specification. Autonomous Specification results from cell-intrinsic properties and it give rise to mosaic development. Conditional Specification is a cell-extrinsic process that relies on cues and interactions between cells or from concentration-gradients of morphogens. Syncytial Specification is a hybrid of the autonomous and conditional specifications that occurs in insects. Since in the newly discovered organism, change in cell concentration (extrinsic factor) at the 100 cell or 1000 cell embryo stage affected the development of kidney, hence the type of specification during commitment stage is conditional.

13. Out of Bacteriophages, Yeast, *Escherichia coli and Bacillus subtilis,* the genome of *Escherichia coli* is the simplest and is well mapped. It is used as a tool for genetic engineering in many recombination experiments. For studying mutations on adjacent pairs of DNA, it is necessary to have a tool that can easily express the results. Thus genome of *Escherichia coli* can be used, modified through genetic recombination for the particular pair of DNA, artificial induction of mutation through mutagenic agents and then reading the expression profile of *Escherichia coli* to analyze the distinction between the mutated pair of adjacent DNAs.

14. RNA stands for ribonucleic acid. It is an important molecule with long chains of nucleotides. The chemical structure of RNA is very similar to that of DNA, with two differences: (a) RNA contains the sugar ribose, while DNA contains the slightly different sugar deoxyribose (a type of ribose that lacks one oxygen atom), and (b) RNA has the base uracil while DNA contains thymine. RNA is a single-stranded molecule in many of its biological roles and has a much shorter chain of nucleotides. While DNA contains deoxyribose, RNA contains ribose (in deoxyribose there is no hydroxyl group attached to the pentose ring in the 2′ position). These hydroxyl groups make RNA less stable than DNA because it is more prone to hydrolysis. There are also 3 types of RNA - mRNA, tRNA, and rRNA. Messenger RNA (mRNA) carries information about a protein sequence to the ribosomes, the protein synthesis factories in the cell. Transfer RNA (tRNA) is a small RNA chain of about 80 nucleotides that transfers a specific amino acid to a growing polypeptide chain at the ribosomal site of protein synthesis during translation. Ribosomal RNA (rRNA) is the catalytic component of the ribosomes. Thus, these 3 forms of RNA contain self complementary sequences that allow parts of RNA to fold and pair with itself to form double helices. This helps to serve RNA to be a genetic material.

15. Progesterone is a female hormone produced by the ovaries during release of a mature egg from an ovary (ovulation). Progesterone helps prepare the lining of the uterus (endometrium) to receive the egg if it becomes fertilized by a sperm. If the egg is not fertilized, progesterone levels drop and menstrual bleeding begins. Estrogens (also called Oestrogens) are steroid compounds that are important for development and functioning of females of the species. They are named so because they play an important role in the oestrous cycle. They are the primary female sex hormones. Prostaglandins are a group of naturally occurring, chemically related fatty acids that stimulate contractility of the uterine and other smooth muscle. Gonadotrophin is any hormone that stimulates the gonads, especially follicle-stimulating hormone and luteinizing hormone. Oestradiol is the most potent naturally occurring ovarian and placental oestrogen in mammals. It prepares the

uterus for implantation of the fertilized ovum and promotes the maturation of and maintenance of the female accessory reproductive organs and secondary sex characters. Prolactin is a hormone released by the pituitary gland that stimulates breast development and milk production in women. Thus, to affect fertilization and ovulation oestrogen and progesterone formulation should be implemented.

16. In sexual reproduction, two parents donate genes to their young, resulting in offspring with a mix of inherited genes. These genes are donated through a process called fertilization. There are two mechanisms by which fertilization can take place. The first is external (the eggs are fertilized outside of the body), and the second is internal (the eggs are fertilized within the female reproductive tract). But behaviour and relationships are governed by both genetics and environmental factors. According to Darwin's theory of evolution, natural selection is a process by which the best traits or the best adapted organisms survive in the prevalent environment while the poorly adapted ones are eliminated. Thus, occurrence of male paternal care through external fertilization results by the process of natural selection over a period of time and generation.

17. Biomagnification is the increasing concentration of a substance, such as a toxic chemical, in the tissues of organisms at successively higher levels in a food chain. As a result of biomagnification, organisms at the top of the food chain generally suffer greater harm from a persistent toxin or pollutant than those at lower levels. It occurs mainly due to the inability of the decomposers (microbes) at the lowest trophic level of food chain to degrade any particular kind of toxin. As such its concentration rises in the food chain and toxicity increases through metabolism of the primary producers present in the chain.

18. Telomerase, also called telomere terminal transferase, is an enzyme made of protein and RNA subunits that elongates chromosomes by adding TTAGGG sequences to the end of existing chromosomes in the telomere region. Reverse transcriptase, also called RNA-directed DNA polymerase, an enzyme encoded from the genetic material of retroviruses that catalyzes the transcription of retrovirus RNA (ribonucleic acid) into DNA (deoxyribonucleic acid). Taq DNA polymerase is a thermo-stable DNA polymerase that possesses a $5'\rightarrow 3'$ polymerase activity and a $5'$ flap endonuclease activity that is used in Polymerase Chain reaction (PCR). Primases are enzymes whose continual activity is required at the DNA replication fork as they catalyze the synthesis of short RNA molecules used as primers for DNA polymerases to perform replication. Since primase produces RNA molecules, the enzyme is a type of RNA polymerase. Thus, all the enzymes except primase catalyze the synthesis of DNA whereas primase catalyzes the synthesis of RNA primers.

19. In juxtacrine interactions, proteins from the inducing cell interact with receptor proteins of adjacent responding cells. The inducer does not diffuse from the cell producing it. There are three types of juxtacrine interactions. In the first type, a protein on one cell binds to its receptor on the adjacent cell. In the second type, a receptor on one cell binds to its ligand on the extracellular matrix secreted by another cell. In the third type, the signal is transmitted directly from the cytoplasm of one cell through small conduits into the cytoplasm of an adjacent cell. Reciprocal signalling occurs between receptors (as in case of integrin and non-integrin). Ligand can be present in the extracellular matrix or may be membrane anchored but both ligand and receptor need not be membrane bound for signalling. Ligands are cleavable by the receptor through proteolytic cleavage during signal transduction (as in case of hormone renin-angiotensin system).

20. Both valine and isoleucine are neutral and essential α-amino acids but valine is hydrophobic whereas isoleucine is hydrophilic. Methionine is a sulphur containing essential amino acid whereas proline is a non-essential amino acid but though aliphatic, it has a ring-like structure. Aspartic acid and glutamic acid are acidic amino acids which play important roles as general acids in enzyme active centres. Histidine, an essential amino acid, has as a positively charged imidazole functional group and arginine is an α-amino acid which can be obtained from food and is necessary for the body to make proteins. Thus, out of all the amino acids, if methionine is replaced by a proline residue it would adversely affect the α-helix because proline has a ring-like structure whereas histidine is linear.

M : FOOD TECHNOLOGY

1. Wheat gluten is the natural protein found in wheat flour that is responsible for the porous and spongy structure of breads. It is a sticky substance obtained by washing out the starch from wheat flour dough. Wheat gluten is added to breads to increase their chewiness. Vital wheat gluten (also called gluten powder or gluten flour) is the dried form of wet wheat gluten. It is added to bakery products to increase dough strength (*e.g.*, durable pizza crust).
2. Mixing can be characterized by analysis of sample compositions and then calculation of the standard deviation, s, of these from the mean composition of the whole mixture. A mixing index M can often be related to the time of mixing by: $[1-(M)] = e^{-Kt}$. Most of the available definitions of the mixing index, which specifies homogeneity or distribution of the composition in a solids mixture, are based on the variance of the concentration of a certain component among spot samples. However, for a solid—solid chemical reaction or any process involving contact between different solid phases, its rate is proportional to the contact points or area among particles of the different phases. Thus a definition of a microscopic and geometric mixing index based on the number of contact points appears to be of practical significance.
3. The main function of fats in the body is to provide energy: By supplying energy, fats save proteins from being used for energy and allow them to perform their more important role of building and repairing tissues. Fats on oxidation provide almost twice as much energy as that given by carbohydrates. Fats are metabolized to release greater amount of energy than would be normally released by other sources like carbohydrates, etc. They are also important to store certain vitamins like vitamin A, D, E and K which are soluble in fats and insoluble in water. It helps protect vital organs such as your heart, kidneys, and liver.
4. The unique ripening of blue-veined cheeses comes from the mould spores *Penicillium roquefortior P. glaucum*, which are added to the milk or to the curds before pressing and are activated by air. Air is introduced by "needling" the cheese with a device that punches about 50 small holes into the top. The hydrolysis of isolated αs1- and β-caseins by *Penicillium roqueforti* aspartyl proteinase produced comparable quantities of pH 4.6 soluble N. The amount of non-protein nitrogen obtained with β-casein was clearly lower than that obtained with αs1-casein, showing that few low molecular weight peptides were released when this casein was hydrolysed. The aroma is due to the formation of methyl ketones.
5. There are two basic types or causes of rancidity that cause and/or contribute to the degradation of stored edible oils: oxidative and hydrolytic. Oxidative rancidity, known as autoxidation, occurs when oxygen is absorbed from the environment. In the presence of oxygen and/or ultraviolet (UV) radiation, most lipids will break down and degrade, forming several other compounds. Oxygen is eight times more soluble in fats than it is in water; it is this exposure that is the main cause of the autoxidation process, increasing the saturation of the oil. Hydrolytic rancidity, also called hydrolysis or enzymatic oxidation, occurs in the absence of air, but with moisture present. This normally is accomplished through enzymatic peroxidation, where enzymes found naturally in plant oils (i.e., lipoxygenase, cyclooxygenase) and animal fats (i.e., lipase) can catalyze reactions between water and oil. Another degradation process is microbial rancidity, in which micro-organisms such as bacteria, moulds and yeast use their enzymes to break down chemical structures in the oil, producing unwanted odours and flavours. Water needs to be present for microbial growth to occur. Rancidification is the decomposition of fats, oils and other lipids by hydrolysis or oxidation, or both. Hydrolysis will split fatty acid chains away from the glycerol backbone in glycerides. These free fatty acids can then undergo further auto-oxidation. Oxidation primarily occurs with unsaturated fats by a free radical-mediated process. These chemical processes can generate highly reactive molecules in rancid foods and oils, which are responsible for producing unpleasant and noxious odours and flavours. These chemical processes may also destroy nutrients in food. Under some conditions, rancidity, and the destruction of vitamins, occurs very quickly.
6. *Shigella* is a genus of bacteria that are a major cause of diarrheoa and dysentery – diarrhoea with blood and mucus in the stools – throughout the world. The bacteria are transmitted by ingestion of contaminated food or water, or through person-to-person contact. In the body, they can invade and destroy the cells lining the large intestine, causing mucosal ulceration and bloody diarrhoea.

Apart from diarrhoea, symptoms of *Shigella* infection include fever, abdominal cramps, and rectal pain. Most patients recover without complications within seven days. Shigellosis can be treated with antibiotics, although some strains have developed drug resistance. Shigellosis can also lead to dehydration and in rare cases, other complications, like arthritis, skin rashes, and kidney failure.

7. Beriberi is a nutritional disorder caused by a deficiency of thiamin (vitamin B1) and characterized by impairment of the nerves and heart. General symptoms include loss of appetite and overall lassitude, digestive irregularities, and a feeling of numbness and weakness in the limbs and extremities. Pellagra is a disease that occurs when a person does not get enough niacin (one of the B complex vitamins) or tryptophan (an amino acid). Anaemia is a condition in which the body does not have enough healthy red blood cells. Red blood cells provide oxygen to body tissues. The body needs certain vitamins, minerals, and nutrients to make enough red blood cells. Iron, vitamin B12, and folic acid are three of the most important ones. The body may not have enough of these nutrients. Scurvy is a disease that occurs when you have a severe lack of vitamin C (ascorbic acid) in your diet. Scurvy causes general weakness, anaemia, gum disease, and skin haemorrhages.

8. Psychrophilic bacteria are adapted to their cool environment by having largely unsaturated fatty acids in their plasma membranes. Some psychrophiles, particularly those from the Antarctic have been found to contain polyunsaturated fatty acids, which generally do not occur in prokaryotes. Thermophiles are adapted to temperatures above 60 degrees in a variety of ways. Often thermophiles have a high G + C content in their DNA such that the melting point of the DNA (the temperature at which the strands of the double helix separate) is at least as high as the organism's maximum T for growth. Considering the total span of temperature where liquid water exists, the prkaryotes may be subdivided into several subclasses on the basis of one or another of their cardinal points for growth. For example, organisms with an optimum temperature near 37 degrees (the body temperature of warm-blooded animals) are called mesophiles.

9. Given, solubility of Sodium bicarbonate in water at

$$20^0C = \frac{9.6g}{100g}$$

Solubility at 60 $^0C = \frac{16.4g}{100g}$

When temperature is dropped from 60^{0}C to 20^{0}C, the amount of Sodium bicarbonate crystallized is:

$$16.4 - 9.6 = \frac{6.8g}{100g}$$

Now, percentage of Sodium bicarbonate crystallized

$$= \frac{6.8}{16.4} \times 100\% = 41.46\%$$

10. The quality of a protein is primarily a function of its essential amino acid composition. To assess the protein quality, Block and Mitchell (1946) introduced the concept of an amino acid or chemical score, in which the amount of the essential amino acid that is in greatest deficit is expressed as a percentage of the amount present in a standard or reference protein. Egg and human milk proteins, for their very high biological value, have been considered as reference standards. Essential amino acids, found in abundance in high-quality dietary protein, are required daily by hospitalized patients and healthy persons to maintain the dynamic process of protein metabolism. One method for assessing dietary protein quality is by determining a diet's chemical score, *i.e.*, the ratio of a gram of the limiting amino acid in a test diet to the same amount of the corresponding amino acid in a reference diet (*e.g.*, whole-egg protein) multiplied by 100.

11. Given, Density of sugar syrup,

$\rho = 1040\ kg/m^3$

Viscosity of the sugar syrup,

$= 1600 \times 10^{-6}$ Pa.s

Diameter of the pipe,

d= 3 cm = 0.03 m

For laminar flow, Reynold's number, $R_e < 2000$

Minimum time required to fill the tank will need maximum velocity (u)

So, for maximum velocity,

$R_e = 2000$

Or $R_e = (\rho \times u \times d)/$

$\Rightarrow$ $(2000 \times\ )/(\rho \times d) = u$

$\Rightarrow$ u= 0.10256 m/s

Time required for the tank to be filled having diameter

= 1.5m and height = 3 m

= Area of the tank/ (velocity × diameter of the pipe)

= 19.3 h

12. It is very important to use the correct amount of salt so that fermentation can take place. Sauerkraut is a salty food. People who must restrict their sodium intake need to take into account the high salt content of sauerkraut when planning their meals. Softness may result from insufficient salt,

high temperatures during fermentation, uneven salt distribution or air pockets caused by improper packing. Pink colour in kraut is caused by the growth of certain types of yeasts on the surface of the kraut. These may grow if there is too much salt, an uneven distribution of salt or if the kraut is insufficiently covered during fermentation. Pink colour may also result from pigments in the cabbage. Rotted kraut is usually found at the surface, where the cabbage has not been covered sufficiently to exclude air during fermentation. Darkness in kraut may be caused by unwashed and improperly trimmed cabbage, insufficient juice to cover the cabbage during fermentation, uneven salt distribution, exposure to air, high temperatures during fermentation, processing or storage, or by a long storage period.

13. Starch blends, including modified high amylose starch derivatives and alpha-amylase converted waxy starch derivatives, together with ingredients such as gelatin and sucrose, have been used in the manufacture of pan coated candies. These and other coatings incorporate a hydroxypropyl derivative of a 70% amylose corn starch. The pectin obtained from the citrus peel is used mainly as a setting agent in the food industry, but also for pharmaceutical and cosmetic products. The use of starch phosphate esters is an expansion and/or texture aid in food or industrial products. It provides the formulations and improved expanded products containing starch phosphate esters, particularly extruded breakfast cereals and snacks. Simple sugars (monosaccharides) and sugar alcohols possess 5-6 hydroxyl sites available for hydrogen bonding with water, making them excellent humectants. Sorbitol, glucose, and fructose are all commonly found in hair-care products.

14. Diacetyl is the main ingredient of the typical butter aroma. It occurs naturally in apples, beans, butter, artichokes, black currants, blueberries, blue cheese and wheat. Limonene, a naturally occurring hydrocarbon, is a cyclic monoterpene with the molecular formula $C_{10}H_{16}$. It is commonly found in the rinds of citrus fruits such as grapefruit, lemon, and lime and, in particular, oranges. Eugenol is sometimes called clove oil because it is the active element in cloves. It causes the aromatic smell typical of cloves and because of this property is often found in perfumes. Menthol ($C_{10}H_{20}$) is a mint-scented solid that is non-hazardous for the ingredients of peppermint candy. Methanol (CH_3OH) is an alcohol-scented liquid.

15. Curd is also a dairy product obtained by curdling milk with rennet or an edible acidic substance such as lemon juice or vinegar and then draining off the liquid portion.The increased acidity causes the milk proteins tangle into solid masses or curds. The process of butter making can be described as an inversion of the original cream emulsion. The system of fat droplets dispersed in water is converted into a continuous phase of fat that contains water droplets. The final product is about 80% milk fat, 18% water, and 2% milk solids, mainly proteins and salts carried in the water. Vegetable soup would be a heterogenous mixture- the various components can be separated out by physical means (such as straining to separate the solid vegetables from the liquid broth). Fresh eggs will achieve the fullest volume as they are slightly acidic and this helps stabilize the proteins. Whipping begins the egg whites on low speed until they become foamy and frothy. Once the egg whites are foamy, the speed is increased to high until they become whipped to the desired stage. The egg whites are still primarily liquid, with some bubbles that may cause the egg whites to look slightly opaque.

16. We have, Mean doubling time for a culture is given by

$$t_d = \frac{t \ln 2}{(\ln N/N_0)}$$

Here, $N = 10^7$ cells; $N_0 = 10^3$ cells, $t = 4$h

$$\text{Therefore, } t_d = \frac{4 \ln 2}{\left(\ln \frac{10^7}{10^3}\right)}$$

$$= \frac{4}{(\ln 10^4)}$$

$$= \frac{0.693}{2.303}$$

$= 0.3009$ h

$= 18.055$ min

17. The Gram stain is a very important preliminary step in the initial characterization and classification of bacteria. It is also a key procedure in the identification of bacteria based on staining characteristics, enabling the bacteria to be examined using a light microscope. The bacteria present in an unstained smear are invisible when viewed using a light microscope. The four basic steps of the Gram Stain are: 1) Application of the primary stain Crystal Violet (CV) to a heat-fixed smear of bacterial culture, 2) Addition of Gram's Iodine, 3) De-colorization with 95% ethyl alcohol and 4) Counter-stain with Safranin.

18. Given, Blanched vegetable weight = 12 kg/min

Initial Moisture content = 50%

Final Moisture content =10%

So, final weight of the blanched vegetable

$$= \frac{(100 - 50)}{(100 - 10)} \times 12$$

= 6.667 kg/min

Weight of water removed

= 12 – 6.67 kg/min

= 5.33 kg/min

Since the continuous dryer cannot handle more than 25% moisture content at one time, so the feed has to be sent two times because of its 50% moisture content.

So, at the end of the 1st drying cycle, moisture removed

$$= 5.33 - \frac{0.50}{0.25}$$

= 3.33 kg/min

So, the required rate of evaporation in the dryer is 3.33 kg/min.

19. Given, From Michaelis Menten equation we have,

$$V = \frac{V_{max} \times [S]}{(K_m + [S])})$$

V_{max} = 22 mol/L/min;

$K_m = 4.7 \times 10^{-5}$M;

$[S] = 2 \times 10^{-4}$M

Therefore,

$$V = \frac{22 \times 2 \times 10^{-4}}{(4.7 \times 10^{-5} + 2 \times 10^{-4})}$$

$= 44 \times 10^{-4}/(2.47 \times 10^{-4})$

= 17.8 mol/L/min.

20. Determining the sterilisation time for foods is based on the same principles as described until now, but there are differences in the way in which the principles are applied. In particular, a property called the decimal reduction time or D-value is defined for an organism and sterilisation times are based on this.

Changing the base of the logarithms in equation:

The D-value is defined as the time to reduce the number of organisms by 1 log cycle

i.e., $\frac{N_0}{N_t} = 10;$

i.e., (log 10 = 1.0)

Since D = *t*, then,

The D value is specific to a temperature. Therefore when quoting D-values for an organism, the temperature must also be quoted.

Given,

F-value = 1.8 min

We know,

$F = D_0 \times$ Reduction fold

Here 99.9999 % reduction takes place which is equivalent to 10 fold (approx.) reduction

So, $D_0 = \frac{1.8}{10} = 0.18$ min.

GATE-2010

XL : LIFE SCIENCES

Time : 3 Hours | *Maximum Marks : 100*

GA : GENERAL APTITUDE

Q.1 - 5 carry one mark each.

1. The question below consists of a pair of related words followed by four pairs of words. Select the pair that best expresses the relation in the original pair.
   Unemployed : Worker
   (*a*) fallow: land (*b*) unaware: sleeper
   (*c*) wit: jester (*d*) renovated: house

2. Choose the most appropriate word from the options given below to complete the following sentence:
   His rather casual remarks on politics ____ his lack of seriousness about the subject.
   (*a*) masked (*b*) belied
   (*c*) betrayed (*d*) suppressed

3. Which of the following options is the closest in meaning to the word below:
   Circuitous
   (*a*) cyclic (*b*) indirect (*c*) confusing (*d*) crooked

4. 25 persons are in a room. 15 of them play hockey, 17 of them play football and 10 of them play both hockey and football. Then the number of persons playing neither hockey nor football is:
   (*a*) 2 (*b*) 17 (*c*) 13 (*d*) 3

5. Choose the most appropriate word from the options given below to complete the following sentence:
   If we manage to____our natural resources, we would leave a better planet for our children.
   (*a*) uphold (*b*) restrain (*c*) cherish (*d*) conserve

Q.6 - Q.10 carry two marks each.

6. 5 skilled workers can build a wall in 20 days; 8 semi-skilled workers can build a wall in 25 days; 10 unskilled workers can build a wall in 30 days. If a team has 2 skilled, 6 semi-skilled and 5 unskilled workers, how long will it take to build the wall?
   (*a*) 20 days (*b*) 18 days (*c*) 16 days (*d*) 15 days

7. Given digits 2, 2, 3, 3, 3, 4, 4, 4, 4 how many distinct 4 digit numbers greater than 3000 can be formed?
   (*a*) 50 (*b*) 51 (*c*) 52 (*d*) 54

8. If 137 + 276 = 435 how much is 731 + 672?
   (*a*) 534 (*b*) 1403 (*c*) 1623 (*d*) 1513

9. Hari (H), Gita (G), Irfan (I) and Saira (S) are siblings (i.e. brothers and sisters). All were born on 15th January. The age difference between any two successive siblings (that is born one after another) is less than 3 years. Given the following facts.
   i. Hari's age + Gita's age > Irfan's age + Saira's age.
   ii. The age difference between Gita and Saira is 1 year. However, Gita is not the oldest and Saira is not the youngest.
   iii. There are no twins.
   In what order were they born (oldest first)?
   (*a*) HSIG (*b*) SGHI (*c*) IGSH (*d*) IHSG

10. Modern warfare has changed from large scale clashes of armies to suppression of civilian populations. Chemical agents that do their work silently appear to be suited to such warfare; and regretfully, there exist people in military establishments who think that chemical agents are useful tools for their cause.
    Which of the following statements best sums up the meaning of the above passage:
    (*a*) Modern warfare has resulted in civil strife.
    (*b*) Chemical agents are useful in modern warfare.
    (*c*) Use of chemical agents in warfare would be undesirable.
    (*d*) People in military establishments like to use chemical agents in war.

H : CHEMISTRY (*Compulsory*)

Q.1 - 5 carry one mark each.

1. For a spontaneous process, the total entropy change ($\Delta S_{system} + \Delta S_{surroundings}$) is
   (*a*) equal to zero
   (*b*) greater than zero
   (*c*) less than zero for endothermic process
   (*d*) less than zero for exothermic process

2. A battery delivers a steady current of 1.25 A for 90 minutes. The total charge 'Q' (in Coulomb units) is
   (*a*) 6750 (*b*) 1012.5 (*c*) 112.5 (*d*) 12.5

3. Molecule that has no lone pair of electrons on the central atom (among the choices) is
   (*a*) XeF_4 (*b*) PF_3 (*c*) ClF_5 (*d*) BF_3

4. The oxidation state of nickel atom in the coordination compound $[Ni(NH_3)_3Cl]Cl$ is
   (*a*) –1 (*b*) 0 (*c*) +1 (*d*) +2

5. The compound that is aromatic, among the choices, is

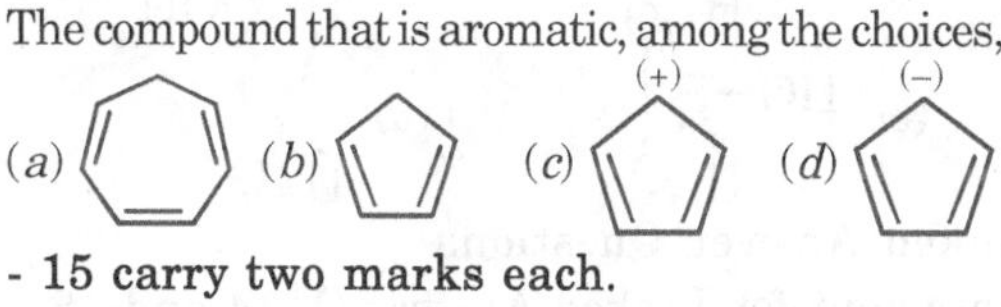

Q.6 - 15 carry two marks each.

6. Consider the following equilibrium reaction:
   $$CO\,(g) + Cl_2\,(g) \rightleftharpoons COCl_2\,(g)$$
   0.60 atm of CO and 1.10 atm of Cl_2 were mixed in a constant volume reaction vessel at a particular temperature. After the equilibrium was established, 0.10 atm of $COCl_2$ was observed. The equilibrium constant for the reaction is
   (*a*) 0.02 (*b*) 0.15 (*c*) 0.2 (*d*) 6.6

7. For a particular reaction, the use of a catalyst reduces the activation energy (E_a) to one-third its original value. The ratio of rate constants ($k_{catalyzed}$ $k_{uncatalyzed}$) is

(*a*) 1 (*b*) $\frac{1}{3}$

(*c*) $\exp\left(\frac{2E_a}{3RT}\right)$ (*d*) $\exp\left(\frac{E_a}{3RT}\right)$

8. Among heptan-1-ol, heptan-2-ol, heptan-3-ol and heptan-4-ol, compounds those exhibit optical activity are

(*a*) heptan-2-ol and heptan-3-ol
(*b*) heptan-2-ol and heptan-4-ol
(*c*) heptan-3-ol and heptan-4-ol
(*d*) heptan-1-ol and heptan-4-ol

9. Structure of the compound Y in the following reaction sequence is

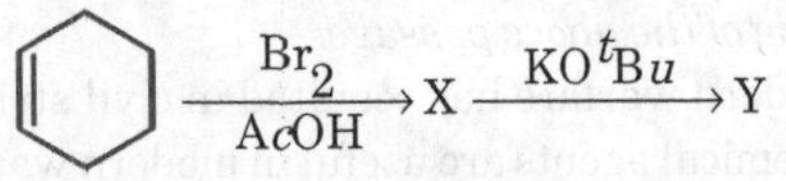

(*a*) 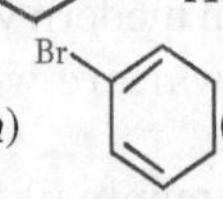 (*b*) 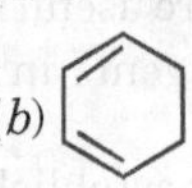 (*c*) 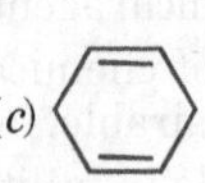 (*d*) 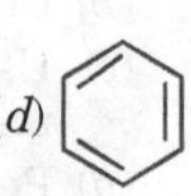

10. The ionization energy follows the order

(*a*) $O_2^+ > O_2 > O_2^- > O_2^{2-}$ (*b*) $O_2 > O_2^+ > O_2^{2-} > O_2^-$
(*c*) $O_2^- > O_2^{2-} > O_2^+ > O_2$ (*d*) $O_2^{2-} > O_2 > O_2^- > O_2^+$

11. Reaction of Na_2SO_3 with 2 equivalents of HCl produces a gas X. Solution of X in water is acidic in nature. X is

(*a*) O_2 (*b*) Cl_2 (*c*) SO_2 (*d*) H_2S

Common Data Questions

Common Data Questions 12 and 13 :

The ionization constants of phosphorous acid (H_3PO_3) are $K_{a1} = 3 \times 10^{-2}$; $K_{a2} = 1.7 \times 10^{-7}$

12. For a dilute solution of phosphorous acid in a pH 5 buffer, the predominant species is

(*a*) H_3PO_3 (*b*) $H_2PO_3^-$ (*c*) HPO_3^{2-} (*d*) PO_3^{3-}

13. The structure of phosphorous acid is

(*a*) 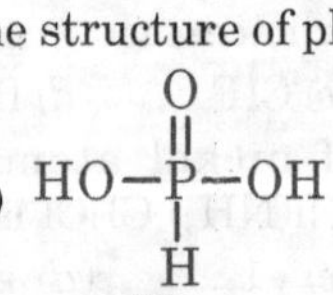 (*b*) 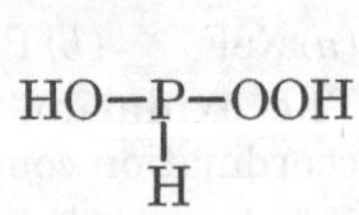

(*c*) 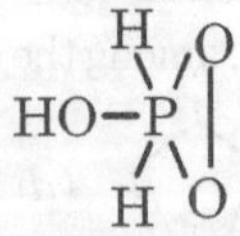 (*d*) 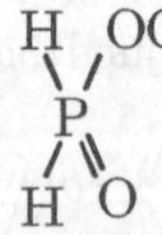

Linked Answer Questions

Statement for Linked Answer Q. 14 and 15

Consider the reaction sequence

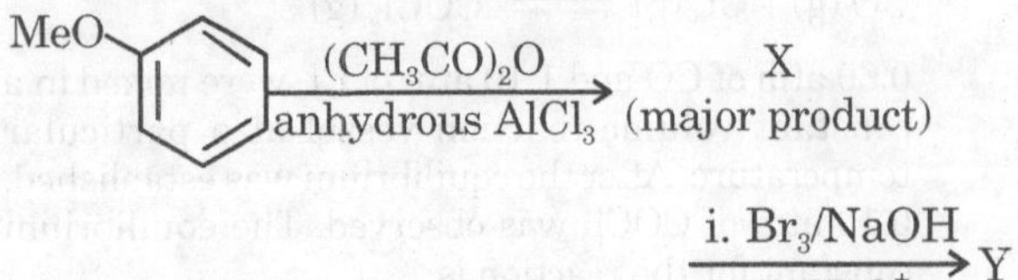

14. The structure of X in the above reaction sequence is

(*a*) 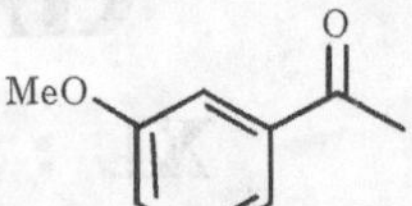 (*b*) 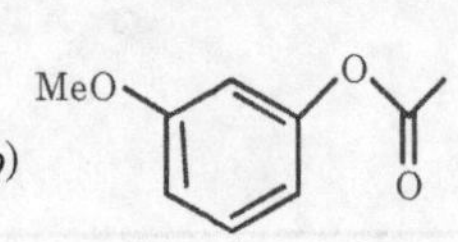

(*c*) 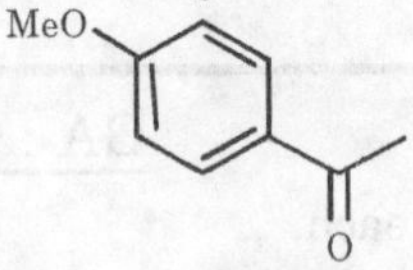 (*d*) 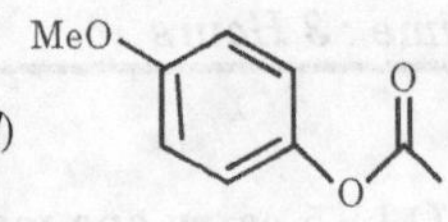

15. The structure of Y in the above reaction sequence is

(*a*) 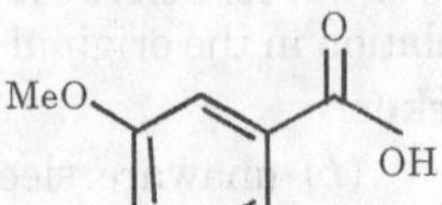 (*b*) 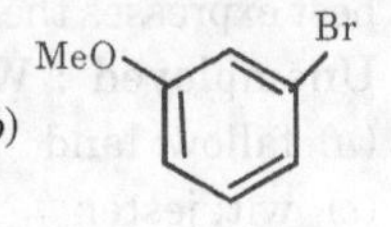

(*c*) 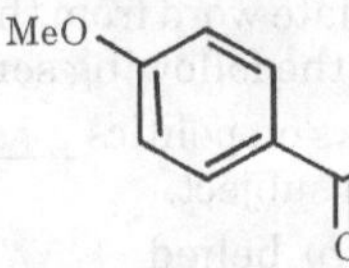 (*d*) 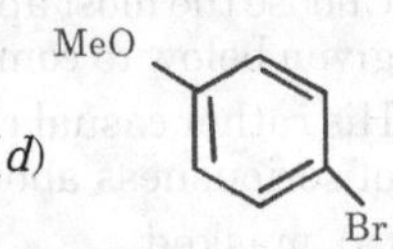

I : BIOCHEMISTRY

Q.1 - 10 carry one mark each.

1. Nucleolus is involved in the synthesis of

(*a*) rRNA (*b*) tRNA (*c*) DNA (*d*) mRNA

2. In tryptophan operon, tryptophan acts as

(*a*) Repressor (*b*) Activator
(*c*) Co-repressor (*d*) Co-activator

3. Positive selection of T–cells ensures

(*a*) MHC restriction
(*b*) Self tolerance
(*c*) TCR engagements
(*d*) Activation by co-stimulatory signal

4. A DNA-binding motif is

(*a*) Helix-loop:-helix (*b*) Helix-turn-helix
(*c*) Helical wheel (*d*) Loop-helix-loop

5. Amino acids responsible for N-linked and O-linked glycosylation of proteins are

(*a*) Asparagine and Aspartic acid
(*b*) Glutamine and Serine
(*c*) Glutamic acid and Serine
(*d*) Asparagine and Threonine

6. One of the following compounds is NOT a neurotransmitter

(*a*) Dopamine (*b*) Glutamic acid
(*c*) Histidine (*d*) Glycine

7. Approximate molecular weight (kDa) of the product after translation of a 390 bases mRNA will be

(*a*) 48 (*b*) 26 (*c*) 39 (*d*) 14

8. Lineweaver-Burk plot is a plot of

(*a*) $\frac{1}{v_0}$ vs $\frac{1}{[S]}$ (*b*) v_0 vs [S]

(*c*) v_0 vs $\frac{1}{[S]}$ (*d*) $\frac{1}{v_0}$ vs [S]

9. A mixture of proteins (W, X, Y, Z) elute from Sephadex G-200 column in the order W, X, Y, Z. The protein with maximum electrophoretic mobility on SDS-PAGE will be
(*a*) W (*b*) X (*c*) Y (*d*) Z

10. Specific precursor for all prostaglandins is
(*a*) Oleic acid (*b*) Arachidonic acid
(*c*) Palmitic acid (*d*) α-Linolenic acid

Q.11 - 20 carry two marks each.

11. Chymotrypsin and lysozyme are involved respectively in
P. Removal of successive carboxyl terminal residues
Q. Hydrolytic cleavage of peptide bond
R. Cleavage of glycosidic C-O bond
S. Oxygen transport in blood
(*a*) P, Q (*b*) Q, R (*c*) Q, S (*d*) R, S

12. Match the items in Group I with those in Group II

Group I	Group II
P. Isotype switching	1. V_H domain
Q. Clonal energy	2. Non responsive to self antigen
R. Class II MHC	3. Non-responsive T_H cells
S. Self tolerance	4. β_2-microglobulin

(*a*) P-1, Q-4, R-3, S-2 (*b*) P-2, Q-4, R-1, S-3
(*c*) P-1, Q-3, R-4, S-2 (*d*) P-2, Q-1, R-3, S-4

13. Multiple RNA polymerase transcribes a DNA template, unwinding about 1.5 turns of DNA template per transcription bubble. From the structural information of classical B-DNA, how many transcription bubbles are possible for a 180 base pair DNA molecule?
(*a*) 12 (*b*) 27 (*c*) 6 (*d*) 270

14. Match the items in Group I with the most appropriate separation techniques in Group II

Group I
P. Mixture of glycine and albumin
Q. Mixture of 20 and 60 kDa proteins
R. Histones from nuclear extract
S. Lectins

Group II
1. Gas chromatography
2. Dialysis
3. Affinity chromatography
4. Size exclusion chromatography
5. Thin layer chromatography
6. Cation exchange chromatography

(*a*) P-1, Q-4, R-3, S-5 (*b*) P-5, Q-3, R-6, S-1
(*c*) P-2, Q-4, R-6, S-3 (*d*) P-6, Q-5, R-2, S-4

15. In the two half reactions
Acetaldehyde + 2 H^+ + 2 e^- → Ethanol
$\Delta E° = -0.16$ V
NADH + H^+ → NAD + $2H^+$ +$2e^-$
$\Delta E° = 0.32$ V
(F = 23,063 cal/V)
The $\Delta G°$ for coupled reaction will be
(*a*) +7,400 cal (*b*) –7,400 cal
(*c*) –22,200 cal (*d*) +22,200 cal

16. Match the parameters in Group I with the correct options in Group II

Group I	Group II
P. K_M	1. Catalytic efficiency of the enzyme
Q. k_{cat}/K_M	2. Affinity of enzyme to the inhibitor
R. pK_a	3. Affinity of enzyme to the substrate
S. K_i	4. Maximum buffering capacity

(*a*) P-3, Q-1, R-2, S-4 (*b*) P-3, Q-1, R-4, S-2
(*c*) P-1, Q-2, R-4, S-3 (*d*) P-1, Q-4, R-2, S-3

17. The rise per residue of α-helix is about 1.5 Å. A protein spans 4 nm bilayer 7 times through its transmembrane α-helical domain. Approximately, how many amino acid residues constitute the transmembrane domain of the protein
(*a*) 105 (*b*) 450
(*c*) 30 (*d*) 190

18. Match the proteins in Group I with their correct functions in Group II

Group I	Group II
P. Shaker protein	1. Inner membrane receptor
Q. Bacteriorhodopsin	2. Active transport
R. Porin	3. Voltage gated K^+ channel
S. ABC transporter	4. Light driven H^+ pump
	5. Membrane fusion
	6. β-barrel simple diffusion channel

(*a*) P-4, Q-2, R-3, S-5 (*b*) P-5, Q-3, R-4, S-6
(*c*) P-6, Q-1, R-5, S-4 (*d*) P-3, Q-4, R-6, S-2

19. The metabolic disorders, Alkaptonuria and Phenylketonuria are caused by defects in the enzymes
P. Glucose- 6-phosphatase
Q. Phenylalanine hydroxylase
R. Homogentisate1 ,2-dioxygenase
S. Tyrosinase
(*a*) Q, R (*b*) P, R (*c*) P, Q (*d*) Q, S

20. Match the metabolic pathways in Group I with the corresponding enzymes in Group II

Group I	Group II
P. β-Oxidation	1. Ribulose bisphosphate carboxylase
Q. Glycolysis	2. Phosphofructo kinase 1
R. Gluconeogenesis	3. Phosphoenol pyruvate carboxykinase
S. Calvin cycle	4. Thiolase
	5. Phosphofructo-kinase 2

(*a*) P-4, Q-2, R-3, S-5 (*b*) P-3, Q-2, R-4, S-1
(*c*) P-3, Q-1, R-5, S-2 (*d*) P-4, Q-2, R-3, S-1

J : BOTANY

Q.1 - 10 carry one mark each.

1. When changes in the phenotype or gene expression occur without changes in the underlying DNA sequence, the phenomenon is called
(*a*) Mutation (*b*) Eugenics
(*c*) Epigenetics (*d*) Epistasis

2. A population growing exponentially can be described by the differential equation dN/dt = rN, where dN/dt represents the rate at which the whole population grows, N is the size of the population, r is the intrinsic rate of increase, and t is time. According to this equation, the per capita rate of growth is
(*a*) Highest at large N (*b*) Constant
(*c*) Lowest at large N (*d*) Highest at small N

3. Which one of the following is NOT a plant hormone?
(*a*) Abscisic acid (*b*) Brassinosteroid
(*c*) Ethylene (*d*) Cytokine

4. *Arabidopsis* and rice have diploid chromosome numbers of 10 and 24, respectively. Assuming no crossing over taking place, genetic variation among F_2 individuals in a genetic cross is likely to be
(*a*) Same in both species but not zero
(*b*) More in *Arabidopsis*
(*c*) More in rice
(*d*) Zero in both the species

5. Which of the following statements is CORRECT?
(*a*) Plants adapted to cold environment have higher ratio of "unsaturated to saturated" fatty acids in their membrane compared to those adapted to hot environment
(*b*) Plants adapted to cold environment have lower ratio of "unsaturated to saturated" fatty acids in their membrane compared to those adapted to hot environment
(*c*) Plants adapted to cold environment have same ratio of "unsaturated to saturated" fatty acids in their membrane compared to those adapted to hot environment
(*d*) Plants do not have any unsaturated fatty acids in the membrane

6. A sign is hammered into a tree trunk 2 meters above the tree's base. If the tree is 10 meters tall and elongates 1 meter each year, how high will the sign be after 10 years?
(*a*) 12 meters (*b*) 7 meters
(*c*) 4 meters (*d*) 2 meters

7. In the arrangement of floral parts in a bud, identify the INCORRECT statement
(*a*) Valvate: where the petals or sepals do not overlap but simply touch one another by their Margins
(*b*) Scabrous: petals rough and harsh to touch
(*c*) Epicalyx: an extra calyx found in some flowers outside the calyx
(*d*) Imbricate: where sepals and petals overlap each other at the margin

8. The possible genotypes of endosperms borne on a heterozygous (Rr) plant will be
(*a*) RRR, RRr, Rrr, rrr (*b*) RRr, Rrr
(*c*) RR, Rr, rr (*d*) Rr

9. The amount of chemical energy available to consumers in an ecosystem is best represented by
(*a*) Gross primary production
(*b*) Net primary production
(*c*) Respiration
(*d*) Photosynthesis

10. Free radical scavenging activity of a medicinally important plant extract can be quantified by
(*a*) ABTS (2,2'-azino-bis-(3-ethyl benzothiozoline- 6-sulphonic acid)) method
(*b*) Bradford method
(*c*) Walkley and Black method
(*d*) Kjeldahl method

Q.11 - 20 carry two marks each.

11. Identify the CORRECT statements from the following
P. Lenticels are the small pores present on the surface of the stem or branches of woody plants
Q. Glyoxysomes contain chlorophyll molecules in their thylakoid membranes
R. The enzyme ribulose 1, 5 bisphosphate carboxylase is otherwise known as carboxydehydratase
S. 18 ATP and 12 NADPH molecules are utilized for fixing 6 molecules of CO_2 in the dark reaction of photosynthesis
(*a*) P, Q (*b*) P, R (*c*) Q, R (*d*) P, S

12. Match the following

Group I	Group II	Group III
P. Sorghum	1. Gossypol	*i.* Protein
Q. Castor	2. Strychnine	*ii.* Glycosidic conjugate
R. Mushroom	3. Dhurrin	*iii.* Alkaloid
S. Cotton	4. Bungarotoxin	*iv.* Polyphenol
	5. Ricin	*v.* Lipid
	6. α-Amanitin	*vi.* Cyclic peptide

(*a*) P-3-ii, Q-5-i, R-6-vi, S-1-iv
(*b*) P-2-iii, Q-4-iv, R-1-ii, S-6-v
(*c*) P-2-vi, Q-5-v, R-1- iv, S-6-ii
(*d*) P-2-i, Q-3-iii, R-4-iv, S-1-v

13. Identify the correct match
Group I (*Anther*)

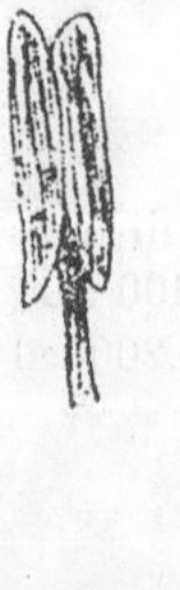
P

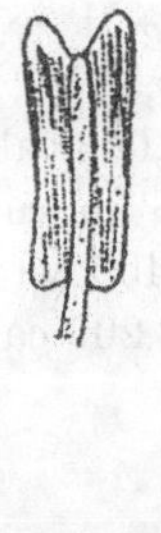
Q

R 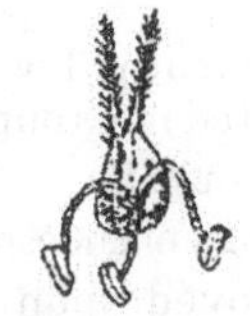 S 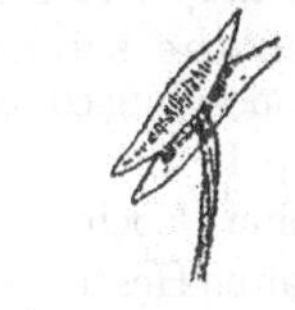

Group II (*Type of fixation*)

1. Basified 2. Longitudinal
3. Dorsifixed 4. Adenate
5. Porous 6. Versatile

(*a*) P-1, Q-4, R-6, S-3 (*b*) P-2, Q-3, R-5, S-6
(*c*) P-1, Q-2, R-6, S-5 (*d*) P-4, Q-3, R-5, S-6

14. From the structures given below, identify the compounds

Group I (*Structure*)

P. 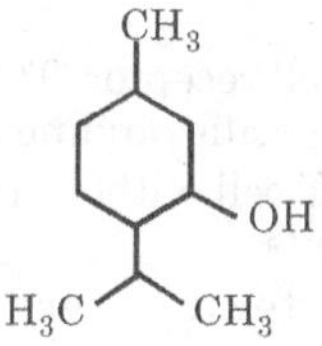 Q. 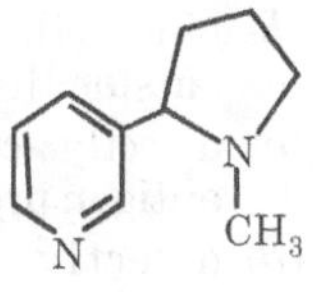

R. 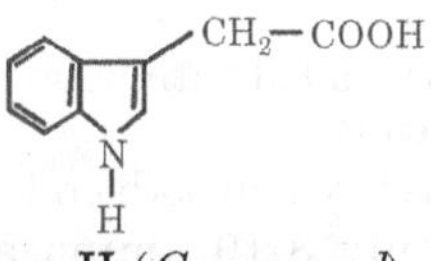 S. $CH_2 = CH_2$

Group II (*Compound*)

1. Ethylene 2. Indole butyric acid
3. Nicotine 4. Indole acetic acid
5. Gibberellic acid 6. Menthol

(*a*) P-6, Q-3, R-4, S-1 (*b*) P-5, Q-2, R-3, S-1
(*c*) P-4, Q-3, R-2, S-6 (*d*) P-1, Q-2, R-5, S-6

15. Regarding the relationships between two organisms in an ecosystem, match the following

Group I (*Relationship*)	**Group II** (*Definition*)
P. Commensalism	1. Both organisms are benefited
Q. Mutualism	2. One impeding the success of the other
R. Parasitism	3. One organism bene-fits but the other is unaffected
S. Amensalism	4. One benefited, other is harmed

(*a*) P-1, Q-2, R-3, S-4 (*b*) P-2, Q-3, R-4, S-1
(*c*) P-3, Q-l, R-4, S-2 (*d*) P-1, Q-4, R-3, S-2

16. Name the structures given below in the order of their appearance and identify corresponding glycosidic linkages

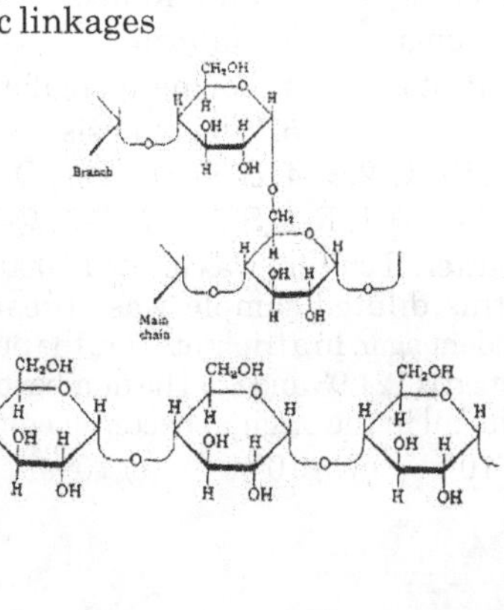

(*a*) Amylose, Cellulose; (α1→4), (β1→6)
(*b*) Cellulose, Dextran; (β2→4), (α3→6)
(*c*) Starch, Cellulose; (α1→6), (α1→4)
(*d*) Amylopectin, Amylose; (α1→6), (α1→4)

17. Identify the CORRECT statements

In *Arabidopsis*, vernalization is associated with

P. Chromatin modification at the FLC (FLOWERING LOCUS C) locus
Q. Degradation of the FLC protein
R. Inactivating the FLC protein by post-translational modification
S. Down-regulation of FLC transcript

(*a*) Q, S (*b*) P, S (*c*) P, R (*d*) Q, R

18. Which of the following statements in plant respiration are CORRECT?

P. The oxidative Pentose Phosphate Pathway can accomplish the oxidation of glucose in the stroma of mitochondria
Q. ATP is produced in the reaction step of TCA cycle catalyzed by succinyl CoA synthatase
R. In addition to Cytochrome c oxidase, an alternative oxidase enzyme resistant to cyanide reduces oxygen molecule in the electron transport system
S. In Glyoxylate cycle acetyl CoA reacts with citrate to form α-keto glutarate

(*a*) P, R (*b*) P, Q (*c*) Q, R (*d*) Q, S

19. Study the following diagram depicting the plant cell cycle and match the following

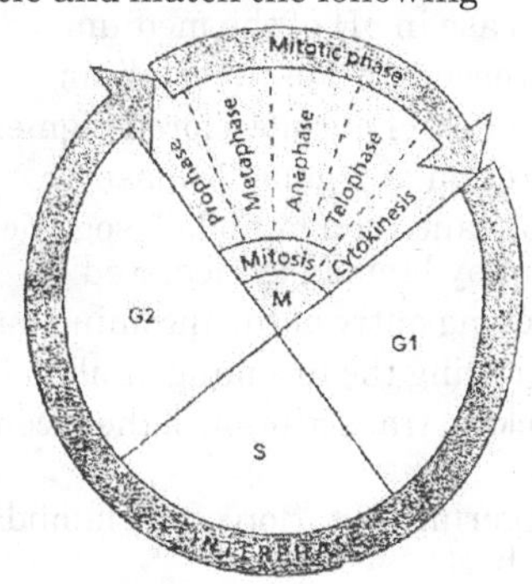

Stages of cell cycle	**Type of cyclin**
P. Late G1-phase	1. Cyclin B
Q. Beginning of S-phase	2. Cyclin E
R. Prior to mitotic phase	3. S-Cyclin
S. Early G1-phase	4. Cyclin D

(*a*) P-4,Q-3, R-1, S-2 (*b*) P-2, Q-3, R-1,S-4
(*c*) P-1,Q-4, R-3, S-2 (*d*) P-3, Q-1, R-2, S-4

20. In the context of plant development, which of the following statements are CORRECT ?

P. Cell migration is absent
Q. Apoptosis plays a major role
R. Pattern formation continues throughout life
S. Homeotic changes are caused by mutations in non-homeodomain proteins

(*a*) P, Q, R (*b*) Q, R, S (*c*) P, Q, S (*d*) P, R, S

K : MICROBIOLOGY

Q.1 - Q.10 carry one mark each.

1. An electron microscope has higher resolution as compared to the light microscope. This is because
(*a*) the wavelength of an electron is longer than the wavelength of light
(*b*) the wavelength of an electron is shorter than the wavelength of light
(*c*) the electrons can penetrate the sample better
(*d*) they use different stains

2. Bacterial cell lysis by lysozyme is due to the
(*a*) hydrolysis of α-1,4-glycosidic bonds between the N-acetylglucosamine and N-acetylmuramic acid
(*b*) inhibition of cell wall synthesis
(*c*) hydrolysis of pentapeptide bridges
(*d*) hydrolysis of β-1,4-glycosidic bonds between the N-acetylglucosamine and N-acetylmuramic acid

3. The recombination frequencies between three genes *x*, *y* and *z* are as follows : *x-y* : 2.6%, *y-z* : 1.4% and *x-z*: 1.2%. Then the gene order is
(*a*) *x-z-y* (*b*) *x-y-z* (*c*) *y-x-z* (*d*) *z-x-y*

4. A mutant phenotype due to a nonsense mutation can be rescued by a mutation in tRNA gene. This rescue is an example of
(*a*) induced mutation (*b*) suppressor mutation
(*c*) spontaneous mutation (*d*) deletion mutation

5. Ames test is performed to detect
(*a*) mutagen (*b*) pH
(*c*) nutrient stress (*d*) salinity

6. Wild type E.*coli forms* purple colored colonies on EMB-lactose plate. This is due to
(*a*) increase in pH of the medium
(*b*) decrease in pH of the medium
(*c*) secretion of purple colored pigment
(*d*) secretion of β-galactosidase

7. The resistance of a lambda lysogenic E.*coli* to re-infection by lambda is mediated by
(*a*) blocking entry of the incoming lambda DNA
(*b*) degrading the incoming lambda DNA
(*c*) blocking transcription of the incoming lambda DNA
(*d*) triggering mutation of the lambda receptor of the host

8. Pasteurization of milk is carried out by
(*a*) boiling for 5 min
(*b*) heating at 72°C for 30 min
(*c*) heating at 63°C for 15 min
(*d*) heating at 63°C for 30 min

9. A growing bacterial culture with a doubling time of 20 min reaches cell density of 2×10^8 cells ml in 3 hours. How much time would it take to reach the cell density of 1×10^8 cells /ml?
(*a*) 200 min (*b*) 180 min (*c*) 160 min (*d*) 90 min

10. The quickest way to determine bacterial growth in terms of viable cells is through
(*a*) Most probable number (MPN) technique
(*b*) Spread plate method
(*c*) Pour plate method
(*d*) Slide culture technique

Q.11- 20 carry two marks each.

11. Match the scientist from Group I with the corresponding contribution listed in Group II

Group I	Group II
P. Robert Koch	1. Discovery of endospores
Q. Walter Hesse	2. Disproved spontaneous generation
R. Louis Pasteur	3. Discovery of caustive agent of tuberculosis
S. Ferdinand Cohn	4. Use of agar as solid media
	5. Invention of microscope

(*a*) P-5,Q-3,R-4,S-2 (*b*) P-3,Q-4,R-1,S-5
(*c*) P-3,Q-4,R-2,S-5 (*d*) P-3,Q-4,R-2,S-1

12. Superantigens elicit a very strong T cell response because they
(*a*) bind to the specific antigen binding site on the T cell receptors (TCR)
(*b*) bind to the site on T cell receptor (TCR)-that is outside the antigen-specific binding site
(*c*) directly activate the T cell without the help of antigen presenting cells
(*d*) directly induce cytokine secretion by macrophages

13. MHC-I groove can be loaded with peptides of only 8-10 amino acids because
(*a*) MHC-I groove is closed on both ends
(*b*) fragments of only 8-10 amino acids are generated in MHC-I bearing cells
(*c*) β_2-microglobulin of MHC-I prevents the binding of large peptides to MHC-I
(*d*) β polypeptides of MHC-I prevents binding of 8-10 amino acid long peptides to MHC-I

14. In a *lac*O^C *lacZ*$^-$ /*lac*O^+ *lacZ*$^+$ partial diploid, of the two lacZ enzymes, only the mutant enzyme (*lacZ*$^-$) is synthesized constitutively. This observation shows that *lac*O^C mutation is
(*a*) *trans*-dominant (*b*) *trans*-recessive
(*c*) *cis*-dominant (*d*) *cis*-recessive

15. Which one of the following events occurs in prokaryotes but NOT in eukaryotes?
(*a*) Protein phosphorylation
(*b*) RNA polymerase and promoter interaction
(*c*) Control of transcription by attenuation
(*d*) Formation of Okazaki fragments

16. Match the pathogen in Group I with the corresponding disease in Group II

Group I	Group II
P. Bacteria	1. Measles
Q. Virus	2. Candidiasis
R. Fungi	3. Malaria
S. Protozoa	4. Bovine spongiform encephalitis
	5. Tuberculosis

(*a*) P-1, Q-2, R-4, S-5 (*b*) P-1, Q-4, R-2, S-3
(*c*) P-5, Q-1, R-4, S-2 (*d*) P-5, Q-1, R-2, S-3

17. A bacterial culture was diluted 1000 fold and 0.1 ml of this diluted sample was spread per plate on nutrient agar. In a triplicate run, the number of colonies formed is 121,93 and 86. The number of colony forming units/ml in the original bacterial culture is
(*a*) 10^6 (*b*) 10^5 (*c*) 10^3 (*d*) 10^2

18. Match the microorganism in Group I with the application in Group II .

Group I	Group II
P. Aspergillus oryzae	1. Metal ore leaching
Q. Brevibacterium flavum	2. Glucoamylase producer
R. Thiobacillus	3. Bread making ferroxidans
S. Saccharomyces	4. Glutamic acid producer cerevisiae
T. Rhizobium meliloti	5. Penicillin producer
	6. Symbiotic nitrogen fixer

(*a*) P-1,Q-6,R-4,S-5,T-2 (*b*) P-2,Q-4,R-1,S-3,T-6
(*c*) P-4,Q-1,R-6,S-3,T-5 (*d*) P-6,Q-2,R-3,S-5,T-1

19. A mutant of E.*coli* grows normally on glucose or on glycerol but not on acetate. The most likely metabolic pathway that is defective in this mutant is
(*a*) Glyoxalate cycle
(*b*) Hexose monophosphate shunt
(*c*) Krebs cycle
(*d*) Entner-Duodoroff pathway

20. Match the resistance mechanism in Group I with the antibiotic in Group II

Group I	Group II
P. β-Lactamases	1. Aminoglycosides
Q. Enhanced folate	2. Penicillins metabolism
R. Drug efflux	3. Sulfa drugs
S. Phosphorylation of the drug	4. Tetracyclins
T. Mutant RNA polymerase	5. Naladixic acid
	6. Rifamycin

(*a*) P-2,Q-3,R-4,S-5,T-6 (*b*) P-3,Q-4,R-1,S-6,T-5
(*c*) P-2,Q-3,R-4,S-1,T-6 (*d*) P-1,Q-2,R-3,S-4,T-6

L : ZOOLOGY

Q.1 - 10 carry one mark each.

1. From the perspective of developmental origin, which of the following structures is homologous to a tortoise shell?
(*a*) Exoskeleton of a lobster
(*b*) Bones of a fish
(*c*) Skull of humans
(*d*) Feathers of birds

2. Acoelomates are characterized by
(*a*) the absence of cavity surrounding the internal organs
(*b*) the presence of huge body cavity, as in case of terrestrial animals
(*c*) the presence of air sacs, as in case of birds
(*d*) the absence of brain in a group of extinct species

3. Identify the phylum that is characterized by the animals that have segmented appendages.
(*a*) Cnideria (*b*) Porifera
(*c*) Arthropoda (*d*) Mollusca

4. Which one of the following is the smallest biological unit capable of evolving over time?
(*a*) A cell (*b*) An individual organism
(*c*) A population (*d*) A species

5. In case of parasites that require multiple hosts to complete their life cycle, what does definitive host mean?
(*a*) It is the host that harbors the sexual stages of the parasite.
(*b*) It is the host in which the parasite reproduces asexually.
(*c*) It is the host in which the parasite feeds.
(*d*) It is the host in which the parasite remains in a dormant stage.

6. Enzymes catalyze biochemical reactions by
(*a*) sequestering the product(s)
(*b*) decreasing the ΔG of the reaction
(*c*) increasing the ΔG of the reaction
(*d*) stabilizing the transition state of the reaction.

7. Which one of the following results from Mendel's monohybrid cross is the strongest evidence against the blending theory?
(*a*) 3:1 ratio of phenotypes in the F1 generation
(*b*) All progeny of the F1 generation exhibited the dominant phenotype
(*c*) The recessive phenotype showed up in the F2 progeny
(*d*) The observation of incomplete dominance

8. In the context of cell differentiation, lateral inhibition is referred to as the
(*a*) formation of two distinct cell types within a uniform field.
(*b*) inhibition of formation of a distinct cell type next to an existing cell type.
(*c*) inhibition of stem cells towards self-renewal.
(*d*) inhibition of erythopoesis in the lateral plate mesoderm.

9. As compared to peptide hormones, steroid hormones take more time to activate a cellular response because
(*a*) steroid hormones show non-specific binding with diverse sets of receptors.
(*b*) steroid hormone acts through a receptor which is a transcription factor.
(*c*) cells that respond to steroid hormones are dormant in nature.
(*d*) peptide hormones are not transported through plasma while steroid hormones are.

10. In allopatric mode of speciation, a new species forms due to
(*a*) Geographic isolation
(*b*) Genetic drift
(*c*) Formation of a few fertile individuals that can not mate with other members of the same species living in the same geographical area
(*d*) The formation of allopolyploid condition

Q. 11- 20 carry two marks each.

11. Neurogen (Ngn) a newly discovered protein in chicken, is produced by the notochord and the floor plate (FP). Ngn induces cells of the neural tube (NT) to become neurons. It is known that from ventral to dorsal direction cells at different levels give rise to distinct types of neuronal cells. Which of the following observations will cast a doubt in the claim that Ngn is a morphogen?

(*a*) Ngn is a cytosolic protein

(*b*) Artificial mis-expression of Ngn at identical level through out NT does not affect the neuronal cell types formed in the NT

(*c*) Ngn is an integral membrane protein

(*d*) All of the above

12. An alien species has been discovered with very similar genetic makeup as that of the existing species on planet earth with certain differences. The genetic material of this new species is referred to as DNA *. The building blocks of the genetic material is known as Nucleotide*. The proteins of the new species (Protein*) is made up of Amino Acids*.

It has also been discovered that the new species has 5 distinct Nucleotide* as opposed to the four for species on planet earth. The new species has 40 different Amino Acids* as opposed to the 20 for species on planet earth. What should be the codon length for this new species (the same for species of planet earth is 3)? It may be assumed that the average codon degeneracy of the new species is very similar to that of species of planet earth.

(*a*) 2 (*b*) 3 (*c*) 4 (*d*) 5

13. Which one of the following options is NOT a viable strategy for developing a female contraceptive? The administration of

(*a*) a combination of synthetic progesterone and estrogen

(*b*) synthetic progesterone alone

(*c*) ormeloxifene-a selective estrogen receptor modulator

(*d*) a synthetic oxytocin

14. In the field of community ecology, the term "competitive exclusion" refers to two species that cannot co-exist

(*a*) in a community if the niches are identical.

(*b*) in two different communities if the niches are identical.

(*c*) if the ecosystem is imbalanced.

(*d*) in the event of a volcanic eruption.

15. During immune response, helper T-cell memory against the antigen appears earlier than the B memory cells. Which one of the following is the primary reason for this phenomenon?

(*a*) Affinity of antibody molecules produced by B - cells is weaker than those of T - cells

(*b*) B memory cells proliferate at a rate slower than that of T cells

(*c*) B-cell activation requires helper T - cells

(*d*) Thymic selection more rapidly enhances the T cell population than B - cell population

16. Oceans have enormous impact on the biosphere. Identify which one of the following factors is NOT influenced by the marine biome.

(*a*) CO_2 level in the atmosphere

(*b*) Climatic change in the terrestrial biome

(*c*) pH of the fresh water bodies

(*d*) Oxygen level in the biosphere

17. Certain lung fishes that live in small stagnant fresh water pools produce urea as a nitrogenous waste. What is the advantage of this adaptation?

(*a*) Urea form precipitates and does not accumulate in the surrounding water.

(*b*) Lung fish do not find enough water for production of ammonia and hence the nitrogenous waste is excreted as urea.

(*c*) The excreted urea makes the pool uninhabitable to the predators of the lung fish.

(*d*) Urea requires much less energy for its synthesis than ammonia.

18. Hamilton's rule measures the probability of whether or not natural selection would favor an altruistic act. Which one of the following statements best explains Hamilton's rule.

Natural selection would favor an altruistic act only when

(*a*) the receiver and not the altruist is benefited.

(*b*) the receiver is an offspring and NOT a sibling of the altruist.

(*c*) the benefit to the receiver, reduced by the coefficient of relatedness, exceeds the cost to the altruist act.

(*d*) the altruist survives in an altruist act to save his/her related individuals.

19. In a cross between plants with purple- and white-colored flowers, the following results were obtained in the F1 generation (assume that both varieties are true breeding):

100 plants with white flowers; 150 straw yellow; 200 yellow; 245 greenish yellow; 500 green; 440 light blue; 400 blue; 300 indigo; 253 purple; and 100 dark purple. These data support which one of the following conclusions?

(*a*) Flower color in this species does not follow Mendelian inheritance

(*b*) Law of incomplete dominance

(*c*) Colors are co-dominant in this species

(*d*) Flower color in this species is determined by multiple genes

20. Which one of the following is most crucial for the success of vaccination?

(*a*) Antigen presentation by T helper cells

(*b*) Complement system

(*c*) Presence of long-lived antigen-specific lymphocytes

(*d*) Selection of B cells in the lymphoid tissue

ANSWERS

GA : GENERAL APTITUDE

1. (*a*)	2. (*a*)	3. (*c*)	4. (*d*)	5. (*b*)	6. (*d*)	7. (*b*)	8. (*a*)	9. (*c*)	10. (*a*)

H : CHEMISTRY

1. (*b*)	2. (*a*)	3. (*d*)	4. (*d*)	5. (*d*)	6. (*c*)	7. (*c*)	8. (*a*)	9. (*b*)	10. (*a*)
11. (*c*)	12. (*b*)	13. (*a*)	14. (*c*)	15. (*c*)					

I : BIOCHEMISTRY

1. (*a*)	2. (*c*)	3. (*a*)	4. (*b*)	5. (*d*)	6. (*c*)	7. (*d*)	8. (*a*)	9. (*d*)	10. (*b*)
11. (*b*)	12. (*c*)	13. (*a*)	14. (*c*)	15. (*b*)	16. (*b*)	17. (*d*)	18. (*d*)	19. (*a*)	20. (*d*)

J : BOTANY

1. (*d*)	2. (*a*)	3. (*d*)	4. (*d*)	5. (*a*)	6. (*d*)	7. (*d*)	8. (*a*)	9. (*b*)	10. (*a*)
11. (*d*)	12. (*a*)	13. (*a*)	14. (*a*)	15. (*c*)	16. (*d*)	17. (*b*)	18. (*c*)	19. (*b*)	20. (*c*)

K : MICROBIOLOGY

1. (*b*)	2. (*d*)	3. (*a*)	4. (*b*)	5. (*a*)	6. (*b*)	7. (*c*)	8. (*d*)	9. (*a*)	10. (*b*)
11. (*d*)	12. (*b*)	13. (*a*)	14. (*c*)	15. (*c*)	16. (*d*)	17. (*a*)	18. (*b*)	19. (*a*)	20. (*c*)

L : ZOOLOGY

1. (*a*)	2. (*a*)	3. (*c*)	4. (*c*)	5. (*a*)	6. (*d*)	7. (*c*)	8. (*b*)	9. (*b*)	10. (*a*)
11. (*b*)	12. (*b*)	13. (*d*)	14. (*a*)	15. (*c*)	16. (*c*)	17. (*b*)	18. (*c*)	19. (*d*)	20. (*a*)

EXPLANATION

GA : GENERAL APTITUDE

1. Follow land is cropland that is not seeded for a season, it may or may not be plowed. The land may be cultivated or chemically treaed for control of weeds and other pests or may be left unaltered.
2. Belied :

   (1) to give a false representation to; misrepresent.

   "He spooke roughly in orderto belie his air of genetility"

   (2) To show tobe fals; contradict : Their laughter
3. Circuitous : marked by obliqueness of indirection in speech or conduct, "the explaination was circuitous and puzzling".
4. Total person = 25

   Number of persons playing only football = 17 – 10 = 7

   Number of person playing only Hockey = 15 – 10 = 5

   ∴ Total number of person playing either Football or Hockey = 22

   ∴ Total number of person playing neither Football or Hockey = 25 – 22 = 3
5. Conserve means to use or manage wisely, preverse save : Conserve the woodlands
6. 5 skilled worker can build a wall in 20 days.

   1 skilled worker can build a wall in

   $$20 \times 5 = 100 \text{ days}$$

   2 skilled worker can build a wall in

   $$\frac{100}{2} = 50 \text{ days}$$

   In 1 day 2 skilled worker can build $\frac{1}{50}$ wall.

   8 semiskilled worker can build a wall in 25 days 1 semiskilled worker can build a wall in

   $$25 \times 8 = 200 \text{ days.}$$

   6 semiskilled worker can build a wall in $\frac{6}{200}$ wall.

   In 1 day 6 semiskilled worker can build $\frac{6}{200}$ wall

   10 unskilled worker can build a wall in 30 days

   5 unskilled worker can build wall in $\frac{300}{5} = 60$ days

   In 1 day 5 unskilled worker can build $= \frac{1}{60}$ wall

   So, together 2 skilled, 6 semiskiled and 5 unskilled worker can build $\left(\frac{1}{50}+\frac{1}{200}+\frac{1}{60}\right)^{th}$ wall.

   $= (.02 + .03 + 0.016)$

   $= (0.066)^{th}$ wall

   ∴ Together 2 skilled, 6 semiskilled and 5 unskilled worker can build the wall in $\left(\frac{1}{0.066}\right)$ days = 15 days.
7. 54
8. Digits have been reversed, so in answer too, the digits have been reversed.
9. Saira, Gita, Hari and Irfan

H : CHEMISTRY

1. A spontaneous process corresponds to a rearrangement of atoms and molecules from a less probable to a more probable situation, as measured by the thermodynamic probability W of the reactants and products. The entropy of a perfectly ordered crystal at absolute zero is zero according to the third law of thermodynamics. Increasing the

temperature, volume, or amount of substance increases the entropy. In general the greater the randomness or disorder of the atoms or molecules the greater the entropy of a substance. Since $\Delta G^\circ = \Delta H^\circ - T\,\Delta S^\circ$, a negative enthalpy change is the most important factor governing spontaneity of a reaction at low temperatures. At high values of T, $-T\,\Delta S$ becomes large and an increase in entropy of the system is essential for a spontaneous process.

2. We know, Current across a battery due to the flow of electrons is given by:

$$I = \frac{q}{t}$$

where q is the charge on the substance carrying the current and t is the time of displacement.

Given, I = 1.25 A; t = 90 min = 90 × 60 s = 5400 s

Therefore, $I = \frac{q}{t}$

or $q = I \times t$
$= 1.25 \times 5400$ C
$= 6750$ C

3. Boron trifluoride is largely used in semiconductor manufacturing. Boron atom is a p-type dopant for epitaxial silicon. It is a useful Lewis acid and a versatile building block for other boron compounds. This pungent colourless toxic gas forms white fumes in moist air. In BF_3, there are 3 valence electrons present in the central atom i.e., Boron. The 3 valence electrons in the molecule participate in bond formation with the electronegative molecule of fluorine. As such, there is no lone pair electron present in BF_3.

4. Given, Coordination compound
$= [Ni(NH_3)_3Cl]Cl$

The net charge on the coordination complex is 0. The complex ion $[Ni(NH_3)_3Cl]^+$ is mononegative because of its counter ion Cl^-.

Let us consider the oxidation state for Ni to be a,

In the complex, the net oxidation state or the charge is 0

So we have:

$a + 3 \times (NH_3) + (Cl^-) + (Cl^-) = 0$

Or $a + 3 \times 0 - 1 - 1 = 0$

Or $a - 2 = 0$ or $a = 2$,

So the oxidation of Ni is +2

5. The compound (d) has a lone pair of electrons on the carbon atom. It has an overall number of 6π electrons in it. This is in accordance with the 4n + 2 rule of Huckel which states that any closed ring structure which satisfies the rule is an aromatic compound. So the compound which is cyclopentadienyl ion is an aromatic compound.

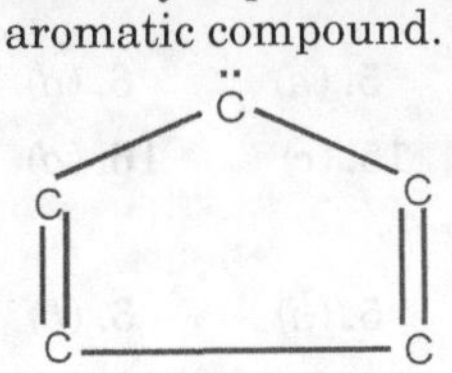

6. Given, the reaction is:

$$CO\,(g) + Cl_2\,(g) \Leftrightarrow COCl_2\,(g)$$

Under initial conditions at the start of the reaction:

(0.60atm) (1.10atm) (0atm)

After equilibrium when the partial pressure has been balanced in the system:

(0.60 – 0.1) (1.10 – 0.1) (0.1atm)

Now, equilibrium constant for the reaction is given by:

$$K_P = \frac{[COCl_2]}{\{[CO]\,[Cl_2]\}}$$

$$= \frac{0.1}{\{0.5 \times 1\}} = 0.2$$

7. Common sense and chemical intuition suggest that higher the temperature, the faster a given chemical reaction will proceed. Quantitatively, the relationship between the rate at which a reaction proceeds and its temperature is determined by the Arrhenius Equation. At higher temperatures, the probability that two molecules will collide is higher. This higher collision rate results in a higher kinetic energy, which has an effect on the activation energy of the reaction. The activation energy is the amount of energy required to ensure that a reaction happens.

$$k = A^* e^{(-Ea/R^*T)};$$

where k is the rate coefficient, A is a constant, Ea is the activation energy, R is the universal gas constant, and T is the temperature (in kelvin)

$$E_{cat} = \frac{1}{3} E_{uncat}$$

Therefore,

$$k_{catalyzed} = A \times e^{-E_{cat}/RT}$$

and $$k_{uncatalyzed} = A \times e^{-3E_{cat}/RT}$$

$$\frac{k_{catalyzed}}{k_{uncatalyzed}} = e^{-E_{cat}/RT + 3E_{cat}/RT}$$

$$= e^{-E_{uncat}/3RT + E_{uncat}/RT}$$

$$= e^{-2E_{uncat}/3RT}$$

$$= e^{-2E_n/3RT}$$

8. Some chemical compounds have optical activity in the sense that these compounds have the ability to rotate the plane of polarized light. Polarized light has light waves all traveling parallel to each other. Ordinary light has light waves traveling in all directions. An optically active organic compound can be identified by finding a chiral carbon. A chiral carbon is one that has four different "groups" attached to it. The groups can be anything from a single H to functional groups to one or more other carbons. In relatively complicated compounds, each carbon must be examined carefully to determine whether it is chiral. In the given varieties of heptanol, heptan-2-ol and heptan-3-ol have chiral centres present.

Heptan-2-ol ⇒ $CH_3CH(OH)(CH_2)_4CH_3$ → the second carbon atom is chiral in nature because of four different groups attached to it.

Heptan-3-ol ⇒ $CH_3CH_2CH(OH)(CH_2)_3CH_3$ → the 3rd carbon atom is asymmetric in nature giving chirality to the compound.

9. In the given reaction:

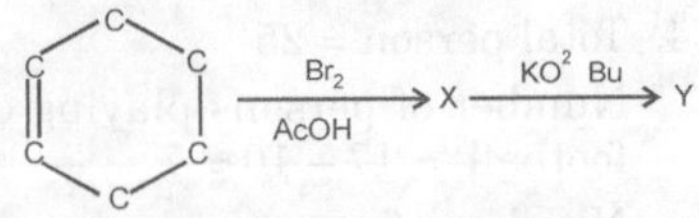

Bromine in presence of acetyl alcohol reacts with the double bond present in the cyclic ring giving rise to an intermediate substitution product:

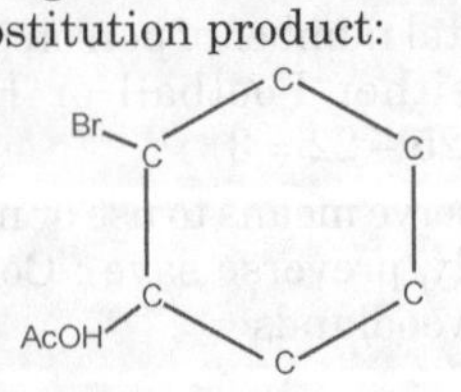

Later, Br and AcOH are removed as HBr and AcOH through a second rate limiting step giving rise to the final product:

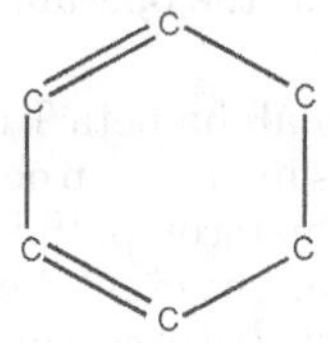

10. Ionisation energy is a measure of the ease in which atoms lose electrons and become positive ions. The first ionisation energy is the energy required to remove one electron from each atom of a mole of gaseous atoms.

$$M(g) - e^- \rightarrow M^+(g)$$

Further electrons may be removed giving successive *i.e.*:

$$M^+(g) - e^- \rightarrow M^{2+}(g)$$

This energy is usually quoted in units of kilojoules per mole (kJ mol^{-1}). Energy is required to remove an electron from any atom because there is an attractive force between the nucleus and the electron being removed which has to be overcome. Ionization energy becomes greater up and to the right of the periodic table. In the given oxidation states of oxygen, ionisation energy would increase with the increase in the bond order of the atoms or ions. In the molecular orbital theory, the following formula is used to find the bond order of a molecule:

$$\frac{\text{(bonding electrons)} - \text{(anti-bonding electrons)}}{2}$$

Now, Bond order of

$$O_2^+ = \frac{(10-5)}{2} = 2.5;$$

$$O_2 = \frac{(10-6)}{2} = 2;$$

$$O_2^- = \frac{(10-7)}{2} = 1.5;$$

$$O_2^{2-} = \frac{(10-8)}{2} = 1.$$

So the decreasing order of bond energy is:

$$O_2^+ > O_2 > O_2^- > O_2^{2-}$$

11. Given, reaction of Na_2SO_3 with 2 equivalents of HCl gives:

$$Na_2SO_3 + 2HCl \rightarrow 2NaCl + SO_2 + H_2O$$

Now, SO_2 when dissolved in water gives rise to an acidic solution due to the formation of sulphurous acid or more dissolution gives rise to sulphuric acid.

$SO_2 + H_2O \rightarrow H_2SO_3$ (acidic, sulphurous acid)

Thus, the product X which is a gaseous molecule is SO_2.

12. Given, Ionisation constants of H_3PO_3,

$$K_{a1} = 3 \times 10^{-2}$$

Ionisation constant of $H_2PO_3^-$,

$$K_{a2} = 1.7 \times 10^{-7}$$

Phosphorous acid dissociates as follows:

$$H_3PO_3 \leftrightarrow H^+ + H_2PO_3^-, K_{a1}$$

$$H_2PO_3^- \leftrightarrow H^+ + HPO_3^{2-}, K_{a2}$$

Now at pH 5,

$$K_{a1} = \frac{[H^+][H_2PO_3^-]}{[H_3PO_3]}$$

or $3 \times 10^{-2} = \dfrac{10^{-5}[H_2PO_3^-]}{[H_3PO_3]}$

or $[H_2PO_3^-] = 3 \times 10^3 [H_3PO_3]$

For

pH 5, $K_{a2} = \dfrac{[H^+][HPO_3^{2-}]}{[H_2PO_3^-]}$

or

$$1.7 \times 10^{-7} = \frac{10^{-5}[HPO_3^{2-}]}{(3 \times 10^3 [H_3PO_3])}$$

Or $[HPO_3^{2-}] = 5.1 \times 10 [H_3PO_3]$

Here, it is clearly evident that concentration of $[H_2PO_3^-]$ is more than $[HPO_3^{2-}]$.

So, $H_2PO_3^-$ is the predominant species.

13. The structure of phosphorous acid consists of three OH^- groups attached covalently to a single centred phosphorous atom. There is a single lone pair of electrons that is present on the phosphorous atom.

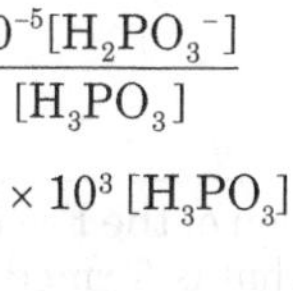

This is the structure of phosphorous acid.

14. An acyl group is an alkyl group attached to a carbon-oxygen double bond. If "R" represents any alkyl group, then an acyl group has the formula RCO–. Acylation means substituting an acyl group into something - in this case, into a benzene ring. The most commonly used acyl group is CH_3CO–. This is called the ethanoyl group, and in this case the reaction is sometimes called "ethanoylation". In the example which follows we are substituting a CH_3CO– group into the ring, but you could equally well use any other acyl group. The most reactive substance containing an acyl group is an acyl chloride (also known as an acid chloride). These have the general formula RCOCl.

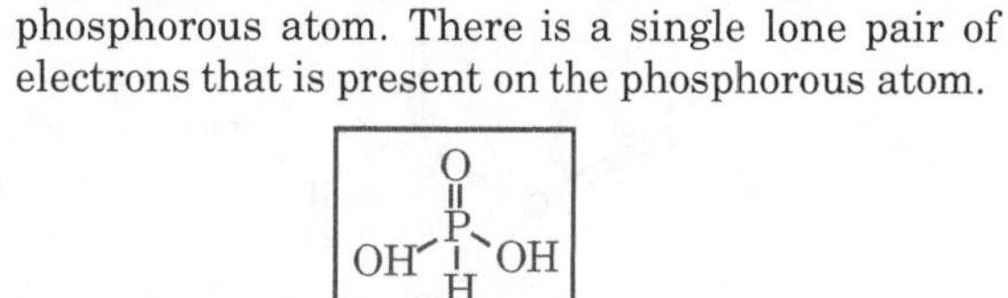

Mechanism of the Friedel-Crafts Acylation

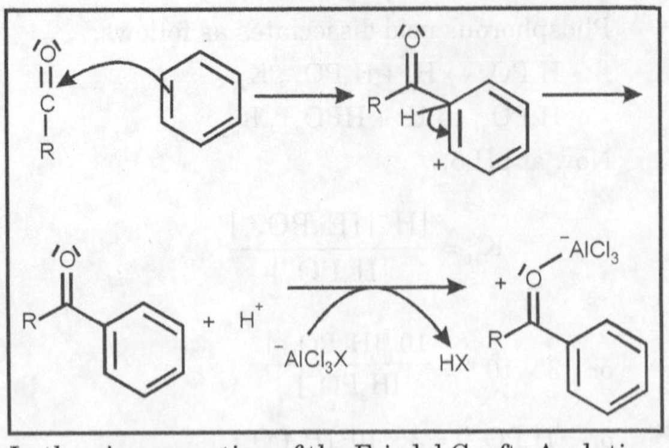

In the given reaction of the Friedel Crafts Acylation, the compound X that is formed is:

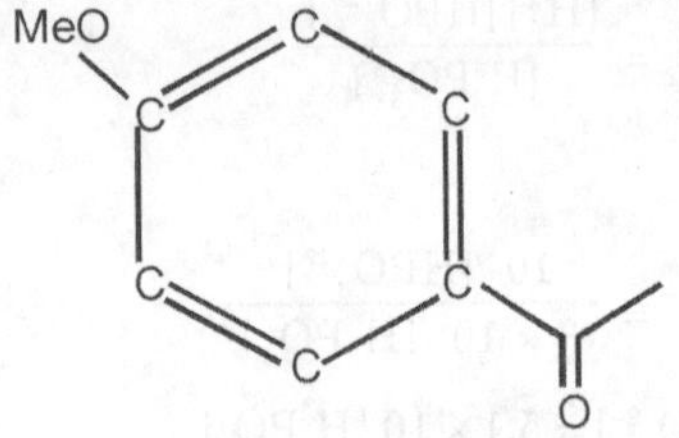

15. The structure of the compound Y that is formed after the addition of Br_2 in presence of NaOH and further addition of H_3O^+ is:

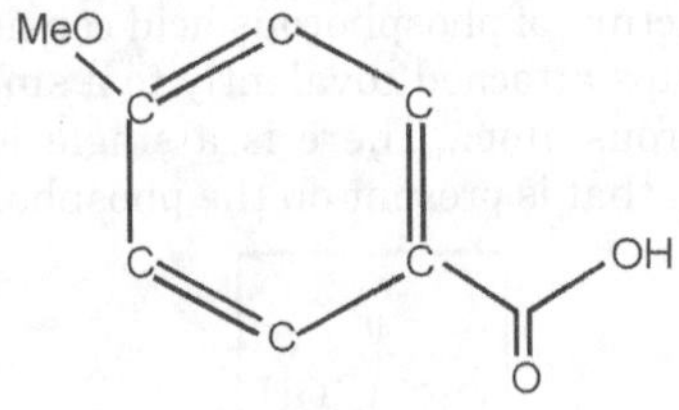

Here, OH group is added after the removal of the methyl group ($-CH_3$).

I : BIOCHEMISTRY

1. The nucleolus is the nuclear sub-domain that assembles ribosomal subunits in eukaryotic cells. The nucleolar organiser regions of chromosomes, which contain the genes for pre-ribosomal ribonucleic acid (rRNA), serve as the foundation for nucleolar structure. The nucleolus disassembles at the beginning of mitosis, its components disperse in various parts of the cell and reassembly occurs during telophase and early G1 phase. Ribosome assembly begins with transcription of pre-rRNA. During transcription ribosomal and non-ribosomal proteins attach to the RNA. Subsequently, there is modification and cleavage of pre-rRNA and incorporation of more ribosomal proteins and 5S rRNA into maturing pre-ribosomal complexes.
2. The tryptophan operon of *E. coli* controls the biosynthesis of tryptophan in the cell from the initial precursor chorismic acid. The tryptophan operon is a repressible system. With repressible systems, the binding of the effector molecule to the repressor greatly increases the affinity of repressor for the operator and the repressor binds and stops transcription. Thus, for the tryptophan operon, the addition of tryptophan (the effector molecule) to the *E. coli* environment shuts off the system because the repressors binds at the operator. Thus, tryptophan is a co-repressor.
3. Differentiation of alpha beta T cell receptor (TCR)-expressing T cells involves an obligatory interaction with self-major histocompatibilty complex (MHC) molecules in the thymus. This process, called positive selection, both rescues thymocytes from programmed cell death and induces their differentiation into mature T cells. Another critical event in thymic development is to prevent maturation of hazardous autoreactive T cells; thus, mechanisms exist to eliminate T cells with self-reactive receptors (negative selection). Both processes are exquisitely MHC-allele specific as they involve MHC-bound peptide recognition, and employ at least some overlapping signal transduction pathways. This pathway of positive selection ensures MHC restriction.
4. The first DNA-binding protein motif to be recognized was the helix-turn-helix. Originally identified in bacterial proteins, this motif has since been found in hundreds of DNA-binding proteins from both eukaryotes and prokaryotes. It is constructed from two α helices connected by a short extended chain of amino acids, which constitutes the "turn". The two helices are held at a fixed angle, primarily through interactions between the two helices. The more C-terminal helix is called the recognition helix because it fits into the major groove of DNA. Thus each protein presents its helix-turn-helix motif to the DNA in a unique way, a feature thought to enhance the versatility of the helix-turn-helix motif by increasing the number of DNA sequences that the motif can be used to recognize.
5. N-linked glycosylation refers to the attachment of oligosaccharides to a nitrogen atom, usually the N4 of asparagine residues. N-glycosylation occurs on secreted or membrane bound proteins, mainly in eukaryotes and archaea. In eukaryotes, N-glycosylation begins as a co-translational event in the endoplasmic reticulum, where preassembled blocks of 14 sugars (including 2 N-acetyl glucosamines, 9 mannoses and 3 glucoses) are first added to the nascent polypeptide chain. After cleavage of 3 glucose and 1 mannose residues, the protein is transferred to the Golgi apparatus where the glycans lose a variable number of mannose residues and acquire a more complex structure during a process called 'terminal glycosylation'. O-linked glycosylation of secreted and membrane bound proteins is a post-translational event that takes place in the cis-Golgi compartment after N-glycosylation and folding of the protein. It refers to the attachment of glycans to serine and threonine, and, to a lesser extent, to hydroxyproline and hydroxylysine. O-linked glycans play important roles in protein localization and trafficking, protein solubility, antigenicity and cell-cell interactions.

6. Neurotransmitters are the brain chemicals that communicate information throughout our brain and body. They relay signals between nerve cells, called "neurons." Dopamine is a neurotransmitter that helps control the brain's reward and pleasure centers. Amino acid transmitters provide the majority of excitatory and inhibitory neurotransmission in the nervous system. Amino acids used for synaptic transmission are compartmentalized. For example, glutamate to be used as a neurotransmitter is compartmentalized from metabolic glutamate used for protein synthesis by packaging the transmitter into synaptic vesicles for subsequent Ca^{2+}-dependent release. Glutamate and aspartate are products of the Kreb's cycle, and both have excitatory effects in the CNS. Glycine is the main neurotransmitter that mediates the inhibitory actions of spinal cord inter-neurons. Histidine is an amino acid which does not act as a neurotransmitter.

7. Given, Number of bases of mRNA = 390

   Since the mRNA forms protein after translation, three codons or bases in the mRNA code for a single amino acid.

   Therefore, the number of amino acids in the protein = $\frac{390}{3}$ = 130.

   Now, we know, average molecular weight of any amino acid residue = 110 Da (approx.)

   Therefore, the average molecular weight of the protein = (130 × 110) Da

   = 14,300 Da

   = 14.30 kDa.

8. The study of the rate at which an enzyme works is called enzyme kinetics. A Lineweaver-Burk plot is used to analyse kinetic data on enzyme-catalysed reactions. The reciprocal of the rate of formation of products (1/v) is plotted against the reciprocal of the substrate concentration (1/[S]). The equation is :

$$\frac{1}{v} = \frac{1}{v_{max}} + \frac{K_M}{v_{max}} \cdot \frac{1}{[S]}$$

   where [S] and K_M have units of mol L^{-1} and v and v_{max} have units of mol L^{-1} s^{-1}. The maximum velocity v_{max} of the enzymolysis is the reciprocal of the y-intercept of the best fit line. The slope of the best fit line is the Michaelis constant K_M divided by v_{max}. This provides a more precise way to determine v_{max} and K_m.

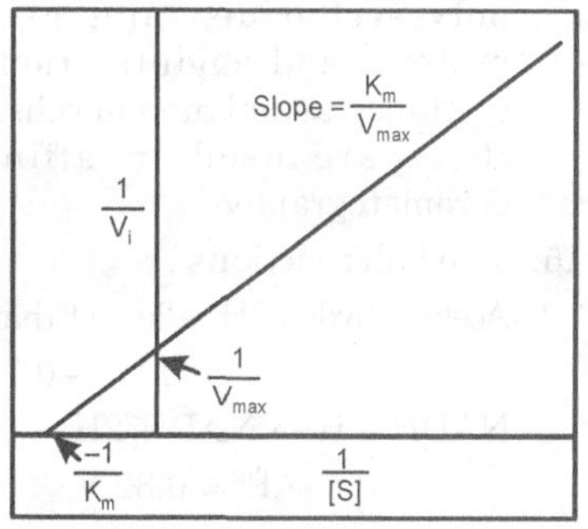

9. After elution of the protein samples using gel filtration chromatography from Sephadex G-200 column, the four proteins appeared on the SDS-PAGE gel in the order W, X, Y, Z. The electrophoretic mobility of a protein is inversely proportional to the molecular weight of the protein. That means a protein with low molecular weight will travel the farthest and the one with a high molecular weight will travel a small distance. Since, the order of appearance of bands on the SDS-PAGE gel is W, X, Y, Z, therefore W is the protein which has travelled the maximum distance and so it has the highest or maximum electrophoretic mobility and the least molecular weight.

10. Arachidonic acid is an essential fatty acid and a precursor for all prostaglandins, thromboxanes, and leukotrienes. Virtually all cellular arachidonic acid is esterified in membrane phospholipids where its presence is tightly regulated through multiple interconnected pathways. Prostaglandin G/H synthase 2 mediates the formation of prostaglandins from arachidonate. It may have a role as a major mediator of inflammation and/or a role for prostanoid signalling in activity-dependent plasticity.

11. Chymotrypsin is a digestive enzyme belonging to a super family of enzymes called serine proteases. It uses an active serine residue to perform hydrolysis on the C-terminal of the aromatic amino acids of other proteins. Chymotrypsin is a protease enzyme that cleaves on the C-terminous phenylalanine (F), tryptophan (W), and tyrosine (Y) on peptide chains. It has specificity for aromatic amino acids because of its hydrophobic pocket. Lysozyme is a small enzyme that attacks the protective cell walls of bacteria. Bacteria build a tough skin of carbohydrate chains, interlocked by short peptide strands, that braces their delicate membrane against the cell's high osmotic pressure. Lysozyme breaks these carbohydrate chains, destroying the structural integrity of the cell wall by breaking the glycosidic linkage. The bacteria burst under their own internal pressure.

12. Immunoglobulin class switching (or isotype switching, or isotypic commutation, or class switch recombination (CSR)) is a biological mechanism that changes a B cell's production of antibody from one class to another; for example, from an isotype called IgM to an isotype called IgG. During this process, the constant region portion of the antibody-heavy chain is changed, but the variable region of the heavy chain stays the same. The clonal anergy theory of induction of immunological tolerance states that differentiating B lymphocytes that encounter multivalent antigen at the pre-B to B cell transition stage can receive and store a negative

signal, which renders them anergic to later triggering stimuli whereas T-cell anergy is induced when TCR stimulation freezes T-cell responses until they receive an adequate subsequent antigenic signal from an antigen presenting cell. The MHC class II molecules, expressed by antigen presenting cells, are heterodimers composed of an alpha and a beta chain, which function to present processed antigen to helper T cells. MHC class I molecules are comprised of two chains: a MHC alpha chain (heavy chain), and a beta2-microglobulin chain (light chain), where only the alpha chain spans the membrane. Tolerance to self is acquired by clonal deletion or inactivation of developing lymphocytes. Tolerance to antigens expressed by grafted tissues can be induced artificially, but it is very difficult to establish once a full repertoire of functional B and T lymphocytes has been produced.

13. DNA in the cell functions as a double-stranded helix of B-form DNA, the structure of which was first determined by Watson and Crick. The polarity of the backbones is antiparallel, with one strand running $3' \rightarrow 5'$ and the other $5' \rightarrow 3'$. The diameter of the B-DNA is ~20 Angstroms, and the distance between base pairs is ~3.4 Angstroms. This means there are 10 bases per turn of the helix. For a 180 base pair DNA molecule, the number of turns possible would be $\frac{180}{10}$ = 18. Given, a multiple RNA polymerase unwinds about 1.5 turns of DNA template per transcription bubble. Therefore, the number of transcription bubbles possible = $\frac{18}{1.5}$ = 12.

14. A mixture of glycine and albumin can be separated using dialysis to filter out the various components based on the diffusion and concentration difference. A mixture of 20 and 60 kDa proteins can be separated using gel filtration or size exclusion chromatography which separates protein based on their molecular weight difference. Histones are basic proteins which can be separated from a nuclear extract based on its charge using ion exchange chromatography (cation resin) supplied with a suitable buffer. Lectins are proteins that interact specifically and reversibly with certain sugar residues. Their specificity enables binding to polysaccharides and glycoproteins and agglutination of erythrocytes and tumour cells. So these are used in affinity chromatography.

15. Two half reactions :

Acetaldehyde + $2H^+$ + $2e^- \rightarrow$ Ethanol,

$\Delta E^0 = -0.16$ V

NADH + H $\rightarrow$ NAD + $2H^+$ + $2e^-$,

$\Delta E^0 = 0.32$ V

We have, $\Delta E^0_{total} = \Delta E^0_{1st} - \Delta E^0_{2nd}$

$= (-0.16 - 0.32)$ V

$= -0.48$ V

Gibb's free energy for a coupled reaction :

$\Delta G^0_{total} = -nF\,\Delta E^0_{total}$

Here, n = 2 (exchange of 2 e^-),

F = 23,063 cal/V,

$\Delta E^0_{total} = -0.48$ V

Therefore,

$\Delta G^0_{total} = -2 \times 23,$

$063 \times (-0.48)$ cal

$= -(-22,140.48)$ cal

= 22,140.48 cal

= 22,200 cal (approx.)

16. *Michaelis-Menten constant K_m*, defined as the substrate concentration with which half the maximum rate is attained determines the affinity of a particular enzyme towards a particular substrate. The ratio $k_{(cat)}/K_{(M)}$—often referred to as the "specificity constant"—is a useful index for comparing the relative rates of an enzyme acting on alternative, competing substrates. The pK_a values (ionization constants) of the active-site residues in an enzyme are of importance to the functionality of the catalytic mechanism of the enzyme. The pK_a values of the proton donor and the catalytic nucleophilic residue are therefore limiting the pH range at which the enzyme can function. pK_a values refer to the maximum buffering capacity of a buffer. K_i is the reaction rate constant when an inhibitor binds to an enzyme or an enzyme substrate complex. It determines the affinity of an enzyme to the inhibitor.

17. Rise per residue of an α-helix

= 1.5 Å

Area spanned by the protein

= 4 nm

= 4×10 Å= 40 Å

Therefore, number of residues per turn of the protein = $\frac{40\text{Å}}{1.5\text{Å}}$

= 26.67 = 27 (approx.)

Now, the transmembrane domain has a span of 7 times in the α-helix. Therefore, number of amino acid residues in the domain = 27 × 7

= 189 =190 (approx.)

18. Potassium voltage-gated channel protein Shaker is a voltage-dependent potassium channel involved in regulation of sleep need or efficiency. It mediates the voltage-dependent potassium ion permeability of excitable membranes. The retinal protein bacteriorhodopsin is the major photosynthetic protein of the archaeon *Halobacterium salinarum*. It converts the energy of "green" light (500-650 nm, max 568 nm) into an electrochemical proton gradient, which in turn is used for ATP production by ATP synthase. It functions as a light-driven proton pump, transporting protons out of the cell, and exemplifies vectorial catalysis. The outer membrane protein F, better known as OmpF porin, is an integral membrane protein located in the outer membrane

of the bacteria, *Escherichia coli.* OmpF porin is a non-specific transport channel that allows for the passive diffusion of small, polar molecules (600-700 Da in size) through the cell's outer membrane. The C termini and strand 16 are essential to trimer formation. Points of contact include the barrel walls and peripheral contacts between L1 and L5. ABC transporters belong to the ATP-Binding Cassette (ABC) superfamily, which uses the hydrolysis of ATP to energise diverse biological systems. The ABC module (approximately two hundred amino acid residues) is known to bind and hydrolyse ATP, thereby coupling transport to ATP hydrolysis in a large number of biological processes through active transport.

19. Alkaptonuria is an inherited condition that causes urine to turn black when exposed to air. Ochronosis, a build up of dark pigment in connective tissues such as cartilage and skin, is also characteristic of the disorder. The HGD gene provides instructions for making an enzyme called homogentisate oxidase. This enzyme helps break down the amino acids phenylalanine and tyrosine, which are important building blocks of proteins. Mutations in the HGD gene impair the enzyme's role in this process. Alkaptonuria is a rare metabolic disorder resulting from loss of homogentisate 1, 2 dioxygenase (HGO) activity. Phenylketonuria (commonly known as PKU) is an inherited disorder that increases the levels of a substance called phenylalanine in the blood. The PAH gene provides instructions for making an enzyme called phenylalanine hydroxylase. This enzyme converts the amino acid phenylalanine to other important compounds in the body. If gene mutations reduce the activity of phenylalanine hydroxylase, phenylalanine from the diet is not processed effectively. As a result, this amino acid can build up to toxic levels in the blood and other tissues.

20. Fatty acid β-oxidation is the process of breaking down a long chain acyl-CoA molecule to acetyl-CoA molecules. This process involves a variety of enzymes, with the four main enzymes involved in fatty acid β-oxidation being, in order, acyl-CoA dehydrogenase, enoyl-CoA hydratase, hydroxyacyl-CoA dehydrogenase, and ketoacyl-CoA thiolase. At the end of each β-oxidation cycle, two new molecules are formed, an acetyl-CoA and an acyl-CoA that is two carbons shorter. Glycolysis begins with phosphorylation of a monosaccharide (generally glucose) on the sixth carbon by a hexokinase, and ends with the production of pyruvate. The most important regulatory step of glycolysis is the phospho-fructokinase reaction. Phosphz-fructokinase is regulated by the energy charge of the cell—that is, the fraction of the adenosine nucleotides of the cell that contain high-energy bonds. Gluconeogenesis occurs mainly in liver. PEP Carboxykinase catalyzes GTP-dependent formation of phosphoenol-pyruvate from oxaloacetate. Oxaloacetate is first decarboxylated to yield a pyruvate enolate anion intermediate. Phosphate transfer from GTP then yields phosphoenolpyruvate (PEP). In Calvin Cycle, carbon molecules from CO_2 are fixed into glucose ($C_6H_{12}O_6$). A five-carbon sugar molecule called ribulose bisphosphate, or RuBP, is the acceptor that binds CO_2 dissolved in the stroma. This process, called CO_2 fixation, is catalyzed by the enzyme RuBP carboxylase, forming an unstable six-carbon molecule.

J : BOTANY

1. Epistasis is the phenomenon of the interaction between two or more genes to control a single phenotype without changing the underlying DNA sequence. In epistasis the expression of one gene depends on the presence of one or more modifier genes.

2. Given the differential equation, $\frac{dN}{dt} = rN$, where $\frac{dN}{dt}$ = rate at which whole population grows. Since N is the size of the population, *r* is the intrinsic rate of increase and t is time, then the per capita rate growth is highest at large value of N as growth rate is directly proportional to size of the population i.e. N.

3. Cytokines are any of a number of substances that are secreted by specific cells of the immune system which carry signals locally between cells, and thus have an effect on other cells. They are a category of signaling molecules that are used extensively in cellular communication. They are proteins, peptides, or glycoproteins and are not a plant hormone.

4. Crossover (CO) is a key process for the accurate segregation of homologous chromosomes during the first meiotic division. In most eukaryotes, meiotic recombination is not homogeneous along the chromosomes, suggesting a tight control of the location of recombination events. Thus if no crossing over takes place in Arabidopsis then genetic variation will be zero in both the species in the F_2 generation.

5. Plants adapted to cold environments would be expected to have more unsaturated fatty acids in their membranes, since those remain fluid at lower temperatures. Plants adapted to hot environments would be expected to have more saturated fatty acids, which would allow the fatty acids to "stack" more closely, making the membranes less fluid and therefore helping them to stay intact at higher temperatures.

6. The sign on the tree trunk will be 2 metres high after 10 years as the increase in the length of tree is due to the activity of the apical meristem.
7. Imbricate overlap does not involve the overlapping of sepals or petals at the margin rather it is an irregular overlap.
8. One sperm nucleus unites with the egg to form the diploid zygote, from which the embryo develops, and the other unites with two polar nuclei to form the triploid, primary endosperm nucleus. Since endosperms are triploid (containing three sets of chromosomes) therefore the possible genotypes of endosperms borne on a heterozygous (Rr) plant will be RRR, RRr, Rrr, rrr.
9. Net primary production is the rate at which all the plants in an ecosystem produce net useful chemical energy. It is equal to the difference between the rate at which the plants in an ecosystem produce useful chemical energy (GPP) and the rate at which they use some of that energy during respiration.

   NPP = GPP – respiration [by plants]
10. Free radical scavenging activity of a medically important plant extract can be quantified by the ABTS method/ assay. In ABTS free radical scavenging assay, the antioxidant activity is measured.
11. Lenticels are one of the small, corky pores or narrow lines on the surface of the stems of woody plants that allow the interchange of gases between the interior tissue and the surrounding air.

    The equation of dark reaction is as follows:

    $$6\ CO_2 + 18\ ATP + 12\ NADPH + 12\ H_2O \longrightarrow C_6H_{12}O_6 + 18\ ADP^+$$

    Thus 18 ATP and 12 NADPH molecules are utilized for fixing 6 molecules of CO_2 in the dark reaction of photosynthesis.
12. Sorghum is a tropical grass with a very high content of the cyanogenic glucoside dhurrin. Dhurrin is a glycosidic conjugate derived from the amino acid tyrosine.

    Castor beans are processed throughout the world to make castor oil. Ricin is a highly toxic, naturally occurring lectin (a carbohydrate -binding protein) which is part of the waste "mash" produced when castor oil is made.

    Alpha-Amanitin or α-amanitin is a cyclic peptide of eight amino acids and it is produced by the poisonous mushrooms.

    Gossypol is a natural phenol derived from the cotton plant. Gossypol is a phenolic aldehyde that permeates cells and acts as an inhibitor for several dehydrogenase enzymes. It is a yellow pigment.
13. Basified fixation: anther attached to their filaments by the base.

    Adenate fixation: anther fixed by its whole length to the filament.

    Versatile fixation: An anther whose attachment is near its middle, thus enabling it to swing free.

    Dorsifixed fixation: Anther attached dorsally and medially to apex of filament.
14. The correct structures are as follows:

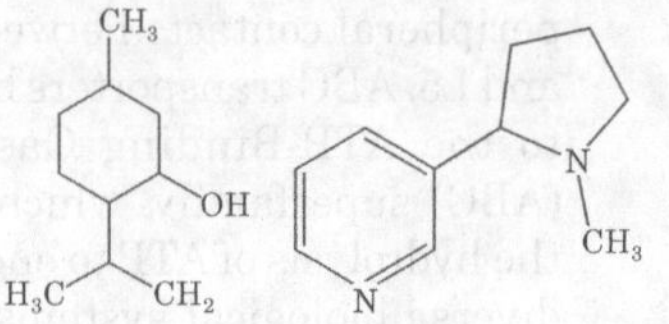

Menthol Nicotine

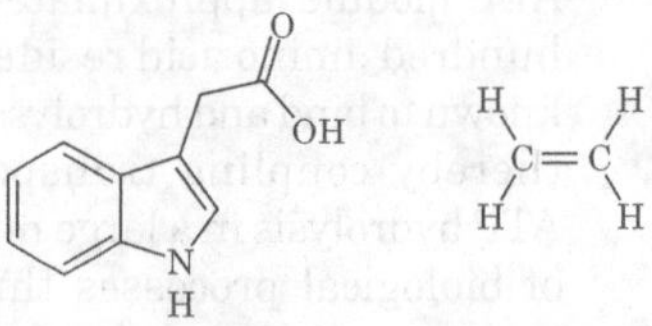

Indol Acetic Acid Ethylene

15. Commensalism is a class of relationship between two organisms where one organism benefits without affecting the other.

    Mutualism is the way in which two organisms of different species exist in a relationship where each individual benefits.

    Parasitism is a non-mutual relationship between organisms of different species where one organism, the parasite, benefits at the expense of the other, the host.

    Amensalism is a relationship in which a product of one organism has a negative effect on another organism means one organism impeding the success of another.
16. The structures in the order of their appearance and identity corresponding glycosidic linkages are as follows:

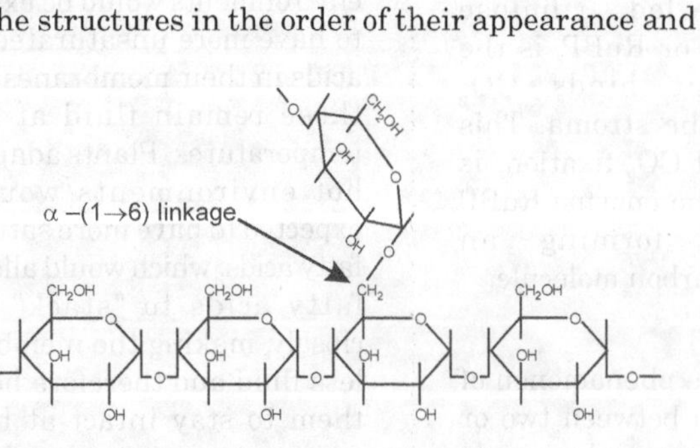

Amylopectin (alpha- 1→ 6 glycosidic linkage)

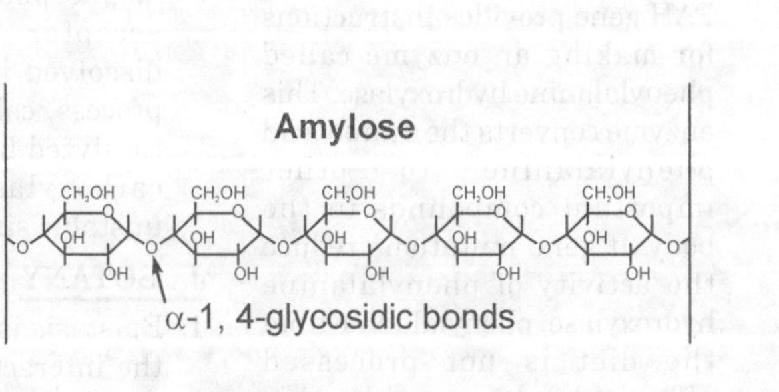

Amylose (alpha- 1 → 4 glycosidic linkage)

17. Vernalization is the artificial exposure of plants (or seeds) to low temperatures in order to stimulate flowering or to enhance seed production. Vernalization quantitatively silences FLC, so relieves the repression on flowering. Chromatin silencing mechanism mediates the epigenetic silencing of FLC. FLC transcription is down regulated in the early phase of cold exposure and this is associated with increased abundance of FLC antisense transcripts.

18. In the TCA cycle the enzyme succinyl co-A synthetase converts ADP → ATP instead of GDP → GTP and leads to generation of 1 ATP.

    In the electron transport system, an alternate oxidase enzyme can also be used which is resistant to cyanide to reduce the oxygen molecule.

19. Cyclin E is found in the later stages of G1 phase which is essential for G1 to S phase transition.

    G1/S Cyclins rise in late G1 and fall in early S phase.

    Cyclin B is a mitotic cyclin which is expressed prior to mitotic phase.

    The synthesis of cyclin D is initiated during G1 and drives the G1/S phase transition.

20. In case of plant development plant cells do not migrate, as do bacteria or animal cells. Apoptosis plays a major role in plant development and in its defence. In plant development the homeotic changes are caused by the mutations in the non-homeodomain proteins.

K : MICROBIOLOGY

1. The electron microscope is a type of microscope that uses a beam of electrons to create an image of the specimen. It is capable of much higher magnifications and has a greater resolving power than a light microscope, allowing it to see much smaller objects in finer detail. Electron microscopes have a higher resolution and are therefore also able of a higher magnification (up to 2 million times). Light microscopes can show a useful magnification only up to 1000-2000 times. This is a physical limit imposed by the wavelength of the light i.e. 0.2 nm which is larger than the wavelength of an electron i.e. 0.005 nm.

2. Lysozyme is an enzyme used to break down bacterial cell walls to improve protein or nucleic acid extraction efficiency. Lysozymes (muramidases) are a family of enzymes with antimicrobial activity characterized by the ability to damage the cell wall of bacteria. The enzyme acts by catalyzing the hydrolysis of 1, 4-beta-linkages between N-acetylmuramic acid and N-acetyl-D-glucosamine residues in peptidoglycans and between the N-acetyl-D-glucosamine residues in chitodextrins.

3. Given, recombination frequency between 3 genes:

   $$x - y = 2.6\%$$
   $$y - z = 1.4\%$$
   and $$x - y = 1.2\%.$$

   Thus the gene order can be:

   $$x - y - z.$$

4. A mutant phenotype due to a non-sense mutation can be rescued by a mutation in tRNA gene. This rescue is an example suppressor mutation. A suppressor mutation is a mutation that partially or completely masks phenotypic expression of a mutation but occurs at a different site from it (i.e., causes suppression); it may be intragenic or intergenic. It is used particularly to describe a secondary mutation that suppresses a nonsense codon created by a primary mutation. It is a mutation that alters the anticodon in a tRNA so that it is complementary to a termination codon, thus suppressing termination of the amino acid chain.

5. Ames test is a test used to determine the mutagenic potential of a substance based on the mutation rate of bacteria that are exposed to the substance. It determines whether a chemical is a mutagen or not. The use of the Ames test is based on the assumption that any substance that is mutagenic for the bacteria used in this test may also turn out to be a carcinogen; that is, to cause cancer.

6. EMB (Eosin Methylene Blue) agar is a differential, selective medium. The dyes (Eosin and Methylene Blue) inhibit the growth of Gram-positive bacteria. The medium contains amino acids and small peptides that support the growth of all Gram-negative rods without significant production of acid. The only carbohydrate is lactose and those organisms capable of lactose fermentation produce acid and become dark green or purple. Lactose-negative colonies are colorless. In a crowded portion of the plate, the local acid concentration may differ from that of an isolated colony, causing a difference in the shade of the pH indicator. Among the lactose fermenters, E. coli, which produces large amounts of acid from lactose, forms colonies with a very dark, metallic sheen. Thus the *E. coli* forms purple colored colonies on EMB- lactose plates due to the decrease in the pH of the medium.

7. The resistance of lambda lysogenic E. coli to re- infection by lambda is mediated by blocking the transcription of the incoming lambda DNA.

8. Batch pasteurization is the simplest and oldest method for pasteurizing milk. Milk is heated to 154.4 degrees Fahrenheit (63 degrees Celsius) in a large container and held at that temperature for 30 minutes. In batch processing, the milk has to be stirred constantly to make sure that each particle of milk is heated.

9. Given, Doubling time, Generation time (G)

   $$= 20 \text{ min} = 0.33 \text{ hrs}$$

We know, $G = t/n$

Where, t = time

n = number of generations

Let X be the no. of bacteria at the beginning of time interval and Y be the no. of bacteria at the end of time interval.

Therefore, we have

$$Y = X * 2^n$$

Taking log on both sides,

$$\log Y = \log X + n \log 2$$

Therefore, $n = \log Y - \log X / \log 2$

$n = 3.3 \log Y/X$ (as log 2 = 0.3010)

But we know,

$$G = t/n \quad ...(i)$$

Therefore, putting the value of n in equation (i), we get,

$$G = t/3.3 \log Y/X \quad ...(ii)$$

We know, $X = 2 * 10^8$

and $t = 3$ hrs (given)

Therefore,

$$n = t/G = 3/0.33 = 9$$

From equation (ii)

$$0.33 = 3/(3.3 \log Y/ 2 * 10^8)$$

Therefore, on solving we get,

$$Y = 10^5$$

Therefore, time required to reach the cell density of $1 * 10^8$ cells/ml can be found as:

$$G = t/3.3 \log Y/X$$

$$0.33 = t/ [3.3(\log 10^8 - \log 10^5)]$$

Therefore on solving we get,

t = 196 min ~ 200 min (approx.)

Therefore, time required to reach the cell density of $1 * 10^8$ cells/ml is 200 min.

10. The quickest way to determine bacterial growth in terms of viable cells is through spread plate method. The spread plate technique is used for the enumeration of aerobic microorganisms from the given sample. This can be done by serial diluting the samples, placing 0.1ml of the diluted sample in the middle of an agar plate and spreading the sample over the surface with a help of an L-rod. After incubating it in a suitable temperature for a period of time the colonies can be counted.

11. Robert Koch worked on anthrax and tuberculosis (TB). Koch and his team developed ways of staining bacteria to improve the bacteria's visibility under the microscope, and were able to identify the bacterial causes of tuberculosis (1882).

    Walter Hesse discovered the use of agar as solid media. He discovered that agar-agar was indeed an ideal agent to gel the beef broth. At 100° C, it could be melted, mixed with the liquid broth and poured into dishes. The new medium was solid at room temperature and well above. Bacteria grew well on it but they could not break it down.

    Louis Pasteur disproved the theory of spontaneous generation. Pasteur proved that life couldn't be spontaneously generated by using various controlled beakers. He boiled half of the special formula and the other halves were autoclaved which removes all life forms. The beakers with lids that were autoclaved showed no life and continue to show no life (they are displayed at a museum) thus proving that life cannot spontaneously generate.

    Ferdinand Cohn was the first to show that Bacillus can change from a vegetative state to an endospore state when subjected to an environment deleterious to the vegetative state.

12. Superantigens are bacterial proteins that generate a powerful immune response by binding to Major Histocompatibility Complex class II molecules on antigen-presenting cells and T cell receptors on T cells.

13. The MHC I molecule consists of a α chain and a β_2-microglobulin. One segment of the β_2-microglobulin is anchored to the membrane, with the rest of the molecule protruding outside the cell. MHC I molecules contain a deep groove in the domain of the molecule farthest away from the membrane and therefore exposed to the environment. This groove is capable of binding short peptides or other antigens that are not part of the MHC molecule. The MHC I groove is closed off (on both ends), thus it can contain only short peptide sequences of 8-10 amino acids only. While the MHC II molecule is open and can bind to peptides of longer lengths.

14. The $lacO^c$ mutation is related to a gene that acts in cis. The lacO gene codes for the operator. The $lacO^c$ mutation alters the DNA sequence of the lacO gene. Whether lactose is present or absent in the medium, the repressor protein is not able to bind the operator. The operator made by any lacO gene in the cell does not diffuse through the cell. Therefore, the RNA polymerase binds to the operator where the $lacO^c$ mutation occurs and transcribes the lac structural genes. Thus the $lacO^c$ mutation is cis- dominant.

15. Attenuation is a mechanism of control in some bacterial operons which results in premature termination of transcription and which are based on the fact that, in bacteria, transcription and translation proceed simultaneously. Thus attenuation is a form of transcriptional regulation which takes place only in prokaryotes. Attenuation does not regulate eukaryotic transcription because eukaryotic cells contain a nuclear envelope, while prokaryotic cells do not. In prokaryotes transcription and translation operate simultaneously, thus the process of attenuation occurs. While transcription and translation occur in separate cellular compartments in eukaryotes attenuation cannot occur.

16. Tuberculosis (TB) is an infectious disease that is caused by a bacterium called Mycobacterium tuberculosis.

    Measles is an infection of the respiratory system caused by a virus, specifically a paramyxo-virus. It is a highly contagious respiratory disease.

Candidiasis also called thrush or moniliasis, is a fungal infection caused by yeasts that belong to the genus Candida. There are over 20 species of Candida yeasts that can cause infection in humans, the most common of which is Candida albicans.

Malaria is a life-threatening blood disease caused by a parasite that is transmitted to humans by the bite of a female Anopheles mosquito.

17. Given,

Culture was diluted 1000 fold

Amount of sample spread per plate = 0.1 ml

Therefore, dilution factor

= 1000/0.1 = 10^4

Number of colonies formed

= 121, 93, 86

Average of colonies formed

$$= \frac{121 + 93 + 86}{3} = 100$$

Therefore, number of colony forming units/ml

= Dilution factor * Average number of colonies

= $10^4 * 100$ or $10^4 * 10^2$

= 10^6.

18. Aspergillus oryzae is an asexual, ascomycetous fungus used for the production of glucoamylase (an amylolytic enzyme) under solid state fermentation.

Brevibacterium flavum is used for the production of a number of amino acids like glutamic acid in the biotechnology industry.

Bioleaching is the extraction of metals from their ores through the use of living organisms. Bioleaching can involve numerous ferrous iron and sulfur oxidizing bacteria, including Acidithiobacillus ferrooxidans and Acidithiobacillus (formerly known as Thiobacillus).

The main purpose of yeast is to serve as a catalyst in the process of fermentation, which is essential in the making of bread. *Saccharomyces cerevisiae* is the yeast that is most commonly used in making bread.

Sinorhizobium meliloti (formerly Rhizobium meliloti) is a soil bacterium that forms nitrogen-fixing nodules on the roots of certain genera of leguminous plants, including Medicago, Melilotus and Trigonella. It forms a symbiotic relationship with legumes.

19. The most likely pathway that is defective in the mutant of *E. coli* is the Glyoxylate cycle. The glyoxylate cycle uses a two-step bypass. The first key enzyme, isocitrate lyase, converts D-threo-isocitrate to form succinate and glyoxylate. The second key enzyme, malate synthase A, condenses glyoxylate and another molecule of acetyl-CoA to form (S)-malate. The subsequent oxidation of malate regenerates the initial acetyl-CoA acceptor molecule of the TCA cycle, oxaloacetate. In *Escherichia coli* the pathway is active when growth on two-carbon compounds requires conservation of four-carbon TCA intermediates. Two acetyl-CoA are taken up per turn. The glyoxylate cycle is repressed during growth on glucose and induced by growth on acetate.

20. Beta-lactamases are enzymes produced by some bacteria that provide resistance to beta-lactam antibiotics like penicillins. Beta-lactamase provides antibiotic resistance by breaking the antibiotics' structure.

Sulfonamides, as antimetabolites, compete with para-aminobenzoic acid (PABA) for incorporation into folic acid. Normally folic acid is synthesized in two steps in bacteria. If a sulfa drug is used, the first enzyme is not too specific and can use the sulfonamide in the first reaction. This reaction produces the product containing pteridine and the sulfa drug. The next and final step is the reaction PABA + with glutamic acid to make folic acid. If the sulfa drug has been substituted for the PABA, then the final enzyme is inhibited and no folic acid is produced.

Tetracycline resistance is attributed to a drug efflux mechanism.

Aminoglycoside phosphotransferases (APHs) catalyze the ATP-dependent phosphorylation of these antibiotics. APH is a modifying enzyme necessary for aminoglycoside resistance.

Mutations in rpoB (RNA polymerase β-subunit) can cause high-level resistance to rifampicin. Rifampicin inhibits bacterial DNA-dependent RNA synthesis by inhibiting bacterial DNA-dependent RNA polymerase.

L : ZOOLOGY

1. There are two parts to the shell of a turtle: the upper portion is called the "carapace" and the bottom half is called the "plastron." Both shells are actually made of many fused bones. The carapace is the fusion of about 50 bones - the ribs and vertebrae. The plastron is the fusion of bones including the clavicles (collar bones), bones between the clavicles, and portions of the ribs. The shells are covered with a layer of keratin and provide protection. Lobsters belong to phylum arthropoda. All lobsters have a hard exoskeleton. Exoskeletons have a role in defence from pests and predators, support, and in providing an attachment framework for musculature. Thus, exoskeleton of lobster is homologous to shell of tortoise on basis of developmental origin.

2. Acoelomate is an animal that lacks a coelom (body cavity or space filled with fluid within the mesoderm). Acoelomates, which include the flatworm, fluke, tapeworm, and ribbon worm, exhibit bilateral symmetry and possess one internal space, the digestive cavity. The term acoelomate literally refers to "without a coelom". As such the class of invertebrates belonging to acoelomates are recognised by the absence of any kind of body cavity around the membranes and internal organs and tissues.

3. Cnidarians may have two basic body forms, polyps and medusae. On their tentacles and sometimes on their body surface, cnidarians bear specialized cells called cnidocytes. Within each cnidocyte is a nematocyst, which is the characteristic of this group. Phylum Porifera refers to sponges which lacks any tissue organization. Porifera refers to the system of pores and belongs to the subkingdom of Parazoa. Arthropods, especially the largest class-insects-are by far the most successful of all animals. Arthropods are segmented protostomes with jointed appendages. Phylum Arthropoda have a coelom, segmented bodies, and jointed appendages. Molluscs (phylum Mollusca) are an extremely diverse animal phylum, second only to the arthropods. Molluscs are the second-largest phylum of animals in terms of named species; molluscs exhibit a variety of body forms and live in many different environments. The body cavity of a mollusc is a coelom, which is completely enclosed within the mesoderm.

4. A population is the smallest biological unit that can evolve. It is a group of individuals of the same species, living in the same place, at the same time. The cell is the basic structural and functional unit of all known living organisms. It is the smallest unit of life that is classified as a living thing. The biological species concept defines a species as members of populations that actually or potentially interbreed in nature, not according to similarity of appearance. An individual organism is the single living organism belonging to a species having all the characteristics of that species.

5. A host in which a parasite develops to an adult or sexually mature stage is known as the definitive host. It is also called the final host. It is any host organism in which a parasite reproduces sexually. The female Anopheles mosquito is the definitive host for malaria. Humans are definitive hosts for pinworms, schistosomes, and tapeworms. A definitive host is very essential in the growth life cycle of a parasite as it is the one in which the parasite would attain sexual maturity.

6. Enzymes are the biochemical catalysts that catalyze the conversion of substrate molecules to product by the lowering of the activation energy required to initiate the reaction and stabilising the transition state. The enzyme-substrate complex that is formed as an intermediate in the reaction stabilises the energy of metabolism during the state of transition of the substrate to product. The enzymes are mostly proteinaceous in nature and are specific in their activities.

7. Mendel's monohybrid cross, also known as the law of segregation, states that every individual possesses a pair of alleles (assuming diploid) for any particular trait and that each parent passes a randomly selected copy (allele) of only one of these to its offspring. Whichever of the two alleles in the offspring is dominant determines how the offspring expresses that trait. The phenotypic ratio of Mendel's monohybrid crosses after first filial generation (F_1 generation) is 3:1 and after second filial generation (F_2 generation) is 9:3:3:1. Every trait or character bred true and there was no blending of the traits in any of the filial generations. Thus, co-dominance was not a suggestive part of the law of segregation. Hence, occurrence of recessive phenotype in the progeny is strong evidence against the theory.

8. The process in which relatively unspecialized cells acquire specialized structural and/or functional features that characterize the cells, tissues, or organs of the mature organism or some other relatively stable phase of the organism's life history is called cell differentiation. Differentiation includes the processes involved in commitment of a cell to a specific fate and its subsequent development to the mature state. Lateral inhibition is a type of cell-to-cell interaction whereby a cell adopting a particular fate prevents its neighbours from developing in the same way. Thus, in the context of cell differentiation, lateral inhibition implies the inhibition of a distinct and particular cell type nearby a well developed lineage of cells.

9. The steroid hormones are all derived from cholesterol. The particular steroid hormone class synthesized by a given cell type depends upon its complement of peptide hormone receptors, its response to peptide hormone stimulation and its genetically expressed complement of enzymes. The receptors for amino acid-derived and peptide hormones are located in the plasma membrane. The hormone-binding signal of most, but not all, plasma membrane receptors is transduced to the interior of cells by the binding of receptor-ligand complexes to a series of membrane-localized GDP/GTP binding proteins known as G-proteins. Steroid hormones bind to nuclear receptors in the cell nucleus for genomic actions. Membrane-associated steroid receptors activate intracellular signaling cascades involved in non-genomic actions. The intracellular cascades are run through transcription and translation (i.e., signalling through protein expression) and so they require a transcription factor. Thus steroid hormones require more time for activation of response.

10. The formation of two or more species often requires geographical isolation of subpopulations of the species. Only then natural selection or genetic drift produce distinctive gene pools. *Allopatric speciation* occurs when a population is separated geographically,

restricting the gene flow between the subpopulations. It is no accident that the various races (or subspecies) of animals almost never occupy the same territory. Their distribution is allopatric ("other country").

11. Morphogens are long-range signaling molecules that pattern developing tissues in a concentration-dependent manner. The graded activity of morphogens within tissues exposes cells to different signal levels and leads to region-specific transcriptional responses and cell fates. Whether neurogen is a morphogen cannot be questioned based on the type of protein it is (membrane anchored or cytosolic). Thus, if artificial mis-expression of Neurogen occurs, if it is a morphogen, it will affect the neuronal cell types produced in the neural tube. But, if neurogen is not a morphogen, it would not affect the formation of neural cell types.

12. As the existing species on planet earth follows the degeneracy of the genetic code, and they have 4 nucleotides present in them, the codons that are generated is given by $4^3 = 64$, which accounts for the genetic codes of all the possible 20 amino acids of the species on earth. Now, for the alien species, which have 5 distinct nucleotides and 40 different amino acids, $5^3 = 125$ possible codons could cover up all the 40 amino acid combinations (since the alien species follows the same average codon degeneracy as in case of existing earth species). Therefore, the most probable codon length would be 3 for the new alien species.

13. Most female contraceptives are based on the formulation strategies of inhibiting or modulating progesterone and oestrogen hormones or receptors. Progesterone is a female hormone produced by the ovaries during release of a mature egg from an ovary (ovulation). Estrogens (also called Oestrogens) are steroid compounds that help in the fertilization process of the ova. Thus, inhibiting their action or modulating their metabolism using synthetic, semi-synthetic and other kinds of drugs or molecules can be formulated as a contraceptive strategy. Oxytocin is a hormone which is released in large amounts after distension of the cervix and uterus during labour, facilitating birth, maternal bonding, and, after stimulation of the nipples, breastfeeding. Thus, synthetic oxytocin cannot be used as a female contraceptive strategy.

14. In community ecology, the term competitive exclusion refers to the principle that when two species compete for the same critical resources within an environment, one of them will eventually outcompete and displace the other. The displaced species may become locally extinct, by either migration or death, or it may adapt to a sufficiently distinct niche within the environment so that it continues to coexist noncompetitively with the displacing species. The competitive exclusion principle also referred to as Gause's Law, states that two species that compete for the exact same resources cannot stably coexist in the same niche.

15. T-cells are activated on account of the entry of a foreign antigen in the body. Then, T-helper cells along with memory cells are generated through differentiation of the T-cells. T-helper cells secrete cytokines (chemical messengers) which stimulate the B-cell on the event of an immune response in the body. Thereafter, B-cells differentiate into plasma cells and memory cells. Plasma B-cells produce antibodies which destroy the foreign antigen and memory cells store the characteristic foreign antigenic encoded protein. That is why helper T-cell memory appears earlier than the B-cell memory against the antigen.

16. The marine biome is the biggest biome in the world. The marine regions are divided between coral reefs, estuaries and oceans. The marine biome has a big influence on the terrestrial climate. Oceans provide rain for crops through evaporation, wind to help circulate air, and affects coastal temperatures. Through photosynthesis, marine plants and algae provide much of the worlds oxygen supply and take in huge amounts of carbon dioxide. This absorption of carbon dioxide may be a useful tool in reducing the severity of climate change. Over 1 million species of plants and animals have been discovered in the oceans. Thus, pH of the fresh water bodies is not influenced by oceans.

17. The lungfish gets the name from the fact that they can breathe atmospheric oxygen by using lungs similar to those found in early amphibians. They belong to the subclass Dipnoi. Lungfish are best known for their ability to breathe air and the presence of lobed fins with a well-developed internal skeleton. They live in fresh water and excrete nitrogenous waste in the form of urea. This is so because of their habitat which is devoid of sufficient water. Hence, they do not excrete ammonia since it is highly toxic and requires adequate quantity of water for dissolving. On the contrary, urea is less toxic and requires minimum amount of water for dissolution. This is the significance of the adaptation.

18. The elements of kin selection (that is, direct fitness and indirect fitness) lead directly to the concept known as Hamilton's rule, which states that aid-giving behaviour can evolve when the indirect fitness benefits of helping relatives compensate the aid giver for any losses in personal reproduction it incurs

by helping. In each behaviour-evoking situation, the individual assesses his neighbour's fitness against his own according to the coefficients of relationship appropriate to the situation. Algebraically, the rule posits that a costly action should be performed if :

C < r x B, where C is the cost in fitness to the actor, r the genetic relatedness between the actor and the recipient or coefficient of relation, and B is the fitness benefit to the recipient.

Now, taking the case of natural selection favouring an altruistic act, if:

C = cost in fitness to the act of altruism, r = coefficient of relatedness and B = benefits to the recipient, then according to Hamilton's rule, C < r x B or r > C/B or B > C/r which gives the statement that benefit to the recipient is reduced by the coefficient of relatedness and it exceeds the cost in fitness to the altruistic act.

19. A variety of colours are produced in the F1 generation from the cross between plants with purple and white coloured flowers. The flower varieties obtained were → white, straw yellow, yellow, greenish yellow, green, light blue, blue, indigo, purple and dark purple flowers. As there is appearance of a large number of flowers with colours different from the parental generation, it can be assumed that the colouring genes in the two plants are present in multiple numbers. Therefore, the two flowering plants are a multi-colouring gene species.

20. Vaccination is the use of vaccines to prevent specific diseases. A vaccine is a biological preparation that improves immunity to a particular disease. A vaccine typically contains an agent that resembles a disease-causing microorganism, and is often made from weakened or killed forms of the microbe, its toxins or one of its surface proteins. T-cells play a vital role in immunity of the body. T-cells differentiate into memory cells and T-helper cells during immunization by any antigen. These T-helper cells have T-cell receptors (TCRs) present on the surface of the cell membrane which help in recognition of the antigen. Antigen recognition by a T-helper cell is done by Major Histocompatibilty complexes (MHC-I and MHC-II) present on TCRs which help in processing and presentation of the antigen. Thus for vaccination to be successful, the T-helper cells must be able to process and present the vaccine (antigen) efficiently using MHC-I and MHC-II.

■■

GATE-2009

XL : LIFE SCIENCES

Time : 3 Hours | *Maximum Marks : 100*

H : CHEMISTRY (Compulsory)

Useful data for Section H : Chemistry

R = 0.08315 L bar K^{-1} mol^{-1}; F = 96490 C mol^{-1}; Atomic Numbers : Fe = 26; Co = 27

Q. 1 to 6 carry one mark each

1. For a second order reaction, $R \xrightarrow{k} P$, the relation between half-life time ($t_{1/2}$) and the initial reactant concentration $[R]_0$ is

(a) $t_{1/2} = \dfrac{\ln 2}{k}$ (b) $t_{1/2} = \dfrac{2}{k[R]_0}$

(c) $t_{1/2} = \dfrac{1}{k[R]_0^2}$ (d) $t_{1/2} = \dfrac{1}{k[R]_0}$

2. The reversible and irreversible entropy changes of a system on going from state '1' to state '2' are ΔS_{12}^{rev} and ΔS_{12}^{irrev} respectively. The correct relationship between the two entropy changes is

(a) $\Delta S_{12}^{irrev} > \Delta S_{12}^{rev}$ (b) $\Delta S_{12}^{irrev} < \Delta S_{12}^{rev}$

(c) $\Delta S_{12}^{irrev} = \Delta S_{12}^{rev}$ (d) $\Delta S_{12}^{irrev} = -\Delta S_{12}^{rev}$

3. Among the following molecules the one that is planar is

(a) $(CH_3)_3N$ (b) $[SO_4]^{2-}$ (c) $[CO_3]^{2-}$ (d) PCl_3

4. Among the following molecules the one that exhibits **only** one isomer is

(a) $[Fe(H_2O)_5OH]^{2+}$ (b) $Pt(NH_3)_2Cl_2$

(c) $[Pt(NH_3)_3Cl_3]^+$ (d) $[CoCl_3(NH_3)_3]$

5. The most stable carbocation among the following is

(a) $CH_3OCH_2CH_2^+$ (b) $CH_3CH = CHCH_2^+$

(c) $CH_3CH_2^+$ (d) $H_3C-\overset{\overset{\displaystyle O}{\|}}{C}-CH_2^+$

6. The carboxylic acid with the lowest *p*Ka value is

(a) $C_6H_5CO_2H$ (b) CH_3CO_2H

(c) p-CH_3O-$C_6H_4CO_2H$ (d) *p*-CH_3-$C_6H_4CO_2H$

Q.7 to 18 carry two marks each

7. If the ground state ionization energy of the hydrogen atom is denoted by ε, then the energy required to ionize an electron from the 3rd energy level of the hydrogen atom is

(a) $\dfrac{2\varepsilon}{3}$ (b) $\dfrac{\varepsilon}{9}$ (c) $\dfrac{\varepsilon}{3}$ (d) $\dfrac{8\varepsilon}{9}$

8. Given the following standard electrode potentials at 25°C :

$$\frac{1}{2}Fe^{2+} + e^- = \frac{1}{2}Fe(s); E^0 = 0.440\ V$$

$$Fe^{3+} + e^- = Fe^{2+}; E^0 = +0.771\ V$$

The standard electrode potential at 25° C for

$$Fe^{3+} + 3e^- = Fe(s) \text{ is}$$

(a) – 0.036 V (b) – 0.331V

(c) – 0.662 V (d) – 2.422 V

9. Identify the major product Q formed in the following reaction:

$$(CH_3)_2CHCH_2Br \xrightarrow[EtOH]{NaOEt} Q$$

(a) $CH_3CH(OEt)\ CH_2CH_3$

(b) $(CH_3)_2\ CHCH_2\ OEt$

(c) $(CH_3)_3\ COEt$

(d) $(CH_3)_2C = CH_2$

10. The reaction of $AgNO_3$ with KCl in an aqueous environment leads to an insoluble product P. Treatment of P with an excess of KCl leads to its dissolution because of the formation of Q.

P and Q respectively are

(a) AgCl and $[AgCl_2]^-$ (b) $[AgCl_2]^-$ and AgCl

(c) AgCl and $[AgCl_3]^-$ (d) $[AgCl_2]^-$ and $[AgCl_3]^{2-}$

11. The major product formed in the nitration of o-methoxybenzoic acid is

(a) 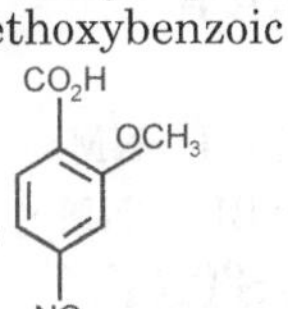

(b) 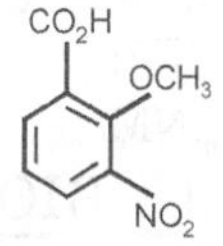

(c) 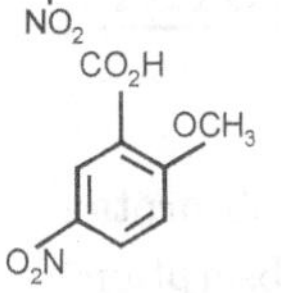

(d) 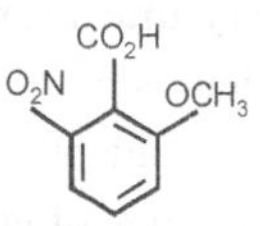

12. Match the following:

P. $[CoCl_4]^{2-}$	1. $\sqrt{15}$ BM
Q. $[Fe(H_2O)_6]^{3+}$	2. 0 BM
R. $[Fe(CN)_6]^{4-}$	3. $\sqrt{35}$ BM

(a) P-2, Q-3, R-1 (b) P-2,Q-1,R-3

(c) P-1, Q-3, R-2 (d) P-3, Q-2, R-1

13. Which one of the following Fischer projections represents (S, S) – tartaric acid?

(a) 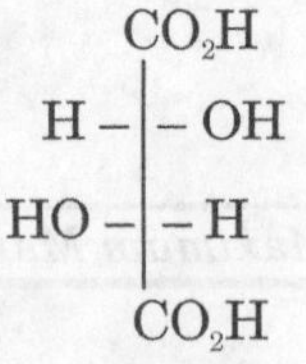
(b) 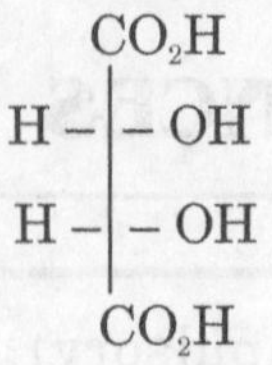
(c) 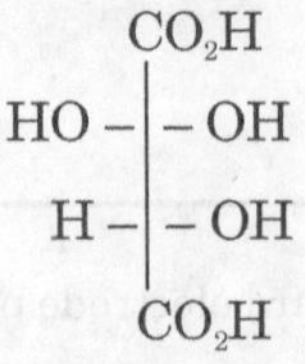
(d) 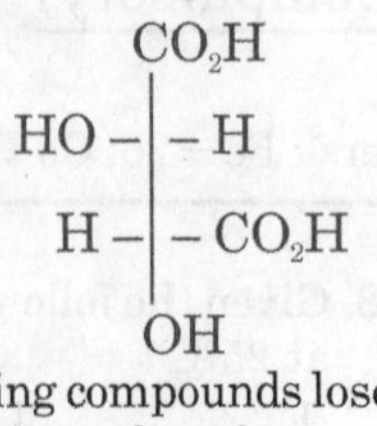

14. Which one among the following compounds loses a proton most readily in a basic medium?
(a) Cyclopentadiene (b) Cycloheptatriene
(c) Cyclopropene (d) 1,3-Cyclohexadiene

Common Data Questions

Common Data for questions 15 and 16:

For the reaction, P(g) = 2Q (g), the equilibrium constant with a standard state pressure of 1 bar is 0.25. Assume ideal gas behaviour.

15. The total pressure (in bar) needed for 50% conversion of P into Q is
(a) 0.1250 (b) 0.1875
(c) 0.5000 (d) 0.7500

16. The amount of P that will be converted to Q at a total pressure of 0.5 bar is approximately
(a) 13% (b) 25%
(c) 33% (d) 55%

Linked Answer Questions

Statements for linked answer Q. 17 and 18:

The reaction of BF_3 with $NaBH_4$ leads to the formation of a stable gaseous boron compound P. The compound P reacts with Me_3N to give Q.

17. Identify P among the following:
(a) BH_3 (b) $Na[B_3H_8]$
(c) B_2H_6 (d) B_4H_{10}

18. The compound Q is
(a) $BH_3.NMe_3$ (b) $B_2H_5.NMe_3$
(c) $B_4H_9.NMe_3$ (d) $BH_3.2NMe_3$

I : BIOCHEMISTRY

Q.1 to carry one mark each.

1. Pernicious anemia is due to
(a) blockage of vitamin B_{12} absorption
(b) blockage of vitamin A absorption
(c) deficiency of vitamin C
(d) deficiency of vitamin B_2

2. Which of these can be an antigen but cannot induce immune responses ?
(a) Hemocyanin (b) Influenza virus
(c) Azobenzene arsonate (d) Corynebacteria

3. In mammals, the second messenger Nitric Oxide (NO) is produced from
(a) Ammonium nitrate (b) Arginine
(c) Urea (d) Nitrous acid

4. Generally, the rate-limiting step of major metabolic pathways is a reaction
(a) in which the availability of the substrate is limited
(b) catalyzed by an allosteric enzyme
(c) catalyzed by an enzyme with very low Km
(d) whose products are not readily consumed by the subsequent step of the pathway.

5. Human DNA (3×10^6 Kb) is replicated in 5 hrs at a rated of 1 Kb/min. The number of origins of replication utilized are
(a) 1 (b) 3 (c) 300 (d) 10,000

6. Phospholipases A1 and A2
(a) play no role in phospholipids synthesis
(b) hydrolyze phosphatidic acid to diglycerate
(c) remove fatty acid from sn-1 and sn-2 of phospholipids
(d) are involved in biosynthesis of phosphatidyl ethanolamine.

7. Equal volumes of two buffers of pH4 and pH6 of identical ionic strengths are mixed. The resultant pH is
(a) close to 4 (b) close to 5
(c) close to 6 (d) exactly 5

Q.8 to 21 carry two marks each

8. An insert (I) of 1 Kb is ligated to a plasmid (P) of 4 Kb in a molar ratio of 4:1 respectively in a final DNA concentration of 10μg/ml. The amounts of insert (I) and plasmid (P) required in μg are
(a) I = 8 and P = 2 (b) I = 2 and P = 8
(c) I = 5 and P = 5 (d) I = 1 and P = 4

9. The formation of ATP from ADP and Pi is not a spontaneous reaction. A reason for this is
(a) ATP readily ionizes
(b) electrostatic repulsion in ATP is lower than that in ADP
(c) ATP is better hydrated than the total hydration levels of ADP and Pi
(d) resonance stabilization of P-O bonds in Pi is higher than that in ATP

10. A beam of light passes through 1 cm of a colored solution. Eighty percent of the incident light is transmitted. If the incident light passes through 2cm of the same solution, the percentage of transmitted light is
(a) 60 (b) 64 (c) 70 (d) 40

11. Lactose uptake in *E.coli* is an example of
(a) Passive transport
(b) Primary active transport
(c) Secondary active transport
(d) Simple diffusion

12. During receptor-mediated endocytosis of LDL bound to its receptor
(*a*) both receptor and ligand are degraded
(*b*) the receptor is degraded and the ligand is recycled
(*c*) both are recycled
(*d*) the ligand is degraded and the receptor is recycled

13. Choose the correct pairs from the following:
A. Isocitrate lyase
B. PEP carboxykinase
C. Pyruvate dehydrogenase complex
D. Phosphofructokinase
E. Pyruvate carboxylase
i. Conversion of amino acids into glucose
ii. Biotin
iii. Synthesis of glucose from acetate
iv. Lipoic acid
v. An allosteric enzyme
(*a*) A-i, B-ii, C-iv, D-v, E-iii
(*b*) A-iii, B-i, C-iv, D-v, E-ii
(*c*) A- iii, B- i, C-iv, D-ii, E-v
(*d*) A-ii, B-v, C- i, D-iv, E-iii

14. The advantage of hemoglobin having a high histidine content is
(*a*) histidine binds to oxygen
(*b*) histidine carries oxygen to the tissues
(*c*) histidine imparts buffering capacity to hemoglobin
(*d*) 'R' group of histidine has low pKa.

15. IgG has four chains. Purified monoclonal IgG was subjected to electrophoresis. The number of bands visible by
A. Reducing SDS-PAGE
B. Isoelectric focusing
C. Native PAGE
(*a*) A-2; B-1; C-1 (*b*) A-1;B-1; C-2
(c) A-2; B-4; C-2 (*d*) A-4; B-2; C-4

16. When *E.coli* is grown in glucose and lactose, the *lac* operon is not expressed. This is because glucose interferes with
(*a*) removal of repressor
(*b*) binding of activator
(*c*) removal of repressor and binding of activator
(*d*) removal of activator.

17. What property of biomembranes is responsible for their self-sealing nature?
(*a*) Hydrophilicity of the phospholipid head group
(*b*) Presence of proteins in biomembranes
(*c*) Presence of cholesterol in biomembranes
(*d*) Hydrophobicity of the fatty acid side chains of phospholipids

18. A mixture of amino acids consisting of glycine, lysine, arginine, histidine, aspartic acid and glutamic acid was placed in the centre of a paper strip, moistened with buffer of pH 6 and electric current applied. The migration of amino acids was as follows:
(*a*) Glycine, lysine and histidine moved towards the anode. Aspartic acid and glutamic acid moved towards the cathode while arginine remained near the origin
(*b*) Aspartic acid and glutamic acid remained near the origin and lysine, histidine and glycine moved towards the anode while arginine moved towards the cathode.
(*c*) Glycine remained near the origin. Lysine, arginine and histidine moved towards the cathode while aspartic acid and glutamic acid moved towards the anode.
(*d*) All amino acids remained near the origin.

19. Cells expressing Epidermal Growth Factor (EGF) receptors were treated (T) or untreated (U) with EGF. The cells were lysed and immunoprecipitated with EGF receptor-specific antibodies. The immunoprecipitate was analyzed by Western blotting with antibodies specific to
i. phosphotryrosine ii. phosphothreonine
iii. tryosine kinases iv. threonine kinases
which of these antibodies would detect a band under T and U conditions?
(*a*) T-i & iii; U - iii (*b*) T - ii & iv; U - iv
(*c*) T-i & ii; U-i (*d*) T - i & iii; U - ii

20. Which of the following would be considered the longest feedback loop?
(*a*) Reproductive steroid hormones .... aminergic neurons
(*b*) Reproductive steroid hormones .... hypothalamic neurons
(*c*) Reproductive steroid hormones........ pituitary gonadotrophs
(*d*) Gonadotropin releasing hormone .... hypothalamic neurons

21. In *myasthenia gravis*, a neuromuscular disorder, the *acetylcholine* receptor becomes dysfunctional because
(*a*) the receptor is mutated
(*b*) antibodies to the receptor inhibit ligand binding
(*c*) of deficiency in acetylcholine transferase
(*d*) of excess of acetylcholine esterase.

K: BOTANY

Q.1 – 7 carry one mark each.

1. Kyoto protocol is related to
(*a*) Acid rain
(*b*) Photochemical smog
(*c*) Ozone hole
(*d*) Global warming

2. Phagotrophs are
   (*a*) Organisms that feed on dead organic matter
   (*b*) Organisms that absorb dissolved organic matter
   (*c*) Organisms that ingest other organisms or particulate organic matter
   (*d*) Organisms that manufacture food from simple inorganic substances

3. Identify the **INCORRECT** statement:
   (*a*) 2,4-dichlorophenoxyacetic acid (2,4-D) is the most commonly used chemical analogue of indole-3-acetic acid.
   (*b*) In somatic embryogenesis, embryo initiation needs a high concentration of 2, 4-D.
   (*c*) Crown-gall disease depends on the presence of Ti-plasmid in *Agrobacterium tumefaciens.*
   (*d*) *Agrobacterium tumefaciens* is responsible for hairy root formation in plants.

4. Choose the correct relation between Angstrom (Å) and nanometer (nm)
   (*a*) 1Å = 10^1 nm (*b*) 1Å = 10^{-1} nm
   (*c*) 1Å = 10^{-2} nm (*d*) 1Å = 10^2 nm

5. In hypogynous flower
   (*a*) Ovary occupies the highest position on the thallamus
   (*b*) Ovary may be partially sunken in the thallamus
   (*c*) Ovary is completely sunken in the thallamus
   (*d*) Ovary is naked

6. Fill up the blanks with appropriate matches.
   The main axis of the inflorescence is known as________and the stalk of the individual flower is called__________.
   (*a*) Pedicel and Panicle (*b*) Panicle and Pedicel
   (*c*) Pedicel and Peduncle (*d*) Peduncle and Pedicel

7. Microorganisms responsible for nitrification are
   (*a*) *Nitrosomonas and Nitrobacter*
   (*b*) *Nostoc and Anabaena*
   (*c*) *Rhizobium and Azotobacter*
   (*d*) *Clostridium and Pseudomonas*

Q.8 to 21 carry two marks each.

8. Identify the amino acids in the following peptide chain :

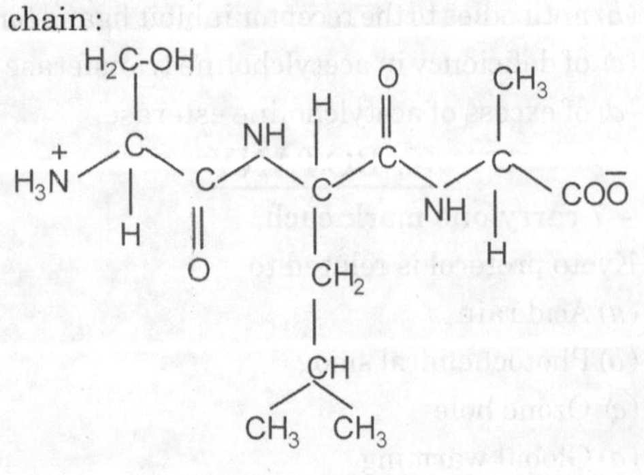

   P. Iso-Leu-Ala Q. Leu-Iso-Asn
   R. Ser-Leu-Ala S. Ser-Pro-Gln
   (*a*) P (*b*) Q (*c*) R (*d*) S

9. Identify the **CORRECT** statements:
   P. Vernalization is the process where flowering is promoted by heat shock
   Q. The four different types of floral organs are initiated as separate whorls
   R. The flowering stimulus is transported to the meristem via the xylem
   S. Abscisic acid synthesis occurs via the carotenoid biosynthetic pathway
   (*a*) P, Q (*b*) Q, S (*c*) R, S (*d*) P, R

10. Which of the following statements are **INCORRECT?**
   P. The frequency of recombination is a measure of linkage between genes on the same chromosome.
   Q. DNA polymerase I is the true DNA replicase in *E. coli.*
   R. The conserved element closest to the transcription initiation site is called the CAAT box.
   S. The introns is the nuclear pre-mRNAs are excised by spliceosomes.
   (*a*) P, Q (*b*) Q, R (*c*) P, R (*d*) P, S

11. Which of the following statements are **TRUE** for transposable genetic elements?
   P. IS elements can be inserted at many different sites in bacterial chromosomes and plasmids.
   Q. In Tn5 the flanking IS elements are in the same orientation.
   R. The *Ac* and *Ds* elements in maize were discovered by Barbara McClintock.
   S. Tn10 consists of two IS elements flanking a gene for streptomycin resistance.
   (*a*) P, Q (*b*) P, R
   (*c*) P, S (*d*) R, S

Direction (Q. 12 – 20) : *In each question, each item P, Q, R and S in Group I matches one of the items in Group II. Choose the correct match from the alternatives a, b, c and d.*

12. Floral formula is a method of describing a plant specimen in which the morphological characters are represented by symbols. Identify the correct matches:

Group I	Group II
P. ♂	1. Zygomorphic
Q. ⊕	2. Male flower
R. CA	3. Epipetalous
S. $\underline{(\ )}$	4. Actinomorphic
	5. Superior ovary
	6. Inferior ovary

   (*a*) P-2, Q-4, R-3, S-5 (*b*) P-1, Q-6, R-5, S-2
   (*c*) P-2, Q-4, R-3, S-6 (*d*) P-6, Q-4, R-1, S-3

13. Identify the pathways where the following reactions occur:

Group I

P. Fatty acid + GTP + Co A $\rightleftharpoons$ Acyl–CoA + GDP+Pi

Q. NH_3 + Glutamate + ATP $\rightleftharpoons$ Glutamine + ADP+Pi

R. Succinate+E–FAD $\rightleftharpoons$ Fumarate + E–$FADH_2$

S. Malonyl-S-CoA + ACP – SH $\rightleftharpoons$ Malonyl–S–ACP + CoA-SH

Group II

1. Fatty acid synthesis
2. Fatty acid oxidation
3. Oxidative phosphorylation
4. Citric acid cycle
5. Gluconeogenesis
6. Amino acid biosynthesis

(*a*) P-5, Q-3, R-4, S-6
(*b*) P-1, Q-2, R-5, S-6
(*c*) P-3, Q-2, K-6, S-1
(*d*) P-2, Q-6, R-4, S-1

14.

Group I	Group II
P. *Ricinus communis*	1. Rice bran oil
Q. *Jatropha curcas*	2. Mahua oil
R. *Pongamia pinnata*	3. Sim-flower oil
S. *Madhuca indica*	4. Castor oil
	5. Karanja oil
	6. Jatropha oil

(*a*) P-4, Q-6, R-5, S-2
(*b*) P-1, Q-6, R-4, S-5
(*c*) P-3, Q-6, R-5, S-2
(*d*) P-1, Q-6, R-5, S-2

15. **Group I**

P. Förster mechanism
Q. Ping-Pong reaction
R. Feed-back inhibition
S. DNA recombination

Group II

1. The initial product inhibit the initial reaction
2. The accumulation of end product inhibit the initial reaction
3. Process of exciton transfer in chromophore molecule
4. Double displacement reaction
5. Michaelis-Menten enzyme kinetics
6. Holliday model

(*a*) P-5, Q-4, R-2, S-6 (*b*) P-2, Q-3, R-4, S-6
(*c*) P-3, Q-4, R-2, S-6 (*d*) P-6, Q-5, R-4, S-1

16.

Group I	Group II
P. AG ↓ CT TC ↑ GA	1. *Eco*RI
Q. GTPy ↓ PuAC CAPu ↑ PyTG	2. *Alu*I
R. C ↓ C G G G G C ↑ C	3. *Hpa*II
S. A ↓ AGCTT TTC GA ↑ A	4. *Hind*III
	5. *Pst*I
	6. *Hinc*II

(*a*) P-1, Q-5, R-6, S-3 (*b*) P-2, Q-6, R-3, S-4
(*c*) P-1, Q-6, R-4, S-2 (*d*) P-1, Q-2, R-6, S-3

17.

Group I	Group II
P. Linnaeus	1. *Flora Indica*
Q. William Roxburgh	2. *Genera Plantarum*
R. Bentham-Hooker	3. Artificial-sexual system
S. Engler	4. Sero diagnostic system
	5. Phylogenetic system
	6. *The Families of Flowering Plants*

(*a*) P-2, Q-4, R-3, S-5 (*b*) P-1, Q-6, R-5, S-2
(*c*) P-3, Q-1, R-5, S-6 (*d*) P-3, Q-1, R-2, S-5

18.

Group I	Group II
P. Monarch butterfly	1. Gene-gene matching
Q. Horizontal resistance	2. Bt. crops
R. Supper weed	3. Polygenic trait
S. Biolistics	4. Tungsten/gold
	5. Herbicide resistance
	6. Pusztai affair

(*a*) P-2, Q-3, R-5, S-4 (*b*) P-2, Q-6, R-5, S-4
(*c*) P-2, Q-6, R-5, S-1 (*d*) P-6, Q-4, R-1, S-3

19.

Group I	Group II
P. Water transport	1. Hydathodes
Q. Guttation	2. Xylem
R. Harting net	3. Arbuscules
S. Secondary active transport	4. Ectotrophic micorrhizal fungi
	5. Proton motive force
	6. Lenticels

(*a*) P-2, Q-1, R-4, S-5
(*b*) P-1, Q-6, R-5, S-2
(*c*) P-2, Q-6, R-4, S-5
(*d*) P-6, Q-4, R-1, S-3

20.

Group I	Group II
P. Tobacco leaf curl *bigeminivirus*	1. *Culex tarsalis*
Q. Cauliflower mosaic *caulimovirus*	2. *Rhopalosiphum maidis*
R. Rice tungro bacilli-form *badnavirus*	3. *Bemisia tabaci*
S. Wheat yellow leaf *closterovirus*	4. *Periplaneta americana*
	5. *Nephotettis sp.*
	6. *Brevicoryne brassicae*

(*a*) P-2, Q-3, R-6, S-4 (*b*) P-3, Q-6, R-5, S-2
(*c*) P-3, Q-4, R-6, S-5 (*d*) P-2, Q-4, R-5, S-6

21. Identify which of the following statements are INCORRECT?
P. *Rhizoctonia solani* causes seedling blight of wheat
Q. *Gebberella zeae* causes root rot of wheat
R. *Phytopthera infestans* causes late blight of potato
S. *Tilletia caries* causes blunt of wheat
(*a*) P, Q (*b*) P, R (*c*) P, S (*d*) Q, S

L : MICROBIOLOGY

Q.1 – 7 carry one mark each.

1. Which of the following scientists are associated with the discoveries listed below?

P. Identification of DNA as the genetic material	1. Fleming
Q. Discovery of penicillin	2. Avery
R. Demonstration of bacterial transformation	3. Beijerink
S. Demonstration of filterable infectious agent	4. Griffith

	P	Q	R	S
(*a*)	2	1	4	3
(*b*)	2	3	1	4
(*c*)	2	4	1	3
(*d*)	2	1	3	4

2. Density of cells of a bacterial culture is routinely measured using Spectrophotometer. This is based on the principle of
(*a*) Light absorption (*b*) Light diffraction
(*c*) Light scattering (*d*) Light reflection

3. Which one of the following life styles does Rhizobium species adopt to fix molecular nitrogen to ammonia?
(*a*) Both symbiotic as well as non symbiotic
(*b*) Only symbiotic
(*c*) Only non-symbiotic
(*d*) Only commensalism

4. A tryptophan auxotrophic Hfr strain of *E. coli* is mixed with F^- histidine auxotroph and plated on to minimal medium to select for prototrophs. The prototrophs are formed due to
(*a*) Conjugation (*b*) Transduction
(*c*) Transformation (*d*) Transfection

5. Identify the correct pair of amino acids which differ only by an atom in the side chain (R) group.
(*a*) Gly-Ala (*b*) Ser-Cys
(*c*) Met-Leu (*d*) Ser-Asp

6. Which one of the following antibiotics inhibits protein biosynthesis precisely by blocking the peptidy transfer stage?
(*a*) Bleomycin (*b*) Rifampicin
(*c*) Chloramphenicol (*d*) Tetracycline

7. Pseudopeptidoglycan is present in the cell wall of
(*a*) *Escherichia coli*
(*b*) *Bacillus subtilis*
(*c*) *Saccharomyces cerevisiae*
(*d*) *Methanococcus jannaschii*

(Q.8 – 21) carry two marks each.

8. A wild type strain of *E.Coli* growing on a mixture of glucose and acetate shows a typical biphasic diauxic growth. A mutant strain was isolated and was found not to exhibit the second phase of diauxic growth. This mutant is likely to be defective in
(*a*) Pyruvate decarboxylase
(*b*) Isocitrate lyase
(*c*) Glucose-6-phosphate dehydrogenase
(*d*) Phosphoglucose isomerase

9. Which one of the following approaches would be appropriate if one wants to cultivate microorganisms under constant physiological conditions?
(*a*) Fed batch culture (*b*) Batch culture
(*c*) Continuous culture (*d*) Discontinuous culture

10. Which one of the following bacterial toxins does NOT have ADP ribosylation activity?
(*a*) Diphtheria toxin
(*b*) Cholera toxin
(*c*) S. aureus α-toxin
(*d*) Pseudomonas exotoxin

11. The high frequency of recombinants obtained from a cross between Hfr and F^- strains is because
(*a*) the F factor integrated into the chromosome mediates transfer of large regions of chromosome into the recipient
(*b*) the strain bears high number of F pilli on its surface
(*c*) there are high number of copies of the F plasmid per cell
(*d*) it induces recombination at high rate

12. A silent mutation is one that
(*a*) results in a truncated polypeptide
(*b*) replaces an amino acid with an equivalent amino acid in polypeptide
(*c*) does not change the amino acid sequence of the polypeptide
(*d*) changes the reading frame of the mRNA leading to an altered polypeptide

13. The rotatory motion of bacterial flagellum is driven by
(*a*) energy obtained through hydrolysis of ATP
(*b*) trans-membrane electrochemical potential linked to proton pumping
(*c*) direct uptake of extra-cellular nutrients
(*d*) concentration gradient of nutrients in the environment

14. Which one of the following metabolic intermediate is involved in the biosynthesis of Phenylalanine and Tyrosine in bacteria?
(*a*) Chorismate (*b*) Pantothenate
(*c*) α-ketobutyrate (*d*) Indole-3-phosphate

15. The DNA mixture containing unlabelled and N^{15} labelled DNA from phage T4 was denatured and allowed to reanneal. How many bands one would observe upon Cs Cl_2 density gradient centrifugation of the above mixture?
(*a*) 0 (*b*) 1
(*c*) 2 (*d*) 3

16. A temperate phage differs from a virulent phage in that, temperate phage
(*a*) can exhibit only lytic cycle
(*b*) can choose between lytic and lysogenic cycle
(*c*) can exhibit only lysogenic cycle
(*d*) engages in lysogenic cycle only at high temperature

17. RecA is a protein involved in
(*a*) Recombinational repair
(*b*) Mismatch repair
(*c*) Nucleotide excision repair
(*d*) Base excision repair

18. In which of the following bacterium, chemical energy is converted to both mechanical as well as light energy?
(*a*) *Vibrio Fischeri*
(*b*) *Bacillus subtilis*
(*c*) *Escherichia coli*
(*d*) *Pseudomonas fluorescence*

19. Initial density of a culture of bacteria with a generation time of 30 minutes was 1×10^5 cells/ml. After 5 hours of incubation, what serial dilution will you have to plate out to get~100 colonies per ml.?
(*a*) 10^3 (*b*) 10^4
(*c*) 10^5 (*d*) 10^6

20. Effective chemotherapeutic agents are difficult to develop for the treatment of fungal infection because
(*a*) Fungi have cell wall
(*b*) Fungi have better mechanisms to inactivate drugs
(*c*) Fungi are eucaryotic cells and their cellular machinery is similar to that of the host
(*d*) Fungal pathogens typically infect organs inaccessible for antibiotic treatment.

21. Which one of the following is NOT the criterion for using ribosomal RNAs as evolutionary chronometers?
(*a*) The large size of Ribosomal RNAs, gives large number of possible sequence combination.
(*b*) Ribosomal RNAs are functionally invariant.
(*c*) Ribosomal RNAs are universally distributed.
(*d*) Ribosomal RNAs have enzyme activity.

M: ZOOLOGY

(Q. 1 – 7) carry one mark each

1. In an normal animal cell, the extra-chromosomal DNA is
(*a*) Single stranded circular
(*b*) Single stranded linear
(*c*) Double stranded circular
(*d*) Double stranded linear

2. Which of the following is NOT a somite derivative?
(*a*) Cardiac muscle (*b*) Skeletal muscle
(*c*) Cartilage (*d*) Tendons

3. During hibernation in a hibernating mammal, its body temperature would be
(*a*) Lower than normal state
(*b*) Same as normal state
(*c*) Higher than normal state
(*d*) Fluctuate between high and low points

4. Mendel's principle of segregation means that the germ cells (egg or sperm) always receive
(*a*) One of the paired alleles
(*b*) One pair of alleles
(*c*) One quarter of the genes
(*d*) Any pair of alleles

5. Cholera toxin acts by
(*a*) Activating a G-protein
(*b*) Blocking an ion channel
(*c*) Activating synaptic transmission
(*d*) Blocking glycolysis

6. Which of the following statements does NOT describe the characteristics of human population in industrialize countries?
(*a*) Relatively small family size
(*b*) Relatively even age structure
(*c*) Rapid reproduction rate
(*d*) Delayed reproduction

7. Sex-linkage refers to
   (*a*) Inheritance of genes linked to sex determination
   (*b*) The ratio of genes on the autosome and sex chromosomes
   (*c*) Inheritance of genes carried on the sex chromosomes
   (*d*) Linkage of genes present on the sex chromosomes

(Q. 8 – 21) carry two marks each.

8. Increase in the emission of fossil is thought to result in global warming. This is possible because an increase in atmospheric CO_2 level would
   (*a*) Increase the amount of sun light entering the earth atmosphere
   (*b*) Increase the amount of infrared radiation entering the earth
   (*c*) Absorb the infrared radiation reflected by the earth
   (*d*) Insulate earth from cold breeze coming from the space

9. Anabolic steroids, taken illegally by sportspersons to enhance their physical strength, are synthetic analogues from natural_____from the_____
   (*a*) testosterone............anterior pituitary
   (*b*) FSH and LH..........posterior pituitary
   (*c*) Cortisol................thyroid
   (*d*) androgen............gonads

10. Holometabolous insects go through a series of larval instars before molting into pupal stage, and into an adult. This developmental is regulated by three key hormones namely, brain hormone, ecdysone, and juvenile hormone. The main function of brain hormones is to
   (*a*) Stimulate the prothoracic gland to secrete ecdysone
   (*b*) Stimulate the corpus allatum to secrete juvenile hormone
   (*c*) Arrest the release of ecdysone by prothoracic gland
   (*d*) Stimulate the release of juvenile hormone by prothoracic gland

11. Homology in anatomical parts helps in determining evolutionary kinship because
   (*a*) Homologous body parts invariably perform similar functions
   (*b*) Display evolutionary adaptations
   (*c*) Undergo similar genetic changes
   (*d*) Have common embryological Origin

12. Which of the following does NOT explain the term "survival of the fittest"?
   (*a*) Fittest animals leave higher number of progeny than those which perish
   (*b*) Fittest group of animals out populates its competitors
   (*c*) Fittest animals are best predators
   (*d*) Fittest group is rich in genetic variation

13. In a coral island in Atlantic Ocean, a natural calamity killed most of its population. The island is repopulated with the surviving individuals and their progeny. The present day population in the island shows high incidence of a rare recessive genetic disorder. What could be the most probable evolutionary force responsible for this phenomenon?
   (*a*) Geographical isolation
   (*b*) Genetic drift
   (*c*) Selective advantage of the recessive disorder
   (*d*) Natural selection

14. The human immune system is able to mount a response when it encounters a novel microorganism for the first time because
   (*a*) White blood cells are able to change their antigen specificity depending upon the microorganism they interact with.
   (*b*) Our body contains million of different kinds of white blood cells, each with a unique type of antigen receptor.
   (*c*) Bone marrow cells make different antigen receptors depending upon the kind of invading microorganism.
   (*d*) Bone marrow cells are able to change their antigen specificity upon physical interaction with the microorganism

15. Acetylcholinesterase is an enzyme that degrades acetylcholine. What would be the effect of administration of an inhibitor of acetylcholinesterase on nerve transmission?
   (*a*) No effect
   (*b*) Synaptic transmission will be prevented
   (*c*) Extra excitatory postsynaptic potentials would occur in the postsynaptic neuron
   (*d*) The presynaptic neuron will be inactivated

16. Which one of the following comparison between oogenesis and spermatogenesis in human is NOT correct?
   (*a*) FSH promotes development of both eggs as well as sperms
   (*b*) LH triggers ovulation in ovary and androgen production in testis
   (c) Primary oocytes and primary spermatocytes follow similar pattern of development through meiosis
   (*d*) An ovum is not produced until it fuses with the sperm whereas sperm is produced even in the absence of the ovum

17. Match the parasitic species with their correct hosts.

P. *Schistosoma mansoni*	1. snails
Q. *Trichinella spiralis*	2. human
R. *Plasmodium*	3. mosquito
S. *Taenia solium*	4. pig

   (*a*) P-1, Q-2, R-3, S-4 (*b*) P-4, Q-3, R-2, S-1
   (*c*) P-2, Q-1, R-3, S-4 (*d*) P-3, Q-4, R-1, S-2

18. Match the embryonic cleavage patterns with the corresponding organisms

P. Isolecithal	1. Chick
Q. Mesolecithal	2. Drosophila
R. Telolecithal	3. Human
S. Centrolecithal	4. Frog

(*a*) P-1, Q-2, R-3, S-4 (*b*) P-2, Q-1, R-3, S-4
(*c*) P-3, Q-4, R-1, S-2 (*d*) P-2, Q-4, R-1, S-3

19. Which combination of the following statements with regard to gene expression is true?
1. Heteronuclear RNA represents contiguous segment of genomic DNA.
2. UTRs are part of heteronuclear RNA but not of mRNA.
3. UTRs are part of exons.
4. Translation start codon MUST be in the first exon.

(*a*) 1-true, 2-false, 3-false, 4-false
(*b*) 1-true, 2-false, 3-true, 4-false
(*c*) 1-true, 2-true, 3-false, 4-true
(*d*) 1-false, 2-true, 3-true, 4-true

20. Which of the following combination of statements regarding Maturation Promoting Factor (MPF) is TRUE?
1. MPF in amphibians regulates cell cycle.
2. MPF in amphibians is composed of cyclins and CDKs.
3. MPF in amphibians undergoes periodic degradation.
4. MPF in amphibians undergoes periodic phosphorylation.

(*a*) 1, 2 and 3 only (*b*) 1 and 4 only
(*c*) 2 and 3 only (*d*) 1, 2, 3 and 4

21. Which of the following combination of statements regarding gastrulation is TRUE?
1. It is marked by coordinated mass cell movement.
2. It results in the formation of organizer.
3. It results in the formation of three germ layers.
4. It marks the end of neurulation.

(*a*) 1 and 3 only (*b*) 1 and 2 only
(*c*) 2 and 3 only (*d*) 1, 2, 3 and 4

ANSWERS

H : CHEMISTRY

1. (*d*)	2. (*a*)	3. (*c*)	4. (*b*)	5. (*b*)	6. (*a*)	7. (*b*)	8. (*a*)	9. (*d*)	10. (*a*)
11. (*c*)	12. (*c*)	13. (*c*)	14. (*a*)	15. (*b*)	16. (*c*)	17. (*c*)	18. (*a*)		

I : BIOCHEMISTRY

1. (*a*)	2. (*a*)	3. (*b*)	4. (*d*)	5. (*d*)	6. (*c*)	7. (*d*)	8. (*c*)	9. (*d*)	10. (*d*)
11. (*c*)	12. (*d*)	13. (*b*)	14. (*c*)	15. (*a*)	16. (*c*)	17. (*d*)	18. (*c*)	19. (*d*)	20. (*b*)
21. (*b*)									

K : BOTANY

1. (*d*)	2. (*c*)	3. (*d*)	4. (*b*)	5. (*a*)	6. (*d*)	7. (*a*)	8. (*c*)	9. (*b*)	10. (*b*)
11. (*a*)	12. (*a*)	13. (*d*)	14. (*a*)	15. (*c*)	16. (*b*)	17. (*d*)	18. (*a*)	19. (*a*)	20. (*b*)
21. (*a*)									

L : MICROBIOLOGY

1. (*a*)	2. (*a*)	3. (*b*)	4. (*a*)	5. (*b*)	6. (*c*)	7. (*d*)	8. (*b*)	9. (*c*)	10. (*c*)
11. (*a*)	12. (*c*)	13. (*b*)	14. (*a*)	15. (*d*)	16. (*b*)	17. (*a*)	18. (*a*)	19. (*d*)	20. (*c*)
21. (*d*)									

M : ZOOLOGY

1. (*c*)	2. (*d*)	3. (*a*)	4. (*a*)	5. (*a*)	6. (*b*)	7. (*c*)	8. (*c*)	9. (*d*)	10. (*a*)
11. (*d*)	12. (*a*)	13. (*c*)	14. (*b*)	15. (*b*)	16. (*d*)	17. (*a*)	18. (*c*)	19. (*a*)	20. (*d*)
21. (*d*)									

EXPLANATIONS

H : CHEMISTRY

1. The half life of any reaction is the amount of time it takes to consume half of the starting material. For a second-order reaction, the half-life is inversely related to the initial concentration of the reactant (A). For a second-order reaction each half-life is twice as long as the life span of the one before. The integrated rate equation for 2nd order is:

$$\frac{1}{[A]_t} - \frac{1}{[A]_0} = kt$$

Since, $[A]_t = \frac{1}{2}[A]_0$ when $t = t_{1/2}$. Therefore, the integrated rate equation becomes:

$$\frac{1}{\frac{1}{2}[A]_0} - \frac{1}{[A]_0} = kt_{1/2}$$

Which can be further simplified to obtain the final equation:

$$\frac{2}{[A]_0} - \frac{1}{[A]_0} = kt_{1/2}$$

$$\Rightarrow \quad \frac{1}{[A]_0} = kt_{1/2}$$

The equation for the half life of the 2nd order reaction will be:

$$t_{1/2} = \frac{1}{k[A]_0}$$

2. The total entropy change (system + surroundings) is always greater than or equal to zero for any change of state of the system. The most efficient processes possible for converting energy from one form to another are processes where the net entropy change of the system and the surroundings is zero. It is stated that the entropy of a system in isolation is greater than zero for an irreversible process while for reversible process, it is zero. This is because entropy is randomness or change in the system. In case of a reversible process, there is no net change in the system. So entropy, S = 0. While, in case of an irreversible system, there is always change in the system. That is why entropy in such a system will always be, S > 0. The correct relation between the two entropy changes ΔS_{12}^{rev} and ΔS_{12}^{irrev} is:

$$\Delta S_{12}^{irrev} > \Delta S_{12}^{rev}.$$

3. One way to predict the way electrons within atoms will repel each other is to apply the VSEPR (valence-shell electron-pair repulsion) model. VSEPR can be used to determine a molecule's general geometry. Bond angles are predicted in the following order: lone pair versus lone pair repulsion > lone pair versus bonding pair repulsion > bonding pair versus bonding pair repulsion. Valence Shell Electron Pair Repulsion Theory (VSEPR) is a molecular model to predict the geometry of the atoms making up a molecule where the electrostatic forces between a molecule s valence electrons are minimized around a central atom. According to VSEPR theory,

$(CH_3)_3N \rightarrow$ pyramidal, $[SO_4]^{2-} \rightarrow$ tetrahedral, $[CO_3]^{2-} \rightarrow$ planar trigonal, $PCl_3 \rightarrow$ pyramidal.

Thus, carbonate ion has planar geometry.

4. There are four things attached to the Pt ion. Since NH_3 is neutral, Cl^- has a negative charge, but the compound is neutral, the Pt ion must have a +2 charge. The presence of the chloride ions indicate that this is Pt (II), which makes platinum d8. While metals with other electron counts usually prefer being 6-coordinate, d-8 metal ions [Ir (I), Pt (II), Pd (II), Rh (I), etc.] often go four-coordinate due to orbital reorganization. This minimizes the energy of all the occupied orbitals (with 8 *d* electrons, four of the five *d* orbitals will be occupied) by minimizing the energy of all orbitals having a *z* component. The z-component results in a single isomer for Pt $(NH_3)_2 Cl_2$.

5. In a primary (1°) carbocation, the carbon which carries the positive charge is only attached to one other alkyl group. In a secondary (2°) carbocation, the carbon with the positive charge is attached to two other alkyl groups, which may be the same or different. In a tertiary (3°) carbocation, the positive carbon atom is attached to three alkyl groups, which may be any combination of same or different. The general stability order of simple alkyl carbocations is: (most stable) $3^0 > 2^0 > 1^0 >$ methyl (least stable). This is because alkyl groups are weakly electron donating due to hyperconjugation and inductive effects. Resonance effects can further stabilise carbocations when present. In the given question, $CH_3OCH_2CH_2^+$ is stabilised by the –I effect of the –OCH_2 group present in it. $CH_3CH{=}CHCH_2^+$ is stabilised by resonance in between CH_2^+ group and the '=' bond. The $CH_3CH_2^+$ molecule is destabilised by the +I effect of the –CH_3 group. In the last compound, $CH_3COCH_2^+$, it is being stabilised by the –I effect of C=O group present in it. Thus, the carbocation with resonance stability renders the maximum stability and minimum reactivity. So, that carbocation is $CH_3CH{=}CHCH_2^+$.

6. The K_a value is a value used to describe the tendency of compounds or ions to dissociate. The K_a value is also called the dissociation constant, the ionisation constant, and the acid constant. The pK_a value is related to the Ka value in a logic way. The pK_a values are easier to remember than K_a values and pK_a values are in many cases easier to use than K_a values for fast approximations of concentrations of compounds and ions in equilibriums. The definition of K_a is: $[H^+].[B]/[HB]$, where B is the conjugate base of the acid HB. In the given question, the lowest pK_a value among the compounds is $C_6H_5CO_2H$. This is because it has the highest K_a value due to its –COOH group which contributes to the highest level of acidity.

7. A Hydrogen atom consists of a proton and an electron which are "bound" together – the proton (positive charge) and electron (negative charge) stay together and continually interact with each other. If the electron escapes, the Hydrogen atom (now a single proton) is positively ionized. Similarly, the Hydrogen atom can sometimes bind another electron to it. Such a Hydrogen atom is negatively ionized. Because the states an electron occur only at discrete energy levels, they are said to be quantized. The word quantum comes from a Latin word meaning "how much". The branch of physics that provides the current model of the Hydrogen atom is called quantum mechanics. The electron in a Hydrogen atom can only have certain energies. These energies are called the Hydrogen's "energy levels". The different energy levels of Hydrogen are denoted by the quantum number n where n varies from 1 for the ground state. With this convention, the different energy levels of a Hydrogen atom are given by the equation:

$$E = -E_0/n^2$$

where E_0 = 13.6 eV (1 eV = 1.602×10^{-19} Joules) and n = 1, 2, 3... and so on so that the ground state has energy E_1= –13.6 eV and the second energy level (the first excited state) has energy E_2 = –13.6/4 eV = –3.4 eV. In this case, $E_0 = \varepsilon$

Therefore, the ionisation energy of the electron of Hydrogen atom at 3rd energy level is given by

$$|E| = \frac{\varepsilon}{3^2} = \frac{\varepsilon}{9}$$

8. Given, $\frac{1}{2}$ $Fe^{2+} + e^- \rightarrow \frac{1}{2}$ Fe (s),

$$E^0 = -0.440V \quad ...(I)$$

$Fe^{3+} + e^- \rightarrow Fe^{2+}$,

$$E^0 = +0.771 \text{ V} \quad ...(II)$$

Multiplying the 1st equation with 2 and adding with second equation we have,

$Fe^{2+} + 2e^- + Fe^{3+} + e^- \rightarrow Fe(s) + Fe^{2+}$

$\Rightarrow Fe^{3+} + 3e^- \rightarrow Fe(s)$

So, the net standard electrode potential,

$$\Delta E^0 = 2 \times E^0(I) + E^0(II)$$
$$= -0.880 + 0.771 \text{ V}$$
$$= -0.109 \text{ V}$$

Therefore, the standard electrode potential at 25°C,

$$\Delta E^0 = -nFE^0$$

Or $-0.109 = -3 \times 1 \times E^0$

$$\Rightarrow \quad E^0 = \frac{0.109}{3} = 0.03633$$

So the required potential is 0.03633 V

9. Given, the reaction

$$(CH_3)_2CHCH_2Br \xrightarrow{NaOEt/\ EtOH} Q$$

Use of alcoholic KOH or NaOEt/ EtOH, will result in elimination (dehydrohalogenation). Elimination converts an alkyl halide into an alkene. In this reaction a halogen atom is lost from one carbon and hydrogen at the next carbon.

Mechanism of nucleophilic substitution reactions → The S_N1 and S_N2 mechanisms

$$R-X \quad + \quad \overset{\ominus}{O}H \rightleftharpoons R-OH \quad + \quad \overset{\ominus}{X}$$

R is an alkyl group X is a halogen

Now, in the given question, the dehydrohalogenation elimination reaction occurs at the bromo position of the 2methyl bromo propane. But because of steric hindrance due to the two bulky methyl groups, the alcohol product is the minor product and the major product is the alkene: which is $(CH_3)_2C = CH_2$ with the elimination of HBr.

10. If a silver nitrate solution is added to a potassium chloride solution and a precipitate forms, the reaction is:

$AgNO_3$ (aq) + KCl (aq) → KNO_3 (aq) + AgCl (s)

A reaction such as this, when potassium chloride is added to a solution of an appropriate metal ion, will cause the potassium chloride to precipitate insoluble chloride salts. Potassium chloride is metal halide salt composed of potassium and chloride. White and odourless in its pure state, potassium chloride has a crystal structure that cleaves easily in three directions. Crystals within potassium chloride are face-centred cubic, meaning that the cubic crystals have lattice points on the faces of the cube that each gives exactly one half contributions, in addition to the corner lattice points, giving a total of four atoms. Potassium chloride can be used as a fertiliser, which often gives it its name muriate of potash. On further reaction of the white precipitate AgCl with KCl, a coordination complex if formed which leads to dissolution of the precipitate

$$KCl + AgCl \rightarrow K[AgCl_2]$$

So, P is AgCl and Q is $[AgCl_2]^-$

11.

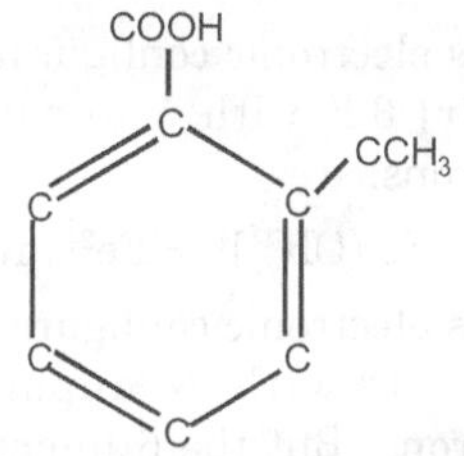

Figure: It is the structure of O-methoxy benzoic acid.

Benzoic acid derivatives substituted by hydroxy group or ether containing oxygen atom have active bacteriostatic and fragrant properties. They are typically used in pharmaceutical and perfumery industry. The destructive metabolic property of oxygen containing benzoic acid derivatives such as protocatechuic acid (3,4-dihydroxybenzoic acid) and veratric acid (3,4-dimethoxybenzoic acid) is used in the application for pharmaceuticals. Protocatechuic acid is a catabolite of epinephrine. Prazosin, a peripheral vasodilator and antihypertensive, is also an example of the application of veratric acid. Hydroxy and ether substituted benzoic acids feature analogue metabolite of aspirin (acetylsalicylic Acid). They are used as intermediates for pharmaceuticals (especially for antipyetic analgesic, antirheumatism) and other organic synthesis. They are used as matrix for ionization of peptides, proteins and carbohydrates. The $-OCH_3$ group is a strongly activating ortho/para directing group while the –COOH group is a moderately deactivating meta directing group. So, the major product of the nitration is:

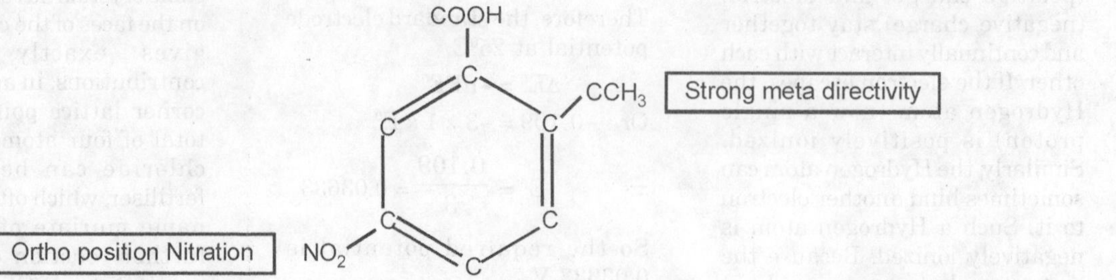

12. Given, $[CoCl_4]^{2-} = Co^{2+}$ atom.

It has an electronic configuration of $[Ar]3d^7$ with 3 unpaired electrons.

$[Fe(H_2O)_6]^{3+} = Fe^{3+}$ atom.

It has electronic configuration of $[Ar]\ 3d^5$ with 5 unpaired electrons.

$[Fe(CN)_6]^{4-} = Fe^{2+}$ atom.

It has electronic configuration $[Ar]\ 3d^6$ with 6 unpaired electrons. But the 6 unpaired electrons pair among themselves because of the strong field ligand CN^-.

We have, Spin magnetic moment,

$$_B = \sqrt{n(n+2)}$$

where n is the number of electrons.

For $[CoCl_4]^{2-}$, $_B = \sqrt{3(3+2)}$

$= \sqrt{15}$ BM

For $[Fe(H_2O)_6]^{3+} = \sqrt{5(5+2)}$

$= \sqrt{35}$ BM

For $[Fe(CN)_6]^{4-} = \sqrt{0(0+2)} = 0$

13. A meso compound contains chirality centres but is identical with its mirror image. This is most easily seen when in a Fischer projection by the fact that the top half of the molecule is the mirror image of the bottom half. For this to be true there must be at least 2 chirality centres because the one in the top half must be the mirror image of the one in the bottom half. Tartaric acid has two chirality centres. Each has an H, an OH, and a carboxyl group, COOH, on it. In Fischer projections, it is customary to have the carbon chain go from top to bottom when possible. The Fisher diagram for tartaric acid is:

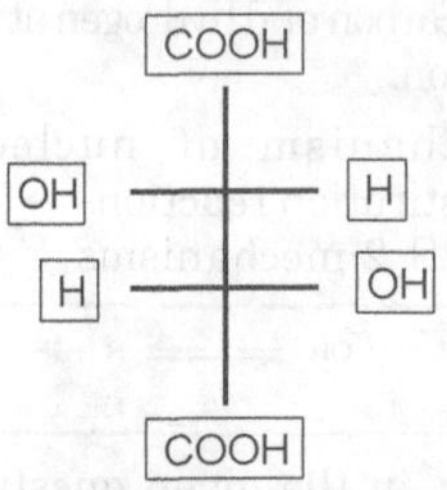

14. Cyclopentadiene is a colourless liquid with an irritating and terpene-like odour. Some properties of it are:

(*i*) Stable at room temperature

(*ii*) Incompatible with oxidizing agents, acids and a wide variety of other compounds

(*iii*) May form peroxides in storage

(*iv*) May undergo spontaneous polymerisation

(*v*) Decomposes on heating

(*vi*) Highly flammable

(*vii*) Mixtures with air are explosive.

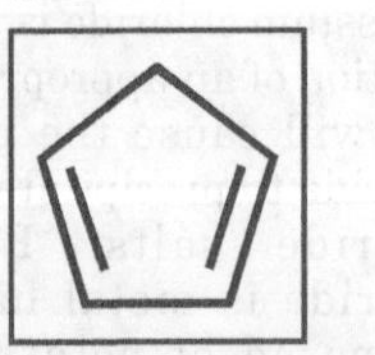

It easily loses a proton from the carbon atom because of the pentacyclic nature of the ring. It is the least stable compound and immediately undergoes deprotonation in a basic medium giving rise to a planar aromatic structure which is more stable (having 6π electrons in the ring).

15. Given, the reaction:

$$P(g) \rightarrow 2\,Q(g)$$

Initially, No. of moles $\rightarrow 1 \quad 0$

At equilibrium, $\rightarrow 1 - x \quad 2x$

Therefore, partial pressure of P,

$$p_P = \frac{(1-x)}{(1+x)} \times P;$$

where P is the total pressure

Partial pressure of Q,

$$p_Q = \frac{2x}{(1+x)} \times P$$

Therefore, equilibrium constant

$$K_p = \frac{[Q]^2}{[P]} = \frac{\left[\frac{2xP}{(1+x)}\right]^2}{\left[\frac{(1-x)P}{(1+x)}\right]}$$

$$= \frac{4x^2P}{(1-x^2)}$$

Given $K_p = 0.25$

When P is converted to 50% Q, $x = 0.5$ moles

Thus, $K_p = 4 \times 0.5^2 \dfrac{P}{(1-0.25)}$

Or $P = 0.25 \times \dfrac{0.75}{(0.25 \times 4)}$

Or $P = 0.1875$

Hence the total pressure is 0.1875 bar.

16. Given, P = 0.5 bar

Therefore, $0.25 = \dfrac{4x^2 0.5}{(1-x^2)}$

$\Rightarrow 0.25 - 0.25\,x^2 = 2x^2$

$\Rightarrow 2.25\,x^2 = 0.25$

$\Rightarrow x^2 = \frac{0.25}{2.25}$

$\Rightarrow x = \frac{0.5}{1.5}$

$\Rightarrow x = 0.3333$

Thus, the conversion of P to Q is 33.33%

17. $NaBH_4$ is a salt, consisting of the tetrahedral BH^{4-} anion. $NaBH_4$ will reduce many organic carbonyls, depending on the precise conditions. It will reduce acyl chlorides, thiol esters and imines. Under typical conditions, it will not reduce esters, amides, or carboxylic acids.

The reaction is $4BF_3 + 3NaBH_4 \rightarrow 2B_2H_6 + 3NaBF_4$. Boron trifluoride on reduction with Sodium tetrahydroborate gives rise to diborane.

18. Diborane, B_2H_6, is a colorless, poisonous, flammable, high-pressure gas mixture. Diborane is largely used in semiconductor manufacturing. Boron atom is a p-type dopant for epitaxial silicon. Boron is introduced in the silicon wafer by diffusion or implantation techniques. Diborane is also used for the production of borophosphosilicate glasses (BPS). Its dominating reaction pattern involves formation of adducts with Lewis bases. Often such initial adducts proceed rapidly to give other products. It reacts with ammonia to form ammonia borane or the diammoniate of diborane, DADB, depending on the conditions used. In the reaction of B_2H_6 with trimethyl amine i.e., Me_3N, the diborane readily forms adduct because of its electron deficiency in the 3d orbital.

$B_2H_6 + Me_3N \rightarrow 2[Me_3N.BH_3]$;

This adduct is the compound Q.

I : BIOCHEMISTRY

1. Pernicious anaemia is a decrease in red blood cells that occurs when the intestine cannot properly absorb vitamin B_{12}. Pernicious anaemia is a chronic illness caused by impaired absorption of vitamin B_{12} because of a lack of intrinsic factor (IF) in gastric secretions. It occurs as a relatively common adult form of anaemia that is associated with gastric atrophy and a loss of IF production and as a rare congenital autosomal recessive form in which IF production is lacking without gastric atrophy.

2. Influenza virus is responsible for causing influenza in human body. *Corynebacterium* affects by causing diphtheria. p-Azobenzenearsonate is a hapten capable of eliciting both antibody formation and delayed hypersensitivity when bound to aromatic amino acids, polypeptides or proteins. It is used as an immunological research tool. These would induce immune response on their entry into the body. Haemocyanin is an oxygen-carrying protein molecule present in certain lower animals, particularly arthropods and molluscs. The molecule is similar to the haemoglobin molecule of human blood but uses copper atoms, rather than iron, and is less efficient than haemoglobin in requiring many more atoms to bind a single molecule of oxygen. Thus, it can be an antigen but it would not induce immune response.

3. Nitric oxide is an important messenger molecule in mammals and other animals. It can be toxic or beneficial, depending on the amount and where in the body it is released. Nitric oxide is produced in the body by an enzyme called nitric oxide synthase, which converts the amino acid L -arginine to nitric oxide and L -citrulline. There are three types of nitric oxide synthase: brain, endothelial, and inducible. Both brain and endothelial enzymes are constitutive, that is, they are always present in cells, while the production of inducible nitric oxide synthase can be turned on or off when a system needs nitric oxide. After nitric oxide is produced in specific areas of the body by nitric oxide synthase, it diffuses to nearby cells. Nitric oxide then reacts preferentially in the interior of these cells with the metal centres of proteins. Nitric oxide binds specifically to the iron (Fe) atom of the heme group in proteins; it can also interact with other metal sites in proteins as well as with the thiol group (SH) of the amino acid cysteine.

4. The Rate Determining Step is the slowest step of a chemical reaction that determines the speed (rate) of the overall reaction. The rate determining step is important in deriving the rate equation of a chemical reaction. For example, consider a multi-step reaction, $A + B \rightarrow C + D$ and assuming the elementary steps for this reaction are :

Step 1 : Slow $A + A \rightarrow C + E$ (with a kinetic constant, k_1)

Step 2 : Fast $E + B \rightarrow A + D$ (with a kinetic constant, k_2)

where E is an intermediate product in step 1 and an intermediate reactant in step 2 that will not show up in the overall reaction. This is because when you add steps 1 and 2, intermediate E will cancel out along with the extra reactant A seen in step 1. In the case of this hypothetical reaction, if step 1 is the slow step and step 2 is the fast step of the reaction, then the overall reaction rate will depend on step 1; this is because the slow step in a reaction is always the rate-limiting step, which is also called the rate determining step. Therefore the rate equation will be, rate = k_1 [A] [A] = k_1 $[A]^2$.

5. Given, size of Human DNA = 3×10^6 Kb.

Rate of replication = 1 Kb/min

Time of replication = 5 hours = 5×60 minutes = 300 minutes

Now, 1 Kb of Human DNA is synthesized in = 1 minute

Therefore, at this rate, 300 Kb of DNA could be synthesized in 300 minutes.

Hence, the number of origins of replication

$$= \frac{\left(3\times10^{6}\right)}{300} = 10^{4} = 10{,}000$$

6. Phospholipase A_1 (PLA_1) is an enzyme that hydrolyzes phospholipids and produces 2-acyl-lysophospholipids and fatty acids and is conserved in a wide range of organisms. Mammals have several enzymes that exhibit PLA1 activity *in vitro*. Phospholipase A2 (PLA2) catalyzes the hydrolysis of the sn-2 position of membrane glycerophospholipids to liberate arachidonic acid (AA), a precursor of eicosanoids including prostaglandins (PGs) and leukotrienes (LTs). The same reaction also produces lysophosholipids, which represent another class of lipid mediators.

7. Given, Buffer-1 having pH = 4 and Buffer-2 having pH = 6.

The volumes of the two buffers are equal = V (say)

When the two buffers are mixed together, their buffering action and pH changes due to the change in volume of the solution = 2V.

$$pH = 4 \Rightarrow [H^+] = 10^{-4}$$

and $pH = 6 \Rightarrow [H^+] = 10^{-6}$.

Net concentration of the H^+ ions $= 10^{-4} + 10^{-6}$

But, since the volume is doubled in the new solution of Buffer-1 and Buffer-2, so the pH will be the mean of the pH of the two buffers.

Therefore, new

$$pH = \frac{\left\{\begin{matrix} pH(\text{for Buffer}-1) \\ +pH(\text{for Buffer}-2) \end{matrix}\right\}}{2}$$

$$= \frac{(4+6)}{2} = \frac{10}{2} = 5.$$

8. Given, an insert I = 1 Kb length and a plasmid P = 4 Kb length.

Molar ratio of ligation = 4 : 1 or concentration

We know, $M_1 \times V_1 = M_2 \times V_2$

where,

M_1 = molarity of the insert,

M_2 = molarity of the plasmid,

V_1 = volume of the insert

and V_2 = volume of the plasmid.

Now, $\frac{M_1}{M_2} = \frac{4}{1}$

$$\Rightarrow \frac{M_1}{M_2} = \frac{V_2}{V_1}$$

$$\Rightarrow \frac{V_2}{V_1} = 4$$

Therefore, $V_2 = 4 \times V_1$.

Now, it is given that the concentration of final DNA is 10 g/mL.

So, we have 10 g of insert + plasmid in 1 mL of the solution.

Let X g be the amount of plasmid that is present.

So, amount of DNA insert required

$$= \frac{\text{Amount of plasmid} \times \text{molar ratio} \times \text{length of insert}}{\text{length of plasmid}}$$

$$= \frac{(X \times 4 \times 1)}{4} = X$$

Therefore, for X g of the plasmid, X g of DNA insert can be ligated. If we consider the volume of the solution to be 1 mL, then amounts of insert and plasmid would be :

$$X + X = 10 \text{ g}$$

$$\Rightarrow 2X = 10$$

$$\Rightarrow X = 5 \text{ g}.$$

Thus, the amount of insert and plasmid is 5 g each for 1 mL solution.

9. ATP is generated from ADP and phosphate ions by a complex set of processes occurring in the cell. These processes depend on the activities of a special group of cofactors called coenzymes. The formation of ATP from ADP and inorganic phosphate (Pi) requires more energy because energy is stored in the covalent bonds between phosphates, with the greatest amount of energy (7 kcal/mole approx.) in the bond between the second and third phosphate groups. The formation of ATP from ADP and Pi reverses the hydrolysis reaction. Because this condensation is energetically unfavourable, it must be coupled to an energetically more favourable reaction to occur. The two outermost phosphates in ATP are held to the rest of the molecule by high-energy phosphoanhydride bonds and are readily transferred. Water can be added to ATP to form ADP and inorganic phosphate (Pi). This instability is due to the strong resonating structures of unbound inorganic phosphate molecules as compared to the bound phosphate in ATP.

10. Given, transmittance (T_1) of a solution through a path length of 1 cm = 80%

We know, Absorbance is inversely proportional to transmittance.

Therefore, $\frac{A_1}{A_2} = \frac{T_2}{T_1}$,

where A_1 = absorbance for solution having path length l_1,

A_2 = absorbance for solution having path length l_2,

T_1 = transmittance of the solution having path length l_1

and T_2 = transmittance of the solution having path length l_1.

Again, according to Lambert Beer's law we have, $A = \varepsilon \times C \times l$ where ε = molar extinction coefficient, C = concentration of the solution and l = path length for the solution. Since the solution remains the same and only path length changes, we have :

$$\frac{A_1}{A_2} = \frac{l_1}{l_2}$$

$$\Rightarrow \frac{T_2}{T_1} = \frac{l_1}{l_2}$$

$$\Rightarrow T_2 = \frac{T_1 \times l_1}{l_2}$$

$$\Rightarrow T_2 = \frac{(80 \times 1)}{2}$$

where $T_2 = 80\%$,

$l_1 = 1$ cm,

$l_2 = 2$ cm

$\Rightarrow T_2 = 40$

The required transmittance is 80%.

11. Secondary active transport involves using energy to establish a gradient across the cell membrane, and then utilizing that gradient to transport a molecule of interest up its concentration gradient. An example of this mechanism is as follows: *E. coli* establishes a proton (H+) gradient across the cell membrane by using energy to pump protons out of the cell. Then those protons are coupled to lactose at the lactose permease transmembrane protein. The lactose permease uses the energy of the proton moving down its concentration gradient to transport lactose into the cell. This coupled transport in the same direction across the cell membrane is known as a symport. *E. coli* uses similar proton driven symports to transport ribose, arabinose, and several amino acids.

12. Receptor mediated endocytosis is an endocytosis process in which cell surface receptors ensure specificity of transport. Cholesterol, a hormone precursor and component of plasma membranes, is synthesized in the liver. Lipoprotein complexes such as LDL (low density lipoprotein) transport the insoluble cholesterol molecules to the body's cells. The LDL receptor binds to LDL complexes and mediates their endocytosis. The events of LDL uptake follow the general steps of receptor-mediated endocytosis: i) The LDL particle binds to the LDL receptor ii) LDL receptors cluster in clathrin-coated pits iii) The coated pits pinch off to form endocytic vesicles and are uncoated iv) The vesicles are directed to an endosome, where the low pH causes a conformational change in the receptors that results in the release of LDL particles v) The receptors recycle to the cell surface vi) The LDL particles are delivered to a lysosome and degraded, releasing free cholesterol.

13. Isocitrate lyase is an enzyme that catalyzes the conversion of isocitrate to succinate and glyoxylate. This is the first step in the glyoxylate bypass, an alternative to the tricarboxylic acid cycle in bacteria, fungi and plants. The unique enzymes of this route are isocitrate lyase (ICL) and malate synthase (MS). ICL cleaves isocitrate to glyoxylate and succinate, and MS converts glyoxylate and acetyl-CoA to malate. The end products of the bypass can be used for gluconeogenesis and other biosynthetic processes. PEP carboxykinase catalyzes the conversion of oxaloacetate (OAA) to phosphoenolpyruvate (PEP), the rate-limiting step in the metabolic pathway that produces glucose from lactate and other precursors derived from the citric acid cycle. The pyruvate dehydrogenase complex links glycolysis to the TCA cycle. The pyruvate dehydrogenase complex oxidizes pyruvate to generate acetyl-coA. Pyruvate dehydrogenase is a multi-enzyme complex that uses three enzymes: 1) E1: Pyruvate dehydrogenase which uses thiamine pyrophosphate (TPP) as its prosthetic group 2) E2: Dihydrolipoyl transacetylase which uses lipoamide and coenzyme A (also known as coASH) as its prosthetic groups 3) E3: Dihydrolipoyl dehydrogenase which uses flavin adenine dinucleotide (FAD) and nicotinamide adenine dinucleotide (NAD^+) as its cofactors. The enzyme-catalysed transfer of a phosphoryl group from ATP is an important reaction in a wide variety of biological processes. One enzyme that utilises this reaction is phosphofructokinase (PFK), which catalyses the phosphorylation of fructose-6-phosphate to fructose-1, 6-bisphosphate, a key regulatory step in the glycolytic pathway. It comprises of two similar (alpha/beta) lobes: one involved in ATP binding and the other housing both the substrate-binding site and the allosteric site (a regulatory binding site distinct from the active site, but that affects enzyme activity). Pyruvate carboxylase catalyzes a 2-step reaction, involving the ATP-dependent carboxylation of the covalently attached biotin in the first step and the transfer of the carboxyl group to pyruvate in the second. It catalyzes in a tissue specific manner, the initial reactions of glucose (liver, kidney) and lipid (adipose tissue, liver, brain) synthesis from pyruvate.

14. Histidine is an essential amino acid that is significant in the growth and repair of tissues. A haeme molecule is a cyclic molecule that consists of nitrogen, carbon and hydrogen atoms with a Fe^{2+} ion located in the center. Within the molecule, four nitrogen molecules hold the iron in the centre. The iron ion also bonds with a histidine side chain from one of the subunits that form the pocket. The iron ion bonds to histidine 87 in the alpha chain and histidine 92 in the beta chain. The histidine 87 and histidine 92 are both part of the F helix in each subunit. Anchoring of the haeme is facilitated by histidine nitrogen that binds to the iron. A second histidine is near the bound oxygen. Histidine helps in maintenance of proper blood pH and so has an action of buffering.

15. IgG antibodies are found in all body fluids. They are the smallest but most common antibody (75% to 80%) of all the antibodies in the body. IgG antibodies are very important in fighting bacterial and viral infections. IgG antibodies are the only type of antibody that can cross the placenta in a pregnant woman to help protect her baby (foetus). In IgG, there are 2 heavy chains and two light chains of different molecular weights. In reducing SDS-PAGE, the molecule of IgG would be electrophoresed based on the mass of the individual chains. So, the gel would have two

different bands for the heavy and light chains of the molecule. In isoelectric focussing gel electrophoresis, samples are separated based on their isoelectric pH. In case of IgG, the net isoelectric pH of the molecule would be the same. So it would appear as a single band in the isoelectric gel. In case of native PAGE, there is no usage of any kind of reducing agent. As such, the protein IgG remains intact and does not separate into its light and heavy chains and so is electrophoresed as a single band in the gel.

16. In the lac operon in the absence of lactose, the repressor protein encoded by the I gene binds to the lac operator and prevents transcription. Binding of allolactose to the repressor causes it to leave the operator. This enables RNA polymerase to transcribe the three genes of the operon. The single mRNA molecule that results is then translated into the three proteins. The lac repressor binds to a specific sequence of two dozen nucleotides called the operator. When the repressor is bound to the operator, RNA polymerase is unable to proceed downstream with its task of gene transcription. Absence of the lac repressor is essential but not sufficient for effective transcription of the lac operon. The activity of RNA polymerase also depends on the presence of another DNA-binding protein called catabolite activator protein or CAP. Like the lac repressor, CAP has two types of binding sites : one binds the nucleotide cyclic AMP and the other binds a sequence of 16 base pairs upstream of the promoter. CAP can bind to DNA only when cAMP is bound to CAP. So when cAMP levels in the cell are low, CAP fails to bind DNA and thus RNA polymerase cannot begin its work, even in the absence of the repressor. So the lac operon is under both negative (the repressor) and positive (CAP) control. Although the presence of lactose removes the repressor, the presence of glucose lowers the level of cAMP in the cell and thus removes CAP.

17. The most abundant lipid components in most membranes are phospholipids, which are amphipathic molecules (i.e., they have a hydrophilic and a hydrophobic part). Phospholipids of the composition present in cells spontaneously form symmetric sheet-like phospholipid bilayers, which are two molecules thick. All cellular membranes are closed structures, surrounding the cell itself or individual compartments. Cellular membranes thus have an internal face (the side oriented toward the interior of the compartment) and an external face (the side presented to the environment). The hydrophobic interior is generated by the fatty acyl side chains. Some of these chains have bends caused by double bonds. In both pure phospholipid bilayers and natural membranes, thermal motion permits phospholipid and glycolipid molecules to rotate freely around their long axes and to diffuse laterally within the membrane leaflet. Because such movements are lateral or rotational, the fatty acyl chains remain in the hydrophobic interior of the membrane and seal the self membrane.

18. An amino acid has both a basic amine group and an acidic carboxylic acid group. There is an internal transfer of a hydrogen ion from the -COOH group to the -NH_2 group to leave an ion with both a negative charge and a positive charge. This is called a zwitterion. Amino acids whose isoelectric points are lower than the pH of the buffer would behave as negatively charged moieties and those with isoelectric points higher than the buffer pH would be positively charged. Now, the isoelectric points of the given amino acids are:
Glycine (5.97 = buffer pH 6), Lysine (9.74>6), Arginine (10.76>6), Histidine (7.59>6), Aspartic acid (2.77<6) and Glutamic acid (3.22<6).
The positively charged amino acids are Lysine, Arginine and Histidine and the negatively charged amino acids are aspartic acid and glutamic acid. While, glycine is a neutral amino acid with no charge as it remains as a zwitterion due to its isoelectric point pH. Thus, the positively charged amino acids→lysine, arginine and histidine will migrate towards the cathode and the negatively charged amino acids→aspartic acid and glutamic acid migrate towards anode. Glycine remains at the origin.

19. The epidermal growth factor receptor family consists of four receptor genes and at least 11 ligands, several of which are produced in different protein forms. They create an interacting system that has the ability to receive and process information that results in multiple outputs. The family has an important role in directing and coordinating many normal processes, including growth and development, normal tissue turnover and wound healing. The epidermal growth factor (EGF) receptor (R) belongs to the ErbB family of receptor tyrosine kinases (RTKs). These receptors possess protein tyrosine kinase (PTK) activity and are found only in metazoans, in contrast to many of the serine/threonine kinase families, which are conserved throughout eukaryotes and are found in both unicellular and multicellular organisms. The four receptor genes, encoding the EGF receptor (EGFR/erbB-1), c-erbB-2/HER2, c-erbB3-/HER3 and c-erbB4/HER4, can be alternatively spliced to give rise to various partial protein products. Receptor tyrosine kinase binds ligands of the EGF family and activates several signalling cascades to convert extracellular cues into appropriate cellular responses. Known ligands include EGF, TGFA/TGF-alpha, amphiregulin, epigen/EPGN, BTC/betacellulin, epiregulin/EREG and HBEGF/heparin-

binding EGF. Those cells which were treated with epidermal growth factor would exhibit phosphotyrosine and tyrosine kinase activity. So, the antibodies prepared for immuni-precipitation would be specific to these two enzymes only. Whereas for untreated cells, the phosphothreonine present in the receptor is not phosphorylated to phosphotyrosine and so antibodies specific to it precipitate it.

20. Hypothalamic neurons in the peri-ventricular region and arcuate nucleus produce reproductive hormones, and sexual behaviour is influenced by the medial preoptic, the ventromedial, and the ventral pre-mammalian nuclei. The pre-optic area also appears to regulate autonomic control over the genitalia (penile erection, secretion of lubrication). Reproduction thus interacts with systems controlling adequate energy stores, fluid balance to insure blood supply to the developing foetus, and thermoregulation. It is also highly arousing. The synthesis and secretion of estrogens is stimulated by follicle-stimulating hormone (FSH), which is, in turn, controlled by the hypothalamic gonadotropin releasing hormone (GnRH). This feedback mechanism of the hypothalamus and the hormones of the reproductive system is the longest loop.

21. Myasthenia gravis (MG) is an autoimmune syndrome caused by the failure of neuromuscular transmission, which results from the binding of auto-antibodies to proteins involved in signalling at the neuromuscular junction (NMJ). These proteins include the nicotinic AChR or, less frequently, a muscle-specific tyrosine kinase (MuSK) involved in AChR clustering. Much is known about the mechanisms that maintain self tolerance and modulate anti-AChR antibody synthesis, AChR clustering, and AChR function as well as those that cause neuromuscular transmission failure upon antibody binding. The condition develops when auto-antibodies attack normal skeletal muscle tissue. Nerve endings that innervate skeletal muscle typically release a chemical, acetylcholine, to induce the muscles to contract. In myasthenia, antibodies attach themselves to the receptors for the acetylcholine on the skeletal muscle. Thus, when acetylcholine is released from a nerve and tries to induce contraction in a muscle, the receptors cannot attach to the acetylcholine so muscle weakness and fatigue results.

K : BOTANY

1. The Kyoto Protocol is an international agreement linked to the United Nations Framework Convention on Climate Change (global warming). The Kyoto Protocol was adopted in Kyoto, Japan, on 11 December 1997 and entered into force on 16 February 2005.

2. Phagotrophs are organisms that obtain nutrients through the ingestion of solid organic matter. This class of organism includes all animals from the simplest, single-celled animal (for example, the protozoa) to the higher life forms.

3. The soil bacterium *Agrobacterium rhizogenes* infects the plant tissues and leads to the formation of adventitious roots or it is called as "hairy roots". *Agrobacterium tumefaciens* is not responsible for hairy root formation rather it is a widespread naturally occurring soil bacterium that causes crown gall, and has the ability to introduce new genetic material into the plant cell.

4. We know,

$$10\ \text{Å} = 1\text{nm}$$

So, $$1\ \text{Å} = \frac{1}{10}\ \text{nm}$$

Therefore, $1\ \text{Å} = 0.1\text{nm}$ or 10^{-1} nm

5. In hypogynous flowers, the perianth and stamens are attached to the receptacle below the gynoecium; the ovary is superior to these organs, and the remaining floral organs arise from below the point of origin of the carpel.

6. The main axis of the inflorescence is known as **peduncle** and the stalk of the individual flower is called **pedicel**.

Peduncle is a stalk supporting an inflorescence, which is the part of the shoot of seed plants where flowers are formed. A pedicel is a stem that attaches single flowers to the main stem of the inflorescence.

7. Nitrobacter plays an important role in the nitrogen cycle by oxidizing nitrite into nitrate in soil. Nitrosomonas bacteria first convert ammonia into nitrites. Nitrobacter convert the nitrites into nitrates, which are readily absorbed by the plants. These are responsible for nitrification.

8. The amino acids present in the polypeptide chain are Serine (Ser), Leucine (Leu) and Alanine (Ala).

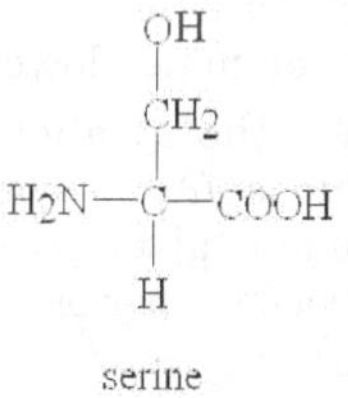

serine

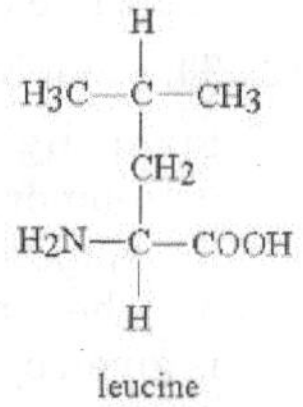

leucine

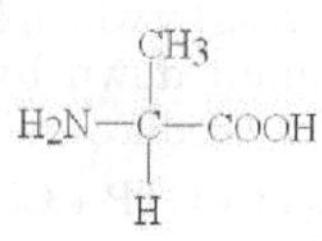

alanine

9. The sepals, petals, stamens, and carpels of angiosperms form four separate whorls within a complete flower.

Abscisic acid is an isoprenoid plant hormone whose biosynthesis occurs indirectly through the production of carotenoids.

10. DNA polymerase I (or Pol I) is an enzyme that participates in the process of DNA replication. DNA Polymerase I removes the RNA primer (created by Primase) from the lagging strand and fills in the necessary nucleotides between the Okazaki fragments (see DNA replication) in $5' \rightarrow 3'$ direction,

proofreading for mistakes as it goes. It is not known as the true DNA replicase rather DNA polymerase III is known as a true DNA replicase in E. Coli.

The conserved element closest to the transcription initiation site is called TATA box and not the CAAT box. A TATA box is a DNA sequence that indicates the point at which a genetic sequence can be read and decoded. Whereas a CAAT box is present about 75 bp upstream of the start of transcription.

11. Insertion sequence (IS) elements are DNA sequences that are capable of independent transposition and they can be inserted at many different sites in bacterial chromosomes and plasmids.

Two insertion sequences flank one or more accessory genes, such as an antibiotic resistance gene (e.g. Tn10, Tn5) and they are in the same orientation.

12. The symbol for male flower is given by ♂, the symbol for actinomorphic is ⊕ the symbol for epipetalous is given by C A and the symbol for superior ovary is given by (_).

13. Fatty acid oxidation is a multi-step process by which fatty acids are broken down by various tissues to produce energy.

$$\text{Fatty acid} + \text{GTP} + \text{Co-A} \rightleftharpoons \text{Acyl Co-A} + \text{GDP} + \text{Pi}$$

Amino acid synthesis is the set of biochemical processes (metabolic pathways) by which the various amino acids are produced from other compounds.

$$NH_3 + \text{Glutamate} + \text{ATP} \rightleftharpoons \text{Glutamine} + \text{ADP} + \text{Pi}$$

Citric acid cycle is a series of chemical reactions used by all aerobic organisms to generate energy through the oxidization of acetate derived from carbohydrates, fats and proteins into carbon dioxide.

$$\text{Succinate} + \text{E-FAD} \rightleftharpoons \text{Fumarate} + \text{E- FADH}_2$$

Fatty acid synthesis is the creation of fatty acids from acetyl-CoA and malonyl-CoA precursors through action of enzymes called fatty acid synthases.

$$\text{Malonyl-S-Co-A} + \text{ACP- SH} \rightleftharpoons \text{Malonyl-S-ACP} + \text{Co-A-SH}$$

14. The castor oil plant, Ricinus communis, is a species of flowering plant in the spurge family, Euphorbiaceae. It belongs to a monotypic genus, Ricinus, and subtribe, Ricininae.

Jatropha Curcas is a non- edible oil crop predominately used to produce bio-diesel.

Non-edible oil contains several unsaponifiable and toxic components, which make them unsuitable for human consumption. Karanja (Pongamia pinnata) is an underutilized plant which is grown in many parts of India.

Madhuca indica also known as Mahua is an Indian tropical tree found largely in the central and north Indian plains and forests.

15. Förster mechanism is a mechanism describing energy transfer between two chromophores. A donor chromophore, initially in its electronic excited state, may transfer energy to an acceptor chromophore through non-radioactive dipole-dipole coupling.

Ping-pong mechanism also called adouble- displacement reaction is characterized by the change of the enzyme into an intermediate form when the first substrate to product reaction occurs.

The term feedback inhibition refers to a situation in which the substances at the end of a long series of reactions inhibit a reaction at the beginning of the series of reactions.

The Holliday Model is a schematic model which predicts the results of the recombination of two duplex DNAs.

16. Alu I cleavage site is given as:

5′A G ↓ C T 3′
3′T C ↑ G A 5′

Hinc III cleavage site is given as:

5′G T Py ↓ Pu A C 3′
3′ C A Pu ↑ Py T G 5′

Hpa II cleavage site is given as:

5′C ↓ C G G 3′
3′G G C ↑ C 5′

Hind III cleavage site is given as:

5′A ↓ A G C T T 3′
3′ T T C G A ↑ A 5′

17. Linnaeus proposed an artificial sexual system of classification containing 24 species.

William Roxburgh was known as the father of Indian botany. In 1820, William Carey edited and published vol. 1 of Dr. William Roxburgh's Flora Indica; or Descriptions of Indian Plants. In 1824, Carey edited and published vol. 2 of Roxburgh's Flora Indica.

George Bentham a great taxonomist and plant explorer Sir Joseph Dalton hooker a great plant geographer and English systematize jointly presented a system of classification. Their classification was published in 3 volumes of genera plantarum.

Adolf Engler was a German botanist. He is notable for his work on plant taxonomy and phytogeography, such as Die natürlichen Pflanzenfamilien (The Natural Plant Families).

18. The pollen from Bt crops affects the Monarch caterpillars.

Horizontal resistance is polygenic and it describes many gene resistances.

A super weed is a weed that has become resistant to a particular herbicide.

A gene gun or a biolistic particle delivery system, originally designed for plant transformation, is a device for injecting cells with genetic information. The payload is an elemental particle of a heavy metal usually gold/tungsten coated with plasmid DNA.

19. The xylem transports water and soluble mineral nutrients from the roots throughout the plant.

Guttation is the loss of water in the form of water droplets from hydathodes (small pores) on the leaf margin of a small herbacious plant.

Hartig net is a hyphal network that extends into the root penetrating between epidermal and cortical cells. This network is a site of nutrient exchange between the fungus and the host plant. Hartig net is typical for ectomycorrhiza.

Proton motive force also can be generated via primary active transport that is, using ATP-driven proton pumps. The resulting force employed for ATP generation via the action of ATP synthase, and to power co-transport, i.e., secondary active transport.

20. Chilli leaf curl is a disease caused by tobacco leaf curl bigeminivirus belonging to bigeminivirus group. The virus is transmitted by whitefly (Bemisia tabaci).

Cauliflower Mosaic Virus (CaMV) is a member of the genus Caulimovirus. CaMV infects mostly plants of the Brassicaceae family (Brevicoryne brassicae).

Rice tungro bacilliform virus (RTBV) is a pararetrovirus, and a member of the family Caulimoviridae in the genus Badnavirus. RTBV is required for the transmission of the two viruses by the leafhopper vector Nephotettix virescens.

Wheat yellow leaf virus (WYLV) is a wheat, barley, rye, and oat pathogenic virus of the family Closteroviridae. The virus, like other members of its genus, is transmitted by aphids. Identified vectors include Rhopalosiphum maidis.

21. Rhizoctonia solani is a plant pathogenic fungus which is known to cause serious plant losses by attacking primarily the roots and lower stems of plants and although it has a wide range of hosts, their main targets are herbaceous plants.

Gibberella zeae is a plant pathogen which causes fusarium head blight, a devastating disease on wheat and barley.

L : MICROBIOLOGY

1. Oswald Theodore Avery (1877-1955) was a distinguished Canadian-born bacteriologist and research physician and one of the founders of immunochemistry. He is best known for his discovery that deoxyribonucleic acid (DNA) serves as genetic material.

In 1928, a Scottish bacteriologist Sir Alexander Fleming made a chance discovery from an already discarded, contaminated Petri dish. The mold that had contaminated the experiment turned out to contain a powerful antibiotic, penicillin.

Griffith's experiment, reported in 1928 by Frederick Griffith was one of the first experiments suggesting that bacteria are capable of transferring genetic information through a process known as transformation.

Martinus W. Beijerinck was a Dutch microbiologist and botanist who was the first to recognize that viruses are reproducing entities that are different from other organisms. He later made other important advances in plant and soil science through his studies of Azotobacter, denitrifying bacteria, nitrogen fixation, and tobacco mosaic virus. He used the term filterable virus to describe the ability of the latter agent to pass through a fine-pored filter. He described the virus as contagium vivum fluidum, thinking it was a fluid rather than a particulate entity.

2. A spectrophotometer is employed to measure the amount of light that a sample absorbs. The instrument operates by passing a beam of light through a sample and measuring the intensity of light reaching a detector. Thus it is based on the principle of light absorption.

3. Rhizobia are Gram-negative bacilli that live freely in the soil (especially where legumes have been grown). However, they cannot fix atmospheric nitrogen until they have invaded the roots of the appropriate legume. Thus symbiotic nitrogen fixation occurs in plants that harbor nitrogen-fixing bacteria within their tissues. The best-studied example is the association between legumes and bacteria in the genus Rhizobium. Each of these is able to survive independently (soil nitrates must then be available to the legume), but life together is clearly beneficial to both. Only together can nitrogen fixation take place.

4. In bacterial conjugation, the transfer of genes is directional, from a donor to a recipient. The donor "male" has a fertility factor (F+) that is itself heritable. Recipient females do not have the F factor and are F-. Bacteria that have the F factor make the pili needed for conjugation. Thus the prototroph are formed due to conjugation when a tryptophan auxotrophic Hfr strain of *E. coli* is mixed with F- histidine auxotroph.

5. Cysteine is one of two sulfur-containing amino acids; the other is methionine. Cysteine differs from serine in a single atom-- the sulfur of the thiol replaces the oxygen of the alcohol.

6. Chloramphenicol is a bacteriostatic antibiotic that binds to the 23S rRNA of the 50S subunit of the bacterial ribosome, inhibiting peptidyl transferase and thus inhibiting protein synthesis at large.

7. Pseudopeptidoglycan is present in the cell wall of *Methanococcus jannaschii* which is a thermophilic methanogenic archaea. It is a major cell wall component of some archaea that differs from bacterial peptidoglycan in chemical structure, but resembles eubacterial peptidoglycan in morphology, function, and physical structure. The basic components are N-acetylglucosamine and N-acetyltalosaminu-ronic acid (peptidoglycan has N-acetylmuramic acid instead), which are linked by β-1,3-glycosidic bonds. Lysozyme, a host defense mechanism, is ineffective against organisms with pseudopeptidoglycan cell walls.

8. Diauxic growth curve of E. coli shows the two distinct phases of active growth. During the first phase of exponential growth, the bacteria utilize glucose as a source of energy until all the glucose is exhausted. Then, after a secondary lag phase, the acetate is utilized during a second stage of exponential growth. This is done by the glyoxylate cycle. The glyoxylate cycle uses a two-step bypass. One key enzyme, isocitrate lyase converts D-threo-isocitrate to form succinate and glyoxylate.

9. Continuous culture is achieved primarily via the use of chemostats where fresh media continuously flows into a growth chamber while spent media continuously flows out. Chemostat is a means of culturing microorganisms under constant physiological conditions over long time frames that involves a constant-rate of input of fresh medium.

10. ADP-ribosylation is the addition of one or more ADP-ribose moieties to a protein. These reactions are involved in cell signaling and the control of many cell processes, including DNA repair and apoptosis. ADP-ribosylation is also responsible for the actions of some bacterial toxins, such as cholera toxin, diphtheria toxin, pertussis toxin, and heat-labile enterotoxin. These toxin proteins are ADP-ribosyltransferases that modify target proteins in human cells.

The best characterized and most potent membrane-damaging toxin of *S. aureus* is alpha toxin. It is expressed as a monomer that binds to the membrane of susceptible cells. Subunits then oligomerize to form heptameric rings with a central pore through which cellular contents leak. Thus the alpha toxin of *S. aureus* does not have ADP ribosylation activity.

11. During conjugation between an Hfr cell and a F– cell a part of the chromosome is transferred with F. Random breakage interrupts the transfer before the entire chromosome is transferred. The chromosomal fragment can then recombine with the recipient chromosome. The Hfr chromosome replicates while it is transferring a single strand to the F– cell; this replication ensures a complete chromosome for the donor cell after mating. The transferred strand is replicated in the recipient cell, and donor genes may become incorporated in the recipient's chromosome through crossovers, creating a recombinant cell. Thus the high frequency of recombinants is obtained.

12. Silent mutations are errors in DNA replication that do not cause a change in the amino acid sequence. For example, the codon UCU might accidentally be translated as UCC, but both codons call for the amino acid serine, so no disruptions in the formation of the protein occur. It is still a mutation in the DNA, but the mutation doesn't change the ultimate structure of the protein and won't have any effect on its function. Therefore, it is "silent".

13. The bacterial flagellar motor is a rotary molecular motor situated in the cell envelopes of bacteria that is driven by a flow of charged ions across the bacterial plasma membrane. The motor powers the rotation of helical flagellar filaments so that bacteria swim, frequently towards a more favorable location.

Rotation of each filament is driven by a motor located in the cell envelope at the base of the filament. This motor is powered by the flux of ions across the plasma membrane – either hydrogen (H^+) or sodium (Na^+) ions, depending on the organism. Ions are driven directly by their electrochemical potential gradient across the membrane; hydrolysis of adenosine triphosphate (ATP) is not necessary for the motor to work.

14. Chorismic acid, more commonly known as its anionic form chorismate, is an important biochemical intermediate in plants and microorganisms. This enzyme participates in phenylalanine, tyrosine and tryptophan biosynthesis. Chorismate synthase catalyzes the last of the seven steps in the shikimate pathway which is used in prokaryotes, fungi and plants for the biosynthesis of aromatic amino acids. It catalyzes the 1,4-trans elimination of the phosphate group from 5-enolpyruvylshikimate-3-phosphate (EPSP) to form chorismate which can then be used in phenylalanine, tyrosine or tryptophan biosynthesis.

15. 3 bands would be observed upon $CsCl_2$ density gradient centrifugation of the mixture containing unlabeled and N^{15} labeled DNA from phage T4.

16. Temperate refers to the life cycle some phages are able to perform. A temperate phage can integrate its genome into its host bacterium's chromosome, becoming a lysogen known as a prophage. A temperate phage is also able to undergo lytic life cycles, where the prophage is expressed, replicates the phage genome and produces phage progeny and the progeny phage leave the bacterium.

The virulent phages have only lytic lifecycles and thus infection results in the host cell's death (due to lytic cell destruction-the phage replicates itself and then bursts the cell, releasing many copies).

Thus the difference between temperate and virulent phage is that a temperate phage can choose between lytic and lysogenic cycle while a virulent phage cannot.

17. The RecA protein is a recombinase functioning in recombinational DNA repair in bacteria. The RecA protein is a critical enzyme in this process, as it catalyzes the pairing of ssDNA with complementary regions of dsDNA. The RecA

monomers first polymerize to form a helical filament around ssDNA. During this process, RecA extends the ssDNA by 1.6 angstroms per axial base pair. Duplex DNA is then bound to the polymer. Bound dsDNA is partially unwound to facilitate base pairing between ssDNA and duplexed DNA. Once ssDNA has hybridized to a region of dsDNA, the duplexed DNA is further unwound to allow for branch migration.

18. Vibrio fischeri, a species of bioluminescent bacterium, is frequently found in symbiotic relationships with marine animals like the bobtail squid. It is an oxidase-positive, Gram-negative bacterium, composed of a cell wall that consists of an outer membrane containing lipopolysaccharides, a periplasmic space with a peptidoglycan layer, and an inner, cytoplasmic membrane. Luminescence is a chemical reaction in which the enzyme, luciferase, oxidizes organic compounds, such as long chain aldehyde and reduced flavin mononucleotide, so as to release free energy in the form of blue-green light at 490nm. Thus in vibrio fischeri chemical energy can be converted to both mechanical as well as light energy.

19. Initial density of culture bacteria,

$N_0 = 1 * 10^5$ cells/ml

Generation time,

G = 30 minutes = 0.5 hrs

Time, t = 5 hrs

$G = t/3.3(\log_{10}N - \log_{10}N_0)$

Therefore, we get,

$N = 10^8$ cells/ml

Thus the dilution required to get 100 colonies per ml or 10^2 cells/ml:

Serial dilution of 10^6 will give 100 colonies per ml.

20. Effective chemotherapeutic agents are difficult to develop for the treatment of fungal infections because fungi are eukaryotic and are composed of rigid cell wall largely made of chitin which is a polymer of N-acetylglucosamine rather than peptidoglycan which is a characteristic component of most bacterial cell walls. The cellular machinery of fungi is similar to the host cells thus it is difficult to develop effective chemotherapeutic agents against them.

21. An evolutionary chronometer (also denoted ED) essentially represents the number of changes between two sequences. DNA segments encoding ribosomes, ATPases and DNA Polymerases are all good evolutionary chronometers because they are universally conserved for the most part. Thus "ribosomal RNAs having enzyme activity" is not a criteria for using ribosomal RNAs as evolutionary chronometers.

M : ZOOLOGY

1. One characteristic of genomic plasticity is the presence of extrachromosomal circular DNA (ecc DNA). Extrachromosomal DNA is contained in cytoplasmic organelles, such as mitochondria (most eukaryotes), and in chloroplasts and plastids (plants). In case of a normal animal cell, they are located in the mitochondria of the cell. Eukaryotic extrachromosomal DNAs have been organized into four major classes: (1) Organelle DNAs, (2) plasmid DNAs, (3) amplified genes, and (4) intermediates and/or by-products of DNA transpositions and rearrangements. Mostly they are circular and double stranded in nature and serve for the semi-autonomous nature of the cytoplasmic organelles of the cell.

2. In the verterbrate embryo, as the primitive streak is regressing, the paraxial mesoderm divides into blocks of cells called somites. These divisions can be seen either side of the notochord. Somites are transient structures that will give rise to cells of the vertebrae and ribs, dermis of the dorsum, skeletal muscle of the body wall, back and limbs. Somites begin to develop at the anterior of the embryo first, and appear at regular intervals. In the developing vertebrate embryo, somites are masses of mesoderm distributed along the two sides of the neural tube and that will eventually become dermis (dermatome), skeletal muscle (myotome), and vertebrae (sclerotome). These somites have four compartments: the sclerotome forms the vertebrae and the rib cartilage; the myotome forms the musculature of the back, the ribs and the limbs; the dermatome forms the skin on the back; and the syndetome forms the tendons and some blood vessels.

3. Hibernation is a state of inactivity and metabolic depression in endotherms. Hibernation refers to a season of heterothermy that is characterized by low body temperature, slow breathing and heart rate, and low metabolic rate. Often associated with cold temperatures, the purpose of hibernation is to conserve energy during a period when sufficient food is scarce. To achieve this energy savings, an endotherm will first decrease its metabolic rate, which then results in a decreased body temperature. Hibernation may last several days, weeks, or months depending on the species, ambient temperature, time of year, and individual animal's body condition.

4. Mendel's monohybrid cross, also known as the law of segregation, states that every individual possesses a pair of alleles (assuming diploid) for any particular trait and that each parent passes a randomly selected copy (allele) of only one of these to its offspring. Whichever of the two alleles in the offspring is dominant determines how the offspring expresses that trait. Thus the germ cells will always receive one of the paired alleles.

5. The action of cholera toxin, secreted by the bacterium *Vibrio cholerae* is to bind receptors in intestinal epithelial cells and

insert an enzymatic subunit that modifies a G protein associated with the adenylate cyclase complex. The consequent stimulated production of cyclic AMP, or other factors such as increased synthesis of prostaglandins by intoxicated cells, initiates a metabolic cascade that results in the excessive secretion of fluid and electrolytes characteristic of the disease. The high cyclic AMP levels activate the cystic fibrosis transmembrane conductance regulator (CFTR), causing a dramatic efflux of ions and water from infected enterocytes, leading to watery diarrhoea.

6. Human population in industrially dominant areas are characterised by the size of the family (small families, concept of micro-family), affect in the reproduction rate, mortality rate, average life span of the individuals and the growth rate of individuals in various genetic and socio-environmental factors. So, industrially developed countries cannot be characterised by even structure of the population.

7. Sex linkage is the phenotypic expression of an allele that is dependent on the gender of the individual and is directly tied to the sex chromosomes. It is the condition in which a gene responsible for a specific trait is located on a sex chromosome, resulting in sexually dependent inheritance of the trait. In such cases there is a homogametic sex and a heterogametic sex. In mammals the homogametic sex is female (XX) and the heterogametic sex is male (XY), thus the sex linked genes are carried on the X chromosome. In birds and in some insects the homogametic sex is male. Mutation of genes on the X chromosome is often apparent only in male offspring, which have only one X chromosome. The mutation may be masked in the female unless the mutation also occurs on the other X chromosome.

8. While CO_2 absorption and release is always happening as a result of natural processes, the recent drastic rise in CO_2 levels in the atmosphere is known to be entirely due to human activity. Burning fossil fuels such as coal and petroleum is the leading cause of increased anthropogenic CO_2. Global warming is mainly the result of CO_2 levels rising in the Earth's atmosphere. Carbon dioxide (CO_2) is the primary greenhouse gas emitted through human activities. It absorbs and emits radiation within the thermal infrared range. This process is the fundamental cause of the greenhouse effect. When energy from the sun reaches the Earth, the planet absorbs some of this energy and radiates the rest back to space as heat. The Earth's surface temperature depends on this balance between incoming and outgoing energy. If this energy balance is shifted, the Earth's surface could become noticeably warmer or cooler, leading to a variety of changes in global climate. This is maintained by the greenhouse gases. Thus, increased levels of CO_2 in the atmosphere would result increased level of penetration of infrared radiation into the earth's atmosphere leading to global warming.

9. Most anabolic steroids are synthetic substances similar to the male sex hormone testosterone. They are taken orally or are injected. Some people, especially athletes, abuse anabolic steroids to build muscle and enhance performance. The gonads contain a powerful androgen called testosterone which is artificially synthesized to produce anabolic steroids. They mimic the effects of testosterone and dihydro-testosterone in the body. The effect of anabolic steroids on muscle mass is caused in at least two ways: first, they increase the production of proteins; second, they reduce recovery time by blocking the effects of stress hormone cortisol on muscle tissue.

10. Holometabolous insects involve the process of holometabolism (undergoing complete metamorphosis) which includes four life stages - as an embryo or egg, a larva, a pupa and an imago or adult. The developmental stage from pupa to an adult is governed by various hormones such as brain hormone, ecdysone hormone and juvenile hormone. Neurosecretory cells in an insect's brain secrete a hormone, the prothoracicotropic hormone (PTTH) that activates prothoracic glands, which secrete a second hormone, usually Ecdysone (a ecdysteroid), that induces ecdysis. PTTH also stimulates the corpora allata, a retrocerebral organ, to produce juvenile hormone (JH), which prevents the development of adult characteristics during ecdysis.

11. Richard Owen defined homology as "the same organ in different animals under every variety of form and function". Homologous traits of organisms are therefore due to descent from a common ancestor. Organs, which have a common fundamental anatomical plan and similar embryonic origin whatever varied functions they may perform are regarded as homologous organs. For instance, the arms of humans and the forelegs of dogs and cats are structurally different but have the same evolutionary or embryological origin. The homologous body parts often have similar functions. The developmental process or the origin of the structure lies in a similar environment. Homologous body parts may or may not exist to perform the same function.

12. The theory of evolution by natural selection was proposed by Charles Darwin. In his theory of natural selection, Charles Darwin suggested that "survival of the fittest" was the basis for organic evolution (the modification of living things with time). The individuals that are best equipped to survive and reproduce perpetuate the highest frequency of genes to descendant populations. This is the principle known colloquially as "survival of the fittest," where fitness denotes an individual's overall

ability to pass copies of his genes on to successive generations. Thus, whether there will be more progeny or not is not explained by the term survival of the fittest.

13. After the natural calamity when the island is re-populated with the surviving individuals, incidence of a rare recessive genetic disorder was high. Recessive genetic disorders are single gene disorders that occur only when an individual carries two malfunctioning copies (mutant alleles) of the relevant gene. Such individuals are described as homozygous, and arise most frequently as the offspring of heterozygous parents - parents who each possess one normal allele and one mutant allele. Examples of recessive diseases include cystic fibrosis, spinal muscular atrophy and phenylketonuria. Thus, the occurrence of the disorder is due to the selective advantage of the recessive disorder.

14. The immune system defends the body against disease. Lymphocytes are one type of white blood cell that helps the body resist infection by recognizing harmful foreign substances, such as bacteria, and eliminating them. The ability of the vertebrate immune system to distinguish self from nonself depends largely on a group of protein makers (antigens) known as the major histocompatibility complex (MHC). These receptor antigens are present on the surface of T-cell lymphocytes. These receptors are different for different types of white blood cells. These receptors help in the processing and presentation of the novel antigens and thus mount the antigenic invasion with an effective response through antibody mediated or cell mediated pathways.

15. Acetylcholine, (ACh), an ester of choline and acetic acid is the transmitter substance at many neural, or nerve, synapses and at the motor end plate of vertebrate muscles. When a nerve impulse arrives at the nerve ending, ACh, which is stored there in vesicles, is released and combines with a receptor molecule in the postsynaptic membrane or the end-plate membrane of a muscle fibre. This bonding changes the permeability of the membrane, and a change in the nature of generator potential results. The ACh is destroyed by an enzyme; acetylcholinesterase at the synaptic cleft (the space between two nerve cells) so the next nerve impulse can be transmitted across the synaptic gap. Inhibitors of the enzyme, however, prolong the lifetime of ACh itself. If an inhibitor of acetylcholinesterase is administered, then acetyl choline will not be degraded and so further transmission of nerve impulse through the synapse will not be possible.

16. Oogenesis (the differentiation of the ovum) differs from spermatogenesis (the origin and development of the sperm cells within the male reproductive organs, the testes) in several ways. Whereas the gamete formed by spermatogenesis is essentially a motile nucleus, the gamete formed by oogenesis contains all the materials needed to initiate and maintain metabolism and development. The process of spermatogenesis and oogenesis is stimulated by follicle stimulating hormone (FSH) present in male and female. While in females, leutinizing hormone (LH) stimulates ovulation in ovary in females, and testosterone production in the testicles of males. Both primary oocytes and spermatocytes are formed through reduction division or meiosis. The production of ovum and sperm are independent of each other and are part of female and male reproductive life cycle.

17. *Schistosoma mansoni* is a significant parasite of humans, a trematode that is one of the major agents of the disease schistosomiasis. The lifecycle of schistosomes includes two hosts: a definitive host (i.e. human) where the parasite undergoes sexual reproduction and a single intermediate snail host where there are a number of asexual reproductive stages. *Trichinella spiralis* is a nematode parasite, occurring in rats, pigs, bears and humans, and is responsible for the disease trichinosis. *Trichinella* species are the smallest nematode parasite of humans, have an unusual life cycle and are one of the most widespread and clinically important parasites in the world. *Plasmodium*, the parasite responsible for human malaria, is among the most researched genera of parasites in the world. All the *Plasmodium* species causing malaria in humans are transmitted by mosquito species of the genus *Anopheles*. *Taenia solium* is a flattened ribbon like tapeworm that is white in color. It infects pigs and humans. The infection is caused by ingestion of eggs shed in the faeces of a human tapeworm carrier. Pigs and humans become infected by ingesting eggs or gravid proglottids. Humans are infected either by ingestion of food contaminated with feces containing eggs, or by autoinfection.

18. Isolecithal refers to the even distribution of yolk in the cytoplasm of ovums of mammals and other vertebrates. In the absence of a large concentration of yolk, four major cleavage types can be observed in isolecithal cells: radial holoblastic, spiral holoblastic, bilateral holoblastic, and rotational holoblastic cleavage. It occurs in case of human. Mesolecithal cleavage pattern is applied to an egg that has a yolk of intermediate size and strongly concentrated in one hemisphere, typical of Petromyzonidae, Acipenseridae, Amiidae, Lepidosirenidae, and Amphibia (frogs). Telolecithal pattern is observed in a medium to large amount of yolk, with the yolk concentrated toward one pole (the vegetal pole). It can be seen in the eggs of fish, amphibians, birds (chick), and reptiles.

Centrolecithal describes the placement of the yolk in the centre of the cytoplasm of ovums. Many arthropod eggs are centrolecithal. Eggs of fruit flies (*Drosophila*) are centrolecithal.

19. Heteronuclear RNA does represent the contiguous segment of the genomic DNA. UTRs or untranslated regions of the gene segment are present in the intron (non-coding region) of the DNA to be transcribed. These UTRs are present before the promoter regions of the DNA sequence and do not code for any protein. Translation start codon or the initiation codon is present in any segment of the exon. The initiation codon for translation in humans is methionine (ATG).

20. Maturation-promoting factor (MPF) is a cell cycle control element able to cause metaphase when injected into amphibian oocytes or when incubated with nuclei in a cell-free system. It is also called mitosis-promoting factor or M-Phase-promoting factor. It is a heterodimeric protein composed of cyclin B and cyclin-dependent kinase (CDK1, also known as Cdc2 or p34 kinase) that stimulates the mitotic and meiotic phases of the cell cycle. MPF promotes the entrance into mitosis (the M phase) from the G2 phase by phosphorylating multiple proteins needed during mitosis. MPF is activated at the end of G_2 by a phosphatase.

21. Gastrulation is a phase early in the embryonic development of most animals, during which the single-layered blastula is reorganized into a trilaminar structure known as the gastrula. These three germ layers are known as the ectoderm, mesoderm, and endoderm. During gastrulation, cell movements result in a massive reorganization of the embryo from a simple spherical ball of cells, the blastula, into a multi-layered organism. During gastrulation, many of the cells at or near the surface of the embryo move to a new, more interior location. The primary germ layers (endoderm, mesoderm, and ectoderm) are formed and organized in their proper locations during gastrulation. Neurulation in vertebrates results in the formation of the neural tube, which gives rise to both the spinal cord and the brain. Neurulation is ended by the beginning of gastrulation.

■■

GATE-2008

XL : LIFE SCIENCES

Time : 3 Hours *Maximum Marks : 100*

J : CHEMISTRY (Compulsory)

Useful Information:

In2 = 0.693; In10 = 2.303; R = 8.314 $JK^{-1} mol^{-1}$ = 0.083 L bar $K^{-1} mol^{-1}$; K_{sp}(AgCI) = 1.8×10^{-10}; K_{sp} (AgI) = 8.3×10^{-17}; Trouton's constant = 85

Q. 1 – 6 carry one mark each.

1. Which of the following will NOT conduct electricity?
   (*a*) Solid metallic Na (*b*) Solid NaCl
   (*c*) Aqueous NaCl (*d*) Fused NaCl
2. The region in which the following spectral lines are observed is
   P. Lyman series Q. Balmer series
   R. Paschen series
   (*a*) P-UV, Q–UV/Vis, R–IR
   (*b*) P–UV/Vis, Q–UV, R–IR
   (*c*) P–IR, Q–UV, R–Vis/IR
   (*d*) P–UV, Q–IR, R–UV/Vis
3. The pH of a 10^{-8} molar hydrochloric acid solution is
   (*a*) exactly 8 (*b*) between 7 and 8
   (*c*) exactly 7 (*d*) between 6 and 7
4. The plot of concentration of A against time is a straight line with negative slope for the reaction:
   $A \rightarrow$ products
   The order of the reaction is
   (*a*) –1 (*b*) 0 (*c*) 1 (*d*) 2
5. Among the following four amines, which one is least basic in aqueous solution?
   (*a*) CH_3NH_2 (*b*) $(CH_3)_2NH$
   (*c*) $(CH_3)_3N$ (*d*) $CH_3NHC_6H_5$
6. Which of the following acids is used for the preparation of cyclohexene from cyclohexanol?
   (*a*) Conc.HNO_3 (*b*) 48% HBr
   (*c*) 85% H_3PO_4 (*d*) $(COOH)_2$

Q. 7 – 24 carry two marks each.

7. An aqueous mixture solution is prepared which contains 0.1 M of *KCl* and 0.1 M *KI*. To this solution, a drop of 0.01 M aqueous solution of $AgNO_3$ is added.
   Which of the following statement is correct?
   (*a*) A precipitate forms which is primarily AgI
   (*b*) A precipitate forms which is primarily AgCl
   (*c*) A precipitate froms which has equimolar amounts of AgCl and AgI.
   (*d*) There will be no precipitation, as there is no common ion between potassium and silver salts.
8. 1 g L^{-1} solution of a protein exerts an osmotic pressure of 8.3×10^{-3} bar at 300 K. Calculate the molar mass of the protein.
   (*a*) 2490 g mol^{-1} (*b*) 3000 g mol^{-1}
   (*c*) 4578 g mol^{-1} (*d*) 6100g mol^{-1}
9. An electrochemical cell of the following representation was found to be a galvanic cell, where 'A' and 'B' represent different metals.
   A(s) | A^{2+} (aq) 1M || B^{2+} (aq) 1M | B(s)
   Which of the following statements with respect to the cell is correct?
   (*a*) The cell converts electrical energy to chemical energy spontaneously.
   (*b*) The cell uses electrical energy to deposit 'A' and dissolve 'B' spontaneously.
   (*c*) (A^{2+}/A) is a stronger reducing agent than (B^{2+}/B).
   (*d*) (A^{2+}/A) is a stronger oxidizing agent than (B^{2+}/B)
10. For a first order reaction at a particular temperature, the half-life was found to be (100 In2) seconds. The specific rate constant of the reaction is
    (*a*) 0.01s^{-1} (*b*) 100 s^{-1} (*c*) 230 s^{-1} (*d*) 693 s^{-1}
11. Liquid bromine boils at 59°C. Assuming it to be a normal liquid, which of the following gives its standard molar enthalpy of vaporization?
    (*a*) (8.314 × 332) J mol^{-1} (*b*) (85 × 332) J mol^{-1}
    (*c*) (332/85) J mol^{-1} (*d*) (332/8.314) J mol^{-1}
12. The limiting molar conductivities of some species are given in (S cm^2 mol^{-1}) units:
    Λ^0 (HCI) = 425.9; Λ^0 (NaCl) =126.4; λ^0 (H^+) = 349.6
    Find the limiting molar conductivity of Na^+ ion.
    (*a*) 50.1 (*b*) 76.3 (*c*) 299.5 (*d*) 476.0
13. The reactivity order for nitration of benzene, chlorobenzene, phenol and nitrobenzene is
    (*a*) Benzene > Chlorobenzene > Phenol > Nitrobenzene
    (*b*) Phenol > Benzene > Chlorobenzene > Nitrobenzene
    (*c*) Nitrobenzene > Phenol > Chlorobenzene > Benzene
    (*d*) Phenol > Chlorobenzene > Benzene > Nitrobenzene

14. 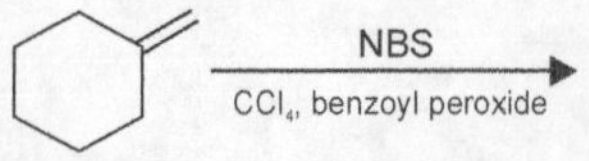

The major product in the above reaction is

(a) 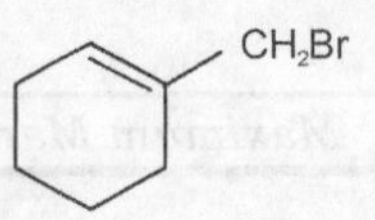 (b) 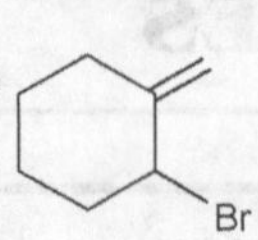

(c) 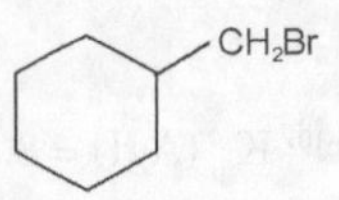 (d) 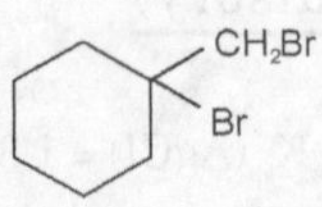

15. When a compound (M) is slowly heated with chloroform in alcoholic KOH solution, it produces an offensive smell. The compound M is

(a) N, N-Diethylaniline
(b) Diethylamine
(c) Ethylamine
(d) Triethylamine

16. Which one of the following will lactonize in presence of acid?

(a) 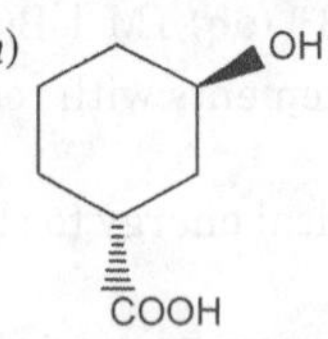 (b) 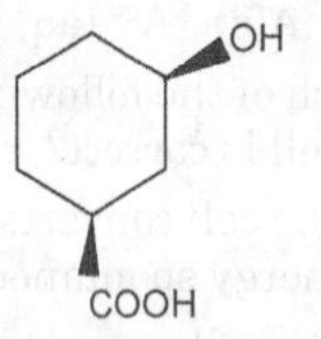

(c) 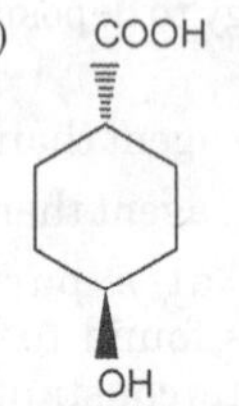 (d) 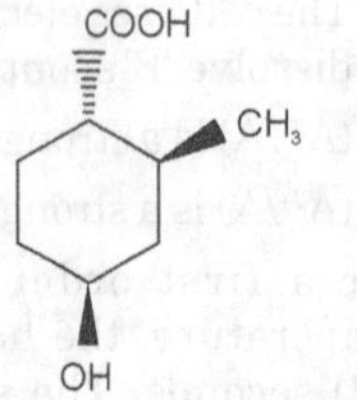

17. The major condensation product in the reaction of benzaldehyde with excess amount of acetone in presence of dilute NaOH solution is

(a) 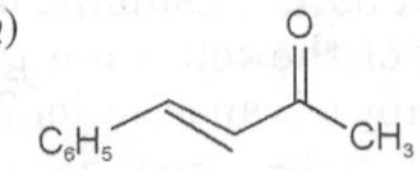

(b) 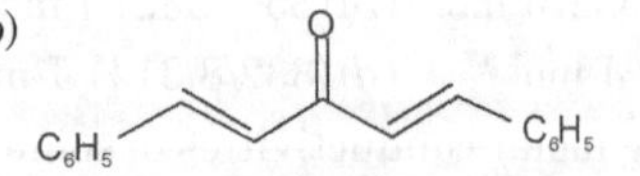

(c) 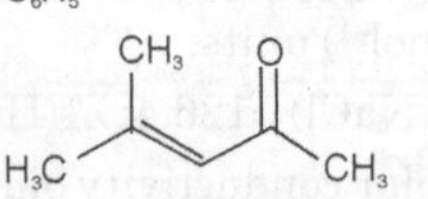

(d) 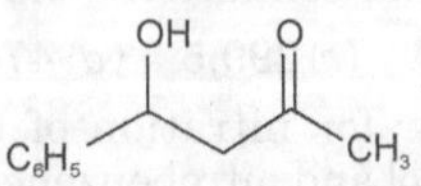

18. Ammonia gas can be dried over

(a) conc. H_2SO_4 (b) anhydrous P_2O_5
(c) anhydrous CaO (d) anhydrous $CaCl_2$

19. Which of the following molecules will have zero dipole moment?

H_2O, $SiCl_4$, CO_2, NH_3, BF_3

(a) H_2O, $SiCl_4$, BF_3 (b) CO_2, NH_3, $SiCl_4$
(c) H_2O, NH_3, BF_3 (d) CO_2, BF_3, $SiCl_4$

20. Which of the following pairs of complexes will NOT show any ligand field d-d transitions?

(a) $K_4[Fe(CN)_6]$, $[Ni(H_2O)_2(NH_3)_4]SO_4$
(b) $[Cu(CH_3CN)_4]Cl$, $Na_3[COCl_2(CN)_4]$
(c) $[Cu(CH_3CN)_4]Cl$, $[Zn(NH_3)_4Cl_2]$
(d) $[Cu(H_2O)_2(NH_3)_4]Cl_2$, $[Zn(H_2O)_4(NH_3)_4]SO_4$

21. Which of the following substances will produce acidic oxides when burnt in excess air? Sodium(P), Sulfur(Q) and Methane(R)

(a) All three (b) Both Q and R
(c) Only Q (d) Both P and R

22. In the ring test for nitrate ion, the brown color is due to the formation of

(a) $[Fe(H_2O)_5(NO)]SO_4$ (b) $[Fe(H_2O)_5(NO_2)]SO_4$
(c) $[Fe(H_2O)_3(NO)_3]SO_4$ (d) $[Fe(H_2O)_5(NO_3)]SO_4$

Common Data Questions

Common Data for Questions 23 and 24:

The compound (N) on treatment with the reagent (O) gives an alkene.

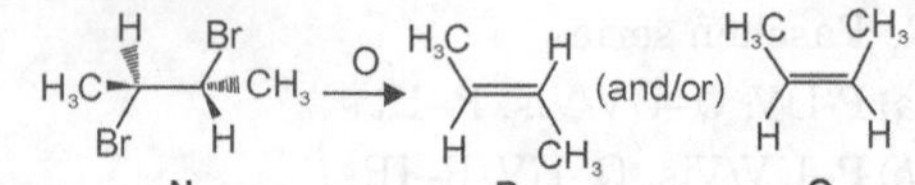

N P Q

23. The appropriate reagent(O) required for this transformation is

(a) KOH/EtOH (b) NaOMe/MeOH
(c) NaI/Acetone (d) $NaNH_2$

24. The alkene will be produced as

(a) P exclusively since it is going through E2 mechanism
(b) Q exclusively since it is going through E2 mechanism
(c) Equal amount of P and Q since it is going through E1 mechanism
(d) P as major amount since it is going through E1cB mechanism

Linked Answer Questions: Q.25 to 28 carry two marks each.

Statement for Linked Answer Q.25 and 26:

$CuSO_4$ solution when treated with aqueous alkali (W) forms a blue precipitate (X), which dissolves on addition of excess W. Another aqueous alkali (Y) precipitates blue solid (Z) when reacted with $CuSO_4$, but the blue precipitate (Z) does not dissolve with excess alkali (Y).

25. Identify W and X

(a) NH_4OH and $Cu(OH)_2$. $CuSO_4$
(b) NH_4OH and $Cu(OH)_2$
(c) NaOH and $Cu(OH)_2$.$CuSO_4$
(d) NaOH and $Cu(OH)_2$

26. Identify Y and Z

(a) NH_4OH and $Cu(OH)_2$. $CuSO_4$
(b) NH_4OH and $Cu(OH)_2$
(c) NaOH and $Cu(OH)_2$.$CuSO_4$
(d) NaOH and $Cu(OH)_2$

Statement for Linked Answer Questions 27 and 28:

For a first order reversible reaction $A \underset{k_b}{\overset{k_f}{\rightleftharpoons}} B$ *at a temperature T, the standard molar free energy* (ΔG^0) *is equal to –2.303RT, and the rate constant of forward reaction* (k_f) *is* $1 \times 10^{-3}\ s^{-1}$

27. The equilibrium constant of the reaction is

(*a*) 23.03 (*b*) 19.09 (*c*) 10 (*d*) 1

28. The rate constant of the backward reaction (k_b) is

(*a*) $5.26 \times 10^{-5}\ s^{-1}$ (*b*) $1 \times 10^{-2}\ s^{-1}$

(*c*) $4.35 \times 10^{-5}\ s^{-1}$ (*d*) $1 \times 10^{-4}\ s^{-1}$

K: BIOCHEMISTRY

Q. 1 – 6 carry one mark each.

1. Which of the following inhibitor uncouples electron transport and oxidative phosphorylation?

(*a*) Azide (*b*) Dinitrophenol

(*c*) Oligomycin (*d*) Rotenone

2. The catalytic efficiency of an enzyme is represented by

(*a*) V_{max} (*b*) K_M (*c*) k_{cat} (*d*) k_{cat}/K_M

3. Which of the following activate protein kinase C?

(*a*) Inositol 1, 4, 5-triphosphate

(*b*) Cyclic AMP

(*c*) Inositol

(*d*) Diacylglycerol

4. Transcription initiation sites can be determined by

(*a*) Footprinting (*b*) Northern blotting

(*c*) Primer extension (*d*) Nick translation

5. One common feature between B and T cells is that

(*a*) both cells produce antibodies

(*b*) both cells possess MHC class II

(*c*) both B cell receptor and T cell receptor undergo rearrangement

(*d*) both cells can produce cytokines

6. In hybridoma technology, the myeloma cells used

(*a*) lack HGPRT ase

(*b*) lack the ability to produce Ig

(*c*) lack both HGPRTase and ability to produce Ig

(*d*) lack thymidine kinase

Q. 7 – Q. 24 carry two marks each.

7. Match the function in Column I with organelle in Column II

Column - I	Column - II
P. Protein synthesis	1. Endoplasmic reticulum
Q. Protein degradation	2. Golgibody
R. Protein glycosylation	3. Lysosome
	4. Peroxisome

	P	Q	R
(*a*)	3	2	1
(*b*)	1	3	2
(*c*)	1	4	3
(*d*)	4	1	2

8. Match the polysaccharides in Column I with their constituent monosaccharide in Column II.

Column - I	Column - II
P. Chitin	1. D-Glucose
Q. Hemicellulose	2. N-Acetyl glucosamine
R. Glycogen	3. D-Xylose
	4. D-Galactose

	P	Q	R
(*a*)	1	3	4
(*b*)	2	4	1
(*c*)	4	2	3
(*d*)	2	3	1

9. The T_m of phosphatidyl choline A is higher than T_m of phosphatidyl choline B because

(*a*) A has shorter chain fatty acid and more unsaturated fatty acid than B

(*b*) A has longer chain fatty acid and more saturated fatty acid than B

(*c*) A has shorter chain fatty acid than B

(*d*) A has more *cis*-unsaturated fatty acid that B

10. A mixture of proteins namely P, Q, R and S having molecular mass 50,80,120, and 150 KDa is applied on the Sephadex-G 200 column. The order of their elution will be

(*a*) P, Q, R, S (*b*) S, R, Q, P

(*c*) Q, P, R, S (*d*) P, Q, S, R

11. Match the transition state or chemical entity of each enzyme that is responsible for their catalytic function

P. Ribonuclease	1. Oxyanion
Q. Lysozyme	2. Pentacovalent phosphorus
R. Chymotrypsin	3. Carbonium ion
S. Carboxypeptidase	4. Mixed anhydride

	P	Q	R	S
(*a*)	3	2	4	1
(*b*)	2	3	1	4
(*c*)	2	1	3	4
(*d*)	4	3	2	1

12. Match the function of following cofactors

P. Thiamine pyrophosphate	1. Acyl group transfer
Q. Coenzyme A	2. Trasfer of one carbon component
R. Pyridoxal phosphate	3. Group transfer to or from amino acid
S. Tetrahydrofolate	4. Aldehyde transfer

	P	Q	R	S
(*a*)	4	3	1	2
(*b*)	4	3	2	1
(*c*)	4	1	3	2
(*d*)	3	1	4	2

13. Match the enzymes in Column I with their metabolic pathways in Column II.

Column I

P. Succinyl CoA synthetase

Q. Acyl CoA dehydrogenase

R. Transketolase

S. Ribulose 1, 5-bisphosphate carboxylase

Column II

1. β-Oxidation
2. Calvin cycle
3. Tricarboxylic acid cycle
4. Pentose phosphate pathway

	P	Q	R	S
(*a*)	1	2	3	4
(*b*)	3	1	2	4
(*c*)	2	4	1	3
(*d*)	3	1	4	2

14. Glycolysis and gluconeogenesis are reciprocally coordinated. Which of the following will activate pyruvate carboxylase in gluconeogenesis?

(*a*) Acetyl CoA

(*b*) Fructose 2, 6-bisphosphate

(*c*) ADP

(*d*) ATP

15. The atoms of pyrimidine ring are derived from

(P) Carbamoyl phosphate

(Q) Inosine mono phosphate

(R) Aspartate

(S) Glutamate

(*a*) PQ (*b*) PR (*c*) PS (*d*) QR

16. Which of the following statements are true for steriod hormones?

(P) increase the enzymatic activity of pre-existing target enzyme

(Q) act at cell nucleus

(R) interact with the plasma membrane receptors of target cell

(S) form a complex with receptor and acts as transcriptional enhancers

(*a*) PR (*b*) QS (*c*) PQ (*d*) RS

17. Match the items on the left with the inhibitors on the right

P. DNA polymerase α	1. Phenyl methyl sulphonyl fluoride (PMSF)
Q. RNA polymerase II	2. Aphidicolin
R. Serine protease	3. α amanitin
	4. Actinomycin

	P	Q	R
(*a*)	2	3	1
(*b*)	3	1	2
(*c*)	2	1	2
(*d*)	1	2	4

18. A nucleic acid sample is resistant to digestion with λ exonuclease. When heated it does not show typical melting curve of a linear double stranded DNA. On CsCl-ethidium bromide equilibrium density centrifugation it settles at the bottom of the centrifuge tube. The nucleic acid is

(*a*) ccc pBR322

(*b*) Bacteriophage P22 DNA

(*c*) rRNA

(*d*) RFII M 13 DNA

19. The following 4 different solutions are prepared by mixing the components of electron transport chain. Which among them is expected to cause a net transfer of electrons to cytochrome c?

(*a*) Reduced ubiquinone and reduced cytochrome c.

(*b*) Reduced ubiquinone, cytochrome b-c_1 complex and reduced cytochrome c.

(*c*) Oxidized ubiquinone and oxidized cytochrome c.

(*d*) Reduced ubiquinone, cytochrome b-c_1 complex and oxidized cytochrome c.

20. Nucleated cells tends to be more resistant to complement mediated lysis than RBC because

(*a*) many nucleated cells can endocytose the membrane attack complex

(*b*) membrane attack complex cannot get inserted in the nucleated cell membrane

(*c*) membrane attack complex can get inactivated by the nucleated cells

(*d*) membrane attack complex get inactivated hence cannot get inserted in the nucleated cell membrane

21. In a fluorescein labeled antibody to heavy chain and rhodamine labeled antibody to δ heavy chain, the fluorescent antibody staining pattern of the progenitor B cells (Pro-B cells) will be

(*a*) anti- staining in cytoplasm and on membrane

(*b*) anti- and anti-δ staining in cytoplasm and on membrane

(*c*) no cytoplasmic or membrane staining with either anti or δ antibody

(*d*) anti- staining on the membrane

22. Serum IgM cannot activate the complement by itself because

(*a*) it does not have complement binding site

(*b*) it is planar in which complement binding sites in the Fc region are not accessible

(*c*) it gets degraded and hence unable to activate the complement

(*d*) it needs metal ions to activate complement

Common Data Questions

Common Data for Questions 23 and 24:

A *Caenorhabditis* contig for one region of *chromosome 2 contains contiguous locations marked 1, 2, 3, 4, 5, 6, 7, 8 and 9. Cosmid clones a, b, c, d and e overlap the locations 2-4, 3-5, 4-6, 5-8, 8-9 respectively. A cloned pBR322-x hybridize to cosmids b, c and d and pUC18-y hybridize to cosmids d and e.*

23. The approximate locations of x and y are

(*a*) 4 and 7 (*b*) 5 and 8

(*c*) 4 and 8 (*d*) 5 and 7

24. Both pBR322-x and pUC18-y will hybridize to cosmids

(*a*) b (*b*) d

(*c*) e (*d*) c

Linked Answer Questions: Q.25 to Q.28 carry two marks each.

Statement for Linked Answer Questions 25 and 26:

In animal cells concentration of sodium ions is higher outside the cell and less inside the cell, yet sodium does not enter the cells.

25. The cellular environment is maintained by generating a gradient and transporting the Na^+ outside the cell through

(*a*) diffusion process

(*b*) passive transport via Na^+-K^+ pump

(*c*) active transport via Na^+-K^+ pump

(*d*) sodium ions not be transported

26. Digitoxigenin, a cardiotonic steroid that inhibits ATPase when applied on extra cellular face of membrane, helps in accumulation of Ca^{2+} inside the cardiac muscle cells by

(*a*) activating Na^+-K^+ pump and blocking Na^+-Ca^{++} exchanger

(*b*) inhibiting Na^+-K^+ pump and blocking Na^+-Ca^{++} exchanger

(*c*) having no effort on Na^+-K^+ pump

(*d*) increasing passive diffusion

Statement for Linked Answer Questions 27 and 28:

Nearly 46% of 45s pre-rRNA is unstable. The remaining portion of it forms mature 5.8s, 18s and 28s rRNA having lengths 160 bases, 1.9 kb and 5.1 kb respectively. The content of pre rRNA per human genome is 7.8×10^{-15} g.

27. The mol.wt. of 45s pre-rRNA is

(*a*) 2×10^6 (*b*) 4.5×10^5

(*c*) 4.5×10^6 (*d*) 3.9×10^7

28. The number of pre-rRNA genes per genome is approximately

(*a*) 10 (*b*) 100

(*c*) 1,000 (*d*) 10,000

M : BOTANY

Q. 1 – 6 carry one mark each.

1. C_4 photosynthesis is a biochemical and structural syndrome that enhances

(*a*) Concentration of CO_2 in the bundle sheath cells

(*b*) Photorespiration

(*c*) Requirement of water and nitrogen

(*d*) Lower radiation use efficiency

2. Pioneering work conducted in green revolution

(*a*) C. Subramanium

(*b*) M. S. Swaminathan

(*c*) E. C. Cocking

(*d*) Norman Bourlag

3. 'Bordeaux mixture' contains

(*a*) Copper nitrate and ferric chloride

(*b*) Copper sulphate and slaked lime

(*c*) Copper sulphate and ferric chloride

(*d*) Ferric chloride and slaked lime

4. The 'Kornberg's enzyme' is now known as

(*a*) DNA polymerase III (*b*) DNA polymerase II

(*c*) DNA polymerase I (*d*) DNA ligase

5. Genome sequencing of rice will help to

(*a*) Characterize genes present in the rice genome

(*b*) Validate the genes available in other plants

(*c*) Control agri-business

(*d*) Control rice germplasm

6. Identify the correct statement

(*a*) Cytokinin does not regulate cell division in plants

(*b*) Kinetin was discovered as a breakdown product of DNA

(*c*) Osmotic adjustment of cells does not help water balance in plants

(*d*) Cytokinin enhances leaf senescence

Q. 7 — 24 carry two marks each.

7. Identify the correct statements

(P) Caryopsis, one-seeded dry indehiscent fruit of Gramineae

(Q) Lithocyst, a cell containing starch

(R) Aleurone layer contains protein granules and enzymes

(S) Embryo development is not of a single cell origin

(*a*) Q, R (*b*) P, S

(*c*) P, R (*d*) Q, S

8. $NADH \rightarrow Q \rightarrow ? \rightarrow Cytc_1 \rightarrow ? \rightarrow Cyt_{(a + a_3)} \rightarrow O_2$

Sequence of electron transfer in oxidative phosphorylation is given above. Complete the missing sequence

(*a*) Cyta and Cytb (*b*) Cyta and Cytc

(*c*) Cytb and Cytc (*b*) Cytb and $Cytb_1$

9. Which of the following statements are true on phytoremediation point of view ?
   P An effective technology that uses plants to tolerate and accumulate metals from the environment
   Q Detoxification of soil phenolic pollutants by plant secretory enzymes
   R Using RT-PCR to quantify gene expression in plants
   S Studies on plant phylogeny and exploiting the biodiversity
   (*a*) P, Q (*b*) P, R (*c*) R, S (*d*) P, S
10. Indentify the correct statements
   P The second law of thermodynamics is also known as the law of conservation of energy
   Q 'Entropy' is a measure of the available energy resulting from transformations
   R The transfer of energy through the food chain of an ecosystem is termed as 'energy flow'
   S The second law of thermodynamics deals with the transfer of energy towards more available state
   (*a*) P, Q (*b*) P, R (*c*) Q, R (*d*) Q, S
11. Red flower (R) dominant to white flower (r) and short pollen grain (I) recessive to long pollen grain (L) are two genes on chromosome number 2 of sweet pea. Plants with red flower and long pollen grains were crossed with plants with white flower and short pollen grains. The hybrids were test crossed and the following progenies were obtained in the F_2.
   a. : Red flower with long pollen grain
   ss. : Red flower with short pollen grain
   35. : White flower with long pollen grain
   350 : White flower with short pollen grain
   What would be the map distance between R and L ?
   (*a*) 16 cM (*b*) 8 cM (*c*) 10 cM (*d*) 30 cM
12. Oryza sativa and Michelia champaca belong to the following families.
   P Gramineae and Chenopodiaceae
   Q Brassicasceae and Malvaceae
   R Gramineae and Magnoliaceae
   S Cyperaceae and Myristicaceae
   (*a*) P (*b*) Q (*c*) R (*d*) S
13. Identify the correct statements
   P Agar is manufactured from Gelidium of Rhodophyceae and algenic acid from Laminaria of Pheophyceae
   Q All mushrooms are edible and coloured mushrooms are poisonous
   R Dioscorea sp. produce diosgenin used as antifertility drugs
   S Gossypium produce high quality jute fibre
   (*a*) P, R (*b*) P, Q (*c*) Q, R (*d*) R, S
14. Identify the correct statements
   P Heterosis is a proven way of increasing productivity of many crop plants
   Q Weed caused considerable yield loss and reduce farmer's income
   R PR (Pathogenesis related) proteins protect plants against bacteria
   S Marker assisted selection can improve crops in field
   (*a*) P, S (*b*) R, S
   (*c*) Q, R (*d*) P, Q
15. Which of the following statements are true on ecological point of view ?
   P Biodiversity is affected by environmental pollution
   Q Alternative agriculture is designed to sustain crop yield while enhancing inputs of fossil fuel, pesticides, etc.
   R Global climate change is caused by human activities
   S Acid rain is caused by excessive CO_2 in the air
   (*a*) P, Q (*b*) P, R
   (*c*) Q, R (*d*) R, S

Direction (Q. 16 - 22) : *In each question, each item P, Q, R and S in Group I matches one of the items in Group II. Choose the correct match from the alternatives a, b, c and d.*

16. **Group I**

P. 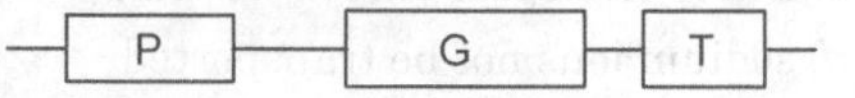

Q. 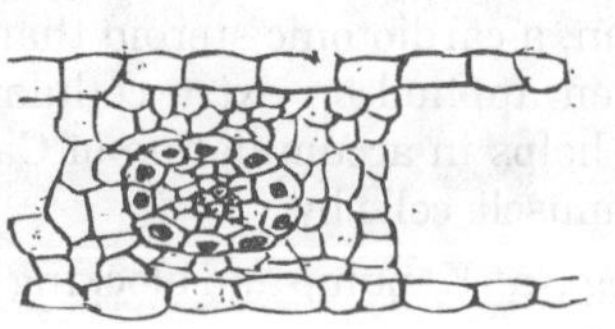

R. 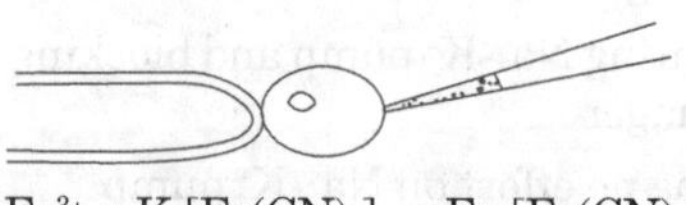

S. $Fe^{3+} + K_4[Fe(CN)_3] \rightarrow Fe_4[Fe(CN)_6]_3 + 4K^+$

Group II
1. Kranz anatomy
2. Single protoplast culture
3. Binary vector
4. Microinjection
5. Partial plasmid map
6. Ferric-Ferro-Cyanide complex

	P	Q	R	S
(*a*)	3	1	4	6
(*b*)	5	1	2	3
(*c*)	5	3	4	6
(*d*)	3	4	1	6

17. **Group I**

P. Foliaceous bracts
Q. Spathe
R. Petaloid bracts
S. Involucre

Group II

1. A large and commonly boat shaped bract enclosing a cluster of flowers
2. One or more whorls of bracteoles developing at the base of a calyx
3. Green, flat and leaf like in appearance
4. Brightly coloured bracts looking somewhat like petals
5. Special bracts - small, dry and scaly
6. One or more whorls of bracts, normally green in colour present around a cluster of flowers

	P	Q	R	S
(*a*)	5	2	3	4
(*b*)	3	1	4	6
(*c*)	3	6	3	2
(*d*)	4	5	2	1

18.

Group I	Group II
P. Atropin	1. Digitalis purpurea
Q. Cocaine	2. Triticum aestivum
R. Digitalis	3. Erythroxylon coca
S. Hops	4. Humulus lupulus
	5. Atropa belladonna
	6. Datura stramonium

	P	Q	R	S
(*a*)	6	5	4	2
(*b*)	3	2	4	1
(*c*)	5	3	1	4
(*d*)	6	5	3	1

19.

Group I	Group II
P. Late blight of potato	1. Synchytrium endobioticum
Q. Early blight of potato	2. Rhizoctonia solani
R. Balck scurf of potato	3. Alternaria solani
S. Wart diseases of potato	4. Phytophthora colocasiae
	5. Phytophthora arecaceae
	6. Phytophthora infestans

	P	Q	R	S
(*a*)	6	3	2	1
(*b*)	6	3	1	2
(*c*)	5	3	2	1
(*d*)	4	3	2	1

20.

Group I	Group II
P. Insect Resistance Rice	1. psy
Q. Non-antibiotic selection	2. crylAb
R. Antibiotic marker gene	3. hpt
S. C_4 photosynthesis	4. PEPC
	5. PMI
	6. Rubisco

	P	Q	R	S
(*a*)	2	1	3	4
(*b*)	5	2	1	6
(*c*)	2	5	3	4
(*d*)	1	2	4	6

21. **Group I**

P. P. Maheshwari
Q. E. Hood
R. B. McClintock
S. S. M. Sarkar

Group II

1. Plant embryology
2. Genetics
3. Agrobacterium transformation
4. Growth hormone
5. Molecular biology
6. Systematic botany

	P	Q	R	S
(*a*)	1	6	3	2
(*b*)	1	3	2	4
(*c*)	1	2	6	5
(*d*)	2	1	5	3

22. **Group I**

P. IPR
Q. Selectable reporter gene
R. Vectorless DNA transfer
S. Selectable market gene

Group II

1. Intellectual property rights
2. International plant registration
3. Protoplast system
4. Agrobacterium system
5. Neomycin phosphotranferase
6. Green fluorescent protein

	P	Q	R	S
(*a*)	1	6	3	5
(*b*)	1	6	4	2
(*c*)	2	6	3	5
(*d*)	2	5	4	6

Common Data Questions

Common Data for Questions 23 and 24:

Union of stamens may involve adhesion or cohesion. Arrangement of stamens of a flower is given below:

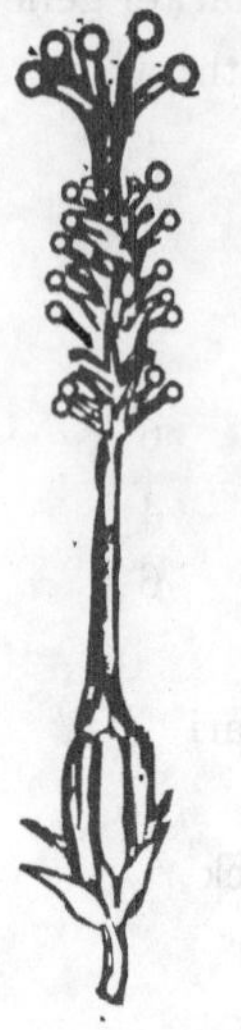

23. Identify the type of stamen
    (*a*) Diadelphous (*b*) Monadelphous
    (*c*) Polydelphous (*d*) Syngenesious
24. Identify the family from the type of stamens
    (*a*) Malvaceae (*b*) Solanaceae
    (*c*) Compositae (*d*) Apiaceae

Linked Answer Questions : Q. 25 to 28 carry two marks each.

Statement for Linked Answer Questions 25 and 26 :

The following reaction is taking place in aerobic organisms

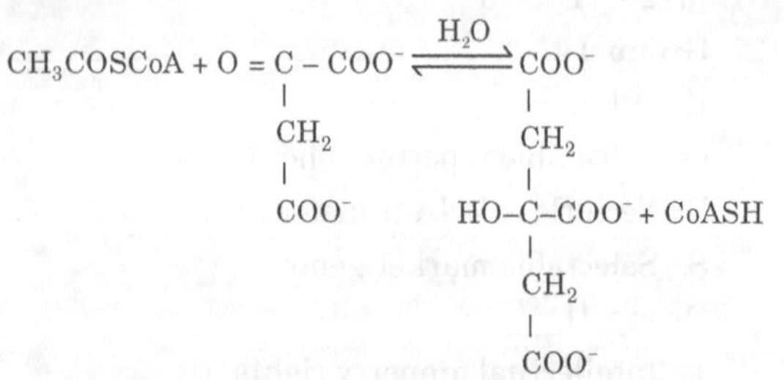

25. Identify the products from the above reaction
    (*a*) Isocitrate and Coenzyme A
    (*b*) Citrate and Coenzyme A
    (*c*) Pyruvate and acetyl CoA
    (*d*) Succinate and acetyl CoA
26. Identify the enzyme and the type of reaction
    (*a*) Citrate synthase and condensation reaction
    (*b*) Citrate synthatase and condensation reaction
    (*c*) Isocitrate dehydrogenase and oxidative decarboxylation
    (*d*) Aconitase and dehydration reaction

Statement for Linked Answer Questions 27 and 28 :

The visible spectrum of light lies between 400-700 nm. The correlation of expression of wavelength is given below :

1m → 10^3 mm → 10^6 m → 10^9 nm → 10^{10} A°

	Colour Spectrum	Wavelength (nm)
P	Blue	1. 55-550
Q	Green	2. 450-500
R	Yellow	3. 650-700
S	Red	4. 550-600

27. Identify the correct combination from the above options

	P	Q	R	S
(*a*)	1	2	4	3
(*b*)	2	1	3	4
(*c*)	2	1	4	3
(*d*)	3	1	2	4

28. For conversion of wavelength from nm to A° and m
    (*a*) Divide the wavelength by 10 and 10^{-3}
    (*b*) Multiply the wavelength by 10 and 10^{-3}
    (*c*) Divide the wavelength by 10 and 10^{-4}
    (*d*) Multiply the wavelength by 10 and 10^{-5}

N : MICROBIOLOGY

Q. 1 – 6 carry one mark each.

1. Which is the most modern method of classification of organisms?
   (*a*) Morphology
   (*b*) Gram staining
   (*c*) Biochemical characterization
   (*d*) 16S rRNA sequence
2. The mode of action of sulfonamides is by inhibition of
   (*a*) Cell wall synthesis (*b*) Folic acid metabolism
   (*c*) DNA replication (*d*) Sulphur metabolism
3. The Ziehl-Neelsen staining technique is used for the detection of
   (*a*) Endospores (*b*) Capsule
   (*c*) Flagella (*d*) Cell wall
4. A solution of ampicillin is
   (*a*) Sterilized by autoclaving
   (*b*) Sterilized by dry heat
   (*c*) Sterilized by membrane filtration
   (*d*) Need not be sterilized
5. Fixation of molecular nitrogen is carried out by
   (*a*) A multi-enzyme complex containing nitrogenase and nitrogenase reductase
   (*b*) Nitrogenase
   (*c*) Nitrogenase reductase
   (*d*) Nitrate reductase

6. The complement fixation test for syphilis was introduced by
(*a*) Theobald Smith
(*b*) Walter Reed
(*c*) Martinus Willem Beijerinck
(*d*) August Von Wassermann

Q. 7 – 24 carry two marks each.

7. You have a culture of metabolically inactive E. coli. To make protoplasts you will use
(*a*) Penicillin
(*b*) Lysozyme
(*c*) Hypertonic solution + penicillin
(*d*) Hypertonic solution + lysozyme

8. The Ames test is carried out on 3 strains of Salmonella typhimurium having 3 different kinds of mutations in the his gene. Two mutagens, acridine orange and ethyl methane sulfonate (EMS), are used in this experiment and the following results are obtained.

Strain	Number of revertants/10^8 cells		
	Acridine orange	EMS	No mutagen
P	10080	1	2
Q	9	101	3
R	2	3	2

Based on the chemical nature of the mutagens, the nature of the mutation in the his gene in the 3 strains is
(*a*) P- silent, Q- insertion, R- base substitution
(*b*) P- insertion, Q- silent, R- frameshift
(*c*) P- frameshift, Q- base substitution, R- insertion
(*d*) P- base substitution, Q- frameshift, R- silent

9. You isolate a natural plasmid from a tetracycline resistant strain of E.coli. You heat denature the plasmid, allow it to self anneal and observe the DNA by electron microscopy. The predominant DNA structure observed is shown schematically below.

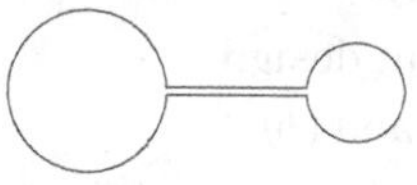

The plasmid is most likely to contain a
(*a*) Phage DNA
(*b*) Transposon
(*c*) Transfer operon
(*d*) T DNA

10. For which of the following diseases does the causative agent NOT strictly obey Koch's postulates?
(*a*) Tuberculosis
(*b*) Cholera
(*c*) Bovine spongifor encephalopathy
(*d*) Bird flu

11. An E. coli culture is mutagenized to obtain leucine auxotrophs. The auxotroph can be identified by plating on medium
(*a*) Containing leucine
(*b*) Lacking leucine
(*c*) Containing leucine followed by replica plating onto (B)
(*d*) Lacking leucine followed by replica plating onto (A)

12. An agent used in the cosmetic treatment of facial wrinkles is isolated from
(*a*) Shigella sp.
(*b*) Bacillus anthracis
(*c*) Clostridium botulinum
(*d*) Aspergillus flavus

13. Three restriction endonucleases P, Q and R recognize 4bp, 6bp and 8bp sequences respectively. The relative frequency of occurrence of these sequences on a bacterial genome is
(*a*) P>Q>R (*b*) P>R>Q
(*c*) R>Q>P (*d*) Q>R>P

14. The alternate pathway of complement-mediated cell lysis is triggered by
(*a*) Bacterial polysaccharide
(*b*) Bacterial polysaccharide + antibody to the polysaccharide
(*c*) Antibody to the polysaccharide
(*d*) All of these

15. Anaphylaxis is initiated by
(*a*) IgE bound to mast cells
(*b*) Antigen bound to IgE on mast cells
(*c*) Antigen bound to mast cells
(*d*) All of these

16. For which one of the following operations are dilution rate and limiting a specific nutrient the important parameters?
(*a*) Batch fermentation
(*b*) Fed batch fermentation
(*c*) Chemostat
(*d*) Turbidostat

17. By doubling the concentration of an enzyme the
(*a*) K_m will remain constant and V_{max} will increase
(*b*) K_m and V_{max} will increase
(*c*) K_m and V_{max} will decrease
(*d*) K_m will increase and V_{max} will remain constant

18. Glycosidic linkages between D-glucose residues in starch and cellulose respectively are
(*a*) (α 1$\rightarrow$4) and (β 1$\rightarrow$4)
(*b*) (α 1$\rightarrow$4) and (α 1$\rightarrow$4)
(*c*) (β 1$\rightarrow$4) and (β 1$\rightarrow$4)
(*d*) (β 1$\rightarrow$4) and (α 1$\rightarrow$4)

19. The enzymes responsible for generation of ATP in E. coli by substrate level phosphory- lation and the electron transport system are located respectively in the

(*a*) Cytoplasm and plasma membrance

(*b*) Plasma membrane and cytoplasm

(*c*) Cytoplasm and outer membrane

(*d*) Outer membrane and cytoplasm

20. Which reducing agent is NOT naturally present in the cell?

(*a*) Ascorbic acid (*b*) Glutathione

(*c*) Cysteine (*d*) Dithiothreitol

21. The TCA cycle begins by the condensation of the two carbon compound (P) with the fou carbon compound (Q) to form the six carbon compound (R). Here P, Q, R represent

(*a*) Oxaloacetate, Citrate, Acetyl~CoA

(*b*) Acetyl~CoA, Oxaloacetate, Citrate

(*c*) Citrate, Oxaloacetate, Acetyl~CoA

(*d*) Acetyl~CoA, Citrate, Oxaloacetate

22. In glycolysis the conversion of glucose to two pyruvate molecules gives a net yield of

(*a*) 2 ATP (*b*) 4 ATP + 2 NADH

(*c*) 2 ATP + 2 NADPH (*d*) 2 ATP + 2 NADH

Common data Questions

Common Data questions 23 and 24 :

A

(P) Retroviridae

(Q) Herpesviridae

(R) Rhabdoviridae

(S) Baculoviridae

B

(1) Linear double stranded DNA

(2) Minus strand RNA

(3) Circular double stranded DNA

(4) Plus strand RNA

23. Match the columns.

	P	Q	R	S
(*a*)	1	2	3	4
(*b*)	2	3	4	1
(*c*)	3	4	1	2
(*d*)	4	1	2	3

24. Which one of the GENOMES listed above is NOT infectious when introduced into host cells by liposomes?

(*a*) Linear double stranded DNA

(*b*) Minus strand RNA

(*c*) Circular double stranded DNA

(*d*) Plus strand RNA

Linked Answer Questions : Q.25 to 28 carry two marks each

Statement for Linked Answer Questions 25 and 26:

A gene is negatively regulated by a repressor that binds to an operator with a dissociation constant (K_D) of 10^{-9} M. There are 100 molecules of repressor per cell and cell volume is 10^{-8} ml.

25. Assuming the Avogadro number (N) to be 10^{23} molecules, what is the concentration of the repressor in the cell?

(*a*) 10^{-8}M (*b*) 10^{-9}M (*c*) 10^{-10}M (*d*) 10^{-11}M

26. At this concentration of the repressor, the gene is

(*a*) Repressed (*b*) Transiently repressed

(*c*) Partially expressed (*d*) Expressed

Statement for Linked Answer questions 27 and 28:

A suspension of temperate phage contains 10^7 particles/ ml. Only 10% of these are capable of infecting bacteria. Hundred microlitres of the phage suspension is mixed with 1000 bacterial cells.

27. What is the multiplicity of infection (MOI)?

(*a*) 10^3 (*b*) 10^2 (*c*) 10^1 (*d*) 10^0

28. At this MOI

(*a*) Lysogeny is favoured

(*b*) Lytic cycle is favoured

(*c*) Both lysogeny and lytic cycle are equally favoured

(*d*) The bacterial cells do not get infected

Q : ZOOLOGY

Q. 1 – 6 carry one mark each

1. In theories of evolution, the example that a giraffe stretching the neck to reach on higher branches has been used to explain the following

(*a*) Use and disuse theory

(*b*) The concept of inheritance of acquired characters

(*c*) Intelligent design

(*d*) Both (*a*) and (*b*)

2. Which of the following statements is true for the systematics of the animal kingdom?

(*a*) Systematics employs a hierarchical system of classification

(*b*) Systematics can also be based on cladistic analysis

(*c*) Systematics can infer phylogeny from molecular data

(*d*) All of these

3. Most modern taxonomists group living organisms into how many kingdoms?

(*a*) 2 (*b*) 3

(*c*) 4 (*d*) 5

4. In many terrestrial vertebrates, including humans, the sensory organ for hearing and equilibrium are closely associated within the inner ear. Which of the following parts in the inner ear represents the organ of equilibrium?
(*a*) Tectorial membrane
(*b*) Tymphanic membrane
(*c*) Semicircular canals
(*d*) Sacule

5. Which combination of mechanisms best explain cross-continental migration of animals?
(*a*) Orientation and navigation
(*b*) Orientation and piloting
(*c*) Navigation and piloting
(*d*) Orientation, navigations and piloting

6. Hemolin is
(*a*) An antibody produced by sponges
(*b*) An antibody produced by annelids
(*c*) A member of the immunoglobulin superfamily
(*d*) A cytotoxic molecule produced by nematodes

Q. 7 – Q. 24 carry two marks each

7. The fossile records suggest evolutionary trends. Choose the correct statement
(*a*) An evolutionary trend does NOT imply that evolution is goal oriented
(*b*) An evolutionary trend implies that evolution is goal oriented
(*c*) Fossil record can NOT be considered as indicators of evolutionary process
(*d*) A fossilized specimen undergoes gradual change over time that "mimics" the evolutionary process

8. Which of the following statements identify the term "biological magnification"?
(*a*) Green house effect will have greater impact on tropical countries
(*b*) Toxins become concentrated in successive trophic levels of food webs
(*c*) Energy is lost at each level in a food chain
(*d*) Primary producers are at the bottom of the food chain

9. Honey bee returning to the hive from a food source performs a "waggle dance". It indicates the
(*a*) Distance between the beehive and the food source
(*b*) Direction to the food resource
(*c*) The type of food available in the source
(*d*) All of these

10. Choose the choice that correctly pairs the following

A. Initial response to antigen	i. Coelomocytes
B. Cytokines	ii. IgM
C. Passive immunity to foetus	iii. IgG
D. Humoral immunity	iv. T cells
E. Phagocytosis	v. B cells

(*a*) A-iv; B-iii; C-ii; D-v; E-i
(*b*) A-i; B-iv; C-v; D-iii; E-ii
(*c*) A-ii; B-iv; C-iii; D-v; E-i
(*d*) A-ii; B-v; C-i; D-iv; E-iii

11. Which of the following is correctly paired?
(*a*) Blastopore - organizer
(*b*) Regulative development - syncytial specification
(*c*) Vegetal pole-mesoderm
(*d*) Spiral cleavage - chick embryo

12. Which of the following is seen in an adult frog?
(*a*) Somite (*b*) Notochord
(*c*) Branchial arches (*d*) None of these

13. Which of the following has all the pairs correct?

A. Ectoderm	i. Heart
B. Mesoderm	ii. Stomach
C. Endoderm	iii. Enteric neuron
D. Ectoderm	iv. Skull
E. Mesoderm	v. Kidney

(*a*) A-iii, B-ii, C-i, D-iv, E-v
(*b*) A-iii, B-i, C-ii, D-iv, E-v
(*c*) A-ii, B-iv, C-v, D-i, E-iii
(*d*) A-ii, B-i, C-v, D-iii, E-iv

14. Which combination of following statements is true?
(i) Hox genes have undergone multiple duplications during animal evolution.
(ii) For some reptiles, sex is determined by environmental factor(s).
(iii) Metamorphosis in amphibians is regulated by nuclear hormone receptor signaling.
(*a*) (i) and (ii) (*b*) (i) and (iii)
(*c*) (ii) and (iii) (*d*) (i) (ii) and (iii)

15. The 5′-untranslated region (5′-UTR) is found
(*a*) Upstream of the promoter
(*b*) Within the first intron
(*c*) Within the first exon
(*d*) Immediately upstream of the splice acceptor site

16. A:T and G:C ratios in a newly discovered organism are 0.63 and 0.8, respectively. Genome of this organism is likely to have
(*a*) Single stranded DNA
(*b*) Double stranded DNA
(*c*) Single stranded RNA
(*d*) Double stranded RNA

17. During enzyme-catalyzed reaction, a competitive inhibitor acts by
(*a*) Reducing activation energy
(*b*) Increasing activation energy
(*c*) Reducing effective substrate concentration
(*d*) Increasing effective substrate concentration

18. Which of the following pairs is NOT correct?
(*a*) Reverse transcriptase - DNA synthesis
(*b*) Primase - RNA synthesis
(*c*) Acetyl transferase - Transcription
(*d*) Reverse transcriptase - transcription

19. In an organism with diploid chromosome number of 8, the cells at anaphase II will display
(*a*) 4 chromosomes
(*b*) 2 chromosomes with 4 chromatids
(*c*) 4 chromatids
(*d*) 8 sister chromatids

20. Symbiotic microbes that help the digestive process in ruminants live in a specialized part of the alimentary canal known as
(*a*) Liver (*b*) Pharynx
(*c*) Stomach (*d*) Cecum

21. In animals, respiration and circulatory systems are often functionally interlinked. Which animal, group represents an exception?
(*a*) Aquatic mammals (*b*) Fish
(*c*) Terrestrial insects (*d*) Amphibians

22. Match the term with the correct description

A. Gene flow	i. Source of new alleles
B. Natural selection	ii. Changes in a population's allele frequencies due to chance alone
C. Mutations	iii. Allele frequencies changes due immigr-ation, emigration or both
D. Genetic drift	iv. Outcome of differences in survival and reproduction among individuals that vary in forms shared traits

(*a*) A - iii, B - iv, C - i, D - ii
(*b*) A - iv, B - iii, C - ii, D - i
(*c*) A - ii, B - i, C - iv, D - iii
(*d*) A - ii, B - iv, C - iii, D - i

Common Data Questions

Common Data for questions 23 and 24 :

Many nematodes are parasites on animals. Ascaris lumbricoides is an example of nematode parasite on human. It infects more than 1 billion people in Africa and Asia. Ascaris passes through several stages of its life cycle inside the human body.

23. Ascaris lumbricoides enters the human host in which stage of its life cycle?
(*a*) Egg (*b*) Larva
(*c*) Adult (*d*) Adult female

24. During its life cycle within the host, Ascaris migrates from
(*a*) Intestine of heart (*b*) Intestine to brain
(*c*) Lungs to throat (*d*) Intestine to liver

Linked Answer Questions : Q.25 to Q.28 carry two marks each

Statement for Linked Answer Questions 25 and 26:

Synthetic progesterone and estrogen are commonly used as birth control pills. Based on your understanding of hormonal regulation of reproduction, answer the following 2 questions.

25. These two hormones act by
(*a*) Negative feedback to stop the release of GnRH
(*b*) Positive feedback by increasing the release of LH and FSH hormones
(*c*) Increasing the level of LH and decreasing the level of FSH
(*d*) Decreasing the level of LH and increasing the level of FSH

26. During a menstrual cycle in human female, elevated levels of progesterone indicates that the process of ovulation is
(*a*) Yet to occur (*b*) Completed
(*c*) Advanced (*d*) Delayed

Statement for Linked Answer Questions 27 and 28:

When an animal of the genotype AaBb was mated with another of the genotype aabb (test cross), the following progeny were observed

AaBb – 980; aabb – 976; Aabb – 287 and aaBb – 291

27. Based on your understanding of the law of independent assortment, what ratios of progeny phenotypes are expected in a test cross (AaBb × aabb)?
(*a*) 1:1:1:1 (*b*) 2:2:1:1
(*c*) 1:2:1:2 (*d*) 1:1:2:2

28. Based on your answer to the previous question, which one of the following statements MOST accurately describes the test cross results mentioned above?
(*a*) Genes A and B are on different chromosomes
(*b*) Genes A and B are probably on the same chromosome
(*c*) Inheritance of A is modified by B
(*d*) Genes A and B assort independently

ANSWERS

J : CHEMISTRY

1. (b)	2. (a)	3. (d)	4. (b)	5. (d)	6. (c)	7. (a)	8. (b)	9. (c)	10. (a)
11. (b)	12. (a)	13. (b)	14. (b)	15. (c)	16. (b)	17. (a)	18. (c)	19. (d)	20. (c)
21. (b)	22. (a)	23. (c)	24. (b)	25. (b)	26. (d)	27. (c)	28. (d)		

K : BIOCHEMISTRY

1. (b)	2. (d)	3. (d)	4. (a)	5. (c)	6. (c)	7. (b)	8. (d)	9. (b)	10. (b)
11. (b)	12. (c)	13. (d)	14. (a)	15. (b)	16. (b)	17. (a)	18. (a)	19. (d)	20. (a)
21. (c)	22. (b)	23. (b)	24. (b)	25. (c)	26. (b)	27. (c)	28. (b)		

M : BOTANY

1. (a)	2. (d)	3. (b)	4. (c)	5. (a)	6. (b)	7. (c)	8. (c)	9. (a)	10. (c)
11. (a)	12. (c)	13. (a)	14. (d)	15. (b)	16. (a)	17. (b)	18. (c)	19. (a)	20. (c)
21. (b)	22. (b)	23. (b)	24. (a)	25. (b)	26. (b)	27. (b)	28. (b)		

N : MICROBIOLOGY

1. (d)	2. (b)	3. (d)	4. (c)	5. (a)	6. (d)	7. (d)	8. (c)	9. (b)	10. (c)
11. (d)	12. (c)	13. (a)	14. (a)	15. (b)	16. (c)	17. (a)	18. (a)	19. (a)	20. (d)
21. (b)	22. (d)	23. (d)	24. (d)	25. (c)	26. (b)	27. (b)	28. (a)		

Q : ZOOLOGY

1. (d)	2. (d)	3. (d)	4. (d)	5. (d)	6. (c)	7. (b)	8. (b)	9. (d)	10. (c)
11. (b)	12. (d)	13. (b)	14. (d)	15. (a)	16. (a)	17. (d)	18. (c)	19. (c)	20. (c)
21. (c)	22. (a)	23. (a)	24. (d)	25. (a)	26. (b)	27. (a)	28. (b)		

EXPLANATIONS

J : CHEMISTRY

1. Electrolytes are able to conduct electricity because the ions in solution are able to carry charge and move it around. A metal conducts because the electrons can move around freely while in an electrolytic solution, the ions move around freely. It is very similar to a metal. The only way that something can conduct is if charged particles such as electrons or ions can move to carry the current. The ions in their lattice form cannot carry charge because they are rigid and unable to move. They are stuck through ionic bonds in their crystal lattice. Their rigidity is a reason why most ionic compounds have incredibly high melting points. An electrolyte solution conducts electricity because of the movement of ions in the solution. The larger the concentration of ions, the better the solution conducts. All electrolytes need to be in fused or aqueous state to conduct electricity. Thus, solid NaCl cannot conduct electricity.

2. The spectrum of H-atom studied by Lyman, Balmer, Paschen, Bracken and Pfund can be explained on the basis of Bohr's Model. When an electron jumps from any of the higher states to the ground state or 1st state ($n = 1$), the series of spectral lines emitted lies in ultra-violet region and are called as Lyman Series. When an electron jumps from any of the higher states to the state with $n = 2$ (IInd state), the series of spectral lines emitted lies in visible region and are called as Balmer Series. When an electron jumps from any of the higher states to the state with $n = 3$ (IIIrd state), the series of spectral lines emitted lies in near infra-red region and are called as Paschen Series. When an electron jumps from any of the higher states to the state with $n = 4$ (IVth state), the series of spectral lines emitted lies in far infra-red region and called as Brackett Series. When an electron jumps from any of the higher states to the state with $n = 5$ (Vth state), the series of spectral lines emitted lies in far infra-red region and are called as Pfund Series.

3. Given, concentration of HCl = 10^{-8} M and concentration of H^+ ion in the solution = 10^{-7} M

Therefore, total concentration of H^+ ion in the solution

$$= [HCl] + [H^+]$$
$$= 10^{-8} + 10^{-7}\ M$$
$$= 10^{-7}(1+10^{-1})$$
$$= 1.1 \times 10^{-7}\ M$$

Now, $pH = -\log[H^+]$

$$= -\log[1.1 \times 10^{-7}]$$
$$= -[\log 1.1 + \log 10^{-7}]$$
$$= -[\log 11 - \log 10 - 7\log 10]$$
$$= -[\log 11 - 8]$$
$$= -[1.04 - 8]$$
$$= -[-6.96] = 6.96$$

Therefore, the pH of the HCl solution lies in between 6 and 7.

4.

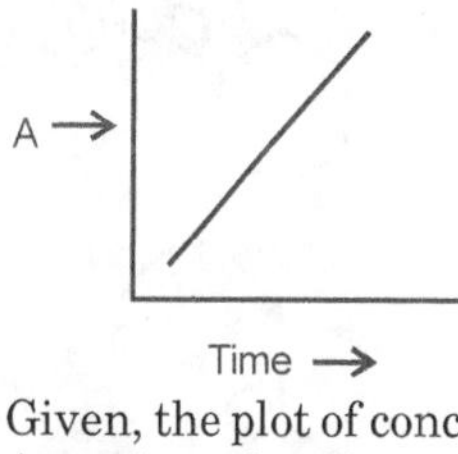

Given, the plot of concentration of A against time is a straight line with negative slope. A zero-order reaction is a reaction that proceeds at a rate that is independent of reactant concentration. In other words, increasing or decreasing the concentration of the reactants will not speed up or slow down the rate of reaction. This means that the rate of the reaction is equal to the rate constant, k, of that reaction. Hence, the order of the reaction is 0.

5. Amines are basic because they possess a pair of unshared electrons, which they can share with other atoms. These unshared electrons create an electron density around the nitrogen atom. The greater the electron density, the more basic is the molecule. Groups that donate or supply electrons will increase the basicity of amines while groups that decrease the electron density around the nitrogen decrease the basicity of the molecule. For alkyl halides in the gas phase, the order of base strength is given as:

$$(CH_3)_3N > (CH_3)_2NH > CH_3NH_2 > NH_3.$$

However, in aqueous solution the order of basicity changes which is given as:

$(CH_3)_2NH > CH_3NH_2 > (CH_3)_3N > NH_3$.

The differences in the basicity order in the gas phase and aqueous solutions are the result of solvation effects. Amines in water solution exist as ammonium ions. Among the four amines, $CH_3NHC_6H_5$ has an aromatic phenyl ring which is an electron accepting group which balances the electron density over nitrogen due to the electron donor CH_3 group present on it. This counter balance occurs due to the resonating structure of C_6H_5 group present. Arylamines are weaker bases than cyclohexylamines because of resonance. Thus, this amine is the least basic.

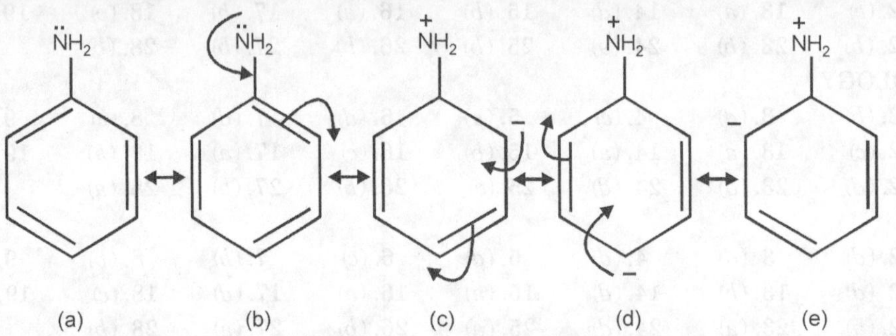

6. The substrate or starting material is cyclohexanol (R-OH). Phosphoric acid is present as a catalyst which promotes the reaction but is not consumed in it. The hydroxyl group in R-OH is a poor-leaving group because it would have to leave as a hydroxide ion (HO^-). Therefore, an acid is used to protonate the alcohol and form $R\text{-}OH_2^+$. Thus, water (a much better leaving group) is the leaving group in this reaction and the product is a secondary carbocation. In the following steps a molecule of water deprotonates the carbocation at either of the adjacent carbons. The remaining electrons flow towards the positive charge producing a p–bond between the carbons and forming a double bond.

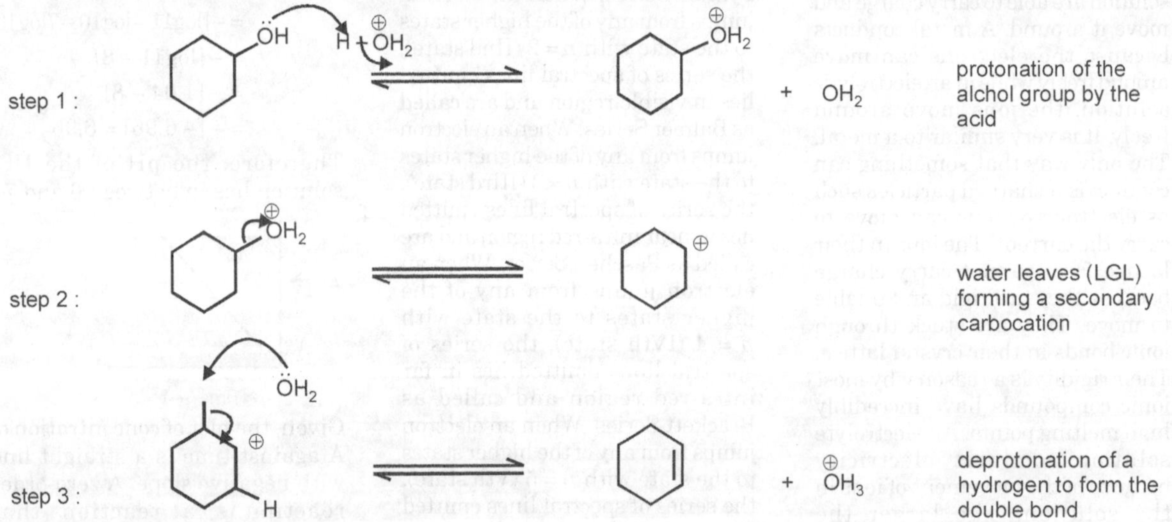

7. When a drop of 0.01 M $AgNO_3$ is added to a solution containing an aqueous mixture of 0.1 M KCl and 0.1 M KI, two types of reactions are possible:

$$KCl + AgNO_3 \rightarrow AgCl + KNO_3$$
$$KI + AgNO_3 \rightarrow AgI + KNO_3$$

The Solubility Product Constant, K_{sp} is the equilibrium constant for a solid substance dissolving in an aqueous solution. It represents the level at which a solute dissolves in solution.

For the product to precipitate, ionic product > K_{sp}.

We know, K_{sp} for AgCl $= 1.77 \times 10^{-10}$

and K_{sp} for AgI $= 8.52 \times 10^{-17}$.

Ionic product for AgCl

$= [KCl] \times [AgNO_3]$

$= 0.1 \times 0.01 = 10^{-3} > K_{sp}$ for AgCl

Ionic product for AgI

$= [KI] \times [AgNO_3]$

$= 0.1 \times 0.01 = 10^{-3} > K_{sp}$ for AgI

Therefore, both AgCl and AgI will precipitate. But, K_{sp} for AgI << K_{sp} for AgCl

So, AgI will precipitate much before AgCl and the solution mixture would contain the precipitate primarily of AgI since it would use a major concentration of $AgNO_3$.

8. Osmotic pressure is expressed by the formula: $\Pi = iMRT$, where Π is the osmotic pressure in atm, i = van't Hoff factor of the solute, M = molar concentration in mol/L, R = universal gas constant = 0.08206 L· atm/mol· K, T = absolute temperature in K.

Given, Concentration of the solution (g/L), C = 1 g/L

Osmotic pressure exerted by the protein,

$$\Pi = 8.3 \times 10^{-3} \text{ bar}$$
$$= 8.3 \times 10^{-3} \times 0.9869 \text{ atm}$$
$$= 8.19 \times 10^{-3} \text{ atm}$$

Now, $\Pi = iMRT = \left(\frac{n}{V}\right)RT$

where i = 1 for calculation purpose,

n = number of moles of the substance,

V = volume of the substance,

$$M = \frac{n}{V} = \left(\frac{w}{MV}\right)RT$$

where $n = \frac{w}{M}$,

w = weight of the substance in grams and

M = molar mass of the substance in g/moles.

$$\Pi = \left(\frac{C}{M}\right)RT$$

where $\frac{w}{V} = C = 1g/L$, T = 300K

$$\Rightarrow 8.19\times10^{-3} = \left(\frac{1}{M}\right)\times0.08206\times300$$

$$\Rightarrow M = \frac{24.618}{\left(8.19\times10^{-3}\right)}$$

$\Rightarrow M = 3.00586 \times 10^3$

$\Rightarrow M = 3005.86$

The molar mass of the protein is 3005.86 g/mol which is 3000 g/mol (approx.)

9. Given an electrochemical cell: A(s) | A^2+ (aq) 1 M||B^2 + (aq) 1 M | B(s), where A and B represent different metals. In an electrochemical cell, the half cell to the left of the salt bridge behaves as the anode and the half cell to the right of the salt bridge behaves as the cathode. Therefore :

A(s) |A^2+ (aq) 1 M $\rightarrow$ anodic cell,
B^{2+} (aq) 1 M|B(s) $\rightarrow$ cathodic cell

In an electrochemical galvanic cell, the anode is negatively charged since the spontaneous oxidation at the anode is the source of the cell's electrons or negative charge. The cathode of a galvanic cell is its positive terminal. Since, the anode has higher negative potential; hence it has a higher power of reducing species than the cathode. Therefore, A^{2+}/A is a stronger reducing agent than B^{2+}/B.

10. We know, Specific rate constant for a 1st order reaction,

$$k = \frac{0.693}{t_{1/2}}$$

Where, $t_{1/2}$ is the half –life of the reactants involved in the reaction

Given, $t_{1/2} = (100 \ln 2)$ s

Therefore, $k = \frac{0.693}{100} \ln 2$

$$= \frac{0.693}{(100\times0.6931)}$$

$= 0.01$

Thus, the specific rate constant for the reaction is 0.01 s^{-1}.

11. Trouton's rule states that for all liquids the entropy of vaporization is same i.e. 87–88 J K^{-1} mol^{-1}. Entropy of vaporization is the ratio of enthalpy of vaporization to the temperature.

The formula is given as:

$$\Delta S_V = \frac{\Delta H_V}{T}$$

$$\Rightarrow \quad 87 = \frac{\Delta H_V}{T}$$

$\Rightarrow \quad \Delta H_V = 87 \times T$

$\Rightarrow \quad \Delta H_V = 87 \times 332;$

where T = 59°C = (273 + 59)°K = 332°K

$\Rightarrow \quad \Delta H_V = 28884$

Therefore, the molar enthalpy of vapourization is (87×332) J/mol = 28,884 J/mol.

12. Kohlrausch's Law states that the molar conductivity, Λ_m of electrolytes increases with increase in dilution till a limiting value Λ_m° is obtained at infinite dilution. In this limit, the positive and negative ions may be thought of as behaving essentially independent of each other. Based up on his exhaustive experimental studies, Kohlrausch gave a generalization, which is known as Kohlrausch law. It states that at infinite dilution, when the dissociation of the electrolyte is complete, each ion makes a definite contribution towards the molar conductivity of electrolyte, irrespective of the nature of the other ion with which it is associated. This implies that the molar conductivity of an electrolyte at infinite dilution can be expressed as the sum of the contributions from its individual ions. If λ°_+ and λ°_- represent the molar conductivities of cation and anion respectively at infinite dilution, then the molar conductivity of electrolyte at infinite dilution Λ°_m is given by :

$$\Lambda_m^\circ = n_+ \lambda^\circ_+ + n_- \lambda^\circ_-.$$

$$\Lambda^\circ_m(NaCl) = \lambda^\circ(Na^+) + \lambda^\circ(Cl^-)$$

$$\Lambda^\circ_m(HCl) = \lambda^\circ(H^+) + \lambda^\circ(Cl^-)$$

Therefore, $\Lambda^\circ_m(NaCl) = \lambda^\circ(Na^+) + \lambda^\circ(Cl^-)$

$\Rightarrow \Lambda^\circ_m(NaCl)$
$= \lambda^\circ(Na^+) + \Lambda^\circ_m(HCl) - \lambda^\circ(H^+)$

[Since, $\lambda^\circ(Cl^-) = \Lambda^\circ_m(HCl) - \lambda^\circ(H^+)$]

$\Rightarrow \lambda^\circ(Na^+) = \Lambda^\circ_m(NaCl) + \lambda^\circ(H^+) - \Lambda^\circ_m(HCl)$

$\Rightarrow \lambda^\circ(Na^+) = 126.4 + 349.6 - 425.9$

[Since, $\Lambda^\circ_m(NaCl) = 126.4$; $\lambda^\circ(H^+) = 349.6$; $\Lambda^\circ_m(HCl) = 425.9$]

$\Rightarrow \lambda^\circ(Na^+) = 50.1$

The limiting molar conductivity of Na^+ is 50.1 S cm^2/ mol.

13. Nitration of benzene firstly involves the formation of a very powerful electrophile, the nitronium ion, which is linear. This occurs following the interaction of two strong acids, sulphuric and nitric acid. Sulphuric acid is the stronger

acid and it protonates the nitric acid on the OH group so that a molecule of water can leave. Benzene attacks the positively charged nitrogen atom of the electrophile, where one of the N=O bonds is broken at the same time. This is followed by rapid loss of a proton to regenerate the aromaticity.

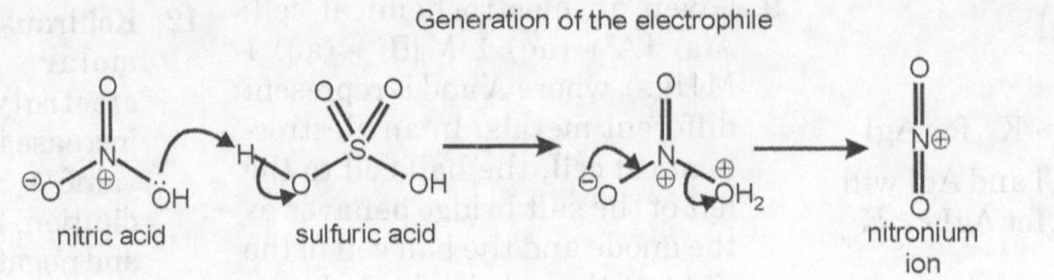

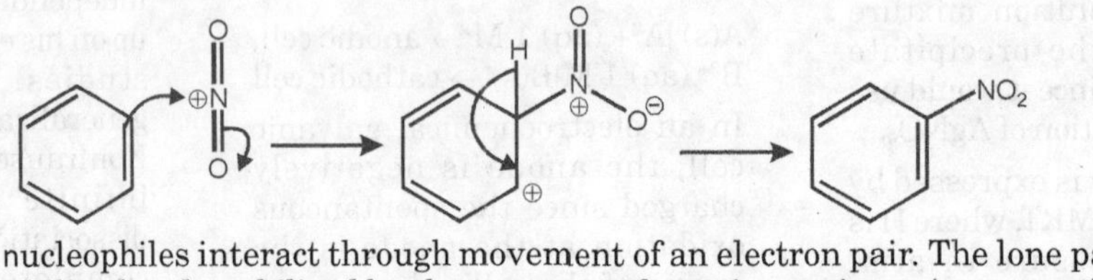

Electrophiles and nucleophiles interact through movement of an electron pair. The lone pair electrons present over NO_2 can be stabilized or destabilized by the presence of certain species or ions over the benzene ring. For example, –OH group of phenol stabilizes the lone pair electrons and thus increases the order of reactivity of phenol over benzene. Also, certain destabilizing species such as NO_2^-, Cl^- present in the benzene ring destabilizes the ring and hinders in the electrophilic substitution of benzene. And, the NO_2^- species has a stronger effect because of its resonating power.

Therefore, the order of reactivity for nitration:

Phenol > Benzene > Chlorobenzene > Nitrobenzene.

14. Allylic bromination is the replacement of hydrogen on a carbon adjacent to a double bond (or aromatic ring, in which case it's called benzylic bromination). NBS (N-bromosuccinimide) is the most commonly used reagent to produce low concentrations of bromine. When suspended in tetrachloride (CCl_4), NBS reacts with trace amounts of HBr to produce a low enough concentration of bromine to facilitate the allylic bromination reaction.

Allylic Bromination Mechanism

Step 1) Initiation

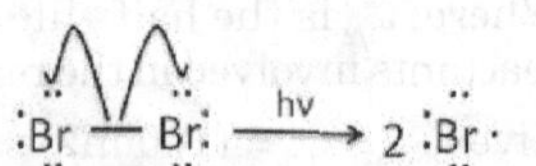

Step 2) Propagation

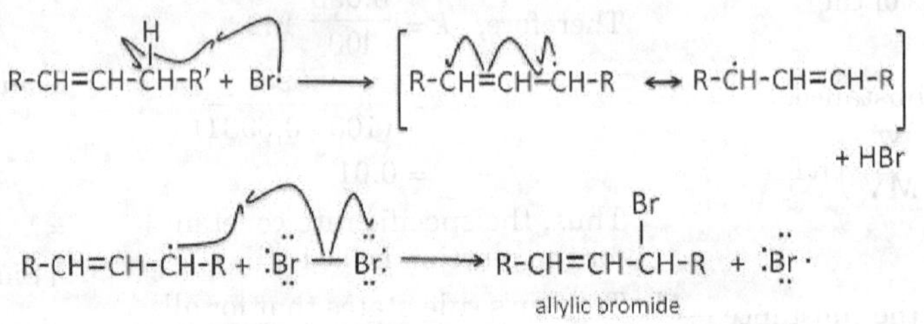

Step 3) Termination

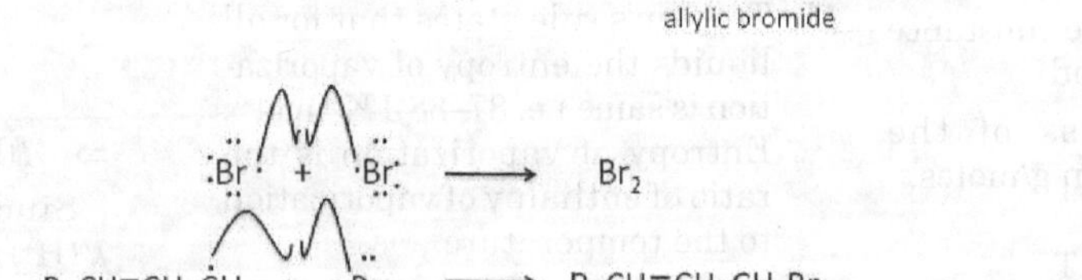

In the reaction :

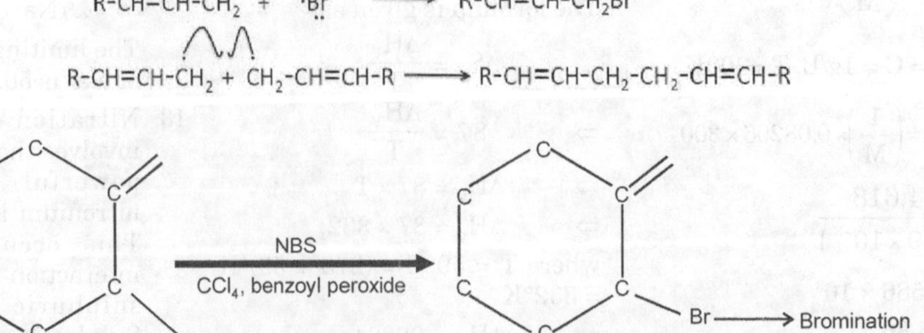

15. When all primary amines react with chloroform and alcoholic KOH, they form isocyanides with bad smell. It is the most versatile test for all primary amines. In this α-elimination occurs. The reaction is known as Hoffmann's Carbylamine Reaction.

$$RNH_2 + CHCl_3 + \text{alc KOH} \longrightarrow R-N \equiv C + 3\,KCl + H_2O$$

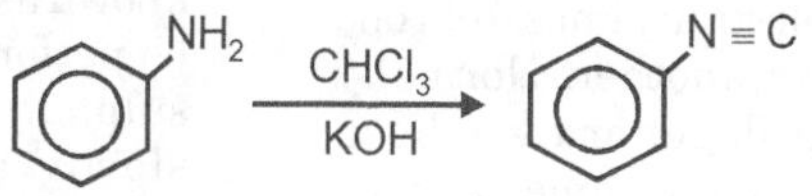

Bad smell of isocyanides

Mechanism :

$$CHCl_3 \xrightarrow{\text{alc.base}} CCl_3^- \xrightarrow{-Cl^-} :CCl_2$$ (Formation of Dichloro Carbene is an example of α-elimination)

$$R\,NH_2 + :CCl_2 \longrightarrow RNH_2 \rightarrow CCl_2 \longrightarrow R-N \equiv C + 2HCl$$

In the given question, ethylamine (CH_3-NH_2) is the only primary amine. So, the compound M is ethylamine.

16. The reaction of carboxylic acids and alcohols to form esters is one of the best known transformations in organic chemistry. This esterification reaction is very slow unless catalyzed by a strong acid. The rate of lactonization is small due to the lower probability of conformations in which the hydroxyl and carboxyl groups are near each other in space (a negative entropy factor). If the concentration of hydroxyl acid is high, dimerization and polymerization is favoured. At low concentrations of hydroxyl acid, lactonization becomes competitive. For lactonization to occur, the –COOH and the –OH groups must be on the same plane for the acid to attack.

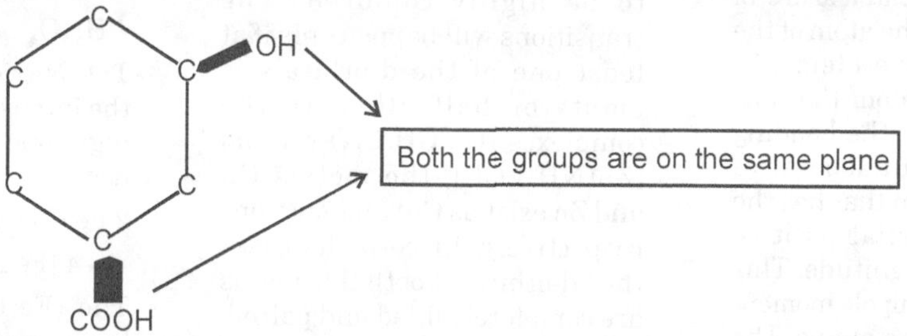

In this compound, both –COOH and –OH groups are on the same plane. So lactonization would occur.

17. The condensation of an aromatic aldehyde with an aliphatic aldehyde or ketone in the presence of a base or an acid to form α, β -unsaturated aldehyde or ketone with high chemo-selectivity is generally known as Claisen–Schmidt condensation.

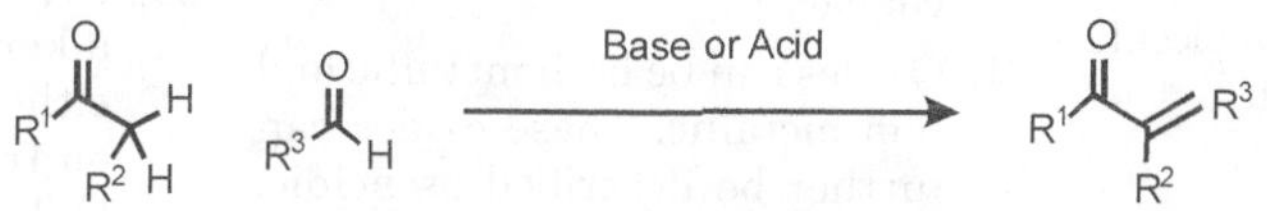

Mechanism:

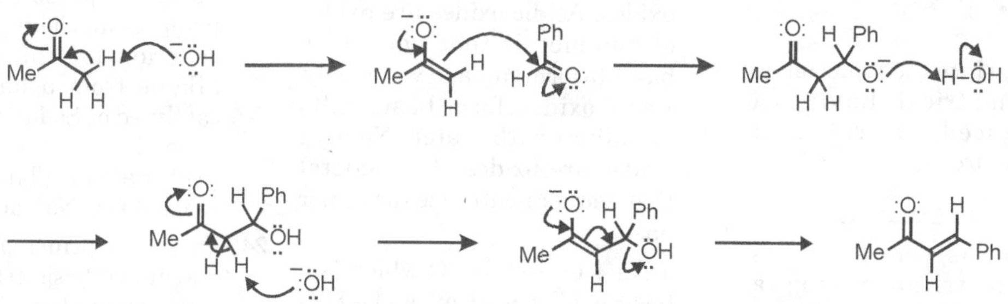

When benzaldehyde reacts with excess amount of acetone in presence of dilute NaOH solution, the product is:

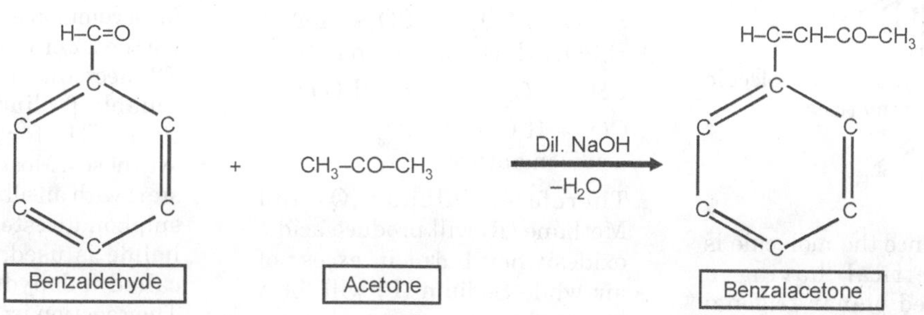

18. The ammonia gas is dried by passing it through the layers of quicklime (CaO). Conventional drying agents like conc. H_2SO_4, phosphorus pentoxide and anhydrous calcium chloride cannot be used since ammonia reacts with the compounds to produce salts. Anhydrous CaO is non-reactive to NH_3 but it reacts with H_2O present on the NH_3 gas resulting in drying of the gas.

$CaO + H_2O \rightarrow Ca(OH)_2$

19. The electrons in a covalent bond connecting two different atoms are not equally shared by the atoms due to the electronegativity difference between the two elements. The atom of the more electronegative element has the greater share of the electrons than the atom of the less electronegative element. Consequently, the atom that has the greater share of the bonding electrons bears a partial negative charge and the atom that has the lesser share a partial positive charge of equal magnitude. This gives rise to a bond dipole moment between two or more atoms. The dipole moments for the given molecules are:

$H_2O \rightarrow$ 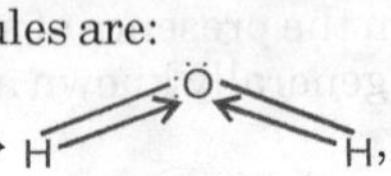

= non-zero, since the molecule is not symmetrical.

$SiCl_4 \rightarrow$ 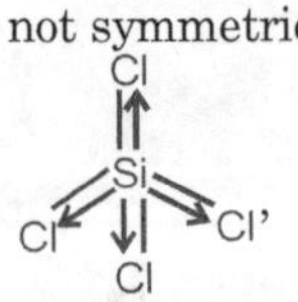

= zero, since the molecule is symmetrical having a balanced tetrahedral structure.

$CO_2 \rightarrow$ 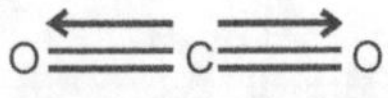

= zero as molecule is symmetrical having a balanced linear structure.

$NH_3 \rightarrow$ 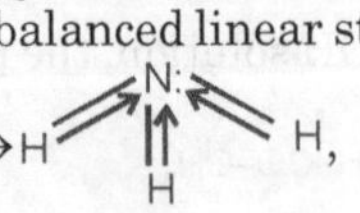

= non-zero, since the molecule is not symmetrical.

$BF_3 \rightarrow$ 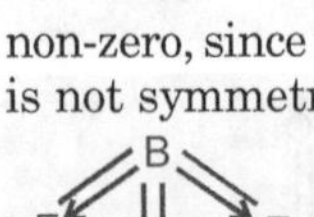

= zero, since the molecule is symmetrical having a balanced planar trigonal structure.

Thus, the molecules having zero dipole moment are: CO_2, BF_3, and $SiCl_4$.

20. The d-d transition is a transition where an electron jumps from one d orbital to another. Normally these are degenerate (the d orbitals have the same energy), but under some conditions, such as the presence of ligand, the degeneracy can be removed so that there is a specific energy (and therefore wavelength) associated with these transitions. These sorts of transitions sometimes have energies located in the visible band, and it is one reason transition metal ions (and complex ions in particular) tend to be highly coloured. The transitions will happen only if at least one of the d-orbitals is empty or half-filled. In the complexes $[Cu(CH_3CN)_4]Cl$ and $[Zn(NH_3)_4Cl_2]$, the metals Cu and Zn exist as Cu^+ and Zn^{2+} ions respectively. In both the cases the 3d-orbital of both the metals are completely filled and paired. As such, there is no chance of ligand transition possible in these two coordinate complexes and they do not show any colour change.

21. Oxides can be both metallic and non metallic. These oxides can further be described as acidic, basic, neutral and amphoteric oxides. Acidic oxides are oxides of non-metals that neutralize bases to form salt and water only. Basic oxides form basic salts (alkaline) with water. Neutral oxides are oxides of non-metal that neither neutralizes acids nor base.

$4 Na + O_2 \rightarrow 2 Na_2O$ which is a basic oxide because $Na_2O + H_2O \rightarrow 2 NaOH$ (basic)

$S + O_2 \rightarrow SO_2$ and $SO_2 + H_2O \rightarrow H_2SO_3$ (which is acidic in nature)

$CH_4 + 2 O_2 \rightarrow CO_2 + 2 H_2O$ and $CO_2 + H_2O \rightarrow H_2CO_3$ (which is acidic in nature)

Therefore, Sulphur (Q) and Methane (R) will produce acidic oxides when burnt in excess of air while Sodium (P) will form basic oxide.

22. A nitrate test is a chemical test used to determine the presence of nitrate ion in solution. A common nitrate test, known as the brown ring test can be performed by adding ferrous sulphate to the solution, then slowly adding concentrated sulphuric acid and watching for a brown ring on the test tube, which will indicate the presence of the nitrate ion. The reaction is as follows:

$$2 Zn(NO_3)_2 + 2 H_2SO_4 \rightarrow 2 ZnSO_4 + 4 HNO_3$$

$$4 FeSO_4 + 2 H_2SO_4 \rightarrow 2 Fe_2(SO_4)_3 + 2H_2.$$

These two reactions happen simultaneously.

$$4 HNO_3 \rightarrow 2 H_2O + 3O_2 + 4 NO.$$

The Nitric Acid decomposes in the intense heat produced by the high concentrate Sulphuric Acid used.

$$2 Fe_2(SO_4)_3 + 2 H_2 + 4 NO \rightarrow 4 [Fe(H_2O)_5NO]SO_4 + 2H_2SO_4.$$

The $[Fe(H_2O)_5NO]SO_4$ forms a brown ring in the middle of the solution produced by the reaction, making it easy to identify the presence of nitrates in the water.

23. Given, a compound N gives an alkene (But-2-ene) which is in either cis or trans form or both on treatment with a compound O. The compound N is 2, 3 Bromo butane represented in Fisher projection. The elimination reaction for the synthesis of alkene from a halo-alkane is catalyzed by Sodium or potassium iodide in presence of acetone for protonation. Therefore, the reagent O is NaI/ acetone.

24. One of the principal methods for alkene synthesis in the laboratory is the elimination of alkyl halides, alcohols, and similar compounds. Most common is the β-elimination via the E2 or E1 mechanism. The E2 mechanism provides a more reliable β-elimination method than E1 for most alkene syntheses. Most E2 eliminations start with an alkyl halide or alkyl sulphonate ester. When an alkyl halide is used, the reaction is called a dehydrohalogenation. The reaction is:

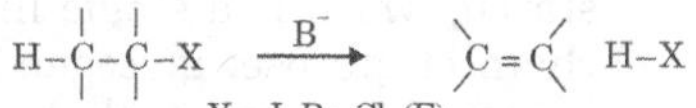

X = I, Br, Cl, (F)

When heated with strong bases, alkyl halides typically undergo a 1, 2-elimination reactions to generate alkenes. Typical bases are NaOH or KOH or NaOR or KOR (alkoxide) especially NaOEt or KOtBu in the alcohol as solvent. The reaction follows E2 mechanism. In the given reaction, the product cis but-2-ene (Q) will be more exclusive than the product trans but-2-ene (P) since the mechanism that follows is E2.

25. Given, $CuSO_4$ + W (aqueous alkali) → X (blue precipitate)

X dissolves on addition of excess of W. The aqueous alkali is ammonium hydroxide which reacts with copper sulphate to form a solid blue precipitate of copper (II) hydroxide. The reaction is:

$CuSO_4 + 2\ NH_4OH\ (aq.) \rightarrow Cu(OH)_2$ [blue ppt.] $+ (NH_4)_2SO_4$

On further addition of ammonium hydroxide, it dissolves cupric hydroxide resulting in a coordinate complex imparting blue colour to the solution. The reaction is:

$Cu(OH)_2 + 2\ NH_4OH\ (aq.) + (NH_4)_2SO_4 \rightarrow [Cu(NH_3)_4]SO_4 + 4\ H_2O$

(blue solution complex)

26. Given, $CuSO_4$ + Y (aqueous alkali)

→ Z (solid blue precipitate)

The solid precipitate Z does not dissolve on addition of excess of the alkali Y. The aqueous alkali is sodium hydroxide which reacts with copper sulphate to form solid blue precipitate Copper (II) hydroxide. The reaction is:

$CuSO_4 + 2\ NaOH\ (aq.) \rightarrow Cu(OH)_2$ [blue ppt.] $+ Na_2SO_4$

But, this solid precipitate of copper hydroxide does not dissolve in excess of sodium hydroxide. Thus, there is no further reaction possible.

$Cu(OH)_2 + NaOH \rightarrow$ No reaction

27. Given, for a 1st order reversible reaction A → B, the rate constant for forward reaction is k_f and the rate constant for backward reaction is k_b. Given, at temperature T, the standard molar free energy,

$\Delta G^0 = -2.303\ RT.$

We know, standard free energy of a reaction is given as:

$\Delta G^0 = -2.303\ RT\ \ln(k_c)$

where R is the universal gas constant, T is the temperature and k_c is the equilibrium gas constant for the reaction.

$\Rightarrow\ -2.303\ RT = -2.303\ RT \ln(k_c)$

$\Rightarrow\ \ln(k_c) = 1$

$\Rightarrow\ \log_{10}(k_c) = 1$

$\Rightarrow\ k_c = 10$

The equilibrium constant for the reaction is 10 s^{-1}.

28. We know, $k_c = \frac{k_f}{k_b}$ for a given 1st order reversible reaction at equilibrium.

Given, $k_c = 10\ s^{-1}$ and

$k_f = 1 \times 10^{-3}\ s^{-1}$

Therefore, $k_c = \frac{k_f}{k_b}$

$\Rightarrow\ k_b = \frac{k_f}{k_c}$

$\Rightarrow\ k_b = \frac{10^{-3}}{10}$

$\Rightarrow\ k_b = 10^{-4}$

Thus, the rate constant for the backward reaction is $1 \times 10^{-4}\ s^{-1}$.

K : BIOCHEMISTRY

1. 2, 4-Dinitrophenol (DNP) is a potent non-selective inhibitor of oxidative phosphorylation, which results in increased metabolism and increased body temperature, and has been used illegally for weight control. It causes uncoupling of oxidative phosphorylation; the classic symptom complex associated with toxicity of phenol-based products such as DNP is a combination of hyperthermia, tachycardia, diaphoresis and tachypnoea, eventually leading to death. It is any of six crystalline compounds, especially a highly toxic compound that increases fat metabolism and was formerly used in weight control.

2. The ratio k_{cat}/k_m → often referred to as the "specificity constant" → is a useful index for comparing the relative rates of enzyme acting on alternative, competing substrates. An alternative description, "catalytic efficiency", is frequently used, to compare the reactivity of two enzymes acting on the same substrate. k_{cat} is called the turnover number of an enzymatic reaction and is defined as the ratio of the moles of product produced per unit time to the moles of the enzyme. Theoretically the maximum value for the catalytic efficiency can be determined by diffusion limit because as soon as enzyme and substrate can come together it can make the products. Catalytic efficiency of enzyme can be used to compare different enzymes or the same enzyme for different substrates.

3. Protein kinase C transduces the cellular signals that promote lipid hydrolysis. This 80kDa enzyme is recruited to the plasma membrane by diacylglycerol and, in many cases, by calcium. The enzyme is activated by diacylglycerol and phospholipid (usually PS) and is thought to undergo a conformational change upon binding to the membrane. PKC phosphorylates a variety of target proteins which control growth and cellular differentiation. The isozymes of PKC are homologous with cAMP-dependent protein kinase (protein kinase A).

4. DNA footprinting is an *in vitro* technique used to examine the binding of proteins to specific regions of DNA. This technique cleverly exploits the fact that when a transcription factor is bound to DNA with a certain affinity, the DNA is protected from degradation by nucleases. The transcription factor of interest thus leaves its "footprint" on the DNA. A typical footprinting experiment involves radioactive labelling of the DNA region of interest-usually a larger chunk of DNA suspected to contain one or more transcription factor binding sites. This fragment is radioactively labelled on one end and then incubated *in vitro* both with and without the transcription factor of interest. Next, the DNA is treated with a nuclease, such

as DNAse I, which digests only unprotected DNA. Finally, the DNA products resulting from the digestion are separated on a polyacrylamide gel, which is dried and placed against X-ray film to enable visualization. The resulting image is referred to as an autoradiograph. Thus, transcription start sites can be determined using footprinting.

5. B cells and T cells are the main types of lymphocytes. B cells work chiefly by secreting substances called antibodies into the body's fluids. Antibodies ambush foreign antigens circulating in the bloodstream. They are powerless, however, to penetrate cells. The job of attacking target cells-either cells that have been infected by viruses or cells that have been distorted by cancer-is left to T cells or other immune cells. Each B cell and T cell is specific for a particular antigen. The specificity of binding resides in a receptor for antigen:-the B cell receptor (BCR) for antigen and the T cell receptor (TCR) respectively. Both BCRs and TCRs share certain properties --> i) They are integral membrane proteins ii) They are encoded by genes assembled by the recombination of segments of DNA iii) They have a unique binding site iv) The binding, like that between an enzyme and its substrate depends on complementarity of the surface of the receptor and the surface of the epitope.

6. Hybridoma technology features effective usage of innate functions of both immune cells and cancers, allowing production of hybridoma cells, which continuously generate monoclonal antibodies specific to antigens of interest. The specific antibody producing B-lymphocytes are mixed with selected myeloma cells and are induced to fuse to form hybrid cells. After cell fusion, selection is aided by the use of HAT medium, which kills HGPRT— myeloma cells, and lymphocytes that have not fused do not survive in culture. This treatment thus selects for the immortalized hybridoma cells that retain the lymphocyte HGPRT. Such hybrid cells are both permanently adapted to growth in culture and capable of forming specific antibody-producing tumours *in vivo*. Thus, the myeloma cells that are selected do not produce antibodies and lack the HGPRT gene for nucleotide biosynthesis.

7. Membranes and their constituent proteins are assembled in the ER. This organelle contains the enzymes involved in lipid synthesis, and as lipids are manufactured in the ER, they are inserted into the organelle's own membranes. The proteins that will be secreted by a cell are also directed to the ER during translation, where they end up in the lumen, the internal cavity, where they are then packaged for vesicular release from the cell. The Golgi apparatus functions as a molecular assembly line in which membrane proteins undergo extensive post-translational modification. Many Golgi reactions involve the addition of sugar residues to membrane proteins and secreted proteins. The carbohydrates that the Golgi attaches to membrane proteins are often quite complex, and their synthesis requires multiple steps called protein glycosylation. Lysosomes break down macromolecules into their constituent parts, which are then recycled. These membrane-bound organelles contain a variety of enzymes called hydrolases that can digest proteins, nucleic acids, lipids, and complex sugars. Thus, these organelles undergo protein degradation.

8. Chitin is a polysaccharide found in the outer skeleton of insects, crabs, shrimps, and lobsters and in the internal structures of other invertebrates. Chitin is composed of β (1-4) linked units of the amino sugar N-acetyl-glucosamine, and is the main source of production of chitosan. Hemicelluloses are polysaccharides in plant cell walls that have β-(1 → 4)-linked backbones with an equatorial configuration. Hemicelluloses include xyloglucans, xylans, mannans and glucomannans, and β-(1 → 3, 1 → 4)-glucans. Glycogen is a chain of glucose subunits held together by a 1, 4 glycosidic bonds, very much like starch (α-amylose). In contrast to starch, which is a single linear chain of glucose, glycogen is a branched structure. At the branch points, subunits are joined by 1, 6 glycosidic bonds. Branches occur at every 8-10 residues.

9. Phosphatidylcholine (once given the trivial name 'lecithin') is usually the most abundant phospholipid in animal and plants, often amounting to almost 50% of the total, and as such it is obviously the key building block of membrane bilayers. In particular, it makes up a very high proportion of the outer leaflet of the plasma membrane. The melting temperature T_m of Phosphatidylcholine A is higher than that of Phosphatidylcholine B. This is because the melting temperature depends on the extent of the carbon fatty acid chain and the content of saturated fatty acids. Both fatty acid chain and saturation content of Phosphatidylcholine A is higher than that of Phosphatidylcholine B.

10. Gel filtration (GF) chromatography separates proteins solely on the basis of molecular size. Separation is achieved using a porous matrix to which the molecules, for steric reasons, have different degrees of access--i.e., smaller molecules have greater access and larger molecules are excluded from the matrix. Hence, proteins are eluted from the GF column in decreasing order of size. Given, four proteins having molecular masses of P = 50 kDa, Q = 80 kDa, R = 120 kDa, and S = 150kDa. The order of elution from the Sephadex G-200 column will be S, R, Q, and P where P comes out first and S will come out at the end because of the decreasing order of molecular mass of the proteins.

11. Ribonuclease is an endonuclease that catalyzes the cleavage of RNA on the 3′ side of pyrimidine nucleotides and acts on single stranded and double stranded RNA. It functions by endonucleolytic cleavage of nucleoside 3′-phosphates and 3′-phosphooligonucleotides ending in Cp or Up

with 2′,3′-cyclic phosphate intermediates. Lysozymes are hydrolytic enzymes, characterized by their ability to cleave the beta-(1, 4)-glycosidic bond between N-acetylmuramic acid and N-acetylglucosamine in peptidoglycan, the major bacterial cell wall polymer. They act through formation of carbonium ion intermediate. Carboxypeptidase is an enzyme synthesized in the pancreas and secreted into the small intestine. This enzyme hydrolyzes the first peptide or amide bond at the carboxyl or C-terminal end of proteins and peptides. It has a stronger preference for those amino acids that have aromatic or branched hydrocarbon chains forming mixed anhydrides. Chymotrypsin is a proteolytic enzyme (Serine protease) acting in the digestive systems of many organisms. It facilitates the cleavage of peptide bonds by a hydrolysis reaction, which despite being thermodynamically favourable occurs extremely slowly in the absence of a catalyst and forming an oxyanion.

12. Thiamine pyrophosphate (TPP) functions as a coenzyme vital to tissue respiration. It is required for the oxidative decarboxylation of pyruvate to form acetyl-coenzyme a, providing entry of oxidizable substrate into the Krebs cycle for the generation of energy. It is also a coenzyme for transketolase, which functions in the pentose phosphate pathway, an alternate pathway for glucose oxidation. Thiamine is most strongly linked with carbohydrate metabolism, but TPP is also required for the oxidative decarboxylation of other alpha-keto acids such as alpha-ketoglutarate and branched-chain alpha-keto acids (i.e., 2-ketocarboxylates) derived from certain amino acids (e.g., valine, isoleucine, leucine). Coenzyme A is a cofactor for 4% of the enzymes in plants. Coenzyme-a is converted into acyl-coenzyme-A (CoA), mainly acetyl-coenzyme-A (CoA), upon reaction with carbohydrate catabolites. Acetyl-coenzyme-A (CoA) is a key substrate in important metabolisms such as citric acid cycle (TCA cycle), fatty acid, some amino acids, flavonoid, wax, isoprenoid, and lignin synthesis and storage lipid degradation. Pyridoxal phosphate is the active form of vitamin B6 (pyridoxine or pyridoxal). PLP enzymes exist in their resting state as a Schiff base, the aldehyde group of PLP forming a linkage with the epsilon-amino group of an active site lysine residue on the enzyme. The alpha-amino group of the substrate displaces the lysine epsilon-amino group, in the process forming a new aldimine with the substrate. This aldimine is the common central intermediate for all PLP-catalysed reactions, enzymatic and non-enzymatic. Enzymes that participate in the transfer of one-carbon units require the coenzyme tetrahydrofolate (THF). Various reactions generate one-carbon derivatives of THF, which can be inter-converted between different oxidation states.

13. Succinyl Co-A synthetase or Succinyl-CoA ligase (GDP-forming) is a mitochondrial enzyme that catalyzes the substrate level phosphorylation step of the tricarboxylic acid cycle: the formation of succinyl-CoA from succinate with a concomitant hydrolysis of GTP to GDP and phosphate. This enzyme is a dimer composed of alpha and beta subunits. Acyl-CoA dehydrogenases are a family of flavoproteins that catalyse the alpha, beta-dehydrogenation of acyl-CoA thioesters to the corresponding trans 2,3-enoyl CoA-products with the concomitant reduction of enzyme-bound FAD. Different family members share a high sequence identity, catalytic mechanisms, and structural properties, but differ in the position of their catalytic bases and in their substrate binding specificity. Transketolase catalyzes the reversible transfer of a two-carbon ketol unit from xylulose 5-phosphate to an aldose receptor, such as ribose 5-phosphate, to form sedoheptulose 7-phosphate and glyceraldehyde 3- phosphate. This enzyme, together with transaldolase, provides a link between the glycolytic and pentose-phosphate pathways. The enzyme ribulose 1, 5-bisphosphate carboxylase/oxygenase (Rubisco) catalyzes the formation of organic molecules from CO_2. The reaction proceeds by the addition of carbon dioxide to the five-carbon compound ribulose 1, 5-bisphosphate (RuBP) and the splitting of the resulting six-carbon compound into two molecules of PGA. This reaction is known as Calvin cycle.

14. The formation of glucose from non-carbohydrate precursors, such as pyruvate, amino acids and glycerol is known as gluconeogenesis. Pyruvate carboxylase is a member of the biotin-dependent enzyme family and it catalyses the ATP-dependent carboxylation of pyruvate to oxaloacetate; thus playing a crucial role in gluconeogenesis. The reaction is : - ATP + pyruvate + HCO_3^- = ADP + phosphate + oxaloacetate. Pyruvate carboxylase catalyzes a 2-step reaction, involving the ATP-dependent carboxylation of the covalently attached biotin in the first step and the transfer of the carboxyl group to pyruvate in the second. It is activated by acetyl Co-A.

15. Pyrimidine nucleotides contain a single ring in the nitrogenous base. In contrast to the synthesis of purines, the pyrimidine ring is synthesized first and then joined to ribose. This pathway is conserved from bacteria to man, occurring in essentially the same manner for all species. The pathway begins with aspartate and carbamoyl phosphate as the first components to build the pyrimidine base. Carbamoyl phosphate is synthesized from bicarbonate ions and nitrogen from glutamine. The condensation of aspartate and carbamoyl phosphate creates carbamoyl aspartate, which goes through ring closure and oxidation to create the precursor pyrimidine orotate. Orotate is joined to ribose phosphate and UMP is finally formed through decarboxylation. CTP is synthesized from UTP through amination using glutamine as the donor in mammals and ammonia in E.coli. This pathway is closely regulated to provide pyrimidines only when they are needed. The pathway is activated by ATP and inhibited by the end product, pyrimidines, providing an example of feedback inhibition.

16. The steroid hormones are derived from cholesterol. They are transported through the bloodstream to the cells of various target organs where they carry out the regulation of a wide range of physiological functions. They act at cell nucleus. All the steroid hormones exert their action by passing through the plasma membrane and binding to intracellular receptors. The mechanism of action of the thyroid hormones is similar; they interact with intracellular receptors. Both the steroid and thyroid hormone-receptor complexes exert their action by binding to specific nucleotide sequences in the DNA of responsive genes. These DNA sequences are identified as hormone response elements, HREs. The interaction of steroid-receptor complexes with DNA leads to altered rates of transcription of the associated genes.

17. Aphidicolin is a selective inhibitor of DNA polymerase alpha. A cell-permeable tetracyclic diterpene antibiotic, it acts as a cell synchronization agent. It blocks the cell cycle at early S-phase and is a specific inhibitor of DNA polymerase α and δ in eukaryotic cells and in some viruses. It potentiates apoptosis induced by arabinosyl nucleosides in leukaemia cell lines. The α-amanitin binding site is beneath a "bridge helix" extending across the cleft between the two largest pol II subunits, Rpb1 and Rpb2 (subunits of RNA polymerase II), in a "funnel"-shaped cavity in the pol II structure. Most RNA polymerase II (pol II) residues interacting with α-amanitin are located almost entirely in the bridge helix and in an adjacent part of Rpb1 on the Rpb2-side of the cleft. Phenylmethanesulfonyl Fluoride (PMSF) is an inhibitor of serine proteases such as trypsin, chymotrypsin, thrombin, and papain. It is routinely added as a supplement to lysis buffers just prior to lysis, to prevent protease degradation.

18. The plasmid pBR322 is one of the most commonly used *E.coli* cloning vectors. pBR322 is 4361 bp in length and contains: (1) the replicon rep responsible for the replication of plasmid (source - plasmid pMB1); (2) rop gene coding for the Rop protein, which promotes conversion of the unstable RNA I - RNA II complex to a stable complex and serves to decrease copy number (source - plasmid pMB1); (3) bla gene, coding for beta-lactamase that confers resistance to ampicillin (source - transposon Tn3); (4) tet gene, encoding tetracycline resistance protein (source - plasmid pSC101). It has sites for restriction endonucleases and thus, cannot be digested by an exonuclease enzyme. That is why it settles at the bottom of the centrifuge tube on performance of density gradient centrifugation because it remains undigested.

19. In the inner mitochondrial membrane, complex I or Nicotinamide adenine dinucleotide (NADH) produced by glycolysis is oxidized (removes electrons) by the enzyme NADH dehydrogenase. The enzyme removes two electrons from NADH and attaches them to an electron carrier, ubiquinone. The transfer of these electrons reduces (adds electrons) ubiquinone into ubiquinol. Complex II (succinate dehydrogenase) is not a proton pump. It serves to funnel additional electrons into the quinone pool (Q) by removing electrons from succinate and transferring them (via FAD) to Q. Complex III (cytochrome bc1 complex) removes in a stepwise fashion two electrons from QH2 at the QO site and sequentially transfers them to two molecules of cytochrome c, a water-soluble electron carrier located within the inter membrane space. The two other electrons are sequentially passed across the protein to the Q_i site where quinone part of ubiquinone is reduced to quinol. Complex IV (cytochrome c oxidase) removes four electrons from four molecules of cytochrome c and transfers them to molecular oxygen (O_2), producing two molecules of water (H_2O). At the same time, it moves four protons across the membrane, producing a proton gradient.

20. Nucleated cells employ several strategies to evade killing by homologous complement. This can happen by 1. Expression and shedding of the membrane complement regulatory proteins (mCRP) CD46, CD55 and CD59; 2. Resistance based on protein phosphorylation; 3. Cell surface expression of sialic acid residues; and 4. Desensitization to complement upon exposure to sublytic complement doses. Resistance of cancer cells to lysis mediated by homologous complement is one of their immune escape strategies that will be a major obstacle to development of immunotherapy based on complement-fixing anti-tumour antibodies.

21. The generation of B lymphocytes from hematopoietic progenitors requires lineage-specific transcription factors that progressively direct cell fate choices. The germ line B-cell or Pro-B-cell helps in the development of the B-cell lymphocytes. During the progenitor stage, the B-cells are present in the germline or germ cell lineage and are not differentiated to Pre-B-cell. Hence, in this stage both the heavy and light chains of B-cell lymphocytes are not formed. So, there would not be any presence of stain in the cytoplasm or the membrane of the cell even if pre-labelled heavy chains of antibodies are being incorporated.

22. IgM antibodies are the largest antibody. They are found in blood and lymph fluid and are the first type of antibody made in response to an infection. They

also cause other immune system cells to destroy foreign substances. IgM antibodies are about 5% to 10% of all the antibodies in the body. Immunoglobulin M (IgM) enhances antibody responses via the complement system, and complement activation by IgM probably starts the chain of events leading to antibody responses to suboptimal antigen doses. The F_c region of IgM is unable to bind to the complement proteins because of its planar structure. This is why IgM immunoglobulin cannot activate the complement on its own.

23. Given, the contiguous locations on chromosome 2 of *Canorhabditis* contig are 1, 2, 3, 4, 5, 6, 7, 8 and 9. There are 5 cosmid clones produced from the contig. The cosmid clones are a, b, c, d and e. It is also given that the overlap regions of the cosmid clones are :

2-4, 3-5, 4-6, 5-8 and 8-9. Arranging the cosmid clones in terms of their overlaps, we have :

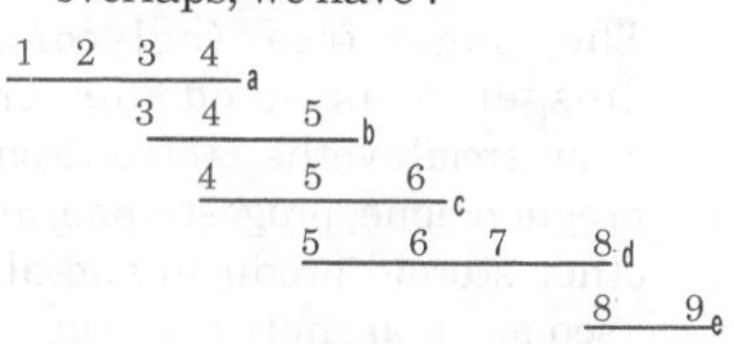

Thus, the overlaps exist amongst a-b, b-c, c-d, b-d and d-e. It is given that pBR322-x hybridizes to b, c and d cosmids and pUC18-y hybridizes to d and e cosmids. Thus, approximate locations of x and y in the chromosome is: 5 and 8 because 5 is the common overlap region of b, c and d cosmids and 8 is the common overlap region of d and e cosmids.

24. If both pBR322 and pUC18 are hybridized together with the cosmids, then the common cosmid for the two vectors would be cosmid d. This is because cosmid d has an overlap with both b, c and also with e. So, d is the common cosmid.

25. The process of moving sodium and potassium ions across the cell membrane is an active transport process involving the hydrolysis of ATP to provide the necessary energy. It involves an enzyme referred to as Na^+/K^+-ATPase. This process is responsible for maintaining the large excess of Na^+ outside the cell and the large excess of K^+ ions on the inside. It accomplishes the transport of three Na^+ ions outside the cell and the transport of two K^+ ions to the inside. This unbalanced charge transfer contributes to the separation of charge across the membrane. The sodium-potassium pump is an important contributor to action potential produced by nerve cells. This pump is called a P-type ion pump because the ATP interaction phosphorylates the transport protein and causes a change in its conformation.

26. Digitoxigenin is cardenolide, obtained especially by hydrolysis of digitoxin (refluxing digitoxin in a mixture of water, alcohol, and hydrochloric acid), which is the aglycon of digitoxin. It is a 5β-cardenolide having hydroxy substituent at the 3β- and 14β-positions. As because it inhibits ATPase, it results in the inhibition of Na^+-K^+ pump which is the main source of ionic balance inside and outside the cell membrane. That is why inhibition of ATPase by digitoxigenin helps in the accumulation of Ca^{2+} ions inside the cardiac muscles and eliminating any chance of Ca^{2+}-Na^+ ion exchange.

27. Given, 46% of pre-rRNA is unstable. So, 54% is stable which comprises of 5.8 S (0.16 kb), 18 S (1.9 kb) and 28 S (5.1 kb).

Total bases in the pre-rRNA

$= \{(0.16 + 1.9 + 5.1) \times 100\}/54$

$= (7.16 \times 100)/54$

$= 13.26$ kb

We have, average molecular weight of one molecule of a ribonucleotide = 321.45 Da.

Therefore, the molecular weight of 45 S pre-rRNA

$= 321.45 \times 13.26$ kDa

$= 4.262 \times 10^3$ kDa

$= 4.3 \times 10^6$ Da

$= 4.5 \times 10^6$ Da (approx.).

28. Given, pre rRNA content of the genome

$= 7.8 \times 10^5$ g

Number of functional bases = 54%

Length of the functional bases

$= 7.16$ kb $= 7.16$ x 103 bases

Number of genes per genome for pre-rRNA

$= (7.8 \times 10^5)/(7.16 \times 10^3)$

$= 1.0893 \times 10^2 = 108.93$

Therefore, the required number of pre-rRNA genes per genome is 109 = 100 (approx.)

M : BOTANY

1. C_4 photosynthesis is one of the most convergent evolutionary phenomena in the biological world, with at least 66 independent origins. The C_4 pathway is the end result of a series of evolutionary modifications to recover photorespired CO_2 in environments where RuBisCO oxygenation is high. The repositioning of mitochondria in the bundle sheath is one of the earliest steps in C_4 evolution, as it establishes a single-celled mechanism to scavenge photorespired CO_2 produced in the bundle sheath cells.

2. Norman Ernest Borlaug (25 March 1914 – 12 September 2009) was an American agricultural scientist, and humanitarian. He was considered as the "father of modern agriculture" and the "father of the green revolution". He won the 1970 Nobel Peace Prize for his life's work.

3. Bordeaux mixture which is a combination of copper sulfate, lime, and water, is an effective fungicide and bactericide that has been used for decades to control diseases of fruit and nut trees, vine fruits, and ornamental plants. These natural minerals, when mixed in the correct order, provide long-lasting protection to plants against diseases. Although there are many formulas for preparing Bordeaux mixture, generally a ratio of 10-10-100 works well for many disease-causing pathogens. It comprises of 10 pounds of copper sulfate, 10 pounds of lime, and 100 gallons of water.

4. Kornberg's enzyme is an alternative name for DNA polymerase I which was first detected in *E. coli* by Arthur Kornberg.
5. Rice was the first cereal to be fully sequenced and it helped to characterize the genes present in the rice genome. The rice genome is well mapped and well characterized, and it is the smallest of the major cereal crop genomes at an estimated 400 to 430 Mb.
6. Kinetin is a type of cytokinin, a class of plant hormone that promotes cell division. Kinetin was originally isolated by Miller and Skoog et al. as a compound from autoclaved herring sperm DNA that had cell division-promoting activity.
7. A caryopsis is a type of simple dry fruit, one that is monocarpellate (formed from a single carpel) and indehiscent (not opening at maturity) and resembles an achene, except that in a caryopsis the pericarp is fused with the thin seed coat.

   The aleurone layer is the outermost layer of the endosperm, followed by the inner starchy endosperm. Aleurone is a protein found in protein granules of maturing seeds and tubers. The homogenous aleurone consists of similar protein bodies (e.g. Phaseolus vulgaris) while the heterogeneous aleurone consists of granules of different shapes and types of proteins covered with a membrane.
8. During oxidative phosphorylation, electrons are transferred from electron donors to electron acceptors such as oxygen, in a series of redox reactions.

   The missing sequence is completed below as:

   NADH → Q → Cyt-b → Cyt-c1

   → Cyt-c → Cyt($a + a_3$) → O_2

   The Cyt-*b* and Cyt-*c* are known as the respiratory enzymes. Electrons are transferred within the inter membrane space by the water-soluble electron transfer protein cytochrome *c*.
9. The use of plants and trees to remove or neutralize contaminants, as in polluted soil or water is known as phytoremediation.

   Phytoremediation consists of mitigating pollutant concentrations in contaminated soils, water, or air, with plants able to contain, degrade, or eliminate metals, pesticides, solvents, explosives, crude oil and its derivatives, and various other contaminants from the media that contain them. It can be used to detoxify the soil phenolic pollutants by using the plant secretory enzymes.
10. Entropy is a measure of the number of specific ways in which a system may be arranged, often taken to be a measure of disorder.

    In ecology, energy flow, also called the calorific flow, refers to the flow of energy through a food chain. The flow of energy is the most important factor that controls what kind of organisms live in an ecosystem and how many organisms the ecosystem can support.
11. When the plant with red flower and long pollen grains (RRLL) was crossed with white flower and short pollen grains (rrll), the F1 progeny resulted in:

    RRLL * rrll → RrLl (Gametes)

    When the hybrids were then test crossed then the F2 progeny resulted in:

    RLrl * rrll (test cross) → RLrl (red flower long pollen), Rlrl (red flower short pollen), rLrl (white flower long pollen), rlrl (white flower short pollen)

    Thus the map distance wbetwen R and L can be given as 16cM.
12. Oryza sativa, commonly known as Asian rice, is the plant species most commonly referred to in English as rice. Oryza sativa is the cereal with the smallest genome, consisting of just 430Mb across 12 chromosomes. It is renowned for being easy to genetically modify, and is a model organism for cereal biology. It belongs to the family Gramineae.

    Michelia champaca is a large evergreen tree, native to the Indomalaya ecozone. It is best known for its strongly fragrant yellow or white flowers. It belongs to the family Magnoliaceae.
13. Agar is a gelatinous substance derived by boiling a polysaccharide in red algae, where it accumulates in the cell walls of agarophyte and serves as the primary structural support for the algae's cell walls. The gelling agent is an unbranched polysaccharide obtained from the cell walls of some species of red algae, primarily from the genera Gelidium (Glelidium of Rhodophyceae) and Gracilaria.

    Diosgenin, a steroid sapogenin, is the product of hydrolysis by acids, strong bases, or enzymes of saponins, extracted from the tubers of Dioscorea sp. The sugar-free (aglycone), diosgenin is used for the commercial synthesis of cortisone, pregnenolone, progesterone, and other steroid products and also used as an antifertility drug.
14. Heterosis refers to the phenomenon that progeny of diverse varieties of a species or crosses between species exhibit greater biomass, speed of development, and fertility than both parents. It is used to increase the productivity of many crop plants.

    Weed causes considerable yield loss and reduces the farmer's income. Weeds compete for water, nutrients & light. Being hardy & vigorous in growth habit, they soon outgrow the crops & consume large amounts of water & nutrients, thus causing heavy losses in yield.
15. Human activities are responsible for most of the loss in biodiversity throughout the world. Toxins and pollution are very harmful to biodiversity. Pollution occurs when substances are released into an environment where they can have a harmful

effect on living and non-living things. Human activities can pollute both on a local and global scale and may affect water, soil and air, three of our most important natural resources.

Human activities are the prime cause for global climatic change. Human-produced particulate pollution, especially reflective sulfur-containing particles, has had a cooling effect on the climate, masking some of the warming effect of greenhouse gases. Human activity is causing the Earth to get warmer, primarily through the burning of fossil fuels, with a smaller contribution from deforestation.

16. Correct marches of figures represented in group I to group II :

A - Binary vector

B - Kranz anatomy

C - C- Microinjection

D - Ferric- ferro- cyanide complex

17. Foliaceous bracts are green, flat and leaf-like in appearance. A bract is generally a modified, usually small, leaf-like structure often positioned beneath a flower or inflorescence.

Spathe is a large bract, often coloured, that surrounds the inflorescence of aroid plants and palms. It encloses or subtends a flower cluster or spadix.

Petaloid bracts are the bracts that resemble petals and are brightly colored bracts.

Involucre is a covering that can be defined as an involucral bract, or a pair, whorl or other collection of such bracts, surrounding a flower or an inflorescence.

18. Atropa Belladonna is a poisonous plant also called deadly nightshade. The substance atropine is extracted by this plant which was prepared by the ointment called witches' whisper.

Erythroxylum coca is a high altitude S. American shrub that's leaves are the source of cocaine.

Digitalis purpurea is a species of flowering plant in the genus Digitalis, in the family Scrophulariaceae, native and widespread throughout most of temperate Europe. The plants are well known as the original source of the heart medicine digoxin, (also called digitalis or digitalin).

Humulus lupulus (hop) is a species of flowering plant in the Cannabaceae family. It is a dioecious, perennial, herbaceous climbing plant which sends up new shoots in early spring and dies back to a cold-hardy rhizome in autumn.

19. Phytophthora infestans is an oomycete that causes the serious potato disease known as late blight or potato blight.

Alternaria solani is a fungal pathogen that produces a disease in tomato and potato plants called early blight.

Black scurf of Potato is a serious disease commonly observed in most potato-producing areas of the world. Caused by Rhizoctonia solani, this disease is favoured by the capacity of fungus to survive in soil as sclerotia and mycelium in plant debris for long periods, and environmental conditions of low soil temperature and high soil moisture.

Synchytrium endobioticum is a chytrid fungus that causes the potato wart disease or black scab.

20. Transgenic rice with a synthetic Cry1Ab gene from Bacillus thuringiensis is highly resistant to eight lepidopteran insects.

An antiplatelet monoclonal antibody is used in the non-antibiotic selection system.

The hygromycin phosphotransferase (hpt) gene is originally derived from Escherichia coli and is an antibiotic marker gene.

In C_4 photosynthesis, Phosphoenolpyruvate carboxylase (PEPC) catalyzes the irreversible carboxylation of phosphoenolpyruvate (PEP) to form oxaloacetate (OAA) and phosphate.

21. The correct matches are as follows:

P Maheshwari- plant embryology

E Hood- Agrobacterium transformation

B McClintock- Genetics

SM Sarkar- Growth hormone

22. Intellectual property rights (IPR) are the rights given to persons over the creations of their minds.

Commonly used reporter genes that induce visually identifiable characteristics usually involve fluorescent and luminescent proteins. Examples include the gene that encodes jellyfish green fluorescent protein (GFP), which causes cells that express it to glow green under blue light.

Transformation using Agrobacterium has several advantages over vectorless systems, although its efficiency on transferring DNA is still low for many species.

Selectable marker gene- International plant registration.

23. The type of stamen in the diagram is Monadelphous. Monadelphous is a term related to stamens whose filaments are united into a single tube-like group. The stamens of flowers of leguminous plants are often monadelphous.

24. The family from the type of stamen is the Malvaceae family. The Malvaceae, or the mallows, are a family of flowering plants containing over 200 genera with close to 2,300 species.

25. The first product in the reaction is citrate and the second product is coenzyme-A. This is the first reaction of the Krebs cycle. The cycle begins with the reaction between acetyl-CoA and the

four-carbon oxaloacetate to form six-carbon citric acid. The reaction is given as:

(1)

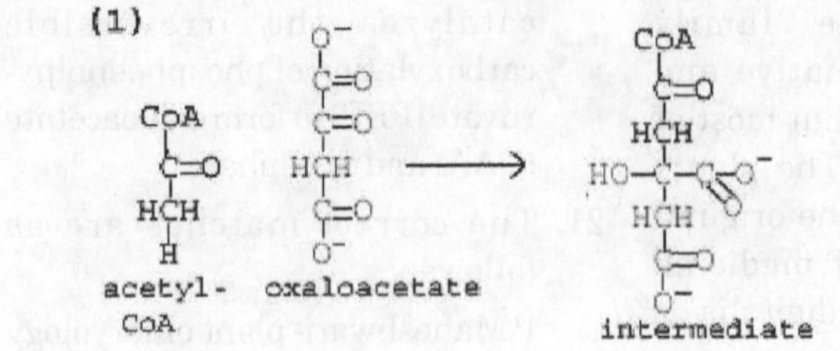

(2)

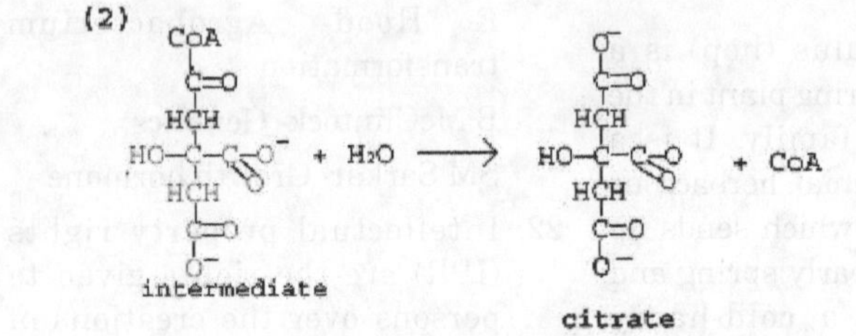

26. The first reaction of the citric acid cycle as given is catalyzed by the enzyme citrate synthetase and it is a condensation reaction as it involves a water molecule.

27. Human eyes perceive blue when observing light which has a wavelength between 450 – 500 nm.

    Green is the color which is seen at light with a wavelength of roughly 520 – 570 nm.

    Light with a wavelength of 650 – 700 nm is yellow, as is light with a suitable mixture of red and green.

    The wavelength of the red color spectrum is 550 – 600 nm.

28. The ångstrom is a unit of length equal to 10 – 10 m (one ten-billionth of a meter) or 0.1 nm.

    Therefore, 1nm = 10Å

    We know, 1 m = 10^3 nm

    Therefore, from the above two equations, we get:
    1nm = 10^{-3} m

N : MICROBIOLOGY

1. 16S Ribosomal RNA sequencing is widely used in microbiology studies to identify the diversities in prokaryotic organisms as well as other organisms and thereby studying the phylogenetic relationships between them. The advantages of using ribosomal RNA in molecular techniques are as follows:
   - Ribosomes and ribosomal RNA are present in all cells.
   - RNA genes are highly conserved in nature.
   - Culturing of microbial cells is absent in the sequencing techniques.
2. Sulfonamides suppress bacterial growth by inhibiting synthesis of folic acid (folate), a compound required by all cells for biosynthesis of DNA, RNA and proteins. The sulfonamides competitively block para-aminobenzoic acid (PABA) to prevent the synthesis of folic acid in susceptible bacteria.
3. Ziehl-Neelsen staining procedure is used to stain mycobacterium tuberculosis and mycobacterium leprae. These bacteria are also called acid fast bacilli. They stain with carbol fuschin, which is a red dye. They retain the dye when treated with acid, which is because of the presence of mycolic acid in their cell wall. Thus it is used for the detection of cell wall.
4. Ampicillin sodium salt is soluble in water (50mg/ml). The Stock solution of ampicillin cannot be autoclaved. Thus, it should be sterilized by filtering through a sterile membrane filter with a porosity of 0.22 micron or less.
5. Nitrogen fixation is carried out by the extremely oxygen labile multi-enzyme complex nitrogenase, that is activated under fixed nitrogen limiting conditions. This enzyme reduces nitrogen gas to ammonia using the following reaction:

   16-24 ATP + 8H+ + 8e- + N_2
   $\rightarrow$ 16-24 ADP + Pi + $2NH_3$ + H_2
6. August Von Wassermann discovered a blood test to detect syphilis known as a complement fixation test which is used to detect antibodies to the syphilis organism treponema; a positive reaction indicates the presence of antibodies and therefore syphilis infection.
7. A protoplast is a bacterial cell which can be prepared by the action of lysozyme in hypertonic solution. Because of the absence of cell wall, the cytoplasmic membrane is directly exposed to the environment in the protoplast, thus it is quiet vulnerable to the change in the environment. The protoplast survives only in the hypertonic solution.
8. The nature of the mutation in the *his* gene in the 3 strains is: P- frame shift, Q- base, and R- insertion. Since the amino acid sequence has been altered due to the change and a normal polypeptide is produced. Thus, strain P shows the frame shift mutation.
9. When a natural plasmid is isolated from a tetracycline resistant strain of E. coli, then after heat denaturing and self- annealing the plasmid, it is most likely that the plasmid would contain a transposon when observed by electron microscopy.
10. Bovine spongiform encephalopathy (BSE), commonly known as mad cow disease, is a fatal neurodegenerative disease in cattle that causes a spongy degeneration in the brain and spinal cord. They are contracted when people eat products contaminated with mad cow disease. It is an exception to Koch's postulates. The hypothesis concerning prions' mode of disease transmission is controversial, because it completely bypasses the more usual bacterial or viral method of infection and seems to violate Koch's postulates.

11. An E. coli culture is mutagenized to obtain leucine auxotrophs. The auxotrophs can be identified by replica plating on a minimal medium with no leucine and a rich medium with leucine.

12. Botulinum toxin is a neurotoxic protein produced by the bacterium Clostridium botulinum. It is one of the most poisonous naturally occurring substances in the world. Though it is highly toxic, it is used in minute doses both to treat painful muscle spasms, and as a cosmetic treatment in some parts of the world. It is sold commercially under the brand names Botox and Dysport for this purpose. The terms Botox and Dysport are trade names and are not used generically to describe the neurotoxins produced by Clostridia species.

13. The three restriction endonucleases P, Q, and R recognize 4bp, 6bp, and 8bp sequences respectively. So the frequency of occurrence of these sequences on a bacterial genome would be P > Q > R as the relative frequency of occurrence of smaller sequence is more as compared to the frequency of larger sequence.

14. The alternative complement pathway constitutes the humoral component of natural defence against infections, which can operate without antibody participation. Six proteins, C3, B, D, H, P, by themselves and I perform the functions of initiation, recognition, and amplification of the pathway, which results in the formation of the activator-bound C3/C5 convertase. A variety of activators of this pathway have been described such as certain particulate polysaccharides, for example, bacterial (LPS), yeast (zymosan), or plant (inulin) polysaccharides, fungi, bacteria, viruses and certain mammalian cells.

15. Anaphylaxis is a potentially deadly allergic reaction that is rapid in onset. In most people, anaphylaxis is caused by the presence of proteins called immunoglobulin E (IgE) antibodies. IgE antibodies are normally produced in the body for the purpose of fighting certain infections. In people with allergies, however, IgE is made in response to non-infectious substances, such as foods, medications, or insect venoms. This IgE then sticks to the outside of mast cells and basophils, a type of white blood cell. The chemicals released from the cells cause the signs and symptoms typical of anaphylaxis.

16. The chemostat is the most popular method in continuous culture. It is based on nutrient limitation. In chemostat fermentation, the nutrient is fed at constant rate. Chemostat is a useful tool for studying the physiology or evolution of a microorganism growing below its maximum specific growth rate. In a chemostat, growth rate is determined by the supply of a single limiting nutrient, the choice of which affects the metabolism and evolution of the microorganism. One of the important features of the chemostat is that it allows the operator to control the cell growth rate. The most common way is controlling the dilution rate.

17. If we double the amount/ concentration of the enzyme, then the V_{max} will double but so will the amount of substrate required to saturate the enzyme. Therefore the K_m of the enzyme will always remain irrespective of the enzyme concentration or substrate concentration.

18. The glycosidic bonds in starch are alpha-1,4 linkages. Starch has two forms that is amylose and amylopectin. Amylose consists of glucose rings hooked together using alpha-1,4 linkages. Amylopectin has chains that are branched in this way. It has alpha-1,4 linkages, but it also has alpha-1,6 linkages where the a-1-OH of one ring links to the #6 OH in another ring.

The glycosidic bonds in cellulose are not alpha-1,4 linkages. That is because the oxygen that's attached to the #1 carbon is in the beta position, but it's still hooked up to the #4 carbon of the second ring. Consequently, the glycosidic bonds in cellulose are referred to as being beta-1, 4 linkages.

19. Electron transport chains are used for extracting energy via redox reactions from sunlight in photosynthesis or, such as in the case of the oxidation of sugars, cellular respiration. In eukaryotes, the electron transport chain can be found in the inner mitochondrial membrane where it serves as the site of oxidative phosphorylation with ATP synthase. It is also found in the thylakoid membrane of the chloroplast in photosynthetic organisms. In bacteria, the electron transport chain is located in their cell membrane.

20. Dithiothreitol is the reducing agent which is not naturally present in the cell. Dithiothreitol (DTT), or Cleland's Reagent, is an important chemical used to reduce disulfide bonds quantitatively and maintain monothiols in the reduced state. At low concentrations, DTT stabilizes enzymes which possess free sulfhydryl groups and has been shown to restore activity lost by oxidation of these groups in vitro. DTT can readily permeate cell membranes allowing it to be used in pharmaceutical applications for high yield isolation and extraction of proteins. At higher concentrations, DTT is an

effective protein denaturant which cleaves disulfide linkages between cysteine groups in proteins and peptides.

21. The TCA cycle consists of eight steps catalyzed by eight different enzymes. The cycle is initiated when acetyl CoA reacts with the compound oxaloacetate to form citrate and to release coenzyme A (CoA-SH). The initiating step of the citric acid cycle occurs when a four carbon compound (oxaloacetic acid) condenses with acetyl CoA (2 carbons) to form citric acid (6 carbons). Thus P is Acetyl CoA, Q is Oxaloacetate and R is Citrate.

22. Glycolysis is a 10 step process. A single glucose molecule in glycolysis produces a total of 2 molecules of pyruvic acid, 2 molecules of ATP, 2 molecules of NADH and 2 molecules of water. Although 2 ATP molecules are used in steps 1-3 (initial steps of glycolysis), 2 ATP molecules are generated in step 7 and 2 more in step 10 (later part of glycolysis). This gives a total of 4 ATP molecules produced. If we subtract the 2 ATP molecules used in steps 1-3 from the 4 generated at the end of step 10, then we end up with a net total of 2 ATP molecules produced.

23. Retroviridae has a positive sense, single-stranded RNA and is linear. It has 3' polyadenylated tail and 5' cap.

All herpes-viruses (herpesviridae) are composed of relatively large double-stranded, linear DNA genomes encoding 100-200 genes encased within an icosahedral protein cage called the capsid.

Rhabdoviruses carry their genetic material in the form of negative-sense single-stranded RNA. They typically carry genes for five proteins: large protein (L), glycoprotein (G), nucleoprotein (N), phosphoprotein (P), and matrix protein (M).

Baculoviruses contain circular double-stranded genome ranging from 80–180 kbp.

24. Retroviral genomes are non-segmented, of positive polarity, and typically between 7 to 12 kb long in size. All retroviral genomes consist of at least 4 genes, gag, pro, pol and env. The gag gene encodes the major structural polyprotein Gag and is all that is necessary and sufficient for the assembly non-infectious and immature viral-like particles.

25. The concentration of the repressor in the cell would be 10^{-10}M assuming the Avogadro number to be 10^{23} molecules.

26. At the concentration of repressor that is 10^{-10}M, the gene would be transiently repressed.

27. Multiplicity of infection (MOI) is the average number of virus particles infecting each cell.

Given,

Phages capable of infecting bacteria = 10% of 10^7 = 10^6/ml

Number of bacterial cells = 1000

Amount of phage suspension = 100 l = 0.1ml

MOI = 0.1 * 10^6/1000 = 10^2.

28. A high multiplicity of infection (MOI) favors the lysogenic pathway: when the MOI is greater than 10, over 95% of the infecting phage forms lysogens. Thus at the MOI of 10^2 lysogeny is favored.

Q : ZOOLOGY

1. The theory of use and disuse of Jean-Baptiste Lamarck, advocated the idea that animals acquired characteristics after using certain physical traits constantly. He believed that the reason why the necks of giraffes were long was because they stretched to reach leaves on high trees. By the same logic, the lack of a human tail could be explained by the fact that humans did not use it. The inheritance of acquired characteristics is a hypothesis that physiological changes acquired over the life of an organism (such as the enlargement of a muscle through repeated use) may be transmitted to offspring. It is also commonly referred to as the theory of adaptation equated with the evolutionary theory known as Lamarckism. The theory of intelligent design holds that certain features of the universe and of living things are best explained by an intelligent cause, not an undirected process such as natural selection. Thus the example of a giraffe stretching its neck is best explained by the concept of inheritance of acquired characters and use and disuse theory.

2. The systematics of animal kingdom is the comparative analysis of living and fossil species, including their discovery, description, evolutionary relationships to other species, and patterns of geographic distribution. Systematics can be divided into four major fields → Taxonomy, often equated with systematics, is the discipline concerned with the discovery, description, and classification of organism groups, termed taxa (singular, taxon). Classification is the clustering of species into a hierarchical arrangement according to some criterion, usually an understanding of their relationships to other species. Phylogenetic analysis, an increasingly important aspect of systematics, is the discovery of the historical, evolutionary relationships among species; this pattern of relationships is termed as phylogeny. The fourth component of systematics is biogeography, the study of species' geographic distributions. Systematic data and interpretations underlie progress in all of biology.

3. Modern taxonomic classification divides the living organisms into 5 kingdoms given by R.H.Whittaker → Kingdom Monera, Kingdom Protista, Kingdom Fungi, Kingdom Plantae, and Kingdom Animalia. This scheme was based on - structure of Cells - {prokaryotic or eukaryotic}, structure of organism - {unicellular or Multicellular} and mode of nutrition - Photosynthesis in green plants, absorption in fungi and ingestion in animals.

4. The sense organs for balance are located near the inner ear, protected by the same hard bones of the skull that surround the cochlea. The vestibular system consists of two main parts with slightly different functions: the semicircular canals (the loops) and two chambers under the canals: the saccule and the utricle. The loops (semicircular canals) and sacs (saccule and utricle) are collectively called the non-auditory labyrinth or just the labyrinth. The entire labyrinth is filled with a fluid called the endolymph, the same fluid found in the cochlea. The semicircular canals are rotary motion detectors. The sacs, the saccule and utricle are linear motion detectors, which mean they detect acceleration and deceleration: movement that can be in a straight line. Within the saccule and utricle are crystals called otoliths (ear stones) surrounding modified hair cells. When the body accelerates or decelerates, the hairs bend under the weight of these crystals.

5. Migration is a cyclic behaviour that involves the regular, seasonal or annual journey of an animal from one place to another and back again. Animals usually migrate to an area that provides a lot of food or a good environment for reproduction. There are three subcategories of migration: piloting, orientation, and navigation. Piloting involves use of familiar landmarks and is used to locate nearby distances. In orientation, an animal detects compass directions and travels in straight-line pathways. Navigation involves being able to determine the current location, and then the use of compass direction to travel in the desired direction.

6. Hemolin, an insect immunoglobulin superfamily member, is a lipopolysaccharide-binding immune protein induced during bacterial infection. It has been isolated from two moths, *Hyalophora cecropia* and *Manduca sexta*. Hemolin is encoded by a single gene, Hemolin. The introns are positioned both within and between the immunoglobulin-like domains, a feature typical for cell-adhesion molecules belonging to the immunoglobulin superfamily. Analysis of the upstream region and introns revealed potential binding sites for the Cecropia immunoresponsive factor (CIF), which recognizes the kappa B-like consensus GGGRA YYYYY.

7. An evolutionary trend can be either directional change within a single lineage or parallel change across lineages, in other words, several lineages undergoing the same sort of change. However, not just any change counts as a trend. For example, titanotheres (a cool, extinct clade related to modern horses and rhinos) exhibit an evolutionary trend. Titanotheres had bony protuberances extending from their noses. The sequence of fossil skulls from these animals shows that evolutionary changes in the size of these "horns" were not random; instead, changes were biased in the direction of increasing horn size. Evolution works by the process of natural selection. Individuals with an advantage compared with others will survive better and leave more offspring. Therefore, evolution works towards a goal. So evolution trend is goal-oriented.

8. Biological magnification, also known as biomagnification or bioamplification, is an increase in the concentration of a substance in organisms that are higher in the food chain. As a result of biomagnification, organisms at the top of the food chain generally suffer greater harm from a persistent toxin or pollutant than those at lower levels. It occurs mainly due to the inability of the decomposers (microbes) at the lowest trophic level of food chain to degrade any particular kind of toxin. As such its concentration rises in the food chain and toxicity increases through metabolism of the primary producers present in the chain.

9. The honeybee waggle dance communicates the distance and direction of good resources (typically pollen and nectar) to nest mates. The waggle dance consists of a looping figure of eight movement with a central, straight 'waggle run'; during which distance and direction information is communicated. During the waggle phase, the dancer moves her body in 15 Hz waggling motions while vibrating her wings in short pulses (20 ms duration) at frequencies ranging from 200 to 300 Hz. Some 5–25% of the workers in the hive are scouts. When food is within 50–75 meters of the hive, the scouts dance the "round dance" on the surface of the comb. But when the food is farther than 75 meters from the hive, the scouts dance the "waggle dance". It is a symbolic expression indicating the distance and direction of a food source and also the type of food available.

10. IgM is the first class of immunoglobulin produced when the body is invaded by a microorganism. As such IgM holds the initial response to an antigen by the B-cells. Cytokines are chemical messengers released by T-helper cell receptors (TCRs) to communicate with the B-cells and the T-cytotoxic cells in the body. Passive immunity to the foetus is provided by antibody IgG. This is because IgG is the only immunoglobulin that can cross the placental barrier. So it crosses the placenta from the mother and reaches the foetus to provide it immunity. Humoral immunity or antibody mediated immunity is performed by B-cells which produce antibodies from its plasma cells after being induced by cytokines released by T-helper cells on account of a foreign antigen. Coelomocytes are considered the immune cells for lower coelomate animals (annelid, mollusca, arthropoda). These cells are type of leucocytes that account for innate immunity of these animals through the process of phagocytosis.

11. Syncytial Specification is a hybrid of the autonomous and conditional specifications that occurs in insects. This method involves the action of morphogen gradients within the syncytium. As there are no cell boundaries in the syncytium, these morphogens can influence nuclei in a concentration-dependent regulative manner. A blastopore is an opening into the archenteron during the embryonic stages of an organism. Spiral cleavage is conserved between many members of the lophotrochozoan taxa, referred to as Spiralia. This group includes annelids, molluscs, and sipuncula. A blastula embryo is divided into two hemispheres: the animal pole and the vegetal pole. The vegetal pole contains large yolky cells that divide very slowly.

12. Frogs are a diverse and largely carnivorous group of short-bodied, tailless amphibians composing the order Anura. At the end of the tadpole stage, frogs undergo metamorphosis in which their bodies make a sudden transition into the adult form. After metamorphosis, young adults may disperse into terrestrial habitats or continue to live in water. Adult frogs are carnivores, eating insects and small invertebrates such as worms and slugs. The principal changes that take place include the development of the lungs and the disappearance of the gills and gill pouch making the front legs visible. They are vertebrates and so notochord present in the embryo develops into the vertebral column. Also, somite and branchial arches seen in the embryo stage disappear in the adult stage.

13. Ectoderm, the outermost of the three germ layers, or masses of cells, appears early in the development of an animal embryo. In vertebrates, ectoderm subsequently gives rise to hair, skin, nails or hooves, skull and the lens of the eye; the epithelia of sense organs, the nasal cavity, the sinuses, and the anal canal; and nervous tissue. Mesoderm, the middle of the three germ layers, or masses of cells (lying between the ectoderm and endoderm), appears early in the development of an animal embryo. In vertebrates it subsequently gives rise to muscle, connective tissue, cardiac tissue, bone, notochord, blood, bone marrow, lymphoid tissue, and the epithelia of blood vessels, lymphatic vessels, body cavities, kidneys. Endoderm, the innermost of the three germ layers, or masses of cells (lying within ectoderm and mesoderm), appears early in the development of an animal embryo. The endoderm subsequently gives rise to the epithelium (tissue that covers, or lines, a structure) of the pharynx; the larynx, trachea, and lungs; the gastrointestinal tract (except mouth and anus), the urinary bladder, the vagina (in females), and the urethra.

14. Hox genes are a group of related genes that provides the basis for anterior-posterior axis specification throughout the animal kingdom and are present in multiple duplicate sets produced through evolution. Hox genes are major regulators of animal development; thus, when one of these genes is missing or defective, there are drastic consequences. Environmental sex determination or ESD is any sex-determination system in which sex is established by a nongenetic cue (e.g. nutrient availability) experienced within a discrete period after conception. Temperature-dependent sex determination is most prevalent and common among amniote vertebrates that are classified under the reptile class. Metamorp-osis in amphibians is regulated by thyroxin concentration in the blood, which stimulates metamorphosis, and prolactin, which counteracts its effect (which are nuclear hormones) and regulated by receptor signalling.

15. The 5′ untranslated region (5′ UTR) is present before the promoter region of the sequence of mRNA. It is present upstream of the promoter region. This is because translation starts from the promoter region and UTRs are having codons which would not code for any protein. So UTRs are part of introns.

16. A double stranded DNA has a high content of A : T and a poor content of G : C. Whereas, a single stranded DNA has a higher content of G : C than A:T. In the newly discovered species, A : T = 0.63 and G : C = 0.8; thus the G :

C content is higher than A : T. Therefore, the newly discovered organism has single stranded DNA in its genome.

17. If a reversible inhibitor can bind to the enzyme active site in place of the substrate, it is described as a "competitive inhibitor." In pure competitive inhibition, the inhibitor is assumed to bind to the free enzyme but not to the enzyme-substrate (ES) complex. In competitive inhibition, a molecule similar to the substrate but unable to be acted on by the enzyme competes with the substrate for the active site. Because of the presence of the inhibitor, fewer active sites are available to act on the substrate. Thus, effective substrate concentration ([S] + [I]) increases because of the presence of the inhibitor.

18. Reverse transcriptase is an enzyme that functions as a RNA-dependent DNA polymerase. It is an enzyme encoded from the genetic material of retroviruses that catalyzes the transcription of retrovirus RNA (ribonucleic acid) into DNA (deoxyribonucleic acid). Primases are enzymes whose continual activity is required at the DNA replication fork as they catalyze the synthesis of short RNA molecules used as primers for DNA polymerases to perform replication. Since primase produces RNA molecules, the enzyme is a type of RNA polymerase. Acetyltransferase (or transacetylase) is a type of transferase enzyme that transfers an acetyl group.

19. Meiosis is a nuclear division which segregates one copy of each homologous chromosome into each new "gamete". Meiosis reduces the number of sets of chromosomes by half, so that when gametic recombination (fertilization) occurs, the ploidy of the parents will be re-established. Two successive nuclear divisions occur, Meiosis I (Reduction) and Meiosis II (Division). Meiosis produces 4 haploid cells. At the end of meiosis I, through reduction division of the chromosome, 2 haploid cells are produced. Through meiosis II, division of the two haploid cells occur resulting in 4 haploid cells. The ploidy number remains reduced in all the 4 haploid cells (i.e., n for chromosome number 2n). Given, diploid organism with chromosome number, 2n = 8. Therefore, n = 4. Hence, at anaphase II of meiosis II, there would be 4 chromatids present in each haploid cell.

20. Symbiosis is a close ecological relationship between the individuals of two or more different species. Vertebrates lack the ability to hydrolyse beta 1, 4 glycosidic bond of plant cellulose due to the lack of an enzyme cellulase. Thus ruminants must completely depend upon the microbial flora, present in rumen or hindgut, so as to digest cellulose. Digestion of food in rumen is primarily carried out by the rumen microflora which contains dense populations of several species of bacteria, protozoa, sometimes yeasts and fungi. As the environment inside a rumen is anaerobic, most of these microbial species are obligate or facultative anaerobes which can decompose complex plant material such ascellulose, hemicellulose, starch, proteins.

21. In all kinds of animals, mostly the higher animals and the vertebrates have their circulatory and respiratory systems inter-linked. This is because in most of the animals the circulatory system is closed in nature. But, in case of arthropods such as terrestrial insects, the circulatory system is of open type. As such there is no connection between the circulatory and the respiratory systems; because circulation is independent of respiration which is not possible in closed type of circulatory system.

22. Gene flow, also called gene migration, is the introduction of genetic material (by interbreeding) from one population of a species to another, thereby changing the composition of the gene pool of the receiving population. The introduction of new alleles through gene flow increases variability within the population and makes possible new combinations of traits. Natural selection is a process in nature in which organisms possessing certain genotypic characteristics that make them better adjusted to an environment tend to survive, reproduce, increase in number or frequency, and therefore, are able to transmit and perpetuate their essential genotypic qualities to succeeding generations. A mutation is a permanent change in the DNA sequence of a gene. Mutations can result from DNA copying mistakes made during cell division, exposure to ionizing radiation, exposure to chemicals called mutagens, or infection by viruses. Genetic drift is the term used in population genetics to refer to the statistical drift over time of gene frequencies in a population due to random sampling effects in the formation of successive generations.

23. *Ascaris lumbricoides* is responsible for the disease ascariasis in humans, and it is the largest and most common parasitic worm in humans. *Ascaris lumbricoides*, or "roundworm", infections in humans occur when an ingested infective egg releases a larval worm that penetrates the wall of the duodenum and enters the blood stream.

24. The life cycle of *Ascaris lumbricoides* takes about three months. Ascariasis starts, when *Ascaris lumbricoides* eggs are accidentally swallowed. Larvae hatch from the eggs, penetrate the intestinal wall and enter the bloodstream. They stop at pulmonary arteries and stay in the lungs for two weeks. They break into the alveoli and travel up the respiratory system to the throat to be swallowed again. The migration is needed for the larvae to develop into adults. Adult worms attach themselves to the intestinal wall ready to mate. Adults survive by eating food digested by the host and live up to 2 years. These adults, through mesenteric vein, enter the hepatic portal vein and into the liver.

25. In the beginning, there is low oestrogen and progesterone circulating in the body. This will trigger the hypothalamus to secrete GnRH. GnRH will act on the anterior pituitary gland to produce LH and FSH. It is a kind of negative feedback mechanism that takes place. The corpus luteum produces oestrogen and progesterone. Thus the level of GnRH in blood will depend on the concentrations of oestrogen and progesterone.

26. The menstrual cycle, under the control of the endocrine system, is necessary for reproduction. It is commonly divided into three phases: the follicular phase, ovulation, and the luteal phase. After ovulation, the ovum only lives for 24 hours or less without fertilization while the remains of the Graafian follicle in the ovary get degenerated to become corpus luteum. Corpus luteum secretes progesterone in large amounts in the blood. If fertilization does not occur within approximately two weeks, the corpus luteum involutes, causing sharp drops in levels of both progesterone and oestrogen.

27. The test cross between AabB and aabb is given by according to law of independent assortment : -

P_1 generation → AabB x aabb

F_1 generation

→ AaBb Aabb aaBb aabb

These four genotypes thus produced would be in the phenotypic ratio of 1 : 1 : 1 : 1 because of independent assortment of the alleles.

28. The test cross for 4 different phenotypes is in the ratio of 1:1:1:1. This indicates that the genes A and B are present in the same chromosome of the pair of alleles. But the loci of the two genes are different as result of which we obtain four different phenotypes of the animal.

GATE-2007

XL : LIFE SCIENCES

Time : 3 Hours **Maximum Marks : 100**

H : CHEMISTRY (Compulsory)

Q. 1 – 6 carry one mark each

1. On the basis of VSEPR theory, the molecule which has a linear structure is

(*a*) SO_2 (*b*) N_2O (*c*) Cl_2O (*d*) NO_2

2. The geometries of $[NiCl_4]^{2-}$ and $[PdCl_4]^{2-}$ respectively are

(*a*) Tetrahedral and square planar

(*b*) Both tetrahedral

(*c*) Both square planar

(*d*) Square planar and tetrahedral

3. The ionization energy of hydrogen atom in ground state is 13.6 eV. The ionization energy of Li^{2+} in ground state would be

(*a*) 1.51 eV (*b*) 4.53 eV

(*c*) 40.8 eV (*d*) 122.4 eV

4. The half-life of ^{14}C is 5730 years. An old sample of wood contains 25% of ^{14}C as would be found in a current living tree. The age of the sample of wood would be

(*a*) 1432 years (*b*) 2865 years

(*c*) 5730 years (*d*) 11460 years

5. The product 'P' formed in the following reaction is

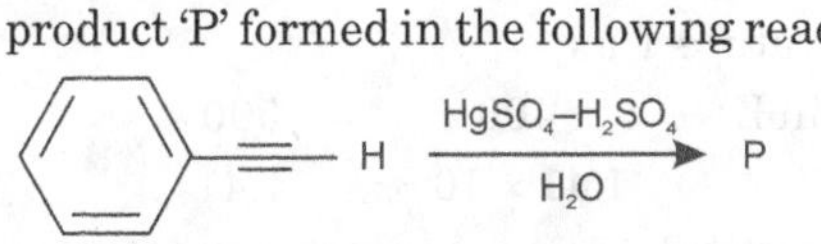

(*a*) 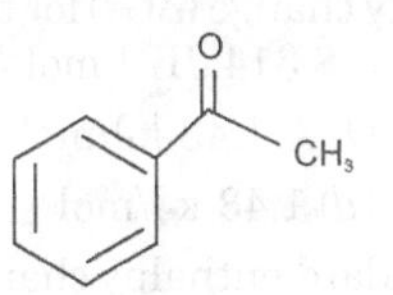 (*b*) 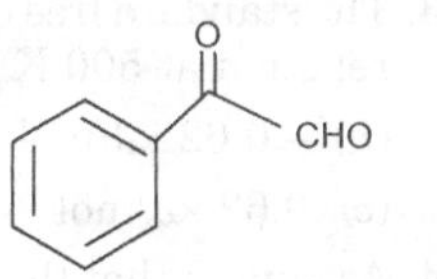

(*c*) 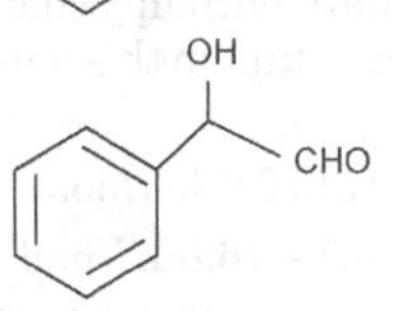 (*d*) 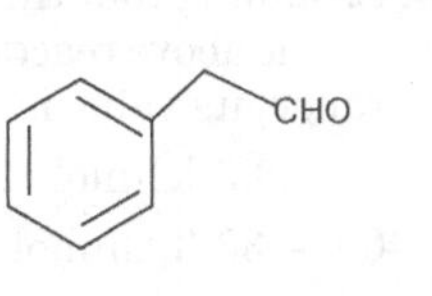

6. The order of reactivity of the following aldehydes with a nucleophile is

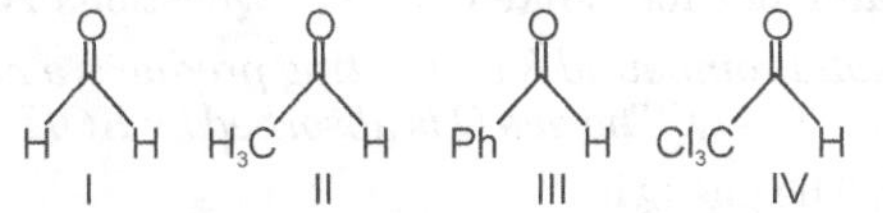

(*a*) I > II > III > IV

(*b*) IV > I > II > III

(*c*) IV > III > II > I

(*d*) I > IV > II > III

Q.7 – Q. 24 carry two marks each

7. In the nuclear reaction of $^{235}_{92}U$ with a neutron, two elements, Kr and 'Y' are formed along with three neutrons.

$$^{235}_{92}U + ^{1}_{0}n \rightarrow ^{91}_{36}Kr + 3\,^{1}_{0}n + \text{'Y'}$$

The element 'Y' is

(*a*) $^{142}_{56}Ba$ (*b*) $^{142}_{55}Cs$ (*c*) $^{142}_{54}Xe$ (*d*) $^{142}_{53}I$

8. Which of the following statements is true about diatomic species He_2 and He_2^+?

(*a*) He_2 is stable AND He_2^+ is stable

(*b*) He_2 is stable AND He_2^+ is unstable

(*c*) He_2 is unstable AND He_2^+ is stable

(*d*) He_2 is unstable AND He_2^+ is unstable

9. For the reaction A $\rightleftharpoons$ B, the activation energy for the forward reaction is 123 kJ/mol. The activation energy for the reverse reaction is 140 kJ/mol. The enthalpy change for the forward reaction is

(*a*) 263 kJ/mol (*b*) – 263 kJ/mol

(*c*) 17 kJ/mol (*d*) – 17 kJ/mol

10. The acid dissociation constant of a weak acid HA is 10^{-5}. A 0.20 M solution of the acid HA also contains 0.10 M of salt MA_2. The pH of the solution is

(*a*) 0.69 (*b*) 1.0 (*c*) 2.85 (*d*) 5.0

11. The attractive part of the van der Waals interaction, $-B/r^6$, where B is a positive coefficient and *r* is the distance between the molecules, is governed by

(*a*) dipole-dipole interaction

(*b*) charge-dipole interaction

(*c*) induced dipole-induced dipole interaction

(*d*) dipole-induced dipole interaction

12. A fuel cell is based on the idea of the reaction $H_2(g) + 1/2\ O_2(g) \rightarrow H_2O(l)$ generating electricity. The standard free energy change ($\Delta G°$) for this reaction at 298 K is – 237.13 kJ/mol.

The standard cell potential for the system at 298 K is (1 Faraday = 96500 coulombs)

(*a*) 2.457 volts (*b*) 1.228 volts

(*c*) – 1.228 volts (*d*) – 2.457 volts

13. The electron-deficient molecule is

(*a*) N_2H_4 (*b*) C_2H_6 (*c*) B_2H_6 (*d*) O_2H_2

14. The complex with crystal field stabilization energy (CFSE) of $-0.4\ \Delta_t$ is

(*a*) $[TiCl_4]$ (*b*) $[MnCl_4]^{2-}$
(*c*) $[CoCl_4]^{2-}$ (*d*) $[CuCl_4]^{2-}$

15. The most stable geometry of BrF_5 is

(*a*) 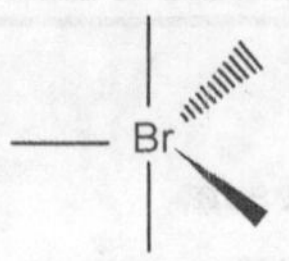 (*b*) 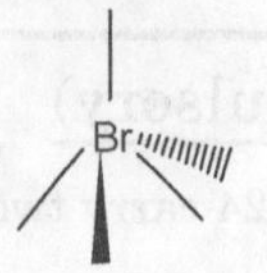

(*c*) 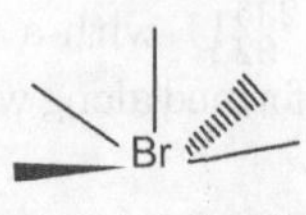 (*d*) 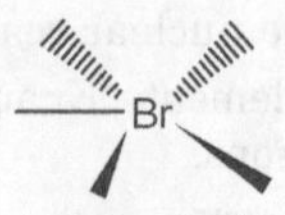

16. The species having three unpaired electrons and tetrahedral geometry is

(*a*) $[Co(CN_6)]^{4-}$ (*b*) $[CoCl_4]^{2-}$
(*c*) $[Ni(CN)_4]^{2-}$ (*d*) $[NiCl_4]^{2-}$

17. The correct arrangement of group 13 elements in terms of increasing average M-Cl bond energy in MCl_3 compounds is

(*a*) Al > Ga > In > Tl (*b*) Tl > In > Ga > Al
(*c*) Al > Ga > Tl > In (*d*) Ga > In > Tl > Al

18. Which of the following olefins leads to a racemic mixture of the diol product upon *cis*-dihydroxylation?

(*a*) $H_2C = CH_2$ (*b*) 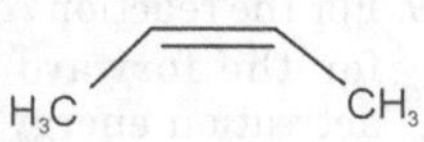

(*c*) 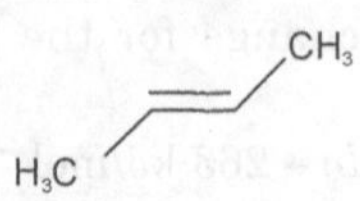 (*d*) 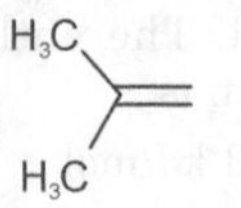

19. The major product 'Q' formed in the following reaction is

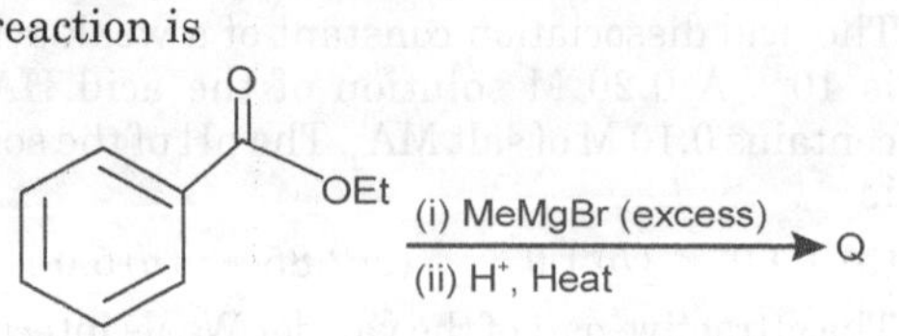

(*a*) 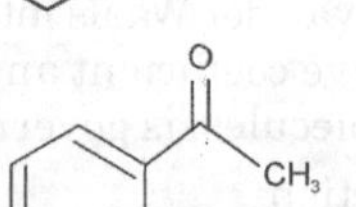 (*b*) 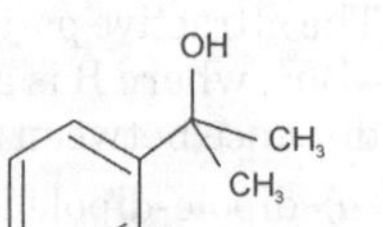

(*c*) 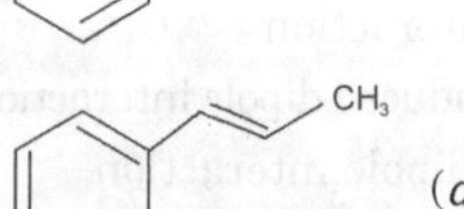 (*d*) 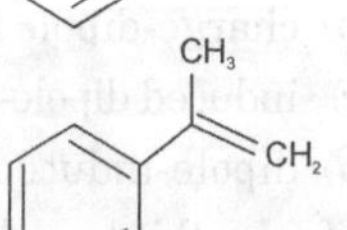

20. The most stable conformation of *cis*-1-*tert*-buty 1-4 methylcyclohexane is

(*a*) 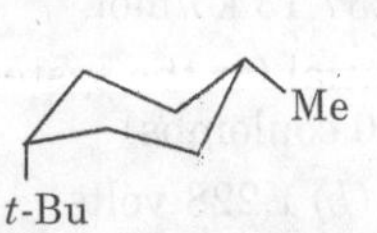 (*b*) 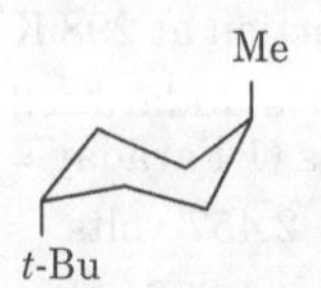

(*c*) 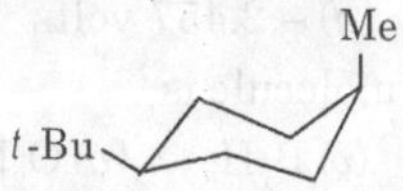 (*d*) 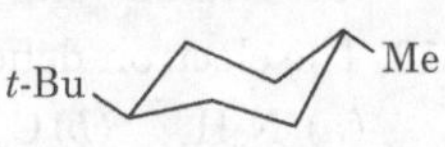

21. The major product 'R' formed in the following reaction sequence is

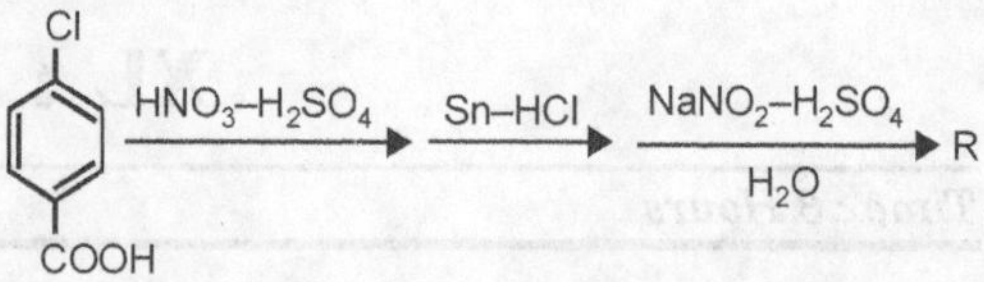

(*a*) 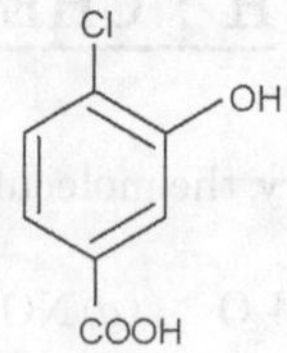 (*b*) 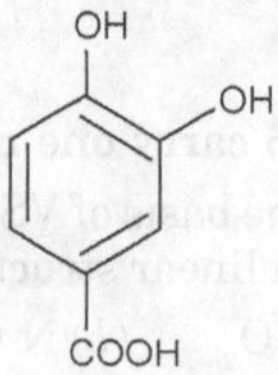

(*c*) 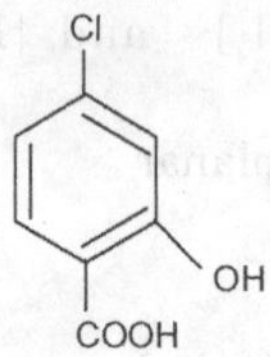 (*d*) 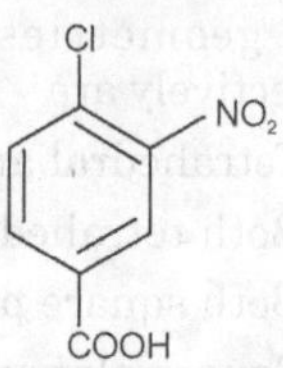

22. The following optically active compound undergoes racemization upon reaction with NaI in acetone

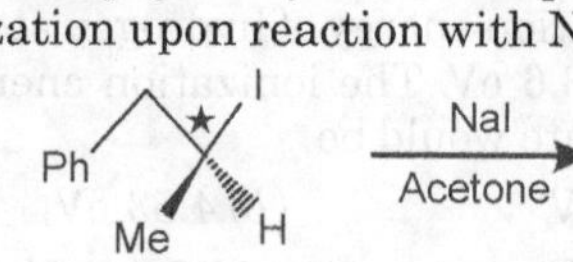

The pathway followed by the reaction is

(*a*) S_N1 (*b*) S_N2 (*c*) E1 (*d*) E2

Common Data Questions

Common Data for Questions 23 and 24 :

The equilibrium constant (K) for the reaction

$Ag_2CO_3(s) \rightleftharpoons Ag_2O(s) + CO_2(g)$ varies with temperature T as

T(in K)	400	500
K	1.41×10^{-2}	1.41

23. The standard free energy change ($\Delta G°$) for the above reaction at 500 K is (R = 8.314 $JK^{-1}\ mol^{-1}$)

(*a*) – 0.62 kJ/mol (*b*) – 1.43 kJ/mol
(*c*) 0.62 kJ/mol (*d*) 1.43 kJ/mol

24. Assuming that the standard enthalpy change ($\Delta H°$) for the above reaction is constant in this temperature range, its value is

(*a*) 33.3 kJ/mol (*b*) 76.6 kJ/mol
(*c*) – 33.3 kJ/mol (*d*) – 76.6 kJ/mol

Linked Answer Questions : Q. 25 to Q. 28 carry two marks each

Statement for Linked Answer Questions 25 and 26 :

A solid compound X on heating produces a new solid P and a gas Q. The gas Q is absorbed by KOH.

25. The gas Q is

(*a*) CO_2 (*b*) O_2 (*c*) N_2 (*d*) NH_3

26. The reaction between P and water forms a new compound R. Compound R gives bleaching powder on reaction with Cl_2. The compound X is

(*a*) NH_4NO_2 (*b*) $KClO_3$ (*c*) $CaCO_3$ (*d*) $CuFeS_2$

Statement for Linked Answer Questions 27 and 28.

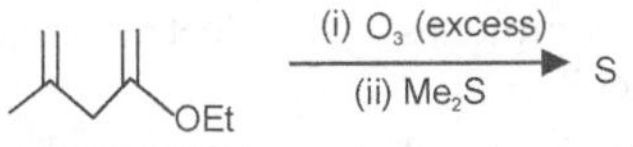

27. The structure of 'S' is

(*a*) 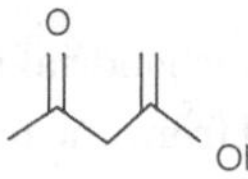 (*b*) 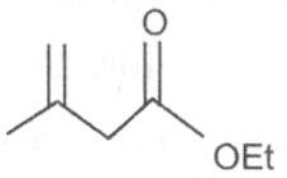

(*c*) 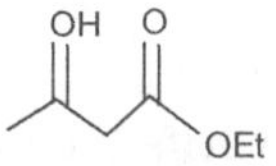 (*d*) 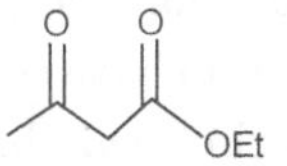

28. The name reaction by which the product 'S' may be readily prepared is
(*a*) Aldol condensation
(*b*) Benzoin condensation
(*c*) Claisen condensation
(*d*) Perkin condensation

I : BIOCHEMISTRY

Q.1 – Q. 6 carry one mark each

1. Deamination of cytosine produces
(*a*) Uracil (*b*) Pseudouracil
(*c*) Hypoxanthine (*d*) 5-Methyluracil

2. Which of the following hormones binds to a cell surface receptor?
(*a*) Estrogen (*b*) Thyroid hormone
(*c*) Insulin (*d*) Aldosterone

3. Systemic lupus erythematosus (SLE), an autoimmune disease, is characterized by the presence of
(*a*) Anti-DNA antibodies
(*b*) Anti-thyroglobulin antibodies
(*c*) Anti-insulin antibodies
(*d*) Anti-collagen antibodies

4. Optical density of 1 means
(*a*) 1% of the incident light is absorbed
(*b*) 1% of the incident light is transmitted
(*c*) 90% of the incident light is absorbed
(*d*) 90% of the incident light is transmitted

5. One of the carbon atoms of a glucose molecule is [^{14}C]-labelled. If $^{14}CO_2$ is released during the conversion of pyruvate to acetyl coenzyme-A, which carbon atom of glucose was radiolabelled?
(*a*) C3 but not C4 (*b*) C3 or C4
(*c*) Cl or C6 (*d*) Cl but not C6

6. When yeast cells are shifted from a medium containing glycerol to glucose, an increase in the transcription of four genes involved in glucose metabolism was reported. Which of the following would be the most appropriate technique to demonstrate increased transcription of these genes?
(*a*) Southern hybridization
(*b*) Northern hybridization
(*c*) Western hybridization
(*d*) Fluorescence *in situ* hybridization

Q. 7 – Q. 24 carry two marks each

7. A mixture containing protein –1, – 2, – 4, and – 5 with molecular weights 5,000, 10,000, 25,000, 65,000 and 100,000, respectively, were separated on a Sephadex G-50 column. The order of elution of these proteins from the column will be
(*a*) Protein-1, protein-2, protein-3, protein-4, and protein-5
(*b*) Protein-5, protein-4, protein-3, protein-2, and protein-1
(*c*) Protein-1, -2, and -3 elute first, followed by protein-5 and -4
(*d*) Protein-4 and -5 elute first, followed by protein-3, -2, and -1

8. The maximum number of hydrogen bonds that a molecule of water can form is
(*a*) 1 (*b*) 2 (*c*) 3 (*d*) 4

9. Match the techniques mentioned in Column A with their applications given in Column B.

Column A
P. PCR
Q. DNA microarray
R. ELISA

Column B
1. Identification of transcription factor binding sites in chromatin
2. Identification of HIV infected patients using serum samples
3. Isolation of mouse homologue of a yeast gene
4. Analysis of differential gene expression in cancer and normal cells

	P	Q	R
(*a*)	4	1	3
(*b*)	3	4	2
(*c*)	4	1	2
(*d*)	3	2	1

10. A nonsense mutation in the gene encoding protein X leading to the synthesis of a truncated protein results in a slow growing strain. Mutagenesis of this strain towards the isolation of extragenic suppressors led to the isolation of a strain which grew normally and synthesized the full-length protein X. The extragenic suppressor is likely to be a gene coding for
(*a*) rRNA
(*b*) RNA polymerase
(*c*) tRNA
(*d*) Ribosomal protein

11. The total radioactivity in 1 ml solution 0.25 mg of glycine is 1 mCi. The specific activity (mCi/millimole) of radiolabelled glycine will be
(*a*) 300 (*b*) 18.75
(*c*) 3000 (*d*) 1875

12. Ten grams of butter was saponified. The non-saponifiable fraction was extracted into 25 ml of chloroform. The absorbance of this solution in a 1 cm cuvette is 0.53 at 328 nm. If the extinction coefficient ($a_{1\%}$) of vitamin A at this wavelength is 1550, calculate the amount of vitamin A present.

(*a*) 3.419×10^{-3} g/100 ml

(*b*) 3.419×10^{-6} g/100 ml

(*c*) 3.419×10^{-5} g/100 ml

(*d*) 3.419×10^{-4} g/100 ml

13. Folate derivatives are required for the synthesis of which deoxynucleotides ?

(*a*) Adenylate and guanylate

(*b*) Cytidylate and thymidylate

(*c*) Adenylate, guanylate and thymidylate

(*d*) Adenylate, guanylate and cytidylate

14. Cytochrome C reductase, also called as Complex III or cytochrome bc_1 complex, localized on the inner mitochondrial membrane receives electrons from ubiquinol and donates to cytochrome C. In one cycle,

(*a*) Two cytochrome C molecules are reduced

(*b*) One ubiquinol is oxidized

(*c*) Two ubiquinols are oxidized and one ubiquinone is reduced

(*d*) One cytochrome C is reduced

15. Match the biological functions mentioned in Column A with the enzymes given in

A	B
P. Diacylglycerol synthesis	(1) Protein kinase A
Q. CREB phosphorylation	(2) Ras
R. GTP hydrolysis	(3) Phospholipase C
	(4) Phospholipase D
	(5) Protein kinase G

	P	Q	R
(*a*)	3	1	5
(*b*)	4	1	2
(*c*)	3	1	2
(*d*)	3	5	2

16. How does haemoglobin carry carbon dioxide generated in tissues back to the lungs ?

(*a*) By coordination with heme

(*b*) By forming N-terminal carbamate

(*c*) By forming C-terminal carbamate

(*d*) By linking to the epsilon-amino group of lysine

17. Which of the following enzyme activities can be detected in the supernatant obtained by centrifugation of liver homogenate at 100,000 g for 1 hr at 4°C ?

(*a*) Succinate dehydrogenase

(*b*) Glyceraldehyde 3-phosphate dehydrogenase

(*c*) Glycogen synthetase

(*d*) Aconitase

18. Which of the following statements about the enzyme complexes of the electron transport system is correct ?

(*a*) They interact with one another via mobile electron carriers

(*b*) They are located in the mitochondrial matrix

(*c*) They can not be separated from one another in a functional form

(*d*) They all have cytochromes

19. Match the DNA binding motifs mentioned in Column A with the proteins given in Column B.

A	B
P. Zinc finger	(1) c-jun
Q. Leucine zipper	(2) Growth hormone receptor
R. Helix-turnhelix motif	(3) Glucocorticoid receptor
	(4) Histone HI
	(5) Lambda repressor

	P	Q	R
(*a*)	4	5	1
(*b*)	2	5	4
(*c*)	2	1	5
(*d*)	3	1	5

20. Which of the DNA polymerases listed below is primarily responsible for the *de novo* synthesis of new DNA strands ?

(*a*) DNA polymerase I

(*b*) DNA polymerase II

(*c*) DNA polymerase III

(*d*) DNA polymerase IV

21. F_1F_0-ATPase in chloroplasts is located on the

(*a*) inner chloroplast membrane with F1 facing the stroma

(*b*) inner chloroplast membrane with F1 facing the inter-membrane space

(*c*) thylakoid membrane with F1 facing the stroma

(*d*) thylakoid membrane with F1 facing the thylakoid lumen

22. In addition to adjuvants, generation of anti-hapten antibodies will require injection of

(*a*) the hapten to a mice

(*b*) a mixture of hapten and protein to a mice

(*c*) the hapten covalently linked to a protein to a mice

(*d*) a mixture of hapten and lipid to a mice

Common Data Questions

Common Data for Questions 23, 24 :

The number of protons translocated by the various vectorial proteins localized on the inner mitochondrial membrane of an organism was determined. They are as follows: NADH dehydrogenase : 4, cytochrome bc_1 complex : 2, cytochrone aa_3 complex : 4 and F_1F_0-ATPase: 3. One proton is also required for the transport of inorganic phosphate into the mitochondrial matrix.

23. The number of ATP molecules that can be synthesized by the oxidation of one NADH moelcule is

(*a*) 2 (*b*) 2.5 (*c*) 3 (*d*) 3.3

24. If the cytosolic NADH is transported to the matrix by the glyceraldehydes 3-phosphate shuttle, then the number of ATPs synthesized is

(*a*) 1.5 (*b*) 2

(*c*) 2.5 (*d*) 3.3

Linked Answer Questions : Q.25 to Q.28 carry two marks each

Statement for Linked Answer Questions 25 and 26 :

Two mammalian cell lines were found to express either epidermal growth factor receptor (EGFR) alone (cell line A) or both EGFR and Ras (cell line B). These cell lines were treated with epidermal growth factor (EGF) and protein phosphorylation was examined in the membrane and cytosolic fractions using anti-phosphotyrosine and antiphosphoserine antibodies.

25. EGF-dependent tyrosine phosphorylation will be detected in

(*a*) Membrane and cytosolic fractions of both the cell lines

(*b*) Only the membrane fraction of only cell line A

(*c*) Only the membrane fraction of both cell lines

(*d*) Only the cytosolic fractions of both cell lines

26. EGF-dependent serine phosphorylation will be detected in

(*a*) membrane and cytosolic fractions of both the cell lines

(*b*) only the membrane fraction of cell line A

(*c*) only the membrane fraction of cell line B

(*d*) only the cytosolic fraction of cell line A

Statement for Linked Answer Question 27 & 28:

$\Delta G°$ is the symbol used to denote standard free-energy change of a chemical reaction in biological systems. The standard conditions are T = 298 K, concentration of water = 55.5 M, pH = 7, and the reactants and products (other than water and proton) are initially present at 1 M concentration.

27. Suppose ΔG denotes the free-energy change for the reaction $A + B \rightleftarrows C + H^+$ at pH 5, all other conditions being the same as the standard conditions specified above. Them

(*a*) $\Delta G = \Delta G°'$ (*b*) $\Delta G = \Delta G°' + 11.5$ RT

(*c*) $\Delta G = \Delta G°' + 4.6$ RT (*d*) $\Delta G = \Delta G°' + 16.1$ RT

28. If $\Delta G°'$ for the reaction is – 11.7 kJ/mol and R = 8.314 kJ/mol, the reaction is

(*a*) Endergonic at both 37°C and 25°C

(*b*) Endergonic at 37°C and exergonic at 25°C

(*c*) Exergonic at both 37°C and 25°C

(*d*) Exergonic at 37°C and endergonic at 25°C

K : BOTANY

Q. 1 – Q. 6 carry one mark each

1. Availability of free energy is maximum in which of the following trophic levels?

(*a*) Producers (*b*) Decomposers

(*c*) Herbivores (*d*) Secondary consumers

2. From the given statements identify the INCORRECT one.

(*a*) GA involves in flowering

(*b*) Ethylene is produced during ripening of the seeds

(*c*) Auxin helps in cell elongation and formation of root

(*d*) Cytokinin helps in embryo development and prevent leaf senescence

3. The correct equation for the reduction of nicotinamide adenine dinucleotide phosphate is

(*a*) $NADP^+ + 2H^+ \rightarrow NADPH^+ + H^+$

(*b*) $NADP^+ + H^+ + e^- \rightarrow NADPH$

(*c*) $NADP^+ + H^+ + 2e^- \rightarrow NADPH$

(*d*) $NADP^+ + 2H^+ + 2e^- \rightarrow NADPH_2$

4. Which of the following factors is critical for haploidy induction?

(*a*) Presence of optimum levels of auxin and cytokinin in the medium

(*b*) Treatment of donor plants with phytohormones

(*c*) Use of colchicine in the medium

(*d*) Induction and proliferation of callus from anther culture

5. Gene transfer method: Choose the correct answer.

(*a*) *Agrobacterium*-mediated transformation was developed by E.C. Cocking

(*b*) Biolistic transformation was first developed by J. C. Sanford

(*c*) Protoplast transformation was first reported by I. Potrykus

(*d*) Pollen tube transformation was demonstrated by Oifa Zhang

6. Identify the mismatch tissue.

(*a*) Periderm (*b*) Phelloderm

(*c*) Phellem (*d*) Pallisade

Q. 7 – Q. 24 carry two marks each.

7. Find out the correct statements for Linnaeus system of classification.

P. It is also known as artificial-sexual system of classification

Q. It was published in the name of "*Genera Plantarum*"

R. In this system plants belonging to widely distant natural groups are placed under one order of a class

S. In this system Gymnospermae and Angiospermae are placed in two taxa of equal ranks

(*a*) P, Q (*b*) Q, R (*c*) R, S (*d*) P, R

8. Which of the following statements are true in case of fluid-mosaic model cell membranes.

P. Between 5-8 nm thick and appear trilaminar when viewed in cross-section under electron microscope

Q. Less than 1 nm thick and consist of a layer of protein sandwitched between two layers of phospholipids

R. In the lipid bilayer, proteins are embedded at irregular intervals and held by hydrophilic interactions between lipids and hydrophilic domains of the proteins

S. The protein domains exposed on one side of the lipid bilayer are different from those exposed on the other side

(*a*) P, Q (*b*) P, S (*c*) Q, S (*d*) P, R

9. Identify the correct statements.

P. Bundle sheath containing chloroplast present in C_4 plants

Q. Annual rings differentiate into barks and woods

R. Sap wood is important for biological functions and heart wood is economically important as it contains gums, resins, oils, tannins, etc.

S. Clonal propagation leads to somaclonal variation

(*a*) P, Q (*b*) Q, R (*c*) R, S (*d*) P, R

10. Which of the following statements are true on ecological point of view?

P. Pyramid of numbers' can sometimes be inverted

Q. Standing crop is not a reliable measure of productivity

R. Primary productivity should always be calculated on dry matter rather than on fresh biomass

S. The total solar energy trapped in the food material by photosynthesis is referred to as net primary production

(*a*) P, Q (*b*) Q, R

(*c*) R, S (*d*) P, R

11. Identify the wheat disease based on the following given symptoms.

- The disease appears when the ears emerges in plants
- Diseased ears emerges out of the boot leaf a little earlier than the healthy ones
- Black powdery mass of spores replace the flowers
- The growth of the plant and its general appearance is not affected

(*a*) Loose smut of wheat

(*b*) Flag smut of wheat

(*c*) Black rust of wheat

(*d*) Powdery mildew of wheat

12. Identify the correct statements from the following with respect to improvement of shelf-life of fruits and vegetables.

P. It should be cooled immediately to slow down the respiration process

Q. The air of the store chamber should pass through charcoal to absorb the ethylene produced during the ripening process

R. It should be treated immediately with silver nitrate and cobalt chloride

S. It should be treated with the low concentration of biotin and nicotinic acid for prolonged preservation

(*a*) P, R (*b*) P, Q (*c*) Q, R (*d*) P, S

13. Heterosis helps in crop improvement. Identify the correct statements.

P. Parental lines improvement by diversification of *cms* and restorer sources for higher yield

Q. Development of fortified food to satisfy market demand

R. Improved hybrid crop developed for dual function-salinity tolerance and fungal resistance

S. Reciprocal crosses of an improved isogenic line for a better yield

(*a*) Q, S (*b*) P, S (*c*) P, Q (*d*) P, R

14. Identify the correct statements.

P. Xylogenesis is defined as the differentiation of parenchyma into specialized xylary cell

Q. First anther culture was reported by Guha and Maheshwari

R. Totipotency was reported by Sundarland

S. *In vitro* fertilization reported by Hofmeister

(*a*) P, S (*b*) P, Q (*c*) P, R (*d*) R, S

15. Encapsulated somatic embryo in alginate beads produce artificial seeds. Identify the correct statements.

(P) Artificial seed is a genetically modified agricultural product

(Q) Artificial seed is a patented product for pharmaceutical industry

(R) Artificial seeds can be stored and transferred to soil for germination

(S) Somatic embryo of single cell origin produce genetically uniform plants

(*a*) P, S (*b*) P, Q (*c*) Q, R (*d*) R, S

Q. 16-22 are matching exercises

Choose the correct one from the alternatives *a, b, c* and *d*.

16.

Group I (*Name of the Fungus*)	**Group II** (*Class*)
P. *Agaricus sp.*	1. Ascomycetes
Q. *Pilobolus sp*	2. Deuteromycetes
R. *Neurospora sp.*	3. Phycomycetes
S. *Rhizoctonia sp.*	4. Actinomycetes
	5. Basidiomycetes
	6. Zygomycetes

	P	Q	R	S
(*a*)	5	4	3	1
(*b*)	4	1	2	6
(*c*)	5	3	1	2
(*d*)	6	1	3	5

17. **Group I** (*Biological activity*)

P. Antibacterial and antifungal
Q. Antibacterial not antifungal
R. Antifungal not antibacterial
S. Antiviral

Group II (*Chemical compound*)

1. Hypericin
2. Aspergillic acid
3. Fulvic acid
4. Ustalagic acid
5. Abscisic acid
6. Terramycin

	P	Q	R	S
(*a*)	1	2	3	4
(*b*)	2	6	4	1
(*c*)	2	1	5	6
(*d*)	5	6	1	2

18.

Group I (*Common name*)	Group II (*Scientific name*)
P. Garden bean	1. *Raphanus sativus*
Q. Oat	2. *Phaseolus vulgaris*
R. Cashew nut	3. *Brassica oleracea*
S. Carrot	4. *Anacardium occidentale*
	5. *Daucus carota*
	6. *Avena sativa*

	P	Q	R	S
(*a*)	2	6	4	5
(*b*)	6	2	4	5
(*c*)	1	3	6	4
(*d*)	5	1	6	4

19.

Group I	Group II
P. Insect resistant cotton	1. Bt
Q. Golden rice	2. Round up
R. 'Flavr-Savr' tomato	3. 2,4-D
S. Herbicide tolerant soyabean	4. Carotenoids
	5. Ferritin
	6. ACC-deaminase

	P	Q	R	S
(*a*)	2	5	1	3
(*b*)	1	4	6	2
(*c*)	1	4	6	3
(*d*)	2	4	6	1

20.

Group I	Group II
P. Funiculus	1. Pea pod
Q. Seed coat dormancy	2. Coconut
R. Reserve food stored in endosperm	3. Rice seed
S. Vivipary germination	4. *Erycibe*
	5. Malvaceae
	6. *Rhizophora*

	P	Q	R	S
(*a*)	1	4	3	5
(*b*)	1	6	5	4
(*c*)	1	5	3	6
(*d*)	1	2	6	3

21. **Group I**

P. Chromosome cycle
Q. G_1 phase
R. Salt glands
S. Tunica-corpus

Group II

1. Interval between mitosis and DNA replication
2. Helps in removing the excess salts
3. Behavior of the cell as they grow and divide
4. Organization of apical meristem based on a single apical cell
5. Concept of tissue differentiation at shoot apical meristem
6. Replication and partitioning of the genome into two daughter cells

	P	Q	R	S
(*a*)	1	6	3	4
(*b*)	2	1	6	5
(*c*)	3	6	4	5
(*d*)	6	1	2	5

22. **Group I**

P.
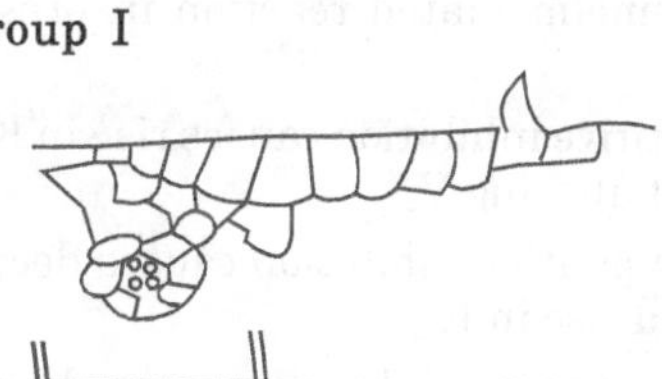

Q.
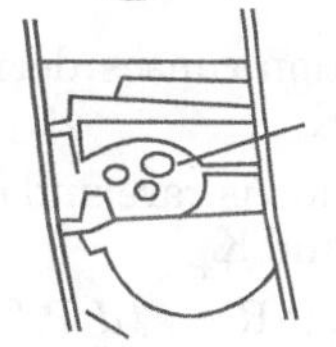

R.
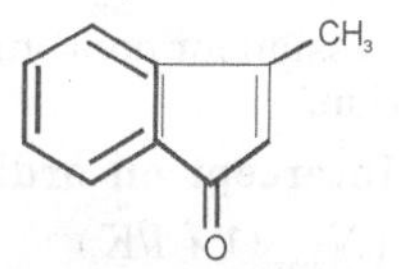

S.
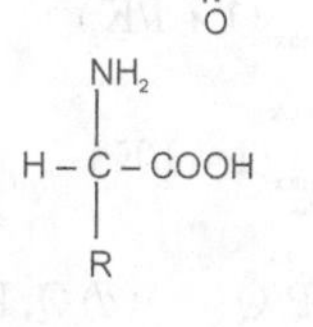

Group II

1. Amino acid
2. Glucose
3. IAA
4. Bulliform cells
5. Tyloses
6. Kinetin

	P	Q	R	S
(*a*)	5	4	6	3
(*b*)	4	5	3	1
(*c*)	5	4	2	3
(*d*)	4	5	3	6

Common Data Questions

Common Data for Questions 23, 24 :

A researcher studied three independently assorting genes in a plant. Each gene has a dominant and a recessive allele. T: tall plant, t: dwarf plant; W: purple flower, w: white flower; C: full pods, c: constricted pods. A cross was conducted between

TTWWCC x tt ww cc

23. How many different kinds of F_1 gamates would be expected from the above cross ?
(*a*) 2 (*b*) 4 (*c*) 8 (*d*) 16

24. How many different kinds of F_2 genotypes would be expected from the above cross ?
(*a*) 8 (*b*) 9 (*c*) 16 (*d*) 27

Linked Answer Questions : Q 25 to 28 carry two marks each

Statement for Linked Answer Questions 25 and 26 :

Enzyme [E] reacts with substrate [S] to form an [ES] complex at normal temperature to produce the product. In the presence of inhibitor the rate of reaction changes.

25. Which of the following statements are **INCORRECT** about enzyme-mediated reaction in presence of inhibitor ?

P. Competitive inhibition causes rise in K_m value without altering V_{max}

Q. Noncompetitive inhibition causes decrease in V_{max} and rise in K_m

R. Uncompetitive inhibition causes decrease in V_{max} without altering K_m

S. Uncompetitive inhibition is rare and causes a decrease in both V_{max} and K_m

(*a*) P, Q (*b*) Q, R (*c*) P, R (*d*) P, S

26. Identify the correct expression for noncompetitive and competitive inhibition.

	Slope	Intercept on ordinate
P.	$K_m/V_{max}(1 + I/K_i)$	$1/V_{max}(1 + I/K_i)$
Q.	$K_m/V_{max}(1 + I/K_i)$	$1/V_{max}$
R.	K_m/V_{max}	$1/V_{max}(1 + I/K_i)$
S.	K_m/V_{max}	$1/V_{max}$

(*a*) P, S (*b*) R, S (*c*) P, Q (*d*) Q, R

Statement for Linked Answer Questions 27 and 28 :

Economically important plants are known for their commercial products and recognized with scientific names.

27. From the given common names, identify sequentially the scientific names of the following plants.

Common names : Cotton, Peanut, Sarpagandha and Tea

P. *Camellia sinensis*

Q. *Arachis hypogea*

R. *Rauwolfia serpentina*

S. *Gossypium arboreum*

(*a*) S

(*a*) P, Q, R, S (*b*) S, R, Q, P

(*c*) S, Q, R, P (*d*) S, P, Q, R

28. Identify the most important commercial products from the above mentioned plants. (Follow the sequence of the common names)

P. Vegetable Oil

Q. Fibre

R. Alkaloid

S. Beverage

(*a*) Q, P, R, S (*b*) S, Q, R, P

(*c*) Q, R, P, S (*d*) R, Q, P, S

L : MICROBIOLOGY

Q.1 – 6 carry one mark each

1. Reverse transcriptase used in genetic engineering was discovered by
(*a*) Temin & Baltimore (*b*) Smith & Arber
(*c*) Smith & Baltimore (*d*) Temin & Arber

2. Infection of *E.coli* by bacteriophage λ is normally detected by
(*a*) Resistance of the bacteria to an antibiotic
(*b*) Growth of single colony on the agar plate
(*c*) The appearance of plaques or lysed bacteria on agar plates
(*d*) Restriction digest of the bacterial DNA

3. A microscope that has a total magnification of 1500X with an oil immersion lens has an ocular of power
(*a*) 1.5 X (*b*) 15 X (*c*) 150 X (*d*) 1500 X

4. Which of the following species shows a high resistance to radiation damage?
(*a*) *Deinococcus* (*b*) *Micrococcus*
(*c*) *Staphylococcus* (*d*) *Planococcus*

5. Peptic ulcers are caused by
(*a*) *Shigella sonei*
(*b*) Giardia lambia
(*c*) *Enterobius vermicularis*
(*d*) *Helicobacter pylori*

6. The evolutionary history of an organism is called
(a) Taxonomy (b) Dendrogram
(c) Phylogeny (d) Cladogram

Q.7 – 24 carry two marks each

7. Which vector would be the most appropriate for cloning a 150 kb fragment of DNA?
(a) pBR322 (b) λ vector (c) YAC (d) BAC

8. Which group of microorganisms have a high level of unsaturated fatty acids in their cell membrane?
(a) Mesophilic (b) Psychrophilic
(c) Thermophilic (d) Hyperthermophilic

9. Complete denitrification of nitrate results in the formation of
(a) N_2 (b) NH_3 (c) N_2O_5 (d) NH_2OH

10. Which of the following disease in **NOT** caused by the Coxsackie virus?
(a) Intestinal infection (b) Meningitis
(c) Gingivitis (d) Myocarditis

11. Bacterial cell wall biosynthesis is inhibited by the antibiotic
(a) Vancomycin (b) Tetracycline
(c) Chloramphenicol (d) Erythromycin

12. Match the correct combination of plasmid DNA to their properties

Plasmid DNA
(P) Conjugative plasmid
(Q) Cryptic plasmid
(R) Episome

Property
(1) can integrate into the chromosome and replicate when the chromosome is copied
(2) capable of transferring itself between prokaryotes
(3) Does not appear to have any function

	P	Q	R
(a)	1	3	2
(b)	2	3	1
(c)	2	1	3
(d)	3	2	1

13. An Hfr bacterium is one that contains
(a) Many unusual plasmids
(b) Chromosomal material acquired from a recipient cell
(c) The ability to undergo transduction
(d) A plasmid integrated into its chromosome

14. Match the following product/process to the microorganism involved

Product/Process	Microorganism
P. Bioplastics	(1) *Beauveria bassiana*
Q. Bioremediation	(2) *Thiobacillus thiooxidans*
R. Bioleaching	(3) *Ralstonia eutropha*
S. Biopesticide	(4) *Pseudomonas putida*

	P	Q	R	S
(a)	3	2	4	1
(b)	1	2	3	4
(c)	3	4	2	1
(d)	1	4	2	3

15. Which of the following enzymes convert glucose-6-phosphate to 6-phosphoglucono-δ-lactone in the Entner-Doudoroff pathway?
(a) Glucose-6-phosphate dehydrogenase
(b) Phosphoglucoisomerase
(c) Phosphoglucolactonase
(d) 6-phosphogluconate dehydrase

16. The process in which a molecule is transported into the cell while being chemically altered is called
(a) Passive transport
(b) Group translocation
(c) Facilitated transport
(d) None of these

17. MacConkey agar is a type of
(a) Selective media
(b) Differential media
(c) Both selective & differential media
(d) None of these

18. Which of the following modes of DNA replication are used by bacteria ?
(a) Rolling circle
(b) Theta replication
(c) Bidirectional replication
(d) All of the above

19. Which of the following is **INCORRECT** about negative staining procedure?
(a) It utilizes a stain such as Nigrosin
(b) Microorganisms stain deeply
(c) Microorganisms repel the dye
(d) An acidic dye is used

20. A mutation in the codon **UCG** to **UAG** is described as
(a) Nonsense mutation
(b) Silent mutation
(c) Mis-sense mutation
(d) Neutral mutation

21. The ineffectiveness of many antibiotics today is closely associated with
(a) Bacteriophages
(b) F plasmids
(c) R plasmids
(d) Bacterial transformations

22. Which type of cells actually secrete antibodies?
(a) T cells (b) Macrophages
(c) Monocytes (d) Plasma cells

Common Data Questions

Common Data for Questions 23, 24 :

The 50μL of competent E.coli cells (10^9 CFU/mL) were transformed using 0.5ng of a 5kb plasmid DNA to which 950 μL of SOC medium was added. Only 50 μL of this was plated on a selective agar plate. A after an 12h incubation at 37°C, 90 colonies were observed

23. Calculate the efficiency of this transformation in CFU/μg of DNA
   (*a*) 3.6×10^5 (*b*) 3.6×10^6
   (*c*) 1.8×10^5 (*d*) 1.8×10^6
24. Calculate the percentage of transformed cells
   (*a*) 0.36% (*b*) 0.72% (*c*) 3.6% (*d*) 7.2%

Linked Answere Questions : Q. 25 To Q. 28 carry two marks each

Statement for Linked Answer Questions 25 and 26 :

An egg sandwich got contaminated with 10 cells of a bacterium. It was left open at 37°C for 4 hours. It was found to contain 40960 cells.

25. What is the generation time of this bacterium?
   (*a*) 15 min (*b*) 20min (*c*) 25 min (*d*) 30 min
26. If the initial inoculum was only 1 cell, then after 10 hours what will be the number of Cells
   (*a*) 2^{20} (*b*) 2^{24} (*c*) 2^{30} (*d*) 2^{40}

Statement for Linked Answer Questions 27 and 28:

A researcher desires to clone a gene (1kb) of a microorganism. Its genome size is 1.5×10^4 kb. The average size of its library fragment is 5 kb.

27. What is the ratio of genome size of the microorganism relative to average size of the fragment in the gene library ?
   (*a*) 3000 (*b*) 1500
   (*c*) 45000 (*d*) None of these
28. The genomic library was created in vectors that were transformed into bacterial cells. If there is a 95% probability of the transformation, how many recombinant bacterial colonies will have to be screened to find this particular gene ?
   (*a*) 7000 (*b*) 8000 (*c*) 9000 (*d*) 10000

M : ZOOLOGY

Q. 1 – 6 carry one mark each

1. Sickle-cell anemia is caused by mutation in
   (*a*) Haemoglobin A (*b*) Haemoglobin B
   (*c*) Haemoglobin F (*d*) Haemoglobin S
2. Each individual antigenic determinant of the variable region of the antibody is referred to as
   (*a*) Paratope (*b*) Epitope
   (*c*) Agretope (*d*) Idiotope
3. Which of the following non covalent interactions is considered as strongest?
   (*a*) Hydrophobic interactions
   (*b*) Ionic bonds
   (*c*) Hydrogen bonds
   (*d*) Van der waals forces
4. Acrosome present on the sperm head is derived from
   (*a*) Golgi apparatus
   (*b*) Nucleus
   (*c*) Endoplasmic reticulum
   (*d*) Centrosome
5. The first site of hematopoiesis in the mouse embryo is
   (*a*) Liver (*b*) Bone marrow
   (*c*) Spleen (*d*) Yolk sac
6. Which of the following fish is considered to be a 'living fossil' ?
   (*a*) Protopterus (*b*) Lepidosiren
   (*c*) Latimeria (*d*) Neoceratodus

Q. 7 – Q. 24 carry two marks each

7. Albinism is controlled by a recessive gene (c). From a marriage between a normal pigmented person carrying genotype Cc and albino cc, what is the chance that an albino child will be born?
   (*a*) 1/2 (*b*) 1/4
   (*c*) 3/4 (*d*) 3/8
8. Many fishes are able to live outside water with the help of special air chambers above the gills. Which one of the following fish does not have same adaptation ?
   (*a*) *Anabas* (*b*) *Saccobranchus*
   (*c*) *Gobius* (*d*) *Clarias*
9. The air sac plays an important role in the aerial life of flying birds. Which of the following is not a function of the air sac?
   (*a*) As a resonator
   (*b*) As a balloon
   (*c*) In perching
   (*d*) Regulator of moisture content of the body
10. Transgenic mice are produced by
   (*a*) *In vitro* fertilization of ova by sperms from a different strain followed by implantation
   (*b*) Transfer of cloned foreign DNA into blastocyst cells followed by implantation
   (*c*) Implantation of mixed blastocyst cells from two different strains
   (*d*) Selection of a given trait by repeated back-crossing
11. Which of the following proteins binds tightly to DNA in the chromatin structure and influences eukaryotic DNA replication ?
   (*a*) Histones
   (*b*) Lamins
   (*c*) Vimentin
   (*d*) Proteasome

12. During DNA replication significant proportion of newly synthesized DNA in the lagging strand exists as small Okazaki fragments. The sizes of these units in bacteria are approximately
(*a*) 100 nucleotides (*b*) 1000 nucleotides
(*c*) 100 base pairs (*d*) 1000 base pairs

13. Which of the following statement is not included in the inductions and deductions of Darwinism?
(*a*) The prodigality or reproduction is very important since over crowdedness results in struggle for existence
(*b*) In the struggle for existence the organisms with variation in structure habits or instincts may be better adapted to new conditions and will have better chance of survival
(*c*) Natural selection operates amongst the fittest and the new forms are established leading to speciation.
(*d*) There is no organism without genotype. The genotype should be changed to give an efficient organism.

14. In case of turtles, the temperature at which the eggs are exposed during development is the deciding factor in sex determination. This is because of the temperature sensitivity of
(*a*) Estrogen (*b*) Testosterone
(*c*) Aromatase enzyme (*d*) Progesterone

15. One of the most remarkable features of evolution is the formation of the amnion and the allantoin, which appeared for the first time in
(*a*) Amphibians (*b*) Fishes
(*c*) Birds (*d*) Reptiles

16. For cloning an animal, which of the following somatic cells would not be suitable?
(*a*) Lymphocytes (*b*) Fibroblasts
(*c*) Epidermal cell (*d*) Neutrophils

17. Differential blood cell counting is carried out routinely not only for assessing the 'general health' of an individual but also for identifying types of infection. Increase in the circulatory eosinophils is likely to be due to infection with
(*a*) Viruses (*b*) Helminths
(*c*) Fungus (*d*) Bacteria

18. Rajesh and Deb while playing in the field got stung by a comparable number of bees. After about 15 minutes, while Rajesh experienced only pain and small swelling, Deb manifested intense swelling, breathlessness and had to be hospitalized. Which of the following reasons would be the most logical explanation for the different reactions ?
(*a*) Deb was on an empty stomach
(*b*) Rajesh is several years younger than Deb
(*c*) Deb had been stung by bees before
(*d*) Deb is several years younger than Rajesh

19. Normally receptors are cell-membrane bound but with few exceptions. Which of the following receptors is present in the cytoplasm ?
(*a*) Thyroid stimulating hormone receptor
(*b*) Epidermal growth factor receptor
(*c*) Progesterone receptor
(*d*) Cytokine receptor

20. During development of the red blood cells from the stem cells of most mammals, the phenomenon of enucleation is observed during the last stage of differentiation. However, the red blood cells of some animals are nucleated :
Identify which one of the following ?
(*a*) Cow (*b*) Rhinoceros
(*c*) Camel (*d*) Polar bear

21. Comparison of the genome sequences of any two animals would reveal evolutionary relatedness. In this context, the similarity between man and chimpanzee is
(*a*) > 95 % (*b*) < 75 % (*c*) < 25 % (*d*) < 50 %

22. Certain types of cancers can be correlated with specific changes in chromosome structure. In patients suffering from myelogenous leukemia, the abnormal chromosome detected was termed Philadelphia chromosome. Which of the following chromosome is altered in this disease?
(*a*) Chromosome 10 (*b*) Chromosome 11
(*c*) Chromosome 20 (*d*) Chromosome 22

Common Data Questions

Common Data for Questions 23 and 24:

The size of mammalian heart is nearly proportional to body size and makes up approximately 0.59% of the body mass. However the heart rate is inversely related to body size. The following graph represents the relationship between the heart rate and body size of the mammals (data are plotted on logarithmic coordinates).

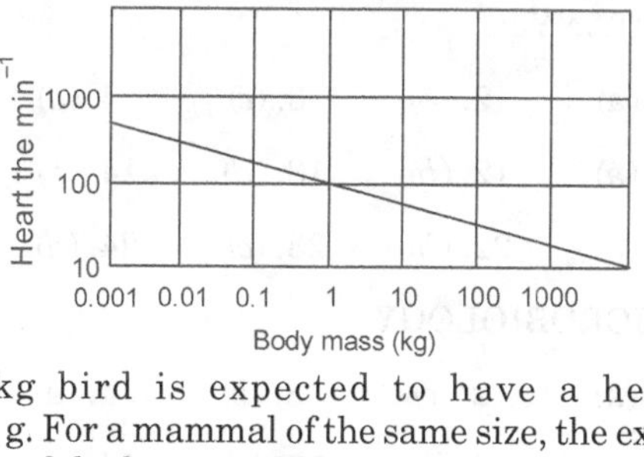

23. 1 kg bird is expected to have a heart of 8.2 g. For a mammal of the same size, the expected size of the heart could be
(*a*) 11.8 g (*b*) 5.9 g (*c*) 2.95 g (*d*) 23.6 g

24. An elephant that weighs 3000 kg has a resting pulse rate of 25 per minute. What would be the possible range of the pulse rate of 3 g shrew (the smallest living mammal)?
(*a*) 25 (*b*) 125 (*c*) 250 (*d*) Above 500

Linked Answer Questions: Q. 25 to Q. 28 carry two marks each

Statement for Linked Answer Questions 25 and 26:

An experiment was carried out to study the immune response to dust mite allergen in two strains of mice viz., BALB/c(b) and Nude (n). The mice were administered the immunogen on days 0 and 8 and allergen specific circulatory antibodies were monitored in the two groups of mice on days 7 and 18.

25. Which of the following class of antibodies would be detected in these strains of mice on day 7?
(*a*) IgM (*b*) IgM (*n*) (*b*) IgG (*b*) IgM (*n*)
(*c*) IgA (*b*) IgM (*n*) (*d*) IgE (*b*) IgM (*n*)

26. Which of the following class of antibodies would be detected in the two strains of mice on day 18?
(*a*) IgG (*b*) IgM (*n*) (*b*) IgE (*b*) IgE (*n*)
(*c*) IgE (*b*) IgE (*n*) (*d*) IgE (*b*) IgG (*n*)

Statement for Linked Answer Questions 27 and 28:

A woman has a rare abnormality of the eye that has been found to be dependent on a single dominant gene (P). The woman's father had abnormal eyes but mother had normal eyes.

27. If the woman marries a man with normal eyes, what proportion of the children will have abnormal eyes?
(*a*) 25% (*b*) 50%
(*c*) 75% (*d*) 100%

28. Which of the following representation does not explain the genotype of the woman's father?
(*a*) Heterozygous for P
(*b*) Homozygous for P
(*c*) Dominant for P
(*d*) Recessive for P

ANSWERS

H : CHEMISTRY

1. (*b*)	2. (*a*)	3. (*d*)	4. (*d*)	5. (*a*)	6. (*b*)	7. (*a*)	8. (*c*)	9. (*c*)	10. (*d*)
11. (*c*)	12. (*b*)	13. (*c*)	14. (*d*)	15. (*c*)	16. (*b*)	17. (*a*)	18. (*c*)	19. (*b*)	20. (*c*)
21. (*a*)	22. (*b*)	23. (*b*)	24. (*b*)	25. (*a*)	26. (*c*)	27. (*d*)	28. (*c*)		

I : BIOCHEMISTRY

1. (*a*)	2. (*c*)	3. (*a*)	4. (*b*)	5. (*a*)	6. (*b*)	7. (*b*)	8. (*d*)	9. (*b*)	10. (*b*)
11. (*a*)	12. (*d*)	13. (*c*)	14. (*c*)	15. (*c*)	16. (*b*)	17. (*c*)	18. (*a*)	19. (*d*)	20. (*a*)
21. (*c*)	22. (*c*)	23. (*c*)	24. (*b*)	25. (*c*)	26. (*c*)	27. (*b*)	28. (*a*)		

K : BOTANY

1. (*a*)	2. (*b*)	3. (*c*)	4. (*d*)	5. (*b*)	6. (*d*)	7. (*a*)	8. (*b*)	9. (*c*)	10. (*d*)
11. (*a*)	12. (*b*)	13. (*d*)	14. (*b*)	15. (*d*)	16. (*c*)	17. (*b*)	18. (*a*)	19. (*b*)	20. (*c*)
21. (*d*)	22. (*b*)	23. (*c*)	24. (*d*)	25. (*b*)	26. (*a*)	27. (*c*)	28. (*a*)		

L : MICROBIOLOGY

1. (*a*)	2. (*c*)	3. (*b*)	4. (*a*)	5. (*d*)	6. (*c*)	7. (*c*)	8. (*b*)	9. (*a*)	10. (*c*)
11. (*a*)	12. (*b*)	13. (*d*)	14. (*c*)	15. (*a*)	16. (*b*)	17. (*c*)	18. (*d*)	19. (*b*)	20. (*a*)
21. (*c*)	22. (*d*)	23. (*a*)	24. (*a*)	25. (*b*)	26. (*c*)	27. (*a*)	28. (*c*)		

M : ZOOLOGY

1. (*d*)	2. (*a*)	3. (*c*)	4. (*a*)	5. (*d*)	6. (*c*)	7. (*a*)	8. (*c*)	9. (*c*)	10. (*b*)
11. (*a*)	12. (*b*)	13. (*d*)	14. (*a*)	15. (*d*)	16. (*a*)	17. (*a*)	18. (*c*)	19. (*c*)	20. (*c*)
21. (*a*)	22. (*d*)	23. (*b*)	24. (*d*)	25. (*b*)	26. (*d*)	27. (*b*)	28. (*d*)		

EXPLANATIONS

H : CHEMISTRY

1. VSEPR stands for Valence Shell Electron Pair Repulsion Theory. VSPER theory is used to predict bent (or angular), linear, octahedral, see-saw, square planar, square pyramidal, tetrahedral, trigonal bipyramidal, trigonal planar, trigonal pyramidal, or T-shaped molecules.

   Steric number = SN

   = the number of bonds + the number of lone pairs.

   For N_2O= SN is 2. Therefore it is a linear molecule with an angle of 180°.

   N :: N :: O. Whereas SN for SO_2 is 3, for Cl_2O is 4 and for NO_2 is 3.

2. $[NiCl_4]^{2-}$ is tetrahedral because it has 4 bonds and no lone pairs of electrons, which means it has 4 regions of electron density.

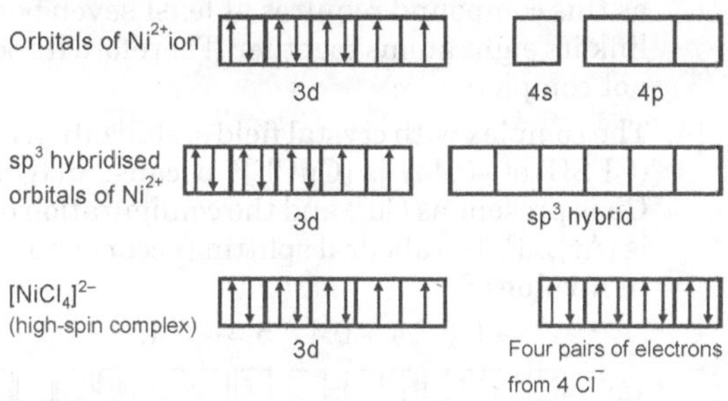

   $[PdCl_4]^{2-}$ has square planar geometry because it has 4 bonds and 2 lone pairs of electrons. Pd is one of those strange elements like S and P that has 6 regions of high electron density.

   $$Pd^{2+} = [Xe]\ 4d^8 5s^0.$$

3. Ionization energy is given by

   $$E_n = E_H * \frac{Z^2}{n^2}.$$

   Where Z = valence,

   E_H = ionization energy of Hydrogen,

   n = energy level.

   We have, E_H = 13.6 eV (given)

   For Li^{2+}, valence (Z) = 3, n =1 (as ground state)

   Therefore, ionization energy of Li^{2+} is:

   $$E_1 = 13.6 * \frac{(3)^2}{(1)^2} = 122.4 \text{ eV}$$

4. Half life of ^{14}C ($t_{1/2}$) is 5730 years.

   We know, $t_{1/2} = \frac{0.693}{k}$

   Where k is the rate constant for the first order reaction and half-life is inversely proportional to the rate constant k.

   Therefore, $k = \frac{0.693}{t_{1/2}}$ (Equation 1)

   Also we know,

   $$T = \frac{2.303}{k} \log \frac{a}{a-x} \quad \text{(Equation 2)}$$

   Where a = concentration at the start and $a-x$ = concentration after given time t.

   Here, a = 100% and $a - x$ = 25%.

   Putting k from equation 1 into equation 2, we get

   $$T = 2.303 * \frac{5730}{0.693} \log \frac{100}{25}$$

   $$= 2.303 * 5x730 * 2\log \frac{2}{0.693}$$

   = 11460 year.

5. The product 'P' formed in the following reaction is:

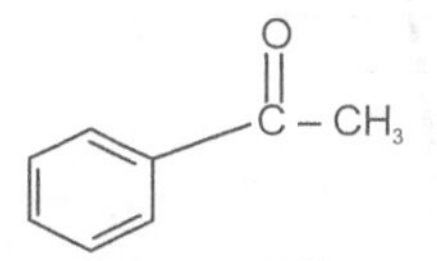

   The given reaction is as follows:

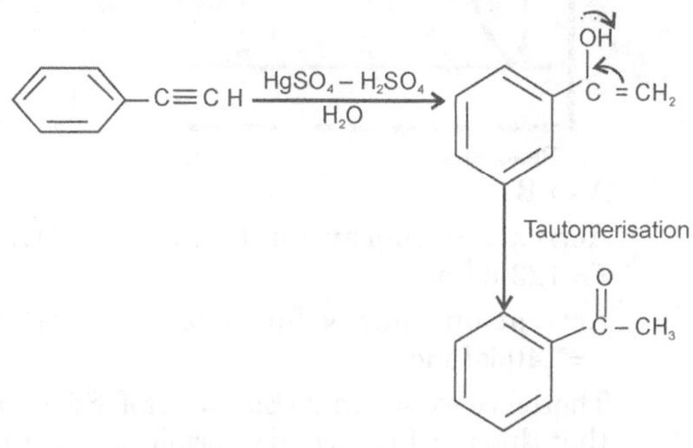

   {Product (P) }

6. The presence of alkyl group increases the crowding near carbonyl group and also increases the electron density at the carbonyl carbon by Inductive effect (+I effect). The size of the alkyl group is more than that of hydrogen. The alkyl groups are larger than a hydrogen atom and these cause hindrance to the attacking group. This is called steric hindrance. In CCl_3CHO, Cl is a withdrawing group thus more inductive.

   Therefore the order of reactivity is,

   IV> I> II> III,

   i.e. CCl_3CHO> HCHO> CH_3CHO> PhCHO.

7. The reaction is:

   $$_{92}U^{235} + {_0n^1} \rightarrow {_{36}Kr^{91}} + 3\,{_0n^1} + Y$$

   The unknown element is 'Y'.

   Mass number of all the elements in the reaction:

   U = 235, n = 1, Kr = 91

   Putting it in the reaction:

   $235 + 1 = 91 + 3 * 1 + Y^A$

   Therefore, $Y^A = 142$.

   Similarly atomic number of all the elements:

   U = 92, n = 0, Kr = 36

   Putting it in the reaction:

   $92 + 0 = 36 + 3 * 0 + {_ZY}$

   Therefore, $_ZY = 56$.

   So, the unknown element $_ZY^A$ is $_{56}Y^{142} = {_{56}Ba^{142}}$.

8. He_2 is not a stable molecule because the number of electrons on the non-bonding sigma orbitals is equal to the number of electrons on the bonding sigma orbital. Hence, the bond order is zero. It has a full octet $1s^2$ and it cannot combine with another He. Therefore in order to gain stability it has to loose its 1 electron (become He^{2+}) so as to combine with another He and gain a conformation of $1s^1$. So, He^{2+} is a stable molecule and not He_2.

9.

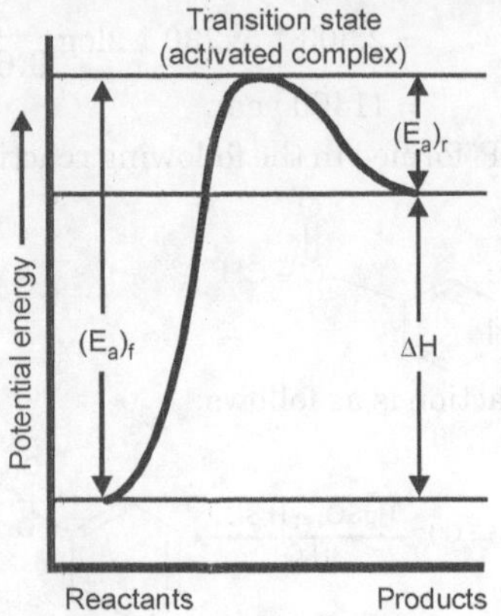

$A \leftrightarrow B$

Activation energy for forward reaction (Ea) f = 123 kJ/mol

Activation energy for reverse reaction (Ea) r = 140 kJ/mol

Therefore we see that (Ea)r > (Ea)f. So, we can say that this reaction is endothermic in nature.

So, we know:

$$E_r = E_f + \Delta H$$

$$\Delta H = 140 - 123 = +17 \text{ kJ/mol}$$

Therefore the enthalpy change for forward reaction is 17 kJ/mol.

10. Acid dissociation constant (pKa) = 10^{-5}

Concentration of solution of weak acid HA [HA] = 0.20M or 0.20N

Concentration of MA_2 salt = 0.10M or 0.20N (As N= nM)

We know,

$$pH = pKa + \log \frac{[salt]}{[Acid]}$$

$$\Rightarrow \quad = -\log Ka + \log \frac{[salt]}{[Acid]}$$

$$= -\log 10^{-5} + \log \frac{0.20}{0.20}$$

We know, $-\log 10^{-5} = 5$

So, $= 5 + 0 = 5$ (as log 1= 0)

Therefore pH of the solution is 5.0

11. The attractive part of van der Waals' interaction is governed by induced dipole- induced dipole interaction. A dipole-induced dipole attraction is a weak attraction that results when a polar molecule induces a dipole in an atom or in a non polar molecule by disturbing the arrangement of electrons in the non polar species.

12. $H_2(g) + \frac{1}{2} O_2(g) \rightarrow H_2O$ (l).

Given,

Standard free energy change (ΔG°)

$= -237.13$ kJ/mol.

T = 298K, 1F = 96500 C.

We know,

$$\Delta G^\circ = -nFE^\circ_{cell}$$

$$E^\circ_{cell} = -\frac{\Delta G^\circ}{nF}$$

Given, n = 2

$$\text{So,} \quad = -\frac{(-237.13 * 10^3 \text{ J})}{2} * 96500)$$

$= 1.228$V.

Therefore, the standard cell potential is 1.228V.

13. The electron deficient molecule is Diborane (B_2H_6) as this compound requires at least seven bonds to link its eight atoms together. Therefore its octet is not complete.

14. The complex with crystal field stabilization energy (CFSE) of $-0.4\ \Delta_t$ is $[CuCl_4]^{2-}$ because in $[CuCl_4]^{2-}$ Cu is present as Cu^{2+} and the configuration of Cu^{2+} is [Ar] $3d^9$. Tetrahedral splitting occurs and results in Δ_t value of:

$$-0.6 * 4 + 0.4 * 5 = -0.4.$$

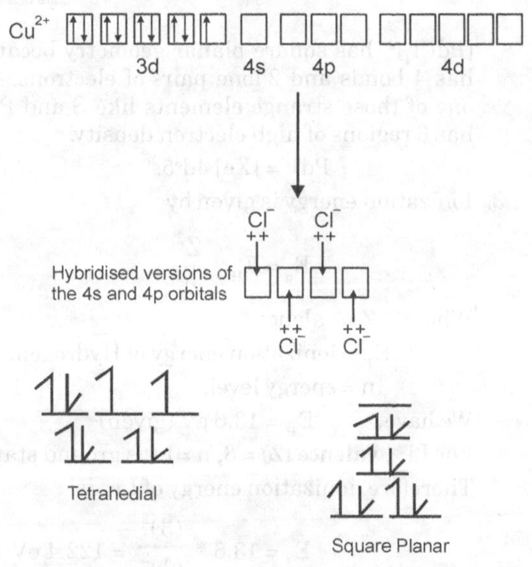

15.

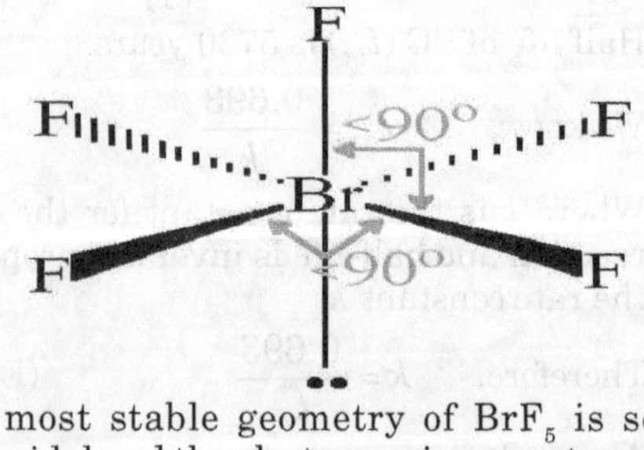

The most stable geometry of BrF_5 is square pyramidal and the electron pair geometry around the central atom is octahedral. In the above picture, 5 bp and 1 lp of electron is present in BrF_5 which makes the molecule stable.

16. The species having 3 unpaired electrons and a tetrahedral geometry is $[CoCl_4]^{2-}$. The coordination number of $[CoCl_4]^{2-}$ is equal to 4; thus, the structure of $[CoCl_4]^{2-}$ is tetrahedral.

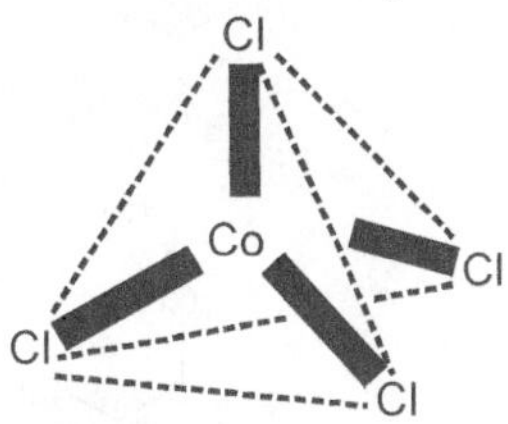

Also, in $[CoCl_4]^{2-}$ Co exists as Co^{2+}. Configuration of Co^{2+} is [Ar] $3d^7$. Therefore 3 unpaired electrons are present in the d orbital. Also as Cl^- is a weak field ligand, so it does not cause pairing.

Whereas in $[Co(CN)_6]^{4-}$ CN is a strong field ligand, which causes pairing, leaving only one unpaired electron. While in $[NiCl_4]^{2-}$ and $[Ni(CN)_4]^{2-}$ there are only 2 unpaired electrons.

17. We know that bond strength is directly proportional to average bond energy. The covalent radius of Aluminium is the least followed by Gallium and then Indium. Also, based upon their position in the Group their ionic radius and associated lattice parameters follows the trend:

Al>Ga>In>Ti

18. The olefins which leads to a racemic mixture of the diol product upon cis- dihydroxylation is:

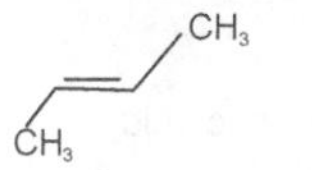

The entire reaction is given as follows:

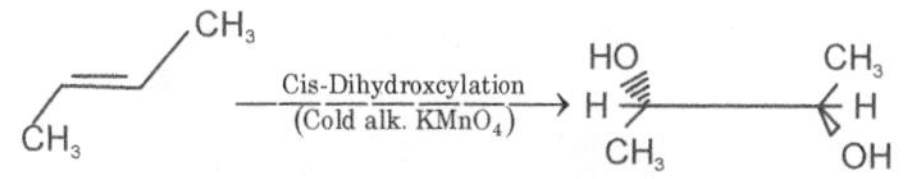

Thus, when 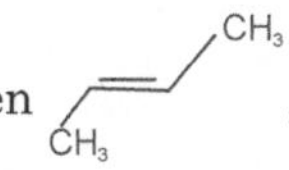 , undergoes cis racemic mixture dihydroxylation, in the presence of Alkaline $KMnO_4$, then it forms a racemic mixture which is of both d and l form.

While the rest of the compounds like

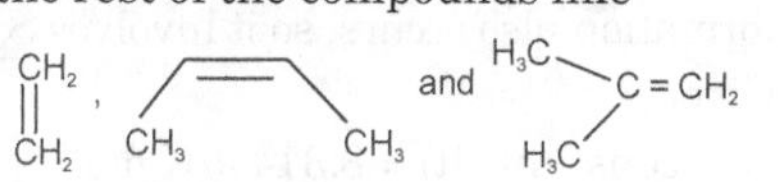

give an optically inactive product.

19. Reaction of 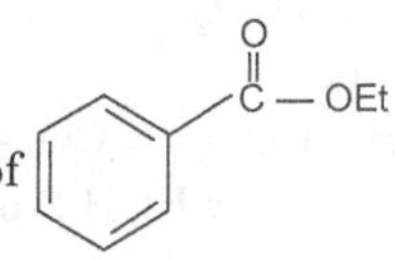 in the presence of H^+ ions, heat and excess of MeMgBr gives a product 'Q'.

The reaction is as follows:

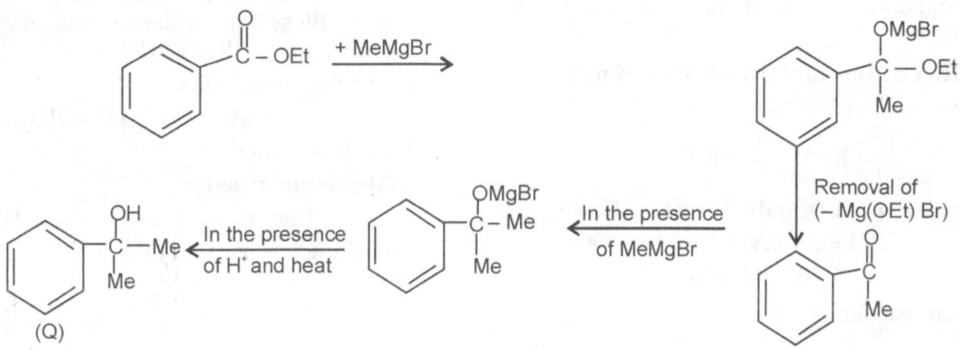

Thus, the product 'Q' formed is:

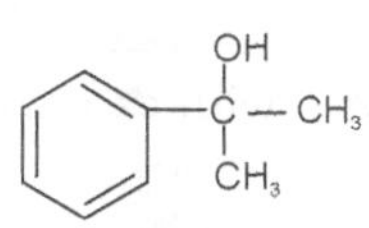

20.

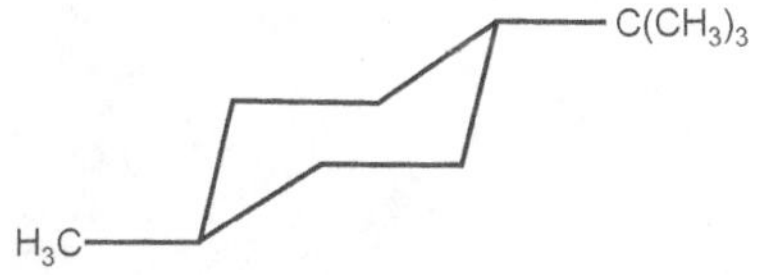

The above conformation is the most stable conformation of cis-1-tert-butyl-4-methylcyclohexane because the largest substituent -t-Butyl is in the equatorial position. However the others are less stable because of axial position of t-Butyl group.

21. When 1-chloro benzoic acid is reacted in the presence of $HNO_3 - H_2SO_4$, then an NO_2 – group is added at its ortho position. This NO_2group is then replaced by an NH_2 group in the presence of Sn-HCl. Finally the NH_2 group is replaced by an OH group in the presence of H_2O. Thus, the compound R formed is 1-chloro, 2-Hydroxybenzoic acid.

Reaction Mechanism:

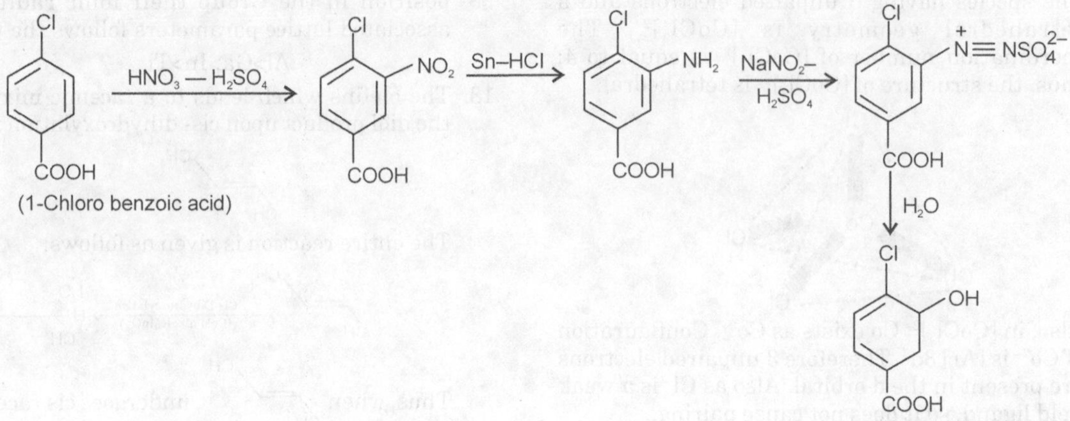

1-Chloro, 2-Hydroxybenzoic acid (Product R).

22. As the product produced is sterically inverted (racemized) and in this reaction an intermediate bond formation also occurs, so it involves S_N2 pathway.

23. Given,

Gas constant (R) = 8.314 J/K mol

Temperature = 500K

Therefore, we know $\Delta G° = -2.303\ RT \log K$

(Where K = equilibrium constant

= 1.41 at T = 500K)

$= -2.303 * 8.314 * 500 \log 1.41$

$= -1.43$ KJ/ mol.

24. Given, Standard enthalpy change ($\Delta H°$) is constant.

$T_1 = 400K$,

$T_2 = 500K$, Gas constant (R) = 8.314 J/K mol

Therefore, we know

$$\log \frac{K_2}{K_1} = \frac{\Delta H}{2.303} * R\left(T_2 - \frac{T_1}{T_2} * T_2\right)$$

Putting all the values and solving for ΔH, we get,

$\Delta H = 2 * 8.314 * 2.303 * 2000$

$= 76.6$ KJ/ mol.

25. When a solid compound X produces a new solid P and a gas Q on heating and also the gas Q is absorbed by KOH, then the gas Q is CO_2.

By the following reaction,

$$CaCO_3 \rightarrow CaO + CO_2$$

Thus here the solid compound $CaCO_3$ produces a solid CaO and a gas CO_2.

In the next reaction,

$$2KOH + CO_2 \rightarrow K_2CO_3 + H_2O.$$

Here, CO_2 is absorbed by KOH producing, $K_2CO_3 + H_2O$.

26. When CaO and water react, they form bleaching powder. Bleaching powder on reaction with Cl_2 gives a compound X called $CaCO_3$.

In the first reaction,

$$CaO + H_2O \rightarrow Ca(OH)_2$$

Lime is obtained.

In the second reaction,

$$Ca(OH)_2 + Cl_2 \rightarrow CaOCl_2 + H_2O$$

Bleaching powder is obtained.

27. The given reaction is

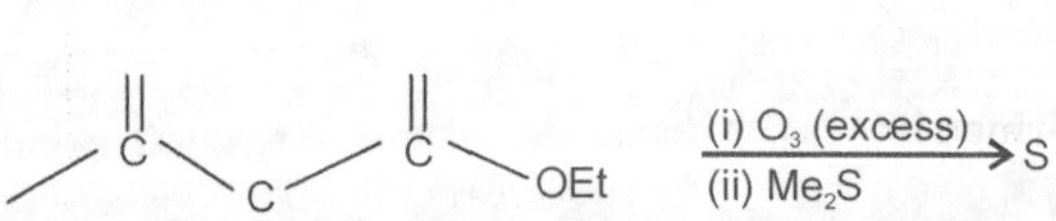

∴ When the above compound is first treated with excess of O_3 and then with Me_2S, then a product 'S' is formed. The structure of 'S' is:

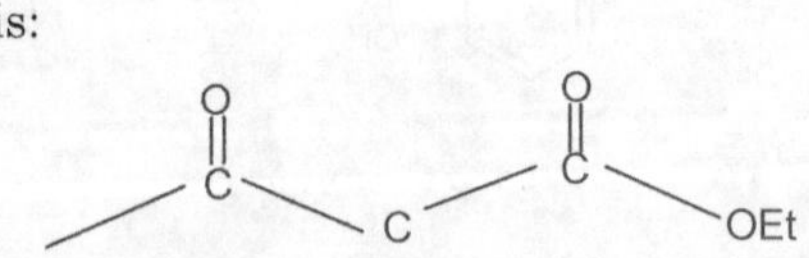

Thus, the product 'S' is known as β-keto ester.

The entire reaction that takes place is as follows:

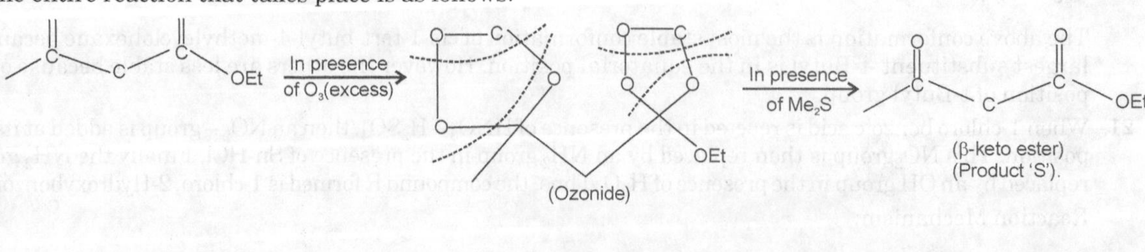

28. In the above reaction, beta- keto ester is obtained. Therefore the reaction should be Claisen condensation. As Claisen condensation is a carbon–carbon bond forming reaction that occurs between two esters or one ester and another carbonyl compound in the presence of a strong base, resulting in a β-keto ester.

I : BIOCHEMISTRY

1. Spontaneous deamination converts cytosine to uracil, which is excised from DNA by the enzyme uracil-DNA glycosylase, leading to error-free repair. 5-Methylcytosine residues are deaminated to thymine, which cannot be excised and repaired by this system. As a result, 5-methylcytosine residues are hotspots for spontaneous transitions, as demonstrated in the lacI gene of *Escherichia coli*. Deamination of cytosine to uracil can occur *in vivo* at the level of nucleotide, in RNA and in DNA. Thus, enzyme-catalyzed deamination of cytidylate to uridylate and of dCTP to dUTP plays a key role in nucleotide metabolism, underpinning the pathway of *de novo* thymidylate synthesis.
2. The behaviour of a cell often relies on the chemical signals it is exposed to in its environment. In general, two types of chemical signals can be found floating through the cellular environment: water-soluble (hydrophilic) molecules or fat-soluble (hydrophobic) molecules. Both are important components of cellular communication and physically interact with cellular structures to facilitate this function. In virtually every case, the cellular structures that these chemical signals interact with are receptor proteins. Insulin is an anabolic hormone, causing cells to take up energy substrates at times of excess. Insulin action is countered by the catabolic hormones glucagon, adrenalin and noradrenalin, and growth hormone. These act primarily through cyclic AMP (cAMP) and protein kinase A. Insulin inhibits breakdown of triglycerides in adipose tissue and gluconeogenesis in the liver. A whole series of intracellular signal substances seemed to be responsible for the many actions of insulin. Insulin's regulation of hepatic metabolism is a major element in control of blood glucose levels. Inappropriate gluconeogenesis in postprandial periods is a key to the hyperglycaemia seen in type 2 diabetes.
3. Systemic lupus erythematosus (SLE) is an autoimmune disease, which means the body's immune system mistakenly attacks healthy tissue. This leads to long-term (chronic) inflammation. Antinuclear antibodies are most characteristic and present in more than 95% of patients. Anti-double stranded DNA (ds-DNA) and anti-Sm antibodies are unique to patients with SLE. Anti-DNA antibodies differ in their properties, including isotype, ability to fix complement, and capacity to bind to the glomeruli causing pathogenicity. SLE is characterised by a myriad of immune system aberrations that involve B cells, T cells, and cells of the monocytic lineage, resulting in polyclonal B cell activation, increased numbers of antibody producing cells, hypergammaglobulinaemia, autoantibody production, and immune complex formation.
4. Optical density is the absorbance of an optical element for a given wavelength λ per unit distance. Optical density is the measure of the transmission of an optical medium for a given wavelength. Higher OD lower transmittance and vice versa e.g., optical density of 1 means 90% of incident light is absorbed and the remaining 10% is transmitted. The optical density is represented in terms of transmittance. It is given by Beer-Lambert Law of Absorbance.
5. Glycolysis begins with phosphorylation of a monosaccharide (generally glucose) on the sixth carbon by a hexokinase, and ends with the production of pyruvate. Pyruvate may be converted to ethanol, lactate, or other small molecules, or fed into the TCA cycle. The reaction is :–

   Pyruvate + CoA + NAD$^+$ → acetyl CoA + CO_2 + NADH

   This irreversible reaction is the link between glycolysis and the citric acid cycle. In the preparation of the glucose derivative pyruvate for the citric acid cycle, an oxidative decarboxylation takes place and high-transfer-potential electrons in the form of NADH are captured. The carbon thus released during CO_2 emission is a C3 carbon, because in glycolysis, the glucose molecule (fructose-1, 6-biphosphate) undergoes a 3 carbon fragmentation into dihydroacetone phosphate and glyceraldehyde-3-phosphate.
6. A northern blot is a laboratory method used to detect specific RNA molecules among a mixture of RNA. Northern blotting can be used to analyze a sample of RNA from a particular tissue or cell type in order to measure the RNA expression of particular genes. When yeast cells underwent a change of medium, it resulted in an increase in the number of genes. Thus, the gene number and expression analysis can be performed using northern blotting. The first step in a northern blot is to denature, or separate, the RNA within the sample into single strands, which ensures that the strands are unfolded and that there is no bonding between strands. The RNA molecules are then separated according to their sizes using a method called gel electrophoresis. Following separation, the RNA is transferred from the gel onto a blotting membrane. Once the transfer is complete, the blotting membrane carries all of the RNA bands originally on the gel. Next, the membrane is treated with a small piece of DNA or RNA called a probe, which has been designed to have a sequence that is complementary to a particular RNA sequence in the sample. Thus, following hybridization, the probe permits the RNA molecule of interest to be detected from among the many different RNA molecules on the membrane.

7. Gel filtration (GF) chromatography separates proteins solely on the basis of molecular size. Separation is achieved using a porous matrix to which the molecules, for steric reasons, have different degrees of access--i.e., smaller molecules have greater access and larger molecules are excluded from the matrix. Hence, proteins are eluted from the GF column in decreasing order of size. Given, five proteins having molecular weights of Protein 1 = 5000 kDa, Protein 2 = 10,000 kDa, Protein 3 = 25,000 kDa, Protein 4 = 65,000 and Protein 5 = 100,000 kDa. Order of elution from the Sephadex G-50 column will be: Protein 5, 4, 3, 2 and 1 based on the decreasing molecular weights.

8. Liquid water is exceptional in having approximately as many hydrogen bonds as it has covalent bonds. In water's hydrogen bonds, the hydrogen atom is covalently attached to the oxygen of a water molecule. Hydrogen bonds within heavy water are stronger. Water's hydrogen bonding holds water molecules up to about 15% closer than if water was a simple liquid with just van der Waals interactions. However, as hydrogen bonding is directional it restricts the number of neighbouring water molecules to about four rather than the larger number found in simple liquids. The hydrogen bond in water is part (about 90%) electrostatic and part (about 10%) covalent and may be approximated by bonds made up of covalent HO-H · · · · OH_2, ionic $HO^{\delta-}$-$H^{\delta+}$· · · · $O^{\delta-}H_2$, and long-bonded covalent HO-· · H--O+H_2 parts with HO-H· · · · OH_2 being very much more in evidence than HO-· · H--O+H_2, where there would be expected to be much extra non-bonded repulsion. In general, a single molecule of water can form 4 hydrogen bonds with four other water molecules.

9. PCR is based on using the ability of DNA polymerase to synthesize new strand of DNA complementary to the offered template strand. Because DNA polymerase can add a nucleotide only onto a pre-existing 3'-OH group, it needs a primer to which it can add the first nucleotide. For isolation of mouse homologue of a yeast gene, we need to undergo PCR for the yeast gene with the mouse homologue and observe for amplification. A DNA microarray (also commonly known as gene chip, DNA chip, or biochip) is a collection of microscopic DNA spots attached to a solid surface. Studying which genes are active and which are inactive in different cell types helps scientists to understand both how these cells function normally and how they are affected when various genes do not perform properly. DNA microarrays are created by robotic machines that arrange minuscule amounts of hundreds or thousands of gene sequences on a single microscope slide. Thus, comparison and analysis of the gene expression between a normal and a cancer cell can be achieved using microarray expression analysis. The ELISA is a fundamental tool of clinical immunology, and is used as an initial screen for HIV detection. Based on the principle of antibody-antibody interaction, this test allows for easy visualization of results and can be completed without the additional concern of radioactive materials use.

10. A suppressor is a second mutation that restores a function lost by the primary mutation. A suppressor mutation that occurs within the same gene is called an "intragenic suppressor", and a suppressor mutation that occurs in a different gene is called an "intergenic suppressor". A suppressor maps at a different site than the mutation it counteracts, either within the same gene or at a more distant locus. Different suppressors act in different ways :

(1) mutation in the same gene that restores the enzyme function.

(2) Mutation in another gene that restores the wild type phenotype.

(3) Bypass suppressor that turns on a new pathway.

(4) Informational suppressor such as tRNA genes.

(5) overproduction/down regulation.

(6) Physiological suppressor.

In the given case of protein X, when the slow growing mutated strain was treated with extragenic suppressors led to a new strain with normal protein X, the suppressor should have revived the slow growing strain of the protein encoding gene X. That means the extragenic suppressor provided was an RNA polymerase which resulted in transcription of the protein X gene leading to the full-length protein X synthesis.

11. We know, Total radioactivity of a substance,

$$A = -dN/dt = \lambda \times N$$

Where, λ = decay constant,

N = amount of the substance,

t = time of decay.

Given, A = 1 mCi,

Amount of substance = 0.25 mg

Molecular weight of Glycine]

= NH_2–CH_2–COOH

= (1×14N+5×1H+12×2C+16×2O)

= 75 g/mol

Amount of glycine in millimoles,

N/N_0 = Amount of the substance/ Molecular weight of the substance

= (0.25 mg)/ (75 g/mol)

= (0.25 mg)/ (75 mg/millimole)

= 0.0033 millimoles where,

N_0 = initial amount of the substance

Therefore, decay constant

$$\lambda = A/N = 1/N$$

We have, Specific activity,

$$S_A = \lambda N_0 = (1/N) \times N_0$$
$$= N_0/N$$
$$= 1/(N/N_0) = 1/0.0033$$
$$= 300.003 \text{ mCi/millimole}$$

Therefore, the required specific activity is 300 mCi/ millimole (approx.)

12. We know, according to Lambert-Beer's law,

Absorbance of any substance, A = $\varepsilon \times C \times l$ where ε = molar extinction coefficient of a substance, C = molar concentration of the substance and l = path length of the light to travel.

Given, A = 0.53 at 328 nm, ε for Vitamin-A ($\varepsilon_{1\%}$) = 1550 per 100 mL, l = 1 cm

Therefore, $A = \varepsilon \times C \times l$

$\Rightarrow C = A/(\varepsilon \times l)$

$\Rightarrow C = 0.53/(1550 \times 1)$

$\Rightarrow C = 0.0003419$

$\Rightarrow C = 3.149 \times 10^{-4}$

The amount of Vitamin-A in the non-saponifiable fraction is 3.149 $\times 10^{-4}$ g/ 100mL.

13. The fidelity and progression of DNA synthesis is critically dependent on the correct balance and availability of the deoxynucleoside triphosphate (dNTP) precursors for the polymerases involved in DNA replication and repair. The enzyme DNA polymerase, which uses deoxynucleotide triphosphate as substrates, makes DNA. To ensure enough precursors for DNA synthesis, two reactions must occur. First, the 2′ position of the ribose ring of ribonucleotides must be reduced from a C-OH to a C-H before the nucleotides can be used for DNA synthesis. Secondly, the thymine ring must be made by addition of a methyl group to uridine. Synthesis of adenylate, guanylate and thymidylate deoxynucleotides require one carbon from folic acid coenzyme for the synthesis of the amino group of the nucleotides followed by the closure of the ring.

14. In the inner mitochondrial membrane, complex I or Nicotinamide adenine dinucleotide (NADH) produced by glycolysis is oxidized (removes electrons) by the enzyme NADH dehydrogenase. The enzyme removes two electrons from NADH and attaches them to an electron carrier, ubiquinone. The transfer of these electrons reduces (adds electrons) ubiquinone into ubiquinol. Complex II (succinate dehydrogenase) is not a proton pump. It serves to funnel additional electrons into the quinone pool (Q) by removing electrons from succinate and transferring them (via FAD) to Q. Complex III (cytochrome bc1 complex) removes in a stepwise fashion two electrons from QH2 at the QO site and sequentially transfers them to two molecules of cytochrome c, a water-soluble electron carrier located within the inter membrane space. The two other electrons are sequentially passed across the protein to the Q_i site where quinone part of ubiquinone is reduced to quinol. Complex IV (cytochrome c oxidase) removes four electrons from four molecules of cytochrome c and transfers them to molecular oxygen (O_2), producing two molecules of water (H_2O). At the same time, it moves four protons across the membrane, producing a proton gradient. In the process, two ubiquinols are oxidized and one ubiquinone is reduced.

15. The involvement of endogenous diacylglycerol production in the stimulation of phosphatidylcholine synthesis was done by exogenous phospholipase C. Phospholipase C treatment of intact cells stimulated CTP : phosphocholine cytidylyltransferase activity significantly more effectively than did maximally effective concentrations of the synthetic diacylglycerol sn-1,2-dioctanoylglycerol. When added to cells together with phospholipase C, oleic acid, but not dioctanoylglycerol, further increased cytidylyltransferase activity with respect to phospholipase C treatment alone, indicating that the enzyme was not maximally activated by the lipase. Cyclic AMP-regulated gene expression frequently involves a DNA element known as the cAMP-regulated enhancer (CRE). Many transcription factors bind to this element, including the protein CREB which is activated as a result of phosphorylation by protein kinase A. This modification stimulates interaction with one or more of the general transcription factors or, alternatively, allows recruitment of a co-activator. The Ras-like GTPases regulate diverse cellular functions via the chemical cycle of binding and hydrolyzing GTP molecules. They alternate between GTP- and GDP-bound conformations. The GTP-bound conformation is biologically active and promotes a cellular function, such as signal transduction, cytoskeleton organization, protein synthesis/ translocation, or a membrane budding/fusion event. GTP hydrolysis turns off the GTPase switch by converting it to the inactive GDP-bound conformation.

16. When carbon dioxide diffuses into the blood plasma and then into the red blood cells (erythrocytes) in the presence of the catalyst carbonic anhydrase most CO_2 reacts with water in the erythrocytes and the following dynamic equilibrium is established.

$$H_2O + CO_2 \rightarrow H_2CO_3$$

Carbonic acid, H_2CO_3, dissociates to form hydrogen ions and hydrogen-carbonate ions. This is also a reversible reaction and undissociated carbonic acid, hydrogen ions and hydrogen-carbonate ions exist in dynamic equilibrium with one another.

$$H_2CO_3 \rightarrow H^+ + HCO^{3-}$$

Inside the erythrocytes negatively charged HCO3- ions diffuse from the cytoplasm to the plasma. This is balanced by diffusion of chloride ions, Cl-, in the opposite direction, maintaining the balance of negative and positive ions either side. This is called the 'chloride shift'. The dissociation of carbonic acid increases the acidity of the blood (decreases its pH). Hydrogen ions, H^+, then react with oxyhaemoglobin to release bound oxygen and reduce the acidity of the blood. This buffering action allows large quantities of carbonic acid to be carried in the blood without major changes in blood pH.

$$Hb.4O_2 + H^+ \rightarrow HHb^+ + 4O_2$$

From tissues, CO_2 generated is carried back to the lungs by the formation of C-terminal carbamates.

17. Glycogen synthase (GS) is the enzyme responsible for the synthesis of 1, 4-linked glucose chains in glycogen. It is the rate limiting enzyme in the synthesis of the polysaccharide, and its activity is highly regulated through phosphorylation at multiple sites and also by allosteric effectors, mainly glucose 6-phosphate (G6P). Liver glycogen is used to buffer the overall blood glucose level; glycogen is synthesized when blood glucose is high, and glycogen is degraded (with the resulting glucose released into the blood stream) when blood glucose is low. Glycogen synthase works efficiently only when it is bound to glycogenin. When blood glucose is low, glycogen is reconverted to glucose in the liver. Glycogen phosphorylase catalyzes the cleavage of terminal glycogen residues by inorganic phosphate. Glycogen phosphorylase requires a covalently bound pyridoxal phosphate cofactor (vitamin B6). Thus, the supernatant obtained after centrifugation of liver will show enzymatic activity of gylcogen synthase.

18. The mitochondrial electron transport chain consists of a series of metallo-proteins bound to the inner membrane of the mitochondria. The metal centres and other cofactors in these proteins act, in essence, as a molecular wire, carrying electrons from the strongly reducing products of the citric acid cycle (NADH, succinate) to highly oxidizing di-oxygen. There are four large proteins associated with mitochondrial electron transport, usually called (strangely enough) Complexes I through IV. The electrons are passed through a series of metal clusters and cofactors, including flavins, iron-sulphur clusters, cytochrome, and copper centres. These groups are embedded in large membrane-bound proteins, and the passage of electrons through them is coupled to the transport of protons across the membrane, from the interior matrix space of the mitochondria to the intermembrane space.

19. Proteins have developed different ways to bind other molecules. Zinc-binding repeats, known as zinc fingers (ZnF), are one such molecular scaffold. ZnF motifs can coordinate one or more zinc atoms. They display considerable versatility in binding modes, even between members of the same class (e.g. some bind DNA, others protein), suggesting that ZnF motifs are stable scaffolds that have evolved specialised functions. Glucocorticoid receptor has ZnF motifs present in it. The basic-leucine zipper (bZIP) domain transcription factors of eukaryotes are proteins that contain a basic region mediating sequence-specific DNA-binding followed by a leucine zipper region required for dimerization. The basic leucine zipper domain of c-Jun, which allows for DNA binding and homo-dimerization, is necessary and sufficient for interaction with TATA-binding protein-associated factor-1 (hsTAF1). Helix-turn-helix (HTH) motifs are found in all known DNA binding proteins that regulate gene expression. The motif consists of approximately 20 residues and is characterised by 2 alpha-helices, which make intimate contacts with the DNA and are joined by a short turn. The HTH motif is very similar in sequence and structure to the N-terminal region of the lambda and other repressor proteins, and has also been identified in many other DNA-binding proteins on the basis of sequence and structural similarity.

20. DNA polymerase I (pol I) processes RNA primers during lagging-strand synthesis and fills small gaps during DNA repair reactions. DNA polymerase I is a DNA-dependent DNA polymerase with inherent $3' \rightarrow 5'$ and $5' \rightarrow 3'$ exonuclease activities. The $5' \rightarrow 3'$ exonuclease activity removes nucleotides ahead of the growing DNA chain, allowing nick-translation. DNA Polymerase I is a template-dependent DNA polymerase and catalyzes $5' \rightarrow 3'$ synthesis of DNA. The enzyme also exhibits $3' \rightarrow 5'$ exonuclease proofreading activity, $5' \rightarrow 3$ exonuclease activity and ribonuclease H activity. Thus it undergoes the *de novo* synthesis of a new DNA strand.

21. Mitochondrial F_1-ATPase is an oligomeric enzyme composed of five distinct subunit polypeptides. The alpha and beta subunits make up the bulk of protein mass of F_1. This represents a group of ATPase F_1F_0-assembly proteins, including ATP_{12} and $ATPAF_2$ (ATP synthase mitochondrial F_1 complex assembly factor 2). These proteins are essential for the assembly of the mitochondrial F_1-F_0 complex. F-ATPases (F_1F_0-ATPases) are found in mitochondria, chloroplasts and bacterial plasma membranes where they are the prime producers of ATP, using the proton gradient generated by oxidative phosphorylation (mitochondria) or photosynthesis (chloroplasts). The thylakoid membrane of chloroplast contains an ATP synthase called the F0F1 complex. Because the thylakoid membrane forms a barrier against proton diffusion, they can only move through the pore of the F_0F_1 complex. The F_0F_1 complex uses the energy released by the protons moving through the pore to add a high-energy phosphate ion (Pi^+) to ADP resulting in ATP formation. For every 4 protons transported through the F_0F_1 complex, one molecule of ATP is created. This process of using the proton gradient to fuel an energy requiring process is known as chemiosmosis.

22. Anti-hapten antibodies are in wide use. For example, anti-BrdU and anti-digoxigen IgGs are common anti-hapten reagents. Hapten immunochemistry forms the basis of a massive clinical, forensic and environmental testing industry. Targeting free aromatic and aliphatic amines to probe cellular expression patterns has also become standard in neurobiology. Few molecules are resistant to hapten detection methods. Even exotic polymeric targets such as C_{60} fullerenes, targets as nonpolar as cholesterol, or as large as vitamin B_{12} have been haptenized. All biologically relevant small molecules are potential haptens. The hapten specific antibodies can be generated through immunization of the mice by injecting the hapten into the mice being bound to a particular protein specific to mice.

23. NADH is oxidized by a series of catalytic redox carriers that are integral proteins of the inner mitochondrial membrane. The free energy change in several of these steps is very exergonic. The redistribution of protons leads to formation of a proton gradient across the mitochondrial membrane. The size of the gradient is proportional to the free energy change of the electron transfer reactions. The result of these reactions is that the redox energy of NADH is converted to the energy of the proton gradient. In the presence of ADP, protons flow down their thermodynamic gradient from outside the mitochondrion back into the mitochondrial matrix. This process is facilitated by a proton carrier in the inner mitochondrial membrane known as ATP synthase. As its name implies, this carrier is coupled to ATP synthesis. The free energy available as a consequence of transferring 2 electrons from NADH or succinate to molecular oxygen is -57 and -36 kcal/mol, respectively. For each pair of electrons originating from NADH, 3 equivalents of ATP are synthesized, requiring 22.4 kcal of energy. Thus, with 31.2 kcal of available energy, it is clear that the proton gradient generated by electron transport contains sufficient energy to drive normal ATP synthesis.

24. The glycerol phosphate shuttle is coupled to an inner mitochondrial membrane, FAD-linked dehydrogenase, of low energy potential like that found in Complex II. Thus, cytosolic NADH oxidized by this pathway can generate only 2 equivalents of ATP. The shuttle involves two different glycerol-3-phosphate dehydrog-enases: one is cytosolic, acting to produce glycerol-3-phosphate, and one is an integral protein of the inner mitochondrial membrane that acts to oxidize the glycerol-3-phosphate produced by the cytosolic enzyme. The net result of the process is that reducing equivalents from cytosolic NADH are transferred to the mitochondrial electron transport system.

25. Epidermal growth factor receptor (EGFR) is a cell surface protein that binds to epidermal growth factor (EGF). Binding of the protein to a ligand induces receptor dimerization and tyrosine auto-phosphorylation and leads to cell proliferation. Mutations in this gene are associated with lung cancer. EGF (Epidermal Growth Factor) is a small 53 amino acid residue protein that is involved in normal cell growth, oncogenesis, and wound healing. This protein shows both strong sequential and functional homology with hTGF-Alpha (human type-Alpha Transforming Growth Factor), which is a competitor for EGF receptor sites. EGF binds to a specific high-affinity, low-capacity receptor on the surface of responsive cells known as EGFR (Epidermal growth factor receptor). EGF-dependent tyrosine phosphorylations are present in cells having EGFR at the membranes of the cells. Since EGFR is present on the surface of both cell line A and B, therefore, the EGF-dependent tyrosine phosphorylation will be detected in membranes of both the cell lines.

26. The epidermal growth factor (EGF) receptor is a transmembrane tyrosine kinase that belongs to the HER/ErbB protein family. Ligand binding results in receptor dimerization, auto-phosphorylation, activation of downstream signalling, internalization, and lysosomal degradation. Phosphorylation of EGFR at specific serine and threonine residues attenuates EGFR kinase activity. Binding of the GRB2 and SOS complex to the EGFR places SOS in proximity to Ras, thus leading to GTP-loading of Ras and subsequent activation of Ras effectors, such as Raf kinases and PI3K (Phosphatidylinositol 3-Kinase). Therefore, EGF-dependent serine phosphorylation will be detected only on the membrane of cell line B because it had a couple of EGFR and Ras.

27. Given, the reaction is :

$A + B \Leftrightarrow C + H^+$ at a pH of 5, ΔG is the free energy change for the reaction at equilibrium.

The initial concentrations of the reactants and products are :

$$[A] = [B] = [C] = 1\text{ M}$$

and $[H^+] = \text{pH } 5 = 10^{-5}$ M.

The equilibrium constant for the reaction,

$$K_{eq} = \{[C] \times [H^+]\}/\{[A] \times [B]\}$$
$$= \{1 \times 10^{-5}\}/\{1 \times 1\} = 10^{-5}$$

Now, we have ΔG for the reaction :

$$\Delta G = \Delta G° + RT \ln (Q_r),$$

where Q_r = reaction quotient

At equilibrium, $\Delta G = 0$,

therefore, $\Delta G° = - RT \ln (K_{eq})$

since, $K_{eq} = Q_r$

$\Rightarrow \quad \Delta G° = - RT \times 2.303 \log (K_{eq})$

$\Rightarrow \quad \Delta G° = - 2.303\ RT \log (10^{-5})$

$\Rightarrow \quad \Delta G° = + 5 \times 2.303\ RT$

$\Rightarrow \quad \Delta G° = 11.515\ RT$

Under standard conditions, the Gibb's free energy change for the reaction is:

$$\Delta G = \Delta G° + \Delta G°'$$

where $\Delta G°'$

= standard Gibb's free energy change

$\Rightarrow \quad \Delta G = \Delta G°' + 11.515\ RT$

28. Given,

$$\Delta G°' = - 11.7\text{ kJ/ mol},$$
$$R = 8.314\text{ kJ/ mol.}$$

At $\quad T = 37°C$

$= (273 + 37)\text{ K} = 310\text{ K},$

$\Rightarrow \quad \Delta G = \Delta G°' + 11.515\ RT$

$\Rightarrow \quad \Delta G = - 11.7 + 11.515 \times 8.314 \times 310$

$\Rightarrow \quad \Delta G = 29,666.37$ kJ/mol

At $\quad T = 25°C$

$= (273 + 25)\text{ K} = 298\text{ K},$

$\Rightarrow \quad \Delta G = -11.7 + 11.515 \times 8.314 \times 298$

$\Rightarrow \quad \Delta G = 28,529.24$ kJ/mol

Since, ΔG is positive in both the cases, therefore, the reaction is endergonic at temperatures of 37°C and 25°C.

K : BOTANY

1. Availability of free energy is maximum in the lowest tropic level i.e. 'producer' because efficiency of utilization of energy is not 100% i.e. always less than 100% therefore availability of free energy decreases in each successive tropic level.

2. Ethylene is ripening hormone and it is produced during the ripening of fruits.
3. NADPH is a reduced form of $NADP^+$. $NADP^+$ differs from NAD^+ in the presence of additional phosphate group on the 2′ position of the ribose ring that carries the adenine moiety.
4. Anther culture is a process of using anther culture haploid plantlets. The technique was discovered in 1964 by Guha and Maheshwari, in experiments using Datura innoxia., induction frequencies of almost 100% and a yield of more than one thousand plantlets or callus have occurred under optimal conditions for one anther. Success can be determined within 24 hours as cell begins to divide.

   Colchicines are used to induce polyploidy while optimum level of auxin and cytokinin are used in plant cell culture for proper growth of both root and shoot.
5. John C Sanford is an American plant geneticist. Sanford is a prolific inventor with more than 32 invented plantlets. At Cornell, Sanford and colleagues developed the 'Biolistic Particle delivery System' or so called Gene Gun.
6. Palisade tissue is composed of photosynthetic, cylindrical cells that are found in a distinct layer under the upper surface of leafs.

   The Periderm is a secondary protective tissue that replaces the epidermis during growth in thickness of stems and roots of gymnosperms and dicotyledons (secondary growths). Periderm is a multilayered tissue, the bulk of which usually constitute the corks, or Phellem, the lateral meristem i.e. cork cambium or phellogen and persistent living cells called Phelloderm.
7. The classification system used by Carolous Linneaus is known as Artificial Sexual System of classification. It was first of all published in the name of 'Genera Plantarum'. Artificial taxonomy was a system of grouping unrelated plant species by a common criteria (on basis of flower sexual organs). This system divided plants into 24 classes. Classes were based largely on the number, union and length of stamens.
8. According to Fluid Mosaic model, plasma membrane consist of lipid bilayer with embedded proteins. In general, there are two groups of proteins associated with membranes. One group called Extrinsic proteins and is not embedded in the hydrophobic core but is weakly bound by ionic bonds and divalent cations salt bridges to the lipid polar head group or intrinsic proteins. The second class of proteins called as Intrinsic proteins is tightly bound to the lipid bilayer by both ionic and hydrophobic forces. Because of the two classes of proteins, Extrinsic and Intrinsic, the outer inner faces of membranes may have markedly different physical, structural and biochemical properties.
9. The growth of plant cells in vitro and their regeneration into whole plants is an asexual process, involving only mitotic division of the cell and theoretically it should not cause any variation. Ideally, clonal multiplication of genetically uniform plants is the expectation but the occurrence of uncontrolled and random spontaneous variation during the culture process is unexpected.

   Sapwood is the outermost, living wood in the growing tree and its principal functions are to conduct water from the roots to the leaves while the heartwood is the dark coloured inner dead wood and it stores gum, resin, oils, tannins etc.
10. In parasitic food chain, the pyramid of number is always inverted. This is because a single plant may support the growth of many herbivore, and each herbivore in turn may provide nutrition to several parasites which supports many hyperparasites. Thus, from the producer towards consumer, there is a reverse position i.e number of organisms gradually shows an increase, making the pyramid inverted in shape.

    To use dry mass instead of fresh mass is useful because among living beings there are differences related to the proportion of water within their body and such differences can distort the quantitative analysis of incorpated organicmaterial.
11. Loose smut of wheat is caused by fungus Ustilago tritici. This is easily recognized at the time of heading by the characteristic dusty black appearance of disease heads. The infected heads emerge from the boot one to three days earlier than those of healthy plants. The spores are loosely held and are easily spread by wind into neighbouring healthy plants. Production of plant growth hormones by fungus result in infected plant heads reaching flowering earlier than healthy heads.
12. It is critical to decrese the temperature of fruits and vegetable as quickly as possible after harvest to slow down their metabolism, unless curing is a pert of plant harvest management. Also for post harvest treatment of fruits and vegetables the storage chamber air is passed continuously through charcoal to adsorb any ethylene produced by ripening fruits and vegetables. Silver nitrate and cobalt chloride are also anti ethylene agents but they are poisonous and hence used in florist industries.
13. Heterosis is a fundamental issue in plant breeding and designates the improved vigour of F_2 hybrids in comparison with their parental homozygous lines. Commercial exploitation of

heterosis has been possible using cytoplasmic male sterility restorer system. Identification and rise of new restorer line is quite essential to know the fertility restoration on new CMS sources and also to diversity the genetic base of the hybrids for increased hybrid vigour.

14. Guha and Maheshwari (1964) developed an anther culture technique for production of haploids in the laboratory.

Xylem cells develop from procambial or cambial initials in sites and they can also be induced from parenchyma cells by wound stress or combination of phyto hormones in vitro. This initiation, progression and development of xylem cell is called Xylogenesis.

15. Alginate hydrogel is frequently selected as matrix for synthetic seeds because of its moderate viscosity and low spinnablity of solution, low toxicity for somatic embryos and quick gellation, low cost and biocompatibility characteristics.

Artificial seed technology involves the production of tissue culture derived somatic embryos encased in a protective coating.

17. Aspergillic acid is most commonly known as an antibiotic antifungal agent that is derived from certain strains of *Aspergillus* flavus.

Hypericin is naturally occurring pigment, is found in certain species of plants from the genus Herberium, the most common of which is Saint John's Wort (*Hypericum perforatum*). Recent interest in hypericin is provoked by the discovery that it possesses extremely high toxicity towards certain viruses such as HIV and towards tumors.

18. *Phaseolus vulgaris*, the common bean, string bean, field bean, flageolet bean, French bean, garden bean, haricot bean, pop bean, or snap bean, is a herbaceous annual plant grown worldwide for its edible fruit, either the dry seed or the unripe fruit, both of which are referred to as beans.

Avena sativa is also known as the common oat. It is a cereal crop of global importance and the species commonly referred to as "oats".

The cashew tree is a tropical evergreen that produces the cashew nut and the cashew apple. Officially classed as *Anacardium occidentale*, it can grow as high as 14 metres (46 ft), but the dwarf cashew, growing up to 6 metres (20 ft), has proved more profitable, with earlier maturity and higher yields. The cashew nut is served as a snack or used in recipes, like other nuts, although it is actually a seed.

Daucus carota (or carrot) is a root vegetable, usually orange in colour, though purple, red, white, and yellow varieties exist. It has a crisp texture when fresh.

19. Golden rice is a variety of Oryza sativa produced through genetic engineering to biosynthesize beta carotene, a precursor of Vitamin A, in the edible part of rice.

Flavr Savr tomato is a genetically modified tomato (GMO), and was made resistant to rotting by adding an antisense gene which infers with the production of the enzyme polygalacturonase.

Insect resistant cotton plant called Bt cotton contained a foreign gene obtained from soil bacterium, *Bacillius thuringenesis.* This Bt gene protect the plant from bollworm, a major pest of cotton.

20. The inside of a pea pod is known as the loculus. Within the loculus are small stems, called 'funiculi', which connect the ovules to the inner wall of the pea pod. Funiculi also deliver nutrients to the ovules.

Seeds of some mangroves are viviparous and begin to germinate while still attached to the parent. They produce large, heavy root which allows the seed to penetrate into the ground when it falls.

21. The salt glands of mangroves are a distinctive multicellular trichome, a glandular hair found on the upper leaf surface and much more densely in the abaxial indumentums. They help in removing the exess salts.

Tunica corpus was proposed by German scientist A. Schmidt in 1924.

22. Indole acetic acid (IAA) is the most common, naturally occurring plant hormone of the auxin class. Bulliform cells are large, bubble shaped epidermal cells that occurs in groups on the upper surface of the leaves of many grasses.

Tyloses are outgrowth on parenchyma cells of xylem vessels. When the plant is stressed by drought or infection, tyloses will fall from the sides of the cells and "Dam" up the vascular tissue to prevent further damage to plants.

23. TTWWCC * ttwwcc

gametes $\rightarrow$ TWC twc

when crossed, 'TWCtwc' is produced in F_1 generation.

Number of gametes = 2^n

where 'n' = number of hetrozygoted

$= 2^3 = 8$

These gametes will be $\rightarrow$ TWC, twc, TWc, TwC, tWC, twC, tWc, Twc respectively.

24. Number of genotype = $3n$,

where 'n' = number of heterozygotes

$= 3^3 = 27$

25. In uncompetitive inhibition both Km and Vmax decreases. In non competitive inhibition Vm decreases but Km remains constant.

In competitibe inhibition Km increases but Vmax remain constant.

26. A linear form of the Michaelis-Menton Equation is used to determine Km and Vmax. The Michaelis-Menton equation may be inverted and written as follows-

$$\frac{1}{Vi} = \frac{K_m}{V_{max}} \times \frac{1}{5} + \frac{1}{V_{max}}$$

28.

COMMON NAME	COMMERCIAL PRODUCT
Cotton	Fibre
Peanut	Vegetable oil
Sarpgandha	Alkaloid
Tea	Beverage

L : MICROBIOLOGY

1. In 1970 David Baltimore found an enzyme, reverse transcriptase that used an RNA template to catalyze the synthesis of DNA. Reverse transcription is the process by which retroviruses infiltrate healthy cells and use the host's cellular machinery to replicate. Baltimore was studying a tumor virus originally discovered at Rockefeller called Rous sarcoma virus (RSV), and the finding had far-reaching implications for cancer research and for molecular biology more generally. In 1975 he was awarded a Nobel Prize for the work, shared with Howard Temin and Renato Dulbecco.

2. When *E. coli* is infected with a lambda phage, two cycles may happen: lytic or lysogenic. The lytic cycle happens when progeny phage particles are produced. The lysogenic cycle, in contrast, does not produce a huge number of progeny phage or break down the host cell. This infection can normally be detected by the appearance of plaques or lysed bacteria on agar plates.

3. The magnification in a normal light microscope is typically a result of two lenses. The ocular lens (the eyepiece) normally has a magnification of 15X. The objective lens would then have to be 100X to obtain a 1500X total magnification. The oil immersion does not act as a lens, but helps to match refractive indices to reduce distortion of the object as viewed through the microscope.

4. Deinococcus is a gram-positive bacterium found to form pink or reddish colored colonies. Deinococcus is known for being the most radiation-resistant vegetative cell. In fact, Deinococcus radiodurans can live through blasts of radiation thousands of times greater than the level that would kill a human being.

5. A peptic ulcer is a sore in the lining of stomach or duodenum, the first part of your small intestine. A burning stomach pain is the most common symptom. Peptic ulcers happen when the acids that help to digest food damage the walls of the stomach or duodenum. The most common cause is infection with a bacterium called Helicobacter pylori. Treatment may include medicines to reduce stomach acids or antibiotics to kill H. pylori.

6. Phylogeny is the evolutionary development and history of a species or higher taxonomic grouping of organisms.

7. Yeast artificial chromosome (YAC) is a human-engineered DNA molecule used to clone DNA sequences in yeast cells. Yeast artificial chromosomes have large insert size (100-1000kb) that is large amount of DNA can be cloned. Thus for cloning a 150 kb fragment of DNA, YAC vectors would be most appropriate.

8. Psychrophilic and psychrotrophic microor-ganisms have the ability to grow at 0 degree C. Psychrotrophic microorganisms have a maximum temperature for growth above 20 degrees C and are widespread in natural environments and in foods. This ability to grow at low temperature may be correlated with a lower temperature characteristic than that of the mesophiles, an increasing proportion of unsaturated fatty acids in the lipid phase of the cell membrane, which makes it more fluid, and a protein conformation functional at low temperature.

9. Complete denitrification of nitrate results in the formation of N_2. Denitrification is the biological conversion of nitrate to nitrogen gas, nitric oxide or nitrous oxide. These compounds are gaseous compounds and are not readily available for microbial growth; therefore they are typically released to the atmosphere. Nitrogen gas makes up over 70% of atmospheric gases, thus the release of N_2 to the atmosphere is benign.

10. Coxsackie viruses are RNA viruses that may cause hand, foot, and mouth disease (HFMD). Occasionally, coxsackieviruses can cause more serious infections that may need to be treated in a hospital, including:
    - viral meningitis, an infection of the meninges (the three membranes that envelop the brain and spinal cord)
    - encephalitis, a brain infection
    - myocarditis, an infection of the heart muscle

    Gingivitis is a form of periodontal disease. Periodontal disease is inflammation and infection that destroys the tissues that support the teeth, including the gums, the periodontal ligaments, and the tooth sockets (alveolar bone). Gingivitis is due to the long-term effects of plaque deposits on the teeth. Thus it is not caused by the Coxsackie virus.

11. Vancomycin inhibits bacterial cell wall synthesis, which stops the bacteria growing and dividing properly. The cell walls are made of strings of sugars, crosslinked by short peptide chains. By binding to D -alanyl-D -alanine groups on the end of

the peptide chains, it stops the crosslinks forming. This prevents the bacteria from building its strong peptidoglycan network.

12. Conjugative plasmid is a plasmid that can move from one cell to another during the process of conjugation. It is a plasmid that can affect its own intercellular transfer by means of conjugation; this transfer is accomplished by a bacterium's being rendered a donor, usually with specialized pili.

Cryptic plasmids are plasmids with no measurable phenotype. They are plasmids that have no known function. They occur in a number of bacterial species.

Episome is a genetic particle of certain cells, especially bacterial cells that can exist either autonomously in the cytoplasm or as part of a chromosome.

13. An Hfr bacterium is one that contains a plasmid integrated into its chromosome. The integrated plasmid must have a functional conjugation system for it to become an Hfr (high frequency recombination) bacterium.

14. *Ralstonia eutropha* is a gram-negative soil bacterium of the betaproteobacteria class. *R. eutropha* is known to produce and sequester polyhydroxyalkanoate (PHA) plastics (bioplastics) when exposed to excess amounts of sugar substrate.

The diverse metabolism of *Pseudomonas putida* may be exploited for bioremediation; for example, it is used as a soil inoculant to remedy naphthalene contaminated soils.

Thiobacillus thiooxidans is a Gram-negative, rod-shaped bacterium that utilizes sulfur as its primary energy source. It is used in the mining technique known as bioleaching, where metals are extracted from their ores through the action of microbes.

Beauveria bassiana is an entomopathogene fungus. It is widely used as bio insecticide for the pest control of agricultural, ornamental and forest plants. Bio pesticides made on the base of *B. bassiana* are effective against various species of thrips and aphids, the glasshouse whitefly, larvae of Colorado beetle and also several species of leaf-gnawing pests.

15. The Entner-Doudoroff pathway begins with the same reactions as the pentose phosphate pathway, the formation of glucose 6-phosphate and }6-phosphogluconate. Glucose 6-phosphate is oxidized by glucose 6-phosphate dehydrogenase to 6-phosphoglucono-δ-lactone (producing NADPH) and this is then hydrolyzed by lactonase to 6-phosphogluconate.

16. Group translocation is a type of active transport in bacteria. The substance being transported passes the cell membrane and during the passing changes its chemical composition. The composition change results in the substance not being able to pass back out of the cell membrane.

17. MacConkey Agar (MAC) is a selective and differential medium designed to isolate and differentiate enterics based on their ability to ferment lactose. Bile salts and crystal violet inhibit the growth of Gram positive organisms. Lactose provides a source of fermentable carbohydrate, allowing for differentiation. Neutral red is a pH indicator that turns red at a pH below 6.8 and is colorless at any pH greater than 6.8.

18. Rolling circle replication describes a process of unidirectional nucleic acid replication that can rapidly synthesize multiple copies of circular molecules of DNA or RNA, such as plasmids, the genomes of bacteriophages, and the circular RNA genome of viroids. Many bacterial plasmids replicate by a rolling-circle (RC) mechanism.

A Theta structure is an intermediate structure formed during the replication of a circular DNA molecule (prokaryote DNA), two replication forks can proceed independently around the DNA ring and when viewed from above it resembles the Greek letter "theta" (θ).

Bacteria are also replicated by bidirectional mode of replication in which replication is moving along in both directions from the starting point. This creates two replication forks, moving in opposite directions.

Thus bacteria can replicate by all the three modes of replication.

19. Negative staining is one of the many staining techniques that can be employed for viewing of bacterial cell morphology and size. The advantages of the negative stain include the use of only one stain and the absence of heat fixation of the sample. Negative staining employs the use of an acidic stain (i.e. Nigrosin) and, due to repulsion between the negative charges of the stain and the bacterial surface; the dye will not penetrate the cell. In negative staining, the results yield a clear cell with a dark background.

Thus microorganisms stain deeply is an incorrect statement about negative staining.

20. A nonsense mutation is the substitution of a single base pair that leads to the appearance of a stop codon where previously there was a codon specifying an amino acid. The presence of this premature stop codon results in the production of a shortened and likely nonfunctional, protein.

Thus a mutation in the codon UCG to UAG is described as nonsense mutation as UAG is a stop codon.

21. Resistance plasmid (R plasmid) is a conjugative factor in bacterial cells that promotes resistance to agents such as antibiotics, metal ions, ultraviolet radiation, and bacteriophages. It confers certain bacterial strain the acquired ability to resist the antimicrobial activity of some drugs.

22. Plasma cells are a type of white blood cell that produces antibodies. As such, they are an important part of the immune system. They are formed from B cells produced in a person's bone marrow. Once produced, B cells mainly stay within the marrow and wait until an antigen appears in the body. Antigens bind to the cell and stimulate it to form plasma cells. These cells then produce antibodies to destroy the pathogen.

23. Number of *E. coli* cells present in 50 l of 10^9CFU/ml or 0.10^9CFU/ l = $5 * 10^7$

1000 l contains $5 * 10^7$ CFU, thus 50 l will contain $25 * 10^5$ CFU

Therefore,

Transformation efficiency (T.E.)

= number of colonies remaining/ number of colonies originally present

$= 90/25 = 3.6 * 10^5$.

The efficiency of this transformation FU/ g of DNA is $3.6 * 10^5$.

24. Since the transformation efficiency is $3.6 * 10^5$ (as calculated above), therefore the percentage of transformed cells can be given as: 0.36%.

25. Given,

Initial number of cells present, $N_0 = 10$

Final number of cells present, N= 40960

Time, t = 4hrs = 4 * 60 min

Therefore generation time can be give as:

$$G = t/3.3(\log_{10}N - \log_{10}N_0)$$

$$= 4 * 60/3.3(\log_{10}40960 - \log_{10}10)$$

On solving, we get,

Generation time,

G = 20 min

26. Now given,

Initial number of cells, $N_0 = 1$

Final number of cells present, N = ?

Generation time, G = 20 min

Time, t = 4 hrs = 4 * 20 min

Therefore,

$$G = t/3.3(\log_{10}N - \log_{10}N_0)$$

$$20 = 4 * 60/3.3(\log_{10}N - \log_{10}1)$$

$$20 = 4 * 60/3.3(\log_{10}N)$$

On solving, we get,

$$N = 2^{30}$$

27. Given,

Genome size = $1.5 * 10^4$ Kb

Average size of library fragment = 5kb

Thus, ratio of genome size of microorganism relative to average size of fragment can be given as:

$1.5 * 10^4/5 = 3000$.

28. Number of recombinant bacterial colonies need to be screened can be given by:

$$N = \ln(1 - P)/\ln(1 - a/b)$$

Where,

N = number of clones required

P = probability that any DNA fragment can be present

a = average size of DNA fragment inserted into vector

b = total size of genome

Therefore, on calculating we get,

N = 9000.

M : ZOOLOGY

1. Sickle cell anaemia is a disease passed down through families in which red blood cells form an abnormal sickle or crescent shape. Red blood cells carry oxygen to the body and are normally shaped like a disc. Sickle cell anaemia is caused by an abnormal type of haemoglobin called haemoglobin S. Haemoglobin is a protein inside red blood cells that carries oxygen. Sickle-cell anaemia is caused by a point mutation in the β-globin chain of haemoglobin, causing the hydrophilic amino acid glutamic acid to be replaced with the hydrophobic amino acid valine at the sixth position. The β-globin gene is found on chromosome 11. The association of two wild-type α-globin subunits with two mutant β-globin subunits forms haemoglobin S (HbS).

2. An antibody is a protein produced by the body's immune system when it detects harmful substances, called antigens. Each type of antibody is unique and defends the body against one specific type of antigen. The paratope is the part of an antibody which recognizes an antigen, the antigen-binding site of an antibody. It is a small region (of 15–22 amino acids) of the antibody's F_{ab} region and contains parts of the antibody's heavy and light chains. An epitope, also known as antigenic determinant, is the part of an antigen that is recognized by the immune system, specifically by antibodies, B cells, or T cells.

3. A hydrogen bond is the attractive force between the hydrogen attached to an electronegative atom of one molecule and an electronegative atom of a different molecule. Usually the electronegative atom is oxygen, nitrogen, or fluorine, which has a partial negative charge. The hydrogen then has the partial positive charge. Hydrogen bonding is usually stronger than normal dipole forces between molecules. Hence, it is the strongest amongst the non-covalent interactions such as hydrophobic, ionic or Vander Waals' interactions.

4. Acrosome is the caplike, membrane-bound structure covering the anterior portion of the head of a spermatozoan and it contains enzymes for penetrating the oocyte. It is bounded by an inner and an outer membrane. It is derived from the Golgi apparatus. Acrosome formation is completed during testicular maturation. Acrosome contains digestive enzymes (including hyaluronidase and acrosin).

5. Haematopoesis is the normal formation and development of blood cells in the bone marrow. In the embryo and fetus it takes place in a variety of sites including the liver, spleen, thymus, lymph nodes, and bone marrow; from birth throughout the rest of life it is mainly in the bone marrow with a small amount occurring in lymph nodes. The yolk sac is the first site of blood-cell production during murine (mice) ontogeny. Primitive erythroid cells originate in the yolk sac and complete their maturation, including enucleation, in the bloodstream. Though species differences exist, the pattern of hematopoietic progenitor cell emergence in the yolk sac is similar in mouse and man.

6. A living fossil is a species (or sometimes a higher group) which was known only from the fossil record, until living specimens were discovered. *Latimeria* is a genus comprising the living species of coelacanth. A living species that was thought to be extinct (e.g. the coelacanth, *Latimeria chalumnae*) could be called a Lazarus taxon (taxon that suddenly reappears, either in the fossil record or in nature) instead of a living fossil. Coelacanths disappeared from the fossil record some 80 million years ago. But later, the Indonesian coelacanth (*Latimeria menadoensis*) and West Indian Ocean coelacanth (*Latimeria chalumnae*), the two living species of coelacanth were identified.

7. Given, Albinism is controlled by the recessive gene c. After sexual reproduction between a normal pigmented person (Cc) and an albino (cc), the cross result would be:-

   Parental generation (gametes) $\rightarrow$ Cc x cc

   F1 generation $\rightarrow$ Cc Cc cc cc [1 : 1 phenotype i.e., ½ normal and ½ albino child]

   Thus, from the genotype obtained in F_1 generation, it can be ascertained that 50% of the children would be normal and 50% would be albino child. Thus, the chance of an albino child to be born is ½.

8. Fishes that are able to leave water for extended periods of time are known as amphibious fish. These fish use a range of terrestrial locomotory modes, such as lateral undulation, tripod-like walking (using paired fins and tail), and jumping. Anabas possesses a labyrinth organ, a structure in the fish's head which allows it to breathe atmospheric oxygen, and therefore can be out of water for an extended period of time (6–8 hours). *Saccobranchus fossilis* is an air-breathing fish which inhabits pools in tropical Asia. The air-breathing organ in it has a posterior diverticulum of the opercular cavity in the form of an air-sac. *Gobius* does not have any special adaptation of the gills for prolonged breathing in air outside water. *Clarias* have a large, accessory breathing organ composed of modified gill arches.

9. The avian respiratory system delivers oxygen from the air to the tissues and also removes carbon dioxide. In addition, the respiratory system plays an important role in thermor-egulation (maintaining normal body temperature). The avian respiratory system is different from that of other vertebrates, with birds having relatively small lungs plus nine air sacs that play an important role in respiration. The air sacs permit a unidirectional flow of air through the lungs. Unidirectional flow means that air moving through bird lungs is largely 'fresh' air & has higher oxygen content. So, in bird lungs, more oxygen is available to diffuse into the blood. Air sacs do not take part in the actual oxygen exchange, but do greatly enhance its efficiency and allow for the high metabolic rates found in birds. As air flows through the air sac system and lungs, there is no mixing of oxygen-rich air and oxygen-poor, carbon dioxide-rich, air as in mammalian lungs. Thus, the partial pressure of oxygen in a bird's lungs is the same as the environment, and so birds have more efficient gas-exchange of both oxygen and carbon dioxide than mammals do.

10. A transgenic mouse contains additional, artificially-introduced genetic material in every cell. A transgenic mouse is a very useful system for studying mammalian gene function and regulation because analysis is carried out on the whole organism. There are two major methods for transgenic mice production $\rightarrow$ In 'pronuclear microinjection', the foreign DNA is introduced directly into the mouse

egg just after fertilisation. Using a fine needle, the DNA is injected into the large male pronucleus, which is derived from the sperm. The second method is the introduction of DNA into embryonic stem cells (ES cells). These are derived from the very early mouse embryo and can therefore differentiate into all types of cell when introduced into another embryo.

11. Histones are highly alkaline proteins found in eukaryotic cell nuclei that package and order the DNA into structural units called nucleosomes. They are the chief protein components of chromatin, acting as spools around which DNA winds, and play a role in gene regulation. Without histones, the unwound DNA in chromosomes would be very long (a length to width ratio of more than 10 million to one in human DNA). For example, each human cell has about 1.8 meters of DNA, but wound on the histones it has about 90 micrometers (0.09 mm) of chromatin, which, when duplicated and condensed during mitosis, result in about 120 micrometers of chromosomes.

12. The double-stranded structure of DNA provides a simple mechanism for DNA replication. Here, the two strands are separated and then each strand's complementary DNA sequence is recreated by an enzyme called DNA polymerase. DNA polymerases can only extend a DNA strand in a 5' to 3' direction, different mechanisms are used to copy the antiparallel strands of the double helix. The leading strand template is the template strand of the DNA double helix that is oriented in a 3' to 5' manner. All DNA synthesis occurs 5'-3'. The lagging strand template is the coding strand of the DNA double helix that is oriented in a 5' to 3' manner. Since the DNA is oriented in a manner that does not allow continual synthesis, only small sections can be read at a time. An RNA primer is placed on the DNA strand 3' to the origin of replication. DNA polymerase reads 3'-5' on the original DNA to produce a 5'-3' nascent strand. These fragments of DNA produced on the lagging strand are called Okazaki fragments. An Okazaki fragment is a relatively short fragment of DNA on the lagging strand during DNA replication. The lengths of Okazaki fragments are between 1,000 to 2,000 nucleotides long in *E. coli* and are generally between 100 to 200 nucleotides long in eukaryotes.

13. Darwinism designates a distinctive form of evolutionary explanation for the history and diversity of life on earth. This entry first formulates 'Darwin's Darwinism' in terms of five philosophically distinctive themes: (i) probability and chance, (ii) the nature, power and scope of selection, (iii) adaptation and teleology, (iv) nominalism vs. essentialism about species and (v) the tempo and mode of evolutionary change. Thus, Darwinism does not speak of genotypic change for an efficient organism.

14. Temperature-dependent sex determination (TSD) is a type of environmental sex determination in which the temperatures experienced during embryonic development determine the sex of the offspring. Synergism between temperature and hormones has also been identified in these systems. Administering estradiol at male-producing temperatures generates females that are physiologically identical to temperature-produced females. In temperature-dependent sex determination, it is the environmental temperature during a critical period of embryonic development that determines whether an egg develops as male or female. In turtles, due to the temperature sensitivity of oestrogen (estradiol), it results in development of varied sexes. Incubation temperature determines the sex of turtles. Female hatchlings are produced at warmer tempera-tures and males at cooler temperatures.

15. In reptiles, birds, and mammals, a membrane forming a fluid-filled cavity (the amniotic sac) that encloses the embryo is called the amnion. The amniotic sac and the fluid it contains are sometimes referred to as the bag of waters. Lined with ectoderm and covered with mesoderm (both are germ layers), the amnion contains a thin, transparent fluid in which the embryo is suspended, thus providing a cushion against mechanical injury. The amnion also provides protection against fluid loss from the embryo itself and against tissue adhesions. Named after the allantois, allantoin is an amniote embryonic excretory organ in which it concentrates during development in most mammals except humans and higher apes, it is a product of oxidation of uric acid by purine catabolism. After birth, it is the predominant means by which nitrogenous waste is excreted in the urine of these animals. These appeared for the first time in reptiles who were the first amphibians.

16. The most common cloning method, known as "somatic cell nuclear transfer" or simply "nuclear transfer," requires two kinds of cell. A somatic cell is any cell other than a sperm cell or egg cell, and contains the complete DNA, or genetic blueprint, of the animal it came from. Somatic cells such as lymphocytes are not suitable for cloning as the lymphocytes are immunogenic cells which produce immunoglobulins or antibodies.

17. The blood differential test measures the percentage of each type of white blood cell (WBC) that you have in the blood. It also reveals if there are any abnormal or immature cells. Five types of white blood cells, also called leukocytes, normally appear in the blood $\rightarrow$ Neutrophils (may indicate bacterial infection), Lymphocytes (B cells and T cells; Higher with some viral infections such as glandular fever), Monocytes (May be raised in bacterial infection, tuberculosis, malaria, Rocky Mountain spotted fever, monocytic leukemia, chronic ulcerative colitis and regional enteritis), Eosinophils (increased in viral and parasitic infections, asthma, or allergic reaction) and Basophils (may be increased in bone marrow related conditions such as leukemia or lymphoma). Any infection or acute stress increases the number of white blood cells.

18. Both Rajesh and Deb were stung by comparable number of bees. Though Rajesh experienced only pain and small swelling, Deb manifested intense swelling, breathlessness and had to be hospitalized. The toxin of bees would be effective with elevated concentrations of the toxin in blood. Thus, for serious symptoms and manifestations, Deb's blood had to have a higher concentration of the bee toxin. Hence, Deb must have been stung before by bees.

19. The Thyroid Stimulating Hormone receptor is found mainly on thyroid follicular cells. Stimulation of the receptor increases T_3 and T_4 production and secretion. The epidermal growth factor receptor (EGFR; ErbB-1; HER1 in humans) is the cell-surface receptor for members of the epidermal growth factor family (EGF-family) of extracellular protein ligand which exists on the cell surface and is activated by binding of its specific ligand. The progesterone receptor is a protein found inside cells. It is activated by the steroid hormone progesterone. It is found in cytoplasm. Cytokine receptors are receptors that bind cytokines. Cytokine receptors may be both membrane-bound and soluble.

20. Nearly all non-mammal vertebrates have nucleated red blood cells (nRBC). Non-nucleated RBC's are a unique feature to mammals. Nucleated RBCs are precursor molecules for erythrocytes. Nucleated RBCs are present in new born babies. But appearance of nucleated RBCs is an indication of certain kind of abnormality of blood in mammals. All mammals, except Camels and Llama have enucleated RBCs.

21. Through comparison with the human genome, a complete catalogue of the genetic differences that have accumulated since the human and chimpanzee species diverged from our common ancestor has been generated, constituting approximately thirty-five million single-nucleotide changes, five million insertion/deletion events, and various chromosomal rearrangements. Human and chimpanzee chromosomes are very similar. The primary difference is that humans have one fewer pair of chromosomes than do other great apes. The human genome shares a 99.5 % similarity with the chimpanzee genome. About 30 percent of all human proteins are identical in sequence to the corresponding chimp protein.

22. Myelogenous leukemia or myelogenic leukemia is the leukemia characterized by proliferation of myeloid tissue in areas such as bone marrow and the spleen and by the abnormal increase of granulocytes, myelocytes, and myeloblasts in tissues and in blood and is also called granulocytic leukemia, myelocytic leukemia and myeloid leukemia. Chronic myelogenous (or myeloid) leukemia (CML) was the first malignancy to be linked to a clear genetic abnormality, the chromosomal translocation known as the Philadelphia chromosome. In this translocation, parts of two chromosomes (the 9th and 22nd by conventional karyotypic numbering) switch places. As a result, part of the BCR ("breakpoint cluster region") gene from chromosome 22 is fused with the ABL gene on chromosome 9. This abnormal "fusion" gene generates a protein of p210 or sometimes p185 weight.

23. Given, size of mammalian heart is nearly proportional to body size and makes up 0.59% of the body mass. Also given, Mass of Bird = 1 kg, Mass of its heart = 8.2 g. Now, given that the size of mammal is same as that of the bird, therefore, Mass of mammal = 1kg = 1000g. Thus, mass or expected size of mammalian heart:-

$\Rightarrow$ 0.59% of body size = Size of heart

$$\Rightarrow \text{Size of heart} = \frac{(0.59 \times 1000)}{100}$$

$\Rightarrow$ Size of heart = 5.9

Therefore, the required size of mammalian heart is 5.9 g.

24. Given, Heart rate of the mammal is inversely proportional to the body size. Also given, Size of an elephant = 3000 kg, heart rate = 25 min^{-1}. Now, since the heart rate bears an inversely proportional or reciprocal relationship, it means that a mammal with smaller body size will have a higher heart rate whereas a mammal with larger body size will have a lower heart rate. Therefore, from the given graph, it can be inferred that the possible range of heart rate or pulse for a 3g shrew would be > 500.

25. BALB/c mice are useful for research into both cancer and immunology. BALB/c substrains are "particularly well known for the production of plasmac-ytomas on injection with mineral oil," an important process for the production of monoclonal antibodies. Nude mice have a spontaneous deletion in the FOXN1 gene. Mice with a targeted deletion in the FOXN1 ("knockout" mice) also show the "nude" phenotype. Because they lack a thymus, nude mice cannot generate mature T lymphocytes. Therefore they are unable to mount most types of immune responses. After 7 days of immunogen administration, IgM immunogl -obulin is first produced by nude cells with the help of T-helper cells from BALB/c strain. This, IgM gets recombinantly converted into IgG to mount the response of the immunogen in the thymal cells of BALB/c strain.

26. On the 18th day of immunogen administration, the cytotoxic cells of BALB/c strain of mice would develop allergic response leading to formation of the antibody IgE. This is a case of hypersensitive reaction of the BALB/c strain. At the same time, the nude strain cells utilize the T-cell receptors of the BALB/c strain for the production of IgG against the hypersensitive reaction for humoral suppression of the antigen.

27. Given, a woman has a rare abnormality of the eye because of a dominant allele P. As a result, if she mates with a normal male having normal eyes, then 50% of her children would bear the dominant gene P for the abnormal eyes while the rest 50% would have normal eyes.

28. The genotype of the father cannot be a recessive for the gene P. This is because the sex-linked trait for abnormal eyes must be present on the X-chromosome of the father for him to transfer it to his daughter. Also, if the trait were recessive, it would not have expressed in the woman, his daughter. Hence, the gene P must be dominant for the trait for it to be expressive in the X-chromosome.

■■

GATE-2006

XL : LIFE SCIENCES

Time : 3 Hours | *Maximum Marks : 100*

H : CHEMISTRY (Compulsory)

Q. 1 – 6 carry one mark each.

1. Which one of the following is not a state function ?

(*a*) Enthalpy (H) (*b*) Internal energy (U)
(*c*) Work done (W) (*d*) Entropy (S)

2. Specify which among the following statements describe uncertainty principle

(*a*) No two electrons in an atom can have the same set of four quantum numbers
(*b*) It is impossible to determine simultaneously the velocity and momentum of an object with certainty
(*c*) Matter like radiation exhibit a dual behaviour
(*d*) It is impossible to simultaneously determine the position and momentum of an object with certainty

3. Among the given compounds, the most stable halogen containing compound of sulfur is

(*a*) SF_6 (*b*) S_2Cl_2 (*c*) SF_4 (*d*) $SOCl_2$

4. The nucleophile among the following is

(*a*) BF_3 (*b*) SO_3
(*c*) $(CH_3)_3N$ (*d*) NO_2^+

5. In the reaction A + B → Products,

If the concentration of A is doubled, the rate of the reaction increases by a factor of 4.

However, if the concentration of B is doubled, the rate remains unaltered. The order of the reaction with respect to A and B will be respectively

(*a*) 2 and 1 (*b*) 2 and 0 (*c*) 1 and 0 (*d*) 1 and 1

6. The major product (X) of the reaction $BrCH_2-CH_2-CH_2Br \xrightarrow{\text{Zinc dust}} (X)$ is

(*a*) 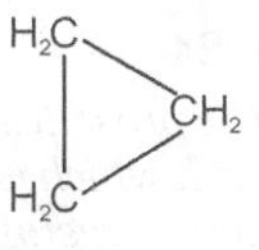 (*b*) $CH_2=CH-CH_2Br$

(*c*) $BrCH_2-CH=CH_2$ (*b*) $CH_2=C=CH_2$

Q. 7 – 24 carry two marks each

7. Which among the following steps is NOT present in the determination of lattice enthalpy of NaI using the Born-Haber cycle

(*a*) $\frac{1}{2}I_2(s) \rightarrow \frac{1}{2}I_2(g)$ (*b*) $Na(s) \rightarrow Na(l)$

(*c*) $\frac{1}{2}I_2(g) \rightarrow I(g)$ (*d*) $I(g) + e^- \rightarrow I^-(g)$

8. The boiling point of pure benzene is 80.0 °C. When a certain amount of benzoic acid was added to it, the boiling point increased to 82.5 °C. If the ebullioscopic constant (K_b) is 2.5 K kg mol^{-1}, then molality of the solution will be

(*a*) 0.02 (*b*) 0.25 (*c*) 1.00 (*d*) 6.25

9. The structure of XeO_2F_2 based on VSEPR theory is best described as

(*a*) See-saw structure with the O-Xe-O angle close to 120°
(*b*) See-saw structure with F-Xe-F angle close to 120°
(*c*) A perfect tetrahedral arrangement of substituents around Xe
(*d*) A square planar structure with the fluorines trans to each other

10. The hydrolysis of which of the following compounds would yield phosphorous acid (H_3PO_3)?

(*a*) PCl_5 (*b*) $POCl_3$ (*c*) P_4O_{10} (*d*) PCl_3

11. The type of hybridization that chromimum show in $Cr(CO)_6$ and $[CrF_6]^{3-}$ are respectively [atomic number of chromium is 24]

(*a*) sp^3d^2 and d^2sp^3 (*b*) sp^3d^2 and sp^3d^3
(*c*) d^2sp^3 and d^2sp^3 (*d*) d^2sp^3 and sp^3d^2

12. Which among the following molecules has the lowest bond dissociation energy?

(*a*) NO (*b*) NO^+ (*c*) NO^- (*d*) N_2

13. A transition metal ion in its +3 oxidation state forms complexes with excess of F^- as well as Cl^-. Given that the ionic radii of the metal ion, F^- and CI^- are 0.64, 1.34 and 1.81 Å respectively, the geometries of the metal complexes formed will be

(*a*) $[MF_6]^{3-}$, octahedral and $[MCl_4]^-$, tetrahedral
(*b*) $[MF_6]^{3-}$, octahedral and $[MCl_6]^{3-}$, octahedral
(*c*) $[MF_4]^-$, tetrahedral and $[MCl_4]^-$, tetrahedral
(*d*) $[MF_4]^-$, tetrahedral and $[MCl_6]^{3-}$, octahedral

14. The reagent required for the conversion

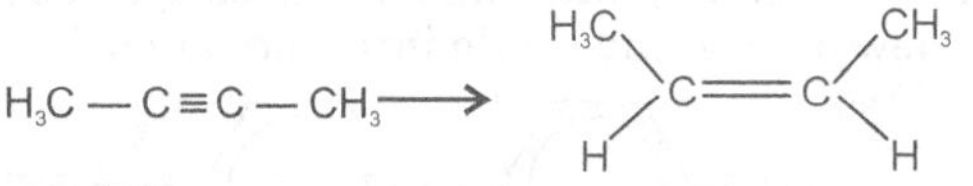

(Cis)

(*a*) Na in liquid ammonia
(*b*) $LiAlH_4$
(*c*) Sn/HCl
(*d*) Pd/$BaSO_4$/Quinoline

15. For the synthesis of

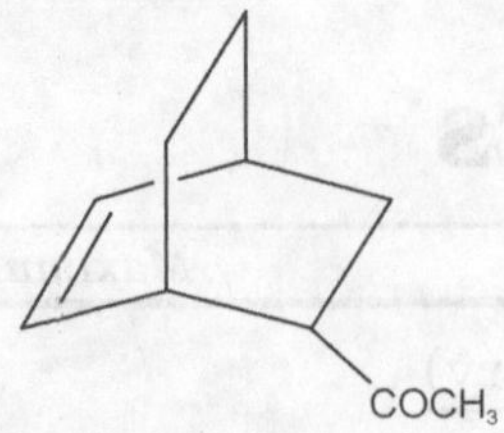

using Diel's-Alder reaction, the reactants required are

(*a*) 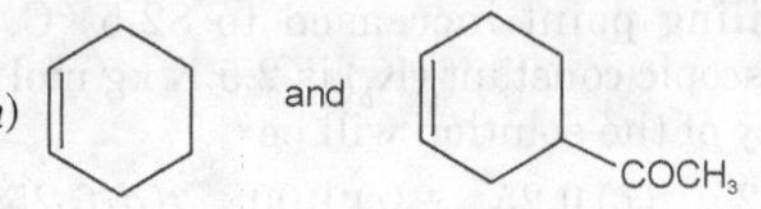

(*b*) 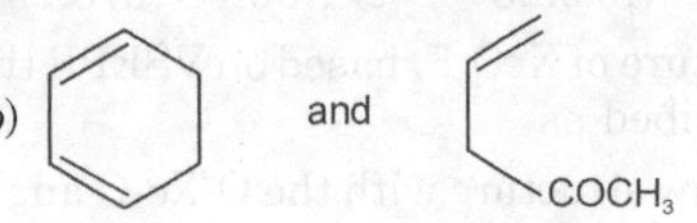

(*c*) 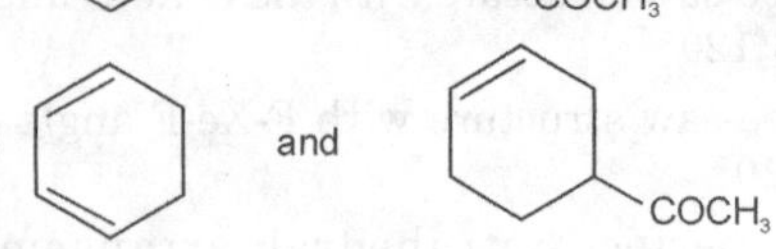

(*d*) 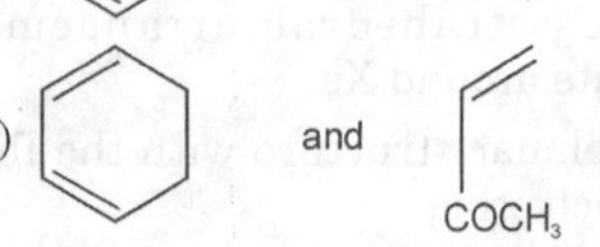

16. Match the values of K_a (given in column 2) with the substituted benzoic acids (given in column 1)

Column 1	Column 2
[P] $P-NO_2$	[X] 36×10^{-5}
[Q] P – OH	[Y] 10×10^{-5}
[R] P – Cl	[Z] 2.6×10^{-5}

(*a*) P – X; Q – Y; R – Z (b) P – Y; Q – X; R – Z

(*c*) P – Z; Q – Y; R – X (*d*) P – X; Q – Z; R – Y

17. The major products (X) and (Y) of the reactions

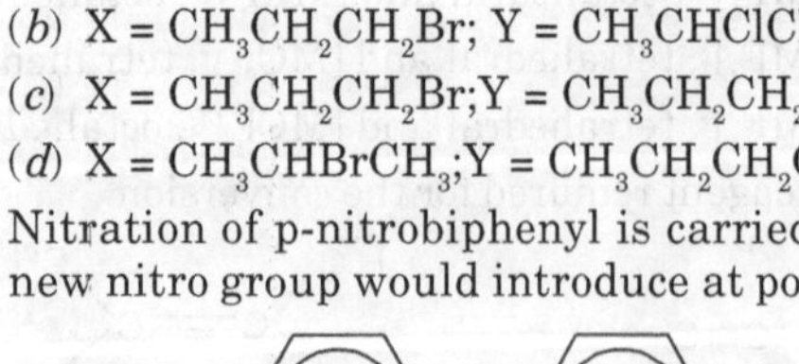

are

(*a*) $X = CH_3CHBrCH_3$; $Y = CH_3CHClCH_3$

(*b*) $X = CH_3CH_2CH_2Br$; $Y = CH_3CHClCH_3$

(*c*) $X = CH_3CH_2CH_2Br$; $Y = CH_3CH_2CH_2Cl$

(*d*) $X = CH_3CHBrCH_3$; $Y = CH_3CH_2CH_2Cl$

18. Nitration of p-nitrobiphenyl is carried out. The new nitro group would introduce at position/s-

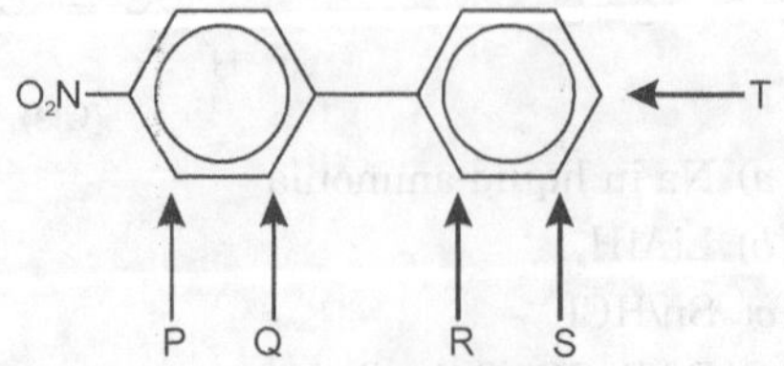

(*a*) P and T (*b*) Only Q

(*c*) R and T (*d*) Q and S

19. In the reaction

$$CH_3(CH_2)_3\underset{\displaystyle X}{\underset{|}{C}H}-CH_3 \xrightarrow{\ominus OCH_3/CH_3OH}$$

If X = F in the first case and X = Br in the second case, the major product formed will be respectively

(*a*) 1-Hexene and 1-Hexene

(*b*) 1-Hexene and 2-Hexene

(*c*) 2-Hexene and 2-Hexene

(*d*) 2-Hexene and 1-Hexene

20. Henderson's equation can be represented as

(*a*) $pH = pK_a + \log \dfrac{[Acid]}{[Salt]}$

(*b*) $pH = pK_a + \log \dfrac{[Salt]}{[Acid]}$

(*c*) $pK_a = pH + \log \dfrac{[Salt]}{[Acid]}$

(*d*) $pK_a = pH - \log \dfrac{[Salt]}{[Acid]}$

21. A concentrated soultion of NaCl is diluted ten times. The specific conductance (K) and molar conductance (Λ_m) will show the following behavior

(*a*) decrease in K and increase in Λ_m

(*b*) increase in K and decrease in Λ_m

(*c*) no change in both

(*d*) increase in both

22. In the reaction

$$2SO_3(g) \rightleftharpoons 2SO_2(g) + O_2(g)$$

taking place at 27° C, K_p is 3.0×10^{-23} atm. The value of K_c (in mol dm^{-3}) for the reaction is [Given R = 0.0821 dm^3 atm K^{-1} mol^{-1}]

(*a*) 74×10^{-23} (*b*) 12×10^{-25}

(*c*) 5×10^{-26} (d) 2×10^{-27}

Common Data Questions

Common Data for Question 23, 24

$KMnO_4$ reacts with oxalic acid in the presence of excess H_2SO_4 to yield a manganese complex X which is colorless in dilute solutions and pale pink in the crystalline form [atomic number of manganese is 25].

23. The number of unpaired electrons present in the complex X is

(*a*) 1 (*b*) 3

(*c*) 4 (*d*) 5

24. The calculated spin only magnetic moment for the compound X is

(*a*) 5.92 BM (*b*) 4.90 BM

(*c*) 3.87 BM (*d*) 1.73 BM

Linked Answer Questions : Q. 25 to Q. 28 carry two marks each

Statement for Linked Answer Questions 25 and 26

Benzene reacts with 1-chloro-2methylpropane in presence of anhydrous $AlCl_3$ at 20 °C to give major product (X).

25. The product (X) is

(*a*) 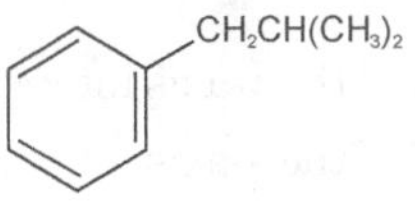

(*b*) 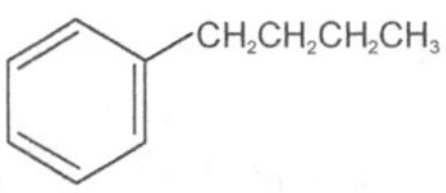

(*c*) 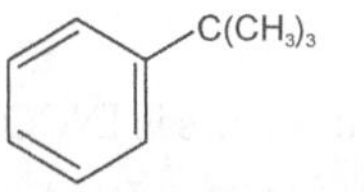

(*d*) 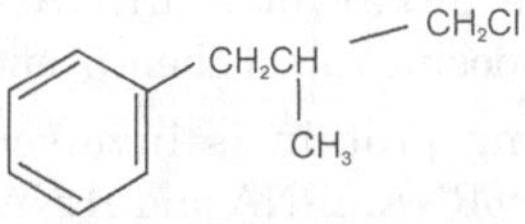

26. Compound (X) on treatment with hot acidic $KMnO_4$ followed by reaction with $LiAlH_4$ gives (Y). Compound (Y) is

(*a*) 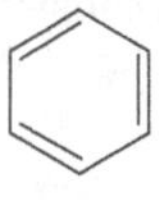 (*b*) 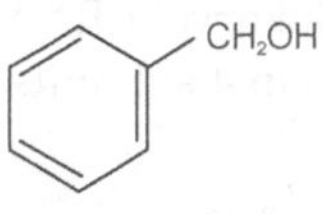

(*c*) 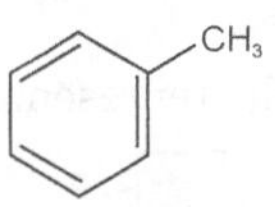 (*d*) 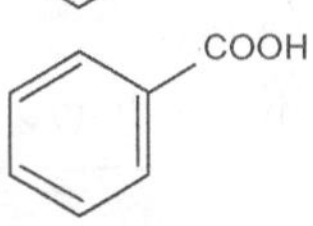

Statement for Linked Answer Questions 27 and 28:

Consider a cell:

Zn(*s*) | Zn^{2+} (*aq*) | | Cu^{2+}(*aq*) | Cu(*s*) operating at 298 K

[Given E° (Zn^{2+}/Zn) = – 0.763 and E° (Cu/Cu^{2+}) = – 0.337 V]

27. The emf of the cell ($E°_{cell}$) will be

(*a*) 1.100V (*b*) 0.426 V

(c) – 1.10 V (*d*) – 0.426 V

28. The value of log K for the cell reaction :

$Zn(s) + Cu^{2+}(aq) \rightleftharpoons Zn^{2+}(aq) + Cu(s)$ where K is the equilibrium constant will be

[Given R = 8.314 JK^{-1} mol^{-1}, F = 96,500 C mol^{-1}]

(*a*) 18.61 (*b*) 14.41 (*c*) – 14.41 (*d*) 37.22

I : BIOCHEMISTRY

Q. 1 – Q. 6 carry one mark each

1. Which of the following amino acids does NOT contribute to fluorescence of a protein?

(*a*) Tyrosine (*b*) Phenylalanine

(*c*) Cysteine (*d*) Tryptophan

2. Immunological memory is manifested during

(*a*) primary immune responses

(*b*) non-specific immune responses

(*c*) innate immune responses

(*d*) secondary immune responses

3. The main function of the pentose phosphate pathway is to

(*a*) supply ribose 5-phosphate and NADPH

(*b*) supply NADH and ATP

(*c*) provide a mechanism to use the carbon skeletons of excess amino acids

(*d*) provide carbon skeletons for oxidation of fatty acids

4. Which one of the following CANNOT be considered as a weak interaction?

(*a*) Van der Waals forces

(*b*) Peptide bonds

(*c*) Hydrogen bonds

(*d*) Ionic interaction

5. Polynucleotide kinase is used

(*a*) to add a nitrogenous base at the 5′ end of DNA

(*b*) to add a nitrogenous base at the 3′ end of DNA

(*c*) to add a phosphate at the 5′ end of DNA

(*d*) to add a phosphate at the 3′ end of DNA

6. The polymer shown below is a component of

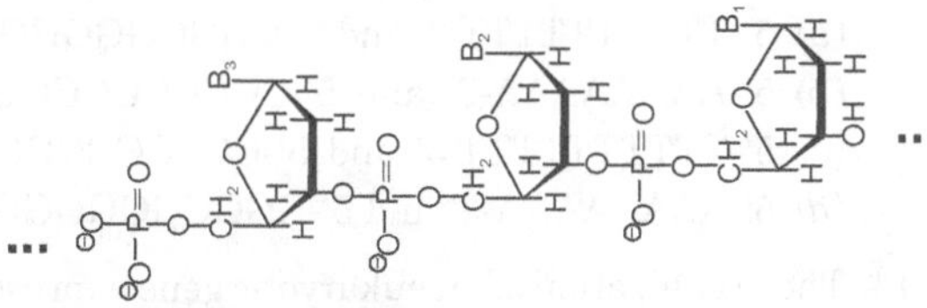

(*a*) polysaccharide

(*b*) polyribonucleotide

(*c*) polyketide

(*d*) polydeoxyribonucleotide

Q. 7 – Q. 24 carry two marks each

7. FOS, JUN and MYC are

(*a*) proteins expressed on the surface of cancerous cells

(*b*) protein kinases that phosphorylate transcription factors in cancerous cells

(*c*) proteins involved in regulation of expression of genes involved in growth promotion

(*d*) proteins involved in ion transport in cancerous cells

8. Using microarray technique it was demonstrated that when a mammalian cell line was exposed to a drug, the expression of 10 genes in increased. Which of the following pairs of techniques could be used to validate microarray data ?

(*a*) Southern blotting and polymerase chain reaction (PCR)

(*b*) Northern blotting and fluorescence *in situ* hybridization

(*c*) Southern blotting and reverse transcriptase (RT)-PCR

(*d*) Northern blotting and RT-PCR

9. Pepsin hydrolysis of IgG molecule will result in the production of

(*a*) one Fc fragment and one F(*ab*′)2 fragment

(*b*) one Fc fragment and one Fab fragments

(*c*) one Fc fragment and one Fab fragment

(*d*) one F (*ab*′) 2 fragment and one Fab fragment

10. Select the correct combination to fill in the blanks.

___are responsible for the production of antibody against free pathogens and soluble products from pathogens while_______destroy pathogen and virally infected cells and abnormal cells.

(*a*) Cytotoxic T cells and B cells

(*b*) Macrophages and T cells

(*c*) B cells and Helper T cells

(*d*) B cells and Cytotoxic T cells

11. Select the correct primer pair for the PCR amplification of the following DNA fragment:

5′-TTTTTTTTTTGTAACTCGTAGGCATT
GAACTATGCGGGGGGGGGG-3′

3′-AAAAAAAAAACATTGAGCCAGCATCC
GTAACTTGATACCCCCCCCCC-5′

(*a*) 5′-TTTTTTTTTT-3′ and 5′-GGGGGGGGGG-3′

(*b*) 5′-AAAAAAAA-3′ and 5′-CCCCCCCCCC-3′

(*c*) 5′-TTTTTTTTTT-3′ and 5′-CCCCCCCCCC-3′

(*d*) 5′-AAAAAAAA-3′ and 5′-GGGGGGGGGG-3′

12. The double-reciprocal transformation of the Michaelis-Menten equation, also called the Lineweaver-Burk plot, is given by

$I/V_0 = K_m/(V_{max}[S]) + 11/V_{max}$

To determine K_m from a double-reciprocal plot, you would

(*a*) take the reciprocal of the *y*-axis intercept

(*b*) take the reciprocal of the *x*-axis intercept

(*c*) multiply the reciprocal of the *x*-axis intercept by – 1

(*d*) multiply the reciprocal of the *y*-axis intercept by – 1

13. Which of the following statements is INCORRECT ?

(*a*) Most of the eukaryotic mRNAs have a 7-methylguanosine cap at their 5′ end

(*b*) TATA binding protein is involved in the synthesis of *m*RNA, *t*RNA and *r*RNA

(*c*) Histones have no other function except in chromatin organization

(*d*) Eukaryotic RNA polymerase II consists of more than 4 subunits

14. The organization of an eukaryotic gene expressed at high levels in liver is diagrammatically represented below:

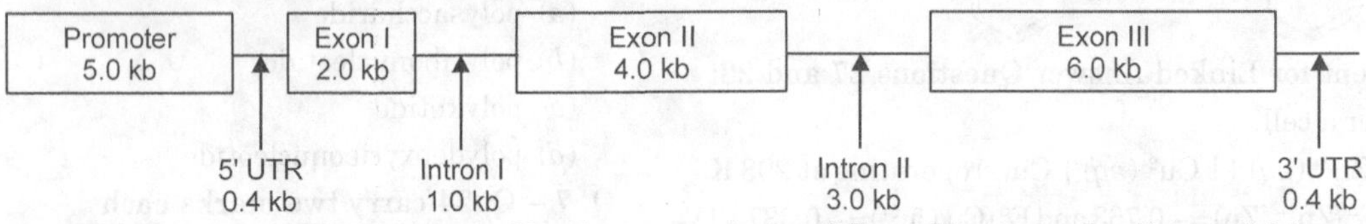

The size of the mature mRNA generated by the transcription followed by normal splicing of this gene will be (assume that this mRNA is not polyadenylated; 5′UTR and 3′UTR refer to the 5′ and 3′ untranslated regions, respectively)

(*a*) 12.4 kb (*b*) 13.0 kb (*c*) 12.0 kb (*d*) 12.6 kb

15. Incubation of a cell extract containing all enzymes of glycolysis with [γ-^{32}P] ATP and unlabeled inorganic phosphate results in the formation of which of the following labelled compounds (assume that pyruvate kinase is inactivated) ?

1. Glucose-6-^{32} Phosphate
2. (3–^{32}P)-Phosphoglycerate
3. (1-Phospho-3-^{32} Phospho) – Bisphosphog lycerate
4. (1-Phospho-6^{32} Phospho) – Fructose isphosphate

(*a*) 1 and 3 (*b*) 1, 2 and 3

(*c*) 2 and 4 (*d*) only 4

16. Electrophoresis of a purified protein named X in the presence of sodium dodecyl sulfate and 2-mercaptoethanol, shows a single band of 45 kDa. In gel filtration column chromatography, protein X elutes between alcohol dehydrogenase (160 kDa) and beta-amylase (190 kDa). How many identical subunits is protein X composed of?

(*a*) One (*b*) Two

(*c*) Three (*d*) Four

17. Identify the correct pairs for the primary functions of the different enzyme classes

P. Kinases	1. cleave bonds by elimination
Q. Lyases	2. make large molecules from small molecules
R. Synthases	3. transfer phosphate group to biomolecules
S. Phosphatases	4. remove phosphate group from biomolecules

	P	Q	R	S
(*a*)	4	2	3	1
(*b*)	3	1	2	4
(*c*)	4	1	2	3
(*d*)	3	2	1	4

18. Which of the following statements about the mitochondrial proton gradient and membrane potential is correct ?

(*a*) Either of them is sufficient to make ATP from ADP + Pi

(*b*) Both are required to make ATP

(*c*) Usually cancel one another since the system is at equilibrium

(*d*) Neither of them is required for ATP synthesis

19. The molecule shown is :

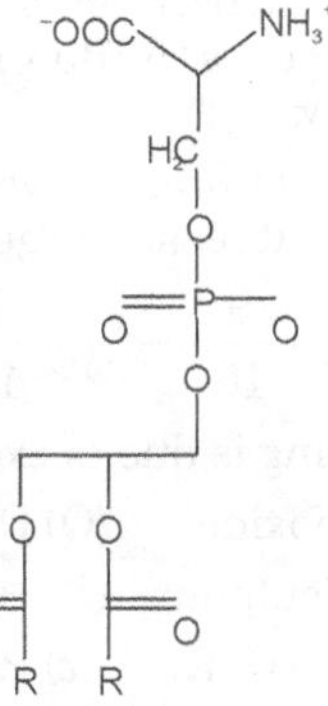

(*a*) Phosphatidylserine

(*b*) Phosphatidylcholine

(*c*) Phosphatidylethanolamine

(*d*) Phosphatidylinositol

20. Melting curve of two DNA specimens X and Y at the same pH and ionic strength have Tm values of 85°C and 80° C, respectively. This means that

(*a*) the AT content of Y is higher than X

(*b*) the GC content of Y is higher than X

(*c*) the AT content is same in X and Y

(*d*) the GC content of X is higher than Y

21. Part of the overall flow in amino acid catabo-lism is shown in the figure. Identify X and Y

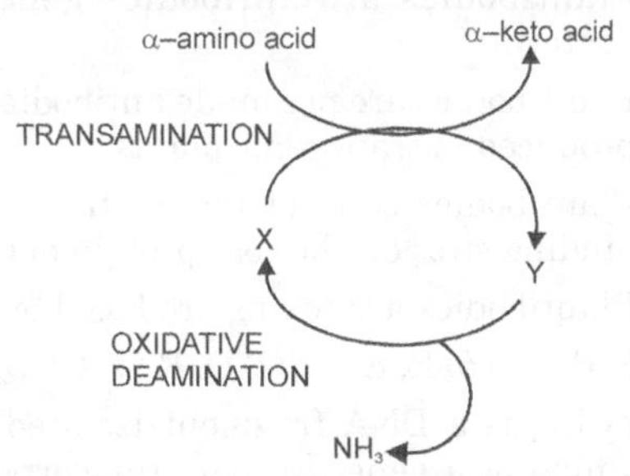

(*a*) X : L-Glutamate; Y: α-Ketoglutarate

(*b*) X : α-Ketoglutarate; Y: L-Glutamate

(*c*) X : α-Ketoglutamate; Y: L-Glutamine

(*d*) X : α-Ketoglutarate; Y:D-Glutamate

22. Which one of the following statements refers to glycogen, and which one refers to cellulose?

I. Branched molecule containing β-1, 4-glycosidic bond

II. Straight chain molecule containing β-1, 4-glycosidic bond

III. Branched molecule containing α-1, 6-glycosidic bond

IV. Straight chain molecule containing α-1, 6-glycosidic bond

(*a*) I = Glycogen; IV = Cellulose

(*b*) II = Glycogen; III = Cellulose

(*c*) III = Glycogen; II = Cellulose

(*d*) IV = Glycogen; I = Cellulose

Common Data Questions

Common Data for Questions 23, 24 :

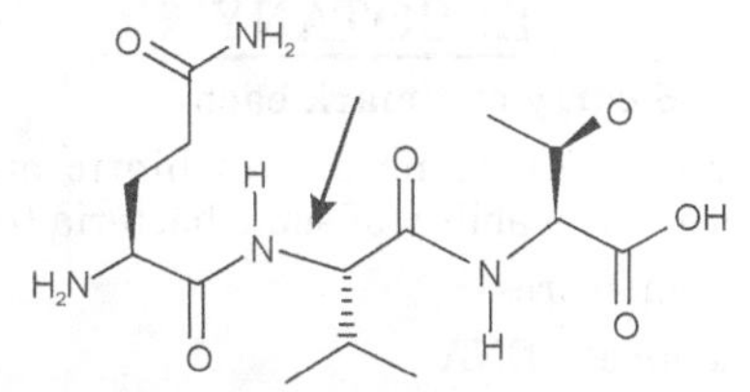

23. The dihedral angle indicated y an arrow in the tripeptide structure corresponds to the

(*a*) psi angle (*b*) phi angle

(*c*) chi angle (*d*) omega angle

24. The amino acid sequence of the above tripeptide is

(*a*) Glutamine-valine-threonine

(*b*) Asparagine-valine-serine

(*c*) Glutamine-leucine-threonine

(*d*) Asparagine-valine-threonine

Linked Answer Questions : Q.25 to Q.28 carry two marks each

Statement for Linked Answer Questions 25 and 26 :

Bind of glucagon to its receptor results in the generation of a specific second messenger.

25. Which of the following second messengers is generated in this case?

(*a*) Calcium

(*b*) cGMP

(*c*) Phosphatidylinositol

(*d*) cAMP

26. Which of the following enzymes is activated by this second messenger ?

(*a*) Protein kinase A (*b*) Protein kinase C

(*c*) Phospholipase C (*d*) Protein phosphatase 2A

Statement for Linked Answer Question 27 & 28:

The figure shows the oxygen binding curves for hemoglobin (Hb) and myoglobin (Mb).

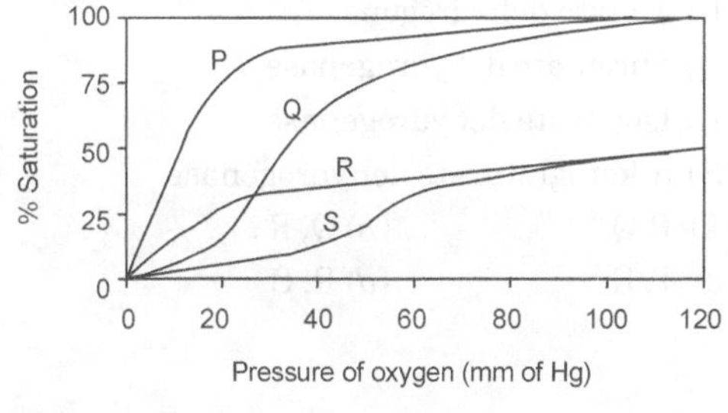

27. Identify the correct curves for Hb and Mb
(*a*) P : Mb; Q : Hb (*b*) Q : Mb; P : Hb
(*c*) R: Mb; Q : Hb (*d*) S : Mb; R: Hb

28. Sickle cell anemia arises due to the formation of a hydrophobic patch in one of the proteins shown in the above curves. This is due to the replacement of
(*a*) Glu 6 by Val 6 in the β subunit of P
(*b*) Glu 6 by Val 6 in the β subunit of Q
(*c*) Glu 6 by Val 6 in the β subunit of R
(*d*) Glu 6 by Val 6 in the β subunit of S

K: BOTANY

Q. 1 – Q. 6 carry one mark each

1. Penicillin functions as antibiotic mainly by inhibiting the ability of some bacteria to
(*a*) Form spores
(*b*) Replicate DNA
(*c*) Synthesize normal cell wall
(*d*) Produce functional ribosome

2. Glyoxylate cycle is used for generating
(*a*) Cyclic adenosine monophosphate
(*b*) Precursors for synthesis of aromatic amino acids
(*c*) 4-carbon intermediates when cells grow on acetate
(*d*) 4-carbon intermediates during growth on hexose

3. Agar-agar is produced by
(*a*) Gelidium, Garacilaria and Gigartina
(*b*) Lamanaria, Lessonia and Eisenia
(*c*) Gelidium, Batrachospermum and Polysiphonia
(*d*) Polysiphonia, Batrachospermum and Sargassum

4. Which of the following pair of tissues has cell walls thickened with lignin ?
(*a*) Collenchyma and cork
(*b*) Collenchyma and selerenchyma
(*c*) Sclerenchyma and cork
(*d*) Sclerenchyma and xylem

5. Identify the mismatched compound.
(*a*) Pectin (*b*) Gum (*c*) Cutin (*d*) Agar

6. The second law of thermodynamics is represented by
(*a*) Energy pyramid (*b*) Number pyramid
(*c*) Food pyramid (*d*) Biomass pyramid

Q. 7 – Q. 24 carry two marks each

7. In Krebs cycle which of the following enzyme reactions release CO_2?
(P) Malate dehydrogenase
(Q) Succinate dehydrogenase
(R) Isocitrate dehydrogenase
(S) α-ketoglutarate dehydrogenase
(*a*) P, Q (*b*) Q, R
(*c*) P, R (*d*) R, S

8. Which of the following statements are features of fasiculated root?
(P) An interesting tuberous root found in Asparagus
(Q) The adventitious roots occur in clusters and all are swollen
(R) It is fusiform with abrupt tapering towards the lower end
(S) The roots grow from the base of the plumules
(*a*) P, Q (*b*) Q, R (*c*) P, R (*d*) R, S

9. Consider a cross between plants heterozygous for two different genes (AaBb × AaBb), each assorting independently.
What fraction of progeny will show the recessive phenotype for at least one gene?
(*a*) $\frac{1}{16}$ (*b*) $\frac{9}{16}$ (*c*) $\frac{7}{16}$ (*d*) $\frac{3}{16}$

10. Global warming is due to excessive emission of
(P) Carbon dioxide (Q) Oxides of nitrogen
(R) Oxides of sulphur (S) Hydrogen sulphide
(*a*) P, Q (*b*) Q, R (*c*) P, R (*d*) Q, S

11. A disease free tomato plant was planted in soil contaminated with *Agrobacterium tumefaciens* harboring Ti plasmid that lacks VirA gene. Provided all other conditions are optimum for the bacterial infection, identify the appropriate consequence
(P) Octapine synthesis by the bacterium will enhance
(Q) Acetylsyringone receptor will not be synthesized
(R) The bacteria will fail to transfer the T DNA to the plant
(S) A fragmented T-DNA will be transferred to the tomato plant
(*a*) P, S (*b*) Q, S (*c*) P, R (*d*) Q, R

12. Identify the correct statements for plantibodies
(P) Plantibodies are antibodies generated by bacteria
(Q) Plantibodies are pre made antibodies that are produced in transgenic plants
(R) Plantibodies can not uncoat the calcium ion binding sites on the coat protein of the virus
(S) Plantibodies are toxins produced by plants
(*a*) P, R (*b*) R, S (*c*) Q, R (*d*) Q, S

13. Following is a DNA fragment isolated from the beginning of a gene. Identify the correct mRNA sequence with proper polarity.
DNA sequence:
-CCC TAC GCC TTT CAG GTT-
-GGG ATG CGG AAA GTC CAA-
(*a*) 3′AUG CGG AAA GUU CAA5′
(*b*) 5′ AUG CGG AAA GUC CAA3′
(*c*) 5′ UAC GCC UUU GUC CAA 3′
(*d*) 3′ UAC GC7C UUU GAG GAA 5′

14. Achyranthus aspera and Delphinium staphisagria belong to the following families

(*a*) Amarantheceae and Rutanceae

(*b*) Amarantheceae and Ranunculaceae

(*c*) Amarantheceae and Tiliaceae

(*d*) Tiliaceae and Ranunculaceae

15. Active transport of ions across the membrane of a root hair cell can be assumed to be taking place if

(P) The cell produces more glutathione

(Q) The cell has mitochondria

(R) The uptake of ions stop when cyanide is added

(S) The uptake of ions is against the concentration gradient

(*a*) P, R (*b*) R, S

(*c*) Q, R (*d*) Q, S

Q 16–22 are matching exercises

Choose the correct one from the alternatives *a*, *b*, *c* and *d*

16. Group I (*Plant disease*)

P Nigrospora disease of rice

Q Loose smut of wheat

R Ring spot of sugarcane

S Leaf blotch of wheat

Group II (*Causal organism*)

1. *Ustilago nuda*
2. *Cercospora concors*
3. *Septoria tritici*
4. *Pyricularia oryzae*
5. *Leptosphaeria sacchari*
6. *Nigrospora oryzae*

	P	Q	R	S
(*a*)	6	1	3	2
(*b*)	6	1	4	3
(*c*)	6	1	5	3
(*d*)	6	4	3	2

17.

Group I (*Fungal toxin*)	**Group II** (*Causal disease*)
P Tabtoxin	1. Canker
Q Phaseolotoxin	2. Leaf blight
R Tentotoxin	3. Chlorosis
S Hv toxin	4. Halo blight
	5. Wild fire
	6. Wheat rust

	P	Q	R	S
(*a*)	1	2	3	6
(*b*)	5	4	3	2
(*c*)	2	4	6	3
(*d*)	4	5	6	1

18. Identify the compounds from the given structure

Group I (*Structure*)

P **Q**

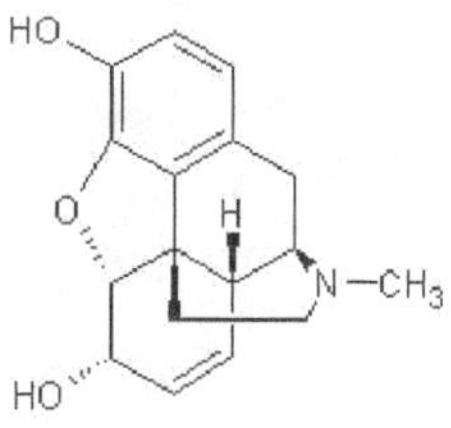

structure of morphine

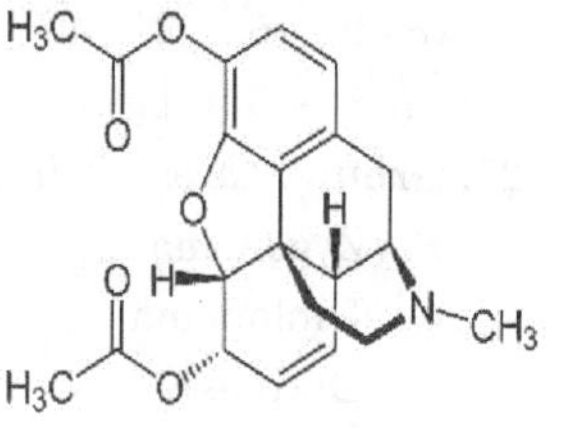

structure of heroin.

Group II (*Alkaloids*)

1. Morphine 2. Vincristine

3. Heroin 4. Cocain

	P	Q
(*a*)	1	2
(*b*)	4	3
(*c*)	3	1
(*d*)	1	3

19. Group I

P Filamentous fungi

Q Gram staining of bacteria

R Agarose gel

S Amino acid

Group II

1. Malachite green
2. Silver staining
3. Lactophenol-cotton blue
4. Crystal violet safranin
5. Ethidium bromide
6. Ninhydrin reagent

	P	Q	R	S
(*a*)	2	4	5	1
(*b*)	3	6	2	5
(*c*)	6	1	3	2
(*d*)	3	4	5	6

20. Group I

P Polysymbiosis

Q Helotism

R Mycobiont

S Crustose lichen

Group II

1. Algal component of a lichen
2. Fungal component of a lichen
3. Pendant forms
4. A combination of algae, fungi and nitrogen fixing bacteria in a lichen thallus
5. Lichen which form a crust closely adpressed to the substrate
6. A partnership between two organisms in which the association is decided at the expense of one

	P	Q	R	S
(*a*)	1	2	3	4
(*b*)	4	6	2	5
(*c*)	2	6	3	4
(*d*)	6	5	1	3

21. Group I (*Meiosis I*)

P Zygonema
Q Diplonema
R Dikinesis
S Metaphase I

Group II (*Event*)

1. Nucleolus and nuclear membrane
2. Replicated chromosomes become visible
3. Assembly of spindle completed
4. Chromatids become fully visible,
5. Homologous chromosomes pair, crossing over occurs
6. Homologous chromosomes pair

	P	Q	R	S
(*a*)	6	2	4	5
(*b*)	1	2	5	4
(*c*)	5	2	1	6
(*d*)	6	4	1	3

22. Group I (*Stress- induced biomolecules*) — **Group II** (*Stress*)

Group I	Group II
P Phytochelatin	1. Heat shock
Q Scytonemin	2. Phosphate limitation
R Proline	3. Carbon limitation
S Chaperonin	4. Metal stress
	5. UV radiation
	6. Osmotic stress

	P	Q	R	S
(*a*)	2	5	6	1
(*b*)	3	4	6	2
(*c*)	4	5	6	1
(*d*)	1	6	4	3

Common Data Questions

Common Data for Questions 23 and 24 :

Nucleotide composition of four molecules is given below :

Molecule	%A	%G	%T	%U	%C
P	33	17	33	0	17
Q	33	33	17	0	17
R	26	24	0	26	24
S	30	20	0	20	30

23. From the above table identify the single stranded RNA molecule

(*a*) P (*b*) Q (*c*) R (*d*) S

24. From the above data find out the double stranded nucleic acid molecule with the lowest T_m

(*a*) P (*b*) Q (*c*) R (*d*) S

Linked Answer Questions : Q 25 to Q. 28 carry two marks each

Statement for Linked Answer Questions 25 and 26 :

Sucrose and maltose are two disaccharides which have the glycosidic linkages and play important role in living system.

25. Which of the following combinations represent the correct structure of maltose and sucrose?

(*a*) O-α-D-glucopyranosyl-(1 → 4)-β-D-glucopyranose and
O-β-D-galactopyranosyl-(1 → 4)-β-D-glucopyranose

(*b*) O-β-D-fructofuranosyl-(2 → 1)-α-D-glucopyranoside and
O-β-D-galactopyranosyl-(1 → 4)-β-D-glucopyranose

(*c*) O-α-D-glucopyranosyl-(1 → 4)-β-D-glucopyranose and
O-α-D-glucopyranosyl-(1 → 2)-β-D-fructofuranoside

(*d*) O-α-D-glucopyranosyl-(1 → 6)-β-D-glucopyranose and
O-β-D- fructofuranosyl- (2 → 1)-α-D-glucopyranoside

26. From the above structure, identify the correct statement for the reducing sugars

(*a*) Maltose is a reducing sugar because the second glucose possesses anomeric carbon atom and its ring can open to give an aldehyde, and sucrose is nonreducing as it has anomeric hydroxyl of α-D glucose which is condensed with the anomeric hydroxyl of β-D-fructose

(*b*) Maltose is a non-reducing sugar as it has anomeric hydroxyl of α-D glucose which is condensed with β-D-fructose, and sucrose is non reducing because the second glucose possesses anomeric carbon atom and its ring can open to give an aldehyde

(*c*) Maltose and sucrose are insoluble in water and thus non-reducing

(*d*) The formation of a glycosidic bond is a condensation reaction in which water molecule is produced which makes the compound non-reducing

Statement for Linked Answer Questions 27 and 28 :

The plant Arabidopsis thaliana has five pairs of chromosomes AA, BB, CC, DD and EE and the plant is self fertilized.

27. Identify the correct chromosomal complement present in the root cells of the offspring

(*a*) ABCDE
(*b*) AAAA BBBB CCCC DDDD EEEE
(*c*) AA BB CC DD EE
(*d*) AAA BBB CCC DDD EEE

28. If the offsprings are selfed, identify the correct genotype of pollen mother cell of F_2 generation
(*a*) AAAA BBBB CCCC DDDD EEEE
(*b*) AA BB CC DD EE
(*c*) ABCDE
(*d*) AAA BBB CCC DDD EEE

L : MICROBIOLOGY

Q.1 – Q.6 carry one mark each

1. Which of the following scientists developed the modern concept of chemotherapy and chemotherapeutic agents ?
(*a*) Robert Koch (*b*) Paul Ehrlich
(*c*) Joseph Lister (*d*) Louis Pasteur

2. The refractive index of the immersion oil used in microscopy to achieve higher resolution is
(*a*) Same as glass (*b*) Less than air
(*c*) Less than glass (*d*) Same as air

3. Which of the following synthetic antibacterial compound inhibit supercoiling of bacterial DNA?
(*a*) Sulfonamide (*b*) p-Fluorophenyl alanine
(*c*) Puromycin (*d*) Rifampin

4. Which one of the following is not a lymphocyte?
(*a*) B-cell (*b*) T-cell (*c*) NK-cell (*d*) Mast-cell

5. Which of the following organism has a single stranded positive sense RNA genome?
(*a*) Influenza virus (*b*) Polio virus
(*c*) Hepatitis B virus (*d*) Pox virus

6. Cyanobacteria comprises a large and morphologically heterogenous group of
(*a*) Chemoautotrophs (*b*) Photoheterotrophs
(*c*) Photoautotrophs (*d*) Chemoheterotrophs

Q.7 – Q.24 carry two marks each.

7. In the peptidoglycan layer of bacterial cell wall, which of the following pair of aminoacids are usually found in D-configuration?
(*a*) Alanine and glutamic acid
(*b*) Alanine and lysine
(*c*) Alanine and arginine
(*d*) Glutamic acid and lysine

8. Which of the following inclusion bodies contains the enzymes responsible for carbon dioxide fixation in bacteria ?
(*a*) Lysosomes
(*b*) Peroxisomes
(*c*) Metachromatic granules
(*d*) Carboxysomes

9. When bacterial cells are placed in a 2 M NaCl solution, the plasmamembrane will
(*a*) Burst
(*b*) Undergo plasmolysis
(*c*) Remain unchanged
(*d*) Swell

10. Which of the following couple will have the maximum tendency to donate electrons? (Redox potentials are given in the parenthesis)
(*a*) $2H^+/H_2$ (–0.42V)
(*b*) $NAD^+/NADH$ (–0.32V)
(*c*) NO_3^-/NO_2^-(+0.42V)
(*d*) $\frac{1}{2}O_2/H_2O$(+0.82V)

11. Match the following group of microorganism with their oxygen requirements.

Group of microorganisms
P. Obligate aerobe
Q. Microacrophile
R. Obligate anaerobe
S. Aerotolerant anaerobe

Oxygen requirement
1. Grows equally well in presence or absence of oxygen
2. Grows only in presence of oxygen
3. Cannot tolerate oxygen
4. Can grow only at reduced oxygen levels

(*a*) P-3; Q-1; R-2; S-4 (*b*) P-4; Q-3; R-2; S-1
(*c*) P-2; Q-4; R-3; S-1 (*d*) P-1; Q-4; R-3; S-2

12. In which of the following cases of microbial growth, lag phase usually does not occur?
(*a*) If inoculum is taken from jole (stationary phase) culture and inoculated into same medium
(*b*) Inoculum consists of damaged cells (but not killed), inoculated into the same medium
(*c*) Inoculum is transferred from a rich culture medium to a poorer one
(*d*) If an exponentially growing culture is inoculated into the same medium under the same conditions of growth

13. Which one of the following statements is INCORRECT about bacterial endospore?
(*a*) Core pH is about 5.5 to 6.0
(*b*) Resistant to lysozyme
(*c*) Dipicolinic acid is present
(*d*) Small acid soluble protein is absent

14. The following reaction of glyoxylate cycle requires two enzymes P and Q

$$\text{Isocitrate} \xrightarrow{P} \text{succinate + glyoxylate}$$

$$\text{Glyoxylate + acetyl CoA} \xrightarrow{Q} \text{malate + CoA}$$

Which of the following combinations is the true representative of P and Q?
(*a*) Isocitrate lyase and malate synthase
(*b*) Isocitrate lyase and malated dehydrogenase
(*c*) Isocitrate dehydroxygenase and malate dehydrogenase
(*d*) Isocitrate dehydrogenase and malate synthase

15. Which of the frollowing statements is NOT included in Koch's postulate?
(*a*) A specific organism can always be found in association with a given disease
(*b*) The organism can be isolated and grown in pure cultures in the laboratory
(*c*) The pure culture will produce the disease when inoculated into susceptible animal
(*d*) It is possible to clone the genome of the organism from the experimentally infected animal

16. The commercially used technique for pasteurization of milk involves low temperature holding (LTH) and high temperature short time (HTST) methods. Which of the following methods is INCORRECT?
(*a*) expose milk to 145″ F for 30 min
(*b*) expose milk to 161″ F for.15 sec
(*c*) expose milk to 143″ F for 30 min
(*d*) expose milk to 71.7″ C for 15 sec

17. The phenomenon in which a prophage is able to make changes in the properties of a host bacterium in lysogeny is termed as
(*a*) Immunity repression
(*b*) Lysogenic induction
(*c*) Lysogenic conversion
(*d*) Lytic infection

18. Phage typing is frequently used in medical diagnosis for the identification of certain strains of pathogens, such as
(*a*) *Staphylococci*
(*b*) *Enteroviruses*
(*c*) *Plasmodium falciparum*
(*d*) *Leishmania donovani*

19. Which of the following virus needs a helper virus for their genome replication?
(*a*) Hepatitis A (*b*) Hepatitis D
(*c*) Hepatitis C (*d*) Hepatitis E

20. Which of the following viruses usually causes 'latent infection' in the human neuronal cells?
(*a*) Poliovirus
(*b*) Japanese Encephalitis virus
(*c*) Herpes simplex virus type I
(*d*) Rabies virus

21. Match the correct combination of toxin and the mode of action

Toxin
P. Pertussis toxin
Q. Diptheria toxin
R. Botulinum toxin
S. Tetanus toxin

Mode of action
1. Prevents release of glycine by nerve end
2. Blocks G-protein signal transduction
3. Induces fluid loss from intestinal cells
4. Inhibits protein synthesis in eukaryotes
5. Causes haemolysis
6. Blocks release of acetylcholin by nerve end

(*a*) P-3, Q-2, R-5, S-4 (*b*) P-2, Q-4, R-6, S-1
(*c*) P-5, Q-6, R-3, S-2 (*d*) P-1, Q-3, R-2, S-5

22. The following antibiotics affects the bacterial protein synthesis with their site of action. Which of the following combinations is correct?

Antibiotic	**Site of action**
P. Streptomycin	1. Aminoacyl tRNA association with ribosome
Q. Tetracyclin	2. Transpeptidation
R. Erythromycin	3. Translocation
S. Chloramphenicol	4. Initiation of protein synthesis

(*a*) P-2; Q-3; R-4; S-1 (*b*) P-4; Q-1; R-3; S-2
(*c*) P-1; Q-4; R-3; S-2 (*d*) P-4; Q-1; R-2; S-3

Common Data Questions

Common Data for Questions 23, 24 :

Besides the repression/derepression control of tryptophan! operon the second level of regulation is known as attenuation. The presence of two tryptophan condons within the trpL controls this phenomenon. The presence of tryptophan-charged $tRNA_{trp}$ causes the premature termination of transcription, yields a 140 nucleotide long leader sequence transcript. By sitedirected mutagenesis the two UGG Trp condons of the trpL sequence were modified to CGG, arginine codon (arg).

23. Which of the following amino acid (*s*) would be able to restore the attenuation control of *trp* operon?
(*a*) Tryptophan alone
(*b*) Arginine alone
(*c*) Tryptophan or arginine
(*d*) Neither arginine nor tryptophan

24. Deletion of part of the *trpL* region will result in
(*a*) Increase in the rate of expression of '*trp*' structural genes
(*b*) Decrease in the rate of expression of '*trp*' structural genes
(*c*) No change in the rate of expression of '*trp*' structural genes
(*d*) Inhibition of the expression of all the genes in the operon

Linked Answere Questions : Q.25 to Q.28 carry two marks each

Statement for Linked Answer Questions 25 and 26 :

The nucleic acid from a microorganism was isolated and the base composition was determined to be as follows:

A = 35%, T = 15%, G = 35%, C = 15%

25. What could be the physical nature of the nucleic acid?
(*a*) Double stranded circular DNA
(*b*) Double stranded linear DNA
(*c*) Single stranded linear DNA
(*d*) Single stranded RNA

26. The optical density of the above nucleic acid was measured at 260 nm wavelength at 37°C and 95°C. What possible changes could you expect in the optical density with the increase in temperature?
(*a*) Significant increase
(*b*) Only two fold increase
(*c*) Significant decrease
(*d*) No significant change

Statement for Linked Answer Questions 27 & 28:

In a bacterial culture initial cell population is 1×10^3 cells. The generation time of the bacterial cell is 20 minutes and the lag phase is 1 hour.

27. If the culture is allowed to grow for 4 hours, then how many generations would take place?
(*a*) 8 (*b*) 12 (*c*) 10 (*d*) 9

28. What will be the cell population after 3 hours?
(*a*) 6.4×10^6 (*b*) 3.2×10^4
(*c*) 3.2×10^6 (*d*) 6.4×10^4

M : ZOOLOGY

Q. 1 – Q. 6 carry one mark each

1. Which one of the following statements about amino acids is true?
(*a*) All amino acids can form hydrogen bonds
(*b*) Only hydrophilic amino acids can form hydrogen bonds
(*c*) Hydrophobic amino acids cannot form hydrogen bonds
(*d*) Amino acids in general do not participate in hydrogen bonds

2. Biological membranes control flow of information between cells and their environment. Which of the following attributes is true for biological membranes?
(*a*) Symmetric
(*b*) Covalent assemblies
(*c*) Fluid structures
(*d*) Electrically depolarized

3. A "leader sequence" in an mRNA of eukaryotes can be found
(*a*) after the "stop" codon
(*b*) between transcriptional start site and translational start site
(*c*) within the first exon
(*d*) in the exon-intron boundaries

4. Most cells are so small and the constraint in the size could be
(*a*) due to the surface-to-volume ratio
(*b*) that the flow of nutrients in larger cells will be much faster and therefore can not be controlled
(*c*) that larger cells might move materials too fast through cytoplasm, leading to inefficient functioning
(*d*) to prevent contacting other cells

5. Which of the following is a population?
(*a*) A spider and flies trapped in its web
(*b*) All the plants that live near each other in a forest
(*c*) The earthworms that live in a grassland plus the earthworm that live in a forest
(*d*) All the sandalwood trees in a forest

6. Which of the following cells are part of the nonspecific, second line of defense?
(*a*) Cytotoxic T cells (*b*) B cells
(*c*) Prostaglandins (*d*) Macrophages

Q. 7 – 24 carry two marks each

7. Mammalian hair evolved from the scales of reptiles. On the other hand, the "hair" on many insects, such as bees, has a completely different origin. These facts mean that the hair of mammals and the hair of insects are
(*a*) congruent structures
(*b*) homologous structures
(*c*) heterologous structures
(*d*) analogous structures

8. Rhodopsin is a transmembrane protein belonging to the large family of G Proteincoupled receptors. It is found in the discs of rod cells of human retina. Activation of rhodopsin is due to
(*a*) phosphorylation of its extracellular tyrosine residue
(*b*) binding of external ligands to its extracellular loops
(*c*) photoisomerization of its prosthetic group
(*d*) binding of calcium ions to its transmembrane aspartic groups

9. In an equilibrium population, thousands of eggs and hundreds of tadpoles are produced by single pair of frogs. On average, about how many offspring per pair will live to reproduce in the next season?
(*a*) 0 (*b*) 2
(*c*) 10 to 20 (*d*) above 100

10. A man is admitted to the hospital suffering from an abnormally low body temperature, loss of appetite, and extreme thirst. A brain scan shows a tumor located in the
(*a*) hypothalamus
(*b*) cerebellum
(*c*) pons
(*d*) right cerebral hemisphere

11. The British geneticist, J.B.S. Haldane, once jokingly said that he would lay down his life for two brothers or eight cousins. In terms of altruistic behavior, Haldane would do this because
(*a*) either two brothers or eight cousins would result in as much representation of Haldane's genes as would two of his own offsprings
(*b*) Haldane's death would enhance the fitness of his brothers and cousins
(*c*) Haldane loved his brothers and cousins
(*d*) none of the above mentioned statements reflect altruistic behavior

12. An unwound DNA and a supercoiled DNA with the same linking number are

(*a*) topologically and geometrically identical
(*b*) topologically and geometrically different
(*c*) topologically identical but geometrically different
(*d*) topologically different buy geometrically identical

13. Evolution is often referred to as speciation. Which is the most correct statement with respect to speciation?

(*a*) Inheritance of the gene pool from one generation to the other
(*b*) Origin of new character in a group of geographically isolated individuals
(*c*) rigin of distinct physical identities amongst races which are located in different geographical locations
(*d*) Origin of reproductive isolation amongst the races of a given species

14. Modern day giraffes are believed to have descended from predecessors with shorter necks. Darwinian theory of survival of fittest would mean the following (select the most likely explanation)

(*a*) Giraffes with longer necks were stronger and therefore they out-populated those with shorter necks
(*b*) Long-necked giraffes foraged better and therefore survived better than those with shorter necks
(*c*) Long-necked giraffes bred more than those with shorter necks
(*d*) During certain physical calamity all the short-necked giraffes perished from the face of the earth

15. Which one of the following choices does NOT correctly pair a biome with some of its characteristics?

(*a*) Temperate deciduous forest: Cold winters moderate to high rainfall
(*b*) Grassland: cool to cold winters, dry summers
(*c*) Taiga: Very cold winters, short growing seasons
(*d*) Savanna: long, cold winters, summer thaws of only the upper layers of soil

16. Uric acid is the nitrogenous waste by birds, insects, and many reptiles. An advantage of excreting uric acid is that it....., but a disadvantage is that it ....

(*a*) saves water.............costs energy
(*b*) saves energy.............is highly toxic
(*c*) is not very toxic......wastes a lot of water
(*d*) saves water...........is highly toxic

17. In animal behavior, the term "imprinting" implies

(*a*) Innate behavior of a given animal which is genetically determined
(*b*) Learned behavior which the animals display during various stages of its life
(*c*) A time-dependent form of learning behavior by exposure to sign stimulus
(*d*) None of the above

18. In a series of immune system experiments, the thymus glands were removed from new born mice. Which of the following would you predict as a likely result?

(*a*) The mice suffered from numerous allergies
(*b*) The mice never developed cancerous tumors
(*c*) The mice suffered from autoimmune diseases
(*d*) The mice readily accepted tissue transplants

19. After eutrophication due to sewage contamination, a lake often becomes inhospitable to fish. Why?

(*a*) Sewage input to a lake reduces the penetration of light into the lake, which results in the death of all the fish
(*b*) Sewage is rich in nutrient and hence results in the explosive growth of algal and cyanobacterial populations. This reduces the penetration of light into the lake, which results in the death of all the fish
(*c*) Sewage input to a lake causes explosive growth of algal and cyanobacterial populations. Bacterial decomposition of dead algae and cyanobacteria results in the depletion of oxygen in the water, which leads to the death of all the fish
(*d*) Sewage input causes the death of algae and cyanobacteria, which eventually reduces the availability of food for fish within the lake

20. A baby is born with the normal number and distribution of rods, but no cones in his eyes. We would expect that the baby's vision would be

(*a*) color-blind, easily blinded by bright light, and capable only of coarse resolving power
(*b*) normal on the left side of the visual field but blurred and gray on the right side
(*c*) normal on the right side of the visual field but totally blind on the left side
(*d*) the baby would be totally blind

21. When body temperature is too......., ... helps to correct the situation because it..........

(*a*) high...........peripheral vasodilation ....dissipates heat at the surface
(*b*) high........sweating.... lowers the metabolic rate by dumping toxic ions
(*c*) low......shivering.....lowers the metabolic rate and conserves blood sugar
(*d*) low.....peripheral vasodilation .... conserves heat in the inner body

22. Blastomeres derived from early stages of cleavage divisions (say second cleavage division) of frog embryo, when separated, can give rise to viable tadpoles. The blastomeres derived from late cleavage stages, however, fail to develop into normal tadpoles when separated from each other. Which is the most correct statement that explains the phenomenon?

(a) Each early blastomere carries the entire genetic information for the development of a tadpole

(b) Each early blastomere carries the entire cytoplasmic constituents necessary for development

(c) Early blastomeres are mirror images of each other

(d) None of the above

Common Data Questions

Common Data for Questions 23, 24:

A major breakthrough in animal science research was achieved when the sheep "Dolly" was born to a foster mother. This represents the first case of cloning in mammals.

23. Dolly was a replica of one of its parents because

(a) She received mitochondrial DNA from the foster mother

(b) she was born out of asexual reproduction

(c) she received entire genetic complement from one of her parents

(d) she completely resembled one of her parents

24. Dolly, however, was distinct from her cousin, a transgenic sheep, due to one of the following reasons

(a) Dolly received stem cells from her parents while her transgenic cousin received only specific gene(s)

(b) Dolly was genetically identical to the donor parent while her transgenic cousin was not

(c) Dolly phenotypically resembled her donor parent while her transgenic cousin did not

(d) None of the above

Linked Answer questions: Q. 25 to Q. 28 carry two marks each

Statement for Linked Answer Questions 25 & 26:

Hormones coordinate the menstrual and ovarian cycles in human females in such a way that growth of the follicle and ovulation are synchronized with the preparation of the uterine lining for possible implantation of an embryo. Five hormones participate in an elaborate scheme, involving both positive and negative feed-back controls.

25. The five critical hormones involved in the menstrual and ovarian cycles are

(a) GnRH, FSH, LH, estrogen and progesterone

(b) Prolactin, FSH, LH, MIS and androgen

(c) Prolactin, FSH, LH, progesterone and oxytocin

(d) GnRH, FSH, LH, estrogen and prolactin

26. Which one of the following statements is correct in explaining the feed-back control mechanisms regulating the reproductive cycles in human female?

(a) Whereas a slow rise of progesterone inhibits the secretion of FSH and LH, high concentrations of progesterone have the opposite effect and stimulate the secretion of FSH and LH from the anterior pituitary

(b) Whereas a slow rise of estrogen inhibits the secretion of pituitary gonadotropins, high concentrations of estrogen have the opposite effect and stimulates the secretion of gonadotropins by acting on the hypothalamus to increase its output of GnRH

(c) Whereas the slow rise of GnRH stimulates the release of LH and FSH, high concentrations of GnRH have the opposite effect and stimulates the secretion of LH and FSH

(d) Whereas the lower concentration of prolactin inhibits the secretion of estrogen, higher concentrations of prolactin have opposite effect and stimulates the release of estrogen

Statement for Linked Answer Questions 27 & 28:

In the fruit fly, *Drosophila* cinnabar and brown refer to two mutant eye colorations in the adult eye which are otherwise dark brown in the wild type flies. In a genetic cross, mutant male flies with cinnabar eye color were mated with females with brown eye color. Following results were seen in F1 and F2 progeny: all F1 flies displayed wild type eye color while of the 465 F2 progeny derived by intercross of F1 progeny, 274 were wild type, 85 were cinnabar, 95 were brown and finally, 11 flies displayed no eye color (white-eyed).

27. F1 progeny display wild type eye color due to

(a) additive effect of two mutations: each mutant version being only part of the wild type eye color

(b) complementation between the two mutations since they represent two separate genes

(c) lack of complementation between the two mutations since they are on the same eye coloration gene

(d) because these mutation represent two different genes which recombine in the progeny

28. What explains the origin of the new eye phenotype (no eye color – white) in the F2 progeny?

(a) Genes, mutated in flies showing brown and cinnabar eye colors, are linked

(b) These two genes (represented by cinnabar and brown eye colorations) DO NOT display dihybrid ratio

(c) The flies displaying no eye color (white) are actually mutant for both cinnabar and brown eye coloration genes

(d) Genes mutated for brown and cinnabar eye colorations display segregation distortion

ANSWERS

H : CHEMISTRY

1. (*c*)	2. (*d*)	3. (*a*)	4. (*c*)	5. (*b*)	6. (*a*)	7. (*b*)	8. (*c*)	9. (*a*)	10. (*d*)
11. (*c*)	12. (*c*)	13. (*a*)	14. (*d*)	15. (*d*)	16. (*d*)	17. (*b*)	18. (*c*)	19. (*b*)	20. (*b*)
21. (*a*)	22. (*b*)	23. (*c*)	24. (*b*)	25. (*c*)	26. (*b*)	27. (*a*)	28. (*d*)		

I : BIOCHEMISTRY

1. (*c*)	2. (*d*)	3. (*a*)	4. (*d*)	5. (*c*)	6. (*b*)	7. (*c*)	8. (*d*)	9. (*a*)	10. (*d*)
11. (*c*)	12. (*c*)	13. (*c*)	14. (*b*)	15. (*b*)	16. (*d*)	17. (*b*)	18. (*b*)	19. (*a*)	20. (*d*)
21. (*b*)	22. (*c*)	23. (*b*)	24. (*a*)	25. (*d*)	26. (*a*)	27. (*a*)	28. (*b*)		

K : BOTANY

1. (*c*)	2. (*c*)	3. (*a*)	4. (*d*)	5. (*c*)	6. (*a*)	7. (*d*)	8. (*a*)	9. (*c*)	10. (*)
11. (*d*)	12. (*c*)	13. (*)	14. (*b*)	15. (*d*)	16. (*c*)	17. (*b*)	18. (*d*)	19. (*d*)	20. (*b*)
21. (*d*)	22. (*c*)	23. (*d*)	24. (*a*)	25. (*)	26. (*)	27. (*)	28. (*)		

L : MICROBIOLOGY

1. (*b*)	2. (*a*)	3. (*a*)	4. (*d*)	5. (*b*)	6. (*c*)	7. (*a*)	8. (*d*)	9. (*b*)	10. (*a*)
11. (*c*)	12. (*d*)	13. (*d*)	14. (*a*)	15. (*d*)	16. (*c*)	17. (*c*)	18. (*a*)	19. (*b*)	20. (*c*)
21. (*b*)	22. (*b*)	23. (*b*)	24. (*a*)	25. (*b*)	26. (*c*)	27. (*d*)	28. (*d*)		

M : ZOOLOGY

1. (*a*)	2. (*c*)	3. (*c*)	4. (*a*)	5. (*d*)	6. (*a*)	7. (*d*)	8. (*c*)	9. (*c*)	10. (*a*)
11. (*a*)	12. (*c*)	13. (*d*)	14. (*b*)	15. (*d*)	16. (*a*)	17. (*b*)	18. (*d*)	19. (*c*)	20. (*a*)
21. (*a*)	22. (*b*)	23. (*c*)	24. (*b*)	25. (*a*)	26. (*c*)	27. (*b*)	28. (*c*)		

EXPLANATIONS

(H) CHEMISTRY

1. Work done (W) is not a state function. Work can't be a state function because it is proportional to the distance an object is moved, which depends on the path used to go from the initial to the final state.

2. The statement which describes uncertainty principle is that it is impossible to simultaneously determine the position and momentum of an object with certainty. As according to Heisenberg uncertainty principle the position and momentum of a particle cannot be simultaneously measured with arbitrarily high precision.

3. SF_6 is the most stable halogen containing compound of sulphur because it is insoluble in water and is inert. Also it has colorless and odorless properties and is a non- flammable gas.

4. The nucleophile among the following is $(CH_3)_3N$ because it has a lone pair of electrons and species with lone pairs of electrons tend to be nucleophiles because they have extra electrons which are attracted to positive charges.

5. The reaction is:

$$A + B \rightarrow \text{Products}$$

Given, rate of reaction increases by a factor of 4 if concentration of A is doubled and no remains unaltered if concentration of B is doubled.

Therefore, $[A] = 2[A]$ and $r' = 4r$

Let the order of reaction with respect to A and B be *a* and *b*.

Therefore according to the rate law,

$$r = k[A]^a[B]^b$$

Putting values of [A] and *r'* in the above equation,

$$4r = k\,(2[A])^a[B]^b$$

Therefore on solving we get,

$$4 = (2)^a$$

$$(2)^2 = (2)^a$$

Therefore $a = 2.$

And on solving $[B'] = 2[B]$ and $r' = r$, we get, $B = 0$

Therefore the order of reaction with respect to A and B is 2 and 0.

6. The major product (X) of the reaction $BrCH_2\text{-}CH_2Br \rightarrow$ is :

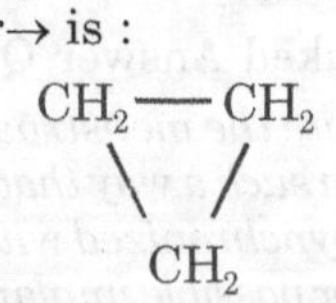

Thus (X) is a Cyclopropane which is formed by reduction of $ZnBr_2$ from $Be\text{-}CH_2\text{-}CH_2\text{-}CH_2Br$.

7. Born Haber Cycle for determining the lattice enthalpy of NaI is given as follows:

$Na\ (s) \rightarrow Na\ (g)\ (\Delta H_{sub}) \rightarrow Na^+\ (g)$

$I_2\ (s) \rightarrow I_2\ (g) \rightarrow \frac{1}{2} I_2\ (g)\ (\Delta H_{diss}) \rightarrow I^-\ (g)$

$Na^+\ (g) + I^-\ (g) \rightarrow Na^+ I^-$

Also, $I_2\ (s) \rightarrow Na^+ I^-\ (\Delta H_\ )$

Therefore the step $Na\ (s) \rightarrow Na\ (l)$ is not present in the Born Haber cycle of NaI.

8. Given, boiling point of pure benzene = 80.0°C
After addition of benzoic acid, boiling point increased to 82.5°C
Ebullioscopic constant (K_b) = 2.5 K-kg/mol.
We know,
$$\Delta T_b = K_b * m$$
Where m = molality
Therefore $$m = \frac{\Delta T_b}{K_b}$$
$$= \frac{2.5}{2.5} = 1$$
Therefore molality (m) of the solution is 1.00 kg/mol.

9. The structure of XeO_2F_2 based on VSEPR theory is best described as see- saw structure with the O-Xe-O angle close to 120°. The XeO_2F_2 molecule uses sp3d type of Xe hybrid orbitals for sigma bonding because Xe forms 2 double bonds between the oxygen's and 2 single bonds between the F's and there's also a lone pair left on the Xe atom. Also the structure of XeO_2F_2 is trigonal bipyramidal because it has one lone pair at equatorial position and has a see- saw geometry.

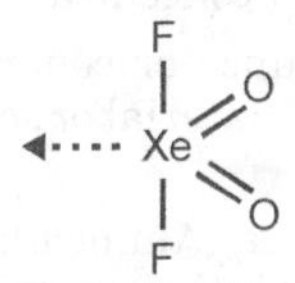

XeO_2F_2

10. The hydrolysis of PCl_3 would yield phosphorous acid (H_3PO_3). While PCl_5, $POCl_3$ and P_4O_{10} would yield phosphoric acid (H_3PO_4).
The reaction is as follows:
$PCl_3 + 3H_2O \rightarrow H_3PO_3$ (phosphorous acid) + 3HCl

11. The hybridization of $Cr(CO)_6$ is d^2sp^3. Carbonyl (CO) is a strong field ligand so it will cause octahedral splitting. So the electrons will pair up. 6 hybrid orbitals are required to form 6 sigma bonds n thus d^2sp^3.

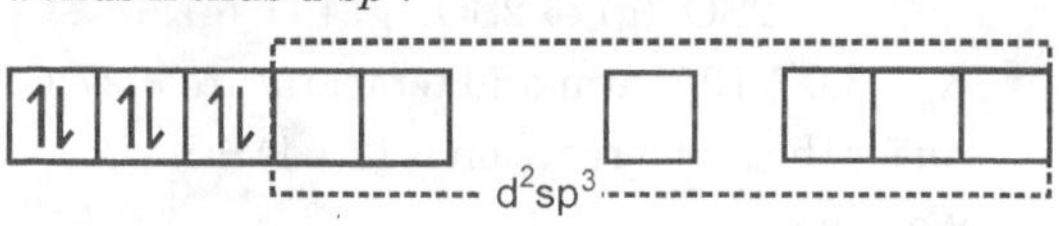

The hybridization of $[CrF_6]^{3-}$ is d^2sp^3 as Cr in $[CrF_6]^{3-}$ is present as Cr^{3+}.
Therefore, $[CrF_6]^{3-}$ = [Ar]

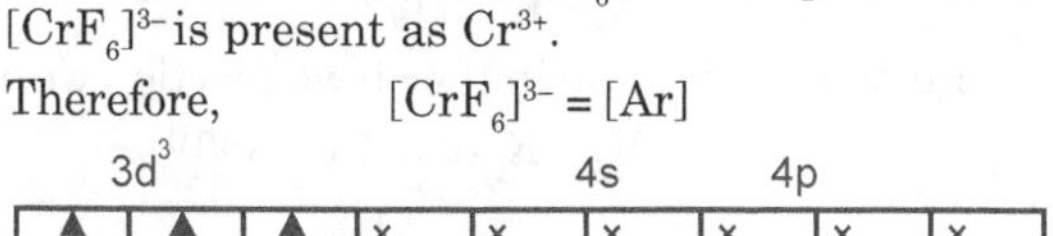

12. NO^- has the lowest bond dissociation energy among NO, NO^+ and N_2 because its bond order (B.O) is the lowest among the four. As lower bond order is directly proportional to lower bond energy.
B.O can be calculated as= $N_b - \frac{N_a}{2}$.
For, NO^- B.O is 10-6/2 = 2. While B.O of NO is 2.5, of NO^+ is 3.

13. Given, ionic radii of metal ion = 0.64Å
Ionic radii of F^- = 1.34 Å
Ionic radii of Cl^- = 1.81 Å
Therefore, the geometry of metal complex formed for F^- is:
$$\frac{r^+}{r^-} = \frac{0.64}{1.34} = 0.4776.$$
The geometry of metal complex formed for Cl^- is:
$$\frac{r^+}{r^-} = \frac{0.64}{1.81} = 0.3536.$$
Therefore the geometry of the metal complex formed for F^- is $[MF_6]^{3-}$ and octahedral and for Cl^- is $[MCl_4]^-$ and tetrahedral, as suggested by the radius ratio. Because the range of radius between 0.255 to 0.414 is indicative of tetrahedral geometry and between 0.414 to 0.732 is indicative of octahedral geometry.

14. The reagent requiired for the conversion of:

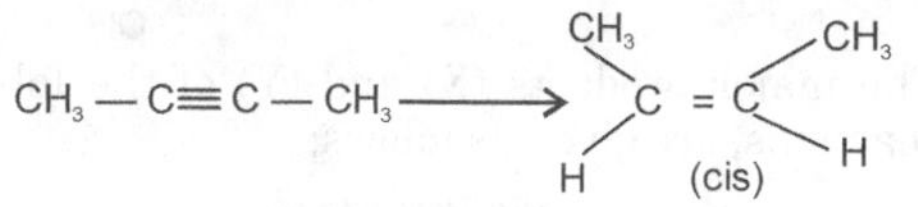

is Pd/$BaSO_4$/Quinoline.
As when alkyne is treated with hydrogen in the presence of Pd and then $BaSO_4$ and partially poisoned quinoline, then only cis-alkene is obtained. The partially poisoned quinoline is known as Lindlar's catalyst.
Therefore, the reaction is

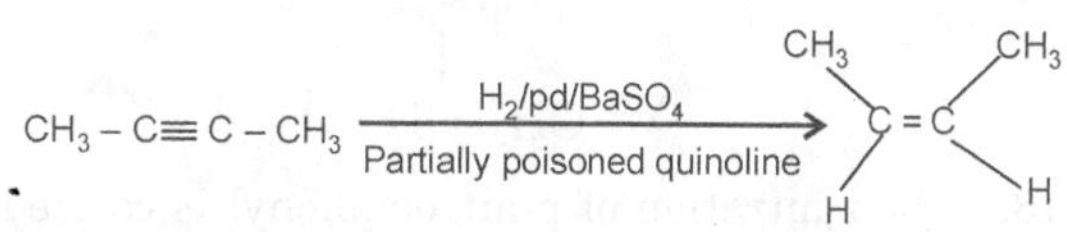

15. The Diels-Alder reaction is an organic chemical reaction between a conjugated diene and a substituted alkene, to form a substituted cyclohexene system. By using Diel's-Alder reaction, the reactants used for the synthesis of

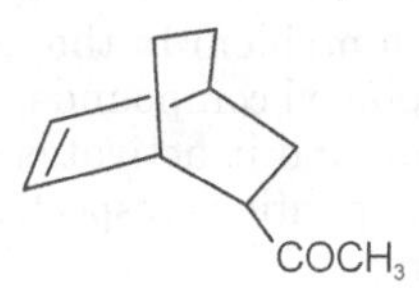

are given in the reaction:

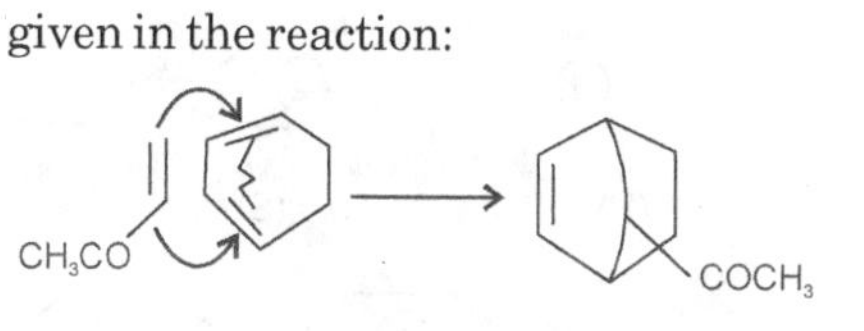

Or

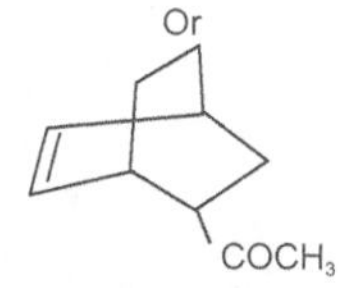

∴ the reactants are:

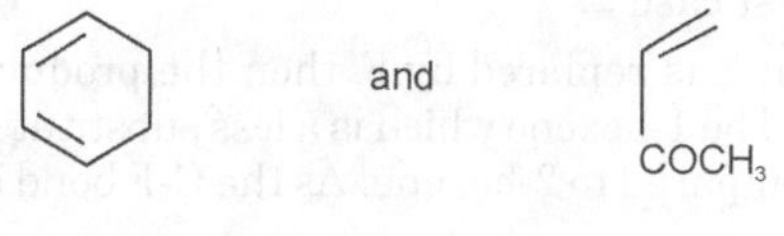

16. The correctly matched values of Ka with substituted benzoic acid is given as:

P.	P-NO_2	–	X.	36×10^{-5}
Q.	P-OH	–	Z.	2.6×10^{-5}
R.	P-Cl	–	Y.	10×10^{-5}

As acidity in the substituted (h) benzoic acid is directly proportional to Ka.

i.e., Acidity α Ka

The compound P-NO_2 shows both-I and – R effect which increases the acidic character. While P – OH and P – Cl show + R and –I effect, thus decreases the acidic strength of benzoic acid. So, order of reactivity is as follows:

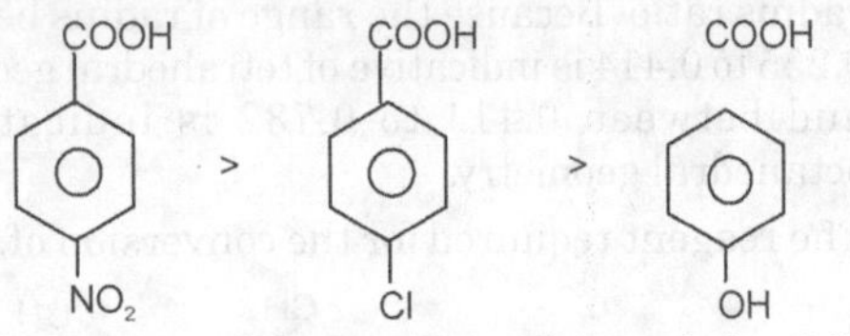

17. The major products (X) and (Y) of the following reactions, are given as folows:

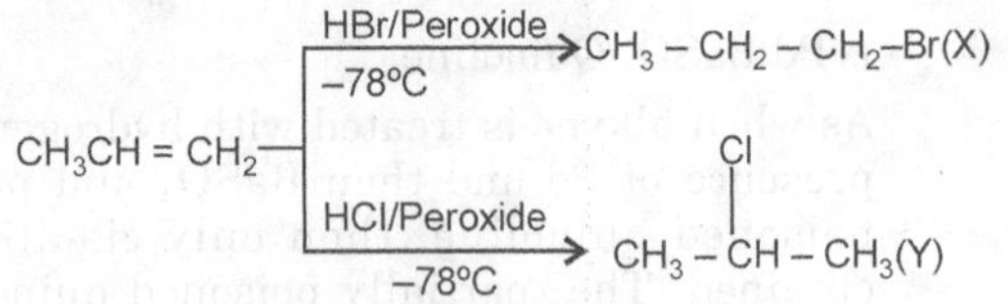

∴ $X = CH_3–CH_2CH_2–Br$

$$Y = CH_3–\underset{|}{\overset{Cl}{C}}H–CH_3$$

18. When nitration of p-nitrobiphenyl is carried out, then the new nitro group would introduce at positions. R and T. As when nitro (–NO_2) group is introduced in the biphenyl compound, then it deactivates the Ist ring as it is an electron with drawing group.

∴ it creates a problem in the activation of other ring. As in biphenyl compounds, one ring acts as a donating group and it activates the other ring at ortho and para–positions respectively. The following reaction occurs:

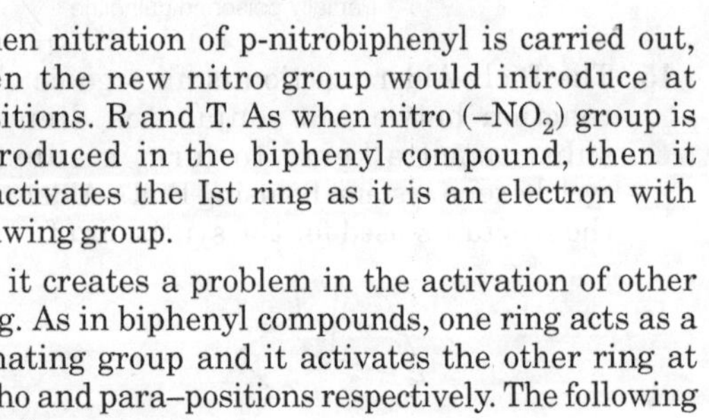

19. In first case ⇒

When X is replaced by F, then the product formed would be 1-hexene which is a less substituted alkene as compared to 2-hexene. As the C-F bond energy is much higher than the C-Br bond energy, so it favours the formation of a less substituted alkene.

The reaction is:

$$CH_3-(CH_2)_3-\underset{\underset{F}{|}}{C}HCH_3 \xrightarrow[CH_3OH]{CH_3O^-} CH_3-(CH_2)_3-CH=CH_2 \text{ (1–Hexone)}$$

In second case ⇒

When X is replaced by Br, then the product formed would be 2-hexene which is a more substituted alkene. Here, the CH_3O^- group is non-bulky so it favours the formation of a more substituted alkene.

The reaction is:

$$CH_3-(CH_2)_3-\underset{\underset{Br}{|}}{C}HCH_3 \xrightarrow[CH_3OH]{CH_3O^-} CH_3-(CH_2)_2CH=CHCH_3 \text{ (2–Hexone)}$$

20. Henderson's equation can be represented as:

$$pH = pKa + \log \frac{[salt]}{[acid]}$$

It can also be written as:

$$pH = pK_a + \log \left(\frac{[A^-]}{[HA]}\right)$$

Where $[A^-]$ = molar concentration of a conjugate base.

21. Specific conductance or conductivity (κ): It is the conductance of a material or solution occupying one cm^3 volume.

Molar conductance (Λm or μ): The conductance of that volume of solution containing one mole of an electrolyte is known as molar conductivity. It is denoted by Λm or μ.

The relation between equivalent conductance, Λ and molar conductance, μ can be given by:

μ = Λ × equivalent factor of the electrolyte.

Therefore when the solution is diluted then specific conductance decreases as number of current carrying particles per cm^3 decreases. So, molar conductance increases.

22. Given reaction is:

$$2SO_3\,(g) \leftrightarrow 2SO_2\,(g) + O_2\,(g)$$

$K_p = 3.0 * 10^{-23}$ atm and temperature = 27°C.

Δn for the given reaction is (2 + 1) = 3.

We know,

$$K_p = K_c\,(RT)^{\Delta n}$$

Putting value of Δn in the above reaction we get,

$$K_p = K_c\,(0.0821 * 300)^1$$

Therefore, $K_c = 3.0 * \frac{10^{-23}}{0.0821} * 300$

$$= 1.2 * 10^{-24} = 12 * 10^{-25}\ mol/dm^3.$$

23. The number of unpaired electrons present in the complex is 4. As when $KMnO_4$ reacts with oxalic acid in the presence of excess H_2SO_4 a complex of manganese (III) oxalate is formed.

The reaction I as follows:

$MnO^-_4 + (COOH)_2 \rightarrow [Mn(ox)_3]^{3-}$

(manganese (III) oxalate)

Here in this complex Mn is present as Mn^{3+}.

There fore Mn^{3+} has [Ar] $3d^4$ configuration and has four unpaired electrons in its d orbital represented as:

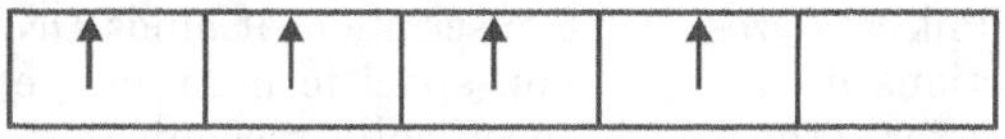

24. Spin only magnetic moment for compound X i.e. $[Mn(ox)_3]^{3-}$ is :

$$\mu = \sqrt{n(n+2)} \text{ B.M}$$

Given, $n = 4$

Therefore, $\mu = \sqrt{4(4+2)} = 4.90\text{B.M}$

25. (*c*) When benzene reacts with 1-Chloro-2-methylpropane in the presence of anhydrous $AlCl_3$ at 20ºC, then the major product (X) formed in given as:

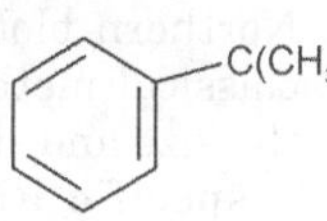

The reaction is:

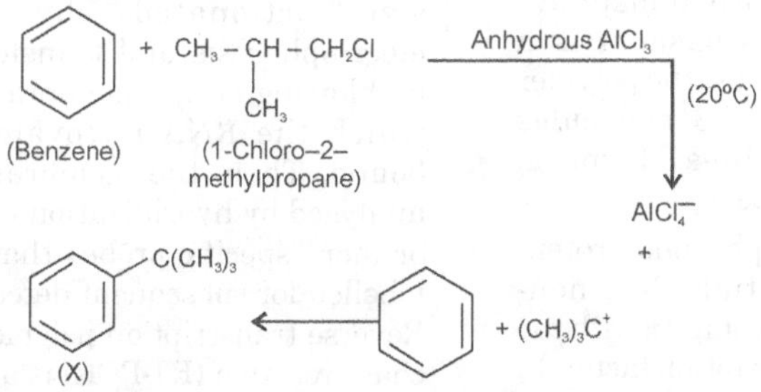

Here in this reaction carbocation of $(CH_3)_2 - CH - CH_2^+$ takes place

$$\underset{(1^\circ\text{-carbocation})}{(CH_3)_2 - CH - CH_2^+} \longleftrightarrow \underset{(3^\circ\text{-carbocation})}{(CH_3)_3 C^+}$$

As, 3°-carbocation is more stable than 1°-carbocation.

26. When the compound (X) i.e. 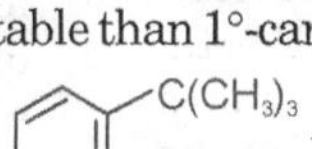 is treated with hot acidic $KMnO_4$ and then with Li Al H_4, then the resulting Y compound is given by the reaction:

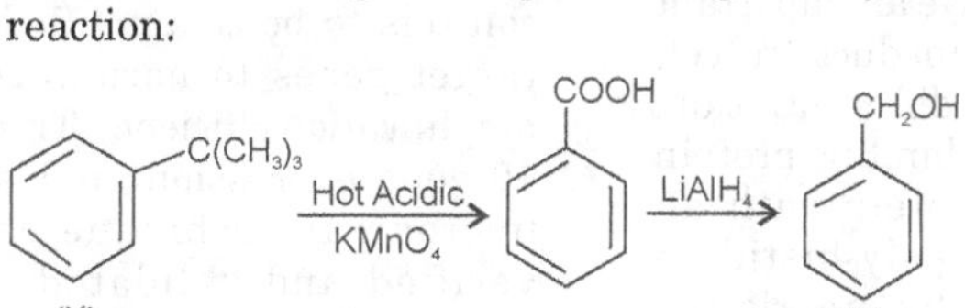

27. Given,

Zn (s) | Zn^{2+} (aq) || Cu^{2+} (aq) | Cu (s) at 298K

$E^\circ (Zn^{2+} / Zn) = -0.763$ V

$E^\circ (Cu / Cu^{2+}) = -0.337$ V

Therefore the emf of the cell is given as:

$$E^\circ_{cell} = E^\circ_{Cu^{2+}/Cu} - E^\circ_{Zn^{2+}/Zn}$$
$$= 0.337 - (-0.763)$$
$$= 1.100 \text{ V}$$

28. Given, the cell reaction:

$$Zn\ (s) + Cu^{2+}\ (aq) \leftrightarrow Zn^{2+}\ (aq) + Cu\ (s)$$

R = 8.314 J/K mol

and F = 96500 C/mol

We know,

$$E^\circ_{cell} = \frac{0.0591}{n} \log k$$

Therefore, $\log k = \dfrac{2.200}{0.0591}$

$= 37.22.$

(I) BIOCHEMISTRY

1. Fluorescent proteins are members of a structurally homologous class of proteins that share the unique property of being self-sufficient to form a visible wavelength chromophore from a sequence of 3 amino acids within their own polypeptide sequence. The property of fluorescence of proteins is attributed to the aromatic amino acids present in the protein. The aromatic amino acids are tyrosine, tryptophan and phenylalanine. Their aromatic structure helps in the electronic transitions responsible for fluorescence. Thus, cysteine does not contribute to the fluorescence of a protein.

2. Immunological memory is the ability of the immune system to respond more rapidly and effectively to pathogens that have been encountered previously, and reflects the preexistence of a clonally expanded population of antigen-specific lymphocytes. Memory responses, which are called secondary, tertiary, and so on, depending on the number of exposures to antigen, also differ qualitatively from primary responses. This is particularly clear in the case of the antibody response, where the characteristics of antibodies produced in secondary and subsequent responses are distinct from those produced in the primary response to the same antigen. Memory is sustained by long-lived antigen-specific lymphocytes that were induced by the original exposure and that persist until a second encounter with the pathogen.

3. The linear portion of the Pentose Phosphate Pathway carries out oxidation and decarboxylation of glucose-6-phosphate, producing the 5-C sugar ribulose-5-phosphate. The pentose phosphate pathway is the major source for the NADPH required for anabolic processes. There are three distinct phases each of which has a distinct outcome. Depending on the needs of the organism the metabolites of that outcome can be fed into many other pathways. Gluconeogenesis is directly connected to the pentose phosphate pathway. Because of the structure of this molecule it readily donates hydrogen ions to metabolites thus reducing them and making them available for energy harvest at a later time. The PPP is the main source of synthesis for NADPH. The pentose phosphate pathway (PPP) is also responsible for the

production of Ribose-5-phosphate which is an important part of nucleic acids. Finally the PPP can also be used to produce glyceraldehyde-3-phosphate which can then be fed into the TCA and ETC cycles allowing for the harvest of energy.

4. Non-covalent molecular interactions are key steps in the dance of life. The three fundamental non-covalent bonds are electrostatic interactions, hydrogen bonds, and van der Waals interactions. They differ in geometry, strength, and specificity. Hydrogen bonds are relatively weak interactions, which nonetheless are crucial for biological macromolecules such as DNA and proteins. These interactions are also responsible for many of the properties of water that make it such a special solvent. The basis of a van der Waals interaction is that the distribution of electronic charge around an atom changes with time. At any instant, the charge distribution is not perfectly symmetric. This transient asymmetry in the electronic charge around an atom acts through electrostatic interactions to induce a complementary asymmetry in the electron distribution around its neighbouring atoms. Peptide bond is the CONH bond between -COOH and $-NH_2$ group of two different amino acids and is a relatively weak bond. Ionic bond, also called electrovalent bond, is type of linkage formed from the electrostatic attraction between oppositely charged ions in a chemical compound. Such a bond forms when the valence (outermost) electrons of one atom are transferred permanently to another atom. Such bonds are strongly interactive bonds.

5. T4 polynucleotide kinase (Pnk) exemplifies a family of bifunctional enzymes with 5′-kinase and 3′-phosphatase activities that play key roles in RNA and DNA repair. T4 Pnk is a homo-tetramer composed of a C-terminal phosphatase domain and an N-terminal kinase domain. The active site is composed of essential side chains that coordinate the β phosphate of the NTP donor and the 3′-phosphate of the 5′-OH acceptor, plus a putative general acid that activates the 5′-OH. T4 Pnk is a homo-tetramer of a 301 amino acid polypeptide. T4 Pnk catalyzes two enzymatic reactions in this pathway: (i) the transfer of the γ-phosphate from ATP to the 5′ OH terminus of RNA; and (ii) the hydrolytic removal of a 3′ PO_4 terminus from RNA.

6. The given polymer has oxygen present at the 3`-position of the carbon ring. The sugar molecule present in the polymer is a pentose sugar and its 3` position is oxygenated. There is sugar phosphate linkage at the 5` ends of the pentose sugar moiety. Also, the 1` carbon atom is bonded with a nitrogenous base. This indicates that the sugar moiety is a ribose sugar and since it forms linkage with both phosphate and nitrogenous base, it is a ribonucleotide. Thus, the polymer having repeats of 3 molecules of ribonucleotides form a polyribonucleotide.

7. FOS is a nuclear phospho-protein which forms a tight but non-covalently linked complex with the JUN/AP-1 transcription factor. In the heterodimer, FOS and JUN/AP-1 basic regions each seems to interact with symmetrical DNA half sites. On TGF-beta activation, forms a multimeric JUN-FOS complex at the AP1/SMAD-binding site to regulate TGF-beta-mediated signalling. It has a critical function in regulating the development of cells destined to form and maintain the skeleton. It is thought to have an important role in signal transduction, cell proliferation and differentiation. JUN is a maltose binding protein (MBP) fusion protein with an amino-terminal poly-histidine tag and purified by proprietary chromatographic techniques. C-JUN is a gene which, in combination with c Fos, forms the AP-1early response transcription factor. C-JUN is activated by the JNK pathway. C-JUN is the putative transforming gene of avian sarcoma virus 17. C-JUN is a protein which is highly similar to the viral protein, and which interacts directly with specific target DNA sequences to regulate gene expression. MYC (Myc proto-oncogene) protein participates in the regulation of gene transcription. It binds DNA in a non-specific manner, yet also specifically recognizes the core sequence 5′-CAC [GA] TG-3′ and seems to activate the transcription of growth-related genes.

8. A northern blot is a laboratory method used to detect specific RNA molecules among a mixture of RNA. Northern blotting can be used to analyze a sample of RNA from a particular tissue or cell type in order to measure the RNA expression of particular genes. Northern blotting analysis is a classical method for analysis of the size and steady-state level of a specific RNA in a complex sample. In short, the RNA is size-fractionated by gel electrophoresis and transferred by blotting onto a membrane to which the RNA is covalently bound. Then, the membrane is analysed by hybridization to one or more specific probes that are labelled for subsequent detection. Reverse transcription-polymerase chain reaction (RT-PCR) is a very sensitive technique to measure and to compare mRNA levels among samples. Since the RT-PCR consists of cDNA synthesis, DNA amplification, and signal detection as sequential steps, the accuracy of quantification is dependent on the efficiency across these steps, especially the RT and the cDNA amplification. Specific genes have been used as baseline controls to be co-amplified with target genes to normalize the amplification efficiency. Thus, the 10 gene expression analysis by microarray technique can be verified and validated using northern blotting and RT-PCR.

9. Pepsin is a nonspecific endo-peptidase that is active only at acid pH. It is irreversibly denatured at neutral or alkaline pH. Digestion of IgG by the enzyme pepsin normally produces one F (ab′) 2 fragment and numerous small peptides of the Fc portion. The resulting F (ab′) 2 fragment is

composed of two disulfide-connected F_{ab} units. The F_c fragment is extensively degraded, and its small fragments can be separated from F (ab') 2 by dialysis, gel filtration or ion exchange chromatography. F (ab') 2 can be separated by mild reduction into two sulfhydryl-containing, univalent F_{ab}' fragments. The advantage of F_{ab}' fragments is that they can be conjugated to detectable labels directly through their sulfhydryl groups, ensuring that the active binding site remains unhindered and active.

10. B cells obtain help from T cells in the antibody response by acting as antigen-specific antigen presenting cells. A direct signal through binding of antigen to membrane Ig can enhance B cell antigen presentation and T-dependent B cell activation, but is not required for a productive interaction between a small resting B cell and a differentiated helper T cell. As a result of helper T cell recognition of antigen on the B cell surface, the T cell becomes activated and in turn activates the B cell. Cytotoxic T lymphocytes (CTLs)—also called killer T cells-perform a different function. These cells directly attack other cells carrying certain foreign or abnormal molecules on their surfaces. CTLs are especially useful for attacking viruses because viruses often hide from other parts of the immune system while they grow inside infected cells. CTLs recognize small fragments of these viruses peeking out from the cell membrane and launch an attack to kill the infected cell.

11. PCR functions because of two essential components - a thermostable DNA polymerase, and a pair of DNA 'primers'. Primers are short stretches of oligonucleotides. The primer directs the polymerase to move 5′ to 3′ because of the 'direction' of DNA. Primers hybridise at a temperature that is affected by their sequence, concentration, length and ionic environment. This annealing temperature is usually referred to as the TM (melting temperature) but is in fact 5–10°C below the T_M. The term T_M describes the temperature at which 50% of the oligonucleotide-target duplexes have formed. The primers hybridise to the 3′ end of the DNA fragment (both lagging and leading strands). The primers for the given DNA strand are :–

5′-TTTTTTTTTT- 3′ (forward primer) and 5′-CCCCCCCCCC- 3′.

12. The study of the rate at which an enzyme works is called enzyme kinetics. A Lineweaver-Burk plot is used to analyse kinetic data on enzyme-catalysed reactions. The reciprocal of the rate of formation of products (1/v) is plotted against the reciprocal of the substrate concentration (1/[S]). The equation is:

$$\frac{1}{V} = \frac{1}{V_{max}} + \frac{K_M}{V_{max}} \cdot \frac{1}{[S]}$$

Where [S] and K_M have units of mol L^{-1} and V and V_{max} have units of mol L^{-1} s^{-1}. The maximum velocity V_{max} of the enzymolysis is the reciprocal of the y-intercept of the best fit line. The slope of the best fit line is the Michaelis constant K_M divided by V_{max}. This provides a more precise way to determine V_{max} and K_M. The value of K_M can be obtained from the graph. The x-intercept in the graph is given by: - ($1/K_M$). So, to obtain the value of K_M, the reciprocal of x-intercept, i.e., - K_M is multiplied by -1. Therefore, the required value of K_M = - 1 x (1/ x-intercept).

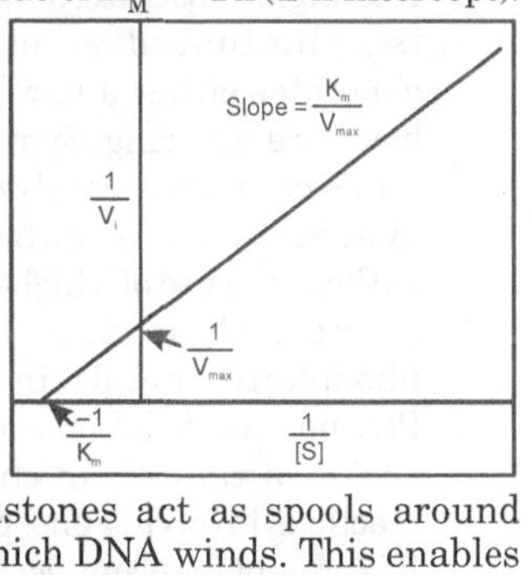

13. Histones act as spools around which DNA winds. This enables the compaction necessary to fit the large genomes of eukaryotes inside cell nuclei: the compacted molecule is 40,000 times shorter than an unpacked molecule. Most well-studied histone modifications are involved in control of transcription. Three histone modifications are particularly associated with repressed genes: Trimethylation of H3 lysine 27, Di and tri-methylation of H3 lysine 9 and Trimethylation of H4 lysine 20. Phosphorylated H2AX (also known as gamma H2AX) is a marker for DNA double strand breaks, and forms part of the response to DNA damage. Gamma H2AX acts as a binding site for the protein MDC1, which in turn recruits key DNA repair proteins. Acetylation of H3 lysine 56 is required for genome stability. Histone modifications act in diverse biological processes such as gene regulation, DNA repair, chromosome condensation (mitosis) and spermatogenesis (meiosis).

14. Given, an eukaryotic gene having 3 exons: Exon I (2 kb), Exon II (4 kb) and Exon III (6 kb) There is one intron in between Exon I and Exon II of size 1 kb and another intron in between Exon II and Exon III of same size. Promoter of 5 kb is upstream of the 5′-UTR (untranslated region). The 5′-UTR is of 0.4 kb length and the 3′-UTR is of 0.6 kb length. After transcription, the mRNA that would be generated would consist of the 5′-UTR...Exon I...Intron I...Exon II...Intron II...Exon III...3′-UTR.

The initial RNA that is transcribed from a gene's DNA template must be processed before it becomes a mature messenger RNA (mRNA) that can direct the synthesis of protein. One of the steps in this processing, called RNA splicing, involves the removal or "splicing out" of certain sequences referred to as intervening sequences, or introns. The final mRNA thus consists of the remaining sequences, called exons, which are connected to one another through the splicing process. So after splicing, the processed mRNA that is generated will be devoid of any introns. The mRNA thus formed :

5′-UTR...Exon I...Exon II...Exon III...3′-UTR as there is no polyadenylation of the spliced mRNA.

Thus the size of the mature mRNA = Size of {(5′-UTR) + (Exon I) + (Exon II) + (Exon III) + (3′-UTR)} = 0.4 kb + 2 kb + 4 kb + 6 kb + 0.6 kb = 13 kb.

15. A cell extract was incubated with ^{32}P labelled ATP molecule and unlabelled inorganic phosphate. The cell extract contains all enzymes of Glycolysis. Given, pyruvate kinase is being inactivated. The overall reaction pathway is given as :

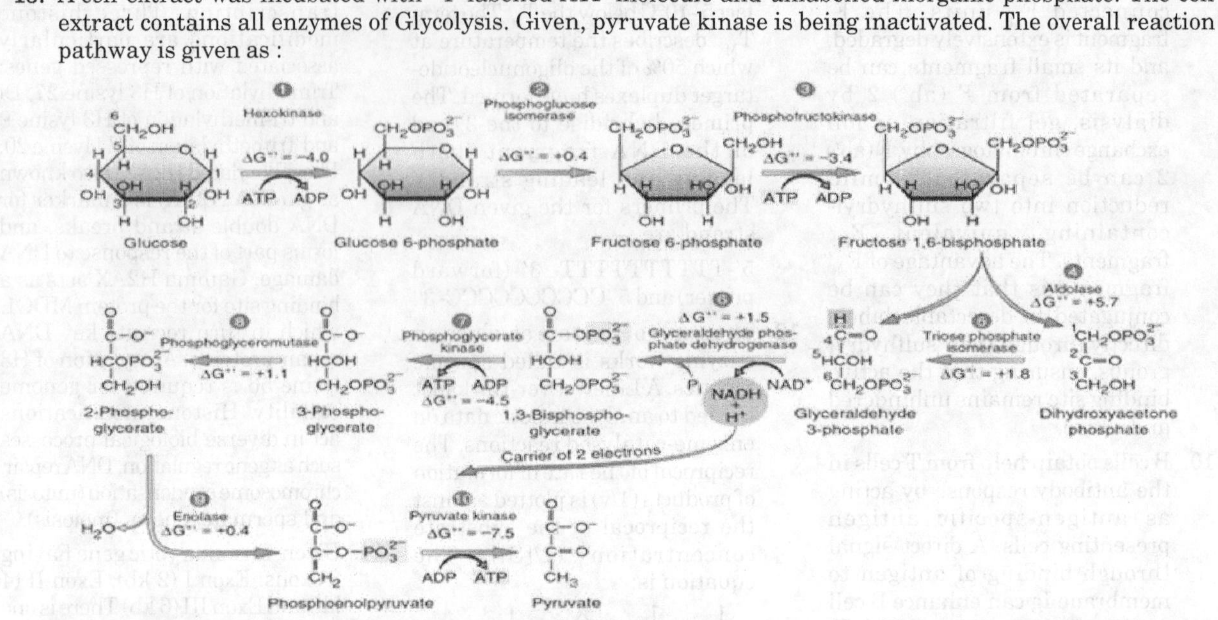

From the pathway, it can be clearly seen that the labelled γ-^{32}P is incorporated through ATP into Glucose-6-phosphate, Fructose-6-phosphate, Fructose-1, 6-biphosphate (both are labelled), glyceradehyde-3-phosphate, 1, 3-Biphosphoglycerate, 3-Phosphoglycerate and 2-Phosphoglycerate. In this reaction, pyruvate is not formed because pyruvate kinase has been inactivated.

16. After running the SDS-PAGE of the protein X, only a single band of 45 kDa could be seen on the electrophoresis gel. This means that either the protein X is a monomeric unit or it has identical subunits. Now, when the protein X was eluted from a gel filtration chromatography column, it was eluted between alcohol dehydrogenase which is 160 kDa in size and beta-amylase which is 190 kDa in size. This implies that protein X is not a monomer. So, for the size of the protein to be in the range of 160-190 kDa, the protein X must have 160/45 or 190/45 = 3.55 or 4.22 subunits present in it. Thus, the protein X has approximately 4 identical subunits.

17. Protein Kinases are key regulators of cell function that constitute one of the largest and most functionally diverse gene families. By adding phosphate groups to substrate proteins, they direct the activity, localization and overall function of many proteins, and serve to orchestrate the activity of almost all cellular processes. Kinases are particularly prominent in signal transduction and co-ordination of complex functions such as the cell cycle. Lyases are enzymes cleaving C-C, C-O, C-N and other bonds by other means than by hydrolysis or oxidation. They differ from other enzymes in that two substrates are involved in one reaction direction, but only one in the other direction. When acting on the single substrate, a molecule is eliminated and this generates either a new double bond or a new ring. Synthase is an enzyme that catalyzes the synthesis of a substance without the use of a high-energy source such as cleavage of a phosphate bond in ATP. Phosphatase is an enzyme that acts as a catalyst in chemical reactions involving phosphorus. It is present in serum, semen, the kidney, and the prostate. It is essential in the calcification of bone. It involves the hydrolytic cleavage of inorganic phosphate from esters.

18. Mitochondria extrude protons across their inner membrane to generate the mitochondrial membrane potential ($\Delta\Psi_m$) and pH gradient (ΔpH_m) that both power ATP synthesis. Mitochondrial uptake and efflux of many ions and metabolites are driven exclusively by ΔpH_m, whose in situ regulation is poorly characterized. As the energy power-plants of the cell, mitochondria generate ATP by utilizing the proton electrochemical gradient potential, or electrochemical proton motive force (Δp), generated by serial reduction of electrons through the respiratory electron transport chain (ETC). Cell membranes in general and membranes of nerve cells in particular, maintain a small voltage or "potential" across the membrane in its normal or resting state. In the rest state, the inside of the nerve cell membrane is negative with respect to the outside (typically about -70 millivolts). The voltage arises from differences in concentration of the electrolyte ions K^+ and Na^+.

Transient current flow and therefore rapid changes in potential are made possible by ion channel, a class of integral proteins that traverse the cell membrane. There is a process called the sodium-potassium pump which utilizes ATP to pump out three Na^+ ions and pump in two K^+ ions.

19. The molecule shown is:

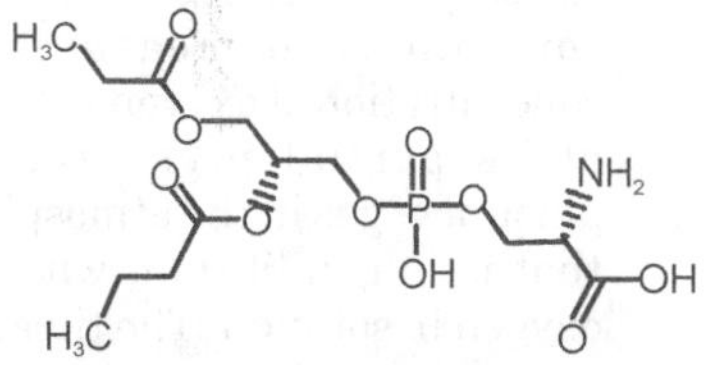

Phosphatidylserine is a structure resembling a triacylglyceride (dietary fat). It possesses a glycerol backbone which attaches to three carbon chain appendages; one of which is a serine molecule bound to the glycerol backbone via a phosphate group. Due to this structure, various compounds may be called phosphatidylserines given they have that one serine containing group; the other two fatty acid chains are irrelevant to the naming, but not necessarily the function. After synthesis, Phosphatidylserine is then used as a structural component of a cell's lipid bilayer (cell membrane) with the serine molecule facing inwards.

20. The melting temperature correlates with how easily a double stranded DNA complex is formed. This, in turn, depends on the likelihood of each pair of nucleotides to bond. The T_m is affected by a number of factors: i) Concentration of DNA ii) Concentration of ions in the solution, most notably Mg^{2+} and K^+ iii) DNA sequence and iv) Length of DNA. The most complex factor is the sequence of the DNA. The sequence has an impact on the T_m for a number of reasons: a) The nucleotide pair 'A-T' has a weaker bond than the nucleotide pair 'G-C' b) Nucleotides on the same strand can interact with each other, forming so-called secondary structures such as internal loops; these structures compete with the formation of the double helix and can thus increase the Tm and c) Neighbouring nucleotide pairs can interact with each other. It is energetically favourable for nucleotide pairs to be neighboured with other nucleotide pairs. This so-called stacking effect decreases the T_m. A simple formula for calculation of the (T_m) is : $T_m = \{4(G + C) + 2(A + T)\}$ °C. Given, T_m for X = 85°C and T_m for Y = 80°C. This implies that X has more content of GC than Y.

21. Glutamate is synthesized from its' widely distributed α-keto acid precursor by a simple 1-step transamination reaction catalyzed by glutamate dehydrogenase. Transaminases (aminotransferases) catalyze the reversible reaction which varies in substrate specificity. Transaminases equilibrate amino groups among available α-keto acids. This permits synthesis of non-essential amino acids, using amino groups derived from other amino acids and carbon skeletons synthesized in the cell. Transaminases funnel amino groups from excess dietary amino acids to those amino acids (e.g., glutamate) that can be deaminated. Carbon skeletons of deaminated amino acids can be catabolized for energy or used to synthesize glucose or fatty acids for energy storage. Glutamate Dehydrogenase catalyzes a major reaction that effects net removal of N from the amino acid pool. Glutamate Dehydrogenase is one of the few enzymes that can utilize either NAD^+ or $NADP^+$ as electron acceptor. The compounds in the reaction flowsheet are : A→α-ketoglutarate and B→L-glutamate.

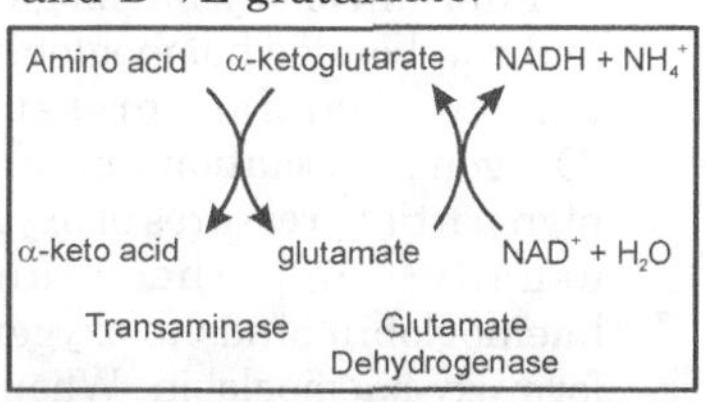

22. Glycogen is a chain of glucose subunits held together by a 1, 4 glycosidic bonds, very much like starch (α-amylose). In contrast to starch, which is a single linear chain of glucose, glycogen is a branched structure. At the branch points, subunits are joined by 1, 6 glycosidic bonds. Branches occur every 8-10 residues. Glycogen is synthesized when blood glucose levels are high. This state is reflected inside liver cells by the presence of high levels of glucose-6-phosphate. G6P is first converted to G1P by phosphoglucomutase. This reaction is analogous to the reaction catalyzed by phosphoglycerate mutase in step 8 of glycolysis, and proceeds by a similar mechanism, with a bi-phosphate intermediate. The major component in the rigid cell walls in plants is cellulose. Cellulose is a linear polysaccharide polymer with many glucose monosaccharides. The structure of cellulose consists of long polymer chains of glucose units connected by α-acetal linkage units. All of the monomer units are β-D-glucose, and all the β-acetal links connect C1 of glucose to C4 of the next glucose.

23. The phi (Φ) angle is the angle of right-handed rotation around N-CA bond, the value being zero if CA-C bond is cis to C-N bond. The psi (ψ) angle is the angle of right-handed rotation around CA-C bond, the value being zero if C-N bond is cis to N-CA bond. The omega (Ω) angle is the angle of right-handed rotation about C-N bond, the value being zero if CA-C bond of the preceding residue is cis to N-CA bond. Most residues in a typical protein are involved in the formation of two peptide bonds. The peptide bond formed by the residues I and I + 1 is assigned to the residue I + 1.

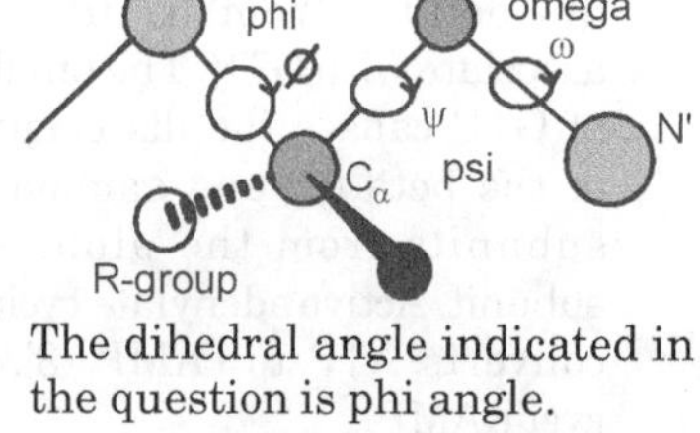

The dihedral angle indicated in the question is phi angle.

24. In the given tri-peptide, the amino acid sequences are that of glutamine-valine-threonine.

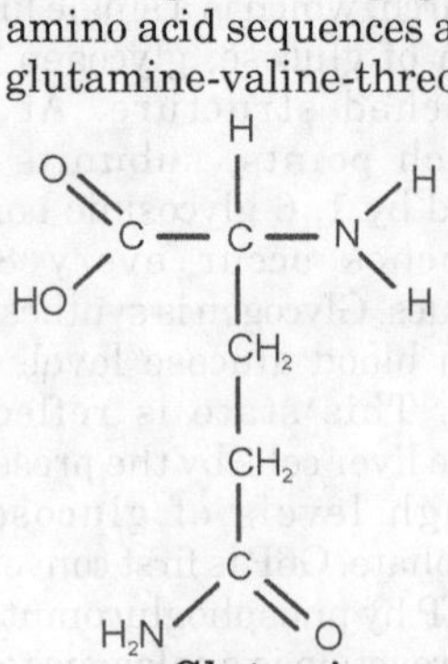

Glutamine

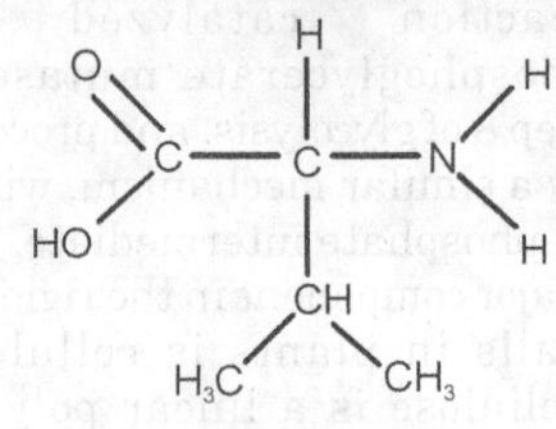

Valine

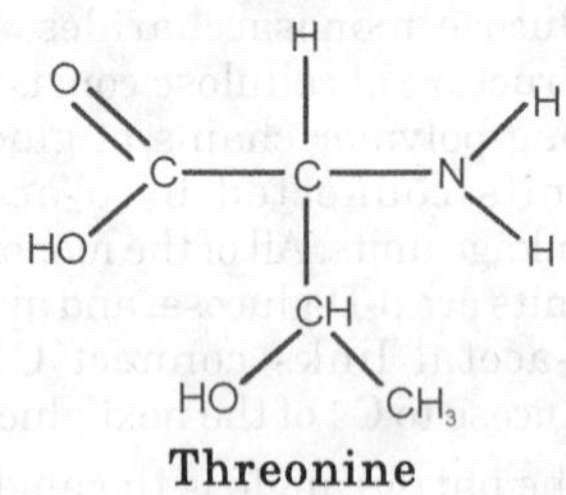

Threonine

25. The cAMP cascade begins when a hormone binds to a receptor on a cell membrane and ends with a change in the rates of many key enzymes reactions and in the concentrations of the key metabolites that they control. The cAMP cascade begins with adrenalin (epinephrine) or glucagon binding to receptors and it ends with the release of glucose from glycogen. Adrenalin binds to a β-adrenergic receptor or glucagon binds to a glucagon receptor and causes a change in conformation. The receptor binds to a heterotrimeric G-protein on the inside of the membrane. Binding causes the G_s protein to dissociate from GDP and associate with GTP. The binding of GTP causes the dissociation of the beta (β) and gamma (γ) subunits from the alpha (α) subunit. Active adenylate cyclase converts ATP to cAMP (3', 5'-cyclic AMP).

26. Active adenylate cyclase converts ATP to cAMP (3', 5'-cyclic AMP). The cAMP diffuses away from the inner membrane and binds to inactive Protein Kinase A. The active subunits cause the phosphorylation of many proteins. Glycogen phosphorylase kinase is eventually inactivated by dephosphorylation by a protein phosphatase. Glycogen phosphorylase-a causes the removal of glucose from glycogen in the form of glucose-1-phosphate. The glucose is used for glycolysis in muscle and to produce blood glucose in the liver.

Hormone + Receptor + G$\alpha\beta\gamma$-GDP

= Hormone -Receptor-G$\alpha\beta\gamma$-GDP

Hormone-Receptor-G$\alpha\beta\gamma$-GDP + GTP

= Hormone-Receptor + GDP + G$\beta\gamma$ + Gα-GTP

Gα-GTP + Adenylate cyclase

= Gα-GTP-Adenylate cyclase

ATP = cAMP + PPi

cAMP + PKARRCC

= 2 cAMP-R + 2 PKA

Inactive phosphorylase kinase + ATP

= active phosphorylase kinase + ADP

Inactive phosphorylase b + ATP

= active phosphorylase a + ADP

Glycogen + Pi

= Glycogen + Glucose-1-P

Glucose-1-P = Glucose-6-P

27. The oxygen dissociation curve is a graph that shows the percent saturation of haemoglobin at various partial pressures of oxygen. The purpose of an oxygen dissociation curve is to show the equilibrium of oxy-haemoglobin and non-bonded haemoglobin at various partial pressures (Oxygen Dissociation Curve). At high partial pressures of oxygen, usually in the lungs, haemoglobin binds to oxygen to form oxy-haemoglobin. When the blood is fully saturated all the erythrocytes are in the form of oxy-haemoglobin. As the erythrocytes travel to tissues deprived of oxygen the partial pressure of oxygen will decrease. Consequently, the oxy-haemoglobin releases the oxygen to form haemoglobin. Each myoglobin molecule is capable of binding oxygen because myoglobin contains one heme per molecule. Even though the reaction of myoglobin and oxygen takes place in solution, it is convenient to measure the concentration of oxygen in terms of its partial pressure, the amount of gas in the atmosphere that is in equilibrium with the oxygen in solution. The titration curve of myoglobin with oxygen is a hyperbola. In the given graph, A is the binding curve for myoglobin and B is the binding curve for haemoglobin.

28. Sickle cell anaemia is an inherited blood disorder characterized primarily by chronic anaemia and periodic episodes of pain. The underlying problem involves haemoglobin, a component of red blood cells. In sickle cell anaemia, the haemoglobin is defective. After haemoglobin molecules give up their oxygen, some may cluster together and form long, rod-like structures. These structures cause red blood cells to become stiff and assume a sickle shape. Sickle cell anaemia is an autosomal recessive genetic disorder caused by a defect in the HBB gene, which codes for haemoglobin. The presence of two defective genes (SS) is needed for sickle cell anaemia. If each parent carries one sickle haemoglobin gene (S) and one normal gene (A), each child has a 25% chance of inheriting two defective genes and having sickle cell anaemia; a 25% chance of inheriting two normal genes and not having the disease; and a 50% chance of being an unaffected carrier like the parents. Structural difference between normal adult haemoglobin and sickle-cell haemoglobin is the replacement of glutamic acid with valine in the β-globin amino acid chain.

(K) BOTANY

1. Penicillin kills susceptible bacteria by specifically inhibiting the transpeptidase that catalyzes the final step in cell wall biosynthesis, the cross-linking of pep-tidoglycan.
2. The glyoxylate cycle, a variation of the tricarboxylic acid cycle, is an anabolic pathway occurring in plants, bacte ria,protists, and fungi. The glyoxylate cycle centers on the conversion of acetyl-CoA to succinate for the synthesis of carbohydrates. In microorganisms, the glyoxylate cycle allows cells to utilize simple carbon compounds as a carbon source when complex sources such as glucose are not available
3. **Agar** or **agar-agar** is a gelatinous substance derived by boiling a polysaccharide in red algae such as *Gelidium, Gracilaria* and *Gigartina*, where it accumulates in the cell walls of agarophyte and serves as the primary structural support for the algae's cell walls.
4. Cork is a suberised tissue while deposition of lignin takes place in xylem and sclerenchyma.
5. Gum, pectin and agar are polysaccharide where as cutin is a waxy substance allied to suberin.
6. Energy pyramid is flow of energy through a food chain.

   At each tropic level in a food chain, energy is used by the organisms at that level to maintain their own life process. Because of the 2nd law of energy, some energy is lost to the surroundings as heat. It is estimated that in going from one tropic level to the next, about 90 % of the energy is lost.

   In moving to the next tropic level, only 10 % of the original energy is available. By the third tropic level only 1% of the energy is available.
7. Kreb cycle is a series of chemical reactions used by all aerobic organisms to generate energy through the oxidization of acetate derived from carbohydrates, fats and proteins into carbon dioxide. In this cycle isocitrate dehydrogenase and α-ketoglutarate dehydrogenase releases CO_2.
8. **Fasciculated root** (tuberous root) occur in clusters at the base of the stem; example: asparagus, dahlia. These roots are generally adventitious and are swollen.
9. Parental generations = 'AaBb' and 'AaBb'

   When both are crossed following genotype and ratio will appear-

GENOTYPE	RATIO
AABB	1:16
AABb	2:16
AAbb	1:16
AaBB	2:16
AaBb	4:16
Aabb	2:16
aaBB	1:16
aaBb	2:16
aabb	1:16

   So recessive traits for atleast one progeny are- AAbb, Aabb, aaBB, aaBb. aabb

$$= \frac{1}{16} + \frac{2}{16} + \frac{1}{16} + \frac{2}{16} + \frac{1}{16}$$

$$= \frac{7}{16}$$

10. Global warming is caused by the emission of greenhouse gases. 72% of the totally emitted greenhouse gases is carbon dioxide (CO_2), 18% Methane and 9% Nitrous oxide (NOx). Thus it is caused by the excessive emission of carbon dioxide and oxides of nitrogen.
11. Since the Agrobacterium tumeficiens lacks Vir A gene in its plasmid thus it will lack the synthesis of acetosyringone receptor as well as the bacteria will fail to transfer the T-DNA to the plant in the absence of Vir A gene.
12. Plantibodies is an antibody produced by genetically engineered crops. Antibodies are part of animal immune systems, and are produced in plants by transforming them with antibody genes from animals. This was first done in 1989, with a mouse antibody made by tobacco plants. Although plants do not naturally make antibodies, plantibodies have been shown to function in the same way as normal antibodies. Also plantibodies cannot uncoat the calcium ion binding sites on the coat protein of the virus.
14. Achyranthus aspera commonly called as 'Prickly Chaff Flower' is a species of plant in the Amarantheceae family whereas Delphinium staphisagria is a species of delphinium or larkspur from the family Ranunculaceae. This plant is also known as Lice-Bane or Stavesacre.
15. Active transport is the movement of a substance across a cell membrane against its concentration gradient (from low to high concentration). In all cells, this is usually concerned with accumulating high concentrations of molecules that the cell needs, such as ions, glucose and amino acids. If the process uses chemical energy, such as from adenosine triphosphate (ATP), it is termed primary active transport. Secondary active transport involves the use of an electrochemical gradient. Active transport uses cellular energy, unlike passive transport, which does not use cellular energy. Active transport is a good example of a process for which cells require energy.
16. Nigrospora oryzae (teleomorph or sexual stage is known as Khuskia oryzae) is a plant pathogen that causes nigrospora disease of rice.

    Loose smut of barley (wheat) is caused by Ustilago nuda. It is a disease that can destroy a large proportion of a barley crop.

    Leptosphaeria sacchari is a plant pathogen which causes ring spot of sugarcane. Ring spot is a minor fungal disease principally affecting the lower leaves of the sugarcane canopy.

Septoria tritici is a species of filamentous fungus. It is a wheat plant pathogen causing septoria leaf blotch that is difficult to control due to resistance to multiple fungicides. The pathogen today causes one of the most important diseases of wheat.

17. Tabtoxin, also known as wildfire toxin, is a simple monobactam biotoxin produced by *Pseudomonas* syringae.

Phaseolotoxin is produced by *Pseudomonas syringae* and leads to the formation of halo lesions of kiwifruit canker disease.

Tentotoxin is produced by *Alternaria* alternate and causes Cholorosis.

18.

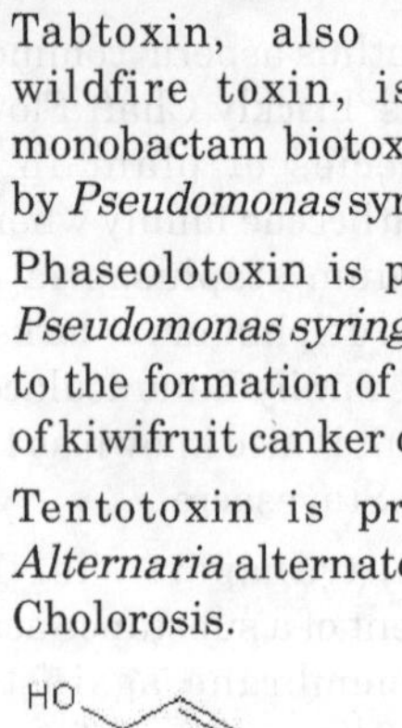

Structure of morphine

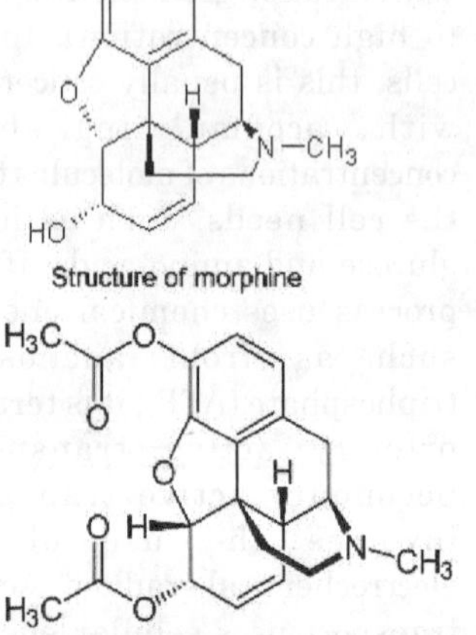

structure of heroin.

19. Lactophenol-cotton blue is used to visualize filamentous fungi. Phenol destroys contaminant compounds that have the fungi; the lactic acid conserves the fungi structures by provoking osmotic gradient change with relation of the interior of the fungi forming a protective "layer". The cotton blue is the one that gives the color and permit to visualize the fungi under optic microscope.

In the Gram staining procedure, Crystal Violet (CV) dissociates in aqueous solutions into CV^+ and Cl^- ions. These two ions then penetrate through the cell wall and cell membrane of both Gram-positive and Gram-negative cells. The CV^+ ions later interacts with negatively charged bacterial components and stains the bacterial cells purple. The decolorized Gram negative cells can be rendered visible with a suitable counter stain, which is usually positively charged safranin, which stains them pink. Pink colour which adheres to the Gram positive bacteria is masked by the purple of the crystal violet.

Ethidium bromide is the most commonly used dye for DNA and RNA detection in agarose gels. Ethidium bromide is a DNA intercalator, inserting itself between the base pairs in the double helix.

Silver staining is used to detect amino acids (proteins) after electrophoretic separation on polyacrylamide gels. It combines excellent sensitivity (in the low nanogram range) whilst using very simple and cheap equipment and chemicals.

20. Polysymbiosis is a combination of algae, fungi and nitrogen fixing bacteria in a lichen thallus.

Helotism is a partnership between two organisms in which the association is decided at the expense of one.

Myocobiont is a fungal component of a lichen whereas Cructose lichen is a lichen which form a crust closely addressed to the substrate.

21. In zygonema, the chromosomes continue to condense, and homologous chromosomes find each other and begin to align to each other in a process known as "rough pairing"

During diplonema, the homologous chromosomes in each tetrad begin to separate, but they remain connected at points of crossing over. Each point of crossing over is known as a chiasma (plural: chiasmata). In the diagram at left, three chiasmata are shown. Also at this stage, the nuclear envelope begins to break down.

Diakinesis is the last stage of prophase I. In this stage, the homologous chromosomes separate further, and the chiasmata terminalize (proceed to the end of the chromatids, then separate).

During metaphase I, assembly of the spindle apparatus is completed, and the chromosome pairs line up across the center of the cell between the two centrioles. This central plane is called the **metaphase plate**.

23. According to Chargoff rule, in RNA,

(*i*) adenine will always make pair with uracil and guanine will always make pair with cytosine.

(*ii*) Concentration of purine = concentration of pyrimidine.

(*iii*) $\frac{(A+U)}{(G+C)}$ = constant for all species.

24. Tm = 2(total A + total T) + 4(total G + total C).

For P, Tm = 2(33 + 33) + 4(17 + 17)
= 132 + 136 = 268

For Q, Tm = 2(33 + 17) + 4(33 + 17)
= 100 + 200 = 300

Thus P will be having lowest Tm

25. Maltose is a disaccharide formed from two units of glucose joined with an α (1→4) bond, formed from a condensation reaction. Its structure is O-α-D-glucopyranosyl-(1→4)-β-D-glucopyranose. Sucrose is a disaccharide composed of the monosaccharides glucose and fructose. The structure of sucrose is O-α-D-glucopyranosyl-(1→2)-β-D-fructofuranoside.

26. Maltose has the ability to reduce the Fehling's solution, due to its free aldehyde. The aldehyde group is oxidized giving a positive result, which means that the maltose is a reducing sugar. In sucrose, the glycosidic bond is formed between the reducing ends of both glucose and fructose, and not between the reducing end of one and the non-reducing end of the other. This linkage inhibits further bonding to other saccharide units. Since it contains no anomeric hydroxyl groups, it is classified as a non-reducing sugar.

(L) MICROBIOLOGY

1. 1907 - A chemotherapeutic cure for sleeping sickness was developed by Paul Ehrlich (1854-915), a German doctor and scientist. Ehrlich's lab also discovered Arsphenamine (Salvarsan), the first treatment for syphilis that was effective, and thus initiated and named the concept of chemotherapy.
2. Typical immersion oils have a refractive index of 1.51 and a dispersion similar to that of glass coverslips.
3. It has been shown to inhibit bacterial DNA synthesis and DNA supercoiling by sulphonamide.
4. A mast cell (also known as mastocyte and labrocyte) is a resident cell of several types of tissues and contains many granules rich in histamine and heparin.
5. A polio virion is composed of a single-stranded positive-sense RNA genome of approximately 7,450 nucleotides enclosed in an icosahedral particle 27nm in diameter. The RNA is the infectious agent for poliomyelitis, while the viral capsid serves as a protective coat for the RNA.
6. Phototrophs are the organisms that carry out photon capture to acquire energy. Cyanobacteria are a large and heterogeneous group of photosynthetic microorganisms, formerly referred to as blue-green algae.
7. Most bacteria have a cell wall containing the polymer peptidoglycan and other ..... There may be up to 40 layers of this polymer making up the cell wall ..... The terminal peptide is D-alanine and D-glutamic although other amino acids are present as D- isomers
8. Carboxysomes are bacterial microcompar-tments that contain enzymes involved in all cyanobacteria and many chemotrophic bacteria that fix carbon dioxide.
9. Plasmolysis. is the osmotic loss of water from a bacterial cell that occurs when it is placed in a hypertonic environment.
10. Reduction potential (also known as redox potential, oxidation/ reduction potential, ORP, pE or E_h) is a measure of the tendency of a chemical species to acquire electrons and thereby be reduced. Reduction potential is measured in volts (V), or millivolts (mV). Each species has its own intrinsic reduction potential; the more positive the potential, the greater the species' affinity for electrons and tendency to be reduced and more negative shows maximum donation of electrons.
11.

Obligate aerobe	Grows only in presence of oxygen
Microaerophilic	Can grow only at reduced oxygen level
Obligate anaerobe	Cannot tolerate oxygen
Aerotolatrent anaerobe	Grow equally well in presence or absence of oxygen

12. A newly inoculated culture usually does not begin growing immediately but rather after of period of no growth which is referred to as the lag phase.

    Conditions that lead to a lag phase –
    - inoculum which is in stationary phase inoculated into the same medium
    - inoculum which is damaged but not killed inoculated into the same medium
    - inoculum transferred from rich to poor medium

    But a lag phase is not necessary when active cells are transferred back to the same medium.
13. Endospores are dormant, non-reproductive and enzymatically inert forms of bacterial vegetative cells. Endospores serve to protect the bacterium from harmful environmental conditions by reducing it into a desiccated, cryptobiotic and highly defensive state which conveys resistance to many environmental conditions that would otherwise harm and kill the vegetative form of the bacterium. These environmental conditions include extreme temperatures, radiation, extreme pH levels, extreme pressures and harmful chemical agents. Small acid-soluble proteins (SASPs) are also only found in endospores. These proteins tightly bind and condense the DNA, and are in part responsible for resistance to UV light and DNA-damaging chemicals.
14. The glyoxylate cycle uses a two-step bypass. One key enzyme, isocitrate lyase, converts D-threo-isocitrate to form succinate and glyoxylate. A second key enzyme, malate synthase, condenses glyoxylate and a second molecule of acetyl-CoA to form (S)-malate. The subsequent oxidation of malate regenerates the initial acetyl-CoA acceptor molecule of the TCA cycle, oxaloacetate.

    Thus in the reaction:

    Isocitrate $\rightarrow$ Succinate + Glyoxylate

    P enzyme is Isocitrate lyase.

    And in the reaction:

    Glyoxylate + Acetyl Co-A $\rightarrow$ Malate + Co-A

    Q enzyme is Malate synthase.
15. Koch's postulates are four criteria designed to establish a causal relationship between a causative microbe and a disease.

    Koch's postulates are the following:
    1. The microorganism must be found in abundance in all organisms suffering from the disease, but should not be found in healthy organisms.
    2. The microorganism must be isolated from a diseased organism and grown in pure culture.
    3. The cultured microorganism should cause disease when introduced into a healthy organism.
    4. The microorganism must be reisolated from the inoculated, diseased experimental host and identified as being identical to the original specific causative agent.

16. Milk can be pasteurized at different time-temperature profiles. A table below illustrates the different time- temperature profiles for mil pasteurization:

63°C (145°F)	30 minutes	Vat Pasteurization
72°C (161°F)	15 seconds	High temperat ure short time Pasteuriz-ation (HTST)
89°C (191°F)	1.0 second	Higher-Heat Shorter Time (HHST)
90°C (194°F)	0.5 seconds	Higher-Heat Shorter Time (HHST)
94°C (201°F)	0.1 seconds	Higher-Heat Shorter Time (HHST)
96°C (204°F)	0.05 seconds	Higher-Heat Shorter Time (HHST)
100°C (212°F)	0.01 seconds	Higher-Heat Shorter Time (HHST)
138°C (280°F)	2.0 seconds	Ultra Pasteuri zation (UP)

Although High-temperature short-time (HTST) pasteurization, or flash pasteurization, is the most common method these days, especially for higher volume processing. This method is faster and more energy efficient than batch pasteurization. Thus exposing milk to 143°F for 30 min is an incorrect method.

17. Loss of the prophage leads to the loss by the bacterium of the properties that originated during the lysogenic conversion.

18. Phage- typing is a procedure for characterizing and detecting bacterial strains by their reaction (susceptibility or resistance) to various known strains of phages. The phage-typing procedure is sometimes employed in epidemiology to identify and trace the progress of an infectious agent. This has been a standard procedure for strains of *Staphylococcus aureus* involved in outbreaks of food poisoning or other infections.

19. Human hepatitis delta virus (HDV) is the smallest RNA virus in genome.The virion particles and DNA or RNA polymerase for replication of the viral genome. but require helper viruses for providing envelopes for assembling mature virions.

20. Herpes simplex virus type 1 (HSV-1) infection in neurons is lifelong and generally asymptomatic.

21.

Toxin	MOA	Disease
Pertusis Toxin	Block G protein signal transduction	Whooping Cough
Diptheria Toxin	Inhibits Protein synthesis in eukaryotes	Diptheria
Botulinum Toxin	Block release of acetyl-choline by nerve end	Botulism
Tetanus Toxin	Cause Haemolysis	Tetanus

22.

Streptomycin	Protein synthesis inhibitor
Tetracyclin	Aminoacyl tRNA association with ribosomes
Erythromycin	Translocation
Chloroamphenicol	Transpeptidation

23. Transcriptional attenuation regulates the expression of *trp* operon in *E. coli* by controlling the ability of RNA polymerase to continue elongation past specific sites. The *trp* operon is regulated in part by a repressor that, when bound to tryptophan, blocks transcription. However, transcriptional attenuation provides an additional level of control that result in more stringent regulation that could be achieved by repression of initiation alone. The site of attenuation is located 162 nucleotides downstream of the transcription start site. Thus arginine alone is able to restore the attenuation control of *trp* operon as tryptophan only controls the attenuation within the *trpL*.

24. because trpL is not related with operator region and do not have any effect on that. But it has effect on structural gens.

25. because it is completing Chargaff's rules state that double stranded linear DNA from any cell of all organisms should have a 1 : 1 ratio (base Pair Rule) of pyrimidine and purine bases.

26. The extent of binding of chlorpromazine to native calf thymus DNA, as measured by spectrophotometric method, is decreased with increasing sodium chloride concentration. A curvature in the scattered plot suggests two types of binding processes. Decreases the optical density at higher temperatures without affecting the Tm of DNA.

27. Given,

Initial cell population (N_0) = 1×10^3 cells

Generation time (G) = 20 minutes = 0.33 hour

Lag phase = 1 hour

Culture is allowed to grow for 4 hours,

Thus, time (t) = 3 hours (since 1 hour is log period)

Thus, number of generations (n)

$= t/G = 3/0.33 = 9$ (approx.)

28. Now, time = 3 hours

Cell population after 3 hours (N) = ?

We know, $G = t/3.3(\log_{10}N - \log_{10}N_0)$

$0.33 = 3/3.3(\log_{10}N - \log 10^3)$

Thus on solving, we get,

$N = 6.4 \times 10^4$

(M) ZOOLOGY

1. Amino acids are organic compounds that combine to form proteins. Amino acids and proteins are the building blocks of life. They are biologically important organic compounds made from amine ($-NH_2$) and carboxylic acid (–COOH) functional groups, along with a side-chain specific to each amino acid. As both the amine and carboxylic acid groups of amino acids can react to form amide bonds, one amino acid molecule can react with another and become joined through an amide linkage. This polymerization of amino acids is what creates proteins. Secondary structure of proteins, i.e., the α-helix and the β-pleated sheet are formed through intra and inter molecular hydrogen bonding between two chains of polypeptide.

2. A biological membrane or biomembrane is an enclosing or separating membrane that acts as a selective barrier, within or around a cell. It consists of a phospholipid bilayer which provides fluidity to cell membrane. The phospholipid bilayer accounts for thequasi-fluid structure of the biological membranes. The biological membranes are also composed of proteins (intrinsic and extrinsic) which help in transport of molecules across the membrane and small chains of oligosachharides that serve as cell-to-cell recognition.

3. Some operons are under attenuator control, in which transcription is initiated but is halted before the mRNA is transcribed. This introductory region of the mRNA is called the leader sequence; it includes the attenuator region, which can fold back on itself, forming a stem-and-loop structure that blocks the RNA polymerase from advancing along the DNA. It is the section of mRNA and DNA beginning at the +1 position up to that region prior to codon sequence, and transcribed into the ribosome-binding site. It is thus located at the site of the first exon of mRNA.

4. The surface-area-to-volume ratio also called the surface-to-volume ratio is the amount of surface area per unit volume of an object or collection of objects. The ratio between the surface area and volume of cells and organisms has an enormous impact on their biology. An increased surface area to volume ratio also means increased exposure to the environment. Surface to volume ratio places a maximum limit on the size of a cell. For example, many aquatic microorganisms have increased surface area to increase their drag in the water. This reduces their rate of sink and allows them to remain near the surface with less energy expenditure.

5. A population is the smallest biological unit that can evolve. It is a group of individuals of the same species, living in the same place, at the same time. They are a group of organisms of one species that interbreed and live in the same place at the same time (e.g. deer population). Thus all the sandalwood trees in the forest represent a population.

6. Non-specific responses are generalized responses to pathogen infection. They do not target a specific cell type. The non-specific response consists of some WBC's and plasma proteins. The second Line of Defense (Innate/Nonspecific Immunity) is comprised of Natural Killer Cells, White Blood Cells (phagocytic), inflammation, fever, and antimicrobial substances. The non-specific type of immunity is governed by the T-cytotoxic cells which are being regulated through cytokines released by T-helper cells. The class of immunity mediated by cytotoxic T-cells is called cell-mediated cytotoxicity. The cell-mediated cytotoxicity can be performed using interferons and complements.

7. The origin of mammalian hair and insect hair (like in bees) has a completely different origin. This implies that hair of mammals and hair of insects are analogous structures. Analogous structures are features of different species that are similar in function but not necessarily in structure and which do not derive from a common ancestral feature and which evolved in response to a similar environmental challenge. An analogy is a trait or an organ that appears similar in two unrelated organisms.

8. The area within the eye that detects light and colour is the called the Retina. The two types of detection cell present, rods and cones, process information coming through the Lens and send it down the optic nerve to the brain. Rod cells (of which there are around 100 million) detect the degree of lightness entering the eye and their sensitivity is dependent on the amount of Rhodopsin present which is itself generated within the cells. Cone cells (of which there are around 3 million) are also sensitive to light levels but retain their function upto high illumination via use of the pigment Iodopsin. The protein Rhodopsin contains the protonated retinal-Schiff's base complex which naturally lies in the inter-membrane pocket formed by the seven trans-membrane α-helical receptors. After the photoisomerisation cascade which occurs via 5 shortlived intermediates, trans retinal diffuses away and is converted back into 11-*cis* retinal before re-entry into the cycle. This process occurs via reduction to all-trans retinol followed by oxidation/isomerisation in the dark. Photoexcited Rhodopsin (4th of the 5 intermediates) triggers an enzymatic cascade process resulting in the hydrolysis of GMP. This in turn closes cation-specific channels within the rod cell membrane which are naturally open to influx of Na^+ in the dark, and due to the effect of hyperpolarisation, the inner synaptic body sends a nerve signal to other neurons in the Retina.

9. The Hardy-Weinberg principle states that both allele and genotype frequencies in a population remain constant-that is, they are in equilibrium-from generation to generation unless specific disturbing influences are introduced. Those disturbing influences include non-random mating, mutations, selection, random genetic drift, gene flow and meiotic drive. This law explains the equilibrium population (a population in which the gene frequencies have reached equilibrium between mutation pressure and selection pressure) of a particular species. Out of 1000 eggs produced by a single pair of frogs, only 100 tadpoles are produced. So, the mortality rate is high despite having a high reproductive rate.

Therefore, on an average $\frac{100}{1000}$ $= \frac{1}{10}$ or 1pair of frogs: 10 pairs of tadpoles are produced which would be capable of reproduction in the next season.

10. The Hypothalamus is an integral part of the brain. About the size of a pearl, the hypothalamus directs a multitude of important functions in the body. It is the control center for many autonomic functions of the peripheral nervous system. Connections with structures of the endocrine and nervous systems enable the hypothalamus to play a vital role in maintaining homeostasis. For example, blood vessel connections between the hypothalamus and pituitary gland allow hypothalamic hormones to control pituitary hormone secretion. As a limbic system structure, the hypothalamus also influences various emotional responses. The hypothalamus is involved in several functions of the body including: (a) Autonomic Function Control (b) Endocrine Function Control (c)Homeostasis (d) Motor Function Control (e) Food and Water Intake Regulation (f) Sleep-Wake Cycle Regulation. Thus, the brain scan would show a tumour present in the hypothalamus.

11. Altruism is a well-documented animal behaviour, which appears most obviously in kin relationships but may also be evident amongst wider social groups, in which an animal sacrifices its own well-being for the benefit of another animal. The apparent altruistic behaviour of many animals is, like some manifestations of sexual selection, a trait that at first seems incompatible with the theory of natural selection. Altruism is a form of behaviour that benefits other individuals at the expense of the one that performs the action; the fitness of the altruist is diminished by its behaviour, whereas individuals those act selfishly. Thus, Haldane would do this because either two or eight cousins would result in as much representation of Haldane's genes as would two of his own.

12. Linking number is a property of a long biopolymer (such as duplex DNA) equal to the number of twists (related to the frequency of turns around the central axis of the helix) plus the writhing number. This is a topological property that determines the degree of supercoiling. It defines the number of times a strand of DNA winds in the right-handed direction around the helix axis when the axis is constrained to lie in a plane. It is the number of times that one DNA strand crosses about the other when the DNA is made to lie flat on a plane. If both strands are covalently intact, the linking number cannot change. Link is thus a topological invariant, remaining unaltered even if the two curves are deformed in space -- as long as neither is cut. Topology theory indicates that the sum of T and W equals to linking number: $L = T + W$. Thus, based on linking theory, an unwound DNA and a supercoiled DNA with the same linking number are topologically identical but geometrically different.

13. Speciation refers to the evolutionary process by which new biological species arise. There are three main ideas concerning the emergence of new species (Modes of Speciation), each based on the degree to which populations undergoing this process are geographically isolated from one another (allopatric speciation, sympatric speciation, parapatric speciation). It is the evolutionary process by which new biological species arise. All forms of natural speciation have taken place over the course of evolution resulting in genetic and reproductive drift amongst species.

14. Darwinism designates a distinctive form of evolutionary explanation for the history and diversity of life on earth. In his theory of natural selection, Charles Darwin suggested that "survival of the fittest" was the basis for organic evolution (the modification of living things with time). The individuals that are best equipped to survive and reproduce perpetuate the highest frequency of genes to descendant populations. This is the principle known colloquially as "survival of the fittest," where fitness denotes an individual's overall ability to pass copies of his genes on to successive generations. Thus, the most likely explanation for modern day giraffes is that long-necked giraffes foraged better and, therefore survived better than those with the shorter necks.

15. Biomes are defined as "the world's major communities, classified according to the predominant vegetation and characterized by adaptations of organisms to that particular environment". Biomes are climatically and geographically defined as similar climatic conditions on the Earth, such as communities of plants, animals, and soil organisms, and are often referred to as ecosystems. Biomes are defined by factors such as plant structures (such as trees, shrubs, and grasses), leaf types (such as broadleaf and needle leaf), plant spacing (forest, woodland, savanna), and climate. A savanna is a grassland ecosystem characterized by the trees being sufficiently small or widely spaced so that the canopy does not close. It is hot, seasonally dry grassland with scattered trees. This environment is intermediate between grassland and a forest. Savannas are located in the dry tropics and the subtropics, often bordering a rainforest. Savannas have an extended dry season and a rainy season.

16. A Uricotelic organism produces uric acid (solid urea) as a result of deamination. An example of such organisms includes birds and insects. Elimination of uric acid as the main nitrogenous waste material is called uricotelism. Animals showing uricotelism are called uricotelic animals. Uric acid is formed from ammonia mostly in the liver and to some extent in the kidneys. The process is highly energy dependant, but is much

less toxic than both ammonia and urea and it is almost insoluble in water and can be eliminated from the body in nearly a solid state, saving a lot of water. Since kidneys can handle the nitrogenous wastes only in solution, reptiles and birds pass a dilute solution of uric acid into the cloaca, where water is absorbed and solid uric acid is eliminated along with faeces.

17. Imprinting, in psychobiology, is a form of learning in which a very young animal fixes its attention on the first object with which it has visual, auditory, or tactile experience and thereafter follows that object. In nature the object is almost invariably a parent; in experiments, other animals and inanimate objects have been used. Imprinting has been intensively studied only in birds, especially chickens, ducks, and geese, but a comparable form of learning apparently occurs in the young of many mammals and some fishes and insects.

18. With the removal of thymus glands from the new born mice, it loses the power of generation and maturation of T-cell lymphocytes since both the processes occurred and were regulated in thymus only. As such, the mice would lose the power of self and non-self recognition which is an attribute of the T-cell. Hence, the mice would readily accept tissue transplants as there would be no tissue rejection phenomena because of absence of Human leucocyte antigens that are present in T-cells.

19. Eutrophication is the process by which a body of water acquires a high concentration of nutrients, especially phosphates and nitrates. These typically promote excessive growth of algae. As the algae die and decompose, high levels of organic matter and the decomposing organisms deplete the water of available oxygen, causing the death of other organisms, such as fish. Eutrophication is defined as an increase in the rate of supply of organic matter in an ecosystem. **Eutrophication** is a syndrome of ecosystem responses to human activities that fertilize water bodies with nitrogen (N) and phosphorus (P), often leading to changes in animal and plant populations and degradation of water and habitat quality. Nitrogen and phosphorus are essential components of structural proteins, enzymes, cell membranes, nucleic acids, and molecules that capture and utilize light and chemical energy to support life. Nutrient enrichment of waters promotes the growth of algae, either as attached multicellular forms (e.g. sea lettuce) or as suspended microscopic phytoplankton, because algae can grow faster than larger vascular plants. As algal biomass builds during blooms it forms aggregates that sink and fuel bacterial growth in bottom waters and sediments. Bacterial metabolism consumes oxygen creating conditions stressful or even lethal for aquatic invertebrates and fish.

20. Rod cells (of which there are around 100 million) detect the degree of lightness entering the eye and their sensitivity is dependent on the amount of Rhodopsin present which is itself generated within the cells. Cone cells (of which there are around 3 million) are also sensitive to light levels but retain their function upto high illumination via use of the pigment Iodopsin. Cone cells, or cones, are photoreceptor cells in the retina of the eye that are responsible for color vision. Cones are less sensitive to light than the rod cells in the retina, but allow the perception of colour. Thus, the baby's vision with no cone cells would be colour-blind, easily blinded by bright light and capable only of coarse resolving power.

21. Vasodilation is the increase in the internal diameter of a blood vessel that results from relaxation of smooth muscle within the wall of the vessel thus causing an increase in blood flow. Vasodilation directly affects the relationship between mean arterial pressure, cardiac output and total peripheral resistance. Vasodilation occurs in superficial blood vessels of warm-blooded animals when their ambient environment is hot. This process diverts the flow of heated blood to the skin of the animal, where heat can be more easily released into the atmosphere.

22. When blastomeres were separated from early stages of cleavage of frog embryo gave viable tadpoles whereas blastomeres from late stages of cleavage, failed to develop into normal tadpoles after separation. This implies that early blastomeres consisted of cytoplasmic factors that governed the further process of embryo development and tadpole generation which was absent in the later stages of cleavage of the blastomeres.

23. Dolly was a female domestic sheep, and the first mammal to be cloned from an adult somatic cell, using the process of nuclear transfer. She was created using the technique of somatic cell nuclear transfer, where the cell nucleus from an adult cell is transferred into an unfertilised oocyte (developing egg cell) that has had its nucleus removed. The hybrid cell is then stimulated to divide by an electric shock, and when it develops into a blastocyst it is implanted in a surrogate mother. So, Dolly was a replica of one of its parents as it received the entire genetic complement from that parent.

24. A transgenic animal is one that carries a foreign gene that has been deliberately inserted into its genome. The foreign gene is constructed using recombinant

DNA technology (RDT). Dolly was different from her cousin who was a transgenic sheep because Dolly received the identical genetic complement of one of her parents while her cousin had a transgene (gene or genetic material that has been transferred naturally or by any of a number of genetic engineering techniques from one organism to another) in its genome.

25. The menstrual cycle, under the control of the endocrine system, is necessary for reproduction. It is divided into three phases: the follicular phase, ovulation, and the luteal phase. In follicular phase, through the influence of a rise in follicle stimulating hormone (FSH) during the first days of the cycle, a few ovarian follicles are stimulated. As they mature, the follicles secrete increasing amounts of estradiol, an oestrogen. The estrogens initiate the formation of a new layer of endometrium in the uterus. During the follicular phase, estradiol suppresses production of luteinizing hormone (LH) from the anterior pituitary gland. In animals, a Gonadotropin-releasing hormone (GnRH) surge has been shown to precede the LH surge, suggesting that estrogen's main effect is on the hypothalamus, which controls GnRH secretion. The release of LH matures the egg and weakens the wall of the follicle in the ovary, causing the fully developed follicle to release its secondary oocyte. The luteal phase is also called the secretory phase. An important role is played by the corpus luteum. After ovulation, the pituitary hormones FSH and LH cause the remaining parts of the dominant follicle to transform into the corpus luteum, which produces progesterone. From the time of ovulation until progesterone withdrawal has caused menstruation to begin, the process typically takes about two weeks, with 14 days considered normal.

26. Gonadotrophin releasing hormone (GnRH) is released from hypothalamus region of the brain. In the beginning, there is low oestrogen and progesterone circulating in the body. This will trigger the hypothalamus to secrete GnRH. GnRH will act on the anterior pituitary gland to produce LH and FSH. It is a kind of negative feedback mechanism that takes place. The corpus luteum produces oestrogen and progesterone. Thus the level of GnRH in blood will depend on the concentrations of oestrogen and progesterone. Hence, progesterone induces the negative feedback mechanism for secretion of LH and FSH.

27. F_1 progeny displays wild type eye colour. This is because the gene for mutant eye colourations is recessive in nature. Also, there occurs complementation of the two mutant genes as they are located in separate loci of two different genes. So they compensate for any loss in the wild type gene and result in wild type eye colours because of the dominance of wild type genes over the mutants.

28. Since, the two colouration genes for cinnabar and brown colours are mutants, in F_2 generation occurrence of the two mutants in an offspring of fruit fly would result in a co-expressive effect of the two mutants resulting in no colour formation (white).

■■

GATE-2005

XL : LIFE SCIENCES

Time : 3 Hours | *Maximum Marks : 100*

H : CHEMISTRY (Compulsory)

Useful data :

F = 96485 C mol^{-1}; R = 8.314 JK^{-1} mol^{-1}; Atomic number; Co = 27

Q. 1 – 10 carry one mark each

1. Elements exhibiting +2 oxidation state in their compounds is

(*a*) Zn and P (*b*) Ca and Al

(*c*) Al and P (*d*) Zn and Ca

2. The paramagnetic species is

(*a*) Na_2 (*b*) NO^+ (*c*) CN (*d*) CO

3. Hydride that readily liberates hydrogen gas on reaction with water is

(*a*) $NaBH_4$ (*b*) CaH_2 (*c*) SiH_4 (*d*) NH_3

4. Which one of the following is aromatic?

(*a*) 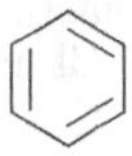 (*b*) 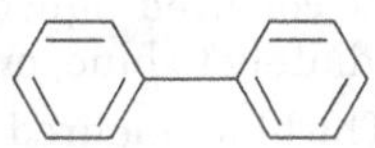

(*c*) 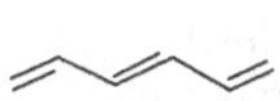 (*d*) 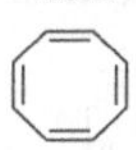

5. Identify the product of the following reaction.

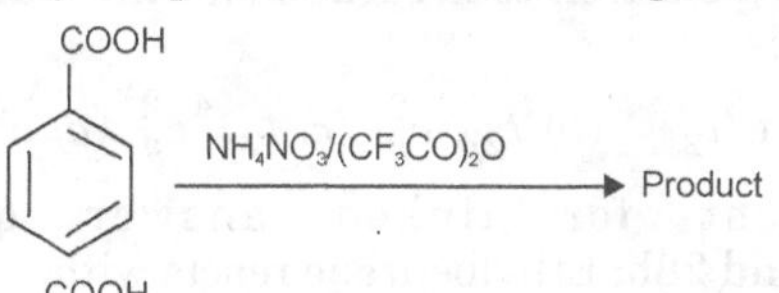

(*a*) 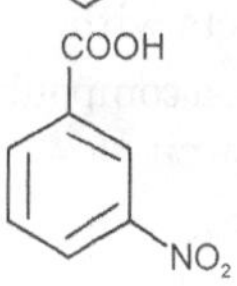

(*b*) 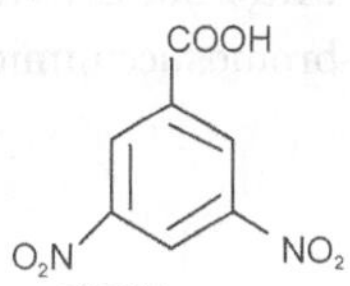

(*c*) 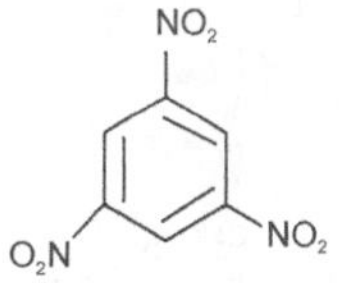

(*d*) 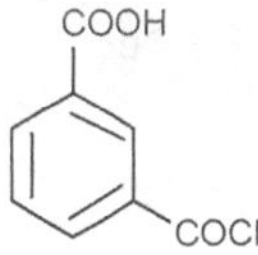

6. Which one of the following is most acidic?

(*a*) Butanoic acid

(*b*) 3-Chlorobutanoic acid

(*c*) 2-Chlorobutanoic acid

(*d*) 4-Chlorobutanoic acid

7. Total number of stereoisomers possible in $CH_3 - CH\,(Ph) - CH = CHCH_3$ is

(*a*) 1 (*b*) 2 (*c*) 3 (*d*) 4

8. The standard EMF of the cell, set up from the reaction $2Cu^+ (aq) \rightarrow Cu(s) + Cu^{2+} (aq)$ is 0.36 V at 298 K. The standard Gibbs free energy in kJ/mol for this reaction is

(*a*) – 34.73 (*b*) – 69.46 (*c*) – 3473 (*d*) – 6946

9. Heisenberg's uncertainty principle is expressed as

(*a*) $\Delta p\,\Delta x \geq h/2\pi$ (*b*) $\Delta p\,\Delta x \leq h/4\pi$

(*c*) $\Delta p\,\Delta x \leq h/2\pi$ (*d*) $\Delta p\,\Delta x \geq h/4\pi$

10. For the reaction, $C_6H_{12}O_6(s) + 6O_2(g) \rightarrow 6CO_2(g) + 6H_2O(l)$, $\Delta U = -2810$ kJ/mol. ΔH in kJ/mol is

(*a*) 845 (*b*) – 890 (*c*) – 2810 (*d*) – 2864

Q. 11 – 26 carry two marks each

11. Which one of the following is a repeating unit of silicone?

(*a*) $Si(CH_3)_4$ (*b*) $Si(CH_3)_2O$

(*c*) SiO_2 (*d*) $Si(OCH_3)_4$

12. The order of lattice energy of NaX is NaI < NaBr < NaCl < NaF. The property of X/X^-, responsible for the trend is

(*a*) ionic radii (*b*) electronegativity

(*c*) atomic radii (*d*) electron affinity

13. Among BF_3, CF_4, PF_3, and OF_2, the molecules that are expected to have a zero dipole moment is

(*a*) OF_2 and CF_4 (*b*) BF_3 and PF_3

(*c*) OF_2 and PF_3 (*d*) BF_3 and CF_4

14. Air oxidation of sodium metal produces a hygroscopic compound 'X', which reacts with CO_2 to produce 'Y'. X and Y respectively are

(*a*) Na_2O_2 and Na_2O_3

(*b*) Na_2O and $NaHCO_3$

(*c*) NaOH and Na_2CO_3

(*d*) Na_2O and Na_2CO_3

15. The product of reaction of HNO_3 with P_4 and P_4O_{10} respectively are

(*a*) N_2O_3 and N_2O_5 (*b*) N_2O_5 and NO_2

(*c*) NO_2 and N_2O_5 (*d*) NO and NO_2

16. Identify the product for the following Diels-Alder reaction.

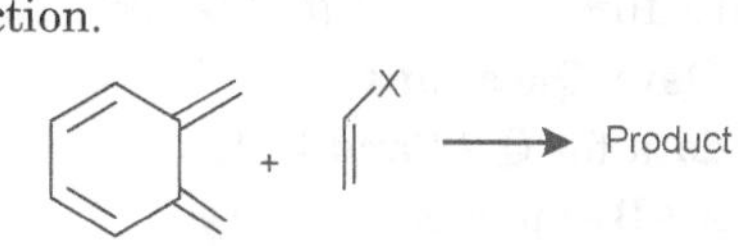

(*a*) 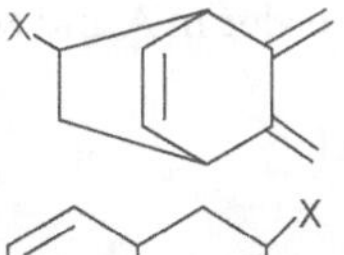

(*b*) 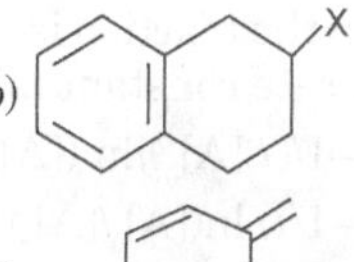

(*c*) 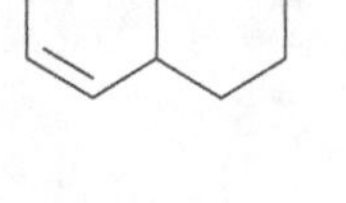

(*d*) 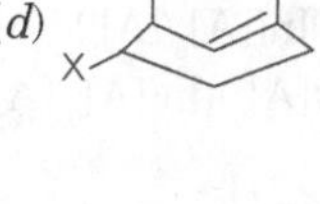

17. Major product of reaction given below is

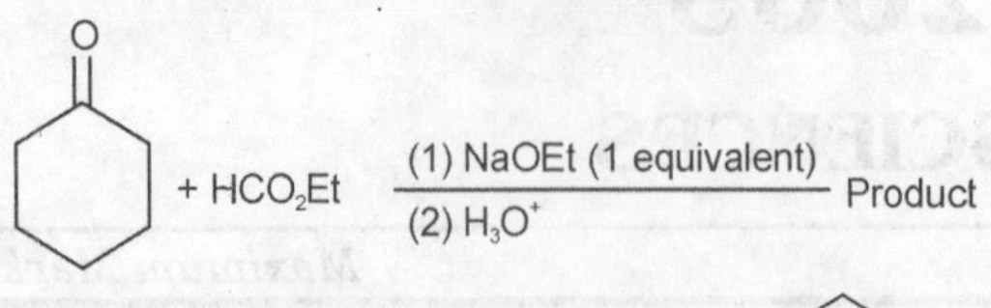

(*a*) 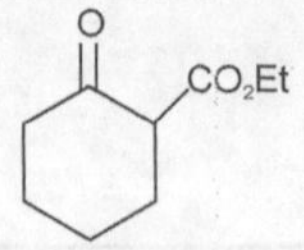 (*b*) 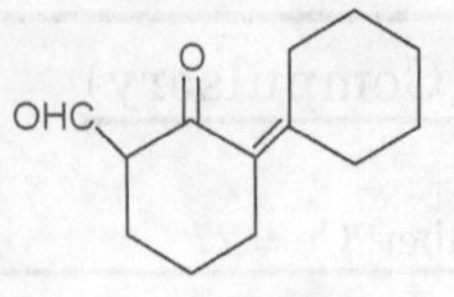

(*c*) 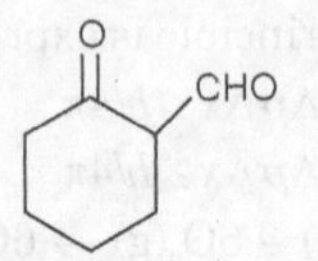 (*d*) 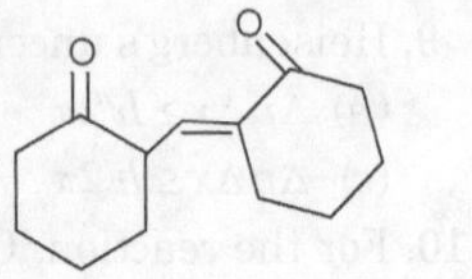

18. 0.050 mol of Ar initially at 25 °C, expands adiabatically and reversibly from 0.50 L to 1.00 L ($C_{v,m}$ for Ar is 12.48 J/Kmol). The work done in this process is

(*a*) 117 J (*b*) – 69 J (*c*) – 138 J (*d*) – 1378 J

19. Efficiency of a reversible cyclic heat engine working between T_c and T_h is

(*a*) $\frac{-T_c}{T_h}$ (*b*) $\frac{T_c - T_h}{T_h}$

(*c*) $\frac{(T_h - T_c)}{T_h}$ (*d*) $\frac{T_c}{T_h}$

20. To prepare one litre of an acetate buffer of 0.1 ionic strength and pH 5, at 25°C, the moles of sodium acetate and acetic acid (dissociation constant = 2.69×10^{-5}) to be added respectively are

(*a*) 0.1 and 0.0372 (*b*) 0.0372 and 0.1

(*c*) 0.01 and 0.372 (*d*) 0.372 and 0.01

21. The EMF of the cell {Pt, H_2 (1 atm) \HCl(*aq*) | | AgCl, Ag |} is 0.332 V and the EMF of AgCl\Ag electrode is 0.277 V. The pH of the solution is

(*a*) 0.926 (*b*) 1.03

(*c*) 3.26 (*d*) 5.61

22. In a saturated aqueous solution of CaF_2, the concentrations of Ca^{2+} and F^- are 3.3×10^{-4} M and 6.7×10^{-4} M, respectively. On adding NaF to this solution, if the concentration of Ca^{2+} changes to 1.5×10^{-4} M, then molar concentration of F^- will be

(*a*) 1.0×10^{-8} (*b*) 1.0×10^{-6}

(*c*) 1.0×10^{-4} (*d*) 1.0×10^{-3}

Common Data Questions

Common data for Q.23 and Q.24:

Reaction: A + B → products

23. When the reaction is first order in A and zero order in B, rate constant is

(*a*) $\{-1/(t)[A]_0\}\ln([A]_0/[A]_t)$

(*b*) $(-1/t)\ln([A]_0/[A]_t)$

(*c*) $(1/t)\ln([A]_0/[A]_t)$

(*d*) $\{1/(t[A]_0)\}\ln([A]_0/[A]_t)$

24. When the reaction is second order in A and zero order in B, rate constant is

(*a*) $(1/t)\{([A]_t)-[A]_0)/(\{A\}_0\{A\}_t\}$

(*b*) $(1/t)\{(1/[A]_t)-(1/[A]_0)\}$

(*c*) $\{[1/(t[A]_0)\}\{([A]/-[A\}_0)/(\{A]_0[A]_t\}$

(*d*) $\{1/(t[A]_0\}\{1/[A]_t-(1/[A]_0)\}$

Common data for Q. 25 and Q. 26:

3, 3-dimethyl-1-butene (Me_3 C–CH = CH_2), on reaction with

25. Hydrochloric acid produces a halogenated compound as major product. The product is

(*a*) Me_3C–CH(Cl)–CH_3 (*b*) Me_3C–CH_2–CH_2Cl

(*c*) Me_2C(Cl)–$CHMe_2$ (*d*) Me_2C(Cl)–$CH_2CH_2CH_3$

26. Hg $(OCOCH_3)_2$ followed by treatment with alkaline $NaBH_4$ produces

(*a*) Me_2C(OH)–$CHMe_2$ (*b*) Me_2C(OH)–$CH_2CH_2CH_3$

(*c*) Me_3C–CH_2–CH_2OH (*d*) Me_3C–CH(OH)–CH_3

Linked Answer Questions Q. 27a to Q. 28b carry two makrs each.

Statement for linked answer Question Q.27a and Q.27b.

A pink coloured aqueous solution of $CoCl_2$, changes immediately to blue, on adding excess of Cl^- ion

27a. The blue coloured species is

(*a*) $[CoCl_6]^{3-}$ (*b*) $[CoCl_4]^{2-}$

(*c*) $[Co(H_2O)_6]^{2+}$ (*d*) $[CoCl_4]^{1-}$

27b. The d-electron configuration for the blue complex ion is

(*a*) $e^3t_2^3$ (*b*) $t_{2g}{}^5e_g^2$ (*c*) $t_{2g}{}^4e_g^2$ (*d*) $e^4t_2^3$

Statement for linked answer question Q. 28a and 28b: Ethylbenzene reacts with.

28a. N-bromosuccinimide to produce a compound 'X'. X is

(*a*) 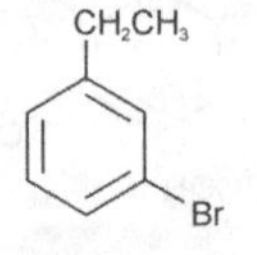 (*b*) 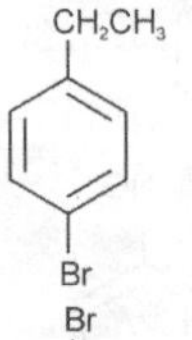

(*c*) 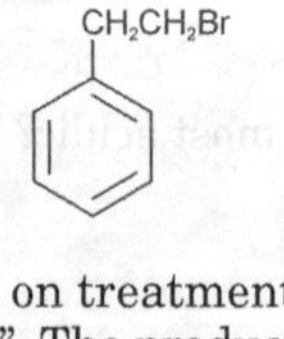 (*d*) 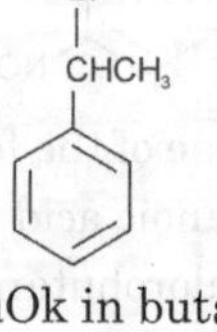

28b. 'X' on treatment with t-BuOk in butanol provides "Y". The product Y is

(*a*) 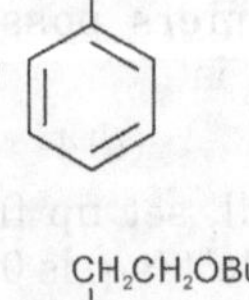 (*b*) 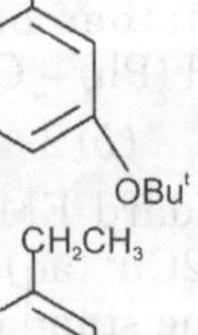

(*c*) 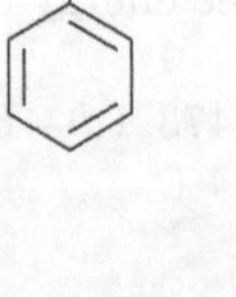 (*d*) 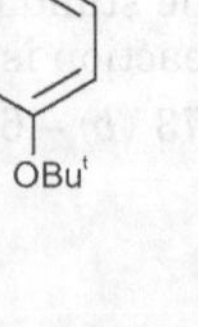

I : BIOCHEMISTRY

Q. 1 – Q. 10 carry one mark each

1. Which pair of amino acid residues can interact in the interior of a protein only through van der Waals forces?
(*a*) Arg, Thr (*b*) Ser, Thr
(*c*) Glu, His (*d*) Val, Leu

2. Okazaki fragments are joined by the enzyme
(*a*) RNA polymerase (*b*) DNA polymerase
(*c*) DNA ligase (*d*) Reverse transcriptase

3. The biosynthetic reactions in a cell mainly take place in
(*a*) Mitochondria
(*b*) Lysosomes
(*c*) Smooth endoplasmic reticulum
(*d*) Golgi apparatus

4. Colchicine inhibits
(*a*) DNA replication
(*b*) Formation of spindle fibers
(*c*) Condensatiosn of chromosomes
(*d*) Cytokinesis

5. The active form of Testosterone is
(*a*) Dihydrotestosterone
(*b*) Dehydrotestosterone
(*c*) Dihydroxytestosterone
(*d*) Dehydroepiandrosterone

6. The sensitivity of a radioimmunoassay depends primarily on
(*a*) Titer of the antibody
(*b*) Specificity of the antibody
(*c*) Specific activity of the ligand
(*d*) Purity of the antigen

7. In eukaryotes, introns can be found in transcripts which are precursors of
(*a*) mRNA (*b*) rRNA
(*c*) tRNA (*d*) All of the above

8. Homologous recombination can be employed to generate
(*a*) Transgenic animals
(*b*) Gene knock-out animals
(*c*) Site specific mutagenesis
(*d*) Specific promoter sequences

9. The mode of action of widely used anticancer drug methotrexate is to inhibit
(*a*) Dihydrofolate reductase
(*b*) Dihydrorotate dehydrogenase
(*c*) Carbamoyl phosphate synthase-2
(*d*) Ribonucleotide reductase

10. For a double stranded DNA which one of the following base-ratios will always be equal to 1?
(*a*) (A+T)/(G+C) (*b*) (A+G)/(C+T)
(*c*) C/T (*d*) A/G

Q. 11. – Q. 26 carry two marks each

11. Activated fatty acyl groups are transported into the mitochondria by
(*a*) Coenzyme A (*b*) Oxaloacetate
(*c*) Carnitine (*d*) Citrate

12. Amixture of Cytochrome-C (MW 11.7 KD) and Myoglobin (MW 17.2 KD) are to be separated by polyacrylamide gel electrophoresis. Their isoelectric pH (pI) values are 9.6 and 7.2 respectively. In which direction will each protein migrate at pH 8.5?
(*a*) Myoglobin will migrate to anode and Cytochrome-C will migrate to cathode
(*b*) Myoglobin will migrate to cathode and Cytochrome-C will migrate to anode
(*c*) Both will migrate to anode
(*d*) Both will migrate to cathode

13. Which one of the following fatty acids will have melting point higher than that of palmitic acid (16:0)?
(*a*) Myristic acid (14:0) (*b*) Palmitoleic acid (16:1)
(*c*) Oleic acid (18:1) (*d*) Stearic acid (18:0)

14. A diabetes mellitus patient excretes glucose in urine even when kept on a carbohydrate free diet. This is because
(*a*) Fats are catabolised in liver to form glucose
(*b*) Amino acids are catabolised in liver to form glucose
(*c*) Increased production of amino acids
(*d*) Increased breakdown of glycogen

15. According to the second law of thermod-ynamics, molecules spontaneously move from region of higher concentration to one of lower concentration. However, sodium ions are present at 143 mM outside the cell and 14 mM inside the cell. Yet sodium cannot pass through the plasma membrane. Transport of sodium into the cell is achieved by
(*a*) Facilitated diffusion
(*b*) Release of acetyl choline
(*c*) Release of norepinephrine
(*d*) Sodium transporter

16. The choice of the enzyme used in ELISA depends on
(*a*) Purity of the enzyme
(*b*) Turnover number
(*c*) Its absence in biological sample which is being analysed
(*d*) Its availability in bulk

17. The T cell antigen receptor
(*a*) Recognises conformational epitopes on the native molecule
(*b*) Has Ig light chains
(*c*) Is made up of heavy chain and β2 microglobulin
(*d*) Recognises epitopes on linear peptides associated with MHC determinants

18. The advantage of degeneracy in codons is that

(*a*) It minimises the deleterious effects of mutations

(*b*) It provides more flexibility

(*c*) It helps to code proteins resistant to proteases

(*d*) It helps to code proteins of very high molecular weight

19. The pK_a's of lysine are given below.
pK_a (COOH) = 2.2, pK_a (α-NH_3^+) = 9.0, pK_a (ε-NH_3^+) = 10.0 The pI of lysine is

(*a*) 7.07 (*b*) 9.50 (*c*) 6.10 (*d*) 5.60

20. The molecular weight of a bacterial DNA molecule is 2.64×10^9. The average molecular weight of a nucleotide pair is 660. Assume that the average protein is made up of a chain of 400 amino acid residues. What is the maximum number of proteins that can be coded by the bacterial DNA molecule?

(*a*) 20000 (*b*) 3333

(*c*) 6667 (*d*) None of the above

21. The coenzymes involved in the formation of Acetyl CoA from Pyruvate are

(*a*) Thiamine pyrophosphate, Lipoic acid and FAD

(*b*) Pyridoxyl phosphate, Biotin and FAD

(*c*) Vitamin B-12, Folic acid and Vitamin C

(*d*) NADH, Lipoic acid and Vitamin E

Common Data Questions

Common Data for Questions 22, 23, 24: A restriction fragment, obtained with a type II endonuclease that recognises a six base pair site, was subjected to Maxam-Gilbert sequence with results as shown in the autoradiogram below.

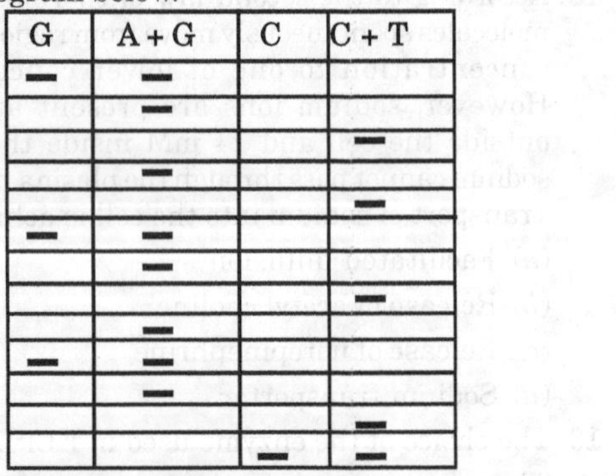

22. The DNA sequence is

(*a*) $^{3'}$CTAGATAGTATAG$^{5'}$

(*b*) $^{5'}$CTAGATAGTATAG$^{3'}$

(*c*) $^{3'}$GATCTATCATATC$^{5'}$

(*d*) $^{5'}$GATCTATCATATC$^{3'}$

23. The restriction site is

(*a*) TAGCTA ATCGAT (*b*) TAGGTA ATCCAT

(*c*) ATCCAT TAGGTA (*d*) GATACC CTATGG

24. Considering this DNA sequence as a template strand, the sequence of the corresponding mRNA is

(*a*) $^{5'}$CTAGATAGTATAG$^{3'}$

(*b*) $^{3'}$GATCTATCATATC$^{5'}$

(*c*) $^{3'}$GAUCUAUCAUAUC$^{5'}$

(*d*) $^{5'}$CUAGAUAGUAUAG$^{3'}$

Common Data for Questions 25, 26: The kinetic data for a enzymatic reaction in the oresence and absence of inhibitors are plotted in the following figure:

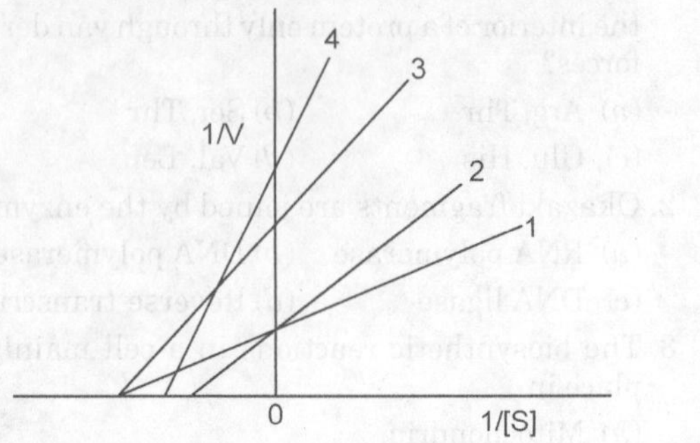

25. Which line represents the kinetics without inhibitor?

(*a*) Line 1 (*b*) Line 2

(*c*) Line 3 (*d*) Line 4

26. Which line represents kinetics of non-competitive inhibition?

(*a*) Line 1 (*b*) Line 2

(*c*) Line 3 (*d*) Line 4

Linked Answer Questions: Q27a to Q28b carry two marks each

Statement for Linked Answer Questions 27a & 27b: Transmission at many synapses in central nervous system is mediated by acetyl choline. Acetyl choline is cleaved to acetate and choline by the enzyme acetyl choline esterase which can be inhibited by disopropyl phosphofluoridate (DIPF).

27a. The mode of action of DIPF is by

(*a*) Modifying histidine residue

(*b*) Covalently modifying a crucial serine residue

(*c*) Inducing a conformational change in the protein

(*d*) Forming a complex with choline

27b. Based on its mode of action, DIPF is used as

(*a*) A therapeutic agent to treat neuro degenerative diseases

(*b*) A nerve gas

(*c*) As an agoni of acetyl choline

(*d*) A reagent to determine the N-terminal amino acid

Staement for Linked Answer Questions 28a & 28b: The following fragments are isolate on partial hydrolysis of a nonapeptide X.

Val-Arg-Pro-Gly, Lys-Phe-Val-Arg, Ala-Gly-Ser-Lys

28a. The correct sequence of X is

(*a*) Ala-Gly-Ser-Lys-Ala-Pro-Val-Arg-Gly

(*b*) Val-Arg-Gly-Lys-Phe-Val-Arg-Ala-Pro

(*c*) Lys-Phe-Val-Arg-Ala-Gly-Ser-Pro-Gly

(*d*) Ala-Gly-Ser-Lys-Phe-Val-Arg-Pro-Gly

28b. The number of fragments obtained when X is digested with trypsin is

(*a*) 0 (*b*) 2

(*c*) 3 (*d*) 4

K: BOTANY

Q. 1 – Q. 10 carry one mark each

1. For the formation of embryo sac the functional megaspore undergoes
   (*a*) Three meiotic division
   (*b*) Three mitotic division
   (*c*) Two mitotic division
   (*d*) Two meiotic division

2. How many nucleosomes per turn are present in a 30 nm chromatin fibre?
   (*a*) 4 (*b*) 8 (*c*) 6 (*d*) 10

3. The process by which water undergoes a phase transition from liquid state to an amorphous 'glassy state' is known as
   (*a*) Desiccation (*b*) Vitrification
   (*c*) Ice nucleation (*d*) Hyperhydricity

4. The term 'somaclonal variation' was coined by
   (*a*) Murashige and Skoog
   (*b*) Karp and Maddock
   (*c*) Gamborg and Phillips
   (*d*) Larkin and Scowcroft

5. Storage and transport of lipid occurs in
   (*a*) Glyoxysomes (*b*) Peroxysomes
   (*c*) Lysosomes (*d*) Spherosomes

6. The drug morphine is obtained from which plant part of *Papaver somniferum?*
   (*a*) Leaf (*b*) Stem
   (*c*) Capsule (*d*) Root

7. The floristic region of the world are determined on the basis of geographical distribution of plant genera. Identify the correct reason for this speciation.
   (*a*) Climate change
   (*b*) Genetic variation
   (*c*) Population distribution
   (*d*) Ecotypic variation

8. Pericycle is regarded as
   (*a*) The origin of lateral root and it is located between the endodermis and vascular bundle
   (*b*) Internal ground tissue present at the central position of the organ limited by the vascular bundles
   (*c*) Parenchymatous ground tissues passing in between the vascular bundles
   (*d*) The layer next to epidermis and solely consists of primary tissues

9. Apospory can be defined as
   (*a*) Development of sporophytes on the gametophytes without any reduction division
   (*b*) Development of gametophytes on the sporophytes without any reduction division
   (*c*) Development of several embryo within the same ovule
   (*d*) Development of an embryo directly from an egg cell or male gamate

10. The synonym of the families Labitae, Umbelliferae, Compositae and Graemineae are:
    (*a*) Leguminaceae, Acantheceae, Asteraceae, Lamiaceae
    (*b*) Solanaceae, Ancaceae, Apiaceae, Poaceae
    (*c*) Lamiaceae, Apiaceae, Asteraceae, Poaceae
    (*d*) Lilliaccae, Cuccrbitaceac, Poaceae, Astciaccac

Q. 11 – Q. 26 carry two marks cach

11. The following features outline a system of plant classification
    – Unisexual flowers are the most primitive within the angiosperms
    – Polyphyletic origin of angiosperms
    – Monocotyledons have been considered more primitive than dicotyledons

    Which one of the following systems of classification represents above features?
    (*a*) Linnaeus (*b*) Engler and Prantl
    (*c*) Rendle (*d*) Hutchinson

12. Following are the features of one type of C4 mechanism
    – The mitochondrion is responsible for malate decarboxylation
    – The mesophyll cell tends to form aspartate rather than malate, from oxaloacetate
    – Presence of double bundle sheath

    Identify the correct one.
    (*a*) NADP-ME type (*b*) PCK-type
    (*c*) NAD-ME type (*d*) CAM-type

13. Which one of the following statements is not true for marker-assisted selection?
    (*a*) The ability to manipulate recessive genes and identify the heterozygotes
    (*b*) A reduction in phenotypic screening and in the number of backcrosses
    (*c*) Without the self-fertilization of individual, heterozygotes cannot be identified
    (*d*) An early detection of superior lines along with the ability to select multiple traits simultaneously

14. Following are the symptoms of a disease in potato
    – Small, isolated, scattered, pale brown spots on the leaflets
    – The lowest leaves are attacked first and the disease progresses upwards
    – In the necrotic spots, concentric rings appear on the older leaves and darkened areas on the stem
    – There is usually a narrow chlorotic zone around the spots which fades into normal green and increases with an increase in the size of the spots

    Identify the disease, which manifests these symptoms
    (*a*) Early blight of potato
    (*b*) Wart disease of potato
    (*c*) Brown rot of potato
    (*d*) Late blight of potato

15. The two important biochemical reactions of nitrogen metabolism are shown below

$$NO_2 + 8H + 6e^- \xrightarrow{\text{ENZYME}} NH_4^+ + 2H_2O$$

$$\text{Glutamate} + NH_3 + ATP + Mg^{2++} \xrightarrow{\text{ENZYME}} \text{Glutamine} + ADP + Pi$$

Which one of the following pairs of enzymes is correct for the above reactions respectively?
(*a*) Nitrite reductase and Glutamate dehydrogenase
(*b*) Nitrate reductase and Glutamine synthetase
(*c*) Nitrite reductase and Glutamine synthetase
(*d*) Nitrite reductase and glutamate synthase

16. The functions of vir D2 protein in plant are
(*a*) Nuclear targeting and protection of 5' end of T-DNA
(*b*) Sensing phenolic kinase and induction of phosphorylation
(*c*) Nicking and processing of T-DNA
(*d*) Synthesis of transfer apparatus and regulation of cell cycle

17. $O_2 \rightarrow {}^1O_2 \rightarrow X \rightarrow Y$
In the given stepwise reduction of O_2, choose the correct sequence of 'reactive oxygen species' formed marked as 'X' and 'Y'
(*a*) ${}^1O_2 \rightarrow {}^1OH$ (*b*) $H_2O_2 \rightarrow {}^1OH$
(*c*) ${}^1O_2 \rightarrow H_2O_2$ (*d*) ${}^1OH \rightarrow {}^1O_2$

18. In a three point test cross XYZ/xyz × xyz/xyz, the following data are obtained:

XYZ	xyz	Xyz	xYZ	XYz	xyZ	XyZ	xYz
476	471	15	18	9	9	1	1

Find out the distance between X and Y genes
(*a*) 5 cM (*b*) 3 cM (*c*) 8 cM (*d*) 2 cM

Q. 19 – 26 are matching exercises. Choose the correct one from among the alternatives A, B, C and D

19. **Group I** (*Type of interaction*) **Group II** (*F_2 Phenotypic ratio*)

P Recessive epistasis.
Q Dominant epistatis
R Duplicate recessive epistatis
S Dominant and recessive epistatis

1. 12:3:1
2. 13:3
3. 9:6:1
4. 9:3:4
5. 9:7
6. 15:1

	P	Q	R	S
(*a*)	2	1	2	5
(*b*)	4	1	5	2
(*c*)	6	3	2	1
(*d*)	1	5	3	4

20. **Group I** (*Secondary metabolite*) **Group II** (*Precursor*)

P Coniine
Q Morphine
R Quinine
S Chalcone

1. Tryptophan
2. Phenylalanine
3. Lysine
4. Tyrosine
5. Ornithine
6. Agmatine

	P	Q	R	S
(*a*)	1	5	3	4
(*b*)	3	4	1	2
(*c*)	2	1	2	3
(*d*)	4	3	6	5

21. **Group I** (*Plant product*) **Group II** (*Plant species*)

P Hing
Q Dalchini
R Saffron
S Kattha

1. *Cinnamomum zeylanicum*
2. *Acacia catechu*
3. *Ferula asafoetida*
4. *Acacia nilotica*
5. *Cinnamomum tamala*
6. *Crocus sativus*

	P	Q	R	S
(*a*)	1	3	6	4
(*b*)	4	2	3	1
(*c*)	3	1	6	2
(*d*)	2	4	5	3

22. **Group I** (*Enzymes*) **Group II** (*Pathways*)

P Glycogen phosphorylase
Q Hexokinase
R Pyruvate carboxylase
S RuBP carboxylase

1. Glycolytic pathways
2. Calvin cycle
3. C_3 cycle
4. C_4 cycle
5. Glycogenolysis
6. C_6 cycle

	P	Q	R	S
(*a*)	5	1	6	3
(*b*)	4	2	5	1
(*c*)	2	1	3	4
(*d*)	6	5	2	1

23. **Group I** (*Inflorescence*) **Group II** (*Plant genera*)

P Raceme
Q Catkin
R Cyathium
S Verticillaster

1. *Poinsettia*
2. *Ocimum*
3. *Raphanus*
4. *Calotropis*
5. *Ficus*
6. *Salix*

	P	Q	R	S
(*a*)	1	4	3	5
(*b*)	3	6	1	2
(*c*)	2	5	3	1
(*d*)	4	3	1	6

24. **Group I** (*Hormone*) **Group II** (*Functions*)

P Gibberellin
Q IAA
R Cytokinin
S Ethylene

1. Phototrophism and gravitrophism
2. Stomatal movement
3. Delay of senesence
4. Combating water deficit
5. Seed germination
6. Ripening of fruits

	P	Q	R	S
(*a*)	6	4	1	2
(*b*)	5	1	3	6
(*c*)	3	4	5	1
(*d*)	4	3	1	5

25.

Group I (*In vitro problems*)	Group II (*Reme.dial measure*)
P Browning of explants	1. Addition of antio xidants in the medium
Q Hyperhydricity of regenerated shoots	2. Nurse culture
R Low frequency of formation of protoplast colonies	3. Osmotic pretreatment of tissues
S Low transformation frequency during biolistic operation	4. Membrane raft culture
	5. Decrease agar concentration
	6. Depletion of CO_2 in the culture vessel

	P	Q	R	S
(*a*)	2	3	5	4
(*b*)	3	2	4	6
(*c*)	1	4	2	3
(*d*)	4	3	1	6

26.

Group I (*Plant disease*)	Group II (*Causal organism*)
P Bunt of rice	1. *Macrophomina phaseolina*
Q Stem rot of jute	2. *Cercospora personata*
R Ergot of rye	3. *Tilletia barclayana*
S Ring rot of potato	4. *Xanthomonas oryzicola*
	5. *Claviceps purpurea*
	6. *Corynebacterium sepidonicum*

	P	Q	R	S
(*a*)	1	4	4	3
(*b*)	3	1	5	6
(*c*)	2	5	3	5
(*d*)	4	3	2	1

Linked Answer Questions: Q. 27a to Q. 28b carry two marks each

Statement for linked answer questions Q. 27a & Q. 27b:

In tomato the following genes are located on chromosome 3:

+ tall plant	*d* dwarf plant
+ normal leaves	*m* mottled leaves
+ smooth fruit	*p* pubescent fruit

Results of the cross

+++/dmp X dmp/dmp were

+++	430	dmp	452	+mp	45	d++	38
++p	16	dm+	17	+m+	1	d+p	1

27a. Which one of the following progeny groups represents double crossovers?

(*a*) +mp / d++ (*b*) ++p / dm+
(*c*) +m+ / d+p (*d*) +++ / dmp

27b. What would be the value of coincidence?

(*a*) 0.25 (*b*) 0.48 (*c*) 0.66 (*d*) 0.82

Statement for linked answer questions Q. 28a & Q. 28b: *Two proteins having same molecular weight of 1,92,000 dalton were identified. During post-translational modification one of the protein is phosphorylated.*

28a. What will be the nature of the band(s) if the mixture of these proteins is separated in electrophoretic gel?

(*a*) Single band
(*b*) Distinct two bands
(*c*) No band(s) at all
(*d*) Bands with a number of subunits

28b. For further separation of these two proteins what method one should adopt?

(*a*) 2-D gel electrophoresis
(*b*) Gel filtration chromatography
(*c*) Native gel electrophoresis
(*d*) Reverse phase chromatography

L: MICROBIOLOGY

Q. 1 – Q. 10 carry one mark each

1. The scientists who discovered restriction endonucleases are

(*a*) Temin and Baltimore
(*b*) Arber and Smith
(*c*) Gilbert and Sanger
(*d*) Lederberg and Tatum

2. The virus responsible for the 'Severe Acute Respiratory Syndrome' (SARS) is a

(*a*) Picomavirus (*b*) Coronavirus
(*c*) Adenovirus (*d*) Influenza virus

3. Denitrification process carried out by a few groups of bacteria reduces nitrate (NO_3) to nitrogen (N_2) gas. How many electrons per nitrogen atom are transferred to nitrate in this process

(*a*) 2 (*b*) 3 (*c*) 4 (*d*) 5

4. Metabolic yield of a product being produced by an industrially important microorganism is defined as

(*a*) gram product formed / gram substrate consumed
(*b*) gram product formed / gram cells formed
(*c*) gram product formed / litre of culture broth
(*d*) gram product formed / (litre . hour)

5. Which of the following features can distinguish Bacteria and Archea?

(*a*) Absence of the membrane-enclosed nucleus
(*b*) Absence of internal membranous organelles
(*c*) The type of glycosidic bonds present in the peptidoglycan layer (or its equivalent) of the cell wall
(*d*) Presence of N-acetylglucosamine in the peptidoglycan layer (or its equivalent) of the cell wall

6. Which of the following feature is not exhibited by green sulphur photosynthetic bacteria
   (*a*) Presence of bacteriochlorphylls
   (*b*) Sulphur deposition outside the cell wall
   (*c*) Oxygenic mode of photosynthesis
   (*d*) Non motile nature of cells
7. The microorganisms which obtain energy from the oxidation of inorganic compounds are known as
   (*a*) Photoautotrophs (*b*) Chemolithotrophs
   (*c*) Photoheterotrophs (*d*) Chemoorganotrophs
8. Neutrophiles exchange potassium for proton using
   (*a*) Antiport transport system
   (*b*) Symport transport system
   (*c*) ABC transport system
   (*d*) Group Translocation
9. Amphotericin B selectively disrupts the cell membrane of fungi because of its high affinity for a compound present in fungal membrane. The name of this compound is
   (*a*) Ergosterol (*b*) Mannitol
   (*c*) Miconazole (*d*) Clotrimazole
10. Which of the following 'hepatitis virus' has DNA genome
   (*a*) Hepatitis A (*b*) Hepatitis B
   (*c*) Hepatitis C (*d*) Hepatitis E

Q. 11 – Q. 26 carry two marks each.

11. Which of the following groups of microorganisms contain both superoxide dismutase and catalase enzymes for growth?
   (*a*) Obligate aerobes only
   (*b*) Facultative anaerobes only
   (*c*) Strict anaerobes only
   (*d*) Both obligate aerobes and facultative anaerobes
12. Which of the following is not responsible for making bacteria resistant to penicillin action
   (*a*) Change in the penicillin binding proteins
   (*b*) Inability of penicillin to reach its site of action
   (*c*) Inability to bind to 30S ribosomal subunit
   (*d*) Presence of plasmid coding for penicillinase
13. Match the correct combination of the antibiotic and the microorganism producing it

Antibiotic	*Microorganism*
P. Vancomycin	1. *Bacillus subtilis*
Q. Bacitracin	2. *Cephalosporium acremonium*
R. Chloramphenicol	3. *Streptomyce orientalis*
S. Streptomycin	4. *Penicillium chrysogenum*
	5. *Streptomyces venezuelae*
	6. *Streptomyces griseus*

	P	Q	R	S
(*a*)	3	1	5	6
(*b*)	1	4	6	3
(*c*)	5	3	6	4
(*d*)	6	3	5	2

14. The pathogenesis associated with *Vibrio cholerae* infection depends on the colonization of the small intestine by the organism and secretion of an enterotoxin. Which of the following statement related to pathogenicity of cholera is incorrect?
   (*a*) *Vibrio cholerae* secretes the enterotoxin choleragen
   (*b*) Choleragen consists of A (active) and B(binding) subunit
   (*c*) Choleragen toxin alone cannot reproduce the symptoms of cholera in the absence of *Vibrio cholerae*
   (*d*) CTX bacteriophage carries the genes of cholera toxin and other virulence factors
15. Prior infection of *Mycobacterium tuberculosis* can be detected by positive tuberculin skin test result. The basis of this test is
   (*a*) Anaphylactic hypersensitivity (Type I)
   (*b*) Antibody dependent cytotoxic hyper-sensitivity (Type II)
   (*c*) Immune complex mediated hyper-sensitivity (Type III)
   (*d*) Cell mediated or delayed hyper-sensitivity (Type IV)
16. A bacterial culture on being transferred from anaerobic to aerobic condition of growth drastically reduce the rate of glucose catabolism. This regulatory phenomenon is know as
   (*a*) Tyndallization (*b*) Pasteurization
   (*c*) Crabtree effect (*d*) Pasteur effect
17. Which of the following statements related to 'High frequency recombination' (Hfr) cells is incorrect
   (*a*) Single strand of DNA that enters into recipient F cell contains a piece of the F factor at the leading end followed by the bacterial chromosomes and then by the remainder of the F factor
   (*b*) Most mating results in the transfer of only a portion of donor chromosome because the attachment between the two cells can break
   (*c*) The bacterial genes adjacent to the leading piece of the F factor are least frequently transferred
   (*d*) The donor cell genes that are transferred vary, since the F plasmid can integrate at several different sites in a bacterial DNA
18. Replication of the positive strand genome of poliovirus requires
   (*a*) Reverse Transcriptase
   (*b*) Virus encoded RNA dependent RNA polymerase
   (*c*) DNA dependent RNA polymerase
   (*d*) DNA polymerase
19. Which of the following statement about bacteriophage λ is incorrect?
   (*a*) It initially produces two proteins; one acts as an inhibitor of λ repressor synthesis and the other acts as a terminator for transcription
   (*b*) It maintains its lysogenic state in the absence of an inducer

(*c*) In switching from the lysogenic to the lytic phase, it turns off the synthesis of λ repressor because cro protein binds to λ operator O_R3

(*d*) It forms N and Q gene products which act as positive regulatory proteins leading to the sequential production of λ encoded proteins

20. While evaluating the effectiveness of a disinfectant (X) against *Salmonella typhi* by the 'Phenol-Coefficient Method' the following data were obtained

	Subculture Tubes			
	Dilution	5 min	10 min	15 min
Disinfectant (X)	1 : 50	0	0	0
	1 : 100	+	0	0
	1 : 150	+	0	0
	1 : 175	+	+	0
	1 : 200	+	+	+
Phenol	1 : 90	+	0	0
	1 : 100	+	+	+

0 = no growth, + = growth

The Phenol-Coefficient of the disinfectant (X) would be

(*a*) 1.66 (*b*) 3.32
(*c*) 0.50 (*d*) 1.00

21. Lactic acid bacteria ferment glucose to produce two moles of lactic acid. What is the net yield of ATP and NADH per mole of glucose?

(*a*) 2 ATP and 2 NADH
(*b*) 2 ATP and 0 NADH
(*c*) 4 ATP and 2 NADH
(*d*) 4 ATP and 0 NADH

Common Data Questions

Common Data for Questions 22, 23, 24: *Analysis of the electron transport system in a newly isolated aerobic Gram-positive bacterium showed the existence of five electron transport molecules. Their redox potentials are as follows:*

Oxidant	Reductant	Electrons transferred	E_0' (volts)
P	PH_2	2	– 0.13
NAD^+	NADH	2	– 0.32
R	RH_2	2	– 0.02
Cytochrome c (+3)	Cytochrome c (+2)	1	+ 0.22
S	SH_2	2	+ 0.63

Faraday constant (F) = 23 kcal/(volt.mole)

22. Which of the following sequence of the electron transport carriers would be involved in the transport of electrons for energy generation?

(*a*) P → NAD^+ → R → Cytochrome c → S
(*b*) NAD^+ → P → R → Cytochrome c → S
(*c*) NAD^+ → P → Cytochrome c → R → S
(*d*) NAD^+ → Cytochrome c → P → R → S

23. If the electrons are transferred from NADH to S, the difference in redox potential would be

(*a*) + 0.95 (*b*) + 0.76 (*c*) – 0.95 (*d*) – 0.76

24. What would be the value of standard free energy change for the transfer of electrons from PH_2 to S?

(*a*) – 17.5 kcal/mol (*b*) – 35.0 kcal/mol
(*c*) + 17.5 kcal/mol (*d*) + 35.0 kcal/mol

Common Data for Questions 25 & 26: *E. coli can metabolize both glucose and lactose sugar as sole source of carbon and energy. While glucose catabolizing enzymes are constitutive lactose catabolizing enzymes are induced in the presence of compounds such as lactose IPTG, etc. Lactose catabolizing enzymes are also regulated by catabolite repression.*

25. Assume that *E. coli* has been grown in a nutrient medium containing lactose only. When the culture has reached the logarithmic phase of growth, the cells are harvested and transferred to a medium containing glucose only. Would you expect the culture to

(*a*) Continue to grow in its logarithmic phase
(*b*) Exhibit a lag phase first and then grow again in its logarithmic phase
(*c*) Undergo lysis
(*d*) Stop growth

26. If the *E. coli* cells are grown in a medium containing both glucose and lactose, what is likely to happen?

(*a*) Both the sugars would be utilized simultaneously
(*b*) The culture will exhibit synchronous growth
(*c*) Lactose will be utilized first followed by glucose
(*d*) Glucose will be utilized first followed by lactose

Linked Answer Questions: Q. 27a to Q. 28b carry two marks each

Statement for Linked Answer Questions 27a & 27b:
Consider a nutrient medium containing 2×10^4 cells. The culture is incubated at 25°C under aerobic conditions for growing the cells. The generation time of the cells is 40 minutes.

27a. If the culture is allowed to grow for 8 hours, how many generations would have taken place?

(*a*) 8 (*b*) 12 (*c*) 16 (*d*) 24

27b. What will be the cell population after 8 hours ?

(*a*) 4.1×10^5 (*b*) 8.2×10^6
(*c*) 4.1×10^7 (*d*) 8.2×10^7

Statement for Linked Answer Questions 28a & 28b:
A mutant of E. coli was found which did not synthesize β-galactosidase in the presence as well as in the absence of the inducer, IPTG. The investigation revealed that the structural genes of the lac operon were unaltered in the mutant, but one of the controlling genes (I or O) was mutated. The different allelic forms of the regulator gene and the operator gene are as follows

I^+ – Wild type regulator gene
I^c – Constitutive regulator
I^s – Repressor form which is insensitive to inducer
O^+ – Wild type operator gene
O^c – Constitutive operator

28a. Which of the following mutation in the controlling genes was responsible for the above mentioned behaviour of the *E. coli* mutant?

(*a*) $I^+ O^+$ (*b*) $I^C O^+$ (*c*) $I^S O^+$ (*d*) $I^+ O^C$

28b. On further mutation, the *E. coli* mutant synthesized β-galactosidase in the presence of the inducer only. Which of the following mutant form would explain this observation?

(*a*) $I^+ O^+$ (*b*) $I^+ O^C$ (*c*) $I^S O^+$ (*d*) $I^S O^C$

M: ZOOLOGY

Q. 1 – Q. 10 carry one mark each

1. The fur color of a newly identified species of dog is either white or red and is controlled by a single gene with two alleles. In a genetic experiment, a red dog was mated with a white dog. The white to red ratio among the offspring was 1 : 1. What is the genotype of the parent with the red fur?
(*a*) Heterozygous
(*b*) Homozygous for the dominant allele
(*c*) Homozygous for the recessive allele
(*d*) Insufficient data to decide

2. Which one of the following is NOT true regarding human reproduction?
(*a*) Oestrogen has both positive and negative feedback effects on the pituitary gland.
(*b*) Corpus luteum produces progesterone.
(*c*) Progesterone is essential to maintain the structure of the endometrium.
(*d*) Chorionic gonadotropin is secreted by corpus luteum if fertilization occurs.

3. Which one of the following statements is true?
(*a*) All vertebrates contain amnion
(*b*) All chordates are vertebrates
(*c*) All tunicates are chordates
(*d*) Cephalochordates are characterized by the presence of a well defined skull.

4. The body plan common to both annelids and insects is ______.
(*a*) Acoelomate (*b*) Pseudocoel
(*c*) Coelom (*d*) Homocoel

5. Which one of the following is an anatomical feature unique to marine and desert mammals?
(*a*) Four-chambered heart
(*b*) Long kidney loops
(*c*) Waterproof skin
(*d*) Very small kidneys

6. Which one of the following is the most useful method to determine the evolutionary distance between two closely related species?
(*a*) Comparison of anatomical structures
(*b*) Comparison of the DNA sequences of the exons of conserved genes
(*c*) Comparison of the intronic sequences
(*d*) Fossil records

7. Hydrostatic skeleton is one of the characteristics of__________.
(*a*) Onychophorans (*b*) Jelly fish
(*c*) Nematodes (*d*) Sponges

8. Rearrange the following taxonomic terms in the correct hierarchical order.
ORDER – FAMILY – PHYLUM – CLASS
(*a*) FAMILY – PHYLUM – CLASS – ORDER
(*b*) PHYLUM – ORDER – CLASS – FAMILY
(*c*) CLASS – PHYLUM – FAMILY – ORDER
(*d*) PHYLUM – CLASS – ORDER – FAMILY

9. The following is a list of animals and their geographical distribution. Among the options, choose the one that matches the animals to their correct geographical distribution.

A. Tardigrades	1. Ocean
B. Snail	2. Leaf litter
C. Peripatus	3. Fresh water
D. Oyster	4. Moist soil

(*a*) A-4, B-3, C-2, D-1 (*b*) A-3, B-2, C-1, D-4
(*c*) A-2, B-2, C-4, D-3 (*d*) A-3, B-4, C-2, D-1

10. Which one of the following anatomical feature enables the sessile life style of sea-squirts?
(*a*) Endostyle (*b*) Otolith
(*c*) Branchial basket (*d*) Solenocytes

Q. 11 – Q. 26 carry two marks each

11. Which one of the following is a true statement?
(*a*) The embryos of higher organisms resemble the adults of lower organisms
(*b*) Intestine develops from the germ layer called endoderm
(*c*) Blood vessels develop from somites
(*d*) All the brain cells develop from mesoderm

12. The following paired terms are not correctly paired. Which one of the four options is the correct pairing?

A. Hedgehog signaling	1. Anterior – posterior axis duplication
B. Wnt signaling.,	2. Cyclopic eye of lambs
C. Notch signaling	3. Vertebrate limb development
D. Hox genes	4. Nematode germ cell proliferation

(*a*) A-1, B-2, C-3, D-4 (*b*) A-3, B-4, C-1, D-2
(*c*) A-4, B-1, C-2, D-3 (*d*) A-2, B-1, C-4, D-3

13. Which one of the following gives rise to bone?
(*a*) Somites (*b*) Osteoclasts
(*c*) Chondrocytes (*d*) Osteocyte

14. The Michaelis-Menton constant K_m is a measure of__________.
(*a*) The rate of the reaction
(*b*) The affinity of the enzyme for the substrate
(*c*) The concentration of the enzyme-substrate (ES) intermediate
(*d*) None of the above

15. Which one of the following is the major force of attraction that stabilizes the three dimensional structure of globular proteins?
(*a*) Peptide bond
(*b*) Van der Waal's interactions
(*c*) Hydrogen bonds
(*d*) Hydrophobic interactions between the side chains

16. The histone H1 is present in the ______.
(*a*) Linker region (*b*) Nucleosome
(*c*) Nucleolus (*d*) hnRNPs

17. Proper execution of cell division cycle is ensured by______.
(*a*) Apoptosis
(*b*) DNA polymerases
(*c*) Cyclins
(*d*) Proteins of the cell cycle checkpoints

18. The following is a list of subcellular structures and their functions. Choose the option that correctly matches the subcellular structures to their functions.

A. Tonoplast	1. Lipid biosynthesis
B. Peroxisomes	2. Protein degradation
C. Endosome	3. Storage of starch
D. Proteasome	4. Removal of free radicals

(*a*) A-1, B-2, C-3, D-4 (*b*) A-3, B-4, C-1, D-2
(*c*) A-3, B-4, C-2, D-1 (*d*) A-1, B-2, C-4, D-3

19. Choose the correct statement.
(*a*) The endosymbiotic theory views that organelles like mitochondria were once free living organisms.
(*b*) Endosymbiotic theory states that bacteria, like *E. coli,* were once endoparasites.
(*c*) Endosymbiotic theory states that endosperms are prone to parasitic bacterial infection.
(*d*) Endosymbiotic theory states that endospores exist in symbiotic association with bacteria.

20. Cohort it defined as________.
(*a*) Individuals in a population with all of very different age.
(*b*) Individuals in a population with approximately same age.
(*c*) Individuals belonging to different species of animals.
(*d*) Individuals exhibiting most diverse behaviour in a population.

21. The neotropic biogeographical region for terrestrial species include_______.
(*a*) India and Indonesia (*b*) Southern Africa
(*c*) South America (*d*) Australia

22. Pseudocoelomate body cavity is found in_____.
(*a*) *Caenorhabditis elegans*
(*b*) *Octopus vulgaris*
(*c*) *Fasciola hepatica*
(*d*) *Lumbricus terrestris*

23. Asexual reproduction by longitudinal binary fission occurs in the protozoan.
(*a*) Paramaecium (*b*) Plasmodium
(*c*) Amoeba (*d*) Trypanosoma

24. According to fossil history, Hyracotherium is an ancestor of______.
(*a*) Hayena (*b*) Horse
(*c*) Elephant (*d*) Lion

25. Immunoglobulin IgG has 4 chains held by disulphide bonds. The maximum number of different amino acids present at the C terminal end of a monoclonal IgG is_____.
(*a*) 1 (*b*) 2 (*c*) 3 (*d*) 4

26. There is a change of concentration of ions during formation of urine, the concentration in urine being higher than that in plasma in healthy humans. The correct order of change in ion concentration between plasma and urine is________.
(*a*) $NH_4^+ > PO_4^{-3} > K^+ > Na^+$
(*b*) $PO_4^{-3} > K^+ > Na^+ > NH_4^+$
(*c*) $NH_4^+ > PO_4^{-3} > Na^+ > K^+$
(*d*) $Na^+ > K^+ > PO_4^{-3} > NH_4^+$

Linked Answer Questions: Q.27a to Q.28b carry two marks each

Statement for Linked Answer Questions 27a & 27b: *Assume genes a, b and c are on the same chromosome. In a mating experiment to map the relative positions of these three genes, the following results were obtained:*

1. Out of 500 progenies of the parents with the genotype *a*(–) *b*(–) /*a*(+) *b*(+), 20 were *a*(–) *b*(–)/*a*(–) *b*(+).
2. Out of 1000 progenies of the parents with the genotype *a*(–) *c*(–)/*a*(+) *c*(+), 80 were *a*(–) *c*(–)/*a*(+) *c*(–).

27a. What are the frequencies of recombination between *a* and *b*, and between *a* and *c*?
(*a*) 8 and 4 (*b*) 24 and 12
(*c*) 4 and 8 (*d*) 12 and 24

27b. Which one of the following is definitely true in terms of the relative map positions?
(*a*) *a* is closer to *c* than to *b*
(*b*) *a* is closer to *b* than to *c*
(*c*) *b* is closer to *a* than to *c*
(*d*) *c* is closer to *b* than to *a*

Statement for Linked Answer Questions 28a & 28b: *Assume that a population meets Hardy-Weinberg conditions, where p and q are dominant and recessive alleles.*

28a. Which of the following equations can be used to determine the genotype frequence
(*a*) $p + q = 1$ (*b*) $p^2 + 2pq + q^2 = 1$
(*c*) $pp \times q = 1$ (*d*) $(p + q)(p - q) = 1$

28b. In a population where 1% of people are homozygous recessive, the percentage of people with heterozygous genotype is ____
(*a*) 90% (*b*) 9% (*c*) 10% (*d*) 18%

ANSWERS

(H) CHEMISTRY

1. (*d*)	2. (*c*)	3. (*b*)	4. (*a*)	5. (*a*)	6. (*c*)	7. (*d*)	8. (*a*)	9. (*d*)	10. (*c*)
11. (*b*)	12. (*a*)	13. (*d*)	14. (*c*)	15. (*c*)	16. (*b*)	17. (*c*)	18. (*b*)	19. (*c*)	20. (*a*)
21. (*a*)	22. (*d*)	23. (*c*)	24. (*b*)	25. (*c*)	26. (*d*)	27a. (*b*)	27b. (*d*)	28a. (*d*)	28b. (*a*)

(I) BIOCHEMISTRY

1. (*d*)	2. (*c*)	3. (*a*)	4. (*b*)	5. (*a*)	6. (*c*)	7. (*d*)	8. (*b*)	9. (*a*)	10. (*b*)
11. (*d*)	12. (*b*)	13. (*d*)	14. (*d*)	15. (*d*)	16. (*b*)	17. (*d*)	18. (*a*)	19. (*b*)	20. (*c*)
21. (*a*)	22. (*b*)	23. (*b*)	24. (*c*)	25. (*a*)	26. (*d*)	27a. (*b*)	27b. (*b*)	28a. (*d*)	28b. (*b*)

(K) BOTANY

1. (*b*)	2. (*c*)	3. (*b*)	4. (*d*)	5. (*d*)	6. (*c*)	7. (*c*)	8. (*a*)	9. (*b*)	10. (*c*)
11. (*b*)	12. (*c*)	13. (*c*)	14. (*a*)	15. (*c*)	16. (*c*)	17. (*b*)	18. (*b*)	19. (*b*)	20. (*b*)
21. (*c*)	22. (*a*)	23. (*b*)	24. (*b*)	25. (*a*)	26. (*b*)	27a. (*b*)	27b. (*c*)	28a. (*a*)	28b. (*a*)

(L) MICROBIOLOGY

1. (*b*)	2. (*b*)	3. (*d*)	4. (*a*)	5. (*c*)	6. (*c*)	7. (*b*)	8. (*a*)	9. (*a*)	10. (*b*)
11. (*d*)	12. (*c*)	13. (*a*)	14. (*c*)	15. (*d*)	16. (*d*)	17. (*c*)	18. (*b*)	19. (*d*)	20. (*a*)
21. (*b*)	22. (*b*)	23. (*c*)	24. (*b*)	25. (*a*)	26. (*d*)	27a. (*b*)	27b. (*d*)	28a. (*c*)	28b. (*a*)

(M) ZOOLOGY

1. (*c*)	2. (*d*)	3. (*c*)	4. (*c*)	5. (*c*)	6. (*b*)	7. (*b*)	8. (*d*)	9. (*a*)	10. (*c*)
11. (*b*)	12. (*d*)	13. (*d*)	14. (*b*)	15. (*d*)	16. (*a*)	17. (*c*)	18. (*b*)	19. (*a*)	20. (*c*)
21. (*c*)	22. (*a*)	23. (*d*)	24. (*b*)	25. (*d*)	26. (*a*)	27a. (*c*)	27b. (*b*)	28a. (*b*)	28b. (*d*)

EXPLANATIONS

(H) CHEMISTRY

1. Elements exhibiting +2 oxidation state in their compounds is Zn and Ca (Zn^{2+} and Ca^{2+}) as they are group 2 elements.
2. The paramagnetic species is CN as it has 1 unpaired electron. As a compound is paramagnetic if it has a lone electron.
3. The reaction is:

   $CaH_2\ (s) + 2H_2O\ (l) \rightarrow Ca(OH)_2\ (aq) + 2H_2\ (g)$

   Thus we see that, CaH_2 (hydrolith) when reacts with water, leads to the formation of hydrogen gas.
4. A compound which has $4n + 2$ *pi* electrons such as in benzene is known as aromatic compound. Aromatic compounds are more stable than aliphatic compounds. The $4n + 2$ electrons (*pi*) rule is known as Huckels' rule of aromaticity.

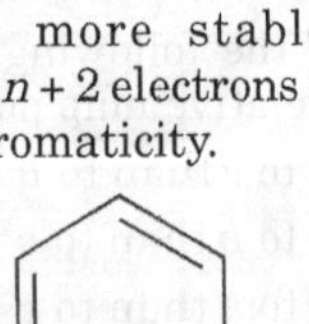

5. When benzoic acid is treated with $NH_4NO_3/CCF_3(O)_2O$, then the product formed is 3-Nitro benzoic acid. Nitro group is present at the meta position as –COOH is a deactivating group.

   The reaction is as follows:

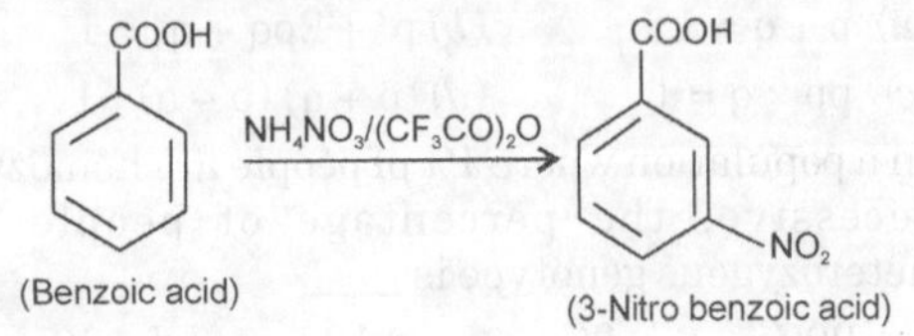

6. 2- chlorobutanoic acid is most acidic as its pKa value is the least of the four. In 2-chlorobutanoic acid, the presence of a chlorine next to the carbonyl, four bonds from the acidic proton, renders this compound much more acidic than butanoic acid; the pKa's are about 2.9 and 4.8, respectively. In 3-chlorobutanoic acid, the pKa is 4.0, whereas in 4-chlorobutanoic acid, with the fluorine all the way at the end of the chain, six bonds away from the acidic position, the pKa is 4.5.

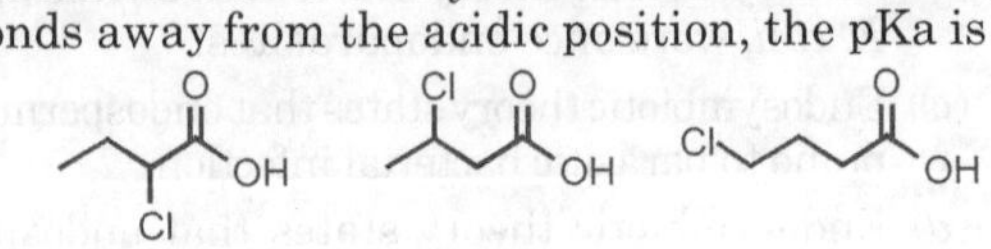

pKa 2.9 pKa 4.0 pKa 4.5

7. The total number of steroisomers possible in $CH_3 - CH(Ph) - CH = CHCH_3$ is 4. The formula for calculating number of optical isomers is 2^n

   where n = number of chiral carbon atoms.

   Here $n = 1$.

   So, number of optical isomers are $2^1 = 2$.

   Similarly, the number of geometrical isomers are $2^n = 2^1 = 2$

   where n = number of double bonds.

   In the above structure only 1 double bond is present.

   Therefore, total number of sterioisomers are 2 + 2 = 4.
8. The given reaction is:

   $$2Cu^+\ (aq) \rightarrow Cu\ (s) + Cu^{2+}\ (aq)$$

   E°= 0.36V, temperature= 298K.

   Therefore, standard Gibbs free energy $(\Delta G) = -nFE°$.

   Where $n = 1$ {as $2Cu^+ \rightarrow Cu + Cu^{2+}$}

   So, $\Delta G° = -1 * 96500 * 0.36$

   $= -34740$ J/mol = –34.740 kj/mol.

9. The Heisenberg's uncertainity principle is expressed as $\Delta x * \Delta p \geq h/(4\pi)$

x = position, Δx = uncertainty in position

p = momentum, Δp = uncertainty in momentum.

This principle states that it is impossible to determine with perfect accuracy both the position and momentum of a particle at any given point in time.

10. The given reaction is:

$C_6H_{12}O_6 (s) + 6O_2 (g) \rightarrow 6CO_2 (g) + 6H_2O (l)$

$\Delta U = -2810$ KJ/mol

We know, $\Delta H = \Delta U + \Delta nRT$

Where $\Delta n = 0$

Therefore, $\Delta H = -2810 + 0 = -2810$ KJ/mol

11. Si $(CH_3)_2O$ is a repeating unit of silicone as suggested by the structure below:

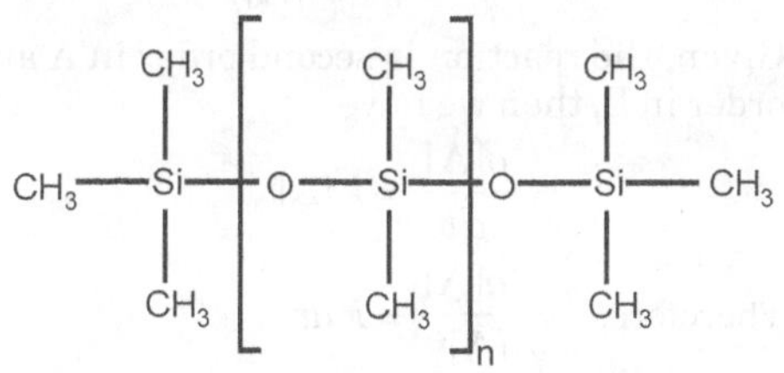

12. The property of X/X⁻ which is responsible for the trend of NaI < NaBr < NaCl < NaF is electron ionic radii as ionic radii is inversely proportional to lattice energy. The smaller the ionic radii, the greater is the lattice energy.

13. Molecules with no dipole are linear, tetrahedral, trigonal planar, trigonal bipyramidal, and octahedral in geometry. Thus BF_3 and CF_4 have zero dipole moment because BF_3 has a trigonal planar geometry while CF_4 has a tetrahedral geometry.

14. When air oxidation of sodium metal occurs a hygroscopic compound X is produced by the reaction:

$4Na + O_2 \rightarrow 2Na_2O + H_2O \rightarrow 2NaOH$ (compound X)

When this compound X reacts with CO_2, then a compound Y is produced as:

$2NaOH + CO_2 \rightarrow Na_2CO_3$ (compound Y)

Therefore the compound X and Y are NaOH and Na_2CO_3 respectively.

15. The reaction of HNO_3 with P_4 is given as:

$$20HNO_3 + P_4 \rightarrow 4H_3PO_4 + 20NO_2 + 4H_2O$$

In this reaction HNO_3 oxidizes P_4 into H_3PO_4 and gets reduced to NO_2.

The reaction of HNO_3 with P_4O_{10} is given as:

$$4HNO_3 + P_4O_{10} \rightarrow 4HPO_3 + 2N_2O_5$$

In this reaction P_4O_{10} produces N_2O_5 by eliminating water from HNO_3.

Thus the two products are NO_2 and N_2O_5.

16. The Diels-Alder reaction is anorganic chemical reaction between a conjugated diene and a substituted alkene, to form a substituted cyclohexene system.

The following Diels-Alder reaction is:

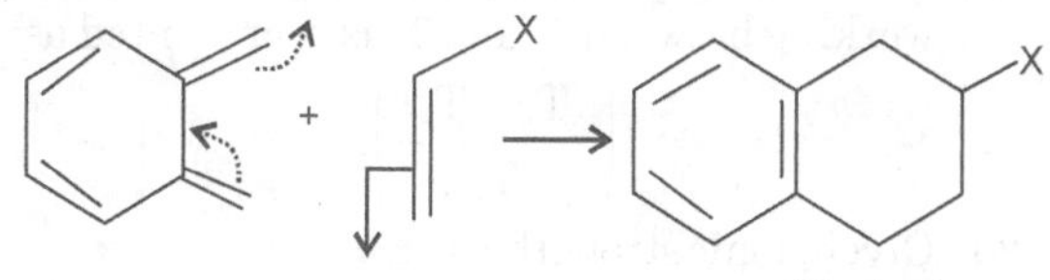

(Product)

17. When 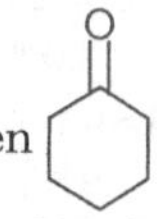 is reacted with HCO_2. Et in the presence of NaOEt first and then H_3O^+, then a-CHO group is added to its ortho position and the product becomes:-

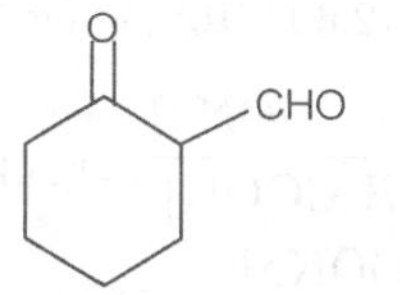

The reaction is given as:

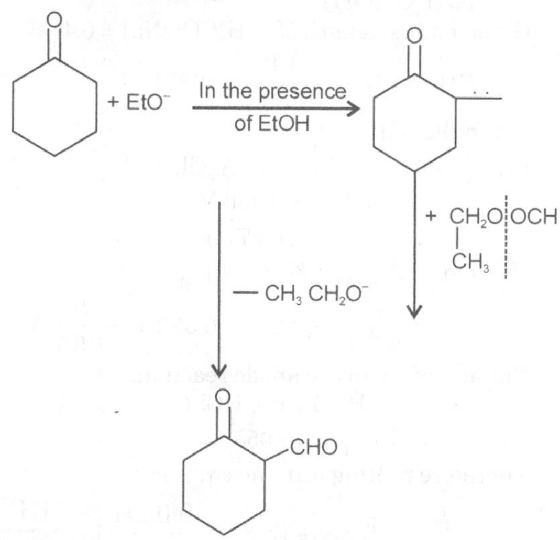

18. Given,

$C_{v,m}$ for Ar = 12.48 J/K mol

Since it is an adiabatic and reversible process, so:

$$T_1/T_2 = (V_2/V_1)^{\gamma-1}$$
$$= (1.00/0.50)^{1.66-1}$$
$$= (2)^{0.66}$$

Therefore, $T_2 = \dfrac{T_1}{1.58}$

We know that,

Work done (W) = $nC_v\Delta T$

Where $\Delta T = T_2 - T_1$, $n = 0.050$

and $C_v = 12.48$

Putting the values, we get

$$W = 0.050 * 12.48 \left(\frac{T_1}{1.58 - T_1}\right)$$

{as $T_2 = T_1/1.58$ in above equation}

On solving this equation we get

$W = -68.2J = -69J$ approx.

19. The efficiency of a reversible cyclic heat engine working between T_c and T_h is represented as: $\left(\frac{(T_h - T_c)}{T_h}\right)$.

20. Given, ionic strength = 0.1

pH = 5, temperature = 25°C

Dissociation constant (Ka) = 2.69 * 10^{-5}

We know, according to Henderson's equation:

$$pH = -\log Ka + \log \frac{[salt]}{[acid]}$$

Therefore putting the values:

$$5 = -\log (2.69 * 10^{-5}) + \log \frac{[CH_3COONa]}{[CH_3COOH]}$$

$$\text{Log} \frac{[CH_3COONa]}{[CH_3COOH]} = 0.43$$

$$\frac{[CH_3COONa]}{[CH_3COOH]} = 2.69$$

Given ionic strength of $[CH_3COONa]$ = 0.1

So, $[CH_3COOH] = \frac{0.1}{2.69} = 0.0371$

21. Given the cell:

Pt, H_2 (1atm) || HCl (aq) || AgCl, Ag |

$E_{cell} = 0.332$ V

$E_{AgCl/Ag} = 0.277$ V

Therefore, $E^\circ_{H^+/H2} = E_{AgCl/Ag} - E_{cell}$

$= 0.277 - 0.332 = -\frac{0}{055}$ V

But according to the anode reaction:

H_2 (1atm)| HCl (aq)

$E_{H^+/H2} = +0.055$

Therefore putting it in the equation:

$$E_{H^+/H2} = E^\circ_{H^+/H2} - \frac{0.0591}{2} \log \frac{[H^2]}{[H^+]^2}$$

Therefore on solving, we get

$-\text{Log}[H^+] = 0.055/0.0591$

We know, $-\text{Log}[H^+] = pH$

So, $pH = \frac{0.055}{0.0591} = 0.930$

22. Given, $[Ca^{2+}] = 3.3 * 10^{-4}$ M

and $[F^-] = 6.7 * 10^{-4}$ M

The reaction is:

$CaF_2 \leftrightarrow Ca^{2+} + 2F^-$

Therefore, $K_{sp} = [Ca^{2+}]. [F^-]^2$

$= (3.3 * 10^{-4}). (6.7 * 10^{-4})^2$

$= 1.48 * 10^{-10}$

Then, when NaF is added to the above solution, the concentration of Ca^{2+} changes as:

$[Ca^{2+}] = 1.5 * 10^{-4}$ M

Now, $[F^-]^2 = \frac{K_{sp}}{[Ca^{2+}]}$

On solving we get,

$[F^-]^2 = 9.876 * 10^{-7}$

Therefore, $[F^-] = 1.0 * 10^{-3}$

23. Given the reaction:

A + B → Products

Assuming that reaction is first order in A and zero order in B, then we have

$$\frac{D[A]}{dt} = k[A]$$

So, $\frac{d[A]}{[A]} = kdt$ {by interchanging}

We get, $\ln[A]_t = -kt + C$

{by integrating both sides}

Now, when $t = 0$ then,

$\ln[A]_t = -kt + \ln[A]_0$

Therefore, $kt = \ln[A]_0 - \ln[A]_t$

Finally, we get $K = \frac{1}{t} \ln \frac{[A]_0}{[A]_t}$

24. Given, the reaction is second order in A and zero order in B, then we have

$$\frac{d[A]}{dt} = k [A]^2$$

Therefore, $\frac{d[A]}{[A]^2} = k\,dt$

We get, $\frac{-1}{[A]} = -kt + C$

{by integrating both sides}

Now at $t = 0$ we have,

$A = [A]_0$ and $\frac{-1}{[A]_0} = C$

Now putting this in equation, we get

$$\frac{-1}{[A]_t} = -kt - \frac{1}{[A]_0}$$

So we get, $kt = \frac{1}{[A]_t} - \frac{1}{[A]_0}$

Therefore on solving,

$$k = \frac{1}{t}\left[\frac{1}{[A]_t} - \frac{1}{[A]_0}\right]$$

25. When 3, 3-dimethyl-1-butene reacts with hydrochloric acid, then a halogenated compound is produced. This halogenated compound is: $Me_2C(Cl)–CHMe_2$.

The reaction is given as:

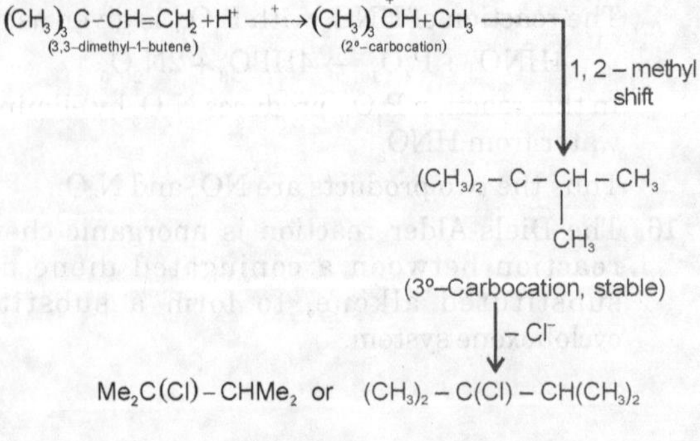

26. When 3, 3-dimethyl-1-butene reacted with $Hg(OCOCH_3)_2$ and then treated with alkaline $NaBH_4$, then it produces:

$Me_3C–CH(OH)–CH_3$

The reaction is given as:

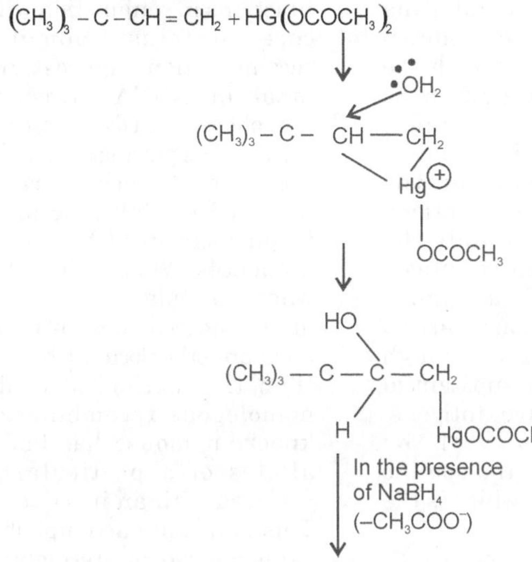

$$(CH_3)_3 - C - CH(OH) - CH_3$$

OR

$$Me_3 - C - CH(OH) - CH_3$$

27a. When the pink colored aqueous solution of $CoCl_2$ immediately changes to blue on adding excess of Cl^- ion then, that blue colored species is $[CoCl_4]^{2-}$. The following reaction takes place:

$$[Co(H_2O)_6]Cl_2 + 4Cl^- \rightarrow [CoCl_4]^{2-} + 6H_2O$$

Therefore in this reaction when excess of Cl^- ions is added then the pink color of $[Co(H_2O)_6]Cl_2$ changes to blue and a blue colored complex is formed as $[CoCl_4]^{2-}$.

27b. The d-electron configuration for the blue colored complex i.e. $[CoCl_4]^{2-}$ is $e^4_g\, t^3_{2g}$. Because in $[CoCl_4]^{2-}$ Co is present as Co^{2+} and its configuration is [Ar] $3d^7\, 4s^0$. As Cl^- is a weak field ligand so tetrahedral splitting occurs in its presence leaving 3 unpaired electrons.

28a. The reaction is carried out as follows:

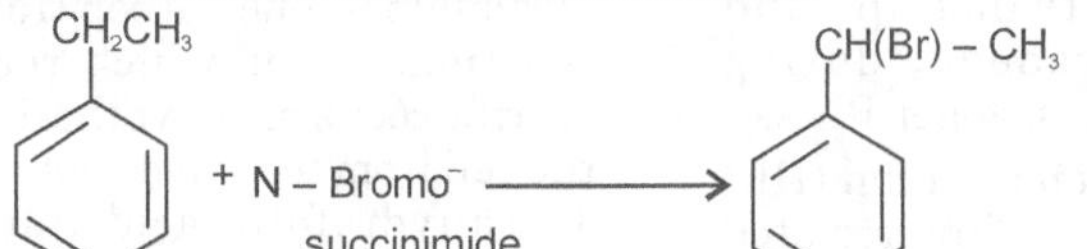

(Ethyl benzene) (NBS) (Compound X)

In the above reaction when ethylbenzene reacts with N-bromosuccinimide then a compound X is produced, given as:

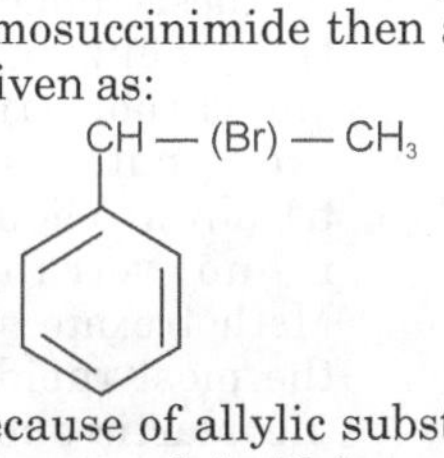

It occurs because of allylic substitution given by NBS (N-Bromosuccinimide).

28b. When compound X i.e.,

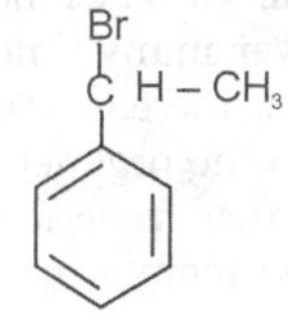

is treated with t-BuOK in the presence of Butanol them it leads to removal of a water molecule and a compound Y is formed.

The reaction is given as:

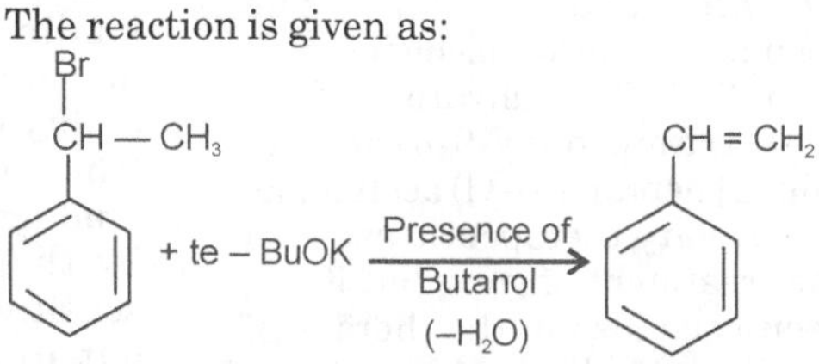

(X) (Compound Y)

Thus, it is an elimination reaction which involves elimination of $1H_2O$ molecule.

(I) BIOCHEMISTRY

1. Van der Waals (dispersion) forces contribute to interactions of proteins with other molecules or with surfaces, but because of the structural complexity of protein molecules, the magnitude of these effects is usually estimated based on idealized models of the molecular geometry, e.g., spheres or spheroids. The beta sheet involves H-bonding between backbone residues in adjacent chains. In the beta sheet, a single chain forms H-bonds with its neighbouring chains, with the donor (amide) and acceptor (carbonyl) atoms pointing sideways rather than along the chain, as in the alpha helix. Beta formers include valine, isoleucine, phenylalanine, tyrosine, tryptophan, and threonine. No relationship is apparent between the chemical nature of the amino acid side chain and the existence of amino acid in one structure or another. Within the complex interior or the hydrophobic patches of the proteins, these amino acids interact mostly by weak Van der Waal's forces.
2. Okazaki fragments are created during DNA replication because DNA polymerase can only add nucleotides in a 5' to 3' direction. This means that one strand (the leading strand) can be continuously created, but the other strand (the lagging strand) runs in the opposite direction. This means that loops must be created and shorter parts of DNA replicated one at a time. This creates fragments on the lagging strand. The RNA primers on this strand are later replaced with DNA by DNA Polymerase I, and joined together with DNA ligase.
3. Mitochondria are known as the power houses of the cell. They are organelles that act like a digestive system that takes in nutrients, breaks them down, and creates energy for the cell. The process of creating cell energy is known as cellular respiration. Most of the chemical reactions involved in cellular respiration happen in the mitochondria. Mitochondria have two membranes (not one as in other organelles). The outer membrane covers the

organelle and contains it. The inner membrane folds over many times (cristae). That folding increases the surface area inside the organelle. Many of the chemical reactions happen on the inner membrane of the mitochondria.

4. Colchicine is an alkaloid prepared from the dried corns and seeds of *Colchicum autumnale*. The chemical name for colchicine is (S) N-(5, 6, 7, 9-tetrahydro- 1, 2, 3, IO-tetramethoxy-9-oxobenzo [alpha] heptaien-7-yl) acetamide. Its primary therapeutic use is in the treatment of gout, but it has been used also in the therapy of familial Mediterranean fever (periodic disease). Colchicine decreases leukocyte chemotaxis and phagocytosis and inhibits the formation and release of a chemotactic glycoprotein that is produced during phagocytosis of urate crystals. Colchicine also inhibits urate crystal deposition, which is enhanced by a low pH in the tissues, probably by inhibiting oxidation of glucose and subsequent lactic acid production in leukocytes. Colchicine has no analgesic or antihyperuricemic activity. Colchicine inhibits microtubule assembly in various cells, including leukocytes, probably by binding to and interfering with polymerization of the microtubule subunit tubulin.

5. Dihydrotestosterone (DHT) is an androgenic hormone formed in peripheral tissue from testosterone. It is thought to be the androgen responsible for development of the male primary sex characters during embryogenesis and of male secondary sex characters at puberty and for adult male sexual function. It is a derivative of testosterone having androgenic activity and anabolic and tumour-suppressing capabilities useful in the treatment of certain breast cancers. DHT is considered to be the active form of testosterone in males.

6. Radioimmunoassay is based upon the competition between labelled and unlabeled antigen for specific antibody sites, forming antigen-antibody complexes. At equilibrium, the radioactive complex (bound) is separated from the radioactive antigen (free). The Bound (B)/ Free (F) ratio is dependent upon the amount of nonradioactive antigen. Antigen concentration in unknown samples is determined by comparing the B/F ratio to the B/F ratios obtained by incubating varying amounts of known nonradioactive antigen with the same amount of antibody as in the unknown sample under similar assay conditions. The measurement depends on the ability of the unlabelled antigen (the unknown) to inhibit the binding of the radioactive antigen by the antibody. To maximize sensitivity, the reaction is carried out in the presence of enough antibodies to achieve substantial binding of radioactive antigens. Thus, the sensitivity of the reaction depends on the specific activity of the ligand which is the unlabelled antigen.

7. Introns have been found in eukaryotic mRNA, tRNA and rRNA, as well as chloroplast, mitochondrial and a phage of *E. coli*. Eubacteria are the only species in which introns have not been found. In general, genes that are related by evolution have related organizations with conservation of the position at least some introns. The amount and size of introns varies greatly. Splicing appears to involve a complex called the spliceosome. This complex consists of RNA and protein, and appears to be composed of a group of small nuclear ribonucleoprotein particles or snRNPs. Introns are non-coding, intervening sequences of DNA that are transcribed, but are removed from within the primary gene transcript and rapidly degraded during maturation of messenger RNA.

8. Homologous recombination (HR) comprises a series of interrelated pathways that function in the repair of DNA double-stranded breaks (DSBs) and inter-strand crosslink (ICLs). In addition, recombination provides critical support for DNA replication in the recovery of stalled or broken replication forks, contributing to tolerance of DNA damage. A central core of proteins, most critically the RecA homolog Rad51, catalyzes the key reactions that typify HR: homology search and DNA strand invasion. The diverse functions of recombination are reflected in the need for context-specific factors that perform supplemental functions in conjunction with the core proteins. Homologous recombination requires a nick or break in dsDNA, invasion of a homologous dsDNA molecule by ssDNA end, pairing of homologous sequences, branch migration to form a Holliday junction, and isomerisation of the flanking sequences. When an investigator wants to replace one allele with an engineered construct but not affect any other locus in the genome, then the method of choice is homologous recombination. A knockout mouse has had both alleles of a particular gene replaced with an inactive allele. This is usually accomplished by using homologous recombination to replace one allele followed by two or more generations of selective breeding until a breeding pair are isolated that have both alleles of the targeted gene inactivated or knocked out.

9. Methotrexate is an antineoplastic anti-metabolite. Anti-metabolites masquerade as purine or pyrimidine - which become the building blocks of DNA. They prevent these substances becoming incorporated in to DNA during the "S" phase (of the cell cycle), stopping normal development and division. Methotrexate inhibits folic acid reductase which is responsible for the conversion of folic acid to tetrahydrofolic acid. At two stages in the biosynthesis of purines and at one stage in the synthesis of pyrimidines, one-carbon transfer reactions occur which require specific coenzymes synthesized in the cell from tetrahydrofolic acid. Tetrahydrofolic acid itself is synthesized in the cell from folic acid with the help of an enzyme, folic acid reductase. Thus, DNA synthesis cannot proceed because the coenzymes needed for one-carbon transfer reactions are not produced from tetrahydrofolic acid because there is no tetrahydrofolic acid. Methotrexate selectively affects the most rapidly dividing cells (neoplastic and psoriatic cells). Methotrexate is also indicated in

the management of severe, active, classical, or definite rheumatoid arthritis.

10. The rules of base pairing (or nucleotide pairing) are: i) A with T: the purine adenine (A) always pairs with the pyrimidine thymine (T) and ii) C with G: the pyrimidine cytosine (C) always pairs with the purine guanine (G). The rules of base pairing explain the phenomenon that whatever the amount of adenine (A) in the DNA of an organism, the amount of thymine (T) is the same (called Chargaff's rule). Similarly, whatever the amount of guanine (G), the amount of cytosine (C) is the same. The (C+G):(A+T) ratio varies from organism to organism (particularly among the bacteria), but within the limits of experimental error, A = T and C = G. Since A = T and C = G, therefore, A + G = C + T which implies that (A + G)/ (C + T) = 1.

11. The fatty acyl group is transported into the mitochondrial matrix, where it undergoes beta-oxidation. In the intermembrane space of the mitochondria, fatty acyl CoA reacts with carnitine in a reaction catalyzed by carnitine acyltransferase I (CAT-I), yielding CoA and fatty acyl carnitine. The resulting fatty acyl carnitine crosses the inner mitochondrial membrane. CAT-I is associated with the inner leaflet of the outer mitochondrial membrane. In liver the CAT-I reaction is rate-limiting; the enzyme is allosterically inhibited by malonyl CoA. Malonyl CoA concentration would be high during fatty acid synthesis. Inhibition of CAT-I by malonyl CoA prevents simultaneous synthesis and degradation of fatty acids. Fatty acids are activated on the outer mitochondrial membrane, whereas they are oxidized in the mitochondrial matrix. A special transport mechanism is needed to carry long-chain acyl CoA molecules across the inner mitochondrial membrane. Activated long-chain fatty acids are transported across the membrane by conjugating them to carnitine, a zwitterionic alcohol. The acyl group is transferred from the sulphur atom of CoA to the hydroxyl group of carnitine to form acyl carnitine. This reaction is catalyzed by carnitine acyltransferase I (also called carnitine palmitoyl transferase I), which is bound to the outer mitochondrial membrane.

12. Given, the molecular weight of Cytochrome-c = 11.7 KD and the molecular weight of myoglobin = 17.2 KD. pH of the gel is kept at 8.5. The two proteins are to be separated using polyacrylamide gel electrophoresis based on their mass/ charge ratio. It is given that pI for cytochrome-c = 9.6 and pI for myoglobin = 7.2. We know, when pH > pI => amino acid is positively charged as H^+ ions are in plenty and protonate the NH_2 (N-terminal) of the amino acid to NH_3^+. Again, when pH < pI, H^+ ions in the solution are less in number, so H^+ ions are donated by the COOH (C-terminal) of the amino acid reducing itself to COO^-. This means that cytochrome-c develops a net positive charge and myoglobin develops a net negative charge on them. Thus, myoglobin migrates toward the positively charged cathode and cytochrome-c migrates toward the negatively charged anode of the electrolytic cell.

13. Stearic Acid is a typical example of a fatty acid, which are essentially long hydrocarbon chains containing a carboxyl group at one end and a methyl group at the other. The chain lengths can vary from 3 (propionic acid) to 24 (lignoceric acid) but the majority of fatty acids found in hydrogenated vegetable or animal oils are around C16-C20 in length. The unsaturated fatty acids have lower melting points than the saturated fatty acids. The tetrahedral bond angles on carbon results in a molecular geometry for saturated fatty acids that is relatively linear although with zigzags. This molecular structure allows many fatty acid molecules to be rather closely "stacked" together. As a result, close intermolecular interactions result in relatively high melting points. The introduction of one or more double bonds in the hydrocarbon chain in unsaturated fatty acids results in one or more "bends" in the molecule. The geometry of the double bond is almost always a cis configuration in natural fatty acids. These molecules do not "stack" very well. The intermolecular interactions are much weaker than saturated molecules. As a result, the melting points are much lower for unsaturated fatty acids. The melting points for the saturated fatty acids follow the boiling point principle observed previously. Melting point principle: as the molecular weight increases, the melting point increases. This is observed in the series as lauric (C12), palmitic (C16), stearic (C18).

14. Following the consumption of food, carbohydrates are broken down into glucose molecules in the gut. Glucose is absorbed into the bloodstream elevating blood glucose levels. This rise in glycaemia stimulates the secretion of insulin from the beta cells of the pancreas. Insulin is needed by most cells to allow glucose entry. Insulin binds to specific cellular receptors and facilitates entry of glucose into the cell, which uses the glucose for energy. If insulin production and secretion are altered by disease, blood glucose dynamics will also change. If insulin production is decreased, glucose entry into cells will be inhibited, resulting in hyperglycaemia. The same effect will be seen if insulin is secreted from the pancreas but is not used properly by target cells. If insulin secretion is increased, blood glucose levels may become very low (hypoglycaemia) as large amounts of glucose enter tissue cells and little remains in the bloodstream. The underlying patho-physiological defect in type 1 diabetes is an autoimmune destruction of pancreatic beta cells. Following this destruction, the individual has an absolute insulin deficiency and no longer produces insulin. The underlying patho-physiological defect in type 2 diabetes does not involve

autoimmune beta-cell destruction.

15. Kidney plays an important role in sodium balance. Almost 99% of filtered sodium is reabsorbed. The absorption occurs via sodium transporters located in the various segments of the nephron. Each of these transporters has unique features and is blocked by a specific diuretic. The activating and inactivating mutations of these transporters are associated with important clinical syndromes. Primary active sodium transport is coupled to an energy-yielding chemical reaction such as ATP hydrolysis. Secondary active transport utilizes the voltage and ion gradients produced by the primary transport to drive the co-transport of other ions or molecules. These may be transported in the same (symport) or opposite (antiport) direction. Thus, sodium balance is maintained in and out of the cell with the help of sodium transporters.

16. ELISAs can be performed with a number of modifications to the basic procedure. The key step, immobilization of the antigen of interest, can be accomplished by direct adsorption to the assay plate or indirectly via a capture antibody that has been attached to the plate. The antigen is then detected either directly (labelled primary antibody) or indirectly (labelled secondary antibody). The most powerful ELISA assay format is the sandwich assay. This type of capture assay is called a "sandwich" assay because the analyte to be measured is bound between two primary antibodies - the capture antibody and the detection antibody. A detection enzyme or other tag can be linked directly to the primary antibody or introduced through a secondary antibody that recognizes the primary antibody. It also can be linked to a protein such as streptavidin if the primary antibody is biotin labelled. The most commonly used enzyme labels are horseradish peroxidase (HRP) and alkaline phosphatase (AP). Enzymes provide a high turnover number for better observation of results.

17. T cell receptors recognise foreign antigens, and then convey the message to the nucleus to induce a response. The body produces many T cells, each with specific TCRs on its surface through the recombination of the genes that encode the receptors, before it has encountered complementary antigens. By having a surplus of T cells carrying different TCRs, the body is able to mount a fast response once an intruder is detected. The antigens that TCRs bind are small peptide fragments, or epitopes, displayed by MHC molecules on the surface of cells. Cytotoxic T lymphocyte TCRs recognise epitopes displayed by MHC class I molecules on the surface of almost every cell in the body, so it can distinguish between 'self'-antigens and foreign antigens (viral-infected cells), as well as being sensitive to the amount of self-antigen presented (increased number of self-antigens in malignant cells). Helper T cell and inflammatory T cell TCRs recognise epitopes displayed by MHC class II molecules on the surface of antigen-presenting immune cells, including: macrophages that engulf foreign particles such as bacteria; dendritic cells that present antigen to T cells; and B cells that produce antibodies. The CD8 and CD4 surface glycoproteins recognise MHC class I and II molecules, respectively. The binding of a TCR to an epitope can result in a signal being sent to the nucleus to induce a response.

18. According to the genetic code, the cell would need tRNAs with 61 different anticodons to complement the available 61 codons. However, due to the degeneracy of the genetic code, the third base is less discriminatory for the amino acid than the other two bases. This third position in the codon is referred to as the wobble position. At this position U's and C's may be read by a G in the anticodon. Similarly, A's and G's may be read by U or y (pseudouridine) in the anticodon. Some amino acids are encoded by more than one codon as there are 64 possible base triplets and only 20 amino acids. In fact, 61 of the 64 possible triplets specify particular amino acids and 3 triplets (called stop codons) designate the termination of translation. Thus, for most amino acids, there is more than one code word. If the code were not degenerate, 20 codons would designate amino acids and 44 would lead to chain termination. The probability of mutating to chain termination would therefore be much higher with a non-degenerate code. Chain-termination mutations usually lead to inactive proteins, whereas substitutions of one amino acid for another are usually rather harmless. Thus, degeneracy minimizes the deleterious effects of mutations. Degeneracy of the code may also be significant in permitting DNA base composition to vary over a wide range without altering the amino acid sequence of the proteins encoded by the DNA.

19. L-Lysine is a basic, genetically coded amino acid. It is essential in human nutrition (probably most limited in the food chain). We have, pK_{a1} = a-carboxyl group, pK_{a2} = a-ammonium ion, and pK_{a3} = side chain group. Since, lysine is a basic amino acid with 2 NH_3^+ groups and one COOH group, the isoelectric point for lysine molecule is the average of the two pK_a values NH_3^+ ions. This is given as:- $(10 + 9)/2 = 9.50$. Therefore, the pI for lysine is 9.50

20. Given, Molecular weight of the bacterial DNA = 2.64×10^9 and the average molecular weight of a nucleotide pair = 660.

Now, Number of nucleotide pairs present in the bacterial DNA

$= (2.64 \times 10^9)/660$

$= 0.004 \times 10^9 = 4 \times 10^6$

Hence, number of nucleotides present in the bacterial DNA

$= 2 \times 4 \times 10^6 = 8 \times 10^6$

Given, 400 amino acids on an average constitute a single protein in the bacteria. Therefore number of nucleotides responsible for coding for a single protein

= 3 × 400 = 1200 nucleotides (since we know 3 nucleotides code for a single amino acid).

Again, 1200 nucleotides are encoding for = 1 protein

Therefore, 8×10^6 nucleotides encode for = $(8 \times 10^6)/1200$ = 0.0066666667×10^6 proteins = 6666.667 proteins.

21. The two pyruvate molecules formed from a single glucose molecule enter the mitochondrion in eukaryotes. There, each is converted to acetyl coenzyme A (acetyl-CoA). First, a molecule of CO_2 is removed from each pyruvate, forming a two-carbon fragment. These two-carbon molecules are oxidized-that is, electrons are removed and used to form a total of two NADH molecules (to be used later). Then, each oxidized, two-carbon fragment-an acetyl group-is attached to coenzyme A, forming acetyl-CoA. The pyruvate dehydrogenase complex is a large, highly integrated complex of three kinds of enzymes. The reaction requires the participation of the three enzymes of the pyruvate dehydrogenase complex, each composed of several polypeptide chains, and five coenzymes: thiamine pyrophosphate (TPP), lipoic acid, and FAD serve as catalytic cofactors, and CoA and NAD+ are stoichiometric cofactors. The conversion of pyruvate into acetyl CoA consists of three steps: decarboxylation, oxidation, and transfer of the resultant acetyl group to CoA. First, pyruvate combines with TPP and is then de-carboxylated. This reaction is catalyzed by the pyruvate dehydrogenase component (E1) of the multi-enzyme complex. Second, the hydroxyethyl group attached to TPP is oxidized to form an acetyl group and concomitantly transferred to lipoamide, a derivative of lipoic acid that is linked to the side chain of a lysine residue by an amide linkage. Third, the acetyl group is transferred from acetyllipoamide to CoA to form acetyl CoA.

22. The Maxam-Gilbert method of nucleotide sequence determination is based on preferential, base-specific methylation followed by chemical cleavage to generate a nested set of end- labelled derivatives. The method requires radioactive labelling at one end and purification of the DNA fragment to be sequenced. Chemical treatment generates breaks at a small proportion of one or two of the four nucleotide bases in each of four reactions (G, A+G, C, and C+ T). Thus a series of labelled fragments is generated, from the radiolabelled end to the first 'cut' site in each molecule. The fragments in the four reactions are arranged side by side in gel electrophoresis for size separation. To visualize the fragments, the gel is exposed to X-ray film for autoradi-ography, yielding a series of dark bands each corresponding to a radiolabelled DNA fragment, from which the sequence may be inferred. The sequence is read from bottom to top which gives the 5' to 3' run of the DNA sequence.

Thus, from the autoradiogram, the DNA sequence is: 5'-CTAGATAGTATAG-3'.

23. The DNA double strand 5'-CTAGATAGTATAG-3' and 3'-GATCTATCATATC-5' makes the DNA duplex. The 1st codons of the DNA from the 3' and the 5' ends are palindromic to each other. So, the endonuclease II used for digesting the DNA has to be palindromic in nature. So, the site of restriction for the endonuclease is: 5'-TAGCTA-3' and 3'-ATCGAT-5'.

24. The DNA strand is considered as the template strand for the process of transcription to generate mRNA molecule. Therefore, the template strand is: 5'-CTAGATAGTATAG-3'. mRNA molecule thus formed in complementary fashion with the change of thymidine nucleotide with a uridine nucleotide is: 3'-GAUCUAUCAUAUC-5'.

25. The study of the rate at which an enzyme works is called enzyme kinetics. K_m is (roughly) an inverse measure of the affinity or strength of binding between the enzyme and its substrate. The lower the value of K_m, the greater is the affinity.

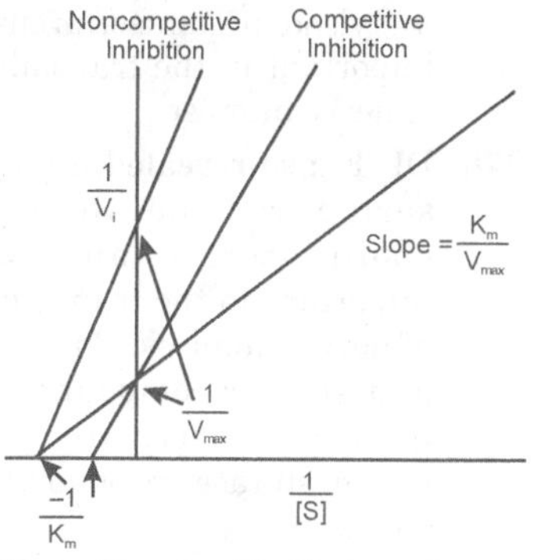

Thus, line 1 with the maximum value of $-1/K_m$ and minimum slope represents the enzymatic reaction with no inhibitor.

26. In the presence of a competitive inhibitor, it takes a higher substrate concentration to achieve the same velocities that were reached in its absence. So while V_{max} can still be reached if sufficient substrate is available, one-half V_{max} requires a higher [S] than before and thus K_m is larger. With non-competitive inhibition, enzyme rate (velocity) is reduced for all values of [S], including V_{max} and one-half V_{max} but K_m remains unchanged because the active site of those enzyme molecules that have not been inhibited is unchanged. In the given figure, line 4 represents non-competitive inhibition.

27a. Irreversible inhibitors that covalently bond to the enzyme provide an alternative and often complementary means for elucidating functional groups at the enzyme active site because they modify the functional groups, which can then be identified. Irreversible inhibitors can be divided into three categories: group-specific reagents, substrate analogs, and suicide inhibitors. Group-specific reagents react with specific R groups of amino acids. Two examples of group-specific reagents are di-isopropylphosphofluoridate (DIPF) and iodoacetamide. DIPF modifies only 1 of the 28 serine residues in the proteolytic enzyme chymotrypsin, implying that this serine residue is especially reactive. DIPF also revealed a reactive serine residue in acetylcholinesterase, an enzyme important in the transmission of nerve impulses.

27b. DIPF also revealed a reactive serine residue in acetylcholinesterase, an enzyme important in the transmission of nerve impulses. Thus, DIPF and similar compounds that bind and inactivate acetylcholinesterase are potent nerve gases.

28a. Partial hydrolysis will produce a mixture of shorter peptides and some amino acids. If the primary structures of these fragments are known, it is sometimes possible to deduce part or all of the original structure by taking advantage of overlapping pieces. For example, if a heptapeptide was composed of three glycines, two alanines, a leucine and a valine, many possible primary structures could be written. On the other hand, if partial hydrolysis gave two known tripeptide and two known dipeptide fragments, simple analysis of the overlapping units identifies the original primary structure. In the given question, the partially hydrolysed fragments are: Val-Arg-Pro-Gly; Lys-Phe-Val-Arg; Ala-Gly-Ser-Lys. Val-Arg is common to both 1st and 2nd fragments and Lys is common to both 2nd and 3rd fragments. Therefore, arranging the three fragments together, the correct sequence of the polypeptide is: Ala-Gly-Ser-Lys- Phe-Val-Arg-Pro-Gly.

28b. Mass spectrometry based proteomics almost invariably involves the enzymatic degradation of proteins to peptides by trypsin. This protease has high cleavage specificity, is very aggressive and stable under a wide variety of conditions. Most importantly, by cleaving C-terminal to arginine or lysine residues, it lead to peptides in the preferred mass range for effective fragmentation by tandem mass spectrometry and it places the highly basic residues at the C-termini of the peptides. Now, the given peptide X: Ala-Gly-Ser-Lys-Phe-Val-Arg- Pro-Gly is cleaved/ digested with trypsin. Since, trypsin cuts at arginine or lysine residues only at the C-terminal, the C-terminal for peptide X is Glycine amino acid. So, trypsin will cut at the arginine residue present near the C-terminal as opposed to the lysine residue present near the N-terminal. So, the peptide X breaks down into two fragments of Ala-Gly-Ser-Lys-Phe-Val-Arg and Pro-Gly.

(K) BOTANY

1. For the production of embryo sac the functional megaspore undergoes 3 mitotic divisions. Initially, it is the megaspore mother cell which divides meiotically forming 4 megaspores. 3 of them abort and remaining one divides mitotically to give rise to haploid cells of embryo sac. 3 divisions of the cell first give rise to 2 megaspore(adyad) and then to 8 nucleated embryo sac.
2. 30nm solenoid appears to be identical with the thick chromatin fibre. When chromatin is visualised in conditions of greater ionic strength the 30nm fibre is obtained. The fibre can be seen to have a coiled structure. It has approx 6 nucleosomes for every turn, which corresponds to a packing ratio of 40 i.e each m along axis of fibre contains 40 m of DNA.
3. Vitrification is a process by which water undergoes a phase transition from liquid state to an amorphous 'glassy state'. It is achieved by cooling a liquid through the glass transition, there occurs certain reactions. An important application of 'vitrification' is the vitrification of an antifreeze like liquid in cryopreservation. It occurs when bonding between particles become higher than a certain threshold values.
4. The term 'somaclonal variation' was coined by Larkin and Scowcroft. It is the variation seen in plants that has been produced by plant tissue culture. Chromosomal rearrange-ments are an important source of this variation. It leads to the creation of an additional genetic variability. The variations can be genotypic or phenotypic, which can be genetic or epigenetic in origin.
5. Storage and transport of lipid occurs in Spherosomes. Spherosomes is a granule found in plant cell. Some regard it as a mass of ribosome and other consider granules to be portion of Endoplasmic reticulum. Spherosomes have greater lipid content. They have a dual function of protein storage and protein catabolism.
6. The drug 'morphine' is derived from capsule of Pepever somniferum. Morphine is a analgesic drug that is used to relieve severe pain. It is most abundant alkaloid found in opium, the dried sap (latex) derieved from slicing the unripe seed pod of *Pepever somniferum* poppy. Morphine accounts 8-14% of dry weight of opium.
7. The floristic regions of the world are determined on the basis of geographical distribution of the plant genera. This is due to Population distribution. The pattern of distribution is not permanent for each species. It can change seasonally in response to availability of resources. Dispersion takes place at the time of reproduction.
8. Pericycle is regarded as the lateral roof and is located between the endodermis and vascular bundles. It is actually a cylinder of parenchyma cells. In plants undergoing secondary growth, the pericycle contributes to the vascular cambium often diverging into a cork cambium. Pericycle is the primary tissue located at the periphery of the root vascular cylinder.

9. Apospory is the development of gametophytes on the sporophytes without any reduction division. Apospory is the opposite of apogamy and involves the development of 2n gametophytes without meiosis from vegetative or non reproductive cells of sporophyte. It is a asexual reproduction through seeds, occurring in flowering plants through many different mechanism.

   Example - fern.

10. Lamiaceae, Apiaceae, Asteraceae and Poaceae are the synonyms of families families Labiatae, Umbelliferae, Compositae and Gramineae respectively. The mints commonly known as Labiatae are a family of flowering plants having cosmopolitan distribution. The Apiaceae commonly known as 'carrots' or Parsley family are of mostly aromatic plants with hollow stem.

    Compositae (aster, daisy or sunflower family) are large and widespread family of angiosperms. The Poaceae (true grasses) are ubiquitous family of monocotyledons flowering plant.

11. Engler and Prantl classification.
    1. Gymnosperms separated and placed before the angiosperms.
    2. Dicotyledons placed after monocotyledons.
    3. Dicotyledons starts with Verticillate with unisexual flowers.
    4. Monocotyledons start with Pandonales.

    Hutchinson system is based in a number of phylogenetic principles and studies a large number of plants.

12. In case of NAD-ME type mechanism aspartate is converted to OAA (oxaloacetic acid) again in the bundle sheath cytosol by aspartate amino transferase. The mitochondria are involved in the decarboxylation process.

13. Marker assisted selection is indirect selection process where a trait of interest is selected not based on the traits itself but on a marker linked to it. The assumption is that linked allele associated with the gene or quantitative trait locus of interest. Marker assisted selection can be useful for traits that are difficult to measure, exhibit low heritability and are expressed low in developments.

    Thus without self fertilization of individual hetrozygotes cannot be identified.

14.

Organisms	Disease in plants
Alternaria solani	Early blight of potatoes
Synchytrium endobioticum	Wort disease of potatoes
Pseudomonas solanacearum	Brown rat of potatoes
Phytophthora infestans	Late blight of potatoes

Symptoms of early blight of potato-

1. Small, isolated, scattered, pale brown spots on the leaflets.
2. In the necrotic spots, concentric rings appear on the older leaves and darkened areas on the stem.
3. The lowest leaves are attacked first and the disease progresses upwards.
4. Tuber symptoms of early blight include circular to irregular lesions that are slightly shunken and often surrounded by a raised purple to dark brown border.

15. Nitrite reductase enzyme accomplishes the six electron reduction of NO_2 to NH_3. It is found in the chloroplast of higher plants where it is associated with the thylakoid membrane.

    Glutamine synthetase is an enzyme that play an essential role in metabolism of nitrogen by catalyzing the condensation of glutamate and ammonia to form glutamine.

16. Vir D2 is one of the key Agrobacterium tumefaciens proteins involved in the T-DNA processing and transfer. In addition to its endonuclease activity, Vir D2 nicks at the T-DNA border sequences generating a single stranded T-DNA molecule to which Vir D2 covalently binds at the 5′end.

17. Reaction is as follows-

$$O_2(e^-) \rightarrow O_2 \rightarrow H_2O_2 \rightarrow OH \rightarrow H_2O.$$

18.

	Genotypes	Considered frequency	Actual frequency
Non cross over	XYZ	a	476
	xyz	b	471
Crossing over (X-Y)	Xyz	c	15
	xYZ	d	18
Crossing over (Y-Z)	XYz	e	9
	xyZ	f	9
Double cross over	XyZ	g	1
	xYz	h	1
			Total (T) = 1000

$$\text{Cross over between (X – Y)} = \frac{c+d+g+h}{T} = \frac{15+18+1+1}{1000} \times 100 = \frac{35}{1000} \times 100 = 3.5\text{cM}$$

19. Recessive epistasis – (9 : 3 : 4)

Supplementary genes are are a pair of non allelic genes of which one produces its phenotype independently in a dominant state, but another cannot produce a phenotypic effect independently.

Dominant epistasis – (12 : 3 : 1)

The dominant allele say 'A' can express itself only in the presence of either 'B' or 'b' allele, such type of epistasis is termed as dominant epistasis.

Duplicate recessive epistasis – (9 : 7)

When the alleles of both genes loci produce the same phenotype without cumulative effect.

Dominant and recessive epistasis – (13 : 3)

When dominant alleles of one gene locus (A) in homozygous (AA)and heterozygous (Aa) condition and the homozygous recessive allele (bb) of another gene locus (B) produce the same phenotype.

20.

Secondary metabolites	Precursor
Coniine	Lysine
Morphine	Tyrosine
Quinine	Tryptophane
Chalcone	Phenyl alanine

21. Heeng → *Ferula asafoetida.*

It is a dried latex extracted from the living underground rhizome or tap root of several species of ferula which is a perennial herb.

Dalchini → Cinnamomum zeylanicum

It is a spice obtained from the inner bark of the tree.

Saffron → Crocus sativus.

Kattha → Acacia catechu. A tree which is deciduous and thorny.

22. Glycogen phosphorylase - It catalyses the rate limiting step in animals by releasing glucose-1-PO_4 from the terminal α-1-4 glycosidic bond. Glycogen phosphorylase is also studied as a model protein regulated by both reversible phosphorylation and allosteric effect.

Hexokinase - It phosphorylate hexoses, forming hexose-PO_4 as in glycolytic pathway, glucose act as substrate and get converted to glucose-6-PO_4.

Pyruvate carboxylase - Usually takes place in C6 cycle, forms oxaloacetate after carboxylation of pyruvate.

RuBP carboxylase- Commonly known as RuBISCO, an enzyme involved in the major step of carbon fixation, a process by which atmospheric CO_2 is converted to glucose by plants.

23. Raceme inflorescence is usually unbranched and indeterminate and bears pedicullate flowers along its axis. Example- Raphanus.

Catkin inflorescence is like spikes, a petalous flowers often pendent and falling as unit. Typically found in Salix.

Cyathium inflorescence forms specialized pseudanthia in plants in the genus Euphorbia and Poinsettia.

Verticillaster inflorescence show groups of flower arranged on the stem where the flowers are born in rings at intervals up the stem. The tip grows and produce more whorls. Example- Ocimum.

24. Gibberlins when purified are white pale yellow solid. It is a pentacyclic diterpene acid promoting growth and elongation of cells.

IAA (indole 3 acetic acid) is a colourless solid native to many plants that serves as potent and important auxin. The molecule is derived from indole containing carboxy methyl group. It is important factor for phototropism and gravitropism of plants.

Cytokine are made in the roots and travel through xylem to leaves and fruits. It promotes cell division and leads to delay of senescence.

Ethylene is related with ripening of fruits.

27b.

Genotype	+++	dmp	+mp	d++	++p	dm+	+m+	d+p
Actual frequency	430	452	45	38	16	17	1	1
Assumed frequency	i	ii	iii	iv	v	vi	vii	viii

Total frequency = sum of all actual frequency = 1000.

Crossing over between '*d*' and '*m*' = $\frac{iii + iv + vii + viii}{1000} \times 100 = \frac{16 + 17 + 1 + 1}{1000} \times 100 = 3.5\%$

Therefore, percentage of double cross = $8.5 \times \frac{3.5}{100} = 0.2975 = 0.3$(approx).

Coefficient of coincidence = observed percentage of double cross over/expected percentage of double cross over.

28a. SDS PAGE (Sodium Dodecyl Sulphate Polyacrylamide Gel Electrophoresis) is the most commonly practised gel electrophoresis. The method provide an easy way to estimate the number of polypeptides on the basis of their molecular weight. SDS denatures the protein and gives negative charge to it, so if two proteins of same molecular weight then only single band in the gel will be visible.

28b. A true determination of the purity of a protein preparation is obtained by 2D gel electrophoresis. It combines of IEF (iso electric focussing) and SDS PAGE. Since, 2D gel electrophoresis is capable of resolving over 2000 proteins in a single gel and it is important as the primary tool of proteonomics research where multiple proteins must be separated for parallel analysis.

(L) MICROBIOLOGY

1. Werner Arber, Daniel Nathans, and Hamilton O. Smith received the Nobel Prize in 1978 for working out the mechanism of restriction enzymes.
2. The SARS coronavirus, sometimes shortened to SARS-CoV, is the virus that causes severe acute respiratory syndrome (SARS)
3. In the denitrification process, nitrate (oxidation number +5) is reduced by organic matter to molecular nitrogen (oxidation number 0), so that 5 electrons are transferred per nitrogen atom.
4. gram product formed / gram substrate consumed
5. The cell walls of Archaea are unusual. Whereas peptidoglycan is a standard component of all bacterial cell walls and the two sugars are bonded with a β, 1-3 glycosidic linkage instead of β,1-4 glycosidic linkage.
6. Green sulphur bacteria are non-motile (except Chloroherpeton thalassium, which may glide) and come in spheres, rods, and spirals. Photos-ynthesis is achieved using bacteriochlorophyll (BChl) *c, d*, or *e*, in addition to BChl a and chlorophyll a not by oxygenic mode.
7. "Oxidation of inorganic nitrogen compounds as an energy source" by chemolithotrophs. Such as sulfide, ammonia and hydrogen.
8. An **antiporter** (also called **exchanger** or **counter-transporter**) is an integral membrane protein involved in secondary active transport of two or more different molecules or ions (i.e., solutes) across a phospholipid membrane such as the plasma membrane in opposite directions.
9. Amphotericin B, an antifungal drug, targets ergosterol. It binds physically to ergosterol within the membrane, and, thus, creates a polar pore in fungal membranes.
10. The genome of HBV is made of circular DNA, but it is unusual because the DNA is not fully double-stranded
11. The action of superoxide dismutase, catalase and peroxidase. These enzymes detoxify oxygen radicals that are inevitably generated by living systems in the presence of O_2. The distribution of these enzymes in cells determines their ability to exist in the presence of O_2

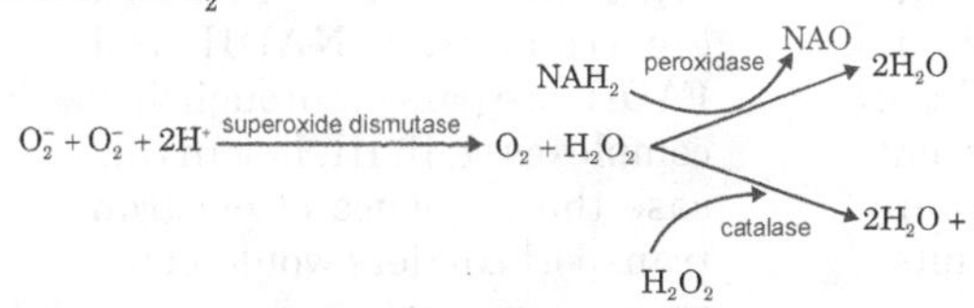

12. Bacterial resistance to penicillin may occur due to diminished permeability of the bacterial cell to the antibiotic; alteration of the penicillin-binding proteins, or production of β-lactamases. But the inability to bind to 30S ribosomal subunit is not responsible for making bacteria resistant to penicillin action
13.

Drug	Producer	Action on
Vancomycin	*Streptomyces orientalis*	Gram +ve bacteira
Bactericin	*Bacillus subtilis*	Food athogens
Chloroamphenicol	*Streptomyces venezuelae*	Bacteria
Streptomycin	*Streptomyces griseus*	Anti TB, Plague

14. The Choleragen (cholera toxin), is the enterotoxin produced by *Vibrio cholerae* which is in large part responsible for the symptomatology of cholera. It stimulates the secretion of electrolytes and water into the small intestine in Asiatic cholera, causing diarrhea and the loss of body fluids and weakening the patient. It is a bacterial toxin consisting of two protomers, A and B, of which the B protomer, composed of five identical polypeptide units, contains the determinants for binding to cells and membranes. Thus choleragen alone can reproduce the symptoms of cholera in the absence of *Vibrio cholerae*.
15. Delayed hypersensitivity reactions are inflammatory reactions initiated by mononuclear leukocytes. Delayed hyper-sensitivity is a major mechanism of defence against various intracellular pathogens, including mycobacteria, fungi, and certain parasites.

    The pathophysiology of the Tuberculin reaction is explained thus: M. tuberculosis are engulfed by macrophages after being identified as foreign, but due to a self- preserving mechanism peculiar to TB it is able to block the fusion of the phagosome within which it is existing with the lysosome which would destroy it. So tuberculin sensitivity test (also known as Mantoux test, Mantoux screening test, Pirquet test, or PPD test for purified protein derivative) is a diagnostic tool for tuberculosis in response as Type 4 hypersensitivity by immune system.
16. The **Pasteur effect** is an inhibiting effect of oxygen on the fermentation process. Under anaerobic conditions, the rate of glucose metabolism is faster, but the amount of ATP produced (as already mentioned) is smaller. When exposed to aerobic conditions, the ATP production increases and the rate of glycolysis slows, because the ATP produced acts as an allosteric inhibitor for phosphofructokinase 1, the third enzyme in the glycolysis pathway.

17. A **high-frequency recombination cell (Hfr cell)** (also called an **Hfr strain**) is a bacterium with a conjugative plasmid (often the F-factor) integrated into its genomic DNA. The Hfr strain was first characterized by Luca Cavalli-Sforza.

18. RNA-dependent RNA polymerase (RdRp) is an essential protein encoded in the genomes of all RNA-containing viruses with synthesis is absolutely required for positive-strand RNA synthesis.

19. The lambda gene N, codes for an antitermination protein (pN) that is necessary to allow RNA polymerase to read through the terminators located at the ends of the immediate early genes. Another antitermination protein, pQ, is required later in phage infection. pN and pQ act on RNA polymerase as it passes specific sites. These sites are located at different relative positions in their respective transcription units.

20. Phenol coefficient is a measure of the bactericidal activity of a chemical compound in relation to phenol. To calculate phenol coefficient, the concentration of the test compound at which the compound kills the test organism in 10 minutes, but not in 5 minutes, is divided by the concentration of phenol that kills the organism under the same conditions.

The formula is given by:

$$N = 1/CT$$

where C is the concentration of agent applied and T is the time for which agent is applied and N is the number of survivors. Thus N is inversely proportional to dose (CT is collectively called dose).

The conc. Pf test compound at which the compound kills the test organism in 10 min, but not in 5 min = 150

The conc. of phenol that kills the organism in 10 min, but not in 5 min = 90

Thus, Phenol coefficient = 150/90 = 1.66

21. The lactic acid bacteria (LAB) are rod-shaped bacilli or cocci characterized by an increased tolerance to a lower pH range. This aspect partially enables LAB to outcompete other bacteria in a natural fermentation, as they can withstand the increased acidity from organic acid production (e.g., lactic acid). This process yields two moles of ATP per mole of glucose consumed.

22. The flow of electrons through the cell's electron transport chain is strictly in the direction of molecules with increasing Standard Reduction Potentials (E_0'). Transfer of electrons in this manner releases energy that can be used to do the work of the cell. In electron transport, electrons from NADH and $FADH_2$ are passed through four complexes (I, II, III, IV). In this case the sequence of electron transport carriers would be:

$$NAD^+ \rightarrow P \rightarrow R \rightarrow \text{Cytochrome-c} \rightarrow S$$

23. Difference in redox potential can be given as:

$$\Delta E = -0.32 - 0.63 = -0.95$$

24. Transfer of electrons from PH_2 to S can be given as:

$$PH_2 + S \rightarrow SH_2 + P$$

$$\Delta E^0 = 0.13 + 0.63 = 0.76V$$

$$\Delta G^0 = -nFE^0 = -2 \times 2.3 \times 0.76 = -35 \text{ kcal/mol}$$

25. continue to grow in its logarithmic phase because it can metabolize both glucose and lactose sugar as sole source of carbon and energy.

26. *E. coli* grows faster on glucose than on any other carbon source. If *E. coli* is placed on an agar plate containing only glucose and lactose, the bacteria will use glucose first and lactose second. When glucose is available in the environment, the synthesis of β-galactosidase is under repression due to the effect of catabolite repression caused by glucose. As it is easier for E.Coli to use glucose sources than lactose sources, and this is related to their energy requirements as they use less energy when they use glucose.

27. (*a*) Given,

Generation time = 40 min

Time = 8 hours

Number of generations

$$= \frac{8 \times 60}{40} \text{min} = 12$$

(*b*) Cell population after 8 hours can be given as:

$$N = 2 \times 10^4 \times 2^{12} = 8.2 \times 10^7$$

28. (*a*) The mutation I^SO^+ in the controlling genes was responsible for the behavior of *E. coli* mutant. As here the regulatory gene is repressor from which it is insensitive to inducer, thus it binds to the wild type operator gene both in the presence and absence of inducer and thus it stops transcription of structural gene.

(*b*) In further mutation, the E. coli mutant synthesized β-galactosidase in the presence of the inducer only. This is possible because of I^+O^+ mutant form as for the synthesis of structural gene both the regulatory and operator gene has to be wild type.

(M) ZOOLOGY

1. Given, a red dog is mated with a white dog and the offsprings were obtained in the ratio of 1 : 1. Since the ratio of offsprings obtained in the F1 generation is 1 : 1, that means one of the two parents is heterozygous for the white colour and the other parent is homozygous for the red colour. Also, the 1 : 1 ratio implies that the homozygous red colour is recessive for the trait.

2. The process of fertilization involves a sperm fusing with an ovum. The most common sequence begins with ejaculation during copulation, follows with ovulation, and finishes with fertilization. Human chorionic gonadotropin (hCG) is a hormone produced during pregnancy that is made by the developing placenta after conception, and later by the placental component syncytiotrophoblast. Human chorionic gonadotropin interacts with the LHCG receptor and promotes the maintenance of the corpus luteum during the beginning of pregnancy, causing it to secrete the hormone progesterone.
3. Tunicates, previously known as Urochordata or urochordates, are members of the Tunicata, a subphylum of the phylum Chordata. Tunicata, are commonly known as "sea squirts." The body of an adult tunicate is quite simple, being essentially a sack with two siphons through which water enters and exits. Water is filtered inside the sack-shaped body. It has a notochord, a dorsal nerve cord, pharyngeal slits, and a post-anal tail. This "tadpole larva" will swim for some time. In many tunicates, it eventually attaches to a hard substrate, it loses its tail and ability to move and its nervous system largely disintegrates.
4. Insects are a class of invertebrates within the arthropod phylum that have a chitinous exoskeleton, a three-part body (head, thorax and abdomen), three pairs of jointed legs, compound eyes and one pair of antennae. They are coelomate in nature. The annelids are a large phylum of segmented worms found in marine environments from tidal zones to hydrothermal vents, in freshwater, and in moist terrestrial environments. They are bilaterally symmetrical, triploblastic, coelomate organisms.They have parapodia for locomotion.
5. Marine mammals, which include seals, whales, dolphins, and walruses, rely on the marine environment for feeding. Marine mammals have developed a number of features for efficient locomotion such as torpedo shaped bodies to reduce drag; modified limbs for propulsion and steering; tail flukes and dorsal fins for propulsion and balance. Marine mammals are adept at thermoregulation using dense fur or blubber to reduce heat loss as well as circulatory adjustments to conserve their body temperature. The two main adaptations that desert animals must make are how to deal with lack of water and how to deal with extremes in temperature. Since water is so scarce, most desert animals get their water from the food they eat: succulent plants, seeds, or the blood and body tissues of their prey. Desert animals prevent water leaving their bodies in a number of different ways. Some, like kangaroo rats and lizards, live in burrows which do not get too hot or too cold and have more humid (damp) air inside. These animals stay in their burrows during the hot days and emerge at night to feed. Other animals have bodies designed to save water. Scorpions and wolf spiders have a thick outer covering which reduces moisture loss. The kidneys of desert animals concentrate urine, so that they excrete less water.
6. Evolutionarily conserved gene is a gene that has remained essentially unchanged throughout evolution. Conservation of a gene indicates that it is unique and essential: There is not an extra copy of that gene with which evolution can tinker, and changes in the gene are likely to be lethal. Conserved sequences are similar or identical sequences that occur within nucleic acid sequences. Highly conserved proteins are often required for basic cellular function, stability or reproduction. Sequence similarities serve as evidence for structural and functional conservation, as well as of evolutionary relationships between the sequences. Consequently, comparative analysis is the primary means by which functional elements are identified. Thus, exons or coding regions of the conserved DNA sequences can be compared for evolutionary distance determination.
7. Hydrostatic skeletons are the most prevalent skeletal system used by animals for movement and support. A minimal hydro skeleton resembles a closed container. The walls are two layers of muscles (antagonists) oriented at right angles to one another; the inside contains an incompressible fluid or gel. Hydrostatic skeletons have a role in the locomotion of echinoderms (starfish, sea urchins), cnidarians (jellyfish), annelids (earthworms), nematodes, and other invertebrates.
8. The hierarchy of biological classification has eight major taxonomic ranks. These are: Domain → Kingdom → Phylum → Class → Order → Family → Genus → Species.
9. Tardigrades are small, water-dwelling, segmented animals with eight legs. They are short and plump with 4 pairs of poorly articulated lobopodial limbs living in moist soil. Snail is a common name that is applied most often to land snails, terrestrial pulmonate gastropod molluscs. When the word "snail" is used in this most general sense, it includes not just land snails but also thousands of species of sea snails and freshwater snails. Peripatus is an invertebrate which gives birth to live young rather than laying eggs and reside mostly on leaf litter. Oyster is a distinct group of bivalve molluscs which live in marine or brackish habitats. The valves are highly calcified.

10. Sea squirt, also called ascidian is any member of the invertebrate class Ascidiacea marine animals with some primitive vertebrate features. Sea squirts are primarily sessile (permanently fixed to a surface), potato-shaped organisms found in all seas, from the intertidal zone to the greatest depths. They commonly reside on pier pilings, ships' hulls, rocks, large seashells, and the backs of large crabs. The body has an outer protective covering, the tunic, which contains a cellulose-like substance. Sea squirts have two large pores, one to guide water into the body cavity (the oral, or branchial, aperture), the other serving as an exit (the atrial, or cloacal, aperture). Water is propelled through the animal by pharyngeal cilia. The branchial basket accounts for the attachment of sea squirt to substratum.

11. Endoderm is the innermost of the three primitive germ layers of the embryo. From it are derived the epithelium of the pharynx, respiratory tract (except the nose), digestive tract, bladder, and urethra. The function of the embryonic endoderm is to construct the linings of two tubes within the body. The first tube, extending throughout the length of the body, is the digestive tube. Buds from this tube form the liver, gallbladder, and pancreas. The second tube, the respiratory tube, forms as an outgrowth of the digestive tube and it eventually bifurcates into two lungs. The digestive and respiratory tubes share a common chamber in the anterior region of the embryo; this region is called the pharynx. Epithelial out pockets of the pharynx give rise to the tonsils and the thyroid, thymus, and parathyroid glands.

12. In *Drosophila*, Hedgehog signalling is initiated by the binding of Hedgehog ligand to Patched (Ptc) which is a 12-transmembrane protein receptor. Ptc acts as an inhibitor of Smoothened (Smo), a 7-transmembrane protein related to the Frizzled family of Wnt receptors and to other 7-transmembrane G protein-coupled receptors. In mammals there are three Hedgehog genes, Sonic, Indian and Desert Hedgehog which result in cyclopic eyes of lambs. The Wnt signaling pathway is a network of proteins that passes signals from receptors on the surface of the cell to DNA expression in the nucleus. Wnt-induced responses result in body axis specification. Notch signaling pathway is a highly conserved cell signaling system referred to as NOTCH1, NOTCH2, NOTCH3, and NOTCH4. The Notch/Lin-12/Glp-1 receptor familywas found to be involved in the specification of cell fates during development in *Drosophila* and *C. elegans* (nematode). Hox genes are a group of related genes that control the body plan of the embryo along the anterior-posterior (head-tail) axis. After the embryonic segments have formed, the Hox proteins determine the type of segment structures (e.g. legs, antennae, and wings in fruit flies or the different vertebrate ribs in humans) that will form on a given segment.

13. Osteocytes descend from osteoblasts. They are formed by the incorporation of osteoblasts into the bone matrix. Osteocyte is a mature osteoblast which no longer secretes matrix yet is surrounded by it. Osteoblasts are commonly called bone-forming cells. They secrete osteoid, which forms the bone matrix. They also begin mineralization, and are unable to divide. Osteoclasts function in resorption and degradation of existing bone, the opposite of osteoblasts.

14. The Michaelis-Menten equation is given by:
$V = (V_{max} S)/(K_m + S)$ where, V = velocity or rate of the reaction at any given time, V_{max} = maximum rate of reaction, S = substrate concentration and K_m = Michaelis-Menten constant. K_m is defined as the substrate concentration when velocity or rate of the reaction is half of the maximum rate or velocity ($V = V_{max}/2$). Thus, K_m is a measure of the affinity of the enzyme for a particular substrate.

15. Globular proteins, also known as spheroproteins, are proteins formed by compacted amino acid chains, which are folded into intricate shapes that often roughly resemble spheres. This type of protein represents one of the three major protein groups. The two other groups are fibrous proteins, which are primarily structural proteins, and membrane proteins, which are usually found attached to the membranes of cells and their organelles. The spherical structure is induced by the protein's tertiary structure. The molecule's apolar (hydrophobic) amino acids are bounded towards the molecule's interior whereas polar (hydrophilic) amino acids are bound outwards, allowing dipole-dipole interactions with the solvent, which explains the molecule's solubility. Non-covalent interactions such as hydrophobic interactions stabilize the structure.

16. Histones are highly alkaline proteins found in eukaryotic cell nuclei that package and order the DNA into structural units called nucleosomes. They are the chief protein components of chromatin, acting as spools around which DNA winds, and play a role in gene regulation. Without histones, the unwound DNA in chromosomes would be very long. Five major families of histones exist: H1/H5, H2A, H2B, H3, and H4. Histones H2A, H2B, H3 and H4 are known as the core histones, while histones H1 and H5 are known as the linker histones. The linker histone H1 binds the nucleosome at the entry and exit sites of the DNA, thus locking the DNA into place and allowing the formation of higher order structure.

17. The cell cycle, or cell-division cycle, is the series of events that take place in a cell leading to its

division and duplication (replication). The cell cycle consists of four distinct phases: G_1 phase, S phase (synthesis), G_2 phase (collectively known as interphase) and M phase (mitosis). Two key classes of regulatory molecules, cyclins and cyclin-dependent kinases (CDKs), determine a cell's progress through the cell cycle. Cyclins form the regulatory subunits and CDKs the catalytic subunits of an activated heterodimer; cyclins have no catalytic activity and CDKs are inactive in the absence of a partner cyclin.

18. Tonoplast is the cytoplasmic membrane that surrounds a vacuole of a plant cell. As a membrane, it is mainly involved in regulating the movements of ions around the cell, and isolating materials that might be harmful or a threat to the cell. The vacuole is the storage house for starch. Peroxisomes are surrounded by only a single membrane, and they do not contain DNA or ribosomes. Peroxisomes are major sites of oxygen utilization. Peroxisomes are so named because they usually contain one or more enzymes that use molecular oxygen to remove hydrogen atoms from specific organic substrates (designated here as R) in an oxidative reaction that produces hydrogen peroxide (H_2O_2). Endosomes are primarily intracellular sorting organelles. They regulate trafficking of proteins and lipids among other subcellular compartments of the secretory and endocytic pathway, specifically the plasma membrane Golgi, trans-Golgi network (TGN), and vacuoles/ lysosomes. Endosomes receive cargo (proteins and lipids) from both the biosynthetic and the endocytic pathways. The proteosome is a multi-subunit structure that degrades protein.

19. The theory of endosymbiosis explains the origin of chloroplasts and mitochondria and their double membranes. Unlike any other organelle, except for chloroplasts, mitochondria appear to originate only from other mitochondria. They contain their own DNA, which is circular as is true with bacteria, along with their own transcriptional and translational machinery. Mitochondrial ribosomes and transfer RNA molecules are similar to those of bacteria, as are components of their membrane. According to this theory, certain organelles originated as free-living bacteria that were taken inside another cell as endosymbionts. Mitochondria developed from proteobacteria or close relatives) and chloroplasts from cyanobacteria.

20. A cohort is a group of animals of the same species, identified by a common characteristic, which are studied over a period of time as part of a scientific or medical investigation. In epidemiology, the word cohort is often used to designate a group of people who share a common experience or condition. A cohort may be defined as the aggregate of individuals (within some population definition) who experienced the same event within the same interval. A recent dictionary by Bégaud defines a cohort as a "Group of subjects selected according to one or more common characteristic(s) and followed over time in order to identify, describe or quantify an event".

21. In biogeography, the Neotropic or Neotropical zone is one of the eight terrestrial ecozones. This ecozone includes South and Central America, the Mexican lowlands, the Caribbean islands, and southern Florida, because these regions share a large number of plant and animal groups. The ecozone also includes temperate southern South America. In contrast, the Neotropical Floristic Kingdom excludes southernmost South America, which instead is placed in the Antarctic Kingdom.

22. Pseudocoelomate is any of a group of invertebrates with a three-layered body that has a fluid-filled body cavity (pseudocoelom) between the endoderm and the mesoderm (the innermost and middle tissue layers). The pseudocoelom is contrasted with the coelom of mollusks, annelid worms, and the more complex animals (including humans and other vertebrates). Pseudocoelomates lack a circulatory system, and the pseudocoelom itself lacks the endothelial lining of a coelom. The hydrostatic pressure of the pseudocoelom gives the body a supportive framework that acts as a skeleton. Most of the pseudocoelomates (e.g., the classes Nematoda and Rotifera) are small and none possess an independent vascular system. *Caenorhabditis elegans* is a free-living, transparent nematode (roundworm).

23. In the process of binary fission (a type of asexual reproduction), an organism duplicates its genetic material, or deoxyribonucleic acid (DNA), and then divides into two parts (cytokinesis), with each new organism receiving one copy of DNA. Binary fission is the primary method of reproduction of prokaryotic organisms. In protists, binary fission is often differentiated into types, such as transverse or longitudinal, depending on the axis of cell separation. Transverse binary fission divides the cell across the short axis (e.g., most bacilli-shaped bacteria), longitudinal binary fission across the long axis (e.g., *Trypanosoma*), and random binary fission across no defined axis (e.g., Amoeba). *Trypanosoma* is a genus of kinetoplastids group of unicellular parasitic flagellate protozoa.

24. *Hyracotherium* is an extinct genus of very small perissodactyl ungulates which was found in the London Clay formation. This small, dog-sized animal was once considered to be the earliest known member of Equidae before the type species,

H. leporinum, was reclassified as a palaeothere, of a perissodactyl family related to both horses and brontotheres. Eohippus (meaning "dawn horse") was the earliest-known horse - it was the size of a tiny dog. Another name for this genus is *Hyracotherium* (meaning "mole beast").

25. IgG or Immunoglobulin Gamma is the only immunoglobin capable of crossing the placental barrier. Given, that IgG has 4 chains held by disulphide bonds. Therefore, the maximum number of different amino acids present at the C terminal end of the IgG would be for generation of the disulphide linkage to yield 4 chains.

26. The change in ion concentration in between the plasma and urine is dependent upon the ion exchange potential of the ions given by: $I = \Sigma C_i Z_i^2$ where, C_i = concentration of ion and Z_i = charge or valency of the ion. This gives the Hoffmeister series of ions. So the correct order of change in ion concentration is:

$NH_4^+ > PO_4^{-3} > K^+ > Na^+$

27a. Out of 500 $\frac{a(-)b(-)}{a(+)b(+)}$, number of $\frac{a(-)b(-)}{a(-)b(+)} = 20$

$$\Rightarrow 500\,\frac{a(-)b(-)}{a(+)b(+)}\text{ population}$$

$$= \frac{20a(-)b(-)}{a(-)b(+)}\text{ frequency}$$

$$\Rightarrow \frac{a(-)b(-)}{a(+)b(+)}\text{ population}$$

$$= \frac{20}{500}\left[\frac{a(-)b(-)}{a(-)b(+)}\right]\text{ frequency}$$

$$\Rightarrow 100\,\frac{a(-)b(-)}{a(+)b(+)}\text{ population}$$

$$= 0.04\left[\frac{a(-)b(-)}{a(-)b(+)}\right]\text{ frequency}$$

$$\Rightarrow \frac{a(-)b(-)}{a(+)b(+)}\text{ population}$$

$$= 4\left[\frac{a(-)b(-)}{a(-)b(+)}\right]\text{ frequency}$$

Therefore, frequency of recombination between a and b is 4.

Out of 1000 progenies of genotype $\frac{a(-)c(-)}{a(+)c(+)}$, number of $\frac{a(-)c(-)}{a(+)c(-)} = 80$

$$\Rightarrow 1000\frac{a(-)c(-)}{a(+)c(+)}\text{ population}$$

$$= 80\frac{a(-)c(-)}{a(+)c(-)}\text{ frequency}$$

$$\Rightarrow \frac{a(-)c(-)}{a(+)c(+)}\text{ population}$$

$$= \frac{80}{1000}\left[\frac{a(-)c(-)}{a(+)c(-)}\right]\text{ frequency}$$

$$\Rightarrow 100\,\frac{a(-)c(-)}{a(+)c(+)}\text{ population}$$

$$= 0.08\left[\frac{a(-)c(-)}{a(+)c(-)}\right]\text{ frequency}$$

$$\Rightarrow \frac{a(-)c(-)}{a(+)c(+)}\text{ population}$$

$$= 8\left[\frac{a(-)c(-)}{a(+)c(-)}\right]\text{ frequency}$$

$\Rightarrow$ Therefore, the frequency of recombination between a and c is 8.

27b. From the previous question, $a \leftarrow\rightarrow b$ = 4 frequency of recombination

And $a \leftarrow\rightarrow c$ = 8 frequency of recombination. Therefore, $c \leftarrow(8)\rightarrow a \leftarrow(4)\rightarrow b$. Thus, it can be seen that a is closer to b than to c.

28a. Hardy-Weinberg law is an algebraic equation that describes the genetic equilibrium within a population. The science of population genetics is based on this principle, which may be stated as follows: in a large, random-mating population, the proportion of dominant and recessive genes present tends to remain constant from generation to generation unless outside forces act to change it. In the simplest case of a single locus with two alleles: allele one is denoted A and allele two a and their frequencies are denoted by p and q; freq (A) = p; freq (a) = q; p + q = 1. If mating is random, then new individuals will have freq (AA) = p^2 for the AA homozygotes in the population, freq (aa) = q^2 for the aa homozygotes, and freq (Aa) = 2pq for the heterozygote. The formula is written as $(p^2) + (2pq) + (q^2) = 1$, representing the fact that probabilities must add up to one.

28b. From Hardy-Weinberg equation given by $(p^2) + (2pq) + (q^2) = 1$, given 1% people are homozygous, *i.e.*, $q^2 = 1\% = 0.01$;

$$q = \sqrt{0.01} = 0.1$$

Therefore, from Hardy-Weinberg's principle, p + q = 1. So, p = 0.9 which is the homozygous dominant genotype.

Now, for the heterozygous genotype, we have 2pq

$$= 2 \times 0.9 \times 0.1 = 0.18 = 18\%.$$

Thus, the % of people with hetero-zygous genotype is 18 %.

GATE-2004

XL : LIFE SCIENCES

Time : 3 Hours | *Maximum Marks : 100*

(H) CHEMISTRY (Compulsory)

Useful data :

Gas constant, R = 8.3143 $JK^{-1}\ mol^{-1}$

Faraday constant, F = 96500 $Cmol^{-1}$

Q. 1 – 10 carry one mark each

1. For a second order reaction, 2B → products, if the initial concentration of the species B is $[B]_0$ and the rate constant is k, then $t_{1/2}$ can he expressed as

(*a*) $1/[B]_0 k$ (*b*) $1/k$ (*c*) $[B]_0/k$ (*d*) $1/2[B]_0 k$

2. If the heats of reaction of the following transformations $C + O_2(g) \rightarrow CO_2(g)$,

$$C+\frac{1}{2}O_2(g)\rightarrow CO(g) \text{ and } CO(g)+\frac{1}{2}O_2(g)$$

$\rightarrow CO_2(g)$ are Q, 11.5 and 10.5 joules respectively, then Q in joules is equal to

(*a*) 120.75 (*b*) 1 (*c*) –1 (*d*) 22

3. The spontaneity of a reaction can be judged from the sign of the emf (E) and the free energy (G) of the cell. The criteria are

(*a*) ΔG = +ve, E = – ve (*b*) ΔG = 0, E = 0

(*c*) ΔG = –ve, E = + ve (*d*) ΔG = – ve, E = – ve

4. The function cos(*ax*) is an eigen function of $\frac{d^2}{dx^2}$ with an eigenvalue of

(*a*) $-a$ (*b*) $-a^2$ (*c*) a (*d*) $-a^{-2}$

5. The heteronuclear diatomic molecule that is isoelectronic to HCN is

(*a*) NO (*b*) CO (*c*) BO (*d*) SO

6. The bond order in Be_2 molecule can be expected to be

(*a*) 0 (*b*) 1 (*c*) 2 (*d*) 3

7. The intense color of $KMnO_4$ is due to

(*a*) electronic transition from one energy level to another in Mn

(*b*) electronic transition from one energy level to another in O

(*c*) charge transfer from Mn to O

(*d*) charge transfer from O to Mn

8. Of the following, the compounds that are aromatic are

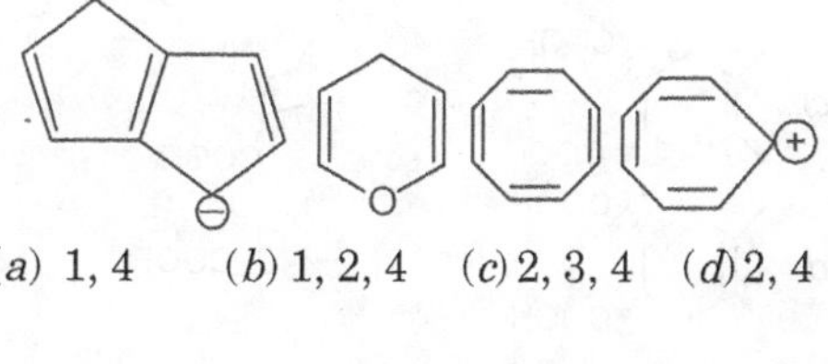

(*a*) 1, 4 (*b*) 1, 2, 4 (*c*) 2, 3, 4 (*d*) 2, 4

9. The hybridization of the atoms indicated by an asterisk in the following compounds in a sequence (from 1 to 4) is given by

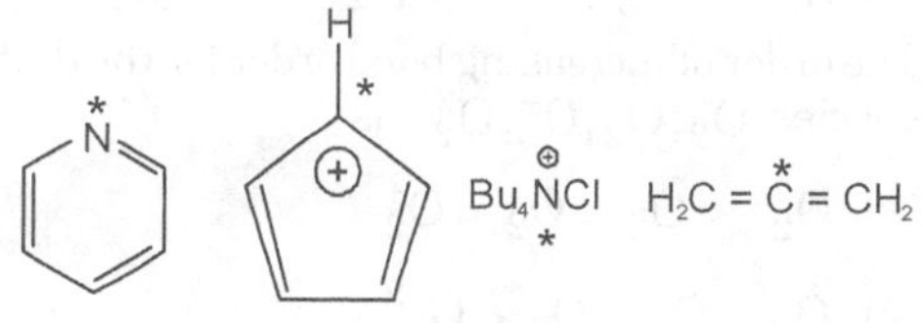

1 2 3 4

(*a*) sp^3, sp^2, sp^3, sp (*b*) sp^2, sp^2, sp^3, sp^2

(*c*) sp^2, sp^2, sp^3, sp (*d*) sp^2, sp^3, sp^3, sp

10. Which of the following compounds can have enantiomers?

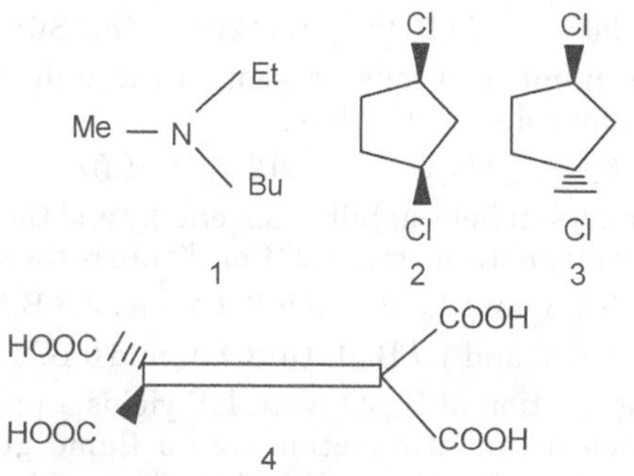

(*a*) 2, 3, 4 (*b*) 1, 3, 4 (*c*) 3, 4 (*d*) 1, 3

Q. 11 – 30 carry two marks each

11. The rate constant for a certain reaction is found to be doubled when the temperature is raised from 27 to 37° C. The activation energy for this reaction in *kJ* is

(*a*) 26.8 (*b*) 107.2 (*c*) 53.6 (*d*) 50.0

12. The standard potential for the electrodes Hg/Hg_2^{+2} and Hg/Hg^{+2} are –0.799 and –0.855 volts at 25° C, respectively. The equilibrium constant for the reaction

$$Hg + Hg^{+2} \rightleftharpoons Hg_2^{+2} \text{ is}$$

(*a*) 85.12 (*b*) 79.12 (*c*) 70 (*d*) 90.20

13. The freezing point of pure benzene is 5.44° C and that of a solution containing 2.092 g of A in 100 g of benzene is 4.44° C. The molal depression constant (k_f) for benzene is 5.1. From this data, the molecular weight of A can be calculated to be

(*a*) 106.7 (*b*) 206.6 (*c*) 213.4 (*d*) 53.2

14. The ion conductance of the alkali metal cations at a given concentration follow the following order

(*a*) $Li^+ > Na^+ > K^+ > Rb^+$ (*b*) $Li^+ < Na^+ < K^+ > Rb^+$

(*c*) $Li^+ < Na^+ < K^+ < Rb^+$ (*d*) $Li^+ \cong Na^+ > K^+ > Rb^+$

15. A system undergoes a certain change in state by path I. The heat absorbed and the work done for this process are 10 kcal mol^{-1}, respectively. The respective quantities for the same change in state by path II are 11 kcal mol^{-1} and 0.5 w_{max}, where w_{max} is the work done, if the change were reversibly carried out. The magnitude of w_{max} in *k*J mol^{-1} (1 cal = 4.2 J) is

(*a*) 4.2 (*b*) 2 (*c*) 1 (*d*) 8.4

16. The total pressure for the reaction $C(s) + CO_2(g) \rightleftharpoons 2CO(g)$ under the equilibrium condition is 15 atm. The value of K_p is

(*a*) 16 (*b*) 10 (*c*) 20 (*d*) 25

17. The order of increasing bond order for the diatomic species $O_2, O_2^+, O_2^-, O_2^{2-}$ is

(*a*) $O_2^{2-} < O_2^- < O_2 < O_2^+$

(*b*) $O_2 < O_2^+ < O_2^- < O_2^{-2}$

(*c*) $O_2^+ < O_2 < O_2^- < O_2^{2-}$

(*d*) $O_2^- < O_2^{2-} < O_2^+ < O_2$

18. The bond angle in I_3^- is

(*a*) 90° (*b*) 104° (*c*) 120° (*d*) 180°

19. The number of ions present in the unit cell of cesium chloride (C*s*Cl) is

(*a*) 6 (*b*) 4 (*c*) 2 (*d*) 8

20. The crystal field stabilization energy and the spin-only magnetic moment of $[CoF_6]^{4-}$ are respectively

(*a*) 0.4 Δ_0 and 4.9 B.M. (*b*) 0.8 Δ_0 and 3.8 B.M.

(*c*) 1.8 Δ_0 and 1.7 B.M. (*d*) 2.4 Δ_0 and 0 B.M.

21. The reaction of H_3BO_3 with HF yields a product, which upon introduction into a flame gives a characteristic green colouration. The product is

(*a*) BH_3 (*b*) B_2H_6 (*c*) B_2O_3 (*d*) BF_3

22. Graphite sublimes at a very high temperature (3700°C). This is due to

(*a*) Weak covalent interactions in the solid and stronger or more covalent interactions in the gas phase

(*b*) Strong covalent interactions in the solid and weaker or fewer covalent interactions in the gas phase

(*c*) Strong covalent interactions in the solid and strong covalent interactions in the gas phase

(*d*) weak covalent interactions in the solid and stronger ionic interactions in the gas phase

23. The nickel (II) complex $\{NiCl_2(PPh_3)_2\}$ is paramagnetic. The analogous complex of palladium (II) is diamagnetic. The number of isomers that will exist for each of these formulations respectively are

(*a*) 1,1 (*b*) 2,2 (*c*) 1,2 (*d*) 2,1

24. The order (from 1 to 3) in which the reactions below follow S_N1 and S_N2 mechanisms is

1. 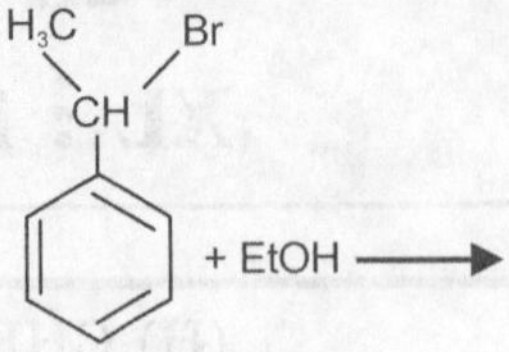

2. $CH_3I + H_3C-C(CH_3)_2-O^- \xrightarrow{\text{t-BuOH}}$

3. 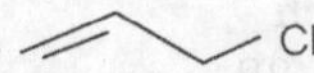 $Cl + CH_3COO^- \xrightarrow[\text{(aprotic solvent)}]{CH_3COCH_3^-}$

(*a*) S_N1, S_N2, S_N2 (*b*) S_N2, S_N1, S_N2

(*c*) S_N1, S_N2, S_N1 (*d*) S_N2, S_N2, S_N1

25. The products 'X' and 'Y' of the following reaction are

$$CH_3CH_2COOEt \xrightarrow[2.H^+/H_2O]{1.2PhMgBr\ ehter} X \xrightarrow{Conc.\,H_2SO_4\cdot\Delta} Y$$

(*a*) $CH_3CH_2-C(OH)Ph_2$ and $H_3CHC = CPh_2$

(*b*) $CH_3CH_2-C(=O)-Ph$ and $CH_3CH_2-C(OH)(H)-Ph$

(*c*) $CH_3CH_2-C(OH)(H)-Ph$ and $CH_3CH_2-C(OH)Ph_2$

(*d*) $CH_3CH_2-C(OH)Ph_2$ and $CH_2 = C = CPh_2$

26. The major products of the following Diels-Alder cycloaddition reaction 1 and 2 with the correct stereochemistry are

1. 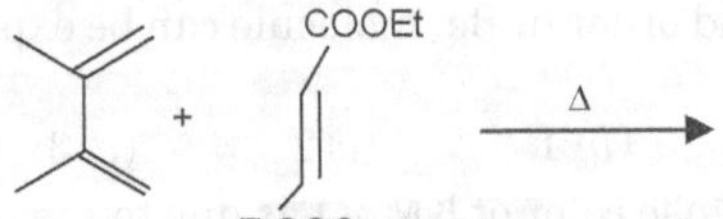

2. 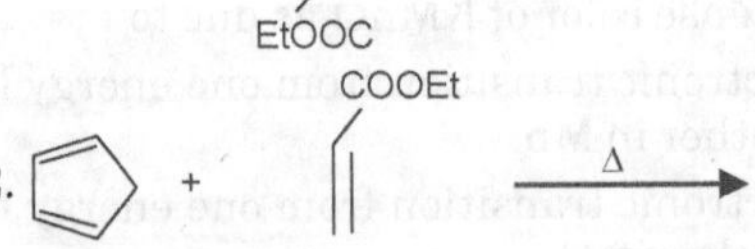

(*a*) 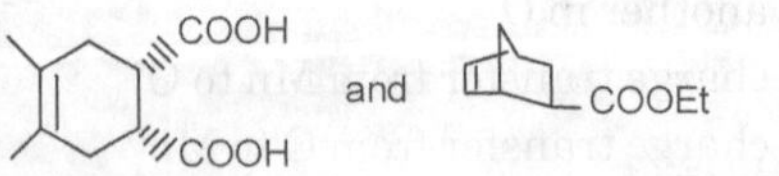

(*b*) 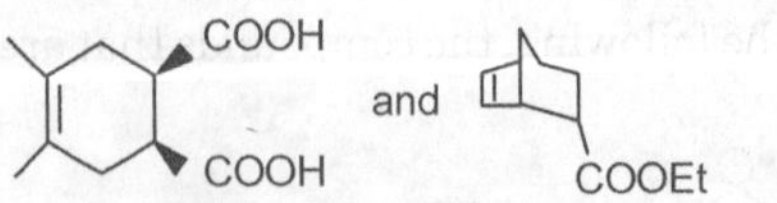

(*c*) 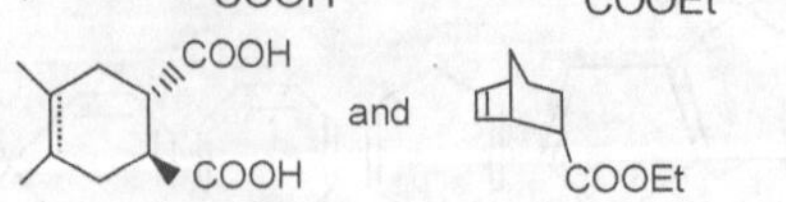

(*d*) 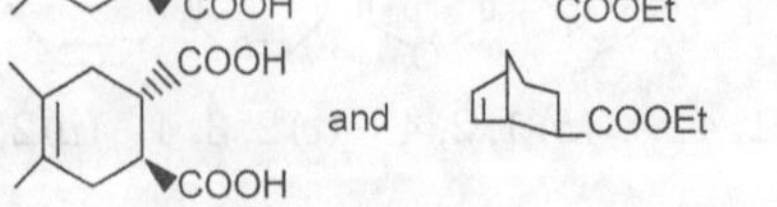

27. *p*-Cresol (4-methylphenol) reacts with two molar equivalents of isobutylene in the presence of HCl and $AlCl_3$ to give a product, which is an excellent antioxidant. The structure of the product is

(*a*) 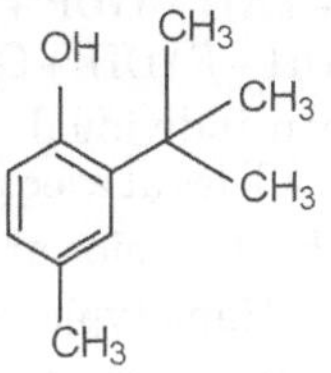

(*b*) 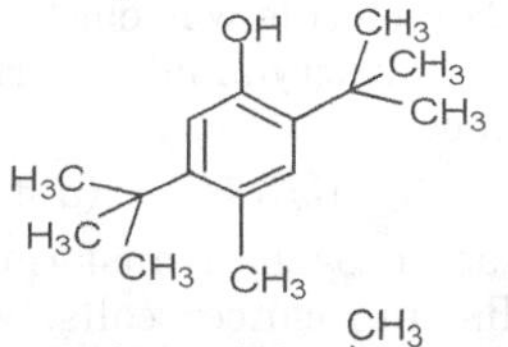

(*c*) 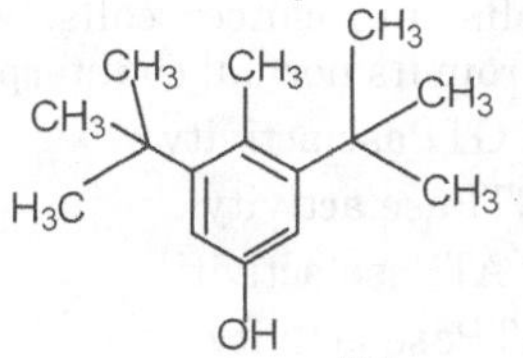

(*d*) 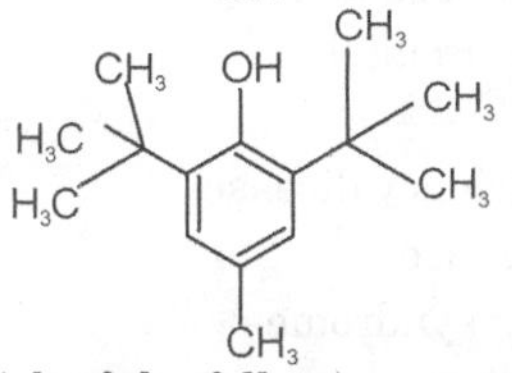

28. Which of the following statement is correct about the elimination given below?

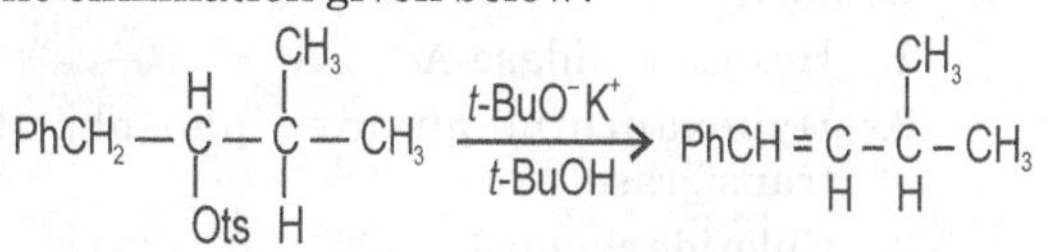

(*a*) the product shown will not be formed, because Saytzeff rule necessitates the formation of the alternative more substituted olefin

(*b*) the product shown will be formed predominantly, because the conjugation of the double bond with the phenyl ring leads to thermodynamic stability

(*c*) the product shown will be formed as a minor one. This follows from Saytzeff rule

(*d*) the product shown is correct and it follows from Saytzeff rule

29. The perhydroxylation of maleic and fumaric acids using $KMnO_4$ leads respectively to the following tartaric acids

(*a*) meso and meso

(*b*) *d,l* racemate and meso

(*c*) meso and *d,l* racemate

(*d*) *d,l* racemate and *d,l* racemate

30. The product of the following reaction and the name reaction that leads to its formation are

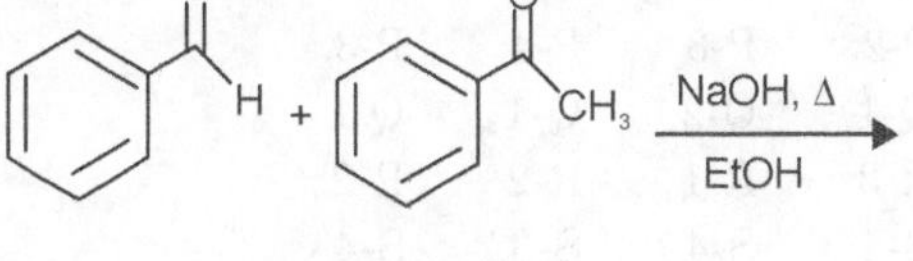

(*a*) 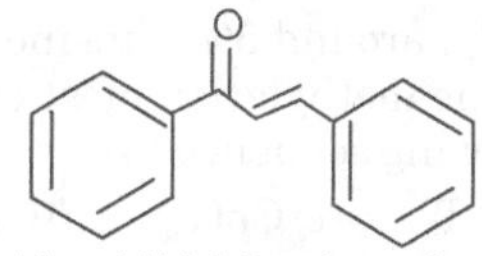

Mixed Aldol Condensation

(*b*) 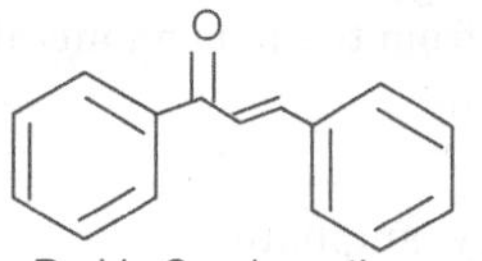

Perkin Condensation

(*c*) 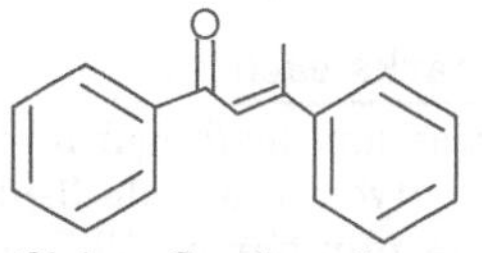

Claisen Condensation

(*d*) 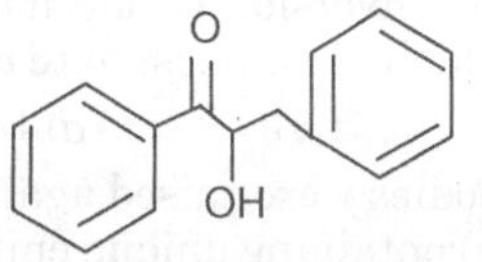

Benzoin Condensation

(I) BIOCHEMISTRY

Q. 1 – 10 carry one mark each

1. The most abundant atom in a living organism is

(*a*) Hydrogen (*b*) Oxygen
(*c*) Nitrogen (*d*) Carbon

2. The coenzyme involved in transfer of carboxyl group is

(*a*) NADH
(*b*) Coenzyme A
(*c*) S-Adenosyl methionine
(*d*) Biotin

3. The unit of length 'Angstrom' equals to

(*a*) 10^{-6} m (*b*) 10^{-8} m (*c*) 10^{-10} m (*d*) 10^{-15} m

4. Which of the following triplet does NOT code for any amino acid

(*a*) UUA (*b*) UCA (*c*) UAA (*d*) UGU

5. Erythrocytes resist shearing forces while travelling through narrow blood vessels because they contain the meshwork of

(*a*) GlycophorinA (*b*) Spectrin
(*c*) Haemoglobin (*d*) Myoglobin

6. Tetrodotoxin, a highly poisonous toxin from Puffer fish acts on

(*a*) Sodium channel (*b*) Potassium Channel
(*c*) Chloride Channel (*d*) Calcium Channel

7. Electron flow in Cytochrome oxidase in the respiratory chain can be blocked by

(*a*) Rotenone (*b*) Amytal
(*c*) Cyanide (*d*) Cycloheximide

8. In case of humans, passive immunity observed in newborn child is due to the passage of the following immunoglobulin from the mother to the child through placenta

(*a*) IgD (*b*) IgE (*c*) IgM (*d*) IgG

9. In eukaryotic cells, around 5% cytosine residues are methylated, the methylation most commonly occurs in the following sequence

(*a*) CpA (*b*) CpT (*c*) CpG (*d*) CpC

10. The following reagent will **NOT** release the integral proteins from the plasma membrane

(*a*) Sodium chloride

(*b*) Triton X-100

(*c*) Sodium dodecyl sulphate

(*d*) NP-40

Q. 11–30 carry two marks each

11. The biochemical reactions leading from glucose to the generation of glyceraldehyde-3-phosphate consume ATP. The number of ATP molecules consumed for the conversion of one molecule of glucose to glyceraldehyde-3-phosphate is

(*a*) 2 (*b*) 1 (*c*) 3 (*d*) 4

12. Monoclonal antibodies were raised against three different proteins containing unique epitopes. All the monoclonal antibodies were mixed together and placed in one of the wells in an Ouchterlony Double Diffusion plate. Similarly all three proteins were mixed together and placed in the adjacent well. The number of precipitin bands observed after incubation are

(*a*) 3 (*b*) 2 (*c*) 1 (*d*) 0

13. L-19 RNA from the protozoan *Tetrahymena* was demonstrated to have two enzymatic activities and these activities are

(*a*) RNA ploymerase, DNA polymerase

(*b*) Ribonuclease, RNA polymerase

(*c*) Ribonuclease, Deoxyribonuclease

(*d*) Ribonulcease, Protease

14. A single stranded DNA of unknown size can **NOT** be distinguished from a double stranded DNA by

(*a*) Analysis of base composition

(*b*) Thermal denaturation

(*c*) Density gradient ultracentrifugation

(*d*) Gel Electrophoresis

15. Telomerase is an enzyme whose macromolecular composition is

(*a*) Lipoprotein only

(*b*) Ribonucleoprotein only

(*c*) Ribonucleic acid only

(*d*) Protein only

16. The molecular weight of IgG-Antigen complex at antigen excess is 300Kd. The molecular weight of antigen is

(*a*) 75 (*b*) 50 (*c*) 100 (*d*) 150

17. The net reaction of the Citric acid cycle is

(*a*) Acetyl CoA + 2NAD$^+$ + FAD + GDP + Pi + $2H_2O$ $\longrightarrow$ $2CO_2$ + 3NADH + $FADH_2$ + GTP + $2H^+$ + CoA

(*b*) Acetyl CoA + 3NAD$^+$ + FAD + GDP + Pi + $2H_2O$ $\longrightarrow$ $2CO_2$ + 3NADH + $FADH_2$ + GTP + $2H^+$ + CoA

(*c*) Acetly CoA + 2NAD$^+$ + 2FAD + 2GDP + Pi + $2H_2O$ $\longrightarrow$ $2CO_2$ + 2NADH + $2FADH_2$ + 2GTP + CoA

(*d*) Acetyl CoA + NAD$^+$ + FAD + GDP + Pi + H_2O $\longrightarrow$ $2CO_2$ + NADH + $FADH_2$ + GTP + CoA

18. Genetic variation between individuals within a species involving different alleles at a locus is called

(*a*) Isotypic variation (*b*) Idiotypic variation

(*c*) Allotypic variation (*d*) Haplotypic variation

19. A pentameric IgM molecule was electrophoresed on a reducing SDS-Polyacrylamide gel. How many bands one can expect

(*a*) 1 (*b*) 2 (*c*) 3 (*d*) 4

20. Viral encoded Ras oncogene transforms normal mammalian cells into cancer cells. Viral Ras protein differs from its normal counterpart by

(*a*) Diminished GTPase activity

(*b*) Increased GTPase activity

(*c*) Diminished ATPase activity

(*d*) Increased ATPase activity

21. Choose the correct match

Group I

P Immunodeficiency disease

Q Tay-Sach disease

R Lesch-Nyhan syndrome

S Cystic fibrosis

Group II

1. Hexosaminidase-A
2. Hypoxanthine-guanine phosphoribosyl-transferase
3. Chloride channel
4. Adenosine deaminase

(*a*)	(*b*)	(*c*)	(*d*)
P-1	P-3	P-4	P-2
Q-3	Q-2	Q-1	Q-4
R-4	R-4	R-2	R-3
S-2	S-1	S-3	S-l

22. Choose the correct match

Group I

P β-ketoacyl-ACP synthase

Q β-ketoacyl-ACP reductase

R Enoyl-ACP-reductase

S Acyl carrier protein (ACP)

Group II

1. Reduces double bond forming saturated acyl-ACP
2. Reduces β-keto group to β-hydroxy group
3. Condenses acyl and malonyl groups
4. Carries acyl group in thioester linkages

(*a*)	(*b*)	(*c*)	(*d*)
P-2	P-3	P-4	P-3
Q-1	Q-2	Q-1	Q-1
R-3	R-1	R-2	R-2
S-4	S-4	S-3	S-4

23. A DNA was labeled at its 5′ end using γ ^{32}P-ATP. Choose the correct combination from the following options to separate the free γ ^{32}P-ATP from γ ^{32}P labeled DNA

P γ ^{32}P-ATP can be removed by treating the sample with phosphatases.

Q The labeled samples can be electro-phoresed and blotted onto nitrocellulose membrane and then labeled DNA can be recovered from nitrocellulose membrane

R Sample can be passed through a gel filtration column to separate free γ ^{32}P-ATP

S DNA can be precipitated using ethanol to separate it from contaminating γ ^{32}P-ATP

(*a*) P, Q (*b*) P, S (*c*) R, S (*d*) R, Q

24. A team of researchers had used the following eluting buffers to prepare an anti albumin IgG from an anti IgG affinity column,

Buffer A : 0.1M Glycine-HCl, pH 3.0

Buffer B : 0.1M Sodium acetate, pH 6.0

Buffer C : 0.1M Sodium phosphate, pH 7.0

Buffer D : 0.1M Tris-HCl, pH 8.0

Which of the above buffers can be used for anti albumin IgG elution?

(*a*) Buffer A (*b*) Buffer B
(*c*) Buffer C (*d*) Buffer D

25. Oligosaccharide chain is added to the Asparagine residue of a newly synthesized protein on the luminal side of the endoplasmic reticulum membrane. The Asparagine of the newly synthesized protein that is linked to oligosaccharide chain is a part of the sequence (x, can be any amino acid other than Proline)

(*a*) Asn-x-Asp (*b*) Asn-x-Thr
(*c*) Asn-x-Ile (*d*) Asn-x-Gly

26. The 'Signal recognition particle' binds to the signal peptide of the protein undergoing synthesis resulting into a pause in the transnational process. The pause in the transnational phenomenon is due to

(*a*) inactivation of aminoacyl-tRNA synthetases
(*b*) inhibits the activity of elongation factor Tu
(*c*) induced confirmational change in the smaller ribosomal subunit
(*d*) blockade of the entry of the next aminoacyl-tRNA for the reaction

27. Which of the following Statement is **NOT** true with respect to the Photosystem II found in the chloroplasts? (Photosystem I = PS I, Photosystem II = PS II)

(*a*) PS II is located in the grana
(*b*) Chlorophyll molecule in the reaction center for the PS II is bound to a 110Kd integral membrane protein
(*c*) A complex of Cytochromes *b* and *f* transports electrons from PS II to PS I
(*d*) PS II reaction center is bound to two Mn^{2+} ions

28. Choose the statement that is **NOT** correct with respect to the Protein Kinase C (PKC)

(*a*) Activated PKC can phosphorylate the specific tryptophan residue on the target protein
(*b*) PKC is a Ca^{2+} dependant kinase
(*c*) PKC can be activated by diacylglycerol
(*d*) Activation of PKC can lead to the activation of MAP kinase

29. 'Enhancer' elements are known to increase the rate of transcription when present at the upstream side of the promoter sequences. If the same enhancer element is placed in reverse orientation,

(*a*) the rate of transcription increases
(*b*) the rate of transcription decreases
(*c*) the rate of transcription remains same
(*d*) no transcription is observed

30. Choose the group containing only the peptide harmones

(*a*) Vasopressin, Oxytocin, Epinephrine
(*b*) Vasopressin, Testosterone, Glucagon
(*c*) Oxytocin, Vasopressin, Thyroxine
(*d*) Oxytocin, Vasopressin, Somatostatin

(K) BOTANY

Q.1 – 10 carry one mark each

1. During seed development, the organelle oleosome functions for storage of

(*a*) Oil Only
(*b*) Oil and starch
(*c*) Oil, starch and protein
(*d*) Oil and protein

2. From the single parent cell how many times the process of mitosis/cell division occur to produce 512 cells

(*a*) 28 (*b*) 10 (*c*) 9 (*d*) 128

3. Two criteria of most cork cells are

(*a*) Suberin and permeable
(*b*) Suberin and impervious
(*c*) Cutin and permeable
(*d*) Cutin and impervious

4. In gynostegium

(*a*) Stamens adnate to corolla
(*b*) Stamens adnate to perianth
(*c*) Stamens adhere to carpels
(*d*) Stamens are united by their filaments

5. Which of the staining procedure is NOT followed to determine the viability of cells?

(*a*) FDA staining
(*b*) TTC staining
(*c*) Evan's blue staining
(*d*) Methyl blue staining

6. In angiosperms adventive embryony develops from

(*a*) Diploid nucellar cells asexually
(*b*) Diploid nucellar cell sexually
(*c*) Megaspore mother cell sexually
(*d*) Any cell of the embryosac asexually

7. Phytoremediation is
   (*a*) Remedial measure in deforestation
   (*b*) Removal of pollutants by plants
   (*c*) Remedial measure in soil erosion using plants
   (*d*) Curing of disease by phytochemicals
8. Given below are the enzymatic reactions of Krebs cycle. In which of the following steps GTP is generated?
   (*a*) Citrate to isocitrate
   (*b*) α-ketoglutarate to succinyl-CoA
   (*c*) Fumarate to malate
   (*d*) Succinyl-CoA to succinate
9. The metal ion required for the enzymatic activity of nitrogenase is
   (*a*) Zinc (*b*) Cobalt
   (*c*) Copper (*d*) Molybdenum
10. The *rol* gene is present in
   (*a*) R_i plasmid (*b*) Both R_i and T_i plasmid
   (*c*) T_i plasmid (*d*) pUC

Q.11 – 30 carry two marks each

11. If A = 1 micrometer, B = 1 nanometer and C = 5 Angstrom, find the product of A/B and B/C
   (*a*) (–) 2000 (*b*) 2000
   (*c*) 5000 (*d*) (–) 5000
12. Identify the correct set of three statements for cytoskeletal protein filaments from the following list
   1. Actin filament is about 8 nm wide
   2. Actin filament is 25 nm wide
   3. Intermediate filaments have size intermediate between actin filaments and microtubules
   4. Protofilaments of microtubules are composed of α/β tubulin heterodimer
   5. Colchicine binds to the tubulin subunits in spindle microtubule causing disassembly to free units.

   (*a*) 3, 4, 5 (*b*) 2, 3, 4 (*c*) 1, 3, 4 (*d*) 1, 2, 3
13. The nucleotide and peptide sequences mentioned in column I were changed after mutation, and now shown in column II. Name the type of mutation.

Column I

DNA 5′..........CCTCGGCCC........3′
3′..........GGAGCCGGG........5′
↓
mRNA 5′..........CCUCGGCCC........3′
↓
Peptide ....Pro Arg Pro...........

Column II

5′........CCTTGGCCC.........3′
3′.......GGAACCGGG.......5′
↓
5′.......CCUUGGCCC......3′
↓
.........Pro Trp Pro............

   (*a*) Frameshift mutation
   (*b*) Non-sense substitution
   (*c*) Same-sense substitution
   (*d*) Mis-sense subsitution
14. A mutant strain (thi^-) of *Neurospora* was crossed with the wild type (thi^+). A total of 132 asci were analyzed.
   First division segregation : 104
   Second division segregation : 29
   Find out the map distance (cM) of *thi* gene from the centromere.
   (*a*) 10.6 (*b*) 21.2 (*c*) 5.3 (*d*) 8.3
15. In pea plants the following cross was made

GGRR x ggrr
(Yellow, round) (Green, wrinkled)
↓
F_1 selfed

Mention the proportion of homozygous: heterozygous yellow, round seeds in F_2.
   (*a*) 1 : 3 (*b*) 1 : 16 (*c*) 1 : 8 (*d*) 9 : 16

Direction (Q. 16–25) : *Following are matching exercises. Choose the correct one from among the alternatives a, b, c and d*

16. **Group 1** (*Pathogen*)
   P *Puccinia graminis*
   Q *Ustilago hordei*
   R *Trichothecium roseum*
   S *Ustilago nuda*

   Group 2 (*Infection site*)
   1. Blossom infection
   2. Seedling infection
   3. Fruit infection
   4. Root infection
   5. Leaf infection
   6. Grain infection

(*a*)	(*b*)	(*c*)	(*d*)
P-5	P-5	P-6	P-1
Q-2	Q-2	Q-5	Q-2
R-4	R-3	R-3	R-3
S-6	S-1	S-1	S-4

17. **Group 1** (*Plant*)
   P Mustard
   Q Pea
   R Cucumber
   S Orchid

   Group 2 (*Floral Formula*)
   1. Zygomorphic, bisexual, $P_{6(3+3)}$, $A_{1 \text{ or } 2}G_{(3)}$
   2. Actinomorphic, ♂, $K_{(5)}$ $C_{(5)}$ $A_{(5)}$
   3. Actinomorphic, bisexual, $P_{(3+3)}$ A_{3+3} $G_{(3)}$
   4. Zygomorphic, bisexual, $K_{(5)}$ C_5 $A_{(9)+1}\underline{G}_1$
   5. Actinomorphic, bisexual, K_{2+2} C_4 A_{2+4} $\underline{G}_{(2)}$
   6. Actinomorphic, bisexual, $K_{(5)}$ C_5 $A(\infty)$ $\underline{G}_{(5)}$

(*a*)	(*b*)	(*c*)	(*d*)
P-5	P-2	P-5	P-5
Q-4	Q-4	Q-6	Q-3
R-2	R-6	R-3	R-4
S-1	S-3	S-2	S-1

18. **Group 1** (*Enzyme*)
P Phosphoglucomutase
Q Hexokinase
R Fructokinase
S Sucrose Phosphatase
Group 2 (*Product*)
1. Fructose-6-PO_4
2. Glucose-1-PO_4
3. Glucose-6-PO_4
4. UDP-glu + PPi
5. Sucrose + Pi
6. Sucrose 6-PO_4

(*a*)	(*b*)	(*c*)	(*d*)
P-3	P-6	P-4	P-2
Q-1	Q-4	Q-6	Q-3
R-4	R-2	R-5	R-1
S-6	S-5	S-3	S-5

19. **Group 1** (*Characteristics*)
P Edible fungi
Q Deadly poisonous fungi
R Alkaloid producing fungi
S Fungi pathogenic to human
Group 2 (*Species*)
1. *Mucor mucedo*
2. *Candida albicans*
3. *Claviceps purpurea*
4. *Amanita verna*
5. *Morchella conica*
6. *Aspergillus flavus*

(*a*)	(*b*)	(*c*)	(*d*)
P-5	P-5	P-5	P-4
Q-3	Q-4	Q-4	Q-1
R-4	R-1	R-3	R-3
S-1	S-2	S-2	S-6

20. **Group 1** (*Property*) — **Group 2** (*Transposon*)

Group 1	Group 2
P Cointegrate	1. Tn5
Q LTRs	2. *P* elements
R Hybrid dysgenesis	3. Tn3
S Controlling elements	4. Ty1
	5. IS elements
	6. Ac/Ds

(*a*)	(*b*)	(*c*)	(*d*)
P-3	P-6	P-4	P-1
Q-4	Q-5	Q-5	Q-3
R-2	R-2	R-2	R-2
S-6	S-1	S-3	S-5

21. **Group 1** — **Group 2**

Group 1	Group 2
P Photochemcial smog	1. Carbon dioxide
Q Ozone hole	2. Ozone
R Global warming	3. Formaldehyde
S Metal pollution	4. Chloroflurocarbons
	5. Phytochelatins
	6. Radon

(*a*)	(*b*)	(*c*)	(*d*)
P-6	P-2	P-3	P-2
Q-4	Q-4	Q-4	Q-4
R-1	R-1	R-1	R-1
S-3	S-5	S-5	S-6

22. **Group 1** (*Pigment*) — **Group 2** (*Absorption maxima*)

Group 1	Group 2
P Chlorophyll *a*	1. 1020 nm
Q C-phycocrythrin	2. 350 nm
R C-phycocyanin	3. 615 nm
S Bacteriochlorophyll *b*	4. 750 nm
	5. 680 nm
	6. 550 nm

(*a*)	(*b*)	(*c*)	(*d*)
P-5	P-1	P-1	P-5
Q-6	Q-2	Q-3	Q-6
R-3	R-3	R-6	R-1
S-1	S-4	S-5	S-2

23. **Group 1** (*Metabolite*) — **Group 2** (*Chemical nature*)

Group 1	Group 2
P Menthol	1. Diterpene
Q Ajmalicine	2. Tetraterpene
R Caffeine	3. Purine alkaloid
S Carotene	4. Phenyl propanoid
	5. Indole alkaloid
	6. Monoterpene

(*a*)	(*b*)	(*c*)	(*d*)
P-6	P-5	P-6	P-1
Q-5	Q-6	Q-5	Q-2
R-2	R-3	R-3	R-3
S-3	S-2	S-2	S-4

24. **Group 1** (*Plant/Organ*) — **Group 2** (*Vascular bundles*)

Group 1	Group 2
P Dicot stem	1. Numerous, scattered in ground tissue
Q Monocot stem	2. Polyarch, xylem exarch
R Dicot root	3. Open, arranged in a ring, xylem endarch.
S Monocot root	4. Diarch to hexarch, xylem exarch

(*a*)	(*b*)	(*c*)	(*d*)
P-3	P-3	P-2	P-2
Q-2	Q-1	Q-4	Q-3
R-1	R-4	R-3	R-1
S-4	S-2	S-1	S-4

25. **Group 1** (*Transgenic plant*) — **Group 2** (*Relevant gene*)

Group 1 (*Transgenic plant*)	Group 2 (*Relevant gene*)
P. Glyphosate resistance	1. psbA
Q. Insect resistance (Bollgard)	2. tfdA
R. Delayed ripening	3. cryI Ac
S. Insect resistance (Yieldgard)	4. pg (Antisense)
	5. cryI Ab
	6. aroA

(*a*)	(*b*)	(*c*)	(*d*)
P-6	P-1	P-6	P-2
Q-3	Q-2	Q-5	Q-3
R-4	R-3	R-1	R-4
S-5	S-4	S-3	S-5

26. With the objective of raising somatic embryos via friable callusing choose the best combination of growth regulators for medium I and II.

Medium I (*Callusing*)	**Medium II** (*Embryogenesis*)
P 2,4-D	1. IAA and TIBA
Q IAA	2. 2,4-D and BAP
	3. IAA and BAP
	4. 2,4-D and ABA

(*a*) Q-2 (*b*) P-1 (*c*) Q-4 (*d*) P-3

27. For cryopreservation of plant cells /tissues, maintaining viability over longest period of time, select the best possible combination of cryoprotectants (I) and temperature (II).

I	II
P Glycerol, DMSO and proline	1. (–)80°C
Q Glycerol, acetic acid and ethanol	2. (–)4°C
	3. (–)196°C
	4. 0°C

(*a*) Q-3 (*b*) P-1 (*c*) P-2 (*d*) Q-4

28. Indentify the inhibitors for the steps 'X' and 'Y' from the following list

$$H_2O \to P_{680} \to Q_A \xrightarrow{X} Q_B \to PQ \xrightarrow{Y} Cyt\ b_6f \to PC \to P_{700}$$

P DCMU
Q CO
R Paraquat
S DBMIB

(*a*) P-R (*b*) Q-R (*c*) P-Q (*d*) P-S

29. Identify the restriction enzyme suitable for the following restriction digestion

5′...........G↓GATCC..............3′
5′...........CCTAG↑G.............5′

(*a*) BamH1 (*b*) EcoR1 (*c*) Alu1 (*d*) HacIII

30. The two scientists who were awarded the Nobel Prize for transposable genetic elements and polymerase chain reaction
(*a*) Barbara McClintock and Susumu Tonegawa
(*b*) Barbara McClintock and Kary Mullis
(*c*) Barbara McClintock and Paul Berg
(*d*) Kary Mullis and Paul Berg

(L) MICROBIOLOGY

Q. 1 – 10 carry one mark each

1. The Scientist who developed aseptic methods using phenol to prevent infections was
(*a*) Robert Koch (*b*) John Tyndall
(*c*) Paul Ehrlich (*d*) Joseph Lister

2. The organism Robert Koch used first to propose Koch's postulates was
(*a*) *Mycobacterium tuberculosis*
(*b*) *Salmonella typhimurium*
(*c*) *Bacillus anthracis*
(*d*) *Klebsiella pneumoniae*

3. The primary strain used for staining endospore is
(*a*) Crystal violet (*b*) Malachite green
(*c*) Safranin (*d*) Carbol fuchsin

4. The engulfment of disease causing bacteria by macrophages was discovered by
(*a*) Emil von Behring
(*b*) Elie Metchnikoff
(*c*) Shibasaburo Kitasato
(*d*) J. Bordet

5. The two key enzymes of glyoxylate cycle are
(*a*) Isocitrate dehydrogenase, α-Ketoglutarate dehydrogenase
(*b*) Isocitrate lyase, α-Ketoglutarate dehydrogenase
(*c*) Isocitrate lyase, Malate synthase
(*d*) Malate synthase, Isocitrate dehydrogenase

6. *Nitrosomonas europaea* is a chemolithotroph in which electron donor and electron acceptor, respectively are
(*a*) NH^+_4, O_2 (*b*) H_2, O_2
(*c*) NO^-_2, O_2 (*d*) H_2S, NO^-_3

7. In Gram negative bacteria, the flagellum is attached to the cytoplasmic membrane by the rings
(*a*) S ring only (*b*) S and M rings
(*c*) P ring (*d*) P and L rings

8. In *Rhizobium*-legume symbiotic nitrogen fixation, oxygen-sensitive nitrogenase is protected by leghemoglobin. The ratio of leghemoglobin-bound O_2 to free O_2 is
(*a*) 10 : 1 (*b*) 100 : 1
(*c*) 1,000 : 1 (*d*) 10,000 : 1

9. Nonphosphorylated Entner Doudoroff pathway (EDP) is operative in species of
(*a*) *Pyrococcus* (*b*) *Streptococcus*
(*c*) *Micrococcus* (*d*) *Staphylococcus*

10. A 'regulon' is defined as
(*a*) A set of operons that are functionally co-ordinated
(*b*) A master gene regulating the function of a set of genes
(*c*) All the regulatory genes of the genome
(*d*) The genes present in the control region of an operon

Q. 11 – 30 carry two marks each

11. In TCA cycle, both carbons of acetyl CoA are oxidized to CO_2 at two steps which are
(*a*) Cis-aconitate → Isocitrate → α-Ketoglutarate
(*b*) α-Ketoglutarate → Succinate → Fumarate
(*c*) Isocitrate → α-Ketoglutarate → Succinate
(*d*) Citrate → Cis-aconitate → Isocitrate

12. Cells of *Escherichia coli* grown on mineral salts medium with glycerol as carbon source, are harvested and exposed to three different inducers of *lac* operon. Their inducing efficiencies are
(*a*) TMG < IPTG < Lactose
(*b*) Lactose < TMG < IPTG
(*c*) IPTG < Lactose < TMG
(*d*) TMG < Lactose < IPTG

13. A bacterial suspension when counted in Petroff-Hausser bacteria counting chamber showed on average 20 bacteria in one large square (each large square = 1/25 mm^2). The number of bacteria/ml of the suspension is
(*a*) 25×10^6 (*b*) 50×10^6 (*c*) 10×10^7 (*d*) 25×10^7

14. *Pseudomonas* species metabolize a wide range of organic compounds through β-ketoadipate whose structure is
(*a*) $CH_3.CH_2.CO.CH_2.COOH$
(*b*) $HOOC.CH_2.CH_2.CO.COOH$
(*c*) $HOOC.CH_2.CH_2.CH_2.CO.COOH$
(*d*) $HOOC.CH_2.CH_2.CO.CH_2.COOH$

15. In a different planet codons have four bases instead of three and there are four termination codons as against three found in our planet. Which of the following statements will <u>**NOT**</u> hold true in 4 base codon planet assuming there is no evolutionary selection?
(*a*) The number of codons will be too few to code for all twenty amino acids
(*b*) There will be greater codon degeneracy than in earth
(*c*) The number of t-RNA genes will be more compared to earth
(*d*) The sizes of proteins will be generally longer

16. In most phototrophic and autotrophic organisms, CO_2 is fixed by RuBisCo via Calvin cycle. The sugar into which CO_2 gets fixed is
(*a*) Ribulose-5-phosphate
(*b*) Glyceraldehyde-3-phosphate
(*c*) 1,3-Bisphosphoglycerate
(*d*) Ribulose-l,5-bisphosphate

17. The genome size of the following organisms are in the order
(*a*) Haemophilus influenzae > Saccharomyces cerevisiae > Escherichia coli > ϕxl74
(*b*) Escherichia coli > Saccharomyces cerevisiae > Haemophilus influenzae > ϕxl74
(*c*) Saccharomyces cerevisiae > Escherichia coli > Haemophilus influenzae > ϕxl74
(*d*) Saccharomyces cerevisiae > Haemophilus influenzae > ϕxl74 > Escherichia coli

18. The following are the number of germ line genes for heavy and light chains in an individual. Calculate the approximate number of diverse IgG (Kappa) molecules that the individual can generate not taking into account somatic mutation

Germline genes	Heavy chain	K chain
V	50	40
D	30	0
J	6	5

(*a*) 131 (*b*) 9,200
(*c*) 18,00,000 (*d*) 36,00,000

19. A strain of *Mycobacterium tuberculosis* was found to be resistant to INH, streptomycin and rifampicin at 10^{-5}, 10^{-6}, 10^{-7} frequencies, respectively. The frequency of appearance of a strain resistance to all three compounds is
(*a*) 10^{-5} (*b*) 10^{-6} (*c*) 10^{-11} (*d*) 10^{-18}

20. In *Escherichia coli* the number of molecules per cell occur in the following order
(*a*) tRNA < mRNA < rRNA < DNA
(*b*) DNA < mRNA < rRNA < tRNA
(*c*) rRNA < mRNA < tRNA < DNA
(*d*) DNA < tRNA < mRNA < rRNA

21. Switch recombination does not take place among the immunoglobulin genes
(*a*) IgM → IgD (*b*) IgM → IgGl
(*c*) IgM → IgE (*d*) IgM → IgA

22. EMB (cosin-methylene blue) agar is used to differentiate *Escherichia coli* from *Enterobacter aerogenes*. The green metallic sheen of the colonies is due to
(*a*) Eosin and methylene blue combine to produce a precipitate under neutral conditions (*E. aerogenes*)
(*b*) Eosin and methylene blue combine to produce a precipitate under acidic-conditions (*E. coli*)
(*c*) Methylene blue gets precipitated under acid conditions (*E. coli*)
(*d*) Eosin gets precipitated under neutral conditions (*E. aerogenes*)

23. UV spectroscopy is not used to quantitate the compounds based on absorbance
(*a*) Nucleic acids have absorbance peak at 260 nm
(*b*) NAD(P)H have absorbance peak at 340 nm
(*c*) Aromatic aminoacids have absorption maxima about 280 nm
(*d*) Sulfur containing aminoacids absorbance at 270 nm

24. Luminous bacterium (*Vibrio fischeri*) and flashlight fish (*Photoblepheron palpebratus*) provide an interesting symbiotic association. In the luciferase reaction, the products are
(*a*) FMN + RCOOH + H_2O
(*b*) RCOOH + H_2O + light
(*c*) FMN + RCOOH + H_2O + light
(*d*) $FMNH_2$ + RCOOH + H_2O + light

25. The flagellate *Monas stigmatica* (6 μm long) swims at the speed of 50 cell lengths per second. The distance it covers in 1 hour is
(*a*) 1.08 cm
(*b*) 10.80 cm
(*c*) 10.8 m
(*d*) 1.08 m

26. The serotypes of *Salmonella* sp. arc due to
(*a*) Lipid A structure
(*b*) Core polysaccharide containing KDO and heptose
(*c*) Unusual sugars in O-side chain
(*d*) Both Lipid A structure and core polysaccharide

27. The property not possessed by Archaeobacteria is
(*a*) They have pseudomurein in their cell walls
(*b*) Their lipids have ether linkage
(*c*) They have N-acetylglucosamine and N-acetyltalosaminuronic acid as repeating alternating units in the backbone
(*d*) They have D and L amino acids in their short peptide chain

28. Which of the following properties of diphtheria toxin is not true
(*a*) The nicked toxin is biologically and immunologically identical to unnicked toxin
(*b*) On reduction with GSH, chains A and B are separable
(*c*) Diptheria toxin inhibits protein synthesis by ADP-ribosylating EF2
(*d*) Chain A alone is toxic to animals and whole cells

29. The following statements are made regarding incorporation of 5-bromodeoxyuridine into DNA
A. 5-bromodeoxyuridine substitutes thymidine in DNA
B. The minimum number of DNA replication cycles required to observe mutation is two
C. 5-bromodeoxyuridine produces GC → AT transition
D. 5-bromodeoxyuridine generates deletion mutants
Which of the above statements are true
(*a*) A and C (*b*) A and B (*c*) C and D (*d*) B and C

30. In a bacterial cell culture the initial cell population (N_o) was 10^3 cells/ml. In 6 hours and 40 minutes, it has gone through 20 generations. The final cell population (N_t) and growth rate constant (K), respectively are

	N_t		K
(*a*)	10^9 cells/ml	and	3
(*b*)	10^8 cells/ml	and	4
(*c*)	10^7 cells/ml	and	5
(*d*)	10^6 cells/ml	and	6

(M) ZOOLOGY

Q.1 – 10 carry one mark each

1. Both birds and bats fly and have wings. Wings of birds and bats represent
(*a*) Analogous structures
(*b*) Homologous structures
(*c*) Vestigial structures
(*d*) Phylogentically conserved structures

2. Which one of the following would you qualify as a holometabolous insect?
(*a*) Cockroach (*b*) Grasshopper
(*c*) Mosquito (*d*) Human body louse

3. All of the following statements about heterochromatin are true except one. Which one?
(*a*) Heterochromatin stains more darkly with DNA dyes than euchromatin
(*b*) Heterochromatin contains more highly condensed DNA than euchromatin
(*c*) Heterochromatin is associated with inactive genes
(*d*) Heterochromatin is more susceptible to DNaseI than euchromatin

4. In human, the cardiac sphincter surrounds the cardiac orifice in the digestive tract. The failure of this sphincter's normal function will result in the
(*a*) regurgitation of food into the esophagus
(*b*) loss of control of defecation
(*c*) movement of the bolus into the trachea rather than the esophagus
(*d*) rapid emptying from the stomach to the small intestine

5. Stroke occurs when
(*a*) the pacemaker becomes defective, producing an irregular heartbeat
(*b*) a blood clot enters and blocks one of the coronary arteries
(*c*) a blood clot dislodges from a vein and moves into the lung where it blocks a pulmonary artery
(*d*) a blood clot enters the cerebral circulation blocking an artery and causing the death of brain tissue

6. Which one of the following statements is true with regard to tissue macrophages?
(*a*) have short life spans because they self-destruct after engulfing foreign invaders
(*b*) originate from monocytes that leave the circulation and enter the tissues
(*c*) are most effective against parasites
(*d*) do not attack microorganisms directly; instead, they destroy virus-infected body cells

7. Which of the following cell types does HIV preferentially infect?
(*a*) cytotoxic T cells (*b*) natural killer cells
(*c*) helper T cells (*d*) memory cells

8. *Trichinella spiralis* infection is most commonly contracted from
   (*a*) Beef products
   (*b*) Eating infested, undercooked pork
   (*c*) Undercooked vegetables
   (*d*) Non-pasteurized milk
9. In three of the four types of animals listed below colonies can be initiated by a single individual. However, the fourth one would need at least a pair (a male and a female) to set up, a colony. Identify which one
   (*a*) Sea anemones (*b*) Frogs
   (*c*) Tapeworms (*d*) Whiptail lizards
10. The synthesis of ATP by chemiosmosis
    (*a*) is endergonic and is coupled to exergonic electron transport
    (*b*) is exergonic and is coupled to endergonic electron transport
    (*c*) is due to electrons shuttled down the electron transport chain to the final electron acceptor, which is NAD+
    (*d*) produces less ATP than the Kreb's cycle and glycolysis combined

Q. 11 – 30 carry two marks cach

11. Presume that you can measure DNA content in a single cell throughout its cell cycle. After measuring the DNA content during G1 phase, at what other points during the remainder of the cell cycle would you find changes in DNA per cell?
    (*a*) Prophase and metaphase
    (*b*) S phase and prophase
    (*c*) S phase and G2
    (*d*) Interphase
12. Frequency of individuals with darkly colored wings in the moth species *Biston bistullaria*, went up during the early days of industrialization in England. This change in the moth population coincided with the darkening of the barks of the trees around the factories. This phenomenon, also referred to as industrial melanism, represents:
    (*a*) Speciation (*b*) Genetic drift
    (*c*) Natural selection (*d*) Allelic variations
13. Consider an island population where a majority of the individuals display hexadactylly of their hands. Evolutionary biologists would readily explain this phenomenon based on
    (*a*) Dominance of the hexadactyl condition
    (*b*) Small size of the founder population
    (*c*) Novel mutations
    (*d*) Improved fitness and adaptation of the hexadactyl individuals
14. Marsupials are naturally found in Australia. The hallmark of the marsupials is:
    (*a*) Ovo-viviparity
    (*b*) Prolonged placental development
    (*c*) Parturition before completion of embryonic development
    (*d*) Incomplete adaptive radiation
15. Imagine that you are examining cosin-haematoxylin stained cross section of a mammalian stomach. Beginning from the outermost to the inner most layers, which of the following description accurately describes the different cell layers of the stomach?
    (*a*) Mucosa-submucosa-serosa-muscularis
    (*b*) Serosa-mucosa-submucosa-muscularis
    (*c*) Serosa-muscularis-submucosa-mucosa
    (*d*) Muscularis-submucosa-mucosa-serosa
16. Animals belonging to the Phylum chordata are unambiguously classified based on only one of the four sets of characteristics described below. Which one?
    (*a*) Notochord, Central nervous system, circulatory system and Segmented muscle
    (*b*) Notochord, dorsal hollow nerve cord, pharyngeal slits and postnatal tail
    (*c*) Notochord, dorsal hollow nerve chord, gills and segmented muscles
    (*d*) Notochord, peripheral nervous system, pharyngeal slits and segmented muscles
17. A female fruit fly, *Drosophila* of the genotype *RrSs* was mated to males with the genotype *rrss*. The progeny obtained in four different situations are displayed on the left column while their probable explanations are displayed on the right. Match the genotypic frequency with the most appropriate explanations.

    Frequency of Progeny
    A. 50% *RS* and the rest *rs*
    B. 50% *RS* & *rs*; the rest *Rs* & *rS*
    C. 90% *RS* & *rs*, the rest *Rs* & *rS*
    D. All the progeny are *RS*

    Explanation
    1. the two loci are not linked
    2. the *r* and *s* gametes in the female were not formed
    3. the two loci are 10 m.u. apart
    4. the two loci are tightly linked

    Codes :
    (*a*) A-4; B-1; C-3; D-2 (*b*) A-1; B-4; C-2; D-3
    (*c*) A-2; B-4; C-3; D-1 (*d*) A-4; B-1; C-2; D-3
18. Diploid chromosome number in human is 46. However, if you count chromatids which are visible during mitotic or meiotic cell divisions, you would be able to count different sets of chromatid numbers depending on the stage and the type of the cell division in question. Match the chromatid numbers given on the left with cell division stage shown on the right

    A. 46 1. Mitotic metaphase
    B. 23 2. Aneuploid meiotic telophase II
    C. 92 3. Meiotic telophase I
    D. 24 4. Meiotic anaphase II

    Codes :
    (*a*) A-3; B-4; C-1; D-2 (*b*) A-2; B-4; C-1; D-3
    (*c*) A-1; B-4; C-2; D-3 (*d*) A-1; B-2; C-3; D-4

19. The transport of molecules of a particular solute from inside an animal cell across the cell membrane to the extracellular fluid always requires energy when
(*a*) the concentration of the solute is higher inside the cell than outside it
(*b*) the concentration of the solute is lower inside the cell than outside it
(*c*) a transport protein is involved in the movement of the molecules
(*d*) the cytoskeleton blocks all available channels

20. Different cell types respond to the same signaling molecule (for example, a hormone like glucagon) in different ways because
(*a*) different cells possess different receptors, which produce signals unique to each cell type
(*b*) different cells possess identical receptors, however, ultimately different sets of targets are activated
(*c*) different cells have membrane receptors that bind to different sides of the signal molecule
(*d*) the signal transduction pathway in cells has a variable length

21. Indicate the order in which the following steps occur in the production of a mature mRNA.
(*a*) initiation of transcription, splicing, addition of 5′ cap, addition of poly A tail, transport to cytoplasm
(*b*) initiation of transcription, addition of 5′ cap, splicing, addition of poly A tail, transport to cytoplasm
(*c*) initiation of transcription, addition of poly A tail, addition of 5′ cap, splicing, transport to cytoplasm
(*d*) initiation of transcription, addition of 5′ cap, addition of poly A tail, splicing, transport to cytoplasm

22. All your cells contain protooncogenes, which can change into cancer-causing genes. Why do cells possess such potential time bombs?
(*a*) Protooncogenes protect cells from infection by cancer-causing viruses
(*b*) Protooncogenes are genetic junk that has not yet been eliminated by natural selection.
(*c*) Protooncogenes are unavoidable environmental carcinogenes
(*d*) Protooncogenes are necessary for normal control of cell division

23. Researchers have found homeotic genes in humans, but they are not yet certain how these genes shape the human phenotype. Considering the functions of homeotic genes are comparable in *Drosophila* and humans, which one of the following statements is most likely to be their function in humans?
(*a*) Determining skin and hair color
(*b*) Regulating the cellular metabolic rate and growth
(*c*) Determining that arms come off the upper portion of the torso and legs from the lower half of the body
(*d*) Regulating the rate and timing of cell division

24. Which one of the pairs of answers provided below will correctly fill the blanks in the statement, "In lakes and ponds, eutrophication occurs when (i)____leading to (ii)____"?
(*a*) (i) levels of dissolved CO_2 rise; (ii) bicarbonate levels too high to support life
(*b*) (i) too much nutrients flow into the water body; (ii) anaerobic conditions in deeper waters
(*c*) (i) pesticides are washed off agricultural land; (ii) decreased aquatic biodiversity
(*d*) (i) primary producers are killed by pollution; (ii) starvation of organisms at higher trophic levels

25. In ecological parlance which of the following can be defined as a population?
(*a*) All the insects that are trapped in a spider web
(*b*) All the plants in a forest
(*c*) All the earthworms that live in a grassland plus those in the forest
(*d*) All the sandalwood trees in a given forest

26. Which one of the following activities does NOT increase the concentration of greenhouse gases in the atmosphere?
(*a*) Increasing the number of cows and sheep to help feed a growing human population
(*b*) Burning tropical rain forests to clear land for grazing
(*c*) Leaving leaks in natural gas pipelines unchecked
(*d*) Spreading salt on roads to prevent ice formation

27. Organism X can see colors we cannot and sense traces of chemicals we cannot. However, if organism X cannot hear very well, then which one of the following statements would be the ultimate explanation for their poor hearing?
(*a*) Organism X is too small to have functional auditory organs
(*b*) Hearing may not contribute much to the reproductive success of organism X
(*c*) If organism X could hear well, its brain would be swamped with unnecessary information
(*d*) This is an example of altruism

28. Every morning a research student turns on the light in a laboratory aquarium to feed the fish. After a couple of weeks of this routine, the student noticed that the fish come to the surface to feed as soon as the lights are turned on. The behavior of the fish is a result of
(*a*) Habituation (*b*) Positive phototaxis
(*c*) Imprinting (*d*) Classical conditioning

29. If an individual were to raise a set of relatives, which one of the following sets would result in a maximal continuation of his own gene pool through successive generations?
(*a*) Eight first cousins
(*b*) One offspring and two nieces
(*c*) One sibling, one grandchild, and two first cousins
(*d*) One offspring, one nephew, and two grandchildren

30. You label a few cells at the tip of the animal pole of a gastrulating frog embryo with a fluorescent dye. At the end of embryogenesis, where would you find the fluorescing cells?
(*a*) The cardiac cells (*b*) The pancreatic cells
(*c*) The neural cells (*d*) The intestinal cells

ANSWERS

(H) CHEMISTRY

1. (*a*)	2. (*d*)	3. (*c*)	4. (*b*)	5. (*b*)	6. (*a*)	7. (*d*)	8. (*a*)	9. (*c*)	10. (*c*)
11. (*c*)	12. (*b*)	13. (*a*)	14. (*c*)	15. (*b*)	16. (*b*)	17. (*a*)	18. (*d*)	19. (*c*)	20. (*b*)
21. (*d*)	22. (*b*)	23. (*c*)	24. (*a*)	25. (*a*)	26. (*c*)	27. (*d*)	28. (*b*)	29. (*c*)	30. (*a*)

(I) BIOCHEMISTRY

1. (*a*)	2. (*d*)	3. (*c*)	4. (*c*)	5. (*b*)	6. (*a*)	7. (*c*)	8. (*d*)	9. (*c*)	10. (*a*)
11. (*a*)	12. (*a*)	13. (*b*)	14. (*a*)	15. (*b*)	16. (*d*)	17. (*b*)	18. (*c*)	19. (*b*)	20. (*a*)
21. (*c*)	22. (*b*)	23. (*a*)	24. (*a*)	25. (*b*)	26. (*b*)	27. (*d*)	28. (*a*)	29. (*a*)	30. (*d*)

(K) BOTANY

1. (*a*)	2. (*c*)	3. (*b*)	4. (*c*)	5. (*d*)	6. (*a*)	7. (*b*)	8. (*d*)	9. (*d*)	10. (*a*)
11. (*b*)	12. (*c*)	13. (*d*)	14. (*b*)	15. (*c*)	16. (*a*)	17. (*a*)	18. (*d*)	19. (*c*)	20. (*a*)
21. (*b*)	22. (*a*)	23. (*c*)	24. (*b*)	25. (*a*)	26. (*a*)	27. (*b*)	28. (*d*)	29. (*a*)	30. (*b*)

(L) MICROBIOLOGY

1. (*d*)	2. (*c*)	3. (*b*)	4. (*b*)	5. (*c*)	6. (*a*)	7. (*a*)	8. (*d*)	9. (*a*)	10. (*a*)
11. (*c*)	12. (*b*)	13. (*a*)	14. (*d*)	15. (*d*)	16. (*b*)	17. (*c*)	18. (*c*)	19. (*d*)	20. (*a*)
21. (*a*)	22. (*b*)	23. (*d*)	24. (*c*)	25. (*d*)	26. (*c*)	27. (*d*)	28. (*a*)	29. (*a*)	30. (*a*)

(M) ZOOLOGY

1. (*b*)	2. (*c*)	3. (*b*)	4. (*a*)	5. (*d*)	6. (*b*)	7. (*c*)	8. (*b*)	9. (*b*)	10. (*d*)
11. (*c*)	12. (*c*)	13. (*c*)	14. (*a*)	15. (*c*)	16. (*b*)	17. (*a*)	18. (*a*)	19. (*b*)	20. (*a*)
21. (*d*)	22. (*d*)	23. (*c*)	24. (*b*)	25. (*d*)	26. (*d*)	27. (*c*)	28. (*d*)	29. (*d*)	30. (*c*)

EXPLANATIONS

(H) CHEMISTRY (Compulsory)

1. Given a second order reaction:
   2B → products with a rate constant k
   Initial concentration of B = $[B]_0$
   Therefore we have,
   $$\frac{d[B]}{dt} = k[B]^2$$
   {as reaction is second order}
   $$\Rightarrow \quad \frac{d[B]}{[B]^2} = k\,dt$$
   After integrating both the sides, we get
   $$\frac{-1}{[B]} = -kt + C$$
   Now, at $t = 0$ and $[B] = [B]_0$ {given}
   We get, $C = -1/[B]_0$
   Put this value in above equation,
   $$\frac{-1}{[B]} = -kt + \left(\frac{-1}{[B]_0}\right)$$
   On solving we get,
   $$T = \frac{1}{k}\left(\frac{1}{[B]} - \frac{-1}{[B]_0}\right)$$
   For $t = t_{1/2}$
   and $[B] = \frac{[B]_0}{2}$
   We get, $$t_{1/2} = \frac{1}{k}\left(\frac{2}{[B]_0} - \frac{1}{[B]_0}\right)$$
   Finally, $$t_{1/2} = \frac{1}{k}[B]_0$$
2. Given, reaction 1 :
   $$C + O_2(g) \rightarrow CO_2(g)$$
   Heat of reaction 1 = Q
   Reaction 2 :
   $$C + \frac{1}{2}O_2(g) \rightarrow CO(g)$$
   Heat of the reaction 2 = 11.5J
   Reaction 3 :
   $$CO(g) + \frac{1}{2}O_2(g) \rightarrow CO_2(g)$$
   Heat of the reaction = 10.5J
   Therefore, adding the heat of all the three reactions:
   Heat of reaction 1
   = Heat of reaction 2
   + Heat of reaction 3
   $\Delta H = 11.5 + 10.5 = 22.0J$
   Therefore, heat of reaction 1 (ΔH) i.e. Q is 22.0 J.
3. When ΔG is negative, a process or chemical reaction proceeds spontaneously in the forward direction. So for ΔG to be negative E must be positive in the equation:
   $$\Delta G = -nEF.$$
   So ΔG = –ve and E = +ve should be the criteria for spontaneity of a reaction.
4. The function cos(ax) is an eigen function of $\frac{d^2}{dx^2}$ with an eigen value of $-a^2$.
   As we know,
   $$f(x) = \cos(ax)$$
   By differentiating both sides, we get
   $$\frac{df(x)}{dx} = -a\sin ax$$
   Squaring both sides,
   $$\frac{d^2 f(x)^2}{dx^2} = -a^2\cos ax.$$
5. The heteronuclear diatomic molecule that is isoelectronic to HCN is CO because it has the same number of electrons i.e. 14 as HCN. While NO has 15, BO has 13 and SO has 24 electrons.
6. Number of electrons in $Be_2 = 4 \times 2 = 8$
   sigma 1s bonding orbital - 2 electrons
   sigma 1s antibonding orbital - 2 electrons
   sigma 2s bonding orbital- 2 electrons
   sigma 2s antibonding - 2 electrons
   Bond order
   $$= \frac{\text{n.o. of } e^- \text{ in bonding orbitals} - \text{n.o. of electrons in antibonding orbitals}}{2}$$
   $$= \frac{(4-4)}{2} = 0$$
   Therefore the bond order (B.O.) of Be_2 is zero.
7. The intense color of $KMnO_4$ solution is due to the presence of MnO_4^- in the solution. The MnO_4^- ion is a transition metal complex, and the color comes from a charge transfer from a ligand to the metal i.e. of charge transfer from Mn to O.
8. The four compounds given are :

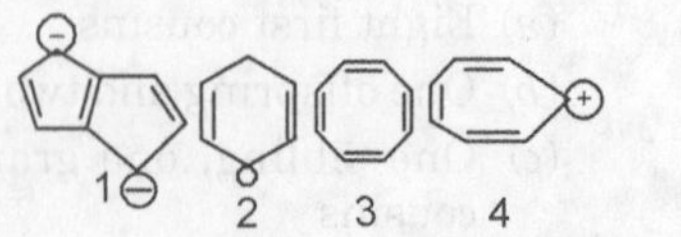

1 2 3 4

   The compounds which are aromatic are: 1 and 4. As 10 π electrons are present in 1 and 6π electrons are present in 4 and it is also planar. So they are aromatic compounds while 8π electrons are present in 3 and 6π electrons are present in 2 but it is non-planar. So they are non-aromatic compounds or anti-aromatic compounds.
9. Hybridisation of compound 1

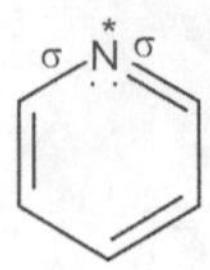

   ⇒1 lone pair of electrons is present. It is sp^2 hybridised as 2σ bonds are also present.
   i.e., 2σ + l.h = 3(sp^2)
   Hybridisation of compound 2

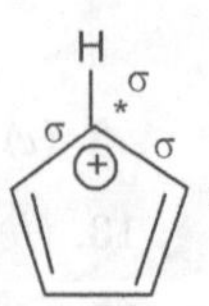

   ⇒ Here 3σ (sigma) bonds are present but no lone pair of electrons. So it is also sp^2 hybridized.
   Hybridisation of compound 3
   $Bu_4\overset{\oplus}{N}Cl$ ⇒ This compound can also be written as:

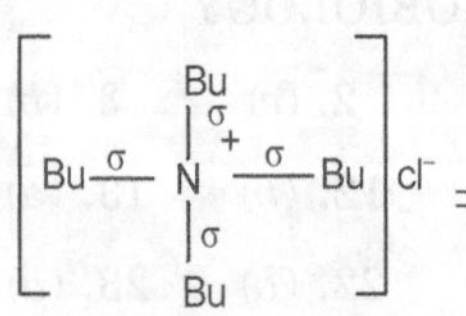

   ⇒ Here 4 σ bonds are present. So it is sp^3 hybridised.
   Hybridisation of compound 4
   $CH_2 \underset{=}{\sigma} \overset{*}{C} \underset{=}{\sigma} CH_2$ ⇒ 2 double bonded sigma bonds are present. So it is sp hybridized.

10. Enantiomers are mirror images of each other that are non-superposable i.e., they are non-identical. The 4 compounds given are:

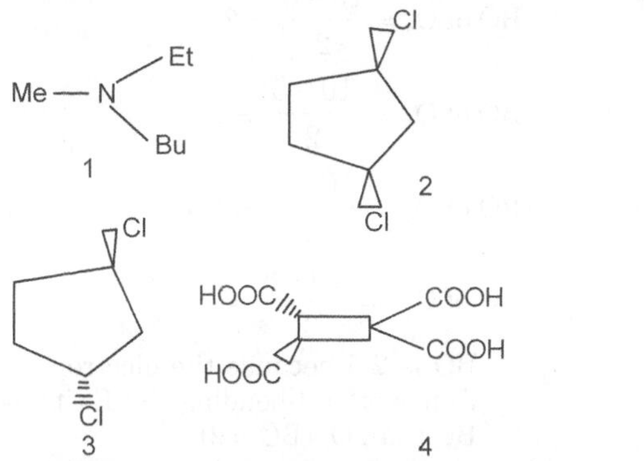

The compounds which can have enantiomers are:

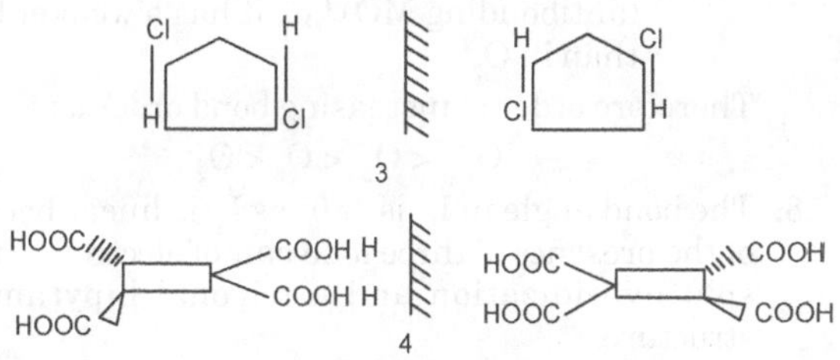

Restricted rotations occur in these two compounds, so they have enantiomers. While compound 1 and 2 cannot have enantiomers because there is no restricted rotation.

11. Given, rate constant (k) gets doubled when temperature is increased from 27 to 37°C i.e.

$$\frac{k_2}{k_1} = 2$$

$$T_1 = 27°C = 27 + 273 = 300\ K$$

$$T_2 = 37°C = 37 + 273 = 310\ K$$

We know,

$$\text{Log}\ \frac{k_2}{k_1} = \frac{E_a}{2.303}\ R\left[\frac{1}{T_1} - \frac{1}{T_2}\right]$$

Putting values in above equation, we get

$$\text{Log}\ 2 = \frac{E_a}{2.303} * 8.314\left[\frac{1}{300} - \frac{1}{310}\right]$$

On solving, we get

$$E_a = 53598.5J = 53.6\ KJ$$

Therefore the activation energy (E_a) for this reaction is 53.6 KJ.

12. Given, the reaction:

$$Hg + Hg^{2+} \leftrightarrow Hg_2^{\ 2+}$$

$$E°_1 \text{ for } \frac{Hg}{Hg_2^{2+}} = -0.799V$$

Therefore, standard free energy change is:

$$\Delta G_1 = -nFE° \qquad \{\text{here } n = 1\}$$
$$= -1 * F * (-0.799)$$
$$= +0.799F$$

$$E°_2 \text{ for } \frac{Hg}{Hg_2^{2+}} = 0.855\ V$$

Therefore, standard free energy change is:

$$\Delta G_2 = -nFE° \qquad \{\text{here } n = 2\}$$
$$\Delta G_2 = -2 * F * (0.855) = -1.71F$$

Therefore, $\Delta G_3 = \Delta G_1 + \Delta G_2$
$= +0.799F - 1.71F = -0.911F$

Now, $\Delta G_4 = \Delta G_3 + \Delta G_1$
$= -0.911F + 0.799F = -0.112F$

Therefore, $\Delta G_4 = -nFE°$

So $E° = +0.112V$

So, $$E° = \frac{0.0591}{1} \log K$$

Therefore, $$\log K = \frac{E°}{0.0591} = \frac{0.112}{0.0591} = 1.895$$

$\Rightarrow$ K = 78.5 = 79.12 approx.

13. Given,

Freezing point of benzene (T_b) = 5.44°C

Freezing point of solution (T_s) = 4.44°C

Molal depression constant (K_f) for benzene = 5.1

Amount of A in 100g benzene = 2.092g

Therefore, depression in freezing point can be calculated as:

$$\Delta T_f = T_b - T_s = 5.44 - 4.44 = 1°C$$

We know,

$$\Delta T_f = K_f * m$$

where, m = molality = $w * \frac{1000}{M.W}$

So, $$1 = 5.1 * 2.092 * \frac{1000}{M.100}$$

Therefore, $$M = 5.1 * 2.092 * \frac{1000}{100} = 106.7$$

Therefore molecular weight of A is 106.7.

14. The ion conductance of the alkali metal cations follows the order of:

$Li^+ < Na^+ < K^+ < Rb^+$ because the size of these metal ions varies inversely with the ionic conductivity. More the size less will be the ionic conductivity of the alkali metal cation.

15. Given, CV = 1.5 R, Cp = 2.5

The reaction is:

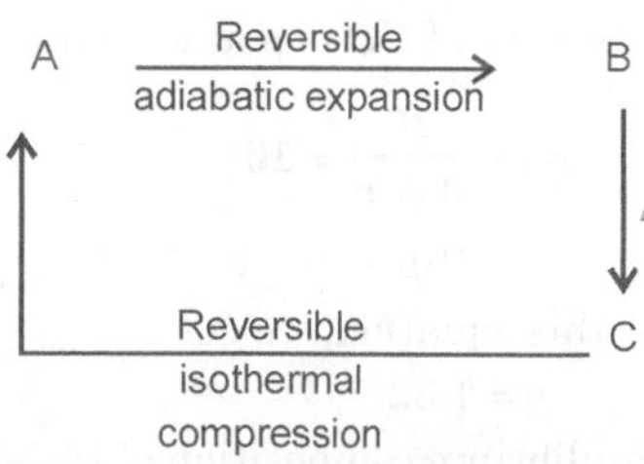

Also given, n = 2 and V = 5/3

Temperature (T) = 500 K, Pressure (P) = 5.0 atm.

As it is a reversible adiabatic reaction so, we have:

$$h_A^{1-r/r} \cdot T_A = h_B^{1-r/r} \cdot T_B$$

$$\Rightarrow \quad T_B = \left(\frac{h_A}{h_b}\right)^{\frac{1-r}{r}} \cdot T_A$$

Putting the values, we get

$$T_B = \left(\frac{5}{2}\right)^{\%} \cdot 500 = 346.57 \text{ K}$$

This adiabatic reversible reaction can be graphically represented as

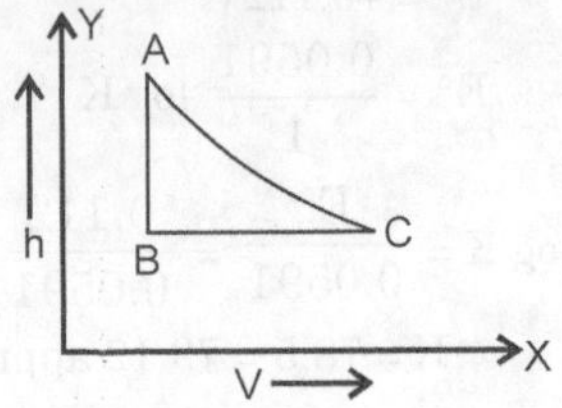

This adiabatic reversible reaction can be graphically represented as

∴ Work done can be calculated as:

$$W_{AB} = n\,Cv\,(T_B - T_A)$$
$$= 2 \times 1.5 \times 153.43 = -3826.85 \text{ J}$$
$$W_{BC} = h\Delta V \text{ or } nR\Delta T$$
$$= -2 \times 8.314 \times 153.43$$
$$= -2551.23 \text{ J}$$
$$W_{CA} = -n\,RT \ln hC/hA$$
$$= -2 \times 8.314 \times 500 \times \ln 2/5 = 7618 \text{ J}$$

So, total work done is

$$W_{total} = W_{AB} + W_{BC} + W_{CA}$$
$$= -3826.85 + (-2551.23) + 7618$$
$$= 1239.92 \text{ J}$$

16. The reaction given is:

$$CO_2\,(g) + C\,(s) \leftrightarrow 2CO\,(g)$$

Temperature = 82°C

K_p = 10 atm

Total pressure = 4.0 atm

We know,

$$K_p = \frac{p_{CO}^2}{p_{CO_2}}$$

Partial pressure of

$$CO_2 = 4 - p$$

{as partial pressure of CO is p at equilibrium}

Therefore, $$K_p = \frac{p^2}{4-p} = 10$$

Therefore, $$p^2 + 10p - 40 = 0$$

After solving this equation, we get

$$p = 1.32$$

Therefore equilibrium composition of

$$CO = \frac{1.32}{4} * 100$$
$$= 33\% \text{ by mol.}$$

17. Bond Order (BO) = ([number of electron in bonding MOs] – [number of electron in antibonding MOs])/2.

$$\text{BO of } O_2 = \frac{10-6}{2} = 2.$$

$$\text{BO of } O_2^+ = \frac{10-5}{2} = 2.5$$

$$\text{BO of } O_2^- = \frac{10-7}{2} = 1.5$$

$$\text{BO of } O_2^{2-} = \frac{10-8}{2} = 1$$

O_2^+ = BO is 2.5 because the electron is removed from a *pi** antibonding MO. So it has a higher BO than O_2 (BO = 2)

O_2^- = BO is 1.5 as extra electron enters a *pi** MO (antibonding MO) i.e., it has a weaker bond than in O_2.

Therefore order of increasing bond order is:

$$O_2^{2-} < O_2^- < O_2 < O_2^+.$$

18. The bond angle in I_3^- is 180° as I_3^- is linear because of the presence of three lone pair of electrons. It has sp^3d hybridization and a trigonal bipyramidal structure.

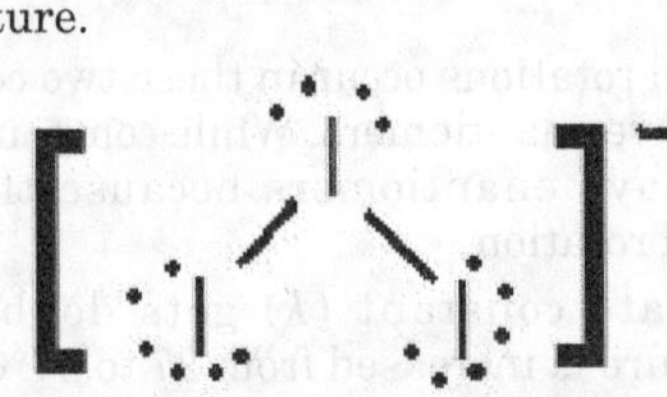

19. The number of ions present in the unit cell of cesium chloride (CsCl) is 2 as the ions present in the unit cell of Cl^- is 1 and of Cs^+ is 1, which gives 1 + 1= 2.

20. Co exists as Co^{2+} in $[CoF_6]^{4-}$

∴ electronic configuration of $[CoF_6]^{4-}$ can be written as :

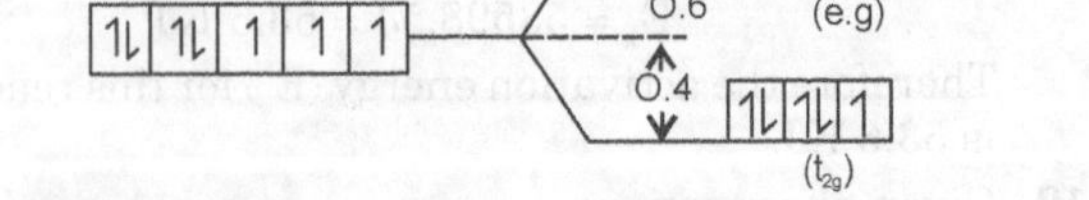

∴ 3 unpaired electrons are present in the 3d orbital as F^- is a weak field ligand, so it does not cause pairing.

In the crystal Field Theory the CFSE (Crystal Field Stabilization Energy) can be calculated as:

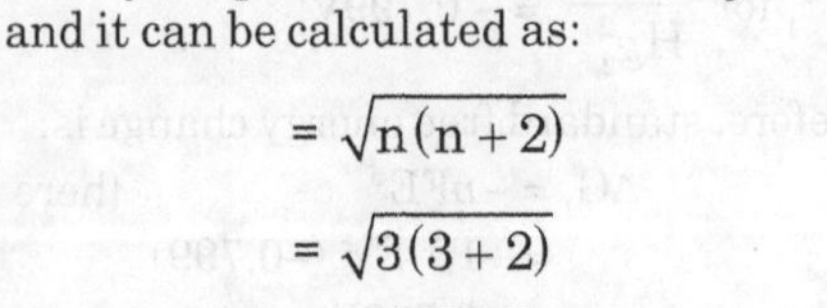

$$\therefore \quad \text{CFSE} = -0.4 \times 5 + 0.6 \times 2$$
$$= -0.8\,\Delta_0.$$

Spin only magnetic moment of $[CoF_6]^{4-}$ is given as ' ' and it can be calculated as:

$$= \sqrt{n(n+2)}$$
$$= \sqrt{3(3+2)}$$
$$= 3.87 \text{ B.M.}$$

21. The product formed after the reaction of H_3BO_3 with HF is BF_3. The reaction is:

$$H_3BO_3 + 3HF \rightarrow 2BF_3 + 3H_2O$$

This BF_3 gives a characteristic green color when it is introduced into a Bunsen burner.

22. Graphite sublimes at a very high temperature around 3700°C because of strong covalent interactions in the solid and weaker or fewer covalent interactions in the gas phase occur. As graphite in solid state so it has strong covalent interactions while in gaseous state has a weaker covalent interaction. A lot of energy is also required to sublime graphite at very high temperature.

23. The nickel (II) complex $[NiCl_2(PPh_3)_2]$ is paramagnetic – and Ni in this complex exists as Ni^{2+}. Only 1 isomer is possible for this complex as it has a tetrahedral geometry, so all 4 ligands are present adjacent to each other.

Also pairing does not occur because Cl^- and PPh_3 present in the complex are weak field ligands.

It can be represented as:

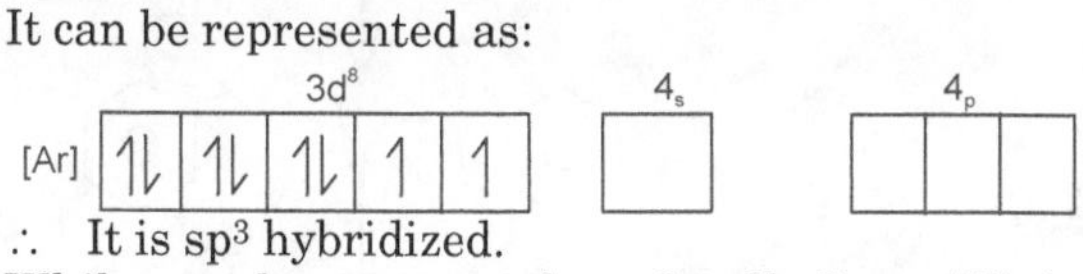

∴ It is sp³ hybridized.

While, analogous complex of palladium (II) is diamagnetic $[Pd\ Cl_2(PPh_3)_2]$. Here 2 isomers are possible for this complex as pairing does occur because size of Pd is large. Thus it has a square planar geometry.

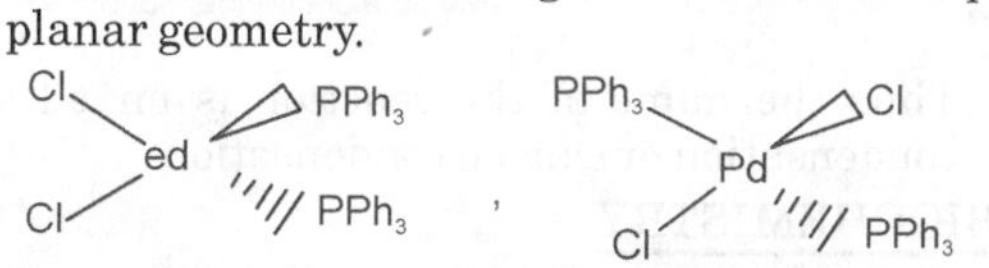

24. The order of the reactions should be SN1, SN2 and SN2

Reaction 1:

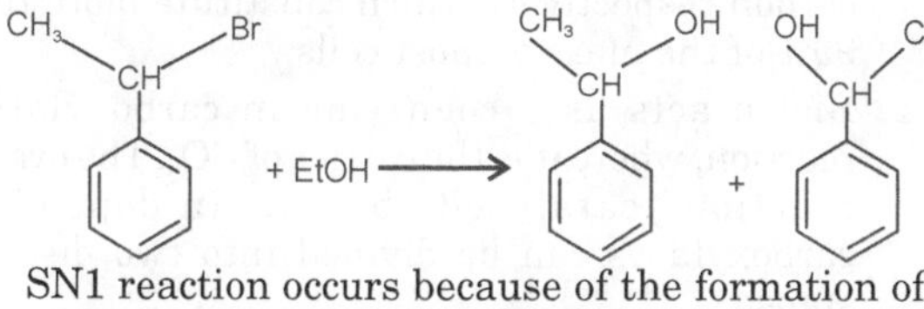

SN1 reaction occurs because of the formation of a stable carbocation. Also, EtOH is present in the reaction, which always undergoes SN1 reaction.

Reaction 2 :

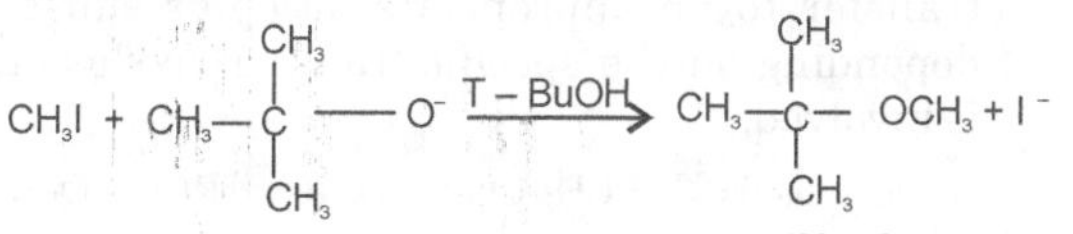

(3° – Carboction)

As 3°–carbocation is formed in this reaction so SN 2 reaction occurs. In reaction 3, an aprotic solvent is present, so SN2 reaction will occur.

25. When CH_3CH_2COOEt reacts with 2Ph MgBr and then with ether, in the prosence of H^+/H_2O, then the compound X formed is :

$$CH_3–CH_2–\underset{\displaystyle OH}{\underset{|}{C}}–Ph_2$$

Further, when this compound X is treated with conc. H_2SO_4 then the compound Y formed is:

$$CH_3 – CH = CPh_2$$

The entire reaction is given as:

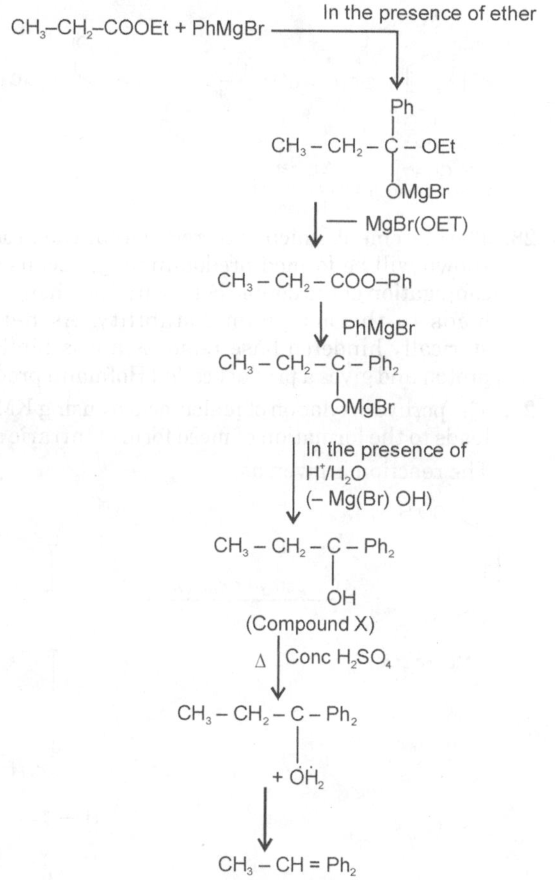

26. The first Diels-Alder cycloaddition reacion is:

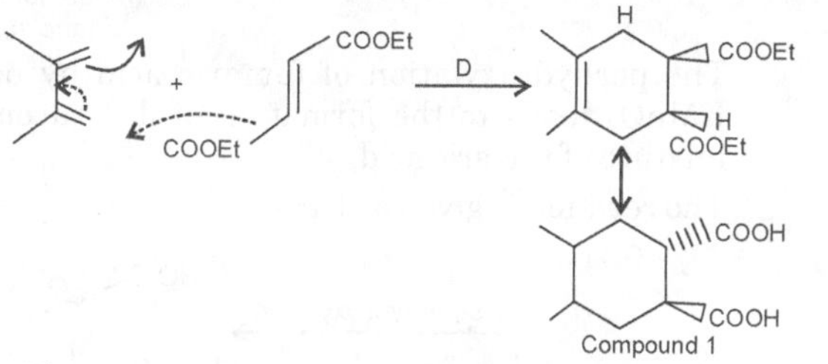

Compound 1

The second Diels-Alder cycloaddition is given as:

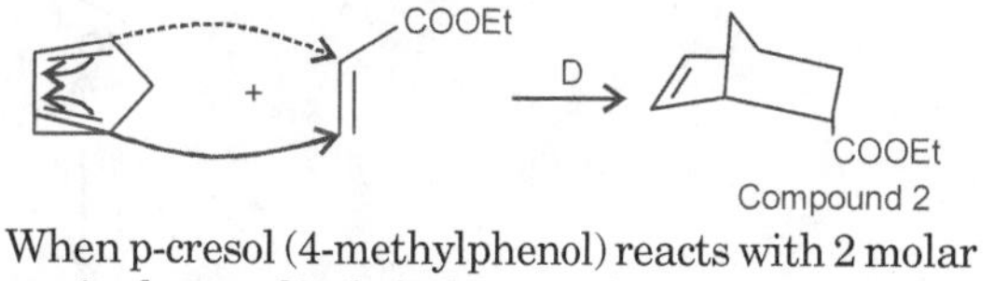

Compound 2

27. When p-cresol (4-methylphenol) reacts with 2 molar equivalents of isobritylene in the presence of HCl and $AlCl_3$ then it forms:

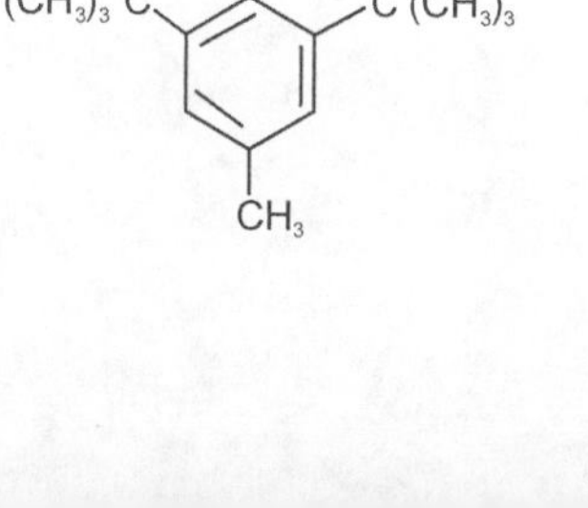

Here, OH is a strongly activating group and CH_3 is a weakly activating group. So OH decides the positioning of the 2 incoming groups.

The reaction is given as:

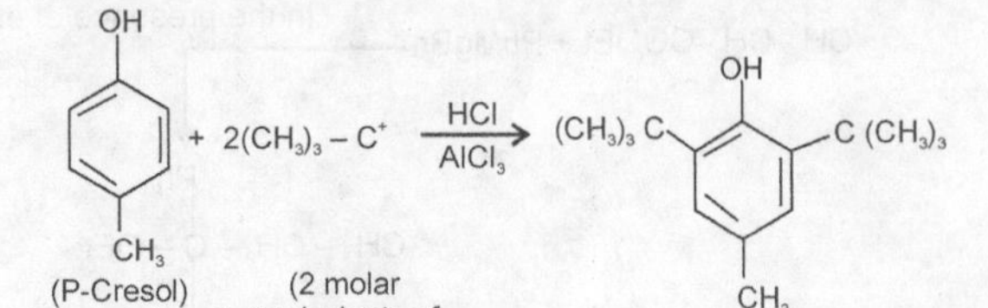

(P-Cresol) (4-methylphenol) (2 molar equivalents of isobitylene)

28. The statement which is correct is that the product shown will be formed predominantly, because the conjugation of the double bond with the phenyl ring leads to thermodynamic stability. As here, a sterically hindered base removes a less hindered proton and gives a product called Hofmann product.

29. The perhydroxylation of maleic acid by using $KMnO_4$ leads to the formation of meso form of tartaric acid.

The reaction is given as:

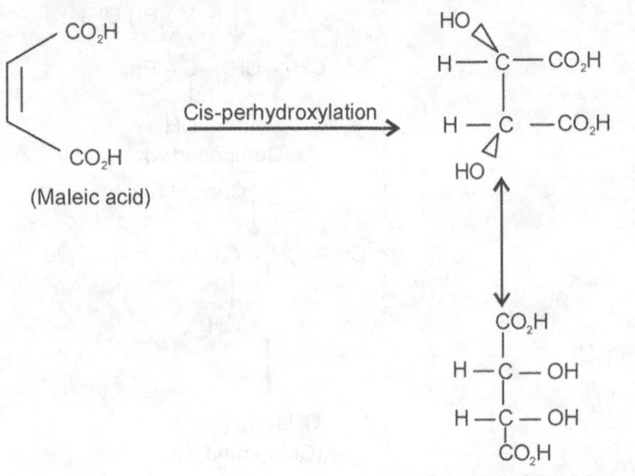

(Meso form of tartaric acid)

The perhydroxylation of fumaric acid by using $KMnO_4$ leads to the formation of d, l racemate mixture of tartaric acid.

The reaction is given as :

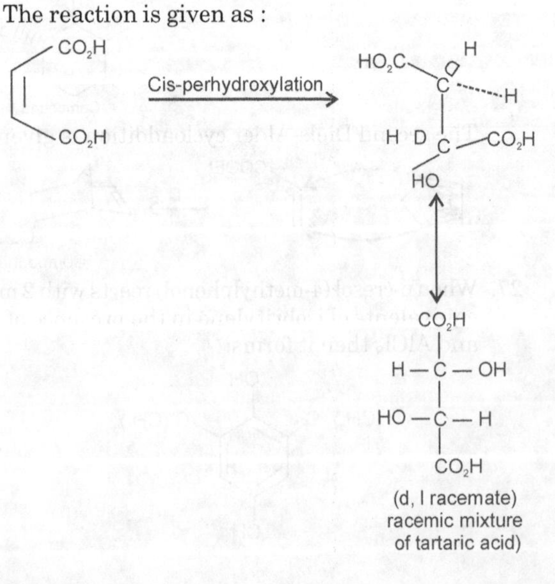

(d, l racemate) racemic mixture of tartaric acid)

30. The reaction is carried out as follows:

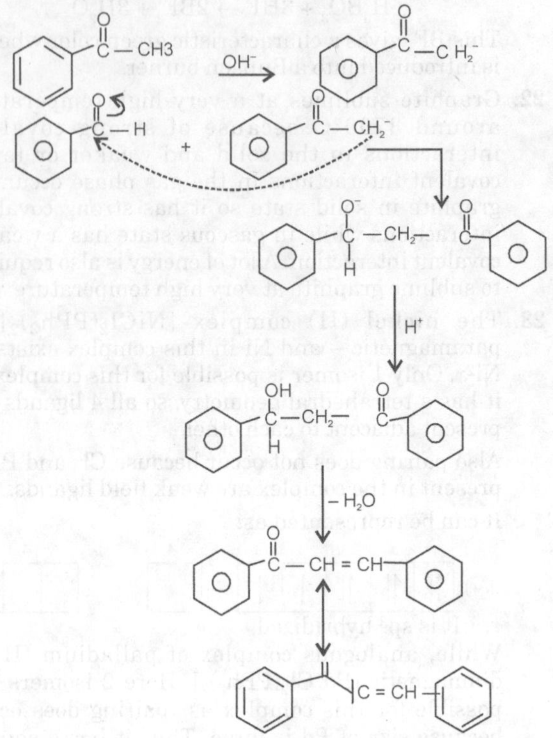

(Mixed aldol condensation)

Thus the name of the reaction is mixed aldol condensation or claisen condensation.

(I) BIOCHEMISTRY

1. The four most abundant elements in living organisms, in terms of percentage of total number of atoms are hydrogen, oxygen, nitrogen and carbon respectively which constitute more than 99% of the mass of most cells.
2. Biotin acts as a coenzyme in carboxylation reaction, where it is the carrier of CO_2. The overall reaction catalyzed by biotin-dependent carboxylases can be divided into two discrete steps.

   The first step involves the formation of carboxyl biotinyl enzyme; the second step involves carboxyl transfer to an appropriate acceptor substrate depending on the specific transcarboxylase that is involved.

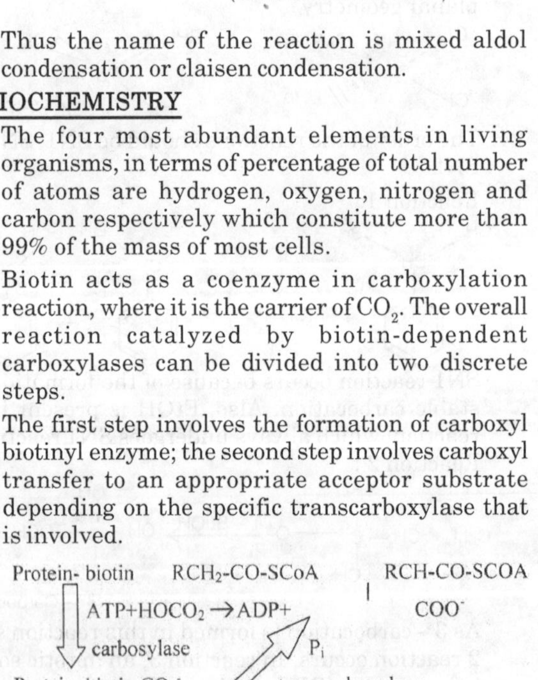

3. Angstrom (A^0) is not an SI unit; however it is used unnecessarily by structural biologist to describe atomic distances. The A^0 is named after the physicist Anders J. Angstrom.

4. Of the 64 triplet possible codons, 61 are employed for encoding amino acids while the 3 codons viz. UAA, UAG, UGA are called stop codon or chain termination codon. Termination occurs by a similar mechanism in eukaryotes as in prokaryotes. A single release factor with an associated GTP recognizes all 3 termination codons. When the release factor binds to the ribosome, termination is affected by the peptidyl transferase activity of the ribosome. GTP hydrolysis is required for termination and dissociation of ribosomal subunits.
5. Spectrin is an actin cross-linking molecular scaffold protein that leaks the plasma membrane to actin cytoskeleton, and functions in the determination of cell shape, arrangement of transmembrane protein and organization of organelles. It is responsible for increasing the plasma membrane elasticity and deformability of red blood cells.
6. Tetrodotoxin is a neurotoxin that is produced by the puffer fish and a number of other animals. Tetrodotoxin is quite specific in blocking the Na^+ ion channels and therefore the flow of Na^+ ions while having no effect on K^+ ions.
7. Cyanide (CN^-), hydrogen sulfide (H_2S), and CO are the inhibitors of electron transfer from Cytochrome C to O_2 by blocking cytoxidase and can therefore totally arrest respiration. Cycloheximide is a protein synthesis inhibitor. It blocks the elongation phase of eukaryotic translation. Rotenone and amytal block NADH dehydrogenase (complex I) in the respiratory chain, stopping the flow of electrons from NADH to CoQ. Therefore no ATP is formed from NADH, but two ATPs are formed from $FADH_2$.
8. IgG is the only antibody isotype that can cross the human placenta, thereby providing protection to the fetus in vitro. IgG is secreted as monomer that is small in size allowing it to easily perfuse tissues.
9. Methylation in the vicinity of promoter inhibits transcription and demethylation is required for gene expression. Critical regions for methylation in vertebrates usually occur in C_pG islands that are found in the 5' region i.e., in or near promoter region of gene. The 'p' in C_pG islands refers to the phosphodiester bond between the cytosine and guanine. CpG islands are detected by the presence of an increased density of the dinucleotide sequence i.e., C_pG [C_pG = 5'-CG-3'].
10. Apart from wide range of use, NaCl is used to preserve some foods (meat, fish, pickles etc.) by inhibiting the growth of microorganisms as it draws water [not protein] from the cells by the process of osmosis. Triton X-100 is non ionic polyoxyethylene surfactant that is most frequently used as component of cell lysis buffers or other solutions intended to extract and solubilized protein. Sodium dodecyl sulphate is a popular anionic detergent for routine protein electrophoresis [e.g. used in SDS PAGE] and cell lysis method. The full name of NP-40 is tergitol type NP-40 which is nonyl phenoxy polyethoxy ethanol. This detergent is used to obtain the cytoplasmic contents of a cellular cut here as it can break the cytoplasmic membrane but not the nuclear membrane.
11. For 1 molecule of glucose, 1 molecule of ATP is consumed to phosphorylate it to Glucose-6-phosphate in the presence of enzyme Hexokinase. The next reaction is reversible isomerisation of G6P to fructose Phosphate in the presence of enzyme phosphoglucoisom-erase. Here no ATP is consumed. In the next reaction, fructose 6 phosphate is phosphorylated to fructose 1, 6 biphosphate by consuming 1 ATP. The next reaction involves the cleavage of fructose 1, 6 biphosphate between C_3 and C_4 to form DHAP and glyceraldehyde 3 phosphate in presence of enzyme Aldolase. Here also no ATP is consumed.

Glucose ⟶ glucose 6 phosphate ⟷ fructose 6 phosphate

ATP→ADP phosphoglucoisomerase ↓ ATP→ADP

phosphofructokinase

DHAP+ glyceraldehydes-3-PO_4 ⟷ Fructose 1,6biphosphate

aldolase

12. Since there are three different antibodies, diffusion rate will be different for each antibody. Also there are three different proteins (antigen), therefore diffusion rate for these three protein will be different. So there will be 3 precipitin bands.
13. One of the best understood of the ribozyme is L19 RNA from the protozoan, *Tetrahymene*. L-19 RNA is involved in the processing of rRNA. L-19 is not only able to cleave itself but is also able to lengthen and shorten the size of the oligoribonucleotide such as pentacytidylate (C_5) in rRNA.

14. The difference between double and single stranded DNA is attributed to difference in linear charge density, chain flexibility and hydrophobicity. DNA absorbs strongly at 260nm and as the DNA melts absorbance will increase until all of the DNA is melted and then remains constant on further heating. This is called hypochromic effect and the absorbance of single stranded DNA is usually 50% greater than that of corresponding duplex DNA. Since the density of double stranded DNA is more than single stranded DNA, it can be distinguished by density gradient ultracentrifugation. Double stranded DNA have trouble squeezing through the gel matrix and are hence retarded while strand migrate easier, hence by gel electrophoresis single stranded DNA and double stranded DNA can be distinguished.

15. Telomerase is a ribonucleoprotein enzyme that catalyzes the cellular synthesis of telomeric DNA during cellular division, resulting in maintenance of telomere length and increased proliferated potential. Several studies suggest that the telomerase may play an important role in the diagnosis and prognosis of cancer because its expression strongly correlates with the potential tumor progression.

16. Since molecular weight of Ig is approximately 150kd, therefore molecular weight of antigen = molecular weight of IgG Ag complex-molecular weight of IgG = 300 – 150 = 150kd.

17. The net reaction of the citric acid cycle is :

$$\text{Acetyl CoA} + 3NAD^+ + FAD + GDP + P_i + 2H_2O \rightarrow 2CO_2 + 3NADH + FADH_2 + GTP + 2H^+ + CoA$$

- Two carbon atoms enter the cycle as acetyl CoA and leaves in the form of CO_2.
- Four pairs of electrons are removed from the substrate, three pairs leave in the form of NADH and one pair leave as $FADH_2$.
- One high energy phosphate is generated in the form of guanosine triphosphate (GTP).

18. Variation observed among the heavy chains of different classes and subclasses of immunoglobulins are known as isotypic variation. The genes for the isotypic variations are present in all the healthy member of a species. For e.g. genes for $\gamma 1$, $\gamma 2$, $\gamma 3$, , $\alpha 1$, $\alpha 2$, δ, ε, W, λ chains are all present in human genome and are therefore isotypes.

Variations in the variable domain, particularly in hyper-variable regions, produce idiotypes, or in other words each individual antigen determinants of the variable region are called idiotype. Haplotype is a combination of alleles at adjacent loci on the chromosome that are transmitted together.

19. Reducing agent (e.g. β mercaptoethanol) used in SDS PAGE reduces the disulphide bond between light and heavy chain of each IgM monomer and disulphide bridges between two IgM and IgM pentamer. This finally yield light chain fragment (Fc) and heavy chain fragment (FaB), as a result these two separate band will be seen on gel.

20. The ras oncogene encodes a protein with normal GTP binding but no GTPase activity. The mutant ras protein is therefore always in its activated (GTP-bound) form, regardless of the signal arriving through normal receptors.

21. Adenosine deaminase deficiency is associated with a severe combined immunodeficiency disease in which both thymus-derived lymphocytes (T cells) and bone marrow derived lymphocytes (B cells) are sparse and dysfunctional. **Tay- Sachs** disease is due to a deficiency of lysosomal hexosaminidase A, which hydrolyses the terminal N- acetyl galactosaminase of GM_2 gangliosides. Its absence leads to the accumulation of the gangliosides in brain tissues. **Lesh Nyhan** syndrome is a hereditary X linked recessive condition that is due to severe or complete deficiency of HGPRT activity. As a result, hypoxanthine and guanine are not salvaged. Also the intracellular levels of PRPD increases, while those of IMP and GMP decreases. This leads to increase de novo synthesis of purines. **Cystis fibrosis** which arises due to a single amino acid deletion in the adenosine triphosphate (ATP) binding domain of a transmembrane conductance regulatory protein that is ATP dependent.

22. β ketoacyl synthase is an enzyme involved in fatty acid synthesis. It catalyses the condensation of malony-ACP with the growing fatty acid chain. β ketoacyl ACP reductase is also an enzyme of fatty acid synthesis. It reduces the β keto group of acetoacetyl ACP to β hydroxyl group forming β hydroxylbutyryl ACP. Enoyl ACP reductase is also an enzyme of fatty acid synthesis. This reduces the double bond of Crotonyl ACP to form butyryl ACP, using NADPH. ACP is a protein that is associated with the fatty acid synthesis system of many organisms from bacteria to plants. They contain one 4'-phosphopantetheine prosthetic group bound covalently by a phosphate ester bond to the hydroxyl group of a serine residue. The sulfahydryl group of the 4'-phosphapantetheine moiety serves as an anchor to which acyl intermediates are (thio) esterified during fatty acid synthesis.

23. The DNA molecules that are labelled with γ ^{32}P-ATP will be easily detected under autoradiogram. But, free molecules of γ ^{32}P-ATP which remained unbound will also be present in the solution. These molecules are required to be removed from the solution using phosphatases which digest labelled ^{32}P-ATP. The DNA molecules can be blotted on nitrocellulose membrane and electrophoresed and the labelled DNA molecules can be extracted and separated from the non-labelled DNA molecules.

24. The most widely used eluting buffer for affinity purification of protein is 0.1M glycine HCl, pH-2.5-3.0. This buffer effectively dissociates most protein -protein and antibody-antigen binding interactions without permanently affecting protein structure. Nevertheless, some antibodies and proteins are damaged by low pH, so eluted fractions are best neutralized immediately after recovered by addition of one tenth volume of alkaline buffer such as 1 M Tris HCl, pH 8.5 to minimize the duration of time in the low pH conditions.

25. Most protein synthesized in endoplasmic reticulum is glycosylated. Much glycosylation, N linked and O linked occurs after protein leaves the ER and enters the golgi apparatus. However, N- linked glycosylation begins in the ER as the proteins are being synthesized. In these oligosaccharides units are attached by N glycosidic bonds to asparagines residues within the sequence Asn-X-Ser or Asn-X-Thr where X can be any amino acid other than proline.

26. The Alu domain of SRP binds the elongation factor binding site of ribosome. All the contact sites used by SRP Alu domain are also used by eEF2, therefore binding of the Alu domain directly competes with elongated factor entering their binding site of ribosomes.

27. Each photo system II contains at least 99 cofactors: 35 chlorophyll, 12 β-carotene, 2 pheophytin, 2 plastoquinone, 2 heme, bicarbonate, 20 lipids, the Mn_4CaO_5 clusters (including Cl^- ion) and 1 non haem Fe^{2+} and 2 putative Ca^{2+} ions per monomer.

28. Diacyl glycerol cooperates with Ca^{2+} in activating PKC. Activation involves the movement of a PKC domain (the pseudo substrate domain) away from its location in the substrate binding region of the enzyme, allowing the enzyme to bind and phosphorylate protein that contain a PKC CONSENSUS SEQUENCE-Ser or Thr residues embedded in an amino acid sequence recognized by PKC.

29. General property of enhancer elements are as follows :
   - Their activity is independent of their orientation relative to the gene.
   - They are functional either upstream or downstream and even at great distances (up to 50kb) from the initiation site.
   - They are cis acting (i.e., they must be linked to the gene)
   - Even though they are called enhancer, some have been found to lead to a repression of transcription.

30. Oxytocin is a peptide of 9 amino acids. Vasopressin is also a peptide consisting of nine amino acids. Somatostatin has 2 active forms produced by alternative cleavage of a single pre pro-protein: one of 14 amino acids, the other of 28 amino acids.

(K) BOTANY

1. Oleosomes are structures found naturally in oil bearing plant seeds and serve as natural storehouses of energy used by the seed until germination. They are found in virtually all crops, including almond and sunflower. Oleosomes are naturally occurring spheres 1-5 feet in diameters which consist of a centre core of emollient plant oils and vitamin E surrounded by a phospholipid membrane and stabilised by protein coat.

2. Number of cells produced from single parent cell = 2n

   Where, n = number of division

   $$512 = 2^n$$
   $$2^9 = 2^n$$
   $$n = 9$$

3. Cork cell consist of a tight web of up to 40 million cells per cubic cm. The cell membrane are filled with an air like gas giving cork its unique capacity to float, insulate and re expand quickly after compression. It is characterized by deposition of suberin which make it impervious to water.

4. Gynostegium condition is a typical feature of membrane of the milkweed family (Asclepiadacae). Gynostegium is formed by the fusion of stamens with stigma.

5. A viability assay is an assay to determine the ability of cells or tissues to maintain or recover its viability. Common viability assays are ATP test, Evans blue, FDA/PI staining, flow cytometry, green fluorescent protein, methyl violet, trypan blue etc.

6. The formation of an embryo in some position other than within an embryo sac. It is a form of apomixes. Adventive embryo may develop from somatic cells of the nucellar chalaza (aposory) and may occur together with a zygotic embryo.

7. Phytoremediation describes the treatment of environmental problems through the use of plants that mitigate the environmental problem without the need to excavate the contaminant material and dispose of it elsewhere.

8. $HSO_2CH_2C\text{-}CH_2\text{-}CO\text{-}S\text{-}CoA + GDP + H_3PO_4 \leftrightarrow HO_2CH_2C\text{-}CH_2CO_2H + GTP + CoASH$

   Succinyl CoA $\rightarrow$ Succinic Acid

   The above reaction of Krebs cycle involves the formation of a new high energy phosphate structure and utilization of a thioester, the total number of high energy structures on each side of the reaction is equal. The GTP formed reacts with ADP to form ATP and GDP in a reaction catalyzed by a nucleoside diphosphokinase located in the mitochondrial intermembrane space.

9. All nitrogenase have an iron and sulphur containing cofactor that includes a heterometal complex in the active site (eg. FeMoCo). In most of the heterometal complex has a central molybdenum atom, though in some species it is replaced by vanadium or iron atom.

10. The plant pathogen Agrobacterium rhizogenes has a large Ri plasmid and induces hairy root disease, causing root proliferation from the infected site.

11. B/C = 1×10^1 A°/ 5 A° = 2 A°

    A/B = 1 m/1nm = 10^4 A°/10 A° = 10^3 A°

    A/B × B/C = 2×10^3 = 2000

12. Actin is an abundant protein found in all eukaryotic cell. Actin polymerizes to form actin filaments, then flexible fibres approx 8nm in diameter and upto several micrometers in length.

    Microtubules are long, hollow cylinder made up of polymerized α and β tubulin dimmers.

    Intermediate filaments have average diameter of 10 nm, which is between that of 8nm actin and 25 nm microtubules.

13. Mis-sense mutation is a point mutation in which single nucleotide is changed, resulting in a codon that codes for different amino acids. A frameshift mutation is a genetic mutation caused by insertion or deletion of a number of nucleotide that is not evenly divisible by three from a DNA sequence.

Same sense mutation, also called silent mutation are DNA mutation that do not result in a change to the amino acid sequence of a protein or that do result in amino acid change but do not results in gradually different property of the changed amino acid hence do not alter the protein function.

Non sense mutation occurs when a premature non sense or stop codon is introduced in the DNA sequence that results in a shorter, unfinished protein product.

14. Map distance = percentage of crossing over

Now, percentage of crossing over

$$= \frac{\text{number of cross over}}{\text{total progeny}} \times 100$$

$$= \frac{28}{132} \times 100 = 21.2$$

15. 1 : 8

16. Puccinia graminis causes black or cereal rust and attacks the part of the plant which are above ground. Stem rust of wheat most frequently affect the leaf sheath but also affect stems, leaves, and glumes.

Covered smut of barley is caused by *ustiligo hordei*. Kernels of infected plants are replaced by masses of dark brown smut spores.

Tricothecium is a filamentous microsporic fungus widely distributed on decaying vegetation and in the soil.

Ustilago *nuda* causes loose smut of barley. The grain heads of barley is replaced by masses of spores called loose smut.

17. A floral formula is a way to represent the structure of flowers using specific letters, numbers and symbols. A floral formula consist of 5 symbols indicatind from left to right-Floral symmetry, number of sepals, number of petals, number of stamens and number of carpels.

18. Glucose enter into the glycolytic pathway by phosphorylation to glucose 6 phosphate accomplished by enzyme 'hexokinase'.

Fructokinase specifically transfers a phosphate group forming fructose 6 phosphate .sucrose 6 phosphate + H_2O

$\rightarrow$ sucrose + phosphate.

Phosphoglucomutase transfer the phosphate group on an α-D glucose monomer from the 1 to 6th position in the forward direction or the 6th to the 1st position in the reverse direction.

19.

Edible fungi	Morchella conica
Deadly poisonous fungi	Amanita verna
Alkaloid producing fungi	Claviceps purpurea
Fungi pathogenic to human	Candida albicans

20. Tn3 transposon is a 4957 base pair mobile genetic element, found in prokaryotes. During its replication in the first step it fuses with the host plasmid and transposon and a short sequence of host DNA are replicated, giving then product 'Cointegrate plasmid' containing two copies of transposon.

LTR(long term repeats) are sequences of DNA that repeats hundred or thousand times. Ty elements are LTR retrotransposon that replicate through an RNA intermediate.

AP element is a transposon that is present specifically in the fruit fly *drosophila melanogaster* and is widely used for mutagenesis and the creation of genetically modified flies for genetic research. The P element give rise to a phenotype called hybrid dysgenesis.

Ac/Ds are transposable genetic element in corn discovered by Barabara Mcclintok.

21. Photochemical smog is unique type of air pollution in which the primary pollutants such as SO_2, CO_2, CO and other volatile organic compounds interact in presence of sunlight to form secondary pollutants, like ozone and additional hydrocarbon. Phytochelatins are found in plants, fungi, nematodes and all group of algae including cyanobacteria and they act as chelators and are important for heavy metals detoxifications.

22.

PIGMENTS	ABSORPTION MAXIMA(nm)
Chlorophyll-a	680
c-phycoethryin	550
c-phycocyanin	615
Bacteriochlorophyll-b	1020

23. Naturally methanol is obtained from cornmint, peppermint or other mint oils. Important terpenoids derieved from monocyclic terpenes are methanol, thymol, carvairol etc. Ajmalicine is indole alkaloid used as hypertensive drugs. Caffeine, theobromine and thiophyline are the main purine alkaloids in plant foods. Structurally carotenes are tetraterpene i.e they are synthesised biochemically from four 10 carbon terpene units which in turn formed from eight 5 carbon isoprene unit.

24. In monocot stem there are numerous vascular bundle scattered in ground tissue while in dicot stem vascular bundle are arranged in a ring. The root of vascular plant (i.e monocot + dicot) are normally considered to have exarch development i.e xylem develops from outside inwards towards centre i.e centripetally. Monocot are usually polyarch.

25.

TRANSGENIC PLANTS	RELEVANT GENES
Glyphosate resistance	areo A
Insect resistance (Bollgard)	cry 1 Ac
Delayed repening	pg (antisense)
Insect resistance (Yeild gard)	Cry i AB

27. Generally we use DMSO, Glycerol and proline all together for preservation at around – 80 °C.

28. DCMU (3 - (3, 4 - dichlorophenyl) - 1, 1 - dimethyl urea) is a very specific herbicide that blocks plastoquinone binding site of

photosystem II. It only blocks electron flow from photosystem II. It replaces Q_B on P_{680} is polypeptide chain.

BDMIB (2,5 – dibromo – 3-methyl – 6 – isopropyl – p – benzoquinone) makes complex with cytochromes at a stochiometry of 2 or 3 per cytochrome molecule.

29. *BamHI* (from Bacillus amyloli) is a type II restriction endonuclease, having the capacity for recognizing short sequences (6 b.p.) of DNA and specifically cleaving them at a target site. This exhibit focuses on the structure-function relations of BamHI . BamHI binds at the recognition sequence 5′ - GGATCC-3. ′ , and cleaves these sequences just after the 5′ -guanine on each strand.

(L) MICROBIOLOGY

1. Carbolic acid, now called phenol, was already known as a deodorizing agent and preservative, and Lister thought it might kill the germs that were causing infections. In 1865 Lister began using carbolic acid as an antiseptic during surgery and in bandaging afterward, publishing his results in 1867.
2. Koch applied host-pathogen relationship criteria to show that anthrax, a common disease of cattle, was caused by the bacterium *Bacillus anthracis*. His postulates provided a framework for proving the role of microbes in disease.
3. A primary stain (malachite green) is used to stain the endospores. Spores are resistant to heat, UV radiation and chemicals because they are comprised of a tough proteinaceous covering called keratin. Because endospores have a keratin covering and resist staining, the malachite green will be forced into the endospores by heating.
4. This process is called as Phagocytosis and Elie Metchnikoff are discoverer of it.
5. Isocitrate lyase that converts isocitrate in to main component of cycle that is glyoxylate and form glyoxylate formation of malate by help of malate synthase enzyme occurs.
6. Some species of Nitrosomonas like N.europaea utilize urea as an ammonia source. Metabolism is aerobic, NH_4^{4+} is the electron donor and O_2 is the electron acceptor.
7. Gram-negative organisms have 4 rings: L ring associates with the lipopolysaccharides, P ring associates with peptidoglycan layer, M ring is imbedded in the cell membrane, and the S ring is directly attached to the cell membrane.
8. Control precise level of oxygen (low and constant). Leghemoglobin-bound O_2. : free O_2. = 10,000 : 1.
9. In pyrococci and, probably, in several other archaea, the main glycolytic flow goes through a different enzyme, glyceraldehyde-3-phosphate : ferredoxin oxidoreductase, whereas glyceraldehyde-3-phosphate dehydrogenase appears to be confined to gluconeogenesis.
10. In cell biology and genetics, a regulon is a collection of genes or operons under regulation by the same regulatory protein. This term is generally used for prokaryotic systems, for example quorum sensing in bacteria. It is a group of operons/genes spread around the chromosome but controlled by a common factor or stimulus. Multiple regulons can form a modulon.
11. Isocitrate $\longrightarrow$ alpha-Ketoglutarate + CO_2. Here enzyme is Isocitrate dehydrogenase (EC 1.1.1.42) and (EC 1.1.1.41), also known as IDH, is an enzyme that participates in the citric acid cycle. It catalyzes the third step of the cycle: the oxidative decarboxylation of isocitrate, producing alpha-ketoglutarate (α-ketoglutarate) and CO_2.

alpha-Ketoglutarate

$\rightarrow$ Succinyl- CoA

$\rightarrow$ Succinate + CO_2

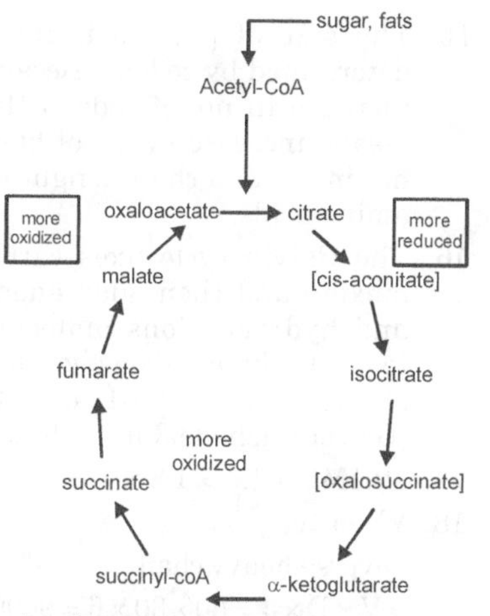

12. In the majority of the cases the gratuitous inducers IPTG or TMG (thiomethyl β-D-galactoside) are used. Lactose is less but natural inducer of lac operon.

IPTG is an effective inducer because of the following reasons:

1. One advantage of IPTG for in vivo studies is that it cannot be metabolized by E. coli, therefore the growth rate of cells (usually maintained with glycerol as the carbon and energy source), is not a variable in the experiment.
2. IPTG is not dependent on permease to enter the cell and is not cleaved by ßgalactosidase. So it is transported efficiently independent of whether the lacY gene is functional. And since cells don't metabolize IPTG, its concentration doesn't change during the course of an experiment.

13. We have,

Total volume

$= 1/25\ mm^2 \times 1/50\ mm$

$= 0.08 \times 10^{-4} mm^3$

$= 8 \times 10^{-7}$ ml

Thus, number of bacteria/ml of suspension

$= 20/8 \times 10^{-7} = 25 \times 10^6$

14. The structure of β- ketoadipate is:

HOOC-CH_2-CH_2-$COCH_2$-COOH

It can also be represented as:

15. The size of protein is never determined by codons. Because increase in no. of codons that means increase in no. of bases not in no. and chain lenghth of amino acids.

16. The Calvin cycle fixes carbon dioxide and then adds energy and hydrogen ions molecules to yield a three carbon phosphate sugar called PGAL or G3P (Glyceraldehyde-3-phosphate).

17. 12.1Mb > 4.6 > 1.8 > 1.77

18. We have,

Diverse heavy chain

$= V \times D \times J = 50 \times 30 \times 6 = 9000$

Diverse light chain $= 40 \times 5 = 200$

Thus, different IgG molecules

$= 200 \times 900 = 18{,}00{,}000$

19. A strain of *Mycobacterium tuberculosis* was found to be resistant to INH, streptomycin and rifampicin at 10^{-5}, 10^{-6}, 10^{-7} frequencies. The frequency of appearance of a strain resistance to all three compounds is 10^{-18} as a cell which has become resistant to one antibiotic is still likely to be inhibited by the other. Thus, $10^{-5} + 10^{-6} + 10^{-7} = 10^{-18}$.

20. In *Escherichia Coli* the number of molecules per cell occurs in the order as follows:

tRNA< mRNA< rRNA< DNA, as *E. coli* has the largest molecules of DNA followed by rRNA, mRNA and tRNA. *E. coli* has one DNA molecule with about 3,000 genes.

21. Immunoglobulin class switching (or **isotype switching** or **isotypic commutation** or **class switch recombination** (CSR)) is a biological mechanism that changes a B cell's production of antibody from one class to another, for example, from an isotype called IgM to an isotype called IgG. Naïve mature B cells produce both IgM and IgD, which are the first two heavy chain segments in the immunoglobulin locus. After activation by antigen, these B cells proliferate. If these activated B cells encounter specific signaling molecules via their CD40 and cytokine receptors (both modulated by T helper cells), they undergo antibody class switching to produce **IgG, IgA or IgE** antibodies and not production of IgD.

22. Eosin methylene blue agar (EMB) is a selective and differential medium used to isolate fecal coliforms. When E.coli grow on medium it produce green metallic sheencolnies due to Eosin Y and methylene blue dyes which combine to form a dark purple precipitate at low pH; they also serve to inhibit the growth of most Gram positive organisms.

23. Cysteine and methionine are the two sulfur containing amino acids which absorb ultraviolet light with an absorbance maximum in the range of 280nm.

24. The reaction catalyzed by bacterial luciferase is also an oxidative process:

$$FMNH_2 + O_2 + RCHO \rightarrow FMN + RCOOH + H_2O + light$$

22. Given,

Speed of flagellate *Monas stigmatica*

= 50 cell lengths/sec

Time = 1 hour

Thus, 50 cell lengths

$= 50 \times 6\ m = 300\ m$

This is distance covered in 1 sec.

Thus distance covered in 1 hour

$= 60 \times 60 \times 300$

$= 10{,}80{,}000\ m = 1.08m$

26. *Salmonella* bacteria are classified into groups according to the Kauffman- White classification scheme. The identification of serotypes is based on:

- "O" (somatic/ cell wall) antigens : The O antigens consist of the lipopolysaccharide-protein chains exposed on the cell surface.
- "H" (flagellar) antigens

27. Archea does not have D and L aminoacids in their short peptides chain. The bacterial cell wall is a unique biopolymer in that it contains both D- and L-amino acids.

28. Nicked diphtheria toxin was used in all experiments and it is more active than un-nicked toxin. Highly purified un-nicked DT does not inhibit protein synthesis, while nicked toxin is effective.

29. Bromodeoxyuridine (5-bromo-2'-deoxyuridine, BrdU, BUdR, BrdUrd) is a synthetic nucleoside that is an analogue of thymidine. BrdU is commonly used in the detection of proliferating cells in living tissues. BrdU can be incorporated into the newly synthesized DNA of replicating cells (during the S phase of the cell cycle), substituting for thymidine during DNA replication. Mutagenesis by 5-bromodeoxyuridine (BrdUrd) can result from base-pairing errors. Replication errors give rise predominantly to AT-to-GC transitions.

30. Given,

Initial cell population (N_0)

$= 10^3$ cells/ml

Time interval, t

= 6hrs 40min or 6.67hrs

Number of generations (n) = 20

Therefore, Generation time (G)

$= t/n = 6.67/20 = 0.33$

By the formula, we know,

$G = t/[3.3(\log_{10}N_t - \log_{10}N_0)]$

$0.33 = 6.67/[3.3(\log N_t - \log 10^{-3})]$

Thus, after solving, we get,

Final cell population (N_t) $= 10^9$

As we know,

Growth constant (K)

= 1/Generation time (G)

Thus, K = 1/0.33 = 3 (approx.)

(M) ZOOLOGY

1. Bat wings and bird wings are analogous as flight structures. Their structure and function have evolved by different routes from a flightless reptilian ancestor. Note for example that a good portion of the flight surface in bats consists of a membrane stretched between the extended digits (chiropatagium), whereas the digits of the bird are relatively small and do not support the flight surface. The bird and bat wings are analogous as wings, but homologous as forelimbs because the organ served as a forearm (not a wing) in the last common ancestor of tetrapods.

2. Holometabolous insects involve the process of holometabolism (undergoing complete metamorphosis) which includes four life stages - as an embryo or egg, a larva, a pupa and an imago or adult. The developmental stage from pupa to an adult is governed by various hormones such as brain hormone, ecdysone hormone and juvenile hormone. Mosquitoes are holometabolous insects and therefore grow through an egg, larva, and pupa to adult stage. The larvae and pupae are aquatic, the adults are free flying.

3. Heterochromatin is that state of chromatin in which it is dark-staining, genetically inactive, and tightly coiled. It is the part of a chromosome that is inactive in gene expression but may function in controlling metabolic activities, transcription, and cell division. It stains most intensely during interphase and usually remains in a condensed state throughout the cell cycle. It consists of two types: constitutive heterochromatin, which is present in all cells and is characteristic of the Y chromosome, and facultative heterochromatin, which is present in the inactivated X chromosome of the mammalian female. Constitutive heterochromatin is the chromatin in which the regions of the chromosomes are invariably heterochromatic. It contains highly repetitive sequences of DNA that are genetically inactive and serves as a structural element of the chromosome. Facultative heterochro-matin is the chromatin in which the regions of the chromosomes become heterochromatic in certain cells and tissues. Heterochromatin does not contain regions of conserved DNA sequences.

4. Cardiac sphincter is the valve between the distal end of the oesophagus and the stomach. It is the physiological sphincter at the oesophagus-gastric junction. This sphincter prevents the acidic contents of the stomach from moving upward into the oesophagus. During peristalsis, the cardiac sphincter allows the food bolus to pass into the stomach. It prevents chyme, a mixture of bolus, stomach acid, and digestive enzymes, from returning up the oesophagus. The cardiac sphincter is aided in the task of keeping the flow of materials in one direction by the diaphragm.

5. A stroke, or cerebrovascular accident (CVA), is the rapid loss of brain function due to disturbance in the blood supply to the brain. Blood flow can be compromised by blockage of an artery and rupture of an artery (haemorrhage). If blood flow is stopped for longer than a few seconds, the brain cannot get blood and oxygen. Brain cells can die, causing permanent damage. There are two major types of stroke: ischemic stroke and hemorrhagic stroke. Ischemic strokes may be caused by clogged arteries. Fat, cholesterol, and other substances collect on the artery walls, forming a sticky substance called plaque. A hemorrhagic stroke occurs when a blood vessel in part of the brain becomes weak and bursts open, causing blood to leak into the brain. High blood pressure is the number one risk factor for strokes.

6. A majority of macrophages are stationed at strategic points where microbial invasion or accumulation of dust is likely to occur. It is a large, mobile, highly phagocytic cell derived from monocytes. Each type of macrophage, determined by its location, has a specific name such as Histiocytes (connective tissue), Kupffer cells (liver), Osteoclasts (bone) etc. When a monocyte enters damaged tissue through the endothelium of a blood vessel, a process known as the leukocyte extravasation, it undergoes a series of changes to become a macrophage.

7. Human immunodeficiency virus (HIV) is a lentivirus (a member of the retrovirus family) that causes acquired immunodeficiency syndrome(AIDS), a condition in humans in which progressive failure of the immune system allows life-threatening opportunistic infections and cancers to thrive. HIV infects vital cells in the human immune system such as helper T cells (specifically $CD4^+$ T cells), macrophages, and dendritic cells. HIV infection leads to low levels of $CD4^+$ T cells through three main mechanisms: First, direct viral killing of infected cells; second, increased rates of apoptosis in infected cells; and third, killing of infected $CD4^+$ T cells by CD8 cytotoxic lymphocytes that recognize infected cells. When $CD4^+$ T cell numbers decline below a critical level, cell-mediated immunity is lost, and the body becomes progressively more susceptible to opportunistic infections.

8. *Trichinella spiralis* is the causative agent of trichinnellosis in humans as well as several animals can be infected. It is a nematode parasite. It is sometimes referred to as the "pork worm" due to it being found commonly in undercooked pork products. *Trichinella spiralis* is a parasitic nematode that has a direct life cycle, meaning it completes all stages of development in one host. The larval forms are encapsulated as a small cystic structure within the infected host. Humans typically become infected when they eat improperly cooked pork or *Trichinella* infected meat. When a human eats the infected meat, the larvae are released from the nurse cell (due to stomach pH) and migrate to the intestine, where they burrow into the intestinal mucosa, mature, and reproduce.

9. Sea anemones can reproduce asexually, by budding, binary fission and pedal laceration, in which small pieces of the pedal disc break off and regenerate into small anemones. When frogs mate, the male climbs on the back of the female and wraps his fore limbs round her body, either behind the front legs or just in front of the hind legs. This position is called amplexus and may be held for several days. So reproduction is sexual and would require a partner. Tapeworms also can reproduce asexually laying eggs and giving rise to an entire colony. In some of the *whiptail lizard* species, there are no males, and they reproduce through parthenogenesis. Those species without males are now known to originate through hybridization, or interspecific breeding. Thus, only frogs require a partner or a mate to set up an entire colony.

10. Chemiosmosis is the diffusion of hydrogen ions (protons) across the biological membrane via the ATP synthase (a transport protein) due to a proton gradient that forms on the other side of the membrane. The proton gradient forms when the hydrogen ions accumulate as they are forcibly moved to the other side of the membrane by carrier proteins while the electrons pass through the electron transport chain in the membrane. Since more hydrogen ions are on the other side they tend to move back across the membrane via the ATP synthase. As they flow through energy is released which is then used to convert ADP to ATP (by a process called phosphorylation). The energy thus produced is less than the amount of energy (ATP) produced in Kreb's cycle and glycolysis combined.

11. The four phases of cell-cylce are G_1-phase,S-phase, G_2-phase and M-phase. The content of DNA gets doubled in the G_1-phase. This is because DNA replication would occur in the S-phase or the synthetic phase. The chromosome is replicated and each chromosome has a pair of sister chromatids. Again, biosynthesis of DNA occurs in G_2-phase due to mitosis. Then, the number or content of DNA is reduced to its original proportion by the end of the M-phase.

12. Industrial melanism is adaptive melanism caused by anthropogenic alteration of the natural environment in terms of industrial pollution. As soot, smoke and other industrial pollutants from factories darken the landscape and because many organisms rely on camouflage to avoid predation, this sudden change in their environment makes them highly vulnerable to predators. This creates a strong selective pressure which will see any organism with a darker colour much more likely to survive and contribute to the gene pool of the next generation. Rare mutations are hence selected for and over time the population will adjust to a new equilibrium. Thus, through natural selection of the environment, survival and selection of the best suited trait was done.

13. The presence of an extra digit, a sixth finger or toe, which is a very common congenital malformation, is called hexadactyly. The word hexadactyly literally means six digits. In medical usage, hexadactyly does not specify whether the six digits are fingers or toes. The 6th digit can be located in three different locations: on either side of the extremity or somewhere in between. This occurrence of hexadectyly on a particular island is an example of novel mutation (a distinct gene alteration that has been newly discovered). Novel mutations are non-lethal and have significant environmental variation.

14. Marsupials are the group of mammals commonly thought of as pouched mammals (like the wallaby and kangaroo). Marsupials are characterized by giving birth to relatively undeveloped young. They lack a complex placenta to protect the embryo from its mother's immune system. They have a front pouch containing multiple nipples for protection and sustenance of the young. Ovoviviparous animals produce eggs, but instead of laying the eggs, the eggs develop within the mother's body. The eggs hatch within the mother and eat unfertilized eggs in the womb for nourishment. Ovoviviparous animals do not have an umbilical cord to attach the embryos to their mother. So, characteristic of marsupials is ovoviviparity.

15. Mucosa consists of the epithelium and the lamina propria (composed of loose connective tissue), with a thin layer of smooth muscle called the muscularis mucosae separating it from the submucosa beneath. Submucosa lies over the mucosa and consists of fibrous connective tissue, separating the mucosa from the next layer. Over the submucosa, the muscularis externa in the stomach differs from that of other Gastro-Intestinal organs in that it has three layers of smooth muscle. Serosa is over the muscularis externa, consisting of layers of connective tissue continuous with the peritoneum.

16. Chordates form a phylum of creatures that are based on a bilateral body plan, and are defined by: (a) a notochord that extends along the inside of the body; among the vertebrate sub-group of chordates, the notochord develops into the spine, and in wholly aquatic species this helps the animal to swim by flexing its tail, (b) a dorsal neural tube that develops into the spinal cord and is the main communication trunk of the nervous system (c) the pharynx is the part of the throat immediately behind the mouth. In fish the slits are modified to form gills, but in some other chordates they are part of a filter-feeding system that extracts particles of food from the water in which the animals live (d) post-anal muscular tail that extends backwards behind the anus and (e) an endostyle which is a groove in the ventral wall of the pharynx.

17. The cross between the female Drosophila with genotype RrSs with male with genotype rrssi given by :

50% RS and the rest rs = the two loci are tightly linked, strongly interlinked allele.

50% RS and rs, the rest Rs and rs = the two loci of the allele are not linked together, they are separate

90% RS and rs, and the res Rs and rS = the two loci must be 10mu apart, i.e, they are very close

All the progeny are RS = some problem with the r and s gamete, may be they were not formed.

18. In mitotic metaphase, all the chromosomes arrange themselves at the equator of the nuclear matrix. The chromosome number doubles as the chromosomes pair with the homologous pair of non-sister chromatids. Thus, chromosome number would be $46 \times 2 = 92$. In meiotic telophase-I, the

reduction division have already occurred in the prophase-I stage of meiosis-I and the reduced chromatids are being pulled towards the poles by the spindle fibres. In this stage, chromosome number is halved, so 46/2 = 23 number of chromosomes. In meiotic anaphase-II, after reduction division, the crossed-over chromatids multiply through division leading to restoration of the original number of chromosome which is 46. Now, in aneuploid meiotic telophase-II, there is loss or gain of one chromatid from the reduced pair of chromosomes. So, the chromosome number would be 24.

19. Movement of solute across a semi-permeable or a selectively permeable membrane is governed by concentration difference across the membrane. The solute molecule would diffuse without any energy through the flux of the movement or diffusion created by the concentration gradient i.e., the inner cytoplasmic matrix has a higher concentration of the solute than the outer environment. However, if the solute concentration is high outside the membrane, then for movement of solute across the membrane, either energy in the form of ATP or carrier molecules like permeases are required for transport of the solute.

20. Different cell types respond to same signalling molecule like a hormone glucagon in different ways. This is because every cell type has a receptor protein which is unique to that particular cell only. Hence, if various cell types are presented with the same ligand, the receptor protein-ligand interaction would be specific for each and every receptor molecule of the cell. Thus, different cell possess different receptor which produce certain signals specific to that receptor interaction.

21. DNA transcription is a process that involves the transcribing of genetic information from DNA to RNA. The transcribed DNA message is used to produce proteins. It controls cellular activity by coding for the production of proteins. The information in DNA is not directly converted into proteins, but must first be copied into mRNA. There are three main steps to the process of DNA transcription $\rightarrow$ (a) Initiation in which RNA Polymerase Binds to DNA. DNA is transcribed by an enzyme called RNA polymerase. Specific nucleotide sequences tell RNA polymerase where to begin and where to end. RNA polymerase attaches to the DNA at a specific area called the promoter region. (b) Elongation in which certain proteins called transcription factors unwind the DNA strand and allow RNA polymerase to transcribe only a single strand of DNA into a single stranded RNA polymer called messenger RNA (mRNA). The strand that serves as the template is called the antisense strand. The strand that is not transcribed is called the sense strand and (c) Termination in which RNA polymerase moves along the DNA until it reaches a terminator sequence. At that point, RNA polymerase releases the mRNA polymer and detaches from the DNA. Since proteins are constructed in the cytoplasm of the cell by a process called translation, mRNA must cross the nuclear membrane to reach the cytoplasm.

22. Proto-oncogenes are a group of genes that cause normal cells to become cancerous when they are mutated. Often, proto-oncogenes encode proteins that function to stimulate cell division, inhibit cell differentiation, and halt cell death. All of these processes are important for normal human development and for the maintenance of tissues and organs. Oncogenes, however, typically exhibit increased production of these proteins, thus leading to increased cell division, decreased cell differentiation, and inhibition of cell death; taken together, these phenotypes define cancer cells. The proto-oncogene can become an oncogene by a relatively small modification of its original function.

23. Homeotic genes are any of a group of genes that control the pattern of body formation during early embryonic development of organisms. These genes encode proteins called transcription factors that direct cells to form various parts of the body. A homeotic protein can activate one gene but repress another, producing effects that are complementary and necessary for the ordered development of an organism. In fruit flies (*Drosophila*), mutation of a particular homeotic gene results in altered transcription, leading to the growth of legs on the head instead of antenna and is known as the antennapedia mutation. Thus, in humans homeotic genes would determine that arms come off the upper portion of the torso and legs from the lower half of the body.

24. Eutrophication is a syndrome of ecosystem responses to human activities that fertilize water bodies with nitrogen (N) and phosphorus (P), often leading to changes in animal and plant populations and degradation of water and habitat quality. Nitrogen and phosphorus are essential components of structural proteins, enzymes, cell membranes, nucleic acids, and molecules that capture and utilize light and chemical energy to support life. Nutrient enrichment of waters promotes the growth of algae, either as attached multicellular forms (e.g. sea lettuce) or as suspended microscopic phytoplankton, because algae can grow faster than larger vascular plants. As algal biomass builds during blooms it forms aggregates that sink and fuel bacterial growth in bottom waters and sediments. Bacterial metabolism consumes oxygen creating conditions stressful or even lethal for aquatic invertebrates and fish as anaerobic conditions are generated at deeper levels of water.

25. A population is the smallest biological unit that can evolve. It is a group of individuals of the same species, living in the same place, at the same time. In ecological parlance, population represents a group of interbreeding species residing at a fixed geographical region at the same event of life and living. Here, all the sandalwood trees in a given forest denote population.

26. While CO_2 absorption and release is always happening as a result of natural processes, the recent drastic rise in CO_2 levels in the atmosphere is known to be entirely due to human activity. Burning fossil fuels such as coal and petroleum is the leading cause of increased anthropogenic CO_2. Global warming is mainly the result of CO_2 levels rising in the Earth's *atmosphere*. Carbon dioxide (CO_2) is the primary greenhouse gas emitted through human activities. It absorbs and emits radiation within the thermal infrared range. This process is the fundamental cause of the greenhouse effect. When energy from the sun reaches the Earth, the planet absorbs some of this energy and radiates the rest back to space as heat. The Earth's surface temperature depends on this balance between incoming and outgoing energy. If this energy balance is shifted, the Earth's surface could become noticeably warmer or cooler, leading to a variety of changes in global climate. This is maintained by the greenhouse gases. Thus, increased levels of CO_2 in the atmosphere would result increased level of penetration of infrared radiation into the earth's atmosphere leading to global warming. Spreading salt on roads to prevent ice formation does not increase the concentration of greenhouse gases.

27. Organism X has better eye-sight as it can see colours that we humans cannot. Organism X also has better perception of sense of traces of chemicals that we are incapable of sensing. But, if Organism X cannot hear, then his brain will be overloaded with information that is not required for processing. That unnecessary information would swamp the brain leading to chaotic decisions and actions. An organism incapable of hearing or disable of hearing sounds would be conditioned in such a way that its brain can pick up only that information relevant to its existence.

28. Classical conditioning is a form of learning in which the conditioned stimulus comes to signal the occurrence of a second stimulus, the unconditioned stimulus. Classical conditioning differs from operant or instrumental conditioning, in which behaviour emitted by the subject is strengthened or weakened by its consequences (i.e. reward or punishment). Here, the fish has been conditioned with the stimulus that switching the lights on is a direct indication that food would be supplied.

29. For continuation of the own gene pool, it is important that the offsprings in future generation develop and give rise to further offspring so that the gene pool is maintained varyingly. So, if a person wants to raise maximum relatives for successive continuation of the gene pool, it is necessary to have one offspring, one nephew, and two grandchildren.

30. A fluorescent dye was used to level the tip of an animal pole of a gastrulating frog embryo. This tip to the animal pole portion is the ectoderm of the embryo. Ectoderm is one of the three primary germ cell layers in the very early embryo. Ectoderm differentiates to form the nervous system (spine, peripheral nerves and brain). As such, at the end of embryogenesis, the fluorescing cells would be found in the neural cells.

■■

GATE-2003

XL : LIFE SCIENCES

Time : 3 Hours | *Maximum Marks : 100*

(H) CHEMISTRY (Compulsory)

Useful data :

Planck's constant, $h = 6.63 \times 10^{-34}$ Js
Mass of electron, $= 9.1 \times 10^{-31}$ kg
Rydberg constant = 109677 cm^{-1}
$\pi = 3.142$

Q. 1 – 10 carry one mark each

1. In ice, each oxygen atom of water molecule is
   (*a*) bonded only covalently to two hydrogen atoms
   (*b*) bonded covalently to two hydrogen atoms and hydrogen-bonded to two other hydrogen atoms
   (*c*) hydrogen-bonded to four hydrogen atoms
   (*d*) bonded obly covalently to four hydrogen atoms

2. I_2 exists in the solid form under normal temperature and pressure. The principal intermolecular forces holding together iodine molecules in solid is
   (*a*) covalent (*b*) metallic
   (*c*) ionic (*d*) Van der Waals

3. Burning of phosphorus in the presence of air produces a highly hygroscopic white compound, which reacts with water to yield
   (*a*) H_3PO_4 (*b*) H_3PO_2 (*c*) $H_4P_2O_7$ (*d*) $H_4P_2O_5$

4. The minimum uncertainty in the speed of an electron in a one dimensional box of length 10^{-10} m is
   (*a*) 580 m/s (*b*) 580 km/s
   (*c*) 1160 km/s (*d*) 5800 km/s

5. Which one of the following explains the origin of colligative properties correctly ?
   (*a*) Increase of the chemical potential of the liquid solvent due to added solute
   (*b*) Reduction of the chemical potential of the liquid solvent due to added solute
   (*c*) Influence of the solute on the chemical potential of the solvent vapour
   (*d*) Influence of the solute on the chemical potential of the solid solvent

6. For a zero order reaction, $A \rightarrow P$, if the initial concentration of species $[A]_0$, then $t_{1/2}$ can be expressed as
   (*a*) $[A]_0/k$ (*b*) $1/k$ (*c*) $2[A]_0/k$ (*d*) $[A]_0/2k$

7. A transition element M forms the oxides MO, M_2O_3, MO and M_2O_7. Which of the following statements about these oxides is true?
   (*a*) MO is the most acidic.
   (*b*) M_2O_3 is the one most likely to be a strong oxidising agent.
   (*c*) MO_3 is the most basic.
   (*d*) M_2O_7 is the one that cannot be a reducing agent.

8. For a compound to be aromatic, how many π electrons must be in the π cloud?
   (*a*) An even number of pairs
   (*b*) An odd number
   (*c*) An even number
   (*d*) An odd number of pairs

9. Which one of the following alkyl halides would be the most stable in water?
   (*a*) Cyclopropenyl bromide
   (*b*) Cyclopentadienyl bromide
   (*c*) Cyclopropyl bromide
   (*d*) Bromobenzene

10. What starting materials must be used in order to have a 1,4-cyclohexadiene to be the product of a Diels Alder reaction?
    (*a*) A conjugated diene and an alkene
    (*b*) A conjugated diene and an alkyne
    (*c*) A 1,4-diene and an alkyne
    (*d*) A 1,2-diene and an alkyne

Q. 11 – 30 carry two marks each

11. The single-bond length between carbon and the elements viz., carbon, nitrogen, oxygen and fluorine follow the order C–C > C–N > C–O > C–F. This trend is due to
    (*a*) increase in electronegativity
    (*b*) increase in bond polarity
    (*c*) increase in atomic weight
    (*d*) decrease in atomic size

12. By applying the VSEPR model on the XeF_4 molecule, which one of the following statements is ture?
    (*a*) Has four bonding pairs and a line pair
    (*b*) Has octahedral geometry and square planar shape
    (*c*) Has square planar geometry and octahedral shape
    (*d*) Has tetrahedral geometry and tetrahedral shape

13. Which one of the following statements is NOT true for borazine and benzene?

(*a*) They are isoelectronic

(*b*) Both are aromatic

(*c*) Both undergo addition reactions

(*d*) Both undergo substitution reactions

14. The action of NH_3 on S_2Cl_2 produces a thermochromic crystalline compound, whose chemical formula is

(*a*) S_3N_3Cl (*b*) S_4N_3Cl (*c*) S_2N_2 (*d*) S_4N_4

15. The oxidation state of Fe and S in $Na_2[Fe(CO)_4Cl_2]$ and $K_2S_2O_8$, respectively are

(*a*) 0 and +5 (*b*) +2 and +7

(*c*) +4 and +5 (*d*) 0 and +4

16. The structure of $Ni(CO)_4$ is

(*a*) square planar (*b*) trigonal pyramidal

(*c*) tetrahedral (*d*) distorted octahedral

17. The reaction of $CuCO_3$ with acetic acid produces a blue crystalline compound with its magnetic moment (μ_{eff}) being ~ 1.4 B.M./Cu. The compound is

(*a*) $Cu(CH_3COO)_2 . 2H_2O$

(*b*) $Cu_2CO_3(CH_3COO)_2 . 2H_2O$

(*c*) $Cu(CH_3COO)_2$

(*d*) $Cu_2(CH_3COO)_2 . 2H_2O$

18. The limiting ionic conductivities of Mg^{2+} and Cl^- in H_2O at 298 K are 10.60 and 7.635 mS m^2 mol^{-1}, respectively. The limiting molar conductivity (in mS m^2 mol^{-1}) of $MgCl_2$ in H_2O at 298 K is

(*a*) 18.235 (*b*) 25.870 (*c*) 28.835 (*d*) 60.893

19. The longest wavelength transition in the Balmer series of atomic hydrogen is

(*a*) 656.5 nm (*b*) 6564.7 nm

(*c*) 15233 nm (*d*) 65647 nm

20. In a liquid vapour phase boundary, a plot of ln vapour pressure against the reciprocal to temperature would yield as slope

(*a*) $\Delta_{vap}H/R$ (*b*) $-\Delta_{vap}H/R$

(*c*) $\Delta_{vap}H/\Delta_{vap}V$ (*d*) $\Delta_{vap}H/R^2$

21. For a first order reaction $A \rightarrow P$, the time required to complete 80% of the reaction is

(*a*) ln 1.25/k (*b*) ln 8/k (*c*) ln 5/k (*d*) ln 80/k

22. If the molar enthalpy the entropy of fusion of water are 6.01 kJ/mol and 22.0 J/.mol K, respectively, then ΔG for the melting of ice at 10° C is

(*a*) – 6220 kJ/mol (*b*) – 214 kJ/mol

(*c*) – 5.79 kJ/mol (*d*) – 0.22 kJ/mol

23. When steady state approximation is applied in enzyme kinetics, which one of the following statements is correct with regard to the concentration of the enzyme substrate complex [ES]

(*a*) $\frac{d[ES]}{dt} = 0$ (*b*) $\frac{d[ES]}{dt} = \text{constant}$

(*c*) $[ES] = 0$ (*d*) $\frac{d[ES]}{dt} = \text{infinity}$

24. The wavelength possessed by a cricket ball of mass 1 kg, travelling with a velocity of 40 m/s is

(*a*) 1.66×10^{-38} m

(*b*) 1.66×10^{-35} m

(*c*) 2.65×10^{-32} m

(*d*) 1.66×10^{33} m

25. Which one of the following reaction sequences will convert toluene to para-chlorobenzoic acid?

(*a*) (*i*) Cl_2/light, (*ii*) hot $KMnO_4/H^+$

(*b*) (*i*) Hot $KMnO_4/H^+$, (*ii*) $Cl_2/FeCl_3$

(*c*) (*i*) $Cl_2/FeCl_3$, (*ii*) hot $KMnO_4/H^+$

(*d*) (*i*) N-chlorosuccinimide, (*ii*) hot $KMnO_4/H^+$

26. For 2, 3-dibromobutane, which one of the following statement is ture?

(*a*) (2S, 3S) and (2R, 3S) is a pair of diastereomers; (2R, 3R) and (2S, 3S) is a pair of enantiomers

(*b*) (2S, 3S) and (2R, 3S) is a pair of diastereomers; (2R, 3S) and (2S, 3R) is a pair of enantiomers

(*c*) (2R, 3R) and (2S, 3S) is a pair of diastereomers; (2S, 3S) and (2R, 3S) is a pair of enantiomers

(*d*) (2R, 3R) and (2S, 3S) is a pair of diastereomers; (2R, 3R) and (2S, 3S) is a pair of enantiomers

27. When trans-1-bromo-2-methylcyclohexane reacts with methoxide ion, what products are formed under $S_N{}^2$ and $S_N{}^1$ conditions?

(*a*) S_N2 and S_N1 both form *cis*and *trans*-1-methoxy-2-methylcyclohexane

(*b*) S_N2 forms *cis*-1-methoxy-2-methyl-cyclohexane and S_N1 forms *cis* and *trans*-1-methoxy-2-methylcyclohexane

(*c*) S_N2 forms *cis*-1-methoxy-2-methyl-cyclohexane, and S_N1 forms *trans*-1-methoxy-2 -methylcyclohexane

(*d*) S_N2 forms *cis*-l-methoxy-2-methylcyclohexane, and S_N1 forms *trans*-1- methoxy-2 methylcyclohexane

28. What product(s) is (are) formed when HBr is eliminated from (2S, 3S)-2-bromo-3-phenylbutane in an E2 reaction?

(*a*) (Z)-2- phenyl-2-butene

(*b*) (Z) and (E)-2-phenyl-2-butene

(*c*) (E)-2-phenyl-2-butene

(*d*) (E)-3-methyl-3-phenyl-l-butene

29. The major product that would be formed in a Diels Alder reaction between (E)-penta-l,3-diene(trans-l-methyl-l,3-butadiene) and methyl acrylate is

(*a*) 1,2-product (*ortho*) with Me and CO_2 Me *cis* to each other

(*b*) 1,2-product (*ortho*) with Me and CO_2Me *trans* to each other

(*c*) 1,3-product (*meta*) with Me and CO_2 Me *cis* to each other

(*d*) 1,3-product {*meta*) with Me and CO_2 Me *trans* to each other

30. How many resonance structure contributors can be written for the carbocation intermediate formed when phenol undergoes electrophilic substitution in the *ortho, meta*, and *para* positions?

(*a*) *ortho*:3, *meta*:3 and *para*:4
(*b*) *ortho*:3, *meta*:3 and *para*:3
(*c*) *ortho*:4, *meta*:3 and *para*:4
(*d*) *ortho*:3, *meta*:3 and *para*:4

(J) BIOCHEMISTRY

Q. 1 – 10 carry one mark each

1. Which amino acid residue is most likely to be found in the interior of a water soluble globular protein?

(*a*) Ser (*b*) Arg (*c*) Val (*d*) Asp

2. Of the peptide sequences given below, which one is the digestive enzyme trypsin most likely to cleave?

(*a*) ---Val-Lys-Pro-Met--- (*b*) ---Arg-Val-Phe-Tyr---
(*c*) ---Trp-Asp-Gln-Pro--- (*d*) ---Glu-Gly-Trp-Gly---

3. Which pair of amino acids will have the highest absorbance at 280 nm? (Assume equimolar concentrations)

(*a*) Thr & His (*b*) Phe & Pro
(*c*) Trp & Tyr (*d*) Phe & His

4. Which one of the following statements about protein secondary structure is correct?

(*a*) An α-helix is primarily stabilized by ionic interactions between the side chains of the amino acids
(*b*) β-sheets exist only in antiparallel form
(*c*) β-turns often contain proline
(*d*) An α-helix can be composed of more than one polypeptide chain

5. The enzymes where catalysis involves transfer of electrons are named as

(*a*) Isomerases (*b*) Transferases
(*c*) Oxidoreductases (*d*) Lyases

6. Vitamin D is derived from which of the following precursors by the action of UV light?

(*a*) 7-Dehydrocholesterol (*b*) Lanosterol
(*c*) Glycocholate (*d*) Squalene epoxide

7. The molecular defect in familial hypercholesterolemia is due to the lack of functional

(*a*) VLDL receptor (*b*) IDL receptor
(*c*) LDL receptor (*d*) HDL receptor

8. Alcaptonuria is an inborn error in metabolism, transmitted as a single recessive Mendelian trait where the enzyme that is absent is

(*a*) Phenylalanine hydroxylase
(*b*) Ornithine decarboxylase
(*c*) Adenosine deaminase
(*d*) Homogentisate oxidase

9. The prokaryotic RNA polymerase holoenzyme has the subunit structure

(*a*) $\alpha_2\beta\beta'\sigma$ (*b*) $\alpha_2\beta_2\sigma$ (*c*) $\alpha_2\beta_2$ (*d*) $\alpha_2\beta\beta'$

10. Given below are four enzymatic reactions involved in glycolysis. In which of the following steps is ATP generated?

(*a*) 2-Phosphoglycerate to Phosphoenol pyruvate
(*b*) Glucose-6-phosphate to Fructose-6-phosphate
(*c*) Phosphoenol pyruvate to Pyruvate
(*d*) Glyceraldehyde-3-phosphate to 1, 3-bisphosphoglycerate

Q. 11 – 30 carry two marks each

11. The correct decreasing order of permeability through a lipid bilayer of the molecules/ions Isoleucine, Tyrosine, O_2 and Na^+ is

(*a*) O_2 > Na^+ > Isoleucine > Tyrosine
(*b*) O_2 > Isoleucine > Tyrosine > Na^+
(*c*) Isoleucine > Tyrosine > O_2 > Na^+
(*d*) Isoleucine > Tyrosine > Na^+ > O_2

12. For the reaction

Fructose-6-phosphate + $P_i \rightleftharpoons$ Fructose. 1,6-bisphosphate + H_2O the equilibrium constant at pH 7 and 300 K is 10^{-3}. The standard free energy change (in kcal per mole) for the reaction is approximately equal to: (R = 2 cal deg^{-1} mol^{-1})

(*a*) + 4.1 (*b*) – 4.1 (*c*) + 2.2 (*d*) – 2.2

13. Of the four statements given below only one is correct. Pick the correct one

(*a*) Progesterone is synthesized in the corpus luteum and it prepares the uterine lining for egg implantation and maintenance of pregnancy
(*b*) Progesterone is synthesized in the ovary and is responsible for female secondary sex characters
(*c*) Progesterone is synthesized in the adrenal cortex and promotes gluconeogenesis and glycogen formation
(*d*) Progesterone is synthesized in testis and is responsible for male secondary sex characters

14. Which one of the following statements about lipoproteins is true?

(*a*) Molecular mass of lipoproteins is directly proportional to their density
(*b*) The percent protein content in lipoproteins increases with molecular mass
(*c*) Density of a lipoprotein decreases with increase in protein content
(*d*) Molecular mass of lipoproteins is inversely proportional to their density

15. Choose the correct common sequence motif of Zn finger proteins from the choices given below. X stands for any amino acid

(*a*) X_3-Cys-X_{2-4}-Cys-X_{1-2}-His-X_{3-4}-His-X_4
(*b*) X_3-Cys-Cys-X_{2-4}-His-His-X_4
(*c*) X_3-Cys-Cys-His-His-X_4
(*d*) X_3-Cys-X_{2-4}-His-X_{1-2}-His-X_{3-4}-Cys-X_4

16. Pick the correct statement

(*a*) In O-linked glycosylation, sugars are attached to the protein via O-glycosidic bonds to the carboxyl groups of Asp and Glu

(*b*) In O-linked glycosylation, preformed oligosaccharides are attached to the relevant protein

(*c*) In O-linked glycosylation, N-acetylgalactosamine is added via O-glycosidic bonds to the OH groups of Ser and Thr after which other sugars are added sequentially

(*d*) O-linked glycosylation is inhibited by the passage of the newly synthesized protein through the Golgi complex

17. Which of the following statements is **NOT** true with regard to photosynthesis?

(*a*) The dark reactions use NADPH and ATP to drive the synthesis of carbohydrate from CO_2 and H_2O

(*b*) The principal photoreceptor, chlorophyll is derived biosynthetically from protoporphyrin IX

(*c*) Photosystem II (PS II) generates a strong reductant capable of reducing $NADP^+$

(*d*) The components involved in the electron transport from H_2O to NADPH are largely organized into three thylakoid membrane-bound particles

18. In the adjoining Ramachandran diagram, which type of secondary structure do the regions marked X, Y and Z represent?

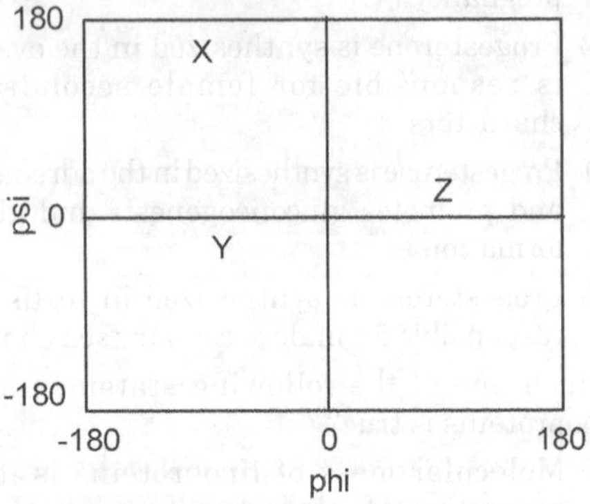

(*a*) X : right handed α-helix
Y : left handed α-helix
Z : β-sheet

(*b*) X : left handed α-helix
Y : right handed α-helix
Z : β-sheet

(*c*) X : β-sheet
Y : right handed α-helix
Z : left handed α-helix

(*d*) X : β-sheet
Y : left handed α-helix
Z : right handed α-helix

19. The RNase A catalyzed hydrolysis of tRNA follows a two-step process with the intermediate formation of a 2′, 3′-cyclic nucleotide. In these steps

(*a*) His 12 acts as a general base in the transphosphorylation step abstracting a proton from an RNA 2′-OH group

(*b*) His 119 acts as a general base in the transphosphorylation step abstracting a proton from an RNA 2′-OH group

(*c*) The 2′, 3′-cyclic intermediate is hydrolyzed when His 12 acts as a general base

(*d*) His 12 acting as a general acid in the transphosphorylation step promotes bond scission by protonating the leaving group

20. Shown below is the autoradiogram of an electrophoresis gel obtained during the sequencing a single stranded DNA by Sanger's method.

The base sequence of the DNA is

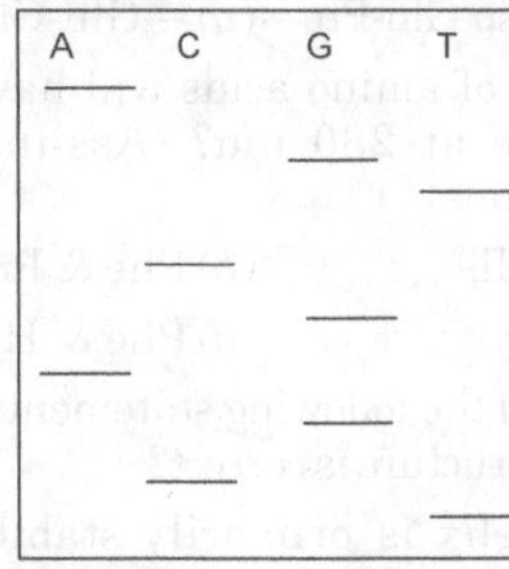

(*a*) 3′-AGTCGAGCT-5′ (*b*) 5′-TCAGCTCGA-3′

(*c*) 3′-TCAGCTCGA-5′ (*d*) 5′-AGTCGAGCT-3′

21. In an antigen antibody interaction, in the zone of equivalence, the isolated antigen IgG complex was found to be in the molar ratio of antigen: IgG, 2 : 1. The number of epitope(s) present on the antigen is

(*a*) 1 (*b*) 2 (*c*) 4 (*d*) 10

22. Class switching occurs in a B cell to produce IgG from IgM. Which one of the following conclusions is correct?

(*a*) Specificity of the IgG and IgM are different from each other

(*b*) Specificity of the IgG is the same as IgM

(*c*) The molecular weight of the new antibody is the same as the old one

(*d*) The valency of the new antibody is the same as the old one

23. Two types of IgMs are produced by the same B cell, one that is secreted and the other that can bind to the membrane. Which one of the following statements is correct?

(*a*) These two antibodies are coded by altogether two different genes

(*b*) The membrane anchor residues are added to the protein by post-translational modification

(*c*) The two different proteins associate, one of which provides the membrane anchor

(*d*) The proteins are produced by alternate splicing of its primary transcript

24. During DNA replication, short RNA primers are synthesized which are then extended by DNA polymerase. These RNA primers in prokaryotes are removed by the enzyme

(*a*) Primase (*b*) RNase H
(*c*) DNA polymerase I (*d*) DNA polymerase III

25. A new antibiotic was discovered which strongly inhibited mRNA precursor transcripts and s_nRNA transcripts. This antibiotic was predicted to be an inhibitor of

(*a*) RNA polymerase I (*b*) RNA polymerase II
(*c*) RNA polymerase III (*d*) Helicase

26. Suppose [4–^{14}C] oxaloacetate is fed to mitochondria. After one turn of the Citric Acid Cycle, which carbon(s) of succinate would be labelled?

(*a*) None
(*b*) Equally distributed between C-l and C-4
(*c*) Equally distributed between C-2 and C-3
(*d*) C-4

27. Two restriction enzymes A and B have eight and four base pairs as their recognition sites respectively. The ratio of the number of fragments that they will generate on restriction digestion of a genomic DNA of *E.coli* is approximately

(*a*) 4 : 8 (*b*) 8 : 4 (*c*) 1 : 64 (*d*) 1 : 256

28. A solution of tryptophan has an absorbance at 280 nm of 0.54 in a 0.5 cm path length cuvette. Given the absorbance coefficient (ε) for tryptophan is $5.4 \times 10^3\ M^{-1}cm^{-1}$, the concentration of the solution is

(*a*) 0.2 mM (*b*) 20 μM
(*c*) 1×10^{-3}M (*d*) 0.1 mM

29. From the data given below, identify the protein pair that would (*a*) give the least mobility band on a sodium dodecyl sulphate polyacrylamide gel electrophoresis (SDS-PAGE) experiment and (*b*) elute last on an anion exchange e.g., DEAE column respectively

Protein	pI	Subunit M.W.	Native M.W.
A	9	10,000	20,000
B	8	35,000	35,000
C	6	15,000	90,000
D	5	20,000	80,000
E	3	30,000	30,000

(*a*) (*a*) Protein C (*b*) Protein A
(*b*) (*a*) Protein A (*b*) Protein E
(*c*) (*a*) Protein B (*b*) Protein E
(*d*) (*a*) Protein B (*b*) Protein A

30. The graph shows a Lineweaver-Burke plot for an enzyme catalyzed reaction

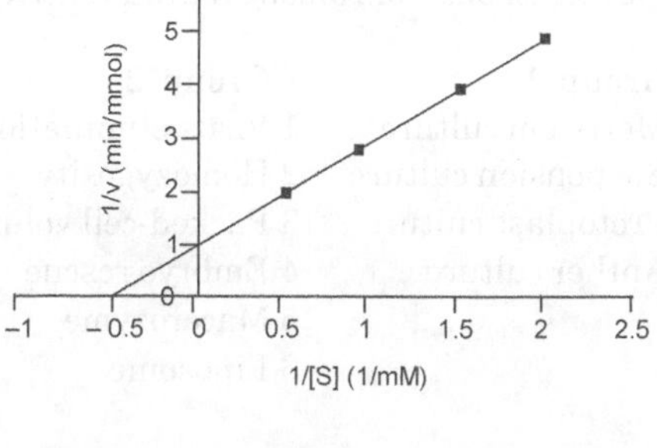

Which of the following statements is correct?

(*a*) The V_{max} is 5 mmol/min and with competitive inhibition V_{max} remains unchanged
(*b*) K_m is 2 mmol/min and with competitive inhibition both K_m and V_{max} decrease
(*c*) K_m is 0.5 mM and with competitive inhibition V_{max} increases but K_m remains unchanged
(*d*) K_m is 2.0 mM and with competitive inhibition K_m increases but V_{max} remains unchanged

(L) BOTANY

Q.1 – 10 carry one mark each

1. The development of embryos from the cells of nucellus or integument is known as

(*a*) Apogamy (*b*) Apospory
(*c*) Parthenogenesis (*d*) Adventive embryony

2. Synthesis of DNA polymerase occurs at

(*a*) G1 (*b*) S (*c*) G2 (*d*) M

3. When the gynoecium is present in the top most position of thalamus the flower is known as

(*a*) Epigynous (*b*) Hypogynous
(*c*) Perigynous (*d*) Inferior

4. Synthetic seed is produced by encapsulating somatic embryo with

(*a*) Sodium alginate (*b*) Sodium nitrate
(*c*) Sodium acetate (*d*) Sodium sulphate

5. Which of the following acts as a precursor of IAA biosynthesis?

(*a*) Tryptophan
(*b*) Methionine
(*c*) Putrescine
(*d*) Geranyl geranyl pyrophosphate

6. Change from purine to pyrimidine or pyrimidine to purine is

(*a*) Transition (*b*) Transversion
(*c*) Frame shift (*d*) Reversion

7. Genetic engineering for male sterility utilizes the gene

(*a*) aroA (*b*) Barnase (*c*) Bt (*d*) CrtI

8. Which plant part of *Crocus sativus* yields saffron, a food colorant?

(*a*) Root (*b*) Leaf (*c*) Stigma (*d*) Seed

9. A form of disease reaction with complete resistance to some races and complete susceptibility to other races is termed as

(*a*) Vertical resistance
(*b*) Polygenic resistance
(*c*) Horizontal resistance
(*d*) Partial resistance

10. Which of the following is a logical sequence of carbon cycle?

(*a*) Producer → Decomposer → Consumer
(*b*) Consumer → Producer → Decomposer
(*c*) Producer → Consumer → Decomposer
(*d*) Decomposer → Consumer → Producer

Q. 11 – 30 carry two marks each

11. A transverse section of monocot stem can be distinguished from that of a dicot stem by observing the

(*a*) Scattered and collateral closed vascular bundle

(*b*) Cortex and collenchymatous hypodermis

(*c*) Collateral open vascular bundle with medullary rays

(*d*) Absence of bundle sheath and presence of pith

12. Choose the right combination for 'Kranz anatomy' from the following features

P Radially arranged parenchymatous cells around each vascular bundle

Q Vascular bundle is enclosed by loosely packed spongy mesophyll cells

R The leaf cells possess one type of chloroplast

S Mesophyll cells differentiated into palisade and spongy parenchyma

(*a*) P, R (*b*) P, Q (*c*) Q, R (*d*) Q, S

13. In the given diagram, fusion of two protoplasts along with the products are presented. Identify which one is the cybrid

Parental Protoplasts:

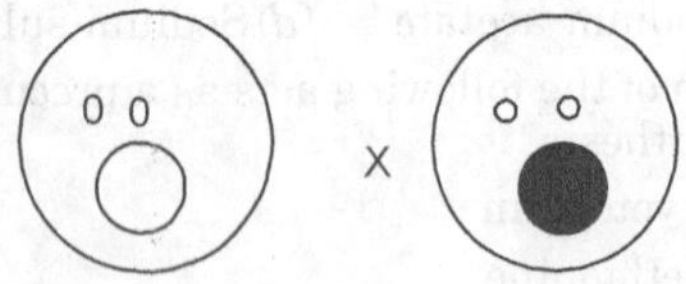

Products:

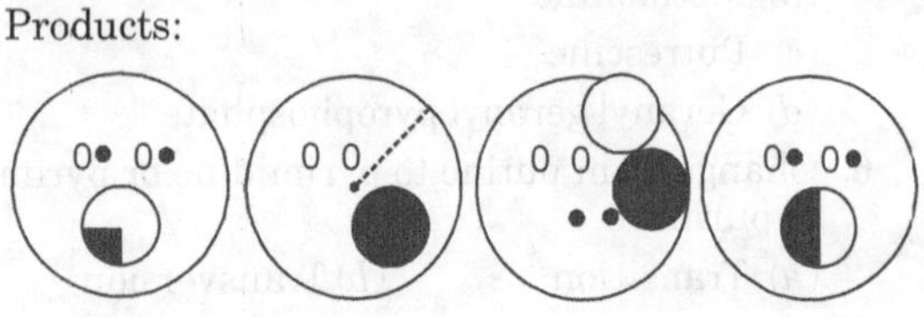

(*a*) (*b*) (*c*) (*d*)

14. The storage protein found in wheat and pea are

(*a*) Glutenin and Patatin (*b*) Glutenin and Vicilin

(*c*) Zein and Vicilin (*d*) Vicilin and Patatin

15. Two cells X and Y are adjacent with each other. The cell X has an osmotic potential of – 20 bars and turgor pressure of 12 bars. Cell Y has an osmotic potential of – 16 bars and turgor pressure of 6 bars. In which direction water will move?

(*a*) From cell X to cell Y

(*b*) From cell Y to cell X

(*c*) There will be no movement of water

(*d*) Water can move either from cell X to cell Y or from Y to X

16. In photorespiration, glycolate and glyoxylate are produced sequentially in the following organelles. Choose the correct sequence

(*a*) Chloroplast and Mitochondria

(*b*) Chloroplast and Peroxisome

(*c*) Peroxisome and Mitochondria

(*d*) Peroxisome and Chloroplast

17. $NH_4^+ \xrightarrow{\text{Nitrosomonas}} I \xrightarrow{\text{Nitrobacter}} II$

In the given reaction sequence, which of the following statement is correct?

(*a*) I is NO_2, II is N_2O (*b*) I is NO_3, II is NO_2

(*c*) I is NO_2, II is NO_3 (*d*) I is N_2O, II is NO_2

18. $NADH \to Q \to Cytb \to Cytc_1 \to Cytc \to Cyt(a+a_3) \to O_2$

Sequence of electron transfer in oxidative phosphorylation is given above. Which of the following pair of inhibitors block the electron transfer in the steps marked with ⊕ ?

(*a*) Rotenone and CO

(*b*) Antimycin-A and CO

(*c*) Antimycin-A and DCMU

(*d*) DCMU and CO

19. Purple leaves (Pl) dominant to green leaves (pl) and pigmy plant (pg) recessive to normal plant size (Pg) are two genes on chromosome number 6 of maize. Hybrids from the cross Plpg / Plpg X plPg/plPg where test crossed and the following progenies were obtained in the F2

419: Normal size plants with green leaves

381: Pigmy plants with purple leaves

79 : Normal size plants with purple leaves

121: Pigmy plants with green leaves

What would be the map distance between Pl and pg?

(*a*) 10 cM (*b*) 15 cM (*c*) 20 cM (*d*) 30 cM

20. Which of the following pairs of DNA sequences could qualify as terminal parts of a bacterial IS elements?

(*a*) 5′-GAATCCGCA-3′ and 5′-ACGCCTAAG-3′

(*b*) 5′-GAATCCGCA-3′ and 5′-CTTAGGCGT-3′

(*c*) 5′-GAATCCGCA-3′ and 5′-GAATCCGCA-3′

(*d*) 5′-GAATCCGCA-3′ and 5 -TGCGGATTC-3′

21. Assume a chromosome with the following gene sequence

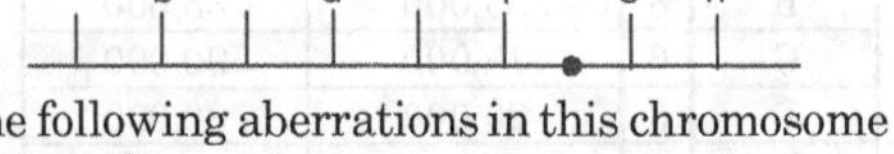

The following aberrations in this chromosome were observed

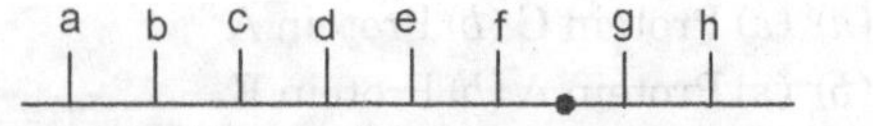

What would be the kind of aberration?

(*a*) Deletion (*b*) Translocation

(*c*) Inversion (*d*) Duplication

Q. 22–25 are "Matching" exercises.

Choose the correct one from among the alternatives a, b, c and d

22.

	Group 1	Group 2
P	Meristem culture	1 Virus elimination
Q	Suspension culture	2 Homozygosity
R	Protoplast culture	3 Packed-cell volume
S	Anther culture	4 Embryo rescue
		5 Macerozyme
		6 Liposome

(a)	(b)	(c)	(d)
P-2	P-1	P-3	P-5
Q-1	Q-3	Q-2	Q-6
R-4	R-5	R-5	R-2
S-6	S-2	S-4	S-1

23.

	Group 1		Group 2
P	Biolistic	1	Gene Pulser
Q	*Agrobacterium*	2	PDS 1000He
R	Electroporation	3	Micromanipulator
S	Microinjection	4	Silicon carbide
		5	*vir* operons
		6	*rol* C

(a)	(b)	(c)	(d)
P-2	P-2	P-5	P-1
Q-5	Q-1	Q-6	Q-5
R-1	R-6	R-2	R-4
S-3	S-4	S-4	S-2

24.

	Group 1		Group 2
P	Reserpine	1	Thea sinensis
Q	Camphor	2	*Taxus brevifolia*
R	Pyrethrin	3	*Rauwolfia serpentina*
S	Catechin	4	*Ocimum americanum*
		5	*Chrysanthemum cinerarifolium*
		6	*Gloriosa superba*

(a)	(b)	(c)	(d)
P-2	P-4	P-3	P-1
Q-3	Q-2	Q-4	Q-6
R-6	R-6	R-5	R-3
S-2	S-3	S-1	S-5

25.

	Group 1		Group 2
P	Early blight of potato	1	*Cercospora personata*
Q	Panama disease of banana	2	*Alternaria solani*
R	Tikka disease of groundnut	3	*Plasmodiophora brassicae*
S	Club root disease of cabbage	4	*Fusarium oxysporum*
		5	*Helminthosporium oryzae*
		6	*Macrophomina phaseolina*

(a)	(b)	(c)	(d)
P-1	P-2	P-4	P-6
Q-3	Q-4	Q-2	Q-5
R-2	R-1	R-5	R-2
S-4	S-3	S-6	S-3

26. Acid rain is due to the emission of

P Oxides of sulphur
Q Oxides of nitrogen
R Chlorofluorocarbons
S Carbon monoxide

Choose the right combination

(*a*) P, Q (*b*) Q, R (*c*) P, R (*d*) Q, S

27. The following statements outline the major features of a system of classification

- Monophyletic origin of angiosperm
- Dicotyledons are the primitive over monocotyledons
- Division of dicotyledonae into Lignosae and Herbaceae

Which of the following system of classifications represents above features?

(*a*) Linnaeus (*b*) Bentham and Hooker
(*c*) Engler and Prantl (*d*) Hutchinson

28. Following are the symptoms of a disease in wheat

- Spikelets transformed into a mass of black or olive green powdery spores
- Spores in young spikelets are covered by a delicate silvery membrane
- After liberation of spores, rachis of the spikelet is left behind as a naked stalk

Identify the disease, which manifests these symptoms

(*a*) Stem rust of wheat (*b*) Loose smut of wheat
(*c*) Bunt of wheat (*d*) Ear rot of wheat

29. Which of the following pair of compounds involved in pathogenecity represents phytoalexin and toxin?

(*a*) Ipomeamarone and Rishitin
(*b*) Piricularin and Victorin
(*c*) Lycomarasmine and Pisatin
(*d*) Medicarpin and Abrin

30. There are three kinds of RNA polymerases (I, II, III) in eukaryotic cells, each specific for one class of RNA molecule

Which of the following is a correct match?

(*a*) RNA pol I - rRNA, RNA pol II - tRNA
(*b*) RNA pol II - mRNA, RNA pol III - rRNA
(*c*) RNA pol I - rRNA, RNA pol II - mRNA
(*d*) RNA pol I - tRNA, RNA pol III - rRNA

(M) MICROBIOLOGY

Q. 1 – 10 carry one mark each

1. Mycoplasmas are different from other prokaryotes by

(*a*) presence of chitin in cell walls
(*b*) presence of murein in cell walls
(*c*) presence of proteins in cell walls
(*d*) absence of cell wall itself

2. Selective media facilitate growth of only one kind of organism. Saboraud's medium is used to selectively isolate

(*a*) Coliform bacteria
(*b*) Gram positive bacteria
(*c*) Yeasts
(*d*) Acid fast organisms

3. The cell walls of Gram positive bacteria contain two modified sugars, viz.,N-acetylglucosamine (NAG) and N-acetvlmuramic acid (NAM). They are covalently linked by
(*a*) α-l,4-glycosidic bond (*b*) β-1,6-glycosidic bond
(*c*) α-l,6-glycosidic bond (*d*) β-1,4-glycosidic bond
4. The metal ion required for the enzymatic activities of nitrogenase and nitrate reductase is
(*a*) Molybdenum (*b*) Iron
(*c*) Copper (*d*) Zinc
5. DNA gyrase is inhibited by
(*a*) Tetracyclin
(*b*) Nalidixic acid
(*c*) Aurintricarboxylic acid
(*d*) Cephalosporin
6. Surface receptor (IgA) on the target cell is the site of binding of
(*a*) Hepatitis B virus (*b*) HIV
(*c*) Rabies (*d*) Influenza A, B viruses
7. In anoxygenic photosynthesis, the green and purple bacteria do not use the following one as electron source
(*a*) H_2O (*b*) H_2
(*c*) H_2S (*d*) S (elemental sulphur)
8. Marcophages are professional antigen-presenting cells. The protein molecule through which they present antigen in humans is
(*a*) Actin (*b*) Interleukin
(*c*) HLA (*d*) CD8
9. The organism used for production of 'BT' bioinsecticide belongs to the genus
(*a*) Borrelia (*b*) Bacillus
(*c*) Bordetella (*d*) Blastobacter
10. The bacteriophage with a single stranded circular DNA, as genome is
(*a*) T4 phage (*b*) λ phage
(*c*) MS2 (*d*) $\phi \times 174$

Q. 11 – 30 carry two marks each

11. A gram negative rod showed on EMB agar colonies with dark centre and greenish metallic sheen. The organism is
(*a*) Salmonella (*b*) Shigella
(*c*) *E. coli* (*d*) Pseudomonas
12. Two antibiotics have different sites of action in a bacterial cell. The frequency of occurrence of resistance to these antibiotics used singly are 10^{-5} and 10^{-6}, respectively. When the antibiotics are used in combination the frequency of occurrence of resistance to both antibiotics are
(*a*) 10^{-5} (*b*) 10^{-6} (*c*) 10^{-30} (*d*) 10^{-11}
13. Species of penicillium, streptomyces and bacteria have been sources of the following group of important biomedical and industrial product(s)
(*a*) Methane and other gases
(*b*) Steroids
(*c*) Antibiotics
(*d*) Insulin, interferon
14. In the normal human being the concentration(s) of various antibodies in the serum is (are) in the order
(*a*) IgM > IgA > IgG > IgE
(*b*) IgG > IgA > IgM > IgE
(*c*) IgE > IgG > IgM > IgA
(*d*) IgA > IgM > IgE > IgG
15. The milk Streptococci produce acetoin that gets spontaneously oxidised yielding a flavoring agent (responsible for aroma of butter) is
(*a*) Acetone (*b*) Acetyl CoA
(*c*) Butyric acid (*d*) Diacetyl
16. Syntrophy is the phenomenon where
(*a*) one microorganism degrades a substance and uses it
(*b*) one microorganism degrades the substance and the other microorganism uses it
(*c*) two or more microorganisms cooperate to degrade a substance which neither can do alone
(*d*) two or more organisms can independently degrade the substance but one inhibits the other from doing so
17. Association coefficient S_{AB} is given by the expression : $2N_{AB}/(N_A + N_B)$
Organism A UCACUUCUG-3′ PO_4
Organism B UAUCUAAUG-3′ PO_4
S_{AB} value for organisms 1 and 2 is
(*a*) 0.25 (*b*) 0.50 (*c*) 0.75 (*d*) 1.00
18. ATP synthetase is a multifunctional enzyme with a subunit constitution of $\alpha_3\beta_3\gamma\delta\varepsilon$. The pair of constituent subunits taking part in nucleotide binding and catalysis are
(*a*) α1β1 (*b*) α2β2 (*c*) α3β3 (*d*) γδ
19. The release of terminal D-ala from Park peptide during cross-linking, is catalyzed by
(*a*) carboxypeptidase (*b*) protease
(*c*) aminopeptidase (*d*) transpeptidase
20. Which one of the following sequences has helped in identifying Eukaryotes, Eubacteria and Archeabacterial cell types?
(*a*) signature sequence
(*b*) signal sequence
(*c*) Shine-Dalgarno sequence
(*d*) aminoacid sequence
21. In photoreactivation of UV-exposed cells the enzyme which synthesizes daughter DNA strand at 70 C and also proof-reads is
(*a*) Klenow fragment
(*b*) DNA pol I (*E. coli*)
(*c*) Pfu pol (*Pyrococcus furiosus*)
(*d*) Taq polymerase
22. Leuconostoc mesenteroides when streaked and grown on sucrose medium produces large mucoid colonies. It is due to the synthesis of dextran layer having a chemical structure of
(*a*) α-glu-β-fru 2 → 6 β-fru
(*b*) α-fru-β-glu 2 → 6 β-glu
(*c*) β-fru-α-glu 1 → 6 α-glu
(*d*) β-glu-α-fru 2 → 6 α-fru

23. Media containing spores and thermolabile constituents are sterilized by
(*a*) Pasteurization (*b*) UV irradiation
(*c*) Dry heat (*d*) Tyndallization

24. A highly aerobic and metabolically versatile organism used in oil-spill-clearing is
(*a*) *Mycobacterium smegmatis*
(*b*) *Azotobacter vinelandii*
(*c*) *Pseudomonas cepacia*
(*d*) *Leuconostoc mesenteroides*

25. Penicillin and lysozyme prevent synthesis and cause lysis, respectively, of cell walls of
(*a*) *Micrococcus lysodeikticus*
(*b*) *Escherichia coli*
(*c*) *Saccharomyces cerevisiae*
(*d*) *Methanobacterium barkeri*

26. In Adansonian numerical taxonomy two organisms (*a*) and (*b*) tested positive and/or negative to a battery of tests
Number of tests positive in both (*a*) and (*b*) = 80
Number of tests positive in (*a*) only = 6
Number of tests positive in (*b*) only = 4
Number of tests negative in both (*a*) and (*b*) = 10
Similarity coefficient S_J is
(*a*) 0.88 (*b*) 0.77 (*c*) 0.66 (*c*) 0.55

27. In Calvin cycle, RubisCO incorporates CO_2 into ribulose 1,5-bisphosphate (1st 6 carbon compound), which rapidly splits into
(*a*) glyceraldehyde-3-P (*b*) 2,3-phosphoglyceric acid
(*c*) 3-phosphoglycerate (*d*) 1,3-diphosphoglycerate

28. A bacterial culture had an initial cell density of 10^3 cells/ml. In 6 hours the cell density reached 10^6 cells/ml. Given the formula for the number of generations,
$n = (\log_{10} N_t - \log_{10} N_0) / 0.301$
The number of generations (n) the cells have undergone is
(*a*) 3 (*b*) 10 (*c*) 15 (*d*) 20

29. Zymomonas mobilis metabolises glucose by Entner-Doudoroff pathway. In this pathway dehydratase converts 6-phosphogluconic acid into
(*a*) phosphogluconic acid
(*b*) 2-keto-6-phosphogluconic acid
(*c*) 2-keto-6-deoxygluconic acid
(*d*) 2-keto-3-deoxyphosphogluconic acid

30. When a 'pseudomonad' is wet-mounted and observed by microscopy, the motility stops after a few minutes. Motility is restored by adding arginine solution because
(*a*) Arginine replenishes amino acid pool
(*b*) Arginine metabolism yields ATP
(*c*) Arginine gets hydrolysed to citrulline and ammonia
(*d*) Arginine metabolism leads to the formation of other amino acids

(N) ZOOLOGY

Q. 1 – 10 carry one mark each

1. Life appeared on earth
(*a*) ≅ 5000 million years ago
(*b*) ≅ 3500 million years ago
(*c*) ≅ 1000 million years ago
(*d*) ≅ 500 million years ago

2. Animals are classified into hierarchical groups. In which of the following, would you find the largest number of species?
(*a*) Genus (*b*) Order (*c*) Class (*d*) Family

3. Human chromosome 1 to 22 are serially numbered
(*a*) In ascending order of their length
(*b*) In descending order of their length
(*c*) Relative position of the centromere from ends of the chromosome
(*d*) In order of their position in the cell

4. Microfilaments are fine protein filaments often abundant in eukaryotic cells. They are made up of the protein
(*a*) Actin (*b*) Albumin (*c*) Globin (*d*) Fibrin

5. The subcellular organelle not bound by a single membrane is
(*a*) Golgi apparatus
(*b*) Lysosomes
(*c*) Endoplasmic reticulum
(*d*) Mitochondria

6. The storage carbohydrate in animal is
(*a*) Starch (*b*) Cellulose
(*c*) Glycogen (*d*) Glucose

7. The hormone testosterone is produced by
(*a*) Leydig cells (*b*) Spermatocyte
(*c*) β cells of Pancreas (*d*) Melanocytes

8. The predominant antibody in saliva is
(*a*) IgG (*b*) IgA (*c*) IgM (*d*) IgD

9. Secondary consumers in ecological parlance are
(*a*) Organisms that are omnivores
(*b*) Organisms that eat only carnivores
(*c*) Organisms that eat only herbivores
(*d*) Organisms that are herbivores

10. In the fish species, where internal fertilization occurs, the parental care is provided by
(*a*) Both parents (*b*) Neither parents
(*c*) Father (*d*) Mother

Q. 11 – 30 carry two marks each

11. Which pair of bases of nucleic acids differ from each other having a hydrogen or a methyl group in 5th position?
(*a*) Adenine and Guanine
(*b*) Cytosine and Thymine
(*c*) Thymine and Uracil
(*d*) Uracil and Cytosine

12. Which is the correct statement of the following pertaining to the mass of bases present in a double stranded DNA with 50% GC content?

(*a*) A = T (*b*) C > G (*c*) A > T (*d*) T > A

13. Nucleosomes contain a core and a linker region. The histones present in the core region and the histones present in the linker region are

(*a*) Core (H1, H2A, H2B, H3)$_2$, Linker H4

(*b*) Core (H2A, H2B, H3, H4)$_2$, Linker H1

(*c*) Core (H2B, H3, H4, H1)$_2$, Linker H2A

(*d*) Core (H4, H2A, H2B, H1)$_2$, Linker H3

14. Two species are considered phylogenetically closer because

(*a*) there was very little difference between a protein they made

(*b*) the base sequence in the messenger RNA they synthesized in a given time were similar

(*c*) they made the same carbohydrate

(*d*) the base sequence of their ribosomal RNA were very similar

15. The secretary IgA was electrophoresed on SDS-PAGE under reduced and denaturing condition. The number of polypeptide bands detected on the gel is (are)

(*a*) 2 (*b*) 3 (*c*) 4 (*d*) 5

16. The following are the primary lymphoid organs in mammals

(*a*) Spleen and Thymus

(*b*) Bone marrow and Thymus

(*c*) Thymus and Lymph node

(*d*) Spleen and Lymph node

17. Telomerase activity was monitored in the following cell types. The highest amount of telomerase activity was found in the combination of

(*a*) Embryonic stem cells and Hematopoitic stem cells

(*b*) Nerve cells and Muscle cells

(*c*) Erythrocytes and Macrophages

(*d*) Hepatocytes and Eosinophiles

18. Apicoplast is a unique organelle in malarial parasite which can be used as a specific drug target. The macromolecular transactions that take place in apicoplast are

(*a*) DNA replication, transcription, fatty acid biosynthesis, nucleotide biosynthesis

(*b*) DNA replication, transcription, translation, fatty acid biosynthesis

(*c*) Translation, fatty acid biosynthesis, nucleotide biosynthesis, protein biosynthesis

(*d*) Nucleotide biosynthesis, fatty acid biosynthesis, amino acid biosynthesis, carbohydrate biosynthesis

19. During oogenesis and spermeogenesis starting from single oocyte or single spermatocyte, the respective number of ovum and sperm generated are

(*a*) two ova and two sperms

(*b*) one ovum and four sperms

(*c*) four ova and four sperms

(*d*) four ova and one sperm

20. A male rabbit was hyperimmunized with sheep red blood cells and produced high titer antibody (1:20,000). The plasma cells of this animal revealed hypermutation of the antibody genes. The animal was crossed with a normal female and a litter containing one male and one female offspring was obtained in F1 generation. The F1 rabbits, when four months old were bled and their serum titer for sheep red blood cells was monitored. The titers that were obtained in the F1 rabbits are

(*a*) F1 male (1:20,000) and F1 female (0)

(*b*) F1 male (1:10,000) and F1 female (1:10,000)

(*c*) F1 male (0) and F1 female (1:20,000)

(*d*) F1 male (0) and F1 female (0)

21. In order for the blood to flow from right ventricle to left atrium in mammalian heart, it must flow through

(*a*) Right ventricle → Pulmonary arteries → Lungs → Pulmonary veins → Left atrium

(*b*) Right ventricle → Pulmonary veins → Lungs → Pulmonary arteries → Left atrium

(*c*) Right ventricle → Right atrium → Lungs → Pulmonary veins → Left atrium

(*d*) Right ventricle → Systemic aorta →Lungs → Pulmonary veins → Left atrium

22. Long limbs are adapted for running. Choose the correct order for the relative length of the limbs in animals evolved for the gaits listed below

(*a*) Plantigrade > Digitigrade > Unguligrade

(*b*) Unguligrade > Digitigrade > Plantigrade

(*c*) Digitigrade > Unguligrade > Plantigrade

(*d*) Digitigrade > Plantigrade > Unguligrade

23. A man found to be suffering from a disorder linked to sex chromosome. All the sons and daughters did not suffer from the disease. This is because

(*a*) The man's father was a carrier of the disease trait

(*b*) The man's paternal grandmother was a carrier of the disease trait

(*c*) The man's paternal grandfather was a carrier of the disease trait

(*d*) The man's mother was a carrier of the disease trait

24. The net order of primary productivity in terms of accumulation of drug organic matter per m^2 per year for various terrestrial communities is

(*a*) Tropical forest > Temperate forest > Boreal forest > Cultivated land

(*b*) Cultivated land > Boreal forest > Temperate forest > Tropical forest

(*c*) Temperate forest > Tropical forest > Cultivated land > Boreal forest

(*d*) Cultivated land > Tropical forest > Temperate forest > Boreal forest

25. When new male lions take over a pride, they often engage in infanticide. The reason attributed for the same is

(*a*) The females of the pride are brought to estrous by killing of suckling infants

(*b*) The infants interfere with hunting

(*c*) They hate the former males of the pride and therefore kill their infants

(*d*) To prove their dominance in the pride

26. The cross over frequency (Cross Over Value = COV) for a four gene loci (P Q R S) on a chromosome are

P – Q = 30; Q – R = 25; Q – S = 15; R – S = 10 and P – R = 5

The sequence in which they occur is

(*a*) PQRS or SRQP

(*b*) SQRP or PRQS

(*c*) RSPQ or QPSR

(*d*) PRSQ or QSRP

27. In a population, the frequency of a recessive allele is 10%. The heterozygotes genotypes (Aa) frequency in the population in percent is

(*a*) 10%

(*b*) 81%

(*c*) 18%

(*d*) 90%

28. Experiments carried out has shown that Rohu and Catla, two common edible fresh water fish have the equal chance of being caught in the net. In a small lake, 100 tagged Rohu were released. Next day, a fisherman caught 10 tagged Rohu, 12 untagged Rohu and 8 Catla in his net. The fish population remaining in the lake is

(*a*) 120 Rohu and 80 Catla

(*b*) 220 Rohu and 80 Catla

(*c*) 198 Rohu and 72 Catla

(*d*) 108 Rohu and 72 Catla

29. Reverse transcriptase is

(*a*) RNA dependant DNA polymerase and DNA dependant DAN polymerase

(*b*) RNA dependant RNA polymerase and DNA dependant RNA polymerase

(*c*) DNA dependant DNA polymerase and DNA dependant RNA polymerase

(*d*) RAN dependant DNA polymerase and RNA dependant RNA polymerase

30. The two scientists who were awarded the Nobel Prize in physiology or medicine for their studies in the area of animal behaviour are

(*a*) B. Benaceraf and Karl von Frisch

(*b*) K. Lorenz and S. Tonegawa

(*c*) Karl von Frisch and K. Lorenz

(*d*) B. Benaceraf and S. Tonegava

ANSWERS

(H) CHEMISTRY

1. (*b*)	2. (*d*)	3. (*c*)	4. (*b*)	5. (*b*)	6. (*d*)	7. (*d*)	8. (*d*)	9. (*d*)	10. (*b*)
11. (*b*)	12. (*c*)	13. (*d*)	14. (*d*)	15. (*a*)	16. (*c*)	17. (*a*)	18. (*b*)	19. (*a*)	20. (*b*)
21. (*c*)	22. (*d*)	23. (*a*)	24. (*b*)	25. (*c*)	26. (*a*)	27. (*b*)	28. (*c*)	29. (*a*)	30. (*c*)

(J) BIOCHEMISTRY

1. (*c*)	2. (*b*)	3. (*c*)	4. (*c*)	5. (*c*)	6. (*a*)	7. (*c*)	8. (*d*)	9. (*a*)	10. (*c*)
11. (*a*)	12. (*a*)	13. (*a*)	14. (*a*)	15. (*a*)	16. (*c*)	17. (*d*)	18. (*c*)	19. (*a*)	20. (*b*)
21. (*a*)	22. (*b*)	23. (*d*)	24. (*b*)	25. (*b*)	26. (*b*)	27. (*a*)	28. (*a*)	29. (*c*)	30. (*d*)

(L) BOTANY

1. (*d*)	2. (*a*)	3. (*b*)	4. (*a*)	5. (*a*)	6. (*b*)	7. (*b*)	8. (*c*)	9. (*a*)	10. (*c*)
11. (*a*)	12. (*b*)	13. (*b*)	14. (*b*)	15. (*d*)	16. (*b*)	17. (*c*)	18. (*b*)	19. (*c*)	20. (*c*)
21. (*c*)	22. (*b*)	23. (*c*)	24. (*c*)	25. (*b*)	26. (*a*)	27. (*d*)	28. (*b*)	29. (*d*)	30. (*c*)

(M) MICROBIOLOGY

1. (*d*)	2. (*c*)	3. (*d*)	4. (*a*)	5. (*b*)	6. (*a*)	7. (*a*)	8. (*d*)	9. (*b*)	10. (*d*)
11. (*c*)	12. (*d*)	13. (*c*)	14. (*b*)	15. (*d*)	16. (*b*)	17. (*)	18. (*c*)	19. (*a*)	20. (*a*)
21. (*c*)	22. (*c*)	23. (*d*)	24. (*c*)	25. (*b*)	26. (*a*)	27. (*c*)	28. (*b*)	29. (*d*)	30. (*b*)

(N) ZOOLOGY

1. (*b*)	2. (*c*)	3. (*a*)	4. (*a*)	5. (*d*)	6. (*c*)	7. (*a*)	8. (*b*)	9. (*c*)	10. (*c*)
11. (*b*)	12. (*a*)	13. (*b*)	14. (*d*)	15. (*a*)	16. (*b*)	17. (*a*)	18. (*b*)	19. (*b*)	20. (*d*)
21. (*a*)	22. (*a*)	23. (*d*)	24. (*a*)	25. (*d*)	26. (*d*)	27. (*c*)	28. (*b*)	29. (*a*)	30. (*c*)

EXPLANATIONS

(H) CHEMISTRY

1. Ice is made from water molecules, H_2O. The structure of water molecules in ice is essentially the same as in the vapour. In ice the Oxygen is "linked" to each other by the combination of a covalent bond + a hydrogen bond. The Oxygen=Oxygen links form the structural framework for all the ice structures. In many ice structures (including normal ice) the hydrogens are distributed at random throughout the Oxygen=Oxygen framework subject to two rules (due to Bernal and Fowler)→1. Only one Hydrogen on each Oxygen=Oxygen link and 2. There must be two Hydrogens associated with Oxygen.

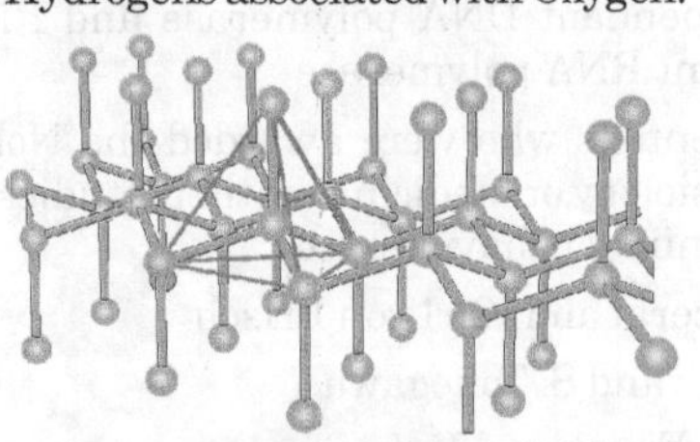

2. Iodine, I_2, is a bluish-black lustrous solid which evaporates (sublimes) to a purple vapour. In its crystalline structure, the covalent I_2 molecules are held together by weak intermolecular bonding. Gently warming a small sample of iodine readily produces the purple vapour. It should be appreciated that as the purple vapour is formed only the weak intermolecular bonds are being overcome. The covalent bonds between the iodine atoms in I_2 molecules are not broken. The forces holding the iodine molecules are the Van der Waals's intermolecular forces.

3. When a piece of phosphorus on an iron deflagrating spoon is kindled by touching it with a hot wire, and it is put into a gas jar containing oxygen, it burns in the oxygen with an exceedingly brilliant white flame, producing a white cloud of phosphorus pentoxide, P_2O_5, which settles in flocks on the inside of the dry jar.

$$P_4 + 5\,O_2 \Rightarrow 2\,P_2O_5$$

When water is poured into the jar the oxide dissolves and phosphoric acid is formed, which changes the colour of blue litmus solution to red:

$$P_2O_5 + 3\,H_2O \Rightarrow 2\,H_3PO_4 \text{ (Phosphoric acid)}$$

4. The uncertainty principle says that we cannot measure the position (x) and the momentum (p) of a particle with absolute precision. The more accurately we know one of these values, the less accurately we know the other. Multiplying together the errors in the measurements of these values (the errors are represented by Δ) has to give a number greater than or equal to half of a constant called "h-bar". This is equal to Planck's constant (usually written as h) divided by 2π. Planck's constant is an important number in quantum theory, a way to measure the granularity of the world at its smallest scales and it has the value 6.626×10^{-34} Joule seconds. The equation is given by:

$$\Delta x * \Delta p = h/4\pi$$

Now, for minimum uncertainty in speed, we have a maximum distance (Δx) and minimum momentum (Δp). Again,

$$\Delta p = m * \Delta v$$

Therefore, we have

$$\Delta x_{max} * \Delta p_{min} = h/4\pi$$

Or $\Delta x * (m * \Delta v_{min}) = h/4\pi$

Or $10^{-10} \times 9.1 \times 10^{-31} \times \Delta v_{min} = 6.626 \times 10^{-34}/(4 \times 3.14)$

Or $\Delta v_{min} = 576.37$ km/s

Therefore, the minimum uncertainty in the speed of an electron is 580 km/s (approx.)

5. Colligative properties are solution properties that have their origin in the fact that the chemical potential of a species in an ideal solution is lower than the chemical potential of the pure component. In ideal solutions all solutes cause identical colligative properties. No solution is completely ideal. Colligative properties are therefore dependent on the identity and the concentration of the solute. The colligative properties are

(*a*) the vapor pressure lowering/ boiling point elevation

(*b*) the freezing point depression and

(*c*) the osmotic pressure.

Thus, the origin of the colligative properties is explained by the reduction in chemical potential of liquid surface due to the addition of solute.

6. For a zero order reaction A→P, the rate is given by

$$d[A]/dt = k$$

Now, $d[A] = kdt$ ...(*i*)

Integrating the equation, we have

$$[A] = -kt + C \quad ...(ii)$$

Now, At $t = 0$, $[A] = [A]_0$; since $[A]_0$ is the initial concentration of the substrate.

Therefore, from equation (*ii*), we have

$$[A]_0 = C \quad ...(iii)$$

Using (*iii*) in equation (*ii*), we have

$$[A] = -kt + [A]_0$$

Or $[A]_0 - [A] = kt$ ...(*iv*)

When half-life of the reaction is reached,

$$t = t_{1/2} \text{ then } [A] = [A]_0/2$$

Using the value of [A] at time $t_{1/2}$, we have

$$[A]_0 - [A]_0/2 = kt_{1/2}$$

$\Rightarrow$ $t_{1/2} = [A]_0/2k$

7. Oxidation state is directly responsible for the acidity or the basicity of any transition metal compound or complex. At its highest oxidation state, a transition element is most acidic. That means the transition element M with oxides at M_2O_7 is the most acidic because it is at its highest oxidation state. MO is the most basic oxide because the element M is at its least transition state. Since, the oxidation states of MO, M_2O_3 and MO_3 are intermediary and these can be oxidized, so they can act as reducing agents. However, since the oxide M_2O_7 has its highest oxidation state, so it cannot be further oxidized and thus it cannot behave as a reducing agent.

8. For monocyclic planar compounds in which each atom has a p orbital (as in benzene) Hückel showed that compounds with $(4n + 2)\,\pi$ electrons, where

$n = 0, 1, 2, 3$ etc, would have closed shells of delocalized p electrons and should show exceptional stability, i.e. planar monocycles with 2, 6, 10, 14.... delocalized π electrons should be "aromatic". That is π electrons are delocalized over the entire ring and the compound is thereby stabilized by the delocalization. So an odd number of pairs must be there in the π-cloud.

9. Bromobenzenes are organic halogen compounds of cyclic aromatics formed by replacing hydrogen atoms in benzene by 1-6 atoms of bromine. They are practically insoluble in water and denser than water. The water solubility is decreasing if more brominated. The flammability of bromobenzenes are very low, the octanol/water partition coefficients are moderate to high, increasing with more brominated, and vapour pressures are low to moderate, decreasing with more bromobenzenes.

10. The Diels-Alder reaction is a conjugate addition reaction of a conjugated diene to an alkene (the dienophile) to produce a cyclohexene. The simplest example is the reaction of 1, 3-butadiene with ethene to form cyclohexene:

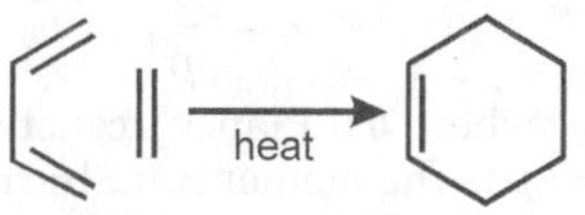

The analogous reaction of 1, 3-butadiene with ethyne to form 1,4-cyclohexadiene is also known:

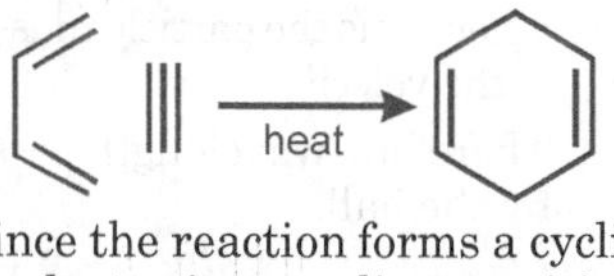

Since the reaction forms a cyclic product, via a cyclic transition state, it can also be described as a "cycloaddition". Due to the high degree of regio- and stereoselectivity (due to the concerted mechanism), the Diels-Alder reaction is a very powerful reaction and is widely used in synthetic organic chemistry. To have a 1, 4-cyclohexadiene to be the product, the starting material should be a conjugated diene and an alkyne.

11. Electronegativity is the strength an atom has to attract a bonding pair of electrons to it. When a chlorine atom covalently bonds to another chlorine atom, the shared electron pair is shared equally. The electron density that comprises the covalent bond is located halfway between the two atoms. The larger the value of the electro negativity, the greater the atom's strength to attract a bonding pair of electrons. A bond in which the electron pair is shifted toward one atom is called a polar covalent bond. The atom that more strongly attracts the bonding electron pair is slightly more negative, while the other atom is slightly more positive. The larger the difference in the electronegativities, the more negative and positive the atoms become. Thus, more the bond polarity, shorter is the bond length.

12. The VSEPR theory assumes that each atom in a molecule will achieve a geometry that minimizes the repulsion between electrons in the valence shell of that atom. In the case of the XeF_4 molecule, the lone pairs will orient themselves in a square plane and the molecule will be linear in shape. In the case of XeF_4, the two lone pairs will locate themselves on opposite sides of the square planar molecule. So XeF_4 has square planar geometry and octahedral shape.

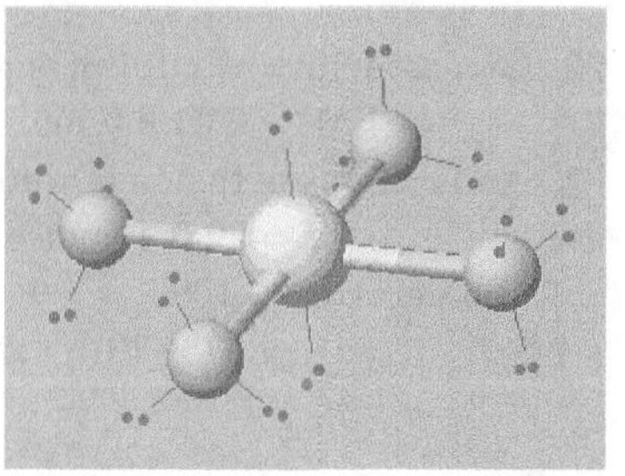

13. Borazine is an inorganic compound with the chemical formula $(BH)_3(NH)_3$. In this cyclic compound, the three BH units and three NH units alternate. The compound is iso-electronic and iso-structural with benzene. For this reason borazine is sometimes referred to as inorganic benzene. Both borazine and benzene undergo addition reactions but are not involved in any kind of substitution reactions.

14. The reaction of ammonia, NH_3 with S_2Cl_2 results in the formation of a thermochromic crystalline compound, S_4N_4 which is given by the following chemical reaction:

$$6S_2Cl_2 + 16\,NH_3 \rightarrow S_4N_4 + 8S + 12NH_4Cl$$

15. The determination of oxidation states is based on knowing which elements can have only one oxidation state other than the elemental state and which elements are able to form more than one oxidation state other than the elemental state.

For $Na_2[Fe(CO)_4Cl_2]$, let us assume that the oxidation state of Fe is x.

Now, the net oxidation state of the complex is 0.

So, we have

$$2 \times 1 + (x) + 0 \times 4 + 2 \times (-1) = 0$$

$$\Rightarrow \ x = 0$$

For, $K_2S_2O_8$, we have $SO_3K - O - O - SO_3K$, and so a peroxide molecule is present.

Assuming that oxidation state of sulphur is y and net oxidation state of the complex is zero

$$2 \times 1 + 2\,y + (-2) \times 6 + (-1) \times 2 = 0$$

[Since peroxide molecules have an oxidation state of -1]

$$\Rightarrow \ 2y = 12$$

$$\Rightarrow \ y = 6$$

So, the oxidation states are 0 and +6.

16. CO is a high spin co-coordinating complex, so it doesn't occupy the inner orbitals (d-orbitals) of Ni. It starts occupying from the s-orbital. Four CO donates 8 electrons to the Ni atom. Starting with s-orbital, 2 electrons go to one s-orbital and the remaining 6 electrons go into three p-orbitals. So the hybridization is sp^3 according to Valence Bond Theory. $Ni\,(CO)_4$ is tetrahedral.

17. Copper atoms can lose one or two electrons to form positively charged ions, Cu^{+1} or Cu^{+2}. They are called cuprous and cupric ions, respectively. Ordinary copper carbonate contains cupric ion and

has the formula $CuCO_3$, but sometimes it has, mixed in, a chemically similar alkaline component, $Cu_2(OH)_2CO_3$. Copper carbonate plus acetic acid (vinegar) produces cupric acetate, water and carbon dioxide. The cupric acetate formed after crystallization is blue coloured and has two waters of crystallization: $Cu(CH_3COO)_2 . 2H_2O$

18. Given, Limiting ionic conductivity of Mg^{2+} ions,

$$\lambda_{Mg}{}^{2+} = 10.60 \text{ mSm}^2/\text{ mol}$$

And Limiting ionic conductivity of Cl^- ions,

$$\lambda_{Cl}{}^{-} = 7.635 \text{ mSm}^2/\text{ mol}$$

Therefore, Molar conductivity of $MgCl_2$,

$$\lambda_{MgCl2} = \lambda_{Mg}{}^{2+} + 2\,\lambda_{Cl}{}^{-}$$
$$= 10.60 + 2 \times 7.635$$
$$= 25.870 \text{ mSm}^2/\text{ mol.}$$

19. A Balmer series provides the wavelengths of the spectral line emissions of the hydrogen atom. A spectral line emission occurs when the photons of a particular wavelength are emitted. The longest wavelength, or lowest energy, photon emitted in the Balmer series is the transition from the $n = 3$ to the $n = 2$ energy level. The Balmer series is defined as the lower energy level being 2, and a transition from higher level than 3 will give a shorter wavelength.

We can use Rydberg's formula:

$\frac{1}{w} = R(1/L^2 - 1/U^2)$ to find the wavelength w,

Where L is the lower energy level (2 for the Balmer series), U the upper energy level, and R is the Rydberg constant, which for hydrogen is 10,967,758 waves per meter. The longest wavelength is for U = 3,

So, $\frac{1}{w} = 10967758\left(\frac{1}{2^2} - \frac{1}{3^2}\right)$

$= 10967758(0.25 - 0.1111111)$

$= 1523299$

So, $w = 1/1523299$

$= 6.564 * 10^{-7}$ meter,

or 656.4 nanometers (red light)

This line is called the Hydrogen-α line in the Balmer series.

20. We have, for a boundary phase between liquid and vapour phases, the vapour pressure is

$$\ln p = \ln A - \frac{\Delta H}{RT}$$

Now, when the equation is compared with the straight line equation

$$y = mx + c$$

The slope m is equivalent to $-\Delta H/R$ where the variables are $\ln p$ and $1/T$.

21. Given, a first order reaction, $A \rightarrow P$

The equilibrium rate constant,

$$k = \frac{1}{t}\ln\left(\frac{x}{x-p}\right)$$

Now, originally substrate concentration,

$$x = 100$$

80% of the reaction is completed, so $p = 80$

Hence, $x - p = 100 - 80 = 20$

Therefore, $t = \ln\frac{\left\{\left(\frac{x}{x-p}\right)\right\}}{k}$

$$= \ln\frac{\left\{\frac{100}{20}\right\}}{k} = \ln\frac{5}{k}$$

22. Given, molar enthalpy of water,

$$\Delta H = 6.01 \text{ kJ/ mol}$$

And entropy of fusion of water,

$$\Delta S = 22.0 \text{ J/ mol-K}$$

Temperature = 10^0C

$$= (273 + 10)\text{K} = 283\text{ K}$$

We have, Gibb's free energy change,

$$\Delta G = \Delta H - T\Delta S$$
$$\Rightarrow \Delta G = 6.01 \times 10^3 - 283 \times 22.0$$
$$\Rightarrow \Delta G = -0.22 \times 10^3$$
$$\Rightarrow \Delta G = -0.22 \text{ kJ/ mol}$$

23. George E. Briggs and John B. S. Haldane applied the Steady-State Approximation method to determine the rate law of the enzyme-catalyzed reaction.

The following assumptions were used:

(*a*) The rate constant of the first step must be slower than the rate constant of the second step ($k_1 <<< k_2$), and

(*b*) Enzyme concentration must be significantly lower than the substrate concentration to keep the first step slower than the second step. The enzyme substrate complex has a concentration of, $d[ES]/dt = 0$.

24. *de* Broglie wave, also called matter wave, is any aspect of the behaviour or properties of a material object that varies in time or space in conformity with the mathematical equations that describe waves.

The wavelength of a particle, given by:

$$\lambda = \frac{h}{p},$$

where h is Planck's constant and p is the momentum. In the non-relativistic limit, this can be written,

$$\lambda = \frac{h}{mv},$$

where m is the particle mass and v is the velocity.

Therefore, wavelength possessed by the ball,

$$\lambda = \frac{h}{1} \times 40$$
$$= 6.6 \times 10^{-34}/\,40m$$
$$= 1.66 \times 10^{-35} m$$

25. 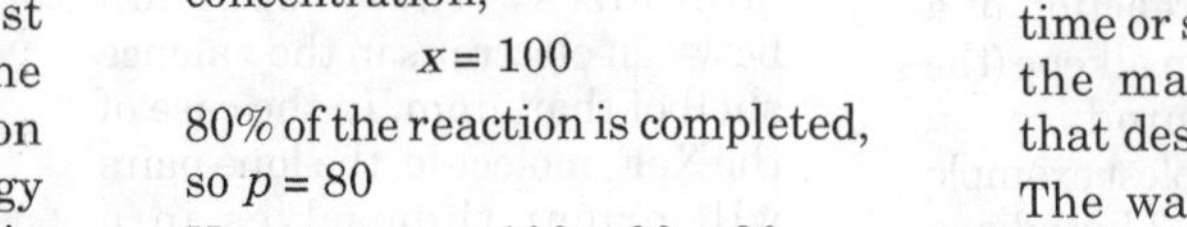

There are two types of reactions: one that would convert toluene to p-chlorobenzoic acid and one that would convert toluene to m-chlorobenzoic acid.

26. In 2, 3-dibromobutane, both stereogenic carbons have a H, a Br, a methyl, and a 1-bromoethyl substituent. In fact there are three stereoisomers, including one achiral stereoisomer. This is because the 2R, 3S molecule is identical to the 2S, 3R molecule, since carbons 2 and 3 are equivalent. In the case of two stereogenic centers ($n = 2$), there are 3 stereoisomers, as it is for 2, 3-dibromobutane.

27. When *trans*-1-bromo-2-methylcyclohexane undergoes S_N2 substitution reaction conditions with methoxide ion (CH_3O^-), it results in the substitution of the halide group (–Br) from the aryl compound and forms *cis*-1-methoxy-2methylcyclohexane due to inversion in the configuration of the *trans*-1-bromo-2-methylcyclohexane. While, in case of S_N1 substitution reaction conditions, there occurs racemization of *trans*-1-bromo-2-methylcyclohexane, which results in the formation of two compounds which are optically inverse to each other at the same time. So, the compounds formed are *trans*-1-methoxy-2-methylcyclohexane and *cis*-1-mthoxy-2-methylcyclohexane.

28. If the β-carbon from which a hydrogen is to be removed is bonded to only one hydrogen, only one alkene product can be formed because there is only one conformer in which the groups to be eliminated are anti. The particular isomer that is formed depends on the configuration of the reactant. Anti-elimination of HBr from (2S, 3S)-2-bromo-3-phenylbutane forms the *E* isomer, whereas anti-elimination of HBr from (2S, 3R)-2-bromo-3-phenylpentane forms the *Z* isomer. So, the product formed after dehydrohalogenation would be (E)-2-phenyl-2-butene.

29. The Diels-Alder reaction is a conjugate addition reaction of a conjugated diene to an alkene (the dienophile) to produce a cyclohexene. Reaction between *trans*-1-methyl-1, 3-butadiene and methyl acrylate gives rise to the major product, a cyclohexene (ortho)-1, 2-addition product with methyl (Me) and carboxymethyl (COOMe) which are cis to each other.

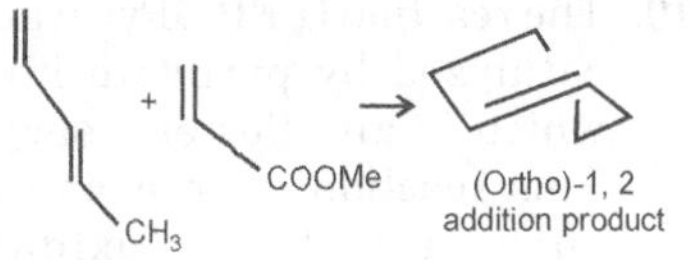

30. The incoming substituent will be directed to the para position, rather than ortho, because of steric strain. If the para position is already occupied, the ortho/para director will direct the incoming group to the ortho position.

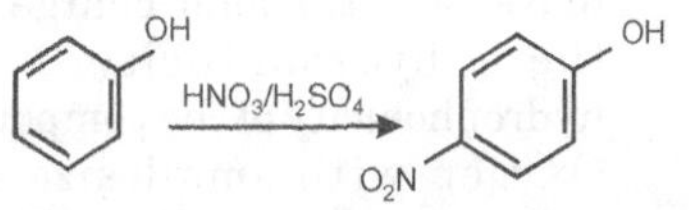

NR_2 , –OR , alkyl, aryl, akenyl groups are o/p directors and activate the ring of phenol.

In case of phenol, during electrophilic substitution at ortho position, there are four resonance contributors, at meta position there are 3 resonance contributors and at para position there are 4 resonance contributors.

(J) BIOCHEMISTRY

1.
- 'Val' usually found in interior of proteins.
- 'Arg' is having basic residue, pka = 12.5, has a strong tendency to be in exterior of protein.
- 'Ser' is having hydroxyl group and has a potential for hydrophobicity and lying on exterior of protein.
- 'Asp' functions as chelators of metal ions. It has a strong preference to be in exterior of protein.

2. Trypsin cleaves the peptide on the C-terminal side of lysine and arginine amino acid residues. If a proline residue is on the carboxyl side of the cleavage site, the cleavage will not occur.

3. Commonly, the optical absorbance of protein is measured at 280 nm. At this wavelength, the absorbance of protein is *mainly* due to the amino acids tryptophan, tyrosine and cysteine with their molar absorption coefficients decreasing in that order. The molar absorption coefficient of the protein itself at 280 nm will depend upon the relative concentrations of these three amino acids.

4. 'Gly' and 'Pro' residues often occur in β-turns. The former, because it is smaller and flexible, the latter, because peptide bonds involving the amino nitrogen of proline readily assumes cis-conformation.

An α-helix is stabilized by H-bond between the >N-H of one amino acid and the >C=O on the 4th amino acid.

β-sheet can exist in both parallel & anti parallel forms.

5. Oxidoreductases are a class of enzymes that catalyze redox reactions Oxidoreductases catalyze the transfer of electrons from one molecule (the oxidant) to another molecule (the reductant). Oxidoreductases catalyze reactions similar to the following, $A^- + B \rightarrow A + B^-$ where A is the oxidant and B is the reductant. Oxidorecuctases can be oxidases or dehydrogenases.

6. Vitamin D_3 (Cholecalciferol) is produced photochemically in the skin from 7-dehydro-cholesterol. 7-dehydro-cholesterol is produced in relatively large quantities, 10,000 and 20,000 IU of vitamin D produced in 30 minutes of whole-body exposure. In the skin of most vertebrate animals, including humans.7-dehydrocholesterol reacts with ultraviolet light of UVB type at wavelengths between 270 and 300 nm, with peak synthesis occurring between 295 and 297 nm. These wavelengths are present in sunlight when the UV index is greater than three, as well as in the light emitted by the UV lamps in tanning beds (which produce ultraviolet primarily in the UVA spectrum, but typically produce 4% to 10% of the total UV emissions as UVB).

7. Patients have mutations in the LDLR gene that encodes the LDL receptor protein, which normally removes LDL from the circulation. Thus there is high amount of LDL (Low Density Lipid) in blood which is also called as 'Bad Cholestrol' causing Hypercholesterolemia.

8. Alkaptonuria is an inherited condition that causes urine to turn black when exposed to air. Ochronosis, a build up of dark pigment in connective tissues such as cartilage and skin, is also characteristic of the disorder. This is an autosomal recessive condition that is due to a defect in the enzyme homogentisate 1, 2-dioxygenase, which participates in the degradation of tyrosine. As a result, homogentisic acid and its oxide, called alkapton, accumulate in the blood and are excreted in urine.

9. When isolated from bacteria, prokaryotic RNA polymerase has two forms: The **core enzyme** and the **holoenzyme**. The core enzyme is a tetramer whose composition is given as $\alpha_2\beta\beta'$ (two α subunits, one β subunit, and one β' subunit). Core RNA polymerase is capable of faithfully copying DNA into RNA but does not initiate at the correct site in a gene. That is, it does not recognize the promoter specifically. Correct promoter recognition is the function of the holoenzyme form of RNA polymerase.

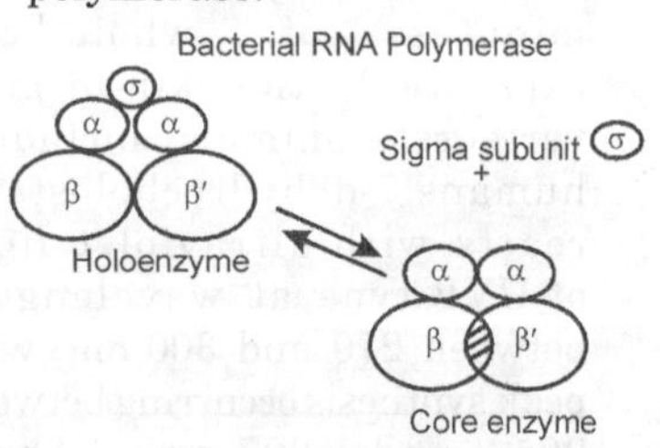

Figure 1

The RNA polymerase holoenzyme contains another subunit, σ (**sigma**), in addition to the subunits found in the core enzyme. Holoenzyme, $\alpha_2\beta\beta'\sigma$, is capable of correct initiation at the promoter region of a gene. σ thus must be involved in promoter recognition. σ subunits are related but distinct in different forms of RNA polymerase holoenzyme. These specialized σ subunits direct RNA polymerase to promoter sequences for different classes of genes.

10. The reaction [PEP→Pyruvate] is catalyzed by pyruvate kinase which is an allosteric enzyme. This reaction is an example of substrate level oxidative phosphorylation in which there is formation of ATP from ADP at the expense of high energy phosphoenol bond of PEP.

11. Permeability through a phospholipid bilayer membrane depends mainly on the molecular mass, size, the ionic charge and the hydrophilicity and hydrophobicity of the compound. Oxygen with small size and molecular mass readily diffuses through the semi-permeable lipid membrane. Na^+ can enter the lipid membrane only when there is a charge redistribution phenomenon under process. Isoleucine has smaller size than tyrosine because tyrosine is an aromatic amino acid. Thus, the decreasing order of permeability is: $O_2 > Na^+ >$ Isoleucine > Tyrosine.

12. $\Delta G = -\,2.303RT\ \log K$

$= -\,2.303 \times 2 \times 300\ \log 10^{-3}$

$= -\,2.303 \times 600 \times (-\,3) \log 10$

$= +\,4145.400\text{Cal}$

$= 4.14\ \text{Kcal}$

13. The corpus luteum is the major source of progesterone for the first 6-8weeks of pregnancy, and then placenta assumes this function. Progesterone is the major hormone of the luteal phase of the menstrual cycle and is required for preparation and maintenance of secretory endometrium that provides early nourishment for the implanted blastocyst.

14. A lipoprotein is a biochemical assembly that contains both proteins and lipids. The lipids or their derivatives may be covalently or non-covalently bound to the proteins. Many enzymes, transporters, structural proteins, antigens, adhesins and toxins are lipoproteins. Examples include the high density (HDL) and low density (LDL) lipoproteins which enable fats to be carried in the blood stream, the transmembrane proteins of the mitochondrion and the chloroplast, and bacterial lipoproteins function of lipoprotein particles is to transport water-insoluble lipids (fats) and cholesterol around the body in the blood. The lipoprotein particles have hydrophilic groups of phospholipids, cholesterol and apoproteins directed outward. Such characteristic makes them soluble in the salt water-based blood pool. Triglyceride-fats and cholesterol esters are carried internally, shielded from the water by the phospholipid monolayer and the apoproteins. Majorly, the lipoproteins have their molecular mass proportional to their density.

15. The Cys_2 His_2 -like fold group is by far the best characterized class of Zinc finger and are extremely common in mammalian transcription factors. These domains adopt a $\beta\beta\alpha$ fold and have the amino acid sequence motif.

16. A protein glycosylation process in which a carbohydrate or carbohydrate derivative unit is added to a protein via the hydroxyl group of peptidyl-serine, peptidyl-threonine, peptidyl-hydroxylysine, or peptidyl-hydroxyproline, or via the phenol group of peptidyl-tyrosine, forming an O-glycan.

17. Photosynthesis is a two stage process. The first process is the Light Dependent Process (Light Reactions), requires the direct energy of light to make energy carrier molecules that are used in the second process. The Light Independent Process (or Dark Reactions) occurs when the products of the Light Reaction are used to form C-C covalent bonds of carbohydrates. The Dark Reactions can usually occur in the dark, if the energy carriers from the light process are present. Recent evidence suggests that a major enzyme of the Dark Reaction is indirectly stimulated by light, thus the term Dark Reaction is

somewhat of a misnomer. The Light Reactions occur in the grana and the Dark Reactions take place in the stroma of the chloroplasts. In the Light Dependent Processes (Light Reactions) light strikes chlorophyll a in such a way as to excite electrons to a higher energy state. In a series of reactions the energy is converted (along an electron transport process) into ATP and NADPH. Water is split in the process, releasing oxygen as a by-product of the reaction.

18. 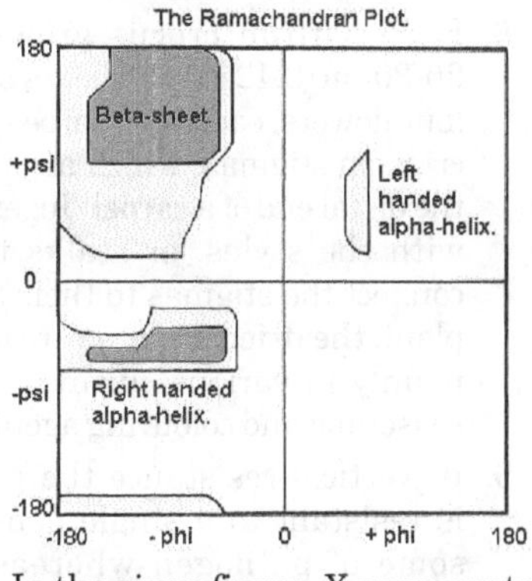

In the given figure, X-represents the β-sheet structure of the polypeptide chain. Y-points to the right handed α-helical structure of the polypeptide chain and Z represents the left handed α-helical structure.

19. RNase A is a non-processive endoribonuclease that catalyzes the cleavage of the bond of RNA specifically on the 3' side of pyrimidine nucleotides. Structural data have implicated Thr45 and Phe120 of the Bl sub-site are acting as mediating this pyrimidine specificity. To investigate this possibility, RNAse A mutants in which all natural amino acids were substituted for Thr45 or Phel20 were screened for the ability to cleave RNA after purine residues. Two mutants were identified as having this ability. T45A and T450 RNAse A cleave polyA, polyC, and polyU efficiently and with increase in purine: pyrimidine specificity. Thus, Thr45 is responsible for the pyrimidine specificity of RNAse A.

20. For determining the pattern of the DNA sequence (5'-3') from the bands formed in the agarose gel read the band from bottom to top of the gel. And it is also important to remember that this sequence is complementary to the template strand of the beginning.

DNA Sequence from gel will be- 5'TCGAGCTGA 3'.

Template strand sequence will be- 3'AGCTCGACT 5'.

21. The zone at which Antibody and Antigen are at optimal concentr-ations and they form a large insoluble lattice together is called the zone of equivalence. So the number of epitopes present will always be 1 in this case.

22. Immunoglobulin class switching is a biological mechanism that changes a B cell's production of antibody from one class to another ,for example, from an isotype called IgM to an isotype called IgG. During this process the constant region portion of the antibody heavy chain is changed, but the variable region of the heavy chain remains same. Since the variable region does not change, class switching does not affect antigen specifically instead the antibody retains affinity for the same antigen, but can interact with different effector molecules.

23. The two forms of IgM are structurally different. The heavy chain of membrane bound IgM has an amino acid sequence at its carboxy terminal end which anchors the molecule into the membrane; the secreted form of IgM has a different C-terminal sequence which lacks a membrane anchoring region. The membrane bound form of IgM is also incapable of associating with J chain and forming its normal pentamere structure: membrane IgM therefore exist exclusively in monomeric form (H_2L_2) also known as IgMs. The two form of chain are synthesized via an alternative splung scheme analogous to that which allows simultaneous IgM and IgD synthesis.

24. The enzyme RNase H is a non specific endonuclease and catalyzes the cleavage of RNA via hydrolytic mechanism. In DNA replication, RNase H is responsible for removing the RNA primer, allowing completion of the newly synthesized DNA.

25. RNA polymerase II is an enzyme found in eukaryotic cells. it catalyzes the transcription of DNA to synthesized precursors of mRNA and most snRNA and microRNA. A 550kDa complex of 12 subunits, RNA polymerase II is the most studied type of RNA polymerase.

26. The carbon lost as CO_2 (at two sites in Kreb cycle) comes from oxaloacetate and not from acetyl CoA. The carbon donated by acetyl CoA become part of the oxaloacetate carbon backbone after the first turn of citric acid cycle. So, during first cycle in succenyl CoA (4C) two carbon will be labeled C3 &C4 and two carbon will not be labelled as it is derived from acetyl CoA and two labelled C is removed as CO_2 before conversion to succunyl CoA. But when succinic acid is formed, randomization of carbon occur and therefore all the carbon (C1 to C4) of succinic acid are equally labelled.

27. Let total base pair of genomic DNA of

(*E.Coli*) = X

Number of fragment produced by restriction

enzyme A = X/8

Number of fragment produced by restriction

enzyme B = X/4

Required ratio of number of fragment

= X/8 : X/4 = 4 : 8

28. Beer -Lambert law is as follows :

$$A = \varepsilon cl$$

$$0.54 = 5.4 \times 10^3 \times C \times 0.5$$

$$C = 0.54/5.4 \times 10^3 \times 0.5 \text{ M}$$

$$= 0.2 \text{ mM}$$

29. To find order of mobility of band on SDS PAGE, subunit molecular weight is considered because before running the gel

proton is denatured. Least mobility band on SDS PAGE will be of protein B, since it has maximum subunit M.W.

Anion exchange chromatography has positively charged resin matrix (stationary phase), so higher the negative charge on protein, more slowly it will travel down to the column and elute last. If buffer of pH -7 is used then relative charge on protein will be (pI - pH) i.e.

A-------- 9 – 7 = + 2

B---------8 – 7 = + 1

C---------6 – 7 = – 1

D---------5 – 7 = – 2

E----------3 – 7 = – 4

Since protein E has higher negative charge, it will elute least.

30. Intercept = – $1/K_m$

$0.5 = -1/K_m$

$K_m = -2mM$

In competitive inhibition, V_{max} remain constant, but K_m increases.

(L) BOTANY

1. Adventive embryony, also called sporophytic apomixis, or nucellar embryony: Here there may be a megagametophyte in the ovule, but the embryos do not arise from the cells of the gametophyte; they arise from cells of nucellus or the integument. Adventive embryony is important in several species of *Citrus, in Garcinia, Euphorbia dulcis, Mangifera indica* etc.
2. The preparation for synthesis of DNA polymerase takes place in S-phase of the cell cycle and the synthesis starts in G_1 phase of cell cycle.
3. In hypogynous flowers, the perianth and stamens are attached to the receptacle below the gynoecium; the ovary is superior to these organs, and the remaining floral organs arise from below the point of origin of the carpel.
4. For synthetic seeds production the somatic embryos isolated are submerged in a solution of sodium alginate, according to the type of encapsulation applied, and subsequently suctioned through a micropipette to provide a protective capsule. In order to seal the capsules, they are then submerged in a complex solution of $CaCl_2$ for a determined period of time followed by washing in sterile water.
5. Indole-3 acetic acid (IAA) is naturally occurring auxin in higher plants. It has been proposed that the biogenesis of IAA proceeds from tryptophan via either tryptamine or indole-3 pyruvic acid. The evidence for this derives from radioactive tracer studies, the isolation of intermediates, and plant growth responses to presumed intermediates.
6. DNA substitution mutations are of two types. Transitions are interchanges of two-ring purines (A ↔ G) or of one-ring pyrimidines (C ↔ T): they therefore involve bases of similar shape. Transversions are interchanges of **purine for pyrimidine bases**, which therefore involve exchange of one-ring and two-ring structures.

   Although there are twice as many possible transversions, because of the molecular mechanisms by which they are generated, transition mutations are generated at higher frequency than transversions.
7. One of the genetic engineering strategy used for male sterility in plants is fulfilled by the use of Barnase gene (isolated from *Bacillus amyloliquifaciens*).
8. Each saffron crocus grows to 20-30 cm (8-12 in) and bears up to four flowers, each with three vivid crimson stigmas, which are each the distal end of a carpel. Together with the styles, or stalks that connect the stigmas to their host plant, **the dried stigmas** are used mainly in various cuisines as a seasoning and colouring agent.
9. In vertical resistance the plant is resistant to a single gene or some of pathogen whereas in horizontal resistance the plant species is resistant to a number of genes or pathogen.
10. In carbon cycle, the atmospheric CO_2 is taken by the plants (autotrophs) and they prepare their food. These plants are also called as Producers. The animals consume the plants and they are called as Consumers. Finally both are decomposed by Decomposers. So the series of cycle is-

    Producers → Consumers → Decomposers.
11. Dicot Stem and Monocot Stem

CHARACTERS	DICOT STEM (e.g., sunflower)	MONOCOT STEM (e.g., Maize)
1. Epidermis		
a) Trichomes	Present	Absent
b) Cuticle	Present	Present
2. Hypodermis	Made up of collenchyma	Made up of sclerenchyma
3. Ground tissue	Differentiated into cortex, endodermis, pericycle, medullary rays and pith	Undifferentiated
4. Vascular bundles		
a) Number	Eight	Numerous
b) Arrangement	In the form of a broken ring	Irregularly scattered
c) Bundle Cap	Present	Absent
d) Bundle Sheath	Absent	Present
5. Nature of the vascular bundles	Conjoint, collateral and open with endarch xylem	Conjoint, collateral and closed with endarch xylem
6. Xylem vessels	Many protoxylem and metaxylem vessels in each bundle	Only two protoxylem vessels in each bundle

12. Kranz anatomy A special structure in the leaves of plants that have a C4 pathway of carbon dioxide fixation. The leaves contain a ring of mesophyll cells, containing a few small chloroplasts concerned with the initial fixing of carbon dioxide, surrounding a sheath of parenchyma cells (the bundle sheath) which has large chloroplasts involved in the Calvin cycle.

13. Cybrid is an artificial hybrid cell produced by introducing nuclear material from one organism into a cell (of the same or different species) from which the nucleus has been removed.

14. In wheat glaidins and glutenin are the storage proteins whereas in pea the storage protein is vicilin.

15. DPD = OP – TP

Where DPD=diffusion pressure defecit, OP=osmotic pressure, TP=turgor pressure

For X, DPD = – 20 + (– 12) = – 32 bars

For Y, DPD = – 16 + (– 6) = – 22 bars

Water moves from low DPD to high DPD. Thus water will move from X to Y.

16. 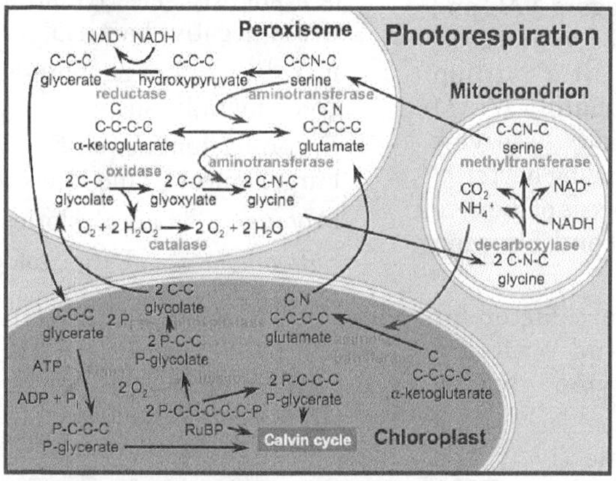

17. Nitrification is a process of nitrogen compound oxidation (effectively, loss of electrons from the nitrogen atom to the oxygen atoms):

1. $2\ NH_3 + 3\ O_2 \rightarrow 2\ NO_2^- + 2\ H_2O + 2\ H^+$ (Nitrosomonas)
2. $2\ NO_2^- + 1\ O_2 \rightarrow 2\ NO_3^-$ (Nitrobacter).

18. Antimycin-A is a respiration inhibitor. It blocks the respiratory chain at complex 3 between cytochrome b and cytochrome c1. It therefore prevents the oxidation of both NADH and succinate, but has no effect on ascorbate + TMPD.

19. Given, parent generations = Plpg(Purple leaves pigmy plant) and plPg(Green leaves normal plant)

Gametes = Plpg and plPg

Test cross = Plpg/plPg * plpg

F1 generation = PlPg (purple leaves normal plant) = 79

Plpg (purple leaves pigmy plant) = 381

plPg (green leaves normal plant) = 419

plpg (green leaves pigmy plant) = 121

Total progeny = 79+381+419+121

= 1000

Parental plants = 381+419 = 800

Recombinants = 79+121=200

% of recombinants = 200/1000 * 100 = 20%

20. Insertion sequence that is inverted terminal repeats are generally present in Bacterial IS element and they usually code for transposase. It is a short DNA sequence that acts as a simple transposable element.

21. An Inversion mutation is a mutation that causes a reversal in the order of a segment of a chromosome within the chromosome, or a gene.

24.

DRUG	ORGANISM
Reserpine	*Rauwolfia serpentine*
Camphor	*Ocimum americanum*
Pyrethin	*Chrysanthemum cinerarifolium*
Catechin	*Thea sinensis*

26. Acid rain is rain consisting of water droplets that are unusually acidic because of atmospheric pollution - most notably the excessive amounts of sulfur and nitrogen released by cars and industrial processes. It is mainly caused by the release of sulfur dioxide and nitrogen oxide during fossil fuel combustion.

27. Hutchinson's classification is based on flowing principles which has been supported by others. The principles are outlined under 24 point which are as follows:

1. The evolution is both upward and downward, the former tending towards preservation and the later to their reduction and degeneration of characters.
2. Evolution does not necessarily involve call organs at one time or simultaneously.
3. Aquatic plants are derived from terrestrial and saprophytes parasites epiphytes are more recent.
4. Trees and shrubs are more primitive than herbs.
5. Perennials are more primitive than biennials and annuals.
6. Plants with vascular bundles arranged in a ring are more primitive those in which vascular bundlers are scattered.
7. Spiral phyllotaxy is primitive than whorled and opposite phyllotaxy.
8. Dioecious plants are more advanced than bisexual flowers.
9. Unisexual flower are more primitive than bisexual flowers.
10. Petalod flowers are more primitive than bisexual flowers.
11. Gamopetally is more advanced than polypetalae.
12. Zygomorphic flower are more advanced than actinomorphic flowers.
13. Hypogyny is more primitive than perigyny and epigyny.
14. Simple leaves are more primitive than compound leaves.
15. Solitary flower is more primitive than infloresceneed flowers.
16. Spirally imbricate floral parts are more primitive than whorled and valvate arrangement.

17. Apocarpy is more primitive than syncarpy.
18. Polycarpy preceedes oligocarpy.
19. Endospermic seeds with small embryo are more primitive than non endospermic seeds with large embryo.
20. Flowers with numerous stamens are more primitive than those with fewer stamens.
21. Free stamens precede the fused ones.
22. Aggregate fruits are more evolved than single fruit and capsule preceedes berry or drupe.
23. Parietal placentation is more primitive than axial and free central placentation.
24. Trees or arboreal habit are more primitive than climbers are twiners in any one family or genus.

28. Symptoms of loose smut and common bunt are not apparent until head emergence. Before heading, dark green, erect leaves may be visible on plants infected by loose smut. Heads of infected plants emerge earlier, are darker in color, and are slightly taller than heads of healthy plants. Spikelets (units of inflorescence) of infected heads may be completely replaced by masses of olive-black spores, which may be removed and blown away by wind, leaving an empty rachis.

29. Medicarpin is a phytoalexin whereas Abrin is a toxin. Abrin works by penetrating the cells of the body and inhibiting cell protein synthesis. By attaching to a carbohydrate chain on the cell surface, the abrin molecule anchors itself to the cell, is subsequently engulfed and enters the inner parts of the cell where it reacts with a ribosomal subunit and interferes with the normal protein synthesis process of the cell. Without these proteins, cells cannot survive. This is harmful to the human body and will be fatal. The severity of the effects of Abrin poisoning vary on the means of exposure to the substance (whether inhaled, ingested, or injected).

30. RNA Polymerase I synthesis rRNA.

RNA Polymerase II synthesis mRNA.

RNA Polymerase III synthesis tRNA.

(M) MICROBIOLOGY

1. Other than mycoplasma, all prokaryotes having cell wall.
2. Sabouraud (pronounced sab-bu-ro′) agar medium selective medium for yeasts Saccharomyces cerevisiae.
3. The alternating sugars NAG and NAM are connected by a β-(1, 4)-glycosidic bond in a million peptidoglycan subunits (NAM NAG + oligopeptide). Lysozyme is known for damaging bacterial cell walls by hydrolysis of the beta (1-4) glycosidic bond between NAM and NAG.
4. The Mo act as a cofactor for nitrogenase and nitrate reductase enzyme during nitrogen fixation.
5. Nalidxic acid selectively and reversibly blocks DNA replication in susceptible bacteria. Nalidixic acid and related antibiotics inhibit a subunit of DNA gyrase and induce formation of relaxation complex analogue. It also inhibits the nicking dosing activity on the subunit of DNA gyrase that releases the positive binding stress on the supercoiled DNA. It is the only FDA approved quinolone for treating UTI infections in children.
6. The hepatitis B virus primarily interferes with the functions of the liver by replicating in liver which begins with the binding to IgA receptor of liver cell.
7. Anoxygenic photosynthesis is the phototrophic process where light energy is captured and converted to ATP, without the production of oxygen. Water is therefore not used as an electron donor.
8. Most cells in the body can present antigen to $CD8^+$ T cells via MHC class I molecules and, thus, act as "APCs"
9. Bacillus *thuringiensis* (or Bt) is a Gram-positive, soil-dwelling bacterium used for the production of BT bioinsecticide.
10. The phi X 174 (or ΦX174) bacteriophage was the first DNA-based genome to be sequenced. This work was completed by Fred Sanger and his team in 1977. This bacteriophage has a [+] circular single-stranded DNA genome of 5386 nucleotides
11. Eosin Methylene Blue (EMB, also known as "Levine's formulation") is a slightly selective stain for Gram-negative bacteria.

    E. coli..........Large, blue-black, green metallic sheen

    Enterobacter/Klebsiella .... Large, mucoid, blue-black

    Proteus..........Large, colorless

    Salmonella..........Large, colorless

    Shigella..........Large, colorless

    Pseudomonas..........Irregular, colorless

    Gram-positive bacteria..........No growth to slight growth

    Organisms that ferment lactose display "nucleated colonies" — colonies with dark centers and the metallic green sheen is an indicator of vigorous lactose and/or sucrose fermentation ability typical of fecal coliforms.
12. Two antibiotics have different sites of action in a bacterial cell. The frequency of occurrence of resistance to these antibiotics used singly is 10^{-5} and 10^{-6} respectively. When the antibiotics are used in combination, the frequencies of occurrence of resistance to both antibiotics are:

    $$10^{-5} + 10^{-6} = 10^{-11}$$
13. Antibiotics provided by these all given organisms that is source of biomedical and industrial products. Penicillin- *Penicillium spp.*, Streptomycin- *Streptomyces griseus*

14. Depends on the healthy human being immunoglobulins concentration IgG> IgA> IgM> IgE.

15. Diacetyl is the compound responsible for buttery or butterscotch flavors that sometimes arise in beer. It is a volatile, colorless liquid with an intensely buttery flavor. In some fermentative bacteria, it is formed from by thiamine pyrophosphate-mediated condensation of pyruvate and acetyl CoA. Sour (cultured) cream, cultured buttermilk, and cultured butter are produced by inoculating pasteurized cream or milk with a lactic starter culture, churning (agitating) and holding the milk until a desired pH drop (or increase in acidity) is attained. Cultured cream, cultured butter and cultured buttermilk owe their tart flavor to lactic acid bacteria and their buttery aroma and taste to diacetyl.

16. Syntrophy, Cross-feeding is the phenomenon that one species lives off the products of another species. (one m.o. degrade and other one use that substances) e.g. many organisms that feast on faeces or dung. Yet another example is the community of micro-organisms in soil that live off leaf litter. Leaves typically last one year and are then replaced by new ones. These micro-organisms mineralize the discarded leaves and release nutrients that are taken up by the plant. Such relationships are called reciprocal syntrophy because the plant lives off the products of micro-organisms. Many symbiotic relationships are based on syntrophy. Finally, anaerobic fermentation/methanogenesis is an example of a syntrophic relationship between different groups of microorganism.

18. Located within the mitochondria, ATP synthetase consists of 2 regions

- The F_0 portion, is within the membrane.
- The F_1 portion of the ATP synthetase is above the membrane, inside the matrix of the mitochondria. A portion of the F_0 (the ring of c-subunits) rotates as the protons pass through the membrane. The c-ring is tightly attached to the asymmetric central stalk (consisting primarily of the gamma subunit), which rotates within the $alpha_3beta_3$ of F_1 causing the 3 catalytic nucleotide binding sites to go through a series of conformational changes that leads to ATP synthesis.

19. The peptidoglycan is a rigid mesh made up of rope like linear polysaccharide chains cross-linked by peptides. The pentapeptide contains a terminal d-alanine-d-alanine unit that is release from here by D-alanine carboxypeptidase.

20. Signature sequences are contiguous patterns of amino acids 10-50 residues long that are associated with a particular structure or function in proteins that are unique to a particular cell type.

21. Pfu DNA Polymerase is a thermostable enzyme that replicates DNA at 75°C. It catalyzes the polymerization of nucleotides into duplex DNA in the 5′ $\rightarrow$ 3′ direction in the presence of magnesium. Pfu DNA polymerase has superior thermo stability and proofreading properties compared to Taq DNA polymerase. The enzyme has a molecular weight of approximately 90,000 Daltons as estimated from the predicted amino acid sequence and exhibits 3′ $\rightarrow$ 5′ exonuclease (proofreading) activity. Unlike Taq DNA polymerase, Pfu DNA polymerase possesses 3' to 5' exonuclease proofreading activity, meaning that it works its way along the DNA from the 5' end to the 3' end and corrects nucleotide-misincorporation errors. Pfu DNA polymerase is recommended for use in PCR and primer extension reactions that require high fidelity.

22. Leuconostoc mesenteroides is a species of bacteria sometimes associated with fermentation, under conditions of salinity and low temperatures. When grown in sucrose solution, they convert it to dextrans, having mostly alpha 1 $\rightarrow$ 6 linkages but 1 $\rightarrow$ 2, 1 $\rightarrow$ 3 and 1 $\rightarrow$ 4 linkages are also present. Therefore, on sucrose medium they produce large colonies because of the chemical structure of dextran layer that is: β- fru- α - glu 1 $\rightarrow$ 6 α- glu.

23. Tyndallization process can be used to destroy the spores. The process is named after its inventor, the 19th century scientist John Tyndall.

24. The use of *Pseudomonas cepacia* var. niagarous to decompose hydrocarbons such as may be found in an oil spill.

25. Action of salivary lysozyme on *Micrococcus* lysodeikticus is effective because Cell wall of *Micrococcus* lysodeikticus as the substrate of lysozyme but it produce penicillinase against penicillin. *Only E.coli* is better sensitive agent for both the substance as *Saccharomyces and Methanobacterium* are resist to Penecillin or reduce its effect.

26. The coefficient S_1 can be given as:

$$S_1 = N_S/N_S + N_D$$

Where, N_S = number of positive features shared by both organisms = 80

N_D = number of positive features in one organism and number of negative features in other organism

$= 6 + 4 + 10$

$= 20$

Thus, $S_1 = 80/80 + 20$

$= 0.88$

27. Ribulose 1, 5-biphosphate + $CO_2 \longrightarrow$ 3-phosphoglycerate

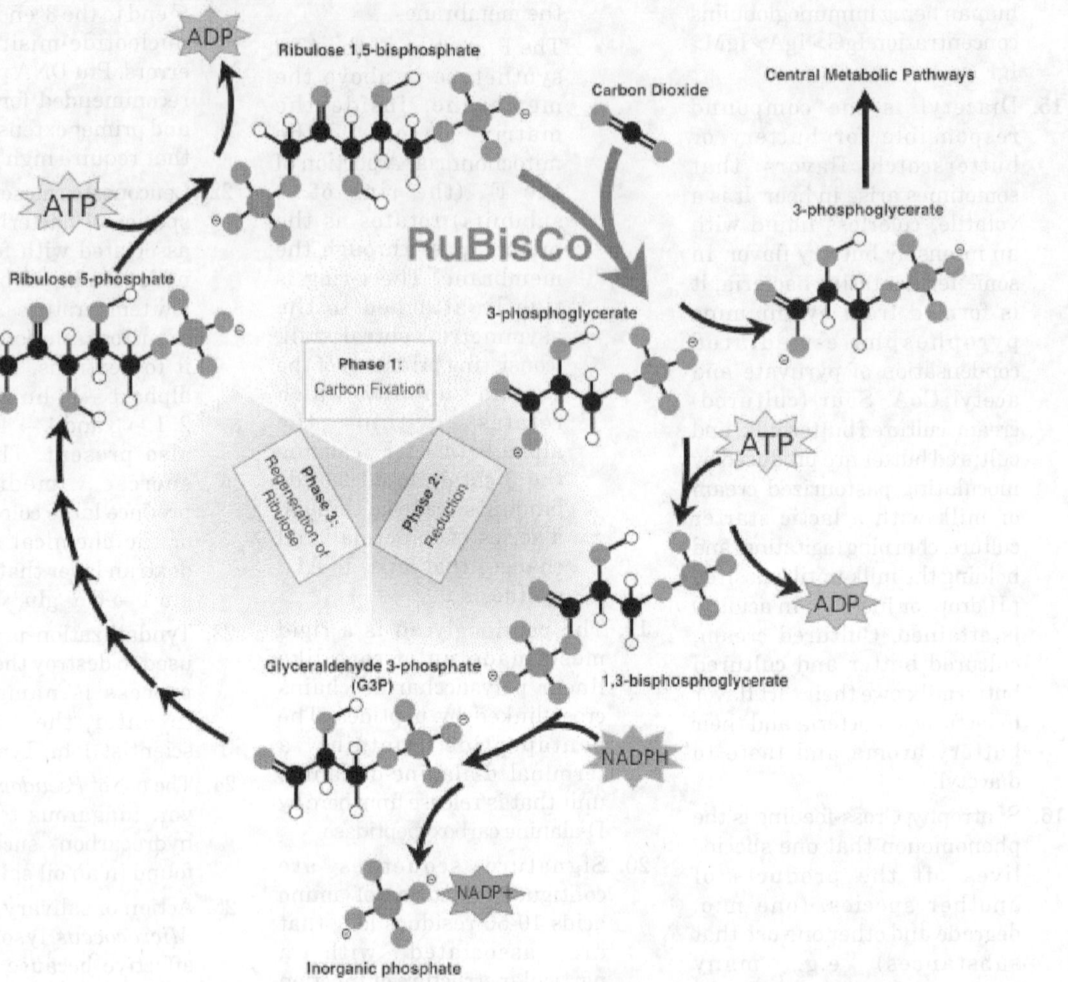

28. Given,

Initial cell density (N_0) = 10^3 cells/ml

Time = 6 hours

Cell density at time $t(N_t) = 10^6$ cells/ml

According to the formula, we have,

$$n = (\log_{10} N_t - \log_{10} N_0)/0.301$$

where n = number of generations.

Thus, $n = (\log_{10} 10^6 - \log_{10} 10^3)/0/301$

On solving, we get,

Number of generations (n) = 10.

29. *Zymomonas mobilis* is a bacterium belonging to the genus Zymomonas. It is notable for its bioethanol-producing capabilities, which surpass yeast in some aspects. *Z. mobilis* degrades sugars to pyruvate using the Entner-Doudoroff pathway. The pyruvate is then fermented to produce ethanol and carbon dioxide as the only products (analogous to yeast).

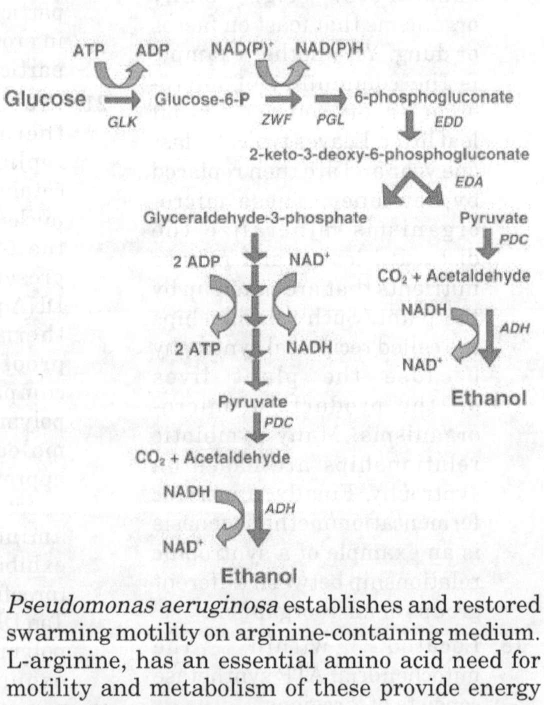

30. *Pseudomonas aeruginosa* establishes and restored swarming motility on arginine-containing medium. L-arginine, has an essential amino acid need for motility and metabolism of these provide energy to tail of bacteria to movement.

(N) ZOOLOGY

1. Although Earth was created around 4.5 billion years ago, life began to exist not long after. Due to the huge timescales involved, there is inconclusive evidence for exact dates, but nonetheless, the eagerness of life to exist was apparent from the beginning. Life on Earth began more than 3 billion years ago, evolving from the most basic of microbes into a dazzling array of complexity over time.
2. The hierarchy of biological classification has eight major taxonomic ranks. These are: Domain $\rightarrow$ Kingdom $\rightarrow$ Phylum $\rightarrow$ Class $\rightarrow$ Order $\rightarrow$ Family $\rightarrow$ Genus $\rightarrow$ Species. As such, class has the maximum number of orders, order has the maximum number of families, family has the maximum number of genus and genus contains the maximum number of species. Therefore, in terms of hierarchy, class has the largest number of species.
3. In humans, each cell normally contains 23 pairs of chromosomes, for a total of 46. Twenty-two of these pairs, called autosomes, look the same in both males and females. The 23rd pair, the sex chromosomes, differs between males and females. Females have two copies of the X chromosome, while males have one X and one Y chromosome. The 22 autosomes are numbered by size. The other two chromosomes, X and Y, are the sex chromosomes. Chromosomes 1-22 are numbered roughly in order of decreasing size. Somatic cells usually have one copy of chromosomes 1-22 from each parent, plus an X chromosome from the mother and either an X or Y chromosome from the father, for a total of 46. There are estimated 20,000-25,000 human protein-coding genes.
4. Microfilaments are solid rods made of a protein known as actin. When it is first produced by the cell, actin appears in a globular form. In microfilaments, however, which are also often referred to as actin filaments, long polymerized chains of the molecules are intertwined in a helix, creating a filamentous form of the protein (F-actin). All of the subunits that compose a microfilament are connected in such a way that they have the same orientation. Due to this fact, each microfilament exhibits polarity, the two ends of the filament being distinctly different. This polarity affects the growth rate of microfilaments, one end (termed the plus end) typically assembling and disassembling faster than the other (the minus end).
5. Mitochondria are structures within cells that convert the energy from food into a form that cells can use. Although most DNA is packaged in chromosomes within the nucleus, mitochondria also have a small amount of their own DNA. This genetic material is known as mitochondrial DNA or mtDNA. Mitochondria are a double membrane bound structure consisting of an outer membrane and an inner membrane. The intra-membrane space is called periplasmic space filled with periplasmic fluid. The inner membrane folds over many times (cristae). That folding increases the surface area inside the organelle. Many of the chemical reactions happen on the inner membrane of the mitochondria.
6. Polysaccharides are carbohydrate polymers consisting of tens to hundreds to several thousand monosaccharide units. All of the common polysaccharides contain glucose as the monosaccharide unit. Polysaccharides are synthesized by plants, animals, and humans to be stored for food, structural support, or metabolized for energy. Glycogen is the storage form of glucose in animals and humans which is analogous to the starch in plants. Glycogen is synthesized and stored mainly in the liver and the muscles. Structurally, glycogen is very similar to amylopectin with alpha acetal linkages, however, it has even more branching and more glucose units are present than in amylopectin.
7. The hormone testosterone is produced by the Leydig cells of testes in males. It is a steroid hormone. Testosterone is necessary for normal sperm development. It activates genes in Sertoli cells, which promote differentiation of spermat-ogonia. It also contributes to the puberty and secondary sexual characters in male.
8. IgA antibodies protect body surfaces that are exposed to outside foreign substances. Immunoglobulin A (IgA), as the major class of antibody present in the mucosal secretions of most mammals, represents a key first line of defence against invasion by inhaled and ingested pathogens at the vulnerable mucosal surfaces. IgA is also found at significant concentrations in the serum of many species, where it functions as a second line of defence mediating elimination of pathogens that have breached the mucosal surface. Receptors specific for the Fc region of IgA, FcαR, are key mediators of IgA effector function. This type of antibody is also found in saliva, tears, and blood. About 10% to 15% of the antibodies present in the body are IgA antibodies. The principal function of secretory IgA may not be to destroy antigen but to prevent passage of foreign substances into the circulatory system.
9. A secondary consumer is part of the food chain. Secondary consumers are animals that eat herbivores. For example, snakes are secondary consumers because they eat rabbits (herbivores), which only eat grass. It is an organism that largely feeds on primary consumers. Carnivores feeding on herbivores or detritivores are called secondary consumers of the food chain.
10. In sexual reproduction, two parents donate genes to their young, resulting in offspring with a mix of inherited genes. These genes are donated through a process called fertilization. There are two mechanisms by which fertilization can take place. The first is external (the eggs are fertilized outside of the body), and the second is internal (the eggs are fertilized within the female reproductive tract). Animals that use internal fertilization specialize in the protection of the developing egg. After the fertilization process, the parental care for internally produced offsprings is provided by the father.

11. The pyrimidine bases have a 6-membered ring with two nitrogens and four carbons. The purine bases have a 9-membered double-ring system with four nitrogens and five carbons. Although both purine and pyrimidine rings have one 6-membered component with two nitrogens and four carbons, they are not related metabolically. Distinct pathways for purine biosynthesis and degradation and for pyrimidine biosynthesis and degradation exist in all organisms. Adenine and guanine are purines while cytosine, thymine and uracil are pyrimidines. Cytosine has hydrogen at its 5th position of the carbon atom. Whereas, thymine has a methyl ($-CH_3$) group at its 5th carbon atom.

12. Given, that the G ≡ C content of a double stranded DNA is 50%. Therefore, the rest 50% is covered by A = T sequences. According to Chargaff's rule, the number of purine is equal to the number of pyrimidine in a double stranded DNA molecule. This means that adenine (A) is equal to thymine (T) and guanine (G) is equal to cytosine (C). This is so because A bonds with T through two hydrogen bonds whereas G bonds with C through three hydrogen bonds. Thus A : T = 1:1 and G : C = 1:1.

13. Histones are highly alkaline proteins found in eukaryotic cell nuclei that package and order the DNA into structural units called nucleosomes. They are the chief protein components of chromatin, acting as spools around which DNA winds, and play a role in gene regulation. Without histones, the unwound DNA in chromosomes would be very long. Five major families of histones exist: H1or H5, H2A, H2B, H3, and H4. Histones H2A, H2B, H3 and H4 are known as the core histones, while histones H1 and H5 are known as the linker histones. The linker histone H1 binds the nucleosome at the entry and exit sites of the DNA, thus locking the DNA into place and allowing the formation of higher order structure. Two of each of the core histones assembles to form one octameric nucleosome core particle, and 147 base pairs of DNA wrap around this core particle 1.65 times in a left-handed super-helical turn. The assembled histones and DNA is called chromatin.

14. Phylogenetic character is determined by the type of evolutionary relatedness. The number and types of differences that accumulate between genes or proteins of two different species can be used to assess their evolutionary relatedness and the amount of time since they diverged from a common ancestor. Ribosomal RNA is used to measure the extent of evolutionary relatedness based on divergent or convergent evolution and substitution or mutation of the base pairs of rRNA. If the predicted amino acid sequence of a newly discovered protein is similar to a known protein in another species, researchers can make guesses about the function of the newly discovered gene based on homology and evolutionary relatedness.

15. Immunoglobulin Alpha (IgA) is composed of α-heavy chain and light chain polypeptides joined together by disulphide linkages between the two. When IgA is electrophoresed, then the two polypeptide chains fragment and break down giving rise to two bands on the gel run. Thus, the number of polypeptide bands detected is 2.

16. Primary lymphoid organs in mammals are those which are directly involved in providing immunity and possessing the power of self and non-self recognition. Primary lymphoid organs originate from the lymphoid progenitor. In mammals, the primary or central lymphoid organs are the thymus and the bone marrow. The thymus gland is a two lobed, glandular organ that lies in the chest under the breast bone. The cells housed within the thymus are primarily white cells called T lymphocytes, along with smaller amounts of other lymphoid cells. All blood cells come from what are called stem cells within the bone marrow. It is in the marrow that the various white blood cells of the immune system form and migrate out into the circulation. The bone marrow is found primarily in the inner, hollow spaces of the flat bones and long bones of the skeleton, and comprises about 5 percent of human body weight.

17. A telomere is a repeating DNA sequence (for example, TTAGGG) at the end of the body's chromosomes. The telomere can reach a length of 15,000 base pairs. Telomerase, also called telomere terminal transferase, is an enzyme made of protein and RNA subunits that elongates chromosomes by adding TTAGGG sequences to the end of existing chromosomes. Telomerase is found in foetal tissues (embryonic cells), adult germ cells (haematopoietic stem cell), and also tumour cells. Telomerase activity is regulated during development and has a very low, almost undetectable activity in somatic (body) cells.

18. Apicomplexan parasites cause severe diseases such as malaria, toxoplasmosis, and coccidiosis (caused by *Plasmodium spp.*, *Toxoplasma*, and *Eimeria*, respectively). These parasites contain a relict plastid-termed "apicoplast"—that originated from the engulfment of an organism of the red algal lineage. The apicoplast has its own genome and expresses a small number of genes, but the vast majority of the apicoplast proteome is encoded in the nuclear genome. The products of these nuclear genes are post-translationally targeted to the organelle via the secretory pathway courtesy of a bipartite N-terminal leader sequence. Apicoplasts are non-photo-synthetic but retain other typical plastid functions such as fatty acid, isoprenoid and heme

synthesis, and products of these pathways might be exported from the apicoplast for use by the parasite. Apicoplast pathways are essentially prokaryotic in nature.

19. The gamete formed by spermatogenesis is essentially a motile nucleus, the gamete formed by oogenesis contains all the materials needed to initiate and maintain metabolism and development. Therefore, in addition to forming a haploid nucleus, oogenesis also builds up a store of cytoplasmic enzymes, mRNAs, organelles, and metabolic substrates. While the sperm becomes differentiated for motility, the egg develops a remarkably complex cytoplasm. When the primary oocyte divides, its nucleus, called the germinal vesicle, breaks down, and the metaphase spindle migrates to the periphery of the cell. At telophase, one of the two daughter cells contains hardly any cytoplasm, whereas the other cell has nearly the entire volume of cellular constituents. The smaller cell is called the first polar body, and the larger cell is referred to as the secondary oocyte. During the second division of meiosis, a similar unequal cytokinesis takes place. Most of the cytoplasm is retained by the mature egg (ovum), and a second polar body receives little more than a haploid nucleus. In spermatogenesis, four motile sperms are produced through meiotic and mitotic divisions.

20. Because of hyperimmunization of the male rabbit with sheep RBCs, antibody of the male rabbit in the plasma cells underwent a hypermutation. As such, the male rabbit is modified in its antigenic response against the sheep RBCs resulting in loss of antigenic response against the foreign antigen. Now, when the mutated male is crossed with a normal female rabbit, the F_1 progeny would possess the mutation resulting in suppression of immunogenic response against the sheep 221RBC. Hence, the titer of the F_1 progeny (both2z male and female) against the sheep RBC would be 1 : 0 or 0.

21. Blood returns to the heart from the body via two large blood vessels, called the superior vena cava and the inferior vena cava. This blood carries little oxygen, as it is returning from the body where oxygen is used. The blood first enters the right atrium. It then flows through the tricuspid valve into the right ventricle. When the heart contracts, the ventricle sends the blood through the pulmonary valve into the pulmonary artery. The pulmonary artery carries blood to the lungs where it picks up oxygen, and leaves the lungs and returns to the heart through the pulmonary vein. The blood enters the left atrium, and then descends through the mitral valve into the left ventricle. The left ventricle then pumps blood through the aortic valve, and into the aorta, the blood vessel that leads to the rest of the body. Thus, the sequence would be Right ventricle → Pulmonary arteries → Lungs → Pulmonary veins → Left autrium.

22. Plantigrade is a position in which an individual is standing flexed at the hips and bearing some weight through the upper extremities. It is a method of locomotion seen in bears, monkeys and humans, in which the animal walks on the phalanges, metacarpal and carpal bones. Digitigrade is an animal that walks so that only the toes touch the ground as e.g. dogs and cats and horses. In mammals, it is like walking on the toes with the posterior part of the foot raised (as cats, dogs, and horses do). Unguligrade animals are several groups of mammals, most of which use the tips of their toes, usually hoofed, to sustain their whole body weight while moving. Therefore, based on the relative length of the limbs, the gaits can be organised as Plantigrade > Digitigrade > Ungligrade.

23. The sex chromosome for the suffering man would have the alleles as X^cY or XY^c where X^cY would be the sex chromosome if the disorder is female sex related (XX^c) so that the man contracted the disease from his mother and XY^c would be the sex chromosome if he inherited it from his father (XY^c) so that the disease is male sex linked. Now, not all the sons and daughters of the man suffer from the disease. This is true if only the disease trait carrier was a female i.e., his mother because if it were his father and the disease trait was Y-linked or male sex linked, then all his sons would have contracted the disease. So, his mother was the carrier of the disease.

24. In terms of productivity due to accumulation of organic matter per m^2 annually, it is given as:

Tropical forest = 45 kg/m^2

Temperate forest = 30–32 kg/m^2

Boreal forest = 20 kg/m^2

Cultivated land = 1kg/m^2

Therefore, decreasing order of productivity is given by: Tropical forest > Temperate forest > Boreal forest > Cultivated land.

25. Male lions kill young cubs to impregnate the females. They will attempt to kill any cubs that are roughly nine months old or younger, though as in other species, the female will attempt to defend her cubs viciously. It is estimated that a quarter of cubs dying in the first year of life are victims of infanticide. Males have, on average, only a two-year window in which to pass on their genes, and lionesses only give birth once every two years, so the selective pressure on them to conform to this behaviour this is strong. So, the dominance of the male lions in the pride is established.

26. Given, the cross over frequency for a four gene loci (PQRS) on a chromosome:-

P – Q = 30, Q – R = 25, Q – S = 15, R – S = 10, P – R = 5.

Since P – Q = 30, this means P and Q are at the 2 terminal ends of the gene. And, P – R = 5, means that P and R are the closest to each other.

Now, adding R – S = 10 and P – R = 5, we have → P – S = 15; So, if we take P at one end, then after P, it would be R and then after R it would be S based on the cross over frequency values. So the gene sequence would be either 'PRSQ' or 'QSRP'.

27. Hardy-Weinberg law is an algebraic equation that describes the genetic equilibrium within a population. In the simplest case of a single locus with two alleles: allele one is denoted A and allele two a and their frequencies are denoted by p and q; freq (A) = p; freq (a) = q; p + q = 1. If mating is random, then new individuals will have freq (AA) = p^2 for the AA homozygotes in the population, freq (aa) = q^2 for the aa homozygotes, and freq (Aa) = 2pq for the heterozygote.

The formula is written as $(p^2) + (2pq) + (q^2) = 1$, representing the fact that probabilities must add up to one. Using the law, we have:-

q = 10% = 0.1; we have p + q = 1, therefore p = 1 – q = 1 – 0.1 = 0.9.

Therefore, dominant allelic frequency is 90%. For heterozygous phenotype, Aa, the frequency of heterozygosity is given by:-

$$2pq = 2 \times 0.9 \times 0.1 = 0.18.$$

Therefore, the % frequency of heterozygous genotype in the population = 18 %.

28. Given, rohu and catla have an equal chance of being caught in the net.

Now,

Number of tagged rohu fish released in the pond = 100

Number of rohu fishes caught = 10

Therefore, percentage of fishes caught = $\left(\frac{10}{100} \times 100\right)\% = 10\%$ which is the chance of getting caught by the tagged rohu fish. Therefore, 10% is the chance of getting caught by the untagged rohu fish and catla fish in the lake.

Therefore, Number of untagged rohu fish caught = 12

So, total number of untagged rohu fish

$$= \frac{(12 \times 100)}{10} = 120$$

Therefore, total number of rohu fish in the lake = 100 + 120 = 220

Number of catla fish caught = 8

Therefore, total number of catla fish in the lake = $\frac{(8 \times 100)}{10} = 80$

29. Reverse transcriptase, also called RNA-directed DNA polymerase, is an enzyme encoded from the genetic material of retroviruses that catalyzes the transcription of retrovirus RNA (ribonucleic acid) into DNA (deoxyribonucleic acid). This catalyzed transcription is the reverse process of normal cellular transcription of DNA into RNA; hence the names reverse transcriptase and retrovirus. Reverse transcriptase is central to the infectious nature of retroviruses, several of which cause disease in humans, including human immunodeficiency virus (HIV), which causes acquired immunodeficiency syndrome (AIDS), and human T-cell lymphotrophic virus I (HTLV-I), which causes leukaemia. Reverse transcriptase is also a fundamental component of a laboratory technology known as reverse transcription-polymerase chain reaction (RT-PCR), a powerful tool used in research and in the diagnosis of diseases such as cancer.

30. The Austrian zoologist Karl von Frisch (1886-1982) is noted for his studies of insect behaviour and sensory physiology. His most famous discovery was that honeybees communicate by waggle dancing. He, along with Konrad Lorenz and Nikolaas Tinbergern, shared the 1973 Nobel Prize for physiology or medicine. Konrad Lorenz was an Austrian zoologist. He is the founder of modern ethology and the study of animal behaviour by means of comparative zoological methods. His ideas contributed to an understanding of how behavioural patterns may be traced to an evolutionary past, and he was also known for his work on the roots of aggression.

■■

GATE-2002

XL : LIFE SCIENCES

Time : 3 Hours **_Maximum Marks : 100_**

(H) CHEMISTRY (Compulsory)

Useful data :

Gas constant, R = 8.314 $JK^{-1} mol^{-1}$

Planck's constant, $h = 6.626 \times 10^{-34}$ Js

I1. For each question given below, four alternative answers are provided of which only one is correct. Write the correct answer in the answeer book by writing *a, b, c* or *d* along with the corresponding sub-question number. (25 × 1 = 25)

1.1 The ground state electronic configuration of iron [Ar] $3d^6 4s^2$. The electronic configuration of ferric iron is

(*a*) [Ar] $3d^6 4s^0$ (*b*) [Ar] $3d^4 4s^2$

(*c*) [Ar] $3d^5 4s^0$ (*d*) [Ar] $3d^3 4s^2$

1.2 In fluorite structure, the coordination number of calcium is

(*a*) 3 (*b*) 4 (*c*) 6 (*d*) 8

1.3 Nickel forms a stable complex with cyanide ion having the composition $[Ni(CN)_4]^{2-}$. The atomic number of nickel is 28. The magnetic moment of the complex in Bohr magneton is

(*a*) 0 (*b*) 1.73 (*c*) 2.83 (*d*) 3.87

1.4 Among the following compounds the one that generates H_2O_2 on acidification is

(*a*) PbO_2 (*b*) MnO_2 (*c*) BaO_2 (*d*) SnO_2

1.5 The complex $[Co(NH_3)_5Cl]Cl_2$ reacts with an aqueous solution of silver nitrate quantitatively. The number of moles of silver chloride formed per mole of the complex is

(*a*) 1 (*b*) 2 (*c*) 3 (*d*) 5

1.6 Among the following the one that is NOT an amphoteric oxide is

(*a*) Al_2O_3 (*b*) MgO (*c*) ZnO (*d*) SnO

1.7 The formula of peroxodisulphuric acid is

(*a*) H_2SO_5 (*b*) $H_2S_2O_3$ (*c*) $H_2S_2O_4$ (*d*) $H_2S_2O_8$

1.8 The oxidation states of sulphur atoms in $Na_2S_2O_3$ are

(*a*) +2, –6 (*b*) +2, +2 (*c*) +2, +6 (*d*) –2, +6

1.9 The pair that shows critical solution temperature in a composition-temperature phase diagram is

(*a*) phenol-water (*b*) phenol-benzene

(*c*) chloroform-water (*d*) methanol-water

1.10 The van't Hoff factor for a completely dissociated aqueous solution of $K_4[Fe(CN)_6]$ is

(*a*) 1 (*b*) 2 (*c*) 3 (*d*) 5

1.11 The solubility product of a sparingly soluble salt, AX_3 in water is 2.7×10^{-31} at 298 K. The solubility of the salt in mol l^{-1} is

(*a*) 5×10^{-16} (*b*) 1×10^{-13} (*c*) 4×10^{-11} (*d*) 1×10^{-8}

1.12 If the standard reduction potential of Fe^{3+}/Fe^{2+} is 0.77 V, then the reduction potential of the electrode Pt/Fe^{3+}(0.1 M), Fe^{2+}(1.0 M) at 298 K is

(*a*) 0.67 V (*b*) 0.71 V (*c*) 0.77 V (*d*) 0.83 V

1.13 Among the following statements the one that is NOT true for a zero order reaction is

(*a*) $t_{1/2}$ is directly proportional to the initial concentration of the reactant

(*b*) the time taken for 75% reaction is 1.5 times that of $t_{1/2}$

(*c*) the rate constant has the dimensions of concentration $time^{-1}$

(*d*) the concentration of the reactant decreases exponentially with time.

1.14 For the gaseous equilibrium $PCl_5 \rightleftharpoons PCl_3 + Cl_2$, the degree of dissociation of PCl_5 is 0.80 at 1 atm. The degree of dissociation at 2 atm is

(*a*) 0.69 (*b*) 0.80

(*c*) 0.85 (*d*) 0.90

1.15 Among the following the one that is an extensive variable is

(*a*) density (*b*) volume

(*c*) specific heat (*d*) temperature

1.16 For an adiabatic irreversible expansion of one mole of an ideal gas

(*a*) ΔS (system) > 0 and ΔS (surroundings) = 0

(*b*) ΔS (system) = 0 and ΔS (surroundings) = 0

(*c*) ΔS (system) < 0 and ΔS (surroundings) > 0

(*d*) ΔS (system) > 0 and ΔS (surroundings) < 0

1.17 Among the following the correct statement is

(*a*) pH of water at 333 K is less than 7

(*b*) pH of 0.1 M NH_4Cl (*aq*) > 0.1 M NaCl (*aq*)

(*c*) pH of 0.1 M CH_3COOH (*aq*) < 0.1 M HCl (*aq*)

(*d*) pH of 10^{-8} M HCl is 8

1.18 Isobutyl alcohol is prepared from the reaction of

(*a*) CH_3CH_2MgBr and CH_3CHO

(*b*) CH_3MgBr and CH_3CH_2CHO

(*c*) $(CH_3)_2CHMgBr$ and HCHO

(*d*) CH_3MgBr and CH_3COCH_3

1.19 The major product obtained by the dehydration of 1-methylcyclohexanol is

(*a*) 1-methylcyclohexene

(*b*) 3-methylcyclohexene

(*c*) 4-methylcyclohexene

(*d*) methylenecyclohexane

1.20 Reaction of aniline with chloroform and KOH produces

(*a*) *ortho*-chloroaniline

(*b*) phenylisocyanide

(*c*) benzoic acid

(*d*) benzenediazonium chloride

1.21 The major product formed on bromination of acetanilide is

(*a*) *ortho*-bromoacetanilide

(*b*) *meta*-bromoacetanilide

(*c*) *para*-bromoacetanilide

(*d*) N-bromoacetanilide

1.22 Among the following the one that is aromatic is

(*a*) cyclohexadienyl cation

(*b*) cycloheptatrienyl cation

(*c*) cyclopentadienyl cation

(*d*) cyclopropyl cation

1.23 The number of stereoisomers possible for 2-bromo-3-chlorobutane is

(*a*) 1 (*b*) 2 (*c*) 3 (*d*) 4

1.24 The solid product formed by the reaction of ammonia with formaldehyde is

(*a*) ammonium formate

(*b*) formaldehyde imine

(*c*) hexamethylenetetramine

(*d*) formamide

1.25 Conversion of benzaldehyde to cinnamic acid is known as

(*a*) Perkin reaction

(*b*) Riemer-Tiemann reaction

(*c*) Cannizzaro reaction

(*d*) Kolbe reaction

I2. (*a*) A metal reacts with hot conc. H_2SO_4 to produce a gas(A) and a blue coloured solution. The gas evolved turns acidified dichromate paper to green colour (B). Identify the chemical species (A) and (B). (2)

(*b*) Calculate the de Broglie wavelength in nm associated with a ball weighing 0.15 kg thrown with a velocity of 30 ms^{-1}. (2)

(*c*) Apply phase rule to show that at the normal bioling point of a liquid, the number of degrees of freedom is zero. (1)

I3. Match each item in Column A with the most appropriate item in Column B.

Column - A	Column - B
(*i*) Sodium aluminium silicate	(*a*) Chelating agent
(*ii*) Titanium dioxide	(*b*) reducing agent
(*iii*) Sodium tripolyphosphate	(*c*) carborundum
(*iv*) Sodium borohydride	(*d*) zeolite
(*v*) Solid carbon dioxide	(*e*) rutile structure
	(*f*) silicon
	(*g*) dry ice

I4. (*a*) The molar conductivity of acetic acid (K_a = 1.8 × 10^{-5}) at infinite dilution is 39.0 × 10^{-3} S m^2 mol^{-1}. Find the molarity of acetic acid, if the measured molar conductivity is 1.56 × 10^{-3} S m^2 mol^{-1}. (2)

(*b*) For a gaseous reaction A + B → C at 300 K, $\Delta U = -12.6$ kJ mol^{-1} and $\Delta S = -42.0$ J K^{-1} mol^{-1}. Calculate ΔG for the reaction. (2)

(*c*) The variation of rate constant for a reaction with temperature is given by the expression

$$\ln K = 30 - [10{,}000/T]$$

Calculate the energy of activation of the reaction. (1)

I5. (*a*) Draw the resonance structures of methoxybenzene (anisole). (2)

(*b*) Explain why optically active 2-iodooctane undergoes racemization when reacted with KI in acetone? (2)

(*c*) Draw the structure of the enol form of acetylacetone. (1)

I6. (*a*) Suggest a suitable method for the synthesis of 3-ethylaniline from acetophenone. (2)

(*b*) Why is it not advisable to use *t*-butyl chloride and sodium ethoxide do prepare *t*-butyl ethyl ether? Suggest an alternative method. (2)

(*c*) Write the structure of the Diels-Alder adduct formed from the reaction of cyclopentadiene with dimethyl acetylenedicarboxylate. (1)

(J) BIOCHEMISTRY

J1. For each of the sub-question given below, four alternatives are given of which only one is appropriate. Write the answer in the answer book by writing *a*, *b*, *c* or *d* along with the corresponding sub-question number. (1 × 25 = 25)

1.1 Proteins maybe separated according to size by,

(*a*) Reverse phase chromatography

(*b*) Ion exchange chromatography

(*c*) Molecular exclusion chromatography

(*d*) Isoelectric focussing

1.2 Which of the following has a quaternary structure?

(*a*) α-chymotrypsin (*b*) Haemoglobin

(*c*) Insulin (*d*) Myoglobin

1.3 Which of the following anti-tumour agent acts by impairing the *de novo* purine synthesis?
(*a*) Cytosine arabinoside
(*b*) 5-fluorouracil
(*c*) Methotrexate
(*d*) Hydroxyurea

1.4 Which of the following is a conservative substitution?
(*a*) Val to Ile (*b*) Asp to Pro
(*c*) Lys to Leu (*d*) Trp to Ala

1.5 cAMP activates all except one of the following molecules,
(*a*) Glycogen phosphorylase
(*b*) Hexokinase
(*c*) 6-Phosphofructokinase-l-kinase
(*d*) Protein kinase A

1.6 Which of the following statements is correct in case of glycoproteins?
(*a*) May contain 95% or more of carbohydrate
(*b*) Have the carbohydrate linked to the protein by either N- or O- glycosidic bonds
(*c*) Found only on cell membranes
(*d*) Always contain a serially repeating carbohydrate unit

1.7 Phospholipids are involved in all except one of the following,
(*a*) Cell-cell recognition
(*b*) Signal transduction
(*c*) Surfactant function in the lungs
(*d*) mediator of hypersensitivity

1.8 Insulin-dependent diabetes mellitus is associated with,
(*a*) High levels of insulin
(*b*) Severe weight gain
(*c*) Destruction of β-cells of pancreas
(*d*) Mutation of insulin receptor

1.9 The z-DNA helix,
(*a*) Has fewer base pairs per turn than the B-DNA
(*b*) Is favoured by an alternating GC sequence
(*c*) Tends to be found at the 3′ end of genes
(*d*) Is the most common conformation of DNA

1.10 Formation of a mature insulin does not include,
(*a*) Removal of a signal peptide
(*b*) Disulfide bond formation
(*c*) Removal of a peptide from an internal region
(*d*) Cyclization of a glutamate residue

1.11 How many energy bonds are expended in the formation of a peptide bond ?
(*a*) 2 (*b*) 4
(*c*) 3 (*d*) 6

1.12 A technique for defining gene arrangement in very long stretches of DNA (50-100 kb) is,
(*a*) RFLP
(*b*) Chromosome walking
(*c*) Nick translation
(*d*) Southern blotting

1.13 Receptors for steroid hormones are found,
(*a*) On cell membranes
(*b*) In cytoplasm
(*c*) In mitochondria
(*d*) On ribosomes

1.14 Platelet aggregation is,
(*a*) Initiated at the site of injury by the conversion of fibrinogen to fibrin
(*b*) Causes release of serotonin
(*c*) Is inhibited by uninjured blood vessels by the secretion of prostacyclins
(*d*) Is inhibited by ADP and thromboxane

1.15 Oral administration of large amounts of tyrosine may interfere with the intestinal absorption of,
(*a*) Leucine (*b*) Glycine
(*c*) Asparatate (*d*) All of the above

1.16 In the 3-dimensional structure of immunoglobulin G,
(*a*) Free SH-groups are conserved to function in binding of antigen
(*b*) C_H and V_H association form the complementary antigen binding sites
(*c*) The predominant secondary structure is α-helix
(*d*) Hinge regions connect the globular domains

1.17 Changes in protein conformation can be detected by,
(*a*) Ultraviolet absorption spectroscopy
(*b*) Fluorescence emission
(*c*) Circular dichroism
(*d*) All of the above

1.18 Endonuclease is an enzyme that hydrolyzes,
(*a*) A nucleotide at the 3′ end of an oligonucleotide
(*b*) A phosphodiester bond located in the interior of a polynucleotide
(*c*) A nucleotide from either terminii of an oligonucleotide
(*d*) A peptide bond located in the interior of a polypeptide

1.19 The Km of an enzyme is,
(*a*) One half of the Vmax
(*b*) A dissociation constant
(*c*) The substrate concentration that gives maximal velocity
(*d*) The substrate concentration that gives half maximal velocity

1.20 The class of immunoglobulins most abundant in body fluids is,

(*a*) IgM (*b*) IgG (*c*) IgA (*d*) IgE

1.21 Which of the following statements is correct in case of chaperone proteins?

(*a*) These do not prevent aggregation

(*b*) They cleave incorrect S-S bonds

(*c*) Act on fully synthesized polypeptides

(*d*) Are involved in the transport of proteins across mitochondria and endoplasmic reticulum

1.22 One of the following participates in phagocytic activities,

(*a*) Neutrophils (*b*) Mast cells

(*c*) T cells (*d*) Thrombocytes

1.23 The basal metabolic rate,

(*a*) Is not influenced by energy intake

(*b*) Increases in response to starvation

(*c*) Increases in direct proportion to energy expenditure

(*d*) Decreases during periods of starvation

1.24 Operons,

(*a*) Are of approximately uniform in size

(*b*) Do not bind proteins

(*c*) Are found in all eukaryotic genes

(*d*) Are shorter and smaller in lower eukaryotes than higher eukaryotes

1.25 In humans, fatty acids,

(*a*) Can be synthesized from excess dietary carbohydrate or protein

(*b*) Must be supplied entirely by diet

(*c*) Are not required at all in the diet

(*d*) Containing double bonds cannot be synthesized

J2. (*a*) Blood groups are determined by the allelic genes A, B and O. These genes code for different enzymes that result in the production of blood group antigens. What is the nature of these enzymes? (2)

(*b*) Where are Rh antigens found? (1)

(*c*) How many genes determine Rh antigens? (1)

(*d*) Name the immunodominant Rh antigen (1)

J3. Match the entries in column I with one appropriate from column II and write matching pairs in the answer books (1 × 5 = 5)

Column - I	Column - II
(A) Apoptosis	(*i*) CD3 complex
(B) T cell receptor	(*ii*) Caspases
(C) 5-Hydroxytrytamine	(*iii*) adenylate cyclase
(D) β-adrenergic receptor	(*iv*) Mitotic spindle
(E) Colchicine	(*v*) Neurotransmitter
	(*vi*) Immunosuppressive
	(*vii*) DNA binding protein

J4. (*a*) What is the possible number of protein sequence that can be read from a genomic sequence? (1)

(*b*) What are the different activities present in the Klenow fragment? Name the enzyme from which Klenow originates? (2)

(*c*) In order to end-label a DNA molecule at its 5′ end, what is the nature of the labeled nucleotide is used? Name the enzyme used. (2)

J5. (1 × 5 = 5)

(*a*) What effect would the removal of the bursa of fabricius have on chickens?

(*b*) Name the primary lymphoid organs in the adult human.

(*c*) Define monoclonal antibodies.

(*d*) Which are the two isotypes of immunoglobulins that can be simultan-eously expressed on naive B cells?

(*e*) What is the precursor of histamine?

J6. A purified enzyme preparation (3 mg/ml) was diluted 10 times. 10 l of the diluted enzyme catalyzed the formation of 30 nmoles of product/min under standard assay conditions.

(*a*) Express the velocity as moles of product/min/mg. (2)

(*b*) What does the velocity expressed in moles/min/mg signify? (1)

(*c*) If the molecular weight of the enzyme is 30,000, calculate its turnover Number. (2)

(L) BOTANY

L1. For each sub-question given below, four alternatives are provided of which only one is correct. Write the correct answer in the answer book by writing *a*, *b*, *c* or *d* along with the sub-question number. (25 × 1 = 25)

1.1 Which of the following cell organelles involved in photorespiration?

(*a*) Peroxisomes (*b*) Ribosomes

(*c*) Dictyosomes (*d*) Lysosomes

1.2 Plasmodesmata connect neighbouring cells, forming a

(*a*) Symplast (*b*) Apoplast

(*c*) Protoplast (*d*) Tonoplast

1.3 Which of the following is wrong for isobilateral leaves?

(*a*) Stomata occur on both the epidermis

(*b*) Mesophyll tissue is of one kind

(*c*) Generally found in monocots

(*d*) Presence of pallisade and spongy cells

1.4 Tyloses are found in

(*a*) Tracheids

(*b*) Xylem vessels

(*c*) Xylem parenchyma

(*d*) Xylem fibers

1.5 The loss of liquid water through hydathode is called
(*a*) Guttation (*b*) Transpiration
(*c*) Secretion (*d*) Bleeding

1.6 In which phase of the cell cycle the drug colchicine exerts its effect?
(*a*) G1 (*b*) S (*c*) G2 (*d*) M

1.7 The condition when anthers mature earlier than stigma is known as
(*a*) Dicliny (*b*) Herkogamy
(*c*) Protandry (*d*) Protogyny

1.8 The stalk with which the ovule remains attached to the placenta is called
(*a*) Funicle (*b*) Hilum
(*c*) Micropyle (*d*) Nucellus

1.9 Viviparous germination is found in
(*a*) *Rhizophora sp.* (*b*) *Mangifera sp.*
(*c*) *Nymphaea sp.* (*d*) *Typha sp.*

1.10 Seed storage proteins of legumes are deficient in
(*a*) Threonine (*b*) Methionine
(*c*) Lysine (*d*) Glycine

1.11 A hormone that controls closure of stomata in response to water stress is
(*a*) Abscisic acid (*b*) Gibberellins
(*c*) Ethylene (*d*) Zeatin

1.12 The process by which a cell secretes macromolecules by fusing a transport vesicle to the plasma membrane is called
(*a*) Pinocytosis (*b*) Phagocytosis
(*c*) Endocytosis (*d*) Exocytosis

1.13 When a cell expends energy to move a solute across its membrane against a concentration gradient, the process is called
(*a*) Diffusion (*b*) Facilitated diffusion
(*c*) Active transport (*d*) Osmosis

1.14 The CO_2 acceptor in C_4 plants is
(*a*) 3-Phosphoglyceric acid
(*b*) Ribulose bis-phosphate
(*c*) Phosphoenol pyruvic acid
(*d*) Xylulose 5-phosphate

1.15 Absorption maxima of phytochrome (P_{fr}) is
(*a*) 660 nm (*b*) 680 nm (*c*) 700 nm (*d*) 730 nm

1.16 Light harvesting complex II is located in the
(*a*) Thylakoid lumen
(*b*) Stroma
(*c*) Thylakoid membrane
(*d*) Outer membrane of chloroplast

1.17 A known uncoupler of the electron transport chain and oxidative phosphorylation is
(*a*) Dinitrophenol (*b*) Ancymidol
(*c*) Triacontanol (*d*) Hexaconazol

1.18 The chromatin fibers at metaphase have an average diameter of
(*a*) 100 A° (*b*) 200 A° (*c*) 300 A° (*d*) 400 A°

1.19 The maximum frequency of a recombination of genes at two loci is
(*a*) 25% (*b*) 50% (*c*) 75% (*d*) 100%

1.20 Symbiotic association between fungi and roots of higher plants is known as
(*a*) Mycorrhiza (*b*) Lichen
(*c*) Coralloid roots (*d*) Epiphytic roots

1.21 Ergot of rye is caused by
(*a*) *Fusarium oxysporum* (*b*) *Claviceps purpurea*
(*c*) *Aspergillus niger* (*d*) *Alternaria solani*

1.22 Production of transgenic cotton resistant to lepidopteran insects utilizes a toxin-producing gene isolated from
(*a*) *Pseudomonas fluorescens*
(*b*) *Bacillus thuringiensis*
(*c*) *Bipolaris maydis*
(*d*) *Clostridium tetani*

1.23 Hutchinson's phylogenetic system of classification appeared in the volume
(*a*) Genera Plantarum
(*b*) Hortus Uplandicus
(*c*) Die Naturlichen Pflanzenfamilen
(*d*) Families of Flowering Plants

1.24 Plants occurring on saline soils are called
(*a*) Hydrophytes (*b*) Epiphytes
(*c*) Mesophytes (*d*) Halophytes

1.25 A group of interconnected food chains is called
(*a*) Pyramid of energy (*b*) Complex food chain
(*c*) Food web(*d*)Food cycle

L2. Write botanical name of the most common plant yielding the following products
(*a*) Menthol (*b*) Nicotine
(*c*) Papain (*d*) Taxol
(*e*) Vanillin (5 × 1 = 5)

L3. (*a*) List two physiological functions of leghaemoglobin in N_2 fixation. (2)
(*b*) Name the precursor, intermediates and enzymes involved in ethylene biosynthesis pathway. (3)

L4. (*a*) How does shoot organogenesis differ from somatic embryogenesis? (2)
(*b*) In what ways are double haploids useful in breeding programme? (3)

L5. (*a*) Diagrammatically represent *cis* and *trans* arrangements for two pairs (A and B are two dominant forms) of linked genes. (2)
(*b*) What functions do telomere provide? (3)

L6. (*a*) Narrate the usefulness of reporter gene and selectable marker in plant transformation studies. (2)
(*b*) Enumerate the role of virA, virB and virDl in T-DNA transfer. (3)

(M) MICROBIOLOGY

M1. For each sub-question given below, four alternatives are provided of which only one is correct. Write the correct answer in the answer book by writing *a*, *b*, *c* or *d* along with the sub-question number. (1 × 25 = 25)

1.1 Which of the statements given below on telomerase is incorrect?
(*a*) Telomerase is a ribonucleoprotein
(*b*) Telomerase can be defined as a reverse transcriptase
(*c*) It is an unusual DNA polymerase as it polymerises in 3′ to 5′ direction.
(*d*) It uses an RNA template to extend the ends of the chromosome

1.2 In order for an electron transport chain (ETC) to function
(*a*) Each component of the ETC should be capable of reduction by the reduced form of previous component and oxidized by the oxidized form of the downstream component
(*b*) Each component of the ETC should be capable of binding oxygen in its active site pocket
(*c*) Each component should be capable of regulating the expression of downstream component
(*d*) Genes of the components of ETC should be located on the same operon

1.3 Electrode potential of hydrogen under physiological conditions is –0.42 V, and that of oxygen is +0.82. If the free energy change is defined by $\Delta Go' = nF\Delta Eo'$, where AGo′ is the free energy change at pH 7.0; n is the number of electrons transferred, F is the Faraday constant (23000 cal/V), and Eo′ is the difference between the electrode potentials. What will be the free energy change upon reduction of oxygen by hydrogen to H_2O.
(*a*) –57,040 cal (*b*) –28,520 cal
(*c*) –23,000 cal (*d*) –104,080 cal

1.4 While facing the minor groove of the right handed double stranded DNA, the left side DNA strand moves up in a
(*a*) 3′ to 5′ direction
(*b*) 5′ to 3′ direction
(*c*) could be either 3′ to 5′ or the 5′ to 3′ direction
(*d*) minor groove does not provide any idea to the direction of strand polarity

1.5 Several eubacterial mRNAs initiate protein synthesis from GUG codon. The initiating amino acid for the proteins encoded by such mRNAs is
(*a*) Met (*b*) fMet (*c*) Val (*d*) fVal

1.6 *Thermus thermophilus* is a
(*a*) Gram negative eubacteria
(*b*) Gram positive eubacteria
(*c*) Gram negative archebacteria
(*d*) Gram positive archebacteria

1.7 Deletion of a single nucleotide from the open reading frame sequence of a mRNA does not result in the following
(*a*) a shorter polypeptide
(*b*) an extended polypeptide
(*c*) an altered N-terminal domain without affecting the C-terminal domain of the polypeptide
(*d*) an altered C-terminal domain without affecting the N-terminal domain of the polypeptide

1.8 Of the following, which component is not required for protein synthesis in archebacteria?
(*a*) Ribosomes (*b*) mRNA
(*c*) release factors (*d*) fMet-tRNA

1.9 A mutant of *E. coli* which expressed lac operon constitutively may have a mutation in the following chromosomal locations,
(*a*) lacI (*b*) lacO
(*c*) lacI or lacO (*d*) lacZ

1.10 What will be the number of antibody specificities in an organism which has 200 V and 5 J genes for the light chain and, 300 V, 10 D and 5 J genes for the heavy chain?
(*a*) 520 (*b*) 1000
(*c*) 15,000,000 (*d*) more than 15,000,000

1.11 Which of the following statements is correct?
(*a*) CD8 binds to an invariant portion of MHC class II molecules
(*b*) CD8 binds to an invariant portion of MHC class I molecules
(*c*) CD8 binds directly to the peptide antigen
(*d*) CD8 binds to the peptide binding site of MHC class I molecules

1.12 Which of the following disease is <u>caused</u> by DNA viruses?
(*a*) Poliomyelitis (*b*) Yellow Fever
(*c*) Measles (*d*) Small pox

1.13 Which of the following disease is <u>not caused</u> by microbial protein toxin?
(*a*) Botulism (*b*) Diptheria
(*c*) Shigella dysentry (*d*) Tuberculosis

1.14 Coxsackie virus B3, a subgroup of enteroviruses, commonly causes:
(*a*) Acute hemorrhagic conjunctivitis
(*b*) Muscular dystrophy
(*c*) Myocarditis
(*d*) Gastroentertitis.

1.15 Immunization with which of the following toxoid induces high titer serum antibody, but does not protect from the corresponding disease?
(*a*) Tetanus (*b*) Botulism
(*c*) Diptheria (*d*) Shigellosis

1.16 All infections do not cause fever and all fevers are not due to infections: which of the following is an example of non-infectious cause of fever?

(*a*) Typhoid
(*b*) Chicken pox
(*c*) Rheumatic disease
(*d*) Malaria

1.17 Which of the following is a primary stain in acid fast staining of mycobacteria?

(*a*) Crystal violet (*b*) Carbol fuchsin
(*c*) Geimsa (*d*) Methylene blue

1.18 Antigenic peptides are presented to T-cells by

(*a*) TCR/CD3 (*b*) CD28
(*c*) CTLA4 (*d*) MHC

1.19 The nature of the poliovirus given for oral vaccination (Sabin vaccine) as part of the irradication program is:

(*a*) Heat killed viruses
(*b*) Live attenuated strains of all three immunological types.
(*c*) Small dosage of wild-type live viruses.
(*d*) Formalin-inactivated viruses

1.20 Which of the following statements on replication in *E. coli* is correct?

(*a*) It occurs in a unidirectional manner
(*b*) It occurs in bidirectional manner
(*c*) Always uses T7 DNA polymerase when infected by T7 phage
(*d*) Occurs only when λ phage has infected *E. coli*

1.21 Retting is a process of biodegradation used for,

(*a*) Degrading retina from dead animals
(*b*) Degrading pectin
(*c*) Degrading cellulose
(*d*) Degrading starch

1.22 Prontosilis

(*a*) an effective antibacterial when used in animals
(*b*) an effective antibacterial when used in *in vitro* cultures
(*c*) an effective antibacterial both in animals as well as in *in vitro* cultures
(*d*) Prontosil can not be used as an antibacterial agent

1.23 Subunit composition of histones in nucleosomes is:

(*a*) (H1)(H2A)(H2B)(H3)(H4)
(*b*) $[(H1)(H2A)(H2B)(H3)(H4)]_2$
(*c*) H1 $[(H2A)(H2B)(H3)(H4)]_2$
(*d*) $[(H2A)(H2B)(H3)(H4)]_2$

1.24 Interval between completion of mitosis and beginning of DNA synthesis is called

(*a*) G1 phase (*b*) G2 phase
(*c*) S phase (*d*) M phase

1.25 During the progression of S-phase cdk2 is partnered by

(*a*) cyclin A
(*b*) cyclin D
(*c*) cyclin E
(*d*) transcription factor E2F

M2. (*a*) Calculate the *writhe* of a covalently closed circular DNA with a linking number of 20 and topological winding number of 22. (2)

(*b*) The chromatin in eukaryotes can exist as a 10 nm or a 30 nm fibre, what is a 10 nm fibre? (1)

(*c*) What is the change in the packaging ratio when a 10 nm fibre is converted to a 30 nm fibre. (2)

M3. Phage Pl lysate was raised on an *E. coli* strain ($Tn10^+$, A^-, B^-, C^-, D^-) and used to transduce a wild type strain of *E. coli.* The transductants were selected on a tetracyclin plate and checked for their phenotypes. Following observations were made. All of the transductants were Tc^R, A^-; 80% were Tc^R, D^-; 20% were Tc^R, B^-; and 5% were Tc^R, C^-. None of the transductants were Tc^R, $A^+B^+C^+D^+$. Assuming that all the markers (A, B, C and D) are downstream of Tn10, answer the following: (1 + 2 + 2)

(*a*) What is the order of A, B, C and D on the chromosome with respect to Tn10?
(*b*) Why do you think that none of the transductants was Tc^R, $A^+B^+C^+D^+$?
(*c*) In a reverse experiment, the Pl lysate was raised on Tc^R, C^- transductants and used to transduce a wild type strain of *E. coli,* what will be the likely frequency of obtaining Tc^R, A^- phenotype.

M4. Of the several DNA polymerases in *E. coli,* DNA polymerase III plays a major role in DNA replication and it is responsible for the synthesis of both the leading strand and the Okazaki fragments in the lagging strand. However, the DNA polymerase I is also required during replication. Answer the following: (1 + 2 + 2)

(*a*) If the DNA polymerase III is mainly responsible for DNA replication, why is DNA polymerase I also needed during replication?
(*b*) While the DNA polymerase III is able to polymerise DNA on its own, it becomes highly processive in the presence of β-subunit, why?
(*c*) Can replication in *E. coli* chromosome begin at any place? If not, what is the exact site where replication begins?

M5. Both the λ, phage and M13 phage infect *E. coli.* Answer the following:

(*a*) λ phage results in the formation of clear plaque, whereas the plaques obtained upon M13 infection are turbid-explain why? (2)
(*b*) How would you separate a mixture of mRNA, biotinylated-tRNA, and rRNA of eukaryotic origin? (3)

M6. Match the name of the cellular processes listed in **panel A** with the specific inhibitors from **panel B.** (5)

Panel A	Panel B
1. Translation in eukaryotes	*a.* α-amanitin
2. Glycosylation	*b.* Cycloheximide
3. Transcription by RNA polymerase II	*c.* Bcl2
4. Bacterial cell wall synthesis	*d.* Tunicamycin
5. Apoptosis	*e.* Penicillin

(N) ZOOLOGY

N1. For each sub-question given below, four alternatives are provided of which only one answer is correct. Write the correct answer in the answer book by writing *a*, *b*, *c* or *d* along with the sub-question number. (1 × 25 = 25)

1.1 Among the following phyla, one evolutionarily closest to the phylum chordata is
(*a*) Annelida (*b*) Arthropoda
(*c*) Echinodermata (*d*) Oncychophora

1.2 The orders Anura, Urodela and Apoda belong to the class
(*a*) Amphibia (*b*) Reptilia
(*c*) Mammalia (*d*) Pisces

1.3 Humans originated in the epoch known as
(*a*) Pleistocene (*b*) Eocene
(*c*) Holocene (*d*) Miocene

1.4 The neotropic biogeographical region per terrestrial species is not bounded by the following biogeographical region is
(*a*) Nearctic (*b*) Afrotropic
(*c*) Antarctic (*d*) Indo-Malayan

1.5 The condition albinism in man is linked to the deficiency of the enzyme
(*a*) Glucose-6-phosphate dehydrogenase
(*b*) Arginase
(*c*) Tyrosinase
(*d*) Xanthin Oxidase

1.6 Of the following, identify the one which is not a stop codon
(*a*) UAA (*b*) UAG (*c*) UGA (*d*) UAC

1.7 In a human cell, the number of moles of which one of the elements is the highest
(*a*) Carbon (*b*) Oxygen
(*c*) Nitrogen (*d*) Hydrogen

1.8 The body temperature of the following groups of animals occur in the order
(*a*) Prototheria > Metatheria > Eutheria > Aves
(*b*) Aves > Eutheria > Metatheria > Prototheria
(*c*) Eutheria > Aves > Metatheria > Prototheria
(*d*) Metatheria > Eutheria > Aves > Prototheria

1.9 The combination of closely linked genetic markers which tend to be transmitted as a unit to the next generation is called
(*a*) Allotype (*b*) Haplotype
(*c*) Karyotype (*d*) Isotype

1.10 The hormone epinephrine is involved in
(*a*) Red blood cell synthesis
(*b*) Stress response
(*c*) Control of blood sugar level
(*d*) Control of metabolic rate

1.11 Which of the following amongst the four is not a respiratory organ
(*a*) Dorsal line (*b*) Trachea
(*c*) Gills (*d*) Lungs

1.12 The hypervariable region of antibody molecule was first demonstrated by
(*a*) Edelman and Porter (*b*) Kabat and Wu
(*c*) Sastry and Pillai (*d*) Milstein and Kholer

1.13 The vector responsible for the spread of Filariasis is
(*a*) Anopheles (*b*) Culex
(*c*) Aedes (*d*) Sandfly

1.14 The following of the four is not a second messenger
(*a*) ATP
(*b*) Inosital 1,4,5 triphosphate
(*c*) Ca^{++}
(*d*) cAMP

1.15 Early pregnancy detection test detects the presence of which one of the following hormones
(*a*) Human chorionic gonodo tropin
(*b*) Lutinizing hormone
(*c*) Follicle stimulating hormone
(*d*) Estrogen

1.16 Selective transfer of which one of the following antibodies is responsible for passive humoral immunity in infants.
(*a*) IgA (*b*) IgM (*c*) IgG (*d*) IgE

1.17 The animal that most recently became extinct is
(*a*) Wooly mammoth (*b*) Giant moa
(*c*) Dodo (*d*) Tasmanian wolf

1.18 The man who championed the theory of evolution of Darwin and often referred to as Darwin's bulldog is
(*a*) Jullian Huxley (*b*) Aldous Huxley
(*c*) T.H.Huxley (*d*) Andrew Huxley

1.19 If you were asked to clone a man from a single cell and you are provided with the following cells, which one you would choose
(*a*) Sperm (*b*) Erythrocyte
(*c*) Lymphocyte (*d*) Kidney fibroblasts

1.20 Community suckling of young ones is found in
(*a*) Cats (*b*) Dogs
(*c*) Lions (*d*) Humans

1.21 The number of complementarity determining region(s) present in human kappa chain are
(*a*) 1 (*b*) 2
(*c*) 3 (*d*) 4

1.22 Transfer RNA genes are transcribed by
(*a*) RNA polymerase I
(*b*) RNA polymerase II
(*c*) RNA polymerase III
(*d*) RNA dependent RNA polymerase

1.23 Shine-Dalgarno sequence is associated with
(*a*) Translation (*b*) Transcription
(*c*) Replication (*d*) Recombination

1.24 Gonadotropin releasing factor is synthesized by
(*a*) Anterior Pituitary (*b*) Hypothalamus
(*c*) Adrenal gland (*d*) Thymus

1.25 In eukaryotic cells, DNA synthesis occurs during the phase of the cell cycle
(*a*) G1 (*b*) G2 (*c*) M (*d*) S

N2. There are major scientific discoveries given in the column A and the names of the discoverers in the column B. Match the discovery with the discoverer. (1 × 5 = 5)

Column A	Column B
(*i*) Base equivalence in DNA	(*a*) J.C.Venter
(*ii*) Human Genome Sequence	(*b*) F.Crick
(*iii*) PCR	(*c*) E.Chargaff
(*iv*) Prions	(*d*) J.Salk
(*v*) Polio Vaccine	(*e*) S.B.Pruisner
	(*f*) K.D.Mullis

N3. Describe the following in one or two sentences. (1 × 5 = 5)
(*a*) Froteasome (*b*) Spliceosome
(*c*) Nucleosome (*d*) Polysome
(*e*) Episome

N4. Define the following (1 × 5 = 5)
(*a*) Autogenic succession
(*b*) Climatic climax
(*c*) Allelomorphs
(*d*) Capacitation
(*e*) Linking number

N5. (*a*) What do you understand by homogametic sex? (1)
(*b*) Is human male is a homogametic sex? Give reason for your answer. (1)
(*c*) What is assertive mating? (1)
(*d*) What is gynendromorph? (1)
(*e*) What is codominance? (1)

N6. (*a*) What do you understand by Non-disjunction? (1)
(*b*) What is the genetic defect present in Down's syndrome? (1)
(*c*) What is co-evolution and what is its implication in host-parasite relationship? (2)
(*d*) What is a cline? (1)

ANSWERS

(H) CHEMISTRY

1.1 (*c*) 1.2 (*d*) 1.3 (*a*) 1.4 (*c*) 1.5 (*b*) 1.6 (*b*) 1.7 (*d*) 1.8 (*d*) 1.9 (*a*) 1.10 (*d*)
1.11 (*d*) 1.12 (*b*) 1.13 (*b*) 1.14 (*a*) 1.15 (*b*) 1.16 (*a*) 1.17 (*a*) 1.18 (*c*) 1.19 (*a*) 1.20 (*b*)
1.21 (*c*) 1.22 (*b*) 1.23 (*d*) 1.24 (*c*) 1.25 (*a*)

(J) BIOCHEMISTRY

1.1 (*c*) 1.2 (*b*) 1.3 (*c*) 1.4 (*a*) 1.5 (*b*) 1.6 (*b*) 1.7 (*a*) 1.8 (*c*) 1.9 (*b*) 1.10 (*d*)
1.11 (*c*) 1.12 (*b*) 1.13 (*b*) 1.14 (*c*) 1.15 (*d*) 1.16 (*d*) 1.17 (*c*) 1.18 (*b*) 1.19 (*d*) 1.20 (*b*)
1.21 (*d*) 1.22 (*a*) 1.23 (*d*) 1.24 (*d*) 1.25 (*d*)

(L) BOTANY

1.1 (*a*) 1.2 (*b*) 1.3 (*d*) 1.4 (*b*) 1.5 (*a*) 1.6 (*d*) 1.7 (*c*) 1.8 (*a*) 1.9 (*a*) 1.10 (*b*)
1.11 (*a*) 1.12 (*d*) 1.13 (*c*) 1.14 (*c*) 1.15 (*d*) 1.16 (*c*) 1.17 (*a*) 1.18 (*c*) 1.19 (*b*) 1.20 (*a*)
1.21 (*b*) 1.22 (*b*) 1.23 (*d*) 1.24 (*d*) 1.25 (*c*)

(M) MICROBIOLOGY

1.1 (*c*) 1.2 (*a*) 1.3 (*a*) 1.4 (*a*) 1.5 (*b*) 1.6 (*a*) 1.7 (*b*) 1.8 (*d*) 1.9 (*c*) 1.10 (*d*)
1.11 (*d*) 1.12 (*d*) 1.13 (*d*) 1.14 (*c*) 1.15 (*d*) 1.16 (*c*) 1.17 (*b*) 1.18 (*d*) 1.19 (*b*) 1.20 (*b*)
1.21 (*b*) 1.22 (*a*) 1.23 (*d*) 1.24 (*a*) 1.25 (*a*)

(N) ZOOLOGY

1.1 (*c*) 1.2 (*a*) 1.3 (*a*) 1.4 (*c*) 1.5 (*c*) 1.6 (*d*) 1.7 (*a*) 1.8 (*b*) 1.9 (*b*) 1.10 (*b*)
1.11 (*a*) 1.12 (*d*) 1.13 (*b*) 1.14 (*a*) 1.15 (*a*) 1.16 (*c*) 1.17 (*c*) 1.18 (*c*) 1.19 (*d*) 1.20 (*b*)
1.21 (*c*) 1.22 (*c*) 1.23 (*a*) 1.24 (*b*) 1.25 (*d*)

EXPLANATIONS

H : CHEMISTRY (COMPULSORY)

1. Given, the ground state electronic configuration of Iron is [Ar] $3d^6$ $4s^2$. For, ferric ions, with an oxidation state of +3, the electronic configuration would be [Ar] $3d^5$ $4s^0$.

2. Calcium fluoride occurs naturally as the mineral fluorite. The calcium ions, which are nearly the same size as the fluoride ion, are inserted into the cubic holes in the fluoride ion array, which expands the array so that no two fluoride ions are in contact with each other. The ionic radius of the calcium ion is 1.26 Å and that of the fluoride ion is 1.17 Å. There is a 1 : 1 ratio of atoms and holes in a simple cubic structure. The Ca^{2+} ion, however, has twice the charge of F^- ion, and thus every hole cannot be filled with a Ca^{2+} without violating electro-neutrality. Consequently, only half of the cubic holes in fluorite are occupied by a Ca^{2+} ion, which results in a 2:1 ratio of F^- to Ca^{2+} ions. So, the FCC structure has 8 cations and 4 anions, meaning coordination number of calcium is 8.

3. The net magnetic moment of an atom is the vector sum of its orbital and spin magnetic moments. It is given by $\mu = \sqrt{(n(n+2)}$, where n is the number of unpaired electrons.

   Normal electronic configuration of Ni in ground state = [Ar] $3d^8$ $4s^2$ [since atomic weight is 28]

   In case of $[Ni(CN)_4]^{2-}$, Ni is present as Ni^{2+} state, so electronic configuration = [Ar] $3d^8$ $4s^0$.

   As we can see, there are no unpaired electrons, so n = 0

   Therefore, Magnetic moment of $[Ni(CN)_4]^{2-}$ is, $\mu = 0$.

4. Barium Peroxide will be the chemical term for BaO_2. In its pure form, Hydrogen Peroxide (H_2O_2) is a faintly bluish, syrupy liquid which boils at 150.2°C. This process was supplanted by an improved version in which the Barium Peroxide is initially treated with Hydrochloric Acid (HCl), followed by addition of Sulfuric Acid (H_2SO_4) to precipitate the Barium Ion (Ba^{2+}) as Barium Sulfate ($BaSO_4$). This leaves a relatively pure aqueous solution of Hydrogen Peroxide:

   $BaO_2(s) + 2\,HCl(aq) \rightarrow H_2O_2(aq) + BaCl_2(aq)$ (Eq. 1)

   $BaCl_2(aq) + H_2SO_4(aq) \rightarrow BaSO_4(s) + 2\,HCl(aq)$ (Eq. 2)

5. Reaction of the complex $[Co(NH_3)_5Cl]Cl_2$ with an aqueous solution of silver nitrate in a quantitative manner is as follows:

   $[Co(NH_3)_5Cl]Cl_2$ (in aqueous solution) → (ionization)

   $$[Co(NH_3)_5Cl]^+ + 2\,Cl^-$$

   And, $2\,Cl^- + 2\,AgNO_3$

   $$\rightarrow 2AgCl + 2\,NO_3^-$$

   So, it is evident that one mole of the complex is responsible for the formation of 2 moles of silver chloride quantitatively from silver nitrate.

6. Only aluminium oxide, zinc oxide and lead oxide are amphoteric oxides. Magnesium oxide is not amphoteric in nature. It is an inorganic oxide. Also, tin oxide is also amphoteric in nature because it has the same amount of ionic and covalent character and thus reacting with both acids such as HCl and bases such as NaOH.

7. The formula for peroxodisulphuric acid is $H_2S_2O_8$. Its gram weight (molecular mass) = 194.14 g/ mol and its Melting point = 65 °C. Its structure is:

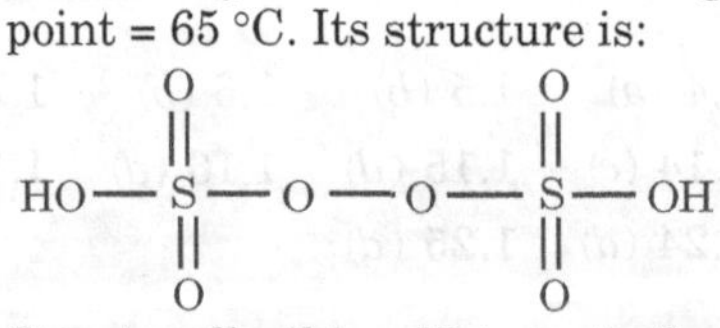

8. Structurally, thiosulfate is similar to sulfate. The molecule has a slightly distorted tetrahedral shape with central and peripheral sulfur (S-SO_3). Sulfur is larger than oxygen and forms weaker pi bonds, so the S-S bond is somewhat longer than the S-O bonds. In hypo Sodium thiosulphate, $Na_2S_2O_3$, the bond between the two sulphur moieties is coordinate bond. So, the donor atom is at +2 oxidation state and the acceptor atom is at –2 oxidation state. Actual oxidation state of the donor S-atom:

   2 × Oxidation state of Na + 3 × Oxidation sate of O + Oxidation state of S_{donor} + Oxidation state of $S_{acceptor}$ = 0

   Or, $2 \times (+1) + 3 \times (-2) + X + (-2) = 0$

   Or, $X = 6$

   So, the two oxidation states of sulphur are +6 and –2.

9. The temperature at which complete miscibility is reached as the temperature is raised or in some cases lowered —used of two liquids that are partially miscible under ordinary conditions —is called critical solution temperature. A binary composition phase diagram shows the phases formed in differing mixtures of two elements over a range of temperatures. So, phenol-water shows the critical solution temperature in the phase diagram.

10. The van't Hoff factor, symbol i, expresses how may ions and particles are formed (on an average) in a solution from one formula unit of solute.

    Now, for $K_4[Fe(CN)_6]$

    $$\rightarrow 4\,K^+ + [Fe(CN)_6]^{4-}$$

    So, number of ions present in the solution = 4 + 1 = 5. Hence the van't Hoff factor, i = 5.

11. Let S be the solubility of the sparingly soluble salt, AX_3

    Now, Solubility product,

    $$K_{sp} = [A^{3+}] \times [3\,X^-]^3 = S \times [3\,S]^3 = 27\,S^4$$

    Given, $K_{sp} = 2.7 \times 10^{-31}$ at 298 K

    Therefore, $2.7 \times 10^{-31} = 27\,S^4$

    $\Rightarrow S = 10^{-32/4} = 10^{-8}$

    Hence, the solubility is 10^{-8} mol/ L

12. At the standard condition of 298 K (25°), the Nernst equation becomes:

    $$\Delta E = \Delta E^\circ - 0.0591\,V/n \log [C]^c[D]^d/[A]^a[B]^b$$

    Here, $\Delta E^0_{cell} = 0.77$ V, number of electrons, n = 1

    Therefore, $\Delta E = \Delta E^\circ - 0.0591/\log [Fe^{2+}]/[Fe^{3+}]$

    $\Rightarrow \Delta E = \Delta E^\circ - 0.0591 \log [1M]/[0.1M]$

    $\Rightarrow \Delta E = 0.77 - 0.0591 \times 1$

    $\Rightarrow \Delta E = 0.7109$

13. A zero-order reaction is a reaction that proceeds at a rate that is independent of reactant concentration, typically with increasing or decreasing reactants concentrations not affecting the observed reaction. This means that the rate of the reaction is equal to the rate constant, k, of that reaction. Zero-order reactions are only applicable for a very narrow region of time. Increasing the concentration of the reacting species will not speed up the rate of the reaction. Zero-order reactions are typically found when a material that is required for the reaction to proceed, such as a surface or a catalyst, is saturated by the reactants. A reaction is zero order if concentration data is plotted versus time and the result is a straight line. A zero-order reaction has a rate that is independent of the concentration of the reactant(s).

We have, the integrated equation for the zero order reaction,

$$t = \{[X]_0 - [X]\}/k$$

At, $t = t_{1/2}$, we have

$$[X] = [X]_0/2;$$

So $t_{1/2} = [X]_0/2k$

And at $t = t_{3/4}$ (after 75% completion of reaction), we have,

$$t_{3/4} = [X]_0/4K$$

So, $t_{1/2} = 2\,t_{3/4}$

$\Rightarrow$ $t_{3/4} = 0.5\,t_{1/2}$.

14. Dissociation of PCl_5 is given by:

$$PCl_5 \Leftrightarrow PCl_3 + Cl_2$$

Initially, at the beginning → 1 0 0

At equilibrium, we have → 1 – x x x

where x is the degree of dissocation

Total moles at equilibrium = 1 – x + x + x = 1 + x

Let P be the total pressure

Now, Partial pressure of PCl_5

= Mole fraction × Total pressure

= (1 – x)/(1 + x) * P

Partial pressure of PCl_3 = x/(1 + x) * P

Partial pressure of Cl_2 = x/(1 + x) * P

Therefore, at equilibrium, Dissociation constant,

$$K_p = P_{PCl_3} * P_{Cl_2}/P_{PCl_5}$$

At P = 1 atm, we have x = 0.80

$\Rightarrow$ $K_p = [x/(1 + x)]*[x/(1 + x)]/[(1 - x)/(1 + x)$

$\Rightarrow$ $K_p = x^2/(1 - x^2)$

$\Rightarrow$ $K_p = (0.8)^2/(1 - (0.8)^2)$

$\Rightarrow$ $K_p = 1.77$

Thus, At P = 2 atm, the value of x will be:

$$1.77 = x^2/(1 - x^2) * 2$$

$\Rightarrow$ $1.77 - 1.77x^2 = 2x^2$

$\Rightarrow$ $3.77x^2 = 1.77$

$\Rightarrow$ $x^2 = \sqrt{(0.4695)}$

$\Rightarrow$ $x = 0.6851$

Hence the dissociation degree at 2 atm is 0.69 (approx.)

15. A variable whose values depend on the quantity of substance under study (e.g., volume V, enthalpy ΔH, entropy ΔS, Gibbs' free energy ΔG, length, mass *m*) is an extensive variable. Extensive variables are additive in nature.

16. Entropy is a function of the state of the system and can be found if any two properties of the system are known,

e.g. $s = s(p, T)$

or $s = s(T, v)$

or $s = s(p, v)$.

The total entropy change (system + surroundings) is always greater than or equal to zero for any change of state of the system. For an adiabatic irreversible expansion of 1 mole of an ideal gas, the total entropy change of the system, $\Delta S_{SYSTEM} > 0$. While, the total entropy change of the surroundings of the ideal gas is, $\Delta S_{SURROUNDING} = 0$, since there is no change in the surroundings due to the system.

17. Normally, the pH of water is 7 at 298 K. But, it has been established that the pH of a substance decreases with rise in temperature. Hence at 333 K, the pH of water will be less than 7. Since NH_4Cl is an acidic salt, so 0.1 M concentration of the salt will have a pH lower than that of the basic salt NaCl of equivalent concentration. CH_3COOH is a very weak organic acid and so its pH will be much higher than that of the strong inorganic acid HCl. HCl is a strong inorganic acid whose pH always lies in the region of 2-3. Hence, its pH cannot be above 7.

18. Isobutanol (isobutyl alcohol) is useful in organic synthesis, as a chemical intermediate and as a solvent in coating applications. Isobutanol is similar in property to n-butyl alcohol and may be used as a supplement or replacement for n-butyl alcohol in many applications. As a relatively slow evaporating latent solvent in lacquers and ambient-cured enamels, isobutanol is effective in reducing the viscosities of many formulations while simultaneously promoting flow and retarding blush. Isobutanol is prepared by:

$(CH_3)_2CHMgBr$ + HCHO → (in presence of H^+/H_3O^+) $(CH_3)_2CH - CH_2OH$ [Isobutanol]

19. A complete mechanism for the acid-catalyzed dehydration of 1-methylcyclohexanol is:

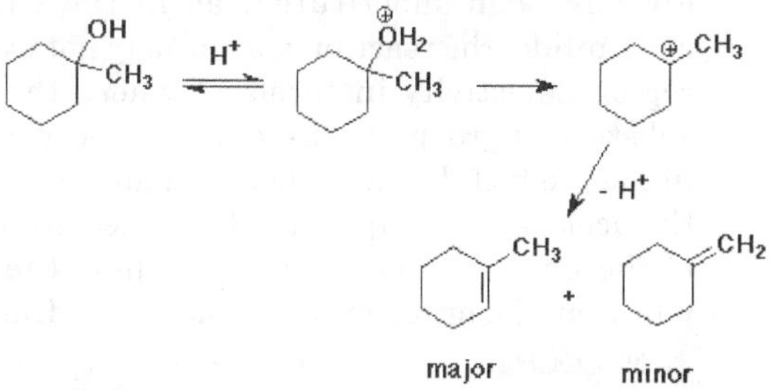

Step 1 - The name for the mechanism of this reaction is E1 method. Step 2 - formation of the carbocation is the slowest step is the rate-determining step. In step 3, loss of H^+ determines the position of the double bond. The major product that is formed is 1-methyl cyclohexene.

20. Carbylamine reaction is used as a test for the identification of primary amines. When aliphatic and aromatic primary amines are heated with chloroform and ethanolic potassium hydroxide, carbylamines (or isocyanides) are formed. These carbylamines have very unpleasant odours. Secondary and tertiary amines do not respond to this test. Heating a mixture of 1° - amine and chloroform with ethanolic potassium hydroxide

$$R\text{-}NH_2 + CHCl_3 + 4KOH \rightarrow RNC + 3KCl + 3H_2O$$

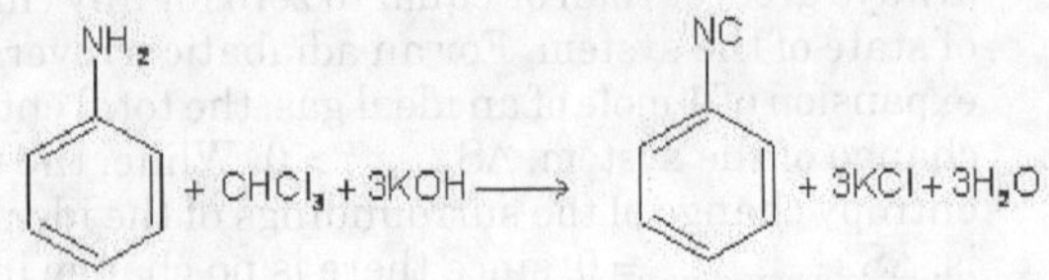

Mechanism proceeds via intermediate formation of dichloromethylene or, dichloro carbene produced from chloroform in alkaline solution.

21. The bromination of acetanilide is an example of electrophilic aromatic substitution. In electrophilic aromatic substitution, an electrophile (in this case, bromine in combination with ferric bromide) will react with a phenyl ring such that the product of the reaction has the electrophile bonded to one of the phenyl carbons, in place of a hydrogen. The mechanism proceeds as follows. First, to generate the electrophile, bromine is complexed with ferric bromide which will generate the bromonium ion (bromine with a positive charge). This is due to ferric bromide's property of being a Lewis acid. Then, one of the pi bonds within the phenyl ring attacks the electrophile, which is electron deficient. This then creates a carbocation on one of the carbons in the phenyl ring. This positive charge, however, is delocalized and can be spread to all six of the carbons in the ring. Finally, deprotonation of one of the phenyl hydrogens restores aromaticity to the ring. In cases where the phenyl ring has already been substituted, as in the case of acetanilide, the reaction may or may not exhibit region selectivity in terms of where the new substituent group (the bromine) will be attached in the product. Because there is a nitrogen (from the acetamido group) directly connected to one of the phenyl carbons in acetanilide, the lone pair from the nitrogen can resonate into the ring.

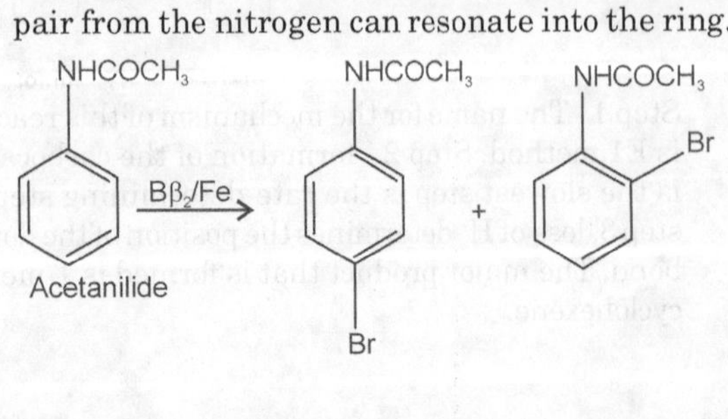

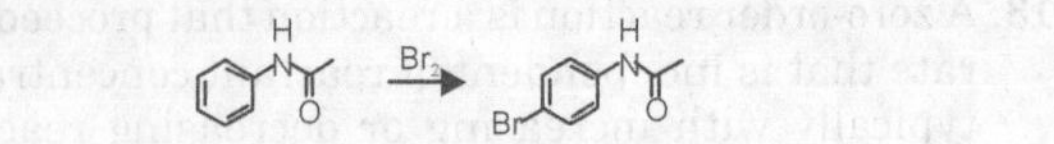

Formation of Bromine :

$5e^- + 6H^+ + BrO_3^- \rightarrow \frac{1}{2}Br_2 + 3H_2O$

$(Br^- \rightarrow \frac{1}{2}Br_2 + 2e^-)\,5$

$BH^+ + 5Br^- + BrO_3^- \rightarrow 3Br_2 + 3H_2O$

Electrophilic Aromatic Substitution :

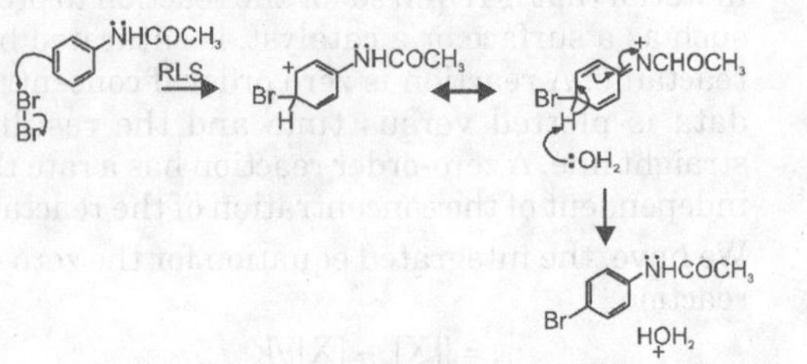

22. The Huckel's Rule for aromaticity says a compound must have 4n + 2 π-electrons. It doesn't say the compound must be electrically neutral. Cycloheptatriene is a seven-carbon atom cyclic compound. It possesses an incorrect number of π-electrons for aromaticity, but by producing from it the cationic structure ($C_7H_7^+$), it gets an appropriate 6 π-electrons. The cycloheptatrienyl cation is quite stable. Another name for the cycloheptatrienyl cation is the tropylium ion.

23. There are two chirality centers in 2-bromo-3-chlorobutane, so there are four stereoisomers for this compound. Each of the four stereoisomers of 2-bromo-3-chlorobutane is chiral. There are two pairs of enantiomers. Any given molecule has its enantiomer; the two other molecules are its diastereomers.

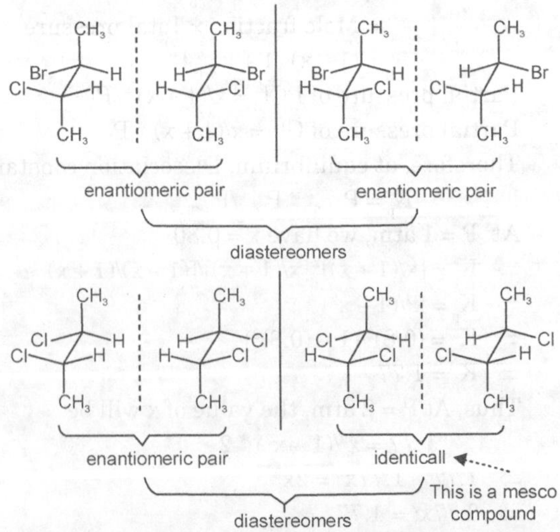

24. Ammonia reacts with formaldehyde to produce a non offensive compound, according to the following:

$$H_2C = O + NH_3 \rightarrow H_2C = N - H + H_2O$$

Then in the second step, it gives rise to hexamethylenetetramine → $(CH_3)_6N_4$

25. The Perkin reaction is an organic reaction used to convert an aromatic aldehyde and an anhydride to α, β-unsaturated carboxylic acid using sodium acetate, a base, and an acid work-up. The regiochemistry of the reaction, the relative position of the carboxylic acid and aromatic ring in the final product, can be either E or Z. The mechanism goes through numerous steps including several additions and eliminations.

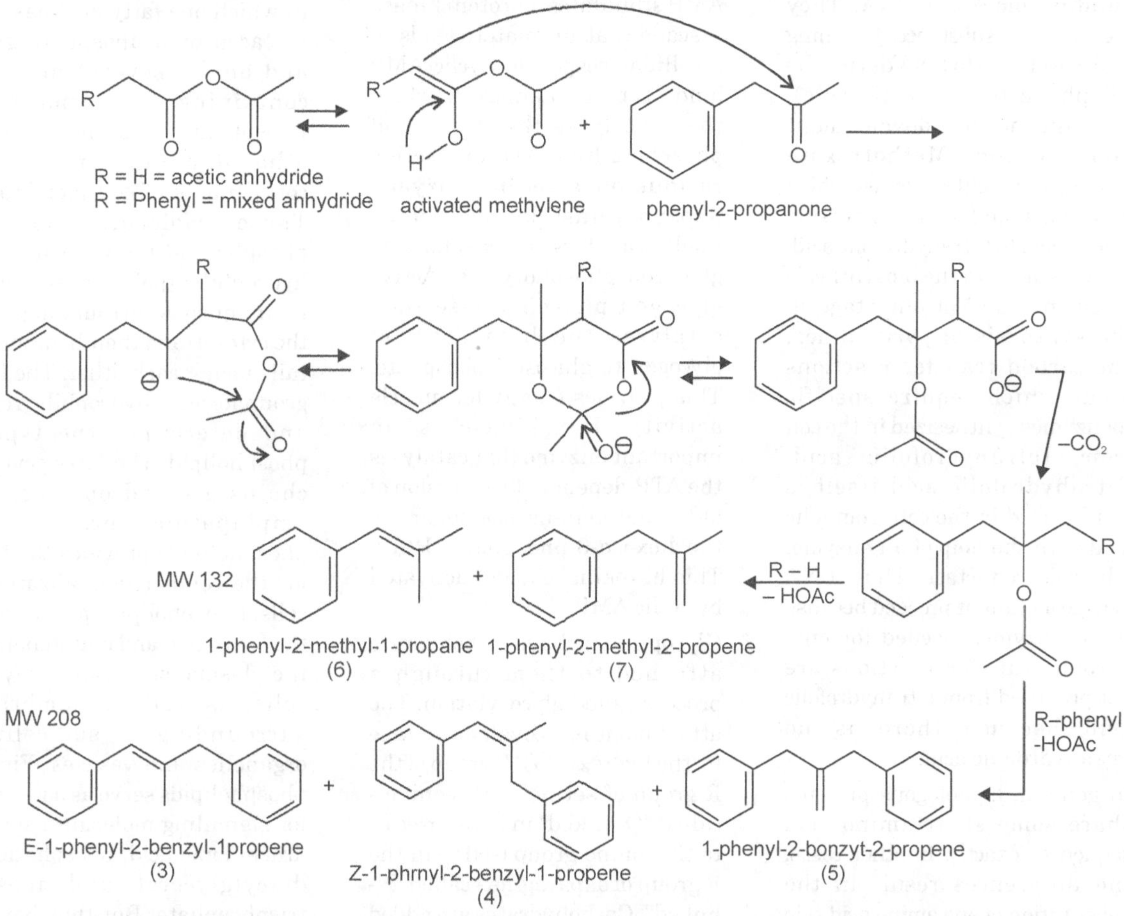

The mechanistic representation of the formation of the Perkin reaction products via the condensation of an activated methylene (anhydride) compound with a molecule of P2P.

(J) BIOCHEMISTRY

1. Size Exclusion Chromatography (SEC) is the separation technique based on the molecular size of the components. Separation is achieved by the differential exclusion from the pores of the packing material, of the sample molecules as they pass through a bed of porous particles. The principle feature of SEC is its gentle non-adsorptive interaction with the sample, enabling high retention of bimolecular activity. Size exclusion chromatography is used primarily for analytical assays and semi-preparative purifications. It is not commonly used for process scale work due to the low capacity of the size exclusion mode. For the separation of biomolecules in aqueous or aqueous/ organic mobile phases, SEC is referred to as gel filtration chromatography (GFC), while the separation of organic polymers in non-aqueous mobile phases is called gel permeation chromatography (GPC).

2. The haemoglobin molecule is a tetramer consisting of 4 polypeptide chains, known as globins, which are usually: 2 α chains that are each 141 amino acids long and 2 β chains that are each 146 amino acids long. Haemoglobin is a protein consisting of four polypeptide chains, two β-chains, and two α-chains folded round each other. The two β-chains of haemoglobin are identical, as are the two β-chains. In haemoglobin, an oxygen transport protein, the binding of oxygen is cooperative and is modulated by ligands such as H^+, CO_2 and BPG (2, 3-bisphosphoglycerate, sometimes referred to as DPG). The Haeme group is a porphyrin derivative containing an iron atom, which undergoes transition from Fe^{2+} to Fe^{3+} on binding O_2, which results in allosteric quaternary structural changes in the globin chains. It is this ferrous iron atom (located centrally within each haeme group) which gives Hb its red appearance. A Haeme group is attached to each of the four chains. All these account for the quaternary structure of haemoglobin.

3. Methotrexate is an antineoplastic anti-metabolite. Anti-metabolites masquerade as purine or pyrimidine - which become the building blocks of DNA. They prevent these substances becoming incorporated in to DNA during the "S" phase (of the cell cycle), stopping normal development and division. Methotrexate inhibits folic acid reductase which is responsible for the conversion of folic acid to tetrahydrofolic acid. At two stages in the biosynthesis of purines and at one stage in the synthesis of pyrimidines, one-carbon transfer reactions occur which require specific coenzymes synthesized in the cell from tetrahydrofolic acid. Tetrahydrofolic acid itself is synthesized in the cell from folic acid with the help of an enzyme, folic acid reductase. Thus, DNA synthesis cannot proceed because the coenzymes needed for one-carbon transfer reactions are not produced from tetrahydrofolic acid because there is no tetrahydrofolic acid.

4. In general, homologous proteins share some short amino acid sequences exactly. In other cases, the differences result in the substitution of one amino acid side chain by another chemically similar one. Six classes of amino acid side chains exist; within a group, the amino acid side chains are chemically similar. Substitution of one amino acid side chain for another one within the same group is known as conservative substitution. Homologous proteins are related by conservative amino acid substitutions. The side chains of glycine, alanine, valine, leucine, and isoleucine contain saturated carbon-carbon and carbon-hydrogen bonds only. Alanine has a methyl group for its side chain, valine a 3-carbon side chain, while leucine and isoleucine have 4-carbon side chains. Both valine and isoleucine have structural conformity which leads to conservative substitution between valine and isoleucine.

5. Cyclic AMP doesn't act directly on its target enzymes; for example, glycogen phosphorylase and glycogen synthase. Instead, cyclic AMP stimulates a protein kinase cascade that ultimately leads to a cellular response. Cyclic AMP binds to protein kinase A, which then catalyzes the transfer of phosphate from ATP to a serine residue on a second enzyme, phosphorylase kinase, which itself transfers a phosphate to glycogen phosphorylase. Active glycogen phosphorylase then catalyzes the breakdown of glycogen to glucose-1-phosphate. This provides energy for muscle activity. Hexokinase is an important enzyme that catalyses the ATP-dependent conversion of aldo- and keto-hexose sugars to the hexose-6-phosphate (H6P). This hexokinase is not activated by cyclic AMP.

6. Glycoproteins have carbohydrate attached to them through a process called glycosylation. The attachment is a covalent linkage to: the hydroxyl (-OH) group of the R group of serine or threonine - called "O-linked" in both cases or to the amino group ($-NH_2$) in the R group of asparagine - called "N-linked". Carbohydrates are added to proteins in a very complicated process which involves two organelles, the endoplasmic reticulum and the Golgi apparatus.CHO addition to proteins occurs both co- and post-translationally. The RNA coding the protein sequence enters the cytoplasm where it binds to ribosomes (large RNA-protein complexes) which are the site for protein synthesis. Cytoplasmic proteins are synthesized on free ribosome, but for future glycoproteins, the ribosome bind to an elongated, extensive organelle in the cell called the endoplasmic reticulum (ER). The most important seems to involve their role in directing proper folding of proteins in the ER which accounts for the observations that glycan addition to proteins in the ER is a co-translational event.

7. Phospholipids are fat derivatives in which one fatty acid has been replaced by a phosphate group and one of several nitrogen-containing molecules. Phospholipids like phosphatidyl ethanolamine are major constituents of cell membranes. These molecules form a phospholipid bilayer with their hydrophilic (polar) heads facing their aqueous surroundings (e.g., the cytosol) and their hydrophobic tails facing each other. The head group forms a hydrophilic region and determines the type of phospholipid. The fatty acyl side chains are hydrophobic; this amphipathic property of phospholipids provides the basis for the compartmentalization of cells. Phospholipids play a role in the formation and maintenance of the plasma membrane bilayer of cells, as well as membranes surrounding sub-cellular organelles and vesicles. Finally, phospholipids serve as a reservoir for signalling molecules, such as arachidonic acid, phosphatidate, diacylglycerol and inositol trisphosphate. But they have no role in cell recognition which is a tribute of glycoproteins (oligosachharides).

8. Insulin-dependent (type I) diabetes mellitus is a chronic disease characterized by hyperglycaemia, impaired metabolism and storage of important nutrients, evidence of autoimmunity, and long-term vascular and neurologic complications. Insulin secretory function is limited. Cell membrane binding is not primarily involved. The goal of treatment is to relieve symptoms and to achieve blood glucose levels as close to normal as possible without severe hypoglycaemia. It is caused by the destruction of β-cells of the pancreatic tissue called the

islets of Langerhans, those cells normally produce insulin, the hormone that helps regulate glucose levels in the blood.

9. Z-DNA is a left-handed double helix wherein the sugar-phosphate backbone has a zigzag pattern due to the alternate stacking of bases in anti-conformation and syn conformation. In Z-DNA only a minor groove is present and the major groove is absent. The residues that allow sequence-specific recognition of Z-DNA are present on the convex outer surface. Z-DNA has a pool of alternating GC sequence present in it. Z-DNA is the first single crystal X-ray structure of a DNA fragment. The formation of Z-DNA invivo is an energy requiring process. Whenever B-DNA transforms into Z-DNA two B-Z, junctions form.

10. The formation of mature insulin occurs by proteolysis of the precursor preproinsulin. The signal sequence is first cleaved from preproinsulin to form proinsulin; proinsulin is then cleaved to release the C peptide, leaving the A and B chains of mature insulin linked by disulfide bridges. Preproinsulin contains an amino-terminal signal sequence that is required in order for the precursor hormone to pass through the membrane of the endoplasmic reticulum (ER) for post-translational processing. The post-translational processing clips away those portions not needed for the bioactive hormone. Upon entering the ER, the preproinsulin signal sequence is proteolytically removed to form proinsulin. Once the post-translational formation of three vital disulfide bonds occurs, specific peptidases cleave proinsulin. The final product of the biosynthesis is mature and active insulin. Finally, insulin is packaged and stored in secretory granules, which accumulate in the cytoplasm, until release is triggered. Thus, formation of mature insulin does not involve any cyclization of glutamate residue.

11. The chemical step of natural protein synthesis, peptide bond formation, is catalysed by the large subunit of the ribosome. A molecule of water must be eliminated for each peptide bond formed. In an aqueous environment, the formation of a peptide bond is not favoured thermodynamically ($\Delta G \approx +10$ kJ/mol at room temperature). Instead, the reverse reaction, hydrolysis of the peptide bond, is favored. Because peptide bond hydrolysis is favoured thermodynamically, not peptide bond formation, additional energy is required to make peptide bonds in cells. Thus, peptide bond formation is coupled to the hydrolysis of high-energy phosphate bonds during the process of translation. The peptide bond is made up of (O=C-N-H) between COOH group of one amino acid and NH_2 group of another amino acid with hydrolysis of one water molecule. In the peptide linkage, there are 3 energy bonds that are present: C=O, C-N and N-H.

12. Chromosome walking is a technique to clone a gene (e.g., a disease gene) from its known closest markers. The closest linked marker (e.g., EST or a known gene) to the gene is used to probe a genomic library. A restriction fragment isolated from the end of the positive clones is used to re-probe the genomic library for overlapping clones. This process is repeated several times to walk across the chromosome and reach the gene of interest. Chromosome walking is a method of positional cloning used to find, isolate, and clone a particular allele in a gene library. To locate a particular disease gene, the walking starts at the closest gene that has already been identified, known as a marker gene. Each successive gene in the sequence is tested repeatedly for what are known as overlap restrictions and mapped for their precise location in the sequence. Eventually, walking through the genes reaches the mutant gene in an unmapped sequence that binds to a fragment of a gene of that particular disease. Once the gene is cloned, its function can be fully identified. To build up a series of overlapping cloned DNA fragments, it begins with one clone from a library, and then identifies a second clone whose insert overlaps with the insert in the first clone.

13. Steroid hormones (SHs) are lipophilic molecules derived from cholesterol and synthesized in the adrenal cortex (glucocorticoids, mineralocorticoids, and adrenal androgens), the testes (testicular androgens, oestrogen), and the ovary and placenta (oestrogens and progestagens or progestins). SHs reach their target cells via the blood, where they are bound to carrier proteins, and because of their lipophilic nature pass the cell membrane by simple diffusion. Within the target cells SHs bind to steroid hormone receptors (SHRs), the key mediators of SH action, which are complexed to chaperones that help other proteins to fold and prevent aggregation. Binding of agonistic or antagonistic ligands leads to different allosteric changes of SHRs making them competent to exert positive or negative effects on the expression of target genes by different mechanisms. Mostly SHRs are present in the matrix of the cytosol.

14. Platelet aggregation is the clustering together of thrombocytes, which are the small, cell-like structures made in the bone marrow that help prevent bleeding. Drugs or agents

which antagonize or impair any mechanism leading to blood platelet aggregation, whether during the phases of activation and shape change or following the dense-granule release reaction and stimulation of the prostaglandin-thromboxane system are the inhibitors of platelet aggregation. Prostacyclin is a prostaglandin. It is a biologically active product of arachidonic acid metabolism in human vascular walls and a potent inhibitor of platelet aggregation. It inhibits the vasoconstrictor effect of angiotensin and stimulates renin release and has been used to treat pulmonary hypertension.

15. L-Tyrosine is a non-essential (or semi-essential), neutral, genetically coded amino acid. It is very little soluble in water. L-Tyrosine is the precursor of the catecholamines; alterations in the availability of L-tyrosine to the brain can influence the synthesis of both dopamine and nor-epinephrine. The main effects of L-tyrosine that have been reported are acute effects in preventing a decline in cognitive function in response to physical stress. Although it is a "natural" product, side effects of tyrosine are still possible. It is a precursor of the neurotransmitters epinephrine, nor-epinephrine and dopamine, all of them extremely important in the brain and transmits nerve impulses and prevents depression. Dopamine is also vital to mental function and seems to play a role in sex drive. The presence of excess amount of L-tyrosine in food or dietary supplements lead to decrease in the rate of absorption of other amino acids in the small intestine.

16. Immunoglobulin G (IgG) molecule has spatial disposition and interaction of the domains. To enable the F_{ab} arms to have the freedom to move and twist so that they can align their hyper-variable regions with the antigenic sites on large immobile carriers, and to permit the F_c structures to adjust spatially in order to trigger their effector functions, it is desirable for IgG to have a high degree of flexibility. The hinge region facilitates the interconnection of the globular domains present in IgG. Structure/function studies on IgG have been aided by the discovery that the proteolytic enzymes pepsin and papain cleave the molecule into specific fragments with specific biological properties. Treatment of an IgG molecule with pepsin generates the F (ab′) 2 fragment, which broadly encompasses the two F_{ab} regions linked by the hinge region. Papain cleaves the IgG molecule in the hinge region between the C_H1 and C_H2 domains to yield two identical F_{ab} fragments, which retain their antigen-binding ability, and one non-antigen–binding fragment—the (F_c) region. The F_c region is glycosylated and has many effector functions (e.g., binding complement, binding to cell receptors on macrophages and monocytes), and serves to distinguish one class of antibody from another.

17. Circular dichroism (CD) spectroscopy is a form of light absorption spectroscopy that measures the difference in absorbance of right- and left-circularly polarized light (rather than the commonly used absorbance of isotropic light) by a substance. It has been shown that CD spectra between 260 and approximately 180 nm can be analyzed for the different secondary structural types: alpha helix, parallel and antiparallel beta sheet, turn, and other. Circularly-polarized light rays will travel through an optically active medium with different velocities due to the different indices of refraction for right- and left-circularly polarized light called optical rotation or circular birefringence. The variation of optical rotation as a function of wavelength is called optical rotary dispersion (ORD). Right- and left-circularly polarized light will also be absorbed to different extents at some wavelengths due to differences in extinction coefficients for the two polarized rays called circular dichroism (CD).

18. Endonuclease is any of a group of enzymes that catalyze the hydrolysis of phosphodiester bonds between nucleic acids in a DNA molecule or RNA sequence. It is an enzyme that cleaves or hydrolyzes phosphodiester bonds within a polynucleotide chain. These are restriction enzymes that cleave large DNA molecules at specific sequences of four to six nucleotides. It is any nuclease specifically catalyzing the hydrolysis of interior bonds of ribonucleotide or deoxyribonucleotide chains.

19. K_m is the concentration of substrate which permits the enzyme to achieve half V_{max}. An enzyme with a high K_m has a low affinity for its substrate, and requires a greater concentration of substrate to achieve V_{max}. The rate of reaction when the enzyme is saturated with substrate is the maximum rate of reaction, V_{max}. The relationship between rate of reaction and concentration of substrate depends on the affinity of the enzyme for its substrate. This is usually expressed as the K_m (Michaelis constant) of the enzyme, an inverse measure of affinity. The K_m of an enzyme, relative to the concentration of its substrate under normal conditions permits prediction of whether or not the rate of formation of product will be affected by the availability of substrate. An enzyme with a low K_m relative to the physiological concentration of substrate is normally saturated with substrate, and will act at a constant rate, regardless of variations in the concentration of substrate within the physiological range. An enzyme with a high K_m relative to the physiological concentration of substrate is not normally saturated with substrate, and its activity will vary as the concentration of substrate varies, so that the rate of formation of product will depend on the availability of substrate.

20. IgG, a monomer, is the predominant Immunoglobulin class present in human serum. Produced as part of the secondary immune response to an antigen, this class of immunoglobulin constitutes approximately 75% of total serum Immunoglobulin. IgG is the only class of Ig that can cross the placenta in humans, and it is largely responsible for protection of the newborn during the first months of life. Because of its relative abundance and excellent specificity toward antigens, IgG is the principle antibody used in immunological research and clinical diagnostics.

21. Molecular chaperones are a ubiquitous class of folding modulators that play a central role in the conformational quality control of the proteome by interacting with, stabilizing and remodelling a wide range of non-native polypeptides. Mechanistically, molecular chaperones rely on the differential exposure of structured hydrophobic domains to the solvent to bind non-polar segments that would normally be buried within the core of their substrates. Chaperones can play an important role in signal transduction, in the maintenance of the organized state of the cytoplasm and other intracellular compartments, in the motions inside the cell, and some other vital functions of the cells.

22. Neutrophils are the most common type of white blood cell, comprising about 50-70% of all white blood cells. They are phagocytic, meaning that they can ingest other cells, though they do not survive the act. Neutrophils are the first immune cells to arrive at a site of infection, through a process known as chemotaxis. Neutrophils inform and shape immune responses, contribute to the repair of tissue as well as its breakdown, use killing mechanisms that enrich our concepts of specificity, and offer exciting opportunities for the treatment of neoplastic, autoinflamm-atory and autoimmune disorders. Neutrophils provide the first line of defence of the innate immune system by phagocytising, killing, and digesting bacteria and fungi. The oxidase pumps electrons into the phagocytic vacuole, thereby inducing a charge across the membrane that must be compensated. The movement of compensating ions produces conditions in the vacuole conducive to microbial killing and digestion by enzymes released into the vacuole from the cytoplasmic granules.

23. The rate at which energy is used by an organism at complete rest, measured in humans by the heat given off per unit time, and expressed as the calories released per kilogram of body weight or per square meter of body surface per hour is known as Basal metabolic rate (BMR). Increase in thyroid hormone (T3 and T4) leads to increase in BMR. More the muscle mass, higher is the BMR and lesser the muscle mass, lower is the BMR. Sedentary lifestyle leads to lower BMR because it leads to less active muscles. During night following a day of strenuous muscular work the BMR is higher than after the inactive day. BMR is highest in 1st two years of life and then it is reduced gradually throughout the childhood and accelerates during puberty. After adolescence stage, BMR declines gradually throughout the life. Women have lower BMR than men because of the production of sex hormones during puberty which retains adipose tissues in women and muscle tissues in men. BMR decreases with the increasing periods of starvation of the body.

24. Operon is a unit of genetic material that functions in a coordinated manner by means of an operator, a promoter, and one or more structural genes that are transcribed together. It is a segment of DNA containing adjacent genes including structural genes and an operator gene and a regulatory gene. There are two different kinds of genes in operons: a) Structural genes code for proteins needed for the normal operation of the cell. The size of operons varies according to the size of the genome of a particular organism. The lower eukaryotes have a smaller size of operon because of the fewer number of genes present in them but higher eukaryotes have more number of operons along with larger sequences because of their large genome structure. But, even though the size of the operons may vary, the exon portion of the operons in higher eukaryotes is much less than that in the lower eukaryotes.

25. Fatty acids are merely carboxylic acids with long hydrocarbon chains. The hydrocarbon chain length may vary from 10-30 carbons (most usual is 12-18). The non-polar hydrocarbon alkane chain is an important counter balance to the polar acid functional group. However, in fatty acids, the non-polar hydrocarbon chain gives the molecule a non- polar character.

When the fatty acid is 16 carbon atoms long, a Thioesterase domain catalyzes hydrolysis of the thioester linking the fatty acid to phosphopantetheine. Fatty acids esterified to coenzyme A serve as substrates. However, fatty acids having double bonds cannot be synthesized in humans.

(L) BOTANY

1. Peroxisomes are small, membrane-enclosed organelles that contain enzymes involved in a variety of metabolic reactions, including several aspects of energy metabolism. Peroxisomes in leaves are involved in photorespiration, which serves to metabolize a side product formed during photosynthesis. Photorespiration involves a complex network of enzyme reactions that exchange metabolites between chloroplasts, leaf peroxisomes and mitochondria.
2. Plasmodesmata connect neighboring cells, forming an apoplast. The apoplast is the "non-living" extracellular space that surrounds the symplast. It consists of cell walls and spaces between cells. Water and solutes can move freely in this framework, except at the endodermis in roots and stems where the apoplastic flow of ions is interrupted by the Casparian strip, forcing water to flow to symplast.
3. The leaves that are oriented parallel to the main axis of the leaf are the isobilateral leaves. The Isobilateral leaves are normally held parallel to the direction of the sunlight. The primary features of an Isobilateral leaf are as follows:
   - The stomata of an Isobilateral leaf are distributed on both the upper and the lower epidermis.
   - There is no such differentiation of the mesophyll tissue into palisade and spongy parenchyma. There is any one type of tissue.
   - The bundle sheath of an Isobilateral leaf contains chloroplasts.
4. Tyloses are outgrowths of the parenchyma contact cells surrounding the xylem vessels that protrude through the pit cavities into the vessel's lumen.
5. Guttation is the loss of water in the form of water droplets from hydathodes (small pores) on the leaf margin of a small herbaceous plant. Plants have hydathodes at the end of the veins, through which this excess water is lost in the form of droplets. It takes place mostly in small plants like banana, rose, etc.
6. The drug colchicine exerts its effect in the M phase of cell cycle. Colchicine is an alkaloid derived from the autumn crocus (Colchicum autumnale). It inhibits mitosis by inhibiting microtubule polymerization. While colchicine is not used to treat cancer in humans, it is commonly used to treat acute attacks of gout.
7. Protandry is a condition related to a flower in which the anthers release their pollen before the stigma of the same flower is receptive. Simply it can be defined as the condition of flowers whose male parts mature before the female ones.
8. The stalk that attaches an ovule or seed to the wall of the ovary is called funicle. It can also be defined as the part that joins the seed to the pod frame. The pod frame is called a replum. The crowning beak of the pod is termed a rostrum.
9. Viriparous germination is that type of germination in which seed germinate inside the fruit. The embryo grows out of the seed and then out of the fruit and projects from it in the form of a green seedling displaying the root and the hypocotyl. This is a special type of germination found in mangrove plants. Mangrove plants are found in marshy areas and on the sea coast. Vivipary is seen in Rhizophora, Cercops, Kandelia and Sonneratia.
10. More than 70% of the proteins consumed by humans are derived from storage proteins of legume and cereal seeds. Seed protein content of legumes varies from 20 to 40%, while in cereals it accounts for 7 – 15% of the dry weight of the seed. The deficiency of certain essential amino acids in the seed proteins may, however, limit their nutritional quality for monogastric animals. In general the cereal storage proteins are deficient in lysine, threonine, and tryptophan while the storage proteins of legumes contain low levels of cysteine and methionine.
11. Abscisic Acid (ABA) is the major hormone that controls plant's ability to survive in a harsh, changing environment. ABA is the hormone that triggers closing of the stomata when soil water is insufficient to keep up with transpiration. It is also known as anti- gibberellic acid hormone.
12. Exocytosis is a process in which an intracellular vesicle (membrane bounded sphere) moves to the plasma membrane and subsequent fusion of the vesicular membrane and plasma membrane ensues.
13. Active transport is the movement of a substance against its concentration gradient (from low to high concentration). In all cells, this is usually concerned with accumulating high concentrations of molecules that the cell needs, such as ions, glucose, and amino acids.
14. Phosphoenol pyruvic acid as the anion is an important chemical compound in biochemistry. In plants, it is also involved in the biosynthesis of various aromatic compounds. However, in C_4

plants, PEP serves as an important substrate in carbon fixation. The reaction is catalyzed by the enzyme phosphoenol pyruvate carboxylase (PEP carboxylase). The reaction is as follows:

PEP + $HCO_3^- \rightarrow$ oxaloacetate

15. Phytochrome has two different chemical structures that are inter-convertible. The forms are named by the color of light that they absorb maximally: Pr is a blue form that absorbs red light (660 nm) and Pfr is a blue-green form that absorbs far-red light (730 nm).

16. The light-harvesting complex II (LHCII) is the main energy absorber for photosynthesis in green plants, and its translocation between photosystems I and II is the primary means of energy redistribution between them. Light harvesting complex II is mainly found in the appressed regions (grana) of the photosynthetic membranes (thylakoids) and light harvesting complex I is mainly found in the non-appressed regions (stroma lamellae).

17. DNP is a chemical uncoupler of electron transport and oxidative phosphorylation. It permeabilizes the inner mitochondrial membrane to protons, destroying the proton gradient and, in doing so, uncouples the electron transport system from the oxidative phosphorylation. In this situation, electrons continue to pass through the electron transport system and reduce oxygen to water, but ATP is not synthesized in the process.

18. Chromatin is the combination of DNA and proteins that make up the contents of the nucleus of a cell. The metaphase structure of chromatin differs vastly to that of interphase. It is optimised for physical strength and manageability, forming the classic chromosome structure seen in karyotypes. The structure of the condensed chromosome is thought to be loops of 30 nm or 300 Å (in diameter) fibre to a central scaffold of proteins.

19. Linkage mapping is done by estimating the recombination fraction between loci, from the genotypes of offspring of particular matings. The further apart two loci are on a chromosome, the greater will be the frequency of recombination between them up to a maximum of 50%, the situation observed when they are sufficiently far apart on a chromosome that recombinant gametes are as frequent as non-recombinant gametes, or when they are on different chromosomes. Also 50% recombination (0.5) is when there is 100% meiosis with single crossovers. Any more crossovers (double) would result in less % recombination as the linked loci became unlinked and linked again.

20. Mycorrhiza are mutualistic/ symbiotic association essential for one or both partners, between a fungus and a root of a living plant that is primarily responsible for nutrient transfer. Mycorrhiza occur in specialized plant organs where intimate contact results from synchronized plant- fungus development.

21. Claviceps purpurea is an ergot fungus that infects various cereal plants forming compact black masses of branching filaments that replace many grains of the plant; a source of medicinally important alkaloids and of lysergic acid. It grows on the ears of rye and related cereal and forage plants.

22. Bacillus thuringiensis (commonly known as 'Bt') is an insecticidal bacterium used for control of many important plant pests - mainly caterpillars of the Lepidoptera (butterflies and moths) but also mosquito larvae. Bt is used for control of Lepidoptera by using a highly potent strain (B. thuringiensis var kurstaki). Also, the toxins produced by B. thuringiensis var aizawai have somewhat different toxins from those of Bt var kurstaki and they are highly specific to lepidoptera, with no effect on other insects.

23. Hutchinson first proposed his classification of angiosperms in his book The Families of Flowering Plants, the first volume on Dicotyledons appearing in 1926 and the second on Monocotyledons in 1934. The classification was revised periodically, second edition in 1959 and third edition in 1973.

24. A plant adapted to living in a saline environment is called halophytes. These are plants which tolerate or even demand sodium chloride concentrations in the soil water they absorb.

25. A food web depicts feeding connections (what-eats-what) in an ecological community and hence is also referred to as a consumer-resource system. Food webs are limited representations of real ecosystems as they necessarily aggregate many species into trophic species, which are functional groups of species that have the same predators and prey in a food web.

(M) MICROBIOLOGY

1. Telomerase enzyme is a ribonucleoprotein, contains RNA and protein. It resembles reverse transcriptases, enzymes that synthesize DNA using an RNA template. Telomerase recognizes the tip of a G- rich strand of an existing telomere DNA repeat sequence and elongates it in the 5'- 3' directions. The telomerase synthesizes a new copy of the repeat, using an RNA template that is a component of the enzyme itself.

2. 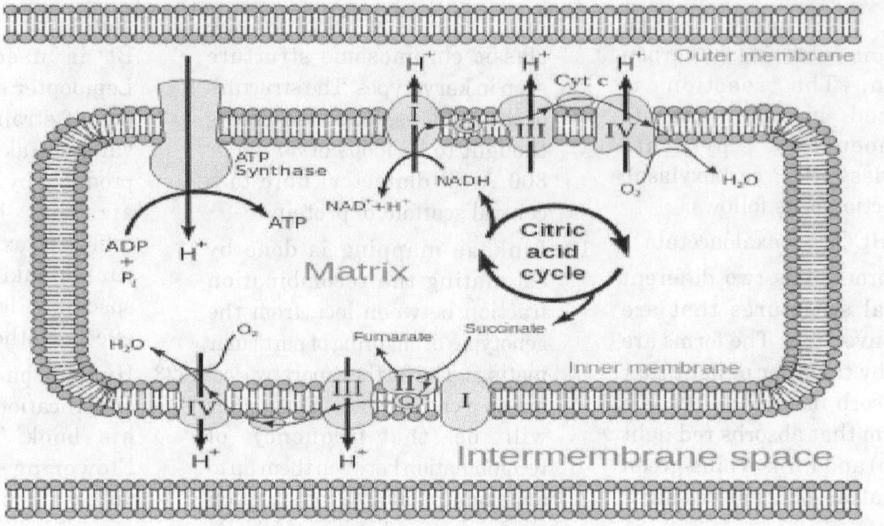

The electron transport chain in the mitochondrion is the site of oxidative phosphorylation in eukaryotes. The NADH and succinate generated in the citric acid cycle are oxidized, providing energy to power ATP synthase.

3. Given,
Faraday constant (F) = 23000 cal/V; $E_0' = +0.82 - (-0.42) = 1.24V$
Number of electrons transferred (n) = 2
Thus, according to the equation:
$\Delta G_0' = nF\Delta E_0'$
Therefore the free energy change G is –57040 cal.

4. When the two parent strands of DNA are separated to begin replication, one strand is oriented in the 5' to 3' direction while the other strand that is left strand is oriented in the 3' to 5' direction.

5. N-Formylmethionine (fMet) is a proteinogenic amino acid. It is a derivative of the amino acid methionine in which a formyl group has been added to the amino group. It is specifically used for initiation of protein synthesis from bacterial and organellar genes, and may be removed post-translationally.

6. Thermus thermophilus is a Gram negative eubacterium used in a range of biotechnological applications, including as a model organism for genetic manipulation, structural genomics, and systems biology. The bacterium is extremely thermophilic, with an optimal growth temperature of about 65°C (149°F)

7. Deletion never extends polypeptides.

8. fMet plays a crucial part in the protein synthesis of bacteria, mitochondria and chloroplasts. It is not used in cytosolic protein synthesis of eukaryotes, where eukaryotic nuclear genes are translated. It is also not used by Archaea. In the human body, fMet is recognized by the immune system as foreign material and stimulates the body to fight against potential infection.

9. The lac repressor (LacI) operates by binding to the major groove of the operator region of the lac operon. This blocks RNA polymerase from binding, and so prevents transcription of the mRNA coding for the Lac proteins. Lac O, the operator is a short region of DNA that lies partially within the promoter and that interacts with a regulatory protein that controls the transcription of the operon. So mutation in locations gives changes. lac Z,Y and A are structural genes of lac operons.

10. More than 15000000 antibody specificities will be present in an organism having 200V and 5J genes for the light chain and 300V, 10D and 5J genes for the heavy chain.

Diverse heavy chain
$= V \times J = 200 \times 5 = 1000$
Diverse light chain
$= V \times D \times J$
$= 300 \times 10 \times 5 = 15000$
Thus number of antibody specificities
$= 1000 \times 15000$
$= 15000000$

11. CD4 and CD8 T cell surface molecules play a role in T cell recognition and activation by binding to their respective class II and class I major histocompatibility complex (MHC)

12. Smallpox was an infectious disease unique to humans, caused by either of two virus variants, Variola major and Variola minor, that is DNA virus and here others are by RNA virus such as measles caused by paramyxovirus, Yellow Fever caused by yellow fever virus and Poliomyelitis caused by Polio virus.

13. Mycobacterium tuberculosis has a very puzzling method of pathogenesis. It seems to defy logic by actually using macrophages, the front line defences of the human immune system, as a safe haven for its reproduction. And apart from its other bacteria do infection due to microbial protein toxin.

14. *Myocarditis* is inflammation of heart muscle (myocardium). It resembles a heart attack but coronary arteries are not blocked. Myocarditis is most often due to infection by common viruses, such as parvovirus B19, less commonly non- viral pathogens such as *Borrelia burgdorferi* (Lyme disease) or *Trypanosoma cruzi*, or as a hypersensitivity response to drugs.
15. Titers of antibodies in serum samples from infected patients were compared with healthy older Vietnamese children and adult's shows have high titers of antibody in case of Shigellosis that caused Shigella.
16. Rheumatic disease are non infectious cause of fever as other are here highly infectious disease.
17. Bacteria with an acid-fast cell wall when stained by the acid-fast procedure, resist decolorization with acid-alcohol and stain red, the color of the primary stain, carbol fuchsin. The genus Mycobacterium and the genus Nocardia are acid-fast. Counterstain is methylene blue.
18. The T cell receptor is restricted to recognizing antigenic peptides only when bound to appropriate molecules of the major histocompatibility complex (MHC).
19. Live attenuated strains (Suspension of living organism with reduce virulence) which has killing effect on all three types of polio virus.
20. DNA replication in prokaryotes is exemplified in E. coli. It is bi-directional and originates at a single origin of replication (OriC).
21. Retting a process for degradation of low esterfied pectin.
22. Prontosil, also called sulfamidochrysoidine was the first commercially available antibacterial drug when used in animals. Prontosil resulted from research, directed by German chemist and pathologist Gerhard Domagk, on the antibacterial action of azo dyes. A red azo dye of low toxicity, Prontosil was shown by Domagk to prevent mortality in mice infected with Streptococcus bacteria. Prontosil was effective not only in combating experimental infections in animals but also against streptococcal diseases in humans, including meningitis and puerperal sepsis.
23. The nucleosome core is formed of two H2A-H2B dimers and a H3-H4 tetramer, forming two nearly symmetrical halves by tertiary structure (C2 symmetry; one macromolecule is the mirror image of the other). The H2A-H2B dimers and H3-H4 tetramer also show pseudo dyad symmetry. The 4 'core' histones (H2A, H2B, H3 and H4) are relatively similar in structure and are highly conserved through evolution, all featuring a 'helix turn helix turn helix' motif (which allows the easy dimerization). Thus the subunit composition of histones in nucleosomes is $[(H2A)(H2B)(H3)(H4)]_2$.
24. G1 is an intermediate phase occupying the time between the end of cell division in mitosis and the beginning of DNA replication during S phase. During this time, the cell grows in preparation for DNA replication, and certain intracellular components, such as the centrosomes undergo replication. Before a cell begins DNA replication, it must ensure that it is biologically ready to take on such a process. G1 is the phase when this cellular monitoring takes place.
25. Association of cyclin A with CDK2 is required for passage into S phase.

(N) ZOOLOGY

1. Echinoderms are eucoelomate deuterostomes. They show a superficial pentamerous radial symmetry. The larvae are bilaterally symmetric, cephalized, and motile but they develop into sessile or sedentary radially symmetric adults. Chordates are eucoelomate deuterostomes and probably share a common ancestor with echinoderms. Three important points unite the Phylum Chordata. At some point in their life cycle, all chordates have a notochord, a dorsal hollow nerve cord and pharyngeal gill slits.
2. Anura is the clade of living frogs and their close fossil relatives. The name Anura refers to the lack of a tail. Some distinctive features are → (a) Shortened vertebral column (nine or fewer presacral vertebrae) (b) Presence of a urostyle formed from developing tail vertebrae (c) Absence of tail in adults and hindlimb longer than forelimb. Urodela is an order of amphibians having the tail well developed and often long. It comprises the salamanders, tritons, and allied animals. To accommodate the earlier and now extinct proto-frogs and proto-salamanders, the group names Salientia and Urodela are used. Apoda is the smallest order (sometimes called Gymnophiona) of the class Amphibia, known as the caecilians. These are wormlike, legless animals with indistinct or even hidden eyes. A series of annular grooves is usually present along the length of the body, heightening the resemblance to an earthworm. Most caecilians lead a burrowing existence, though members of one genus, Typhlonectes, are aquatic.
3. The evolutionary surge that led to *Homo habilis* began during the transition between the Pliocene and Pleistocene Epochs around 2.5 million years ago when climates were becoming cooler and drier. All later species of *Homo* evolved during the Pleistocene (2,600,000-11,700 years ago). This was generally a time of more extremeworld cooling and recurrent glaciations (ice ages). Human evolution was very likely affected strongly by the dramatic climate swings of the Pleistocene. The Holocene is a geological epoch which began at the end of the Pleistocene. The Holocene also encompasses

within it the growth and impacts of the human species world-wide, including all its written history and overall significant transition toward urban living in the present.

4. Neotropical region, also called South American region, one of the six major biogeographic areas of the world defined on the basis of its characteristic animal life. It includes such animals as the llama, tapir, deer, pig, jaguar, puma, a variety of opossums, many rodents and fishes, and extremely rich insect and bird populations. The vegetation division roughly corresponding to the region is called the Neotropical kingdom. This region is bound to Afrotropic, Indo-Malayan, and Nearctic regions. But neotropical region is not bound by the Antarctic region.

5. Albinism occurs when one of several genetic defects makes the body unable to produce or distribute melanin, a natural substance that gives colour to your hair, skin, and iris of the eye. There are two main types of albinism: a) Type 1 albinism is caused by defects that affect production of the pigment, melanin and b) Type 2 albinism is due to a defect in the "P" gene. People with this type have slight colouring at birth. There are two different forms of albinism: a partial lack of the melanin is known as hypomelanism, or hypomelanosis and the total absence of melanin is known as amelanism or amelanosis. It is a congenital disorder characterized by the complete or partial absence of pigment in the skin, hair and eyes due to absence or defect of tyrosinase, a copper-containing enzyme involved in the production of melanin.

6. Stop codons are any of three codons in a molecule of messenger RNA that do not code for an amino acid and thereby signal the termination of the synthesis of a protein. The three stop codons are UAA, UAG, and UGA, where U is uracil, A is adenine, and G is guanine. These are also called termination codon. Stop codons are any of three mRNA sequences (UGA, UAG, and UAA) that do not code for an amino acid and thus signal the end of protein synthesis. UAC is the codon for translation into the first amino acid produced during protein synthesis, i.e., methionine (ATG).

7. In a human cell, the basic constituents are carbohydrates, lipids and fats, proteins, vitamins and minerals. Most of the biochemical compounds are organic in nature. That means carbon is an integral part of a majority of the biological compounds. So, the number of moles of carbon is the highest in a human cell.

8. Aves are the name of the class to which birds belong in taxonomy. They belong to the subphylum Vertebrata of the Phylum Chordata. They have a highly efficient cardiopulmonary system with an endothermic heart (they are warm-blooded). Eutheria is the clade consisting of primates and all other mammals. Since Placentalia includes all living eutherians, the nonplacental eutherians are necessarily extinct. Prototheria is a group of mammals that comprises the monotremes and their extinct relatives. Metatheria is a grouping within the animal class Mammalia including a single order, the Marsupialia and are distinguished by a small braincase, a total of 50 teeth, the inflected angular process of the mandible, and a pair of marsupial bones articulating with the pelvis. Aves have the highest body temperature due to the insulation from the environment provided by their feathers and fur. Amongst the classes of Mammalia, Eutherians have the highest body temperature followed by methatherians and prototherians.

9. A haplotype is a group of genes within an organism that was inherited together from a single parent. The word "haplotype" is derived from the word "haploid," which describes cells with only one set of chromosomes, and from the word "genotype," which refers to the genetic makeup of an organism. A haplotype can describe a pair of genes inherited together from one parent on one chromosome, or it can describe all of the genes on chromosomes that were inherited together from a single parent. This group of genes was inherited together because of genetic linkage, or the phenomenon by which genes that are close to each other on the same chromosome are often inherited together.

10. Epinephrine is a hormone that is secreted by the adrenal glands. Epinephrine is derived from tyrosine, an amino acid. Epinephrine is sometimes referred to as a catecholamine as it contains the catechol moiety. This is a part of the molecule that contains the group $C_6H_4\ (OH)_2$. Epinephrine is involved in the fight or flight response in humans. The fight or flight response occurs when a person is subject to a threat. This causes a signalling process to occur, which causes the body to react to the potential danger. When the nerve signal reaches the adrenal gland, chromaffin cells, in the medulla of the adrenal gland, release epinephrine. Epinephrine then enters the bloodstream. It is thus carried around the body to cells in various locations, where it initiates several responses.

11. In general, trachea is the respiratory organ in insects, gills are present in fishes for respiration and lungs are respiratory organs for mammals. Dorsal line relates to the back or spinal part of the body. It also relates to the back or upper surface of an animal. It means belonging to or on or near the back or upper surface of an animal or organ or part. For example, “the dorsal fin is the vertical fin on the back of a fish and certain marine mammals”.

12. The hypervariable region of antibody was first demonstrated by Milstein and Kholer. The hypervariable region of an antibody represents the highly varying variable regions present on both the heavy and light chains. These highly varying regions are composed of varying sequences of amino acids. These regions are responsible for binding to the foreign antigen. These are also known as the complementarity determining sequences and contribute to the specificity of the antibody.

13. Filariasis is a disease group affecting humans and animals caused by nematode parasites of the order Filariidae, commonly called filariae. Filarial parasites may be classified according to the habitat of the adult worms in the vertebral host. It has been observed (especially in endemic areas), that the prevalence of microfilaremia increases with age, as adult worms are gradually acquired over years. As with most helminths, adult filarial parasites replicate in a secondary host. The adult worm burden in an individual cannot increase unless the host is exposed to additional microfilaria. Because the mosquito vector is inefficient, a relatively prolonged stay in an endemic area is usually required to acquire the infection. The genus Culex is a carrier of viral encephalitis and, in tropical and subtropical climates, of filariasis. It holds its body parallel to the resting surface and its proboscis is bent downward relative to the surface. The wings, with scales on the veins and the margin, are uniform in colour.

14. Second messengers are molecules that relay signals received at receptors on the cell surface - such as the arrival of protein hormones, growth factors, etc. — to target molecules in the cytosol and/or nucleus. There are 3 major classes of second messengers: (1) cyclic nucleotides (e.g., cAMP and cGMP) (2) inositol trisphosphate (IP_3) and diacylglycerol (DAG) and (3) calcium ions (Ca^{2+}). ATP or adenosine triphosphate is a trinucleotide phosphate molecule whose breakdown gives energy that can be utilised in various biochemical pathways.

15. Human chorionic gonadotropin (hCG) is the principal hCG immunoreactivity in early pregnancy urine. It is the principal hCG-related molecule in pregnancy urine in the 2 weeks following the missed menses. Human chorionic gonadotropin interacts with the LHCG receptor and promotes the maintenance of the corpus luteum during the beginning of pregnancy, causing it to secrete the hormone progesterone. Like other gonadotropins, hCG can be extracted from urine or by genetic modification.

16. Passive immunity to the foetus is provided by antibody IgG. This is because IgG is the only immunoglobulin that can cross the placental barrier. So it crosses the placenta from the mother and reaches the foetus to provide it immunity. IgM is the first class of immunoglobulin produced when the body is invaded by a microorganism. As such IgM holds the initial response to an antigen by the B-cells. IgE is meant for allergic response. IgA is present in saliva and secretions.

17. First seen by Europeans in 1598, the Dodo was extinct shortly after 1640. Mauritius, an island in the Indian Ocean was its only home. Human activity is to blame for its extinction. Dodo (*Raphus cucullatus*) was a flightless bird. Its closest genetic relative was the also extinct *Rodrigues solitaire*, the two forming the subfamily Raphinae of the family of pigeons and doves.

18. Darwin's 'The Origin of Species' was published in 1859. It provoked a storm of controversy because it challenged the Christian belief that God created life on Earth. Huxley's repeated and passionate defence of the book earned him the nickname of 'Darwin's Bulldog'. In 1863, he published his own book on evolution, 'Evidence as to Man's Place in Nature'. Unlike Darwin's Origin, this book focused on man's ancestry and was short and populist in style.

19. Firstly, no man can be cloned from a single cell lineage or tissue. The totipotent power of the zygote is lost once it gets converted to the embryo after fertilization. That is why humans are called pleuripotent animals and plants are called totipotent animals because of their power to generate the entire plant from a single cell at any time of life. But, in the given case, sperm cannot be used for cloning as these are reduced in their chromosome number because of their reproductive nature. Erthrocytes are non-nucleated cells with short life span of 120 days and so they are not a good option for cloning. Lymphocytes are differentiated cells developed for fibroblasts, the lymphoid progenitor. Already differentiated cells cannot be induced to give rise to an entire organism in mammals. Kidney fibroblasts are stem cells which are unorganised and can be used to develop a man *in vitro*.

20. Communal suckling is the process of nursing and feeding of a number of offsprings by a single mother. Communal suckling is present whenever there is multiple breeding giving rise to a lot of offsprings. This phenomenon is seen in cows, buffalos and dogs.

21. There are two types of light chain in humans → kappa (κ) chain and lambda (λ) chain. The complementarity determining sequences or regions present in the kappa (κ) chain are 3. These regions render specificity to the antibody and also help in determining the antigen binding capacity of the antibody or immunoglobulin.

22. Transfer RNA (tRNA) is involved in the translation of the nucleic acid message into the amino acids of proteins. tRNA itself is an RNA molecule with a conserved inverted L structure. One end of the tRNA contains an anticodon loop which pairs with an mRNA specifying a certain amino acid. The other end of the tRNA has the amino acid attached to the 3′ OH group via an ester linkage. In eukaryotic cells, tRNAs are transcribed by RNA polymerase III as pre-tRNAs in the nucleus. Pre-tRNAs undergo extensive modifications inside the nucleus. Some pre-tRNAs contain introns that are spliced to form the functional tRNA molecule.

23. Shine-Dalgarno sequence is a part of the leader sequence preceding the start codon of mRNA that is AGGAGGU or a variant thereof that binds the mRNA to a complementary sequence in the 16S component of rRNA so that translation of the mRNA can proceed. The Shine-Dalgarno sequence is a purine-rich tract of 3-10 nucleotides and precedes the start AUG codon by approximately 10 nucleotides upstream on the 5′ side. The Shine-Dalgarno sequence forms base pairing with a highly conserved, pyrimidine-rich region of the 16S rRNA which is part of the 30S ribosomal subunit. This base-pairing properly aligns the start AUG codon in the P site of the 30S ribosomal subunit. In eukaryotes, protein synthesis usually begins with the first AUG codon from the 5′ end. Eukaryotic mRNA has a special cap at the 5′ end of the mRNA which is recognized by a cap-binding protein.

24. Gonadotropin-releasing factor is a substance produced by the hypothalamus that stimulates the release of gonadotropin by the anterior lobe of the pituitary gland. It is also called gonadoliberin. A key area for production of Gonadotropin-releasing hormone (GnRH) is the preoptic area of the hypothalamus, which contains most of the GnRH-secreting neurons. GnRH neurons originate in the nose and migrate into the brain, where they are scattered throughout the medial septum and hypothalamus. The portal blood carries the GnRH to the pituitary gland, which contains the gonadotrope cells, where GnRH activates its own receptor, gonadotropin-releasing hormone receptor (GnRHR), a seven-transmembrane G-protein-coupled receptor that stimulates the synthesis and secretion of the gonadotropins LH and FSH.

25. The four phases of cell cycle are $\rightarrow G_1$, S, G_2 and M-phase. DNA synthesis takes place in the S-phase or the synthetic phase of the cell cycle. DNA is doubled in content in this phase. The G_1, S, G_2 phases are together called the interphase or the preparatory phase of the cell cycle and M-phase is called the mitotic phase of the cell cycle.

■■

GATE-2001

XL : LIFE SCIENCES

Time : 3 Hours **Maximum Marks : 100**

(H) CHEMISTRY (Compulsory)

Useful data :

Gas constant, R = 8.314 J mol^{-1} K^{-1}

I1. For each question given below, four alternative answers are provided of which only one is correct. Write the correct answer in the answeer book by writing *a*, *b*, *c* or *d* along with the corresponding sub-question number. (25 × 1 = 25)

1.1 In CsCl crystal structure, each Cs^+ ion is surrounded by

(*a*) 4 Cl^- (*b*) 6 Cl^- (*c*) 8 Cl^- (*d*) 12 Cl^-

1.2 $Cr(NH_3)_5Cl_3$ reacts with $AgNO_3$ solution quantitatively. The number of moles of $AgNO_3$ consumed by one mole of the metal complex is

(*a*) 1.0 (*b*) 2.0 (*c*) 3.0 (*d*) 4.0

1.3 Bohr model can explain

(*a*) the spectrum of hydrogen atom only

(*b*) the solar system

(*c*) the spectrum of hydrogen molecule

(*d*) the spectrum of an atom or an ion containing only one electron.

1.4 The hybridization of oxygen in the molecule OF_2 is

(*a*) *sp* (*b*) sp^2 (*c*) sp^3 (*d*) dsp^2

1.5 The correct increasing order of electronegativity of the following elements is

(*a*) F < O < N < S (*b*) S < N < O < F

(*c*) N < S < O < F (*d*) O < N < S < F

1.6 Which of the following trihalides of nitrogen is least basic?

(*a*) NF_3 (*b*) NCl_3 (*c*) NBr_3 (*d*) NI_3

1.7 Which of the following compounds has the highest pH when dissolved in water?

(*a*) CH_3COONa (*b*) NH_4Cl

(*c*) NaCN (*d*) NaCl

1.8 Which of the following reactions will give oxygen?

(*a*) NaOH + F_2 (*b*) NaOH + Cl_2

(*c*) NaOH + Br_2 (*d*) NaOH + I_2

1.9 When I-butyne is treated with sulphuric acid in the presence of mercuric sulphate, then stable product formed is

(*a*) Butyl sulphate (*b*) Butan-2-one

(*c*) 2-Buten-1-ol (*d*) Butynediol

1.10 The compound that will not give chloroform on treatment with Cl_2/NaOH is

(*a*) Propanone (*b*) Ethanol

(*c*) Ethanal (*d*) Propanol

1.11 Most reactive compound towards formation of cyanohydrin on treatement with KCN followed by acidification is

(*a*) Benzaldehyde (*b*) *p*-Nitrobenzaldehyde

(*c*) Phenylacetaldehyde (*d*) *p*-Hydroxy benzaldehyde

1.12 The compound with highest pK_a is expected to be

(*a*) *p*-Nitrophenol (*b*) *p*-Chlorophenol

(*c*) *p*-Methylphenol (*d*) *p*-Methoxyphenol

1.13 The method that would provide the highest yield of pure ethylbenzene is the reaction of benzene with

(*a*) ethanol and sulphuric acid

(*b*) ethyl chloride in the presence of aluminium chloride

(*c*) acetyl chloride in the presence of aluminium chloride followed by reduction with $LiAlH_4$

(*d*) ethanoyl chloride in the presence of aluminium chloride.

1.14 Most reactive halide towards SN_1 reaction is

(*a*) *n*-Butyl chloride (*b*) *sec*-Butyl chloride

(*c*) *tert*-Butyl chloride (*d*) Allyl chloride

1.15 Aldol condensation will not be observed in

(*a*) Chloral (*b*) Phenyl acetaldehyde

(*c*) Cyclohexenal (*d*) Nitromethane

1.16 The predominant product of reduction of α-ketoester with sodium borohydride is

(*a*) Primary alcohol (*b*) Secondary alcohol

(*c*) Alkane (*d*) Vinyl borane

1.17 Toluene on reaction with N-bromo-succinimide gives

(*a*) *p*-Bromomethyl benzene

(*b*) *o*-Bromomethyl benzene

(*c*) Phenyl bromomethane

(*d*) *m*-Bromomethyl benzene

1.18 $CaCO_3(s) = CaO(s) + CO_2(g)$

The number of degrees of freedom for the above equilibrium reaction is

(*a*) 0 (*b*) 1 (*c*) 2 (*d*) 3

1.19 A catalyst is one which speeds up the reaction by

(*a*) decreasing the enthalpy of the reactants

(*b*) decreasing the free energy of the reaction

(*c*) increasing the kinetic energy of the reactants

(*d*) decreasing the activation energy of the reaction

1.20 In a chemical reaction, the fraction of the reactant consumed per unit time is independent of the initial concentration. The order of the reactions is

(*a*) Indeterminate (*b*) two

(*c*) one (*d*) zero

1.21 If q is the amount of heat suplied by the system and w is the magnitude of the work done on the system, then change in internal energy of the system equals

(*a*) $-q+w$ (*b*) $q-w$ (*c*) $q+w$ (*d*) $-q-w$

1.22 A drop of ink put in a glass of water mixes uniformly with the passage of time. This is due to

(*a*) gravitational force

(*b*) minimization of potential energy

(*c*) maximization of entropy

(*d*) osmotic pressure of pure water

1.23 A 0.2 M solution of sugar is isotonic with a solution of common salt. Both solutions have the same volume and are at the same temperature. The concentration of the common salt solution is

(*a*) 0.1 M (*b*) 0.2 M (*c*) 0.3 M (*d*) 0.4 M

1.24 The molar conductivity of a strong electrolyte varies

(*a*) linearly with concentration

(*b*) linearly with the square root of concentration

(*c*) inversely with concentration

(*d*) as the square of the concentration

1.25 That the specific heat of a stable solid is positive, can be derived from

(*a*) Gibbs-Helmholtz equation

(*b*) Kirchoff's equation

(*c*) the first law of thermodynamics

(*d*) the second law of thermodynamics

I2. Explain the following observations.

(*i*) $[CoF_6]^{3-}$ is paramagnetic while $[Co(CN)_6]^{3-}$ is diamagnetic. (1)

(*ii*) $AgNO_3$ gives a white precipitate with aqueous solutioon of $Na_2S_2O_3$ which dissolves in excess of $Na_2S_2O_3$. If the precipitate is heated with water, it turns black and the supernatant liquid gives a white precipitate with acidified $Ba(NO_3)_2$. Write the balanced chemical equations involved. (4)

I3. (*i*) Why is electron affinity of fluorine less than that of chlorine? (2)

(*ii*) Why is ammonia more soluble in aqueous ammonium chloride than it is in pure water? (2)

(*iii*) Why is cyclopentadiene an extra-ordinarily acidic hydrocarbon? (1)

I4. (*i*) Bromoalkenes are usually converted to alkynes by treatment with KNH_2 but 1-bromocyclohexene does not undergo dehydrohalogenation under these conditions. Explain. (2)

(*ii*) Write steps involved in the conversion of benzene to 2, 6 dinitrochlorobenzene.

(*iii*) Draw a Fischer projection formula for the diastereoisomer of 2R, 3R-2-chloro-3-bromobutane. (1)

I5. (*i*) Diels Alder reaction between 2, 5-dimethyl-3, 4-diphenylfuran and dimethylfumarate does not take place. Explain why. (2)

(*ii*) Calcualte pH of the solution at equivalence point of a titration between 0.1 M sodium acetic acid and 0.1 M sodium hydroxide solution. (Apparent dissociation constant of acetic acid at this ionic strength is equal to 2.7×10^{-5}). (2)

(*iii*) Assuming that there is no change in pressure and temperature, estimate the change is entropy when two cylinders containing equal volumes of an ideal gas are interconnected.

I6. (*i*) Derive the thermodynamic equation of state, $(\partial U/\partial V)_T = \{T(\partial P/\partial T)_v - P\}$ (2)

(*ii*) When the concentration of both Zn^{2+} and Cu^{2+} ions is 1.0 M, the emf of a Daniel cell is 1.10 V. Calculate the emf of the cell if the concentrations of Zn^{2+} ions and Cu^{2+} ions are changed to 2.0 M and 0.5 M respectively. (2)

(*iii*) Why absolute alcohol cannot be prepared from aqueous alcohol by distillation? (1)

(J) BIOCHEMISTRY

J1. For each sub-question given below, four alternatives are provided of which only one is appropriate. Write the answer in the answer book by writing *a, b, c* or *d* along with the corresponding sub-question number. (1 × 25 = 25)

1.1 The pH of 1 mM HCl is

(*a*) 1 (*b*) 2 (*c*) 0 (*d*) 3

1.2 The length of an α helical section of a plypeptide chain of 20 residues would be

(*a*) 30 Å (*b*) 20 Å (*c*) 5.4 Å (*d*) 3.6 Å

1.3 Which one of these reagents is best suited for identification of the amino terminal residue of a peptide of which you have less than 0.1 μg.

(*a*) performic acid (*b*) dansyl chloride

(*c*) fluoro dinitrobenzene (*d*) cyanogen bromide

1.4 If a solution of double stranded DNA is heated above its melting temperature, its absorbance will,

(*a*) decrease

(*b*) increase

(*c*) remain unchanged

(*d*) initially increase and then decrease

1.5 β-amylase cleaves

(*a*) α (1-4) glycosidic bonds

(*b*) β (1-4) glycosidic bonds

(*c*) α (1-6) glycosidic bonds

(*d*) β (1 – 6) glycosidic bonds

1.6 Gangliosides contain

(*a*) a ceramide structure (*b*) glucose or galactose

(*c*) sialic acid (*d*) all of the above

1.7 A southern transfer of *E. coli* DNA after complete digestion with ECOR1 was probed with labeled cDNA probe of a gene which occurs only once in the *E. coli* genome. If the gene contains one ECOR1 cleavage site near its centre, the number of radioactive bands you are most likely to find on autoradiography would be

(*a*) 0 (*b*) 1 (*c*) 2 (*d*) 3

1.8 The largest energy reserve (kilocalories) in humans is

(*a*) blood glucose
(*b*) liver glycogen
(*c*) muscle glycogen
(*d*) adipose tissue triacylglycerol

1.9 Both strands of DNA serve as templates concurrently in

(*a*) replication (*b*) mismatch repair
(*c*) excision repair (*d*) all of the above

1.10 In which of the following does the inner surface of a closed membrane or vesicle become the outer surface of a closed membrane or vesicle

(*a*) fusion of two intracellular vesicles
(*b*) transfer of an endoplasmic reticular membrane into golgi membrane via vesicle
(*c*) exocytosis of a secretory vesicle
(*d*) division of a bacterial cell

1.11 Enzyme linked immunosorbent assay used to detect antigens or antibodies utilizes those enzymes that

(*a*) have a high turnover rate
(*b*) yield a stable colored product
(*c*) are stable on conjugation to proteins
(*d*) all of the above

1.12 Which of the following hormones uses cyclic AMP as the second messenger

(*a*) follicle stimulating hormone
(*b*) insulin
(*c*) progesterone
(*d*) gonadotropin releasing hormone

1.13 IgM class of antibodies are more effective that IgG in bringing about complement mediated lysis because

(*a*) IgM has higher affinity for complement components
(*b*) IgM has higher affinity for antigen binding
(*c*) IgM is a pentamer
(*d*) IgM is present in higher concentration

1.14 Which of the following statements is false

(*a*) MHC class II molecules are present on all nucleated cells
(*b*) MHC class II molecules are made up of two polypeptides
(*c*) MHC class I molecules are present on all nucleated cells
(*d*) T cell response is MHC - restricted

1.15 Which of these substrats is best suited for measuring RNA systhesis by RNA polymerase

(*a*) γ P^{32} ATP (*b*) α P^{32} d ATP
(*c*) γ P^{32} d ATP (*d*) α P^{32} UTP

1.16 The tripeptide sequence encoded by the following polydeoxyribonucleotide sequence, 5′ CCC AAA TAC 3′, would be

(*a*) pro lys tyr (*b*) met phe gly
(*c*) met gly lys (*d*) met phe lys

1.17 All of the following are true about transposons except

(*a*) transposons move from one location to a different one within a chromosome
(*b*) both donors and target sites must be homologous
(*c*) transposons may activate a gene
(*d*) transposons may inactivate a gene

1.18 The class of immunoglobulins that can get transported across epithelial cells is

(*a*) IgG (*b*) IgE (*c*) IgA (*d*) IgM

1.19 A muscle extract is dialysed exhaustively against 10 mM sodium phosphate buffer, pH 7.0. The extract does not contain any ATPase activity. If ATP is now added, the following cofactor that also must be added to convert glucose to glucose-6-phosphate is

(*a*) NAD^+ (*b*) $FADH_2$ (*c*) Mg^{2+} (*d*) Fe^{3+}

1.20 Injection of dinitrophenol (DNP) into a rat causes an immediate increase in its body temperature, because

(*a*) DNP acts as an inhibitor of mitochondrial ATPase
(*b*) DNP blocks the electron transport chain
(*c*) DNP inhibits succinic dehydrogenase
(*d*) DNP uncouples electron transport from oxidative phosphorylation

1.21 A rat liver extract is treated with avidin. Which of the following conversion in gluconeogenesis will not occur

(*a*) glyceraldehyde 3-P $\rightarrow$ glucose 6 P
(*b*) malate $\rightarrow$ oxaloacetate
(*c*) pyruvate $\rightarrow$ phosphoenolpyruvate
(*d*) fumarate $\rightarrow$ phosphoenolpyruvate

1.22 The direct effect of cyclic AMP in the protein Kinase A pathway is to

(*a*) activate adenylate cyclase
(*b*) dissociate regulatory subunits from protein Kinase A
(*c*) phosphorylate protein Kinase A
(*d*) release hormones from target tissue

1.23 The active site amino acid residue that could be involved in a reaction catalyzed by an enzyme with a pH optimum of 4 would be

(*a*) arginine (*b*) cysteine
(*c*) serine (*d*) glutamate

1.24 The isoelectric pH of γ globulin, human serum albumin (HSA) ribonuclease (RNAase) and hen egg lysozyme (HEL) are 6.6,4.9,7.8 and 11.0 respectively. The order in which these proteins will be eluted from a CM cellulose ion exchange column by an increasing salt gradient at *p*H 7.0 would be

(*a*) HSA, γ globulin, RNAase and HEL

(*b*) HEL, RNAase, γ globulin, HSA

(*c*) HEL, γ globulin, RNAase, HSA

(*d*) HSA. RNAase, HEL, γ globulin

1.25 A solution contains DNA polymerase I, Mg^{2+} salts and dNTPs. Which of these molecules would act as template and lead to DNA synthesis

(*a*) single stranded RNA base paired with a primer with a free 3′ OH group

(*b*) single stranded DNA base paired with a primer with a free 5′ OH group

(*c*) single stranded DNA base paired with a primer with a free 3′ OH group

(*d*) double stranded DNA base paired with a free 3′ OH group at each end

J2. Give correct answers to the following: (1 × 5 = 5)

(*a*) Which of the following amino acids are likely to have their side chains on the inside of globular proteins in solution, val, pro, phe, asp, lys, ile, his

(*b*) Which of the following ion exchangers would be suitable for purification of a DNA binding protein and why?

(*i*) CM cellulose (*ii*) DEAE cellulos

(*c*) What is the coenzyme form of vitamin B6? Name the reactions in which this coenzyme is involved.

(*d*) In a preparation of mitochondria, oxidation of fatty acids is carried out in presence of CoA, O_2, ADP and P_i.

(*i*) How many molecules of ATP will be produced per two carbon fragments converted to CO_2?

(*ii*) What will this number be if amytal is added to the preparation?

(*e*) Northern analysis of nuclear RNA and cytoplasmic RNA from liver when probed with aldolase genomic clone showed that the nuclear RNA specific to aldolase had a molecular weight higher than that of cytoplasmic RNA. Explain why?

J3. Answer the following in one sentence each (Do not exceed) (1 × 5 = 5)

(*a*) What are RAG genes?

(*b*) What are recombination signal sequences?

(*c*) How does simultaneous expression of IgM and IgD occur in mature B cells?

(*d*) Name any four members of the immunoglobulin superfamily other than immunoglobulin?

(*e*) Define monoclonal antibodies.

J4. State true or false against each of the following: (1 × 5 = 5)

(*a*) Methylation of lysine ε-amino group occurs in histones to modulate their interaction with DNA

(*b*) In all cases of diabetes mellitus, circulatory levels of insulin are low or negligible.

(*c*) While bone marrow is the primary lymphoid organ, thymus and spleen are secondary lymphoid organs.

(*d*) Both in the liver and muscle, glycogen functions as a glucose reserve for maintenance of blood glucose concentration.

(*e*) Type I topoisomerases create transient single stranded breaks in DNA, whereas type II topoisomerases make transient double stranded breaks in DNA

J5. Match the entries in column 1 with the appropriate one in the column 2 and write matching pairs in the answer book

(*a*) ionophore	(*i*) cathepsin
(*b*) oubain	(*ii*) Na^+K^+ – ATPase
(*c*) malonate	(*iii*) Homogentisic acid oxidase
(*d*) alkaptonuria	(*iv*) phenylalanine hydroxylase
(*e*) protein hydrolyzing enzymes	(*v*) penicillin
	(*vi*) gramicidine A
	(*vii*) competitive inhibitor of succinic dehydrogenase

J6. (*a*) The Km of a certain enzyme is 1 μM. At a substrate concentration of 1mM, the Vmax is 50 μmoles/min. However the Vmax remained the same, even at a ten fold lower concentration of the substrate. Explain (2)

(*b*) Restriction analysis of a fragment of dsDNA with Hind III gave fragments of sizes 2.8 kb and 1.2 kb. The same DNA upon digestion with BamH1, yielded fragment sizes of 1.8 kb, 1.3 kb and 0.9 kb Double digestion of the DNA with both these enzymes yielded fragment sizes 1.8 kb, 1.0 kb, 0.9 kb and 0.3 kb Making use of this data draw a restriction map of the DNA fragment (2)

(*c*) Define isoenzymes. (1)

(L) BOTANY

L1. For each sub-question given below, four alternatives are provided of which only <u>one</u> is correct. Write the correct answer in the answer book by writing *a,b,c* or *d* along with the sub-question number. (25 × 1 = 25)

1.1 Which of the following proteins is a major component of cytoskeleton?

(*a*) Tubulin (*b*) Fibrin (*c*) Osmotin (*d*) Porin

1.2 The specialized tissue in the roots of epiphytic orchids is known as

(*a*) Haustoria (*b*) Laticifer

(*c*) Velamen (*d*) Periderm

1.3 Lenticel originates from

(*a*) Guard cells (*b*) Subsidiary cells

(*c*) Complimentary cells (*d*) Companion cells

1.4 Plant cell suspension culture is easily initiated from
(*a*) Shoot apex (*b*) Root apex
(*c*) Protoplast (*d*) Friable callus

1.5 The process by which the pollen tube enters the ovule through micropyle is
(*a*) Chalazogamy (*b*) Basigamy
(*c*) Porogamy (*d*) Mesogamys

1.6 Germplasm preservation through tissue culture is
(*a*) *In situ* conservation
(*b*) *Ex situ* conservation
(*c*) Protected area conservation
(*d*) Both *in situ* and *ex situ* conservation

1.7 The taxa in danger of extinction is termed as
(*a*) Extinct (*b*) Rare
(*c*) Vulnerable (*d*) Endangered

1.8 The best definition of biodiversity is variability
(*a*) Within species only
(*b*) Between species only
(*c*) Both within and between species
(*d*) Within species, between species and of ecosystem

1.9 The diploid number of an organism is 12. How many chromosomes would be expected in its nullisomic?
(*a*) 10 (*b*) 11 (*c*) 13 (*d*) 14

1.10 The vascular bundle having xylem and phloem strands in alternate radii is known as
(*a*) Collateral (*b*) Bicollateral
(*c*) Radial (*d*) Concentric

1.11 The average number of chiasma in one pair of homologous chromosome is 1.4. The total length (in map units) for the linkage group is expected to be
(*a*) 90 (*b*) 70 (*c*) 50 (*d*) 30

1.12 A functional unit of gene which specifies one polypeptide is known as
(*a*) Codon (*b*) Muton (*c*) Cistron (*d*) Recon

1.13 How many base pairs are present per complete nucleosome?
(*a*) 166 (*b*) 156 (*c*) 146 (*d*) 136

1.14 Which of the following plants is a member of evergreen coniferous forest?
(*a*) *Acacia* (*b*) *Shorea*
(*c*) *Cryptomeria* (*d*) *Rhizophora*

1.15 Choose the correct statement about phylogenetic system of classification
(*a*) Proposed by John Hutchinson
(*b*) Evolutionary sequence is not considered
(*c*) One or a few superficial character(s) is /are considered
(*d*) Proposed by Linnaeus

1.16 Koch's postulates pertain to
(*a*) Disease and causal organism
(*b*) Bacterial metabolism
(*c*) Viral replication
(*d*) Fungal disease resistance

1.17 Aflatoxins are toxic chemicals produced by
(*a*) *Aspergillus flavus* (*b*) *Alternaria alternata*
(*c*) *Fusarium oxysporum* (*d*) *Clostridium tetani*

1.18 Late blight of potato is caused by
(*a*) Potato virus Y
(*b*) Alternaria solani
(*c*) Phytophthora infestans
(*d*) Phytophthora megasperma

1.19 Which one of the following is an essential ingredient in Bordeaux mixture?
(*a*) Mercuric chloride (*b*) Arsenic oxide
(*c*) Lead nitrate (*d*) Copper sulfate

1.20 The most widely used chemical for protoplast fusion, as fusogen, is
(*a*) Mannitol (*b*) Polyethylene glycol
(*c*) Sorbitol (*d*) Glycerol

1.21 How many molecules of ATPs are produced during oxidation of each molecule of NADH?
(*a*) 1 (*b*) 2 (*c*) 3 (*d*) 4

1.22 Photosystem II has an absorption maximum at
(*a*) 450 nm (*b*) 660 nm (*c*) 680 nm (*d*) 700 nm

1.23 CO_2 fixation during C_4 pathway occurs in the chloroplast of
(*a*) Bundle sheath cell (*b*) Palisade parenchyma
(*c*) Spongy parenchyma (*d*) Guard cell

1.24 The growth retardant cycocel (CCC) inhibit sub-apical cell division by blocking the biosynthesis of
(*a*) Abscisic acid (*b*) Kinetin
(*c*) Traumatic acid (*d*) Gibberellin

1.25 Pollination effected by wind is called
(*a*) Ornithophily (*b*) Anemophily
(*c*) Entomophily (*d*) Hydrophily

L2. Write botanical name of the most common plant yielding the following products (A) Ephedrine (B) Caffeine (C) Azadirachtin (D) Atropine (E) Theophylline (5 × 1 = 5)

L3. (*a*) List three major advantages of micropropagation. (3)
(*b*) Define cybrid and state its application in crop breeding. (2)

L4. (*a*) Outline the reaction sequences in nitrate reduction, indicating name of the enzymes and their locations in the leaf cell. (3)
(*b*) C_4 plants have been reported to use nitrate more efficiently than C_3 plants. Explain the reason. (2)

L5. (*a*) Give a simplified diagram for a composite transposon. (2)
(*b*) Mention three applications of transposons. (3)

L6. (*a*) Depict the structure of a wild type Ti-plasmid. Label the diagram. (3)
(*b*) Describe the basic principle of microprojectile bombardment mediated DNA delivery. (2)

(M) MICROBIOLOGY

M1. For each question given below there are four alternatives, of which only one is the correct answer. Write the correct answer in the answer book by writing *a*, *b*, *c* or *d* along with the corresponding sub-question number. (1 × 25 = 25)

1.1 Which of the following organells contains DNA, divides and possesses some degree of autonomy.
(*a*) Golgi apparatus (*b*) Ribosome
(*c*) Chloroplast (*d*) Peroxisomes

1.2 Which of the following microorganisms is classified as a member of archaebacteria
(*a*) Cyanobacteria (*b*) Methanobacteria
(*c*) Trichomonads (*d*) Mycoplasma

1.3 Archaeal cells usually do not contain peptidoglycan, rather contain pseudo-peptidoglycan which is mainly composed of
(*a*) N-acetylmuramic acid and L-amino acids
(*b*) N-acetyltalosaminuronic acid and D-amino acids
(*c*) N-accetylmuramic acid and D-amino acids
(*d*) N-acetyltalosaminuronic acid and L-amino acids

1.4 Some bacteria contain extensive internal membranes that are involved with specific functions. One example of such membranes is chromatophores, which are
(*a*) Photosynthetic membranes where light is converted to chemical energy in the form of ATP
(*b*) Convolutions of the inner membrane that extend into the interior of the mitochondrion
(*c*) Internal membranes where inorganic nitrogen containing compounds oxidize to generate ATP
(*d*) Interior compartment of chloroplast where fixation of CO_2 occurs

1.5 In establishing proton gradient for chemiosmotic ATP generation by 'aerobic respiration' the terminal electron acceptor is :
(*a*) Nitrate (*b*) Oxygen (*c*) Sulfate (*d*) CO_2

1.6 In which of the following splicing events, the intermediates do not form the lariat or the branched structure?
(*a*) Trans splicing
(*b*) Group I intron splicing
(*c*) Group II intron splicing
(*d*) hnRNA splicing

1.7 Which of the following statements is incorrect for the life cycle of bacteriophage MS2?
(*a*) The phage RNA is (+) stranded and it can act as mRNA
(*b*) Negative strand RNA is synthesized by the phage encoded RNA replicase
(*c*) Ribosomal frame shifting occurs to control the expression of lysis gene
(*d*) MS2 encoded repressor protein allows this virus to undergo lysis

1.8 Which of the following sets of surface associated microorgansims are populated in the upper respiratory tract (nasal cavity and nasopharynx)?
(*a*) Lactobacillus, Escherichia, Enterobacter
(*b*) Streptococcus, Staphylococcus, Neisseria
(*c*) Streptococcus, Lactobacillus, Candida
(*d*) Klebsiella, Staphylococus, Enterobacter

1.9 Autoimmune diseases result from failure of the immune system to recognize self antigen as self. Following are the sets of autoimmune diseases with the corresponding antigens, which one is the incorrect one.
(*a*) Myasthenia gravis - platelets
(*b*) Rheumatoid arthritis - collagen
(*c*) Systematic lupus erythematosus - La nucleo-protein
(*d*) Hashimoto thyroiditis - Thyroglobulin

1.10 The basis for tuberculin test used to detect *Mycobacterium tuberculosis* infection is
(*a*) Anaphylactic hypersensitivity (Type 1)
(*b*) Antibody dependent cytotoxic hyper-sensitivity (Type 2)
(*c*) Immune complex mediated hyper-sensitivity (Type 3)
(*d*) Cell mediated delayed hypersensitivity (Type 4)

1.11 One of the post replication modification in DNA is the methylation of the bases. In this context which of the following statements is incorrect.
(*a*) Methylation protects cell's own DNA from digestion by its own restriction endonuclease(s)
(*b*) Methylation may result in the localized conversion of B-DNA to Z-DNA
(*c*) Methyl groups are added predominantly to cytosines in bacterial cells and to adenines in eukaryotes
(*d*) Methylation of bases is important in some aspects of DNA repair in bacteria

1.12 Where in the cells of the eukaryotic organisms are the ribosomes assembled?
(*a*) Nucleolus (*b*) Cytoplasm
(*c*) Lysosomes (*d*) Golgibodies

1.13 In a mitotically dividing cell, G2 phase occurs at the
(*a*) Beginning of interphase
(*b*) Towards the end of interphase
(*c*) Just before the DNA synthesis
(*d*) Interphase of a mitotically dividing cells is too short to be sub-divided

1.14 Malt used to ferment beer is prepared by
(*a*) Roasting barley
(*b*) Washing the barley with water and drying it in air
(*c*) Barley is soaked in water, germinated and dried
(*d*) Barley is treated with bovine amylase and roasted

1.15 Which of the following equations is correct for double stranded DNA ?
(*a*) $A + T = G + C$ (*b*) $\frac{G}{A} = \frac{T}{C}$
(*c*) $A + C = G + T$ (*d*) $\frac{A}{G} = \frac{C}{T}$

1.16 There are five classes of the antibodies (IgM, IgD, IgG, IgE, IgA). What determines the class to which an antibody belongs?

(*a*) Structure of the light chain

(*b*) Variable region of the antibody

(*c*) Structure of the heavy chain constant region

(*d*) Stage of the infection

1.17 Antigen binding sites of an immunoglobulin are located in

(*a*) Light chain alone

(*b*) Heavy chain alone

(*c*) F_c region of the antibody

(*d*) F_{ab} regions of the antibody

1.18 Pasteurization of milk is done by

(*a*) Boiling the milk for 20 minutes

(*b*) Heating the milk at 72°c for 30 minutes

(*c*) Heating the milk at 72°c for 20 minutes

(*d*) Heating the milk at 62°c for 30 minutes

1.19 The resolving limit of a microscope is defined by which of the following equations. In the equation, '*d*' defines the resolving limit, 'λ' is the wavelength of the light source, 'N' is the refractive index of the medium between the lens and object, 'α' is the half angle of the objective lens

(*a*) $d = \frac{\lambda}{N \cdot \alpha}$ (*b*) $d = \frac{\lambda}{N \cdot \sin\alpha}$

(*c*) $d = \frac{0.5\lambda}{N \sin\alpha}$ (*c*) $d = \frac{0.5N}{\lambda \cdot \sin\alpha}$

1.20 Mode of action of rifampicin in *E. coli* is through inhibiting

(*a*) Cell division

(*b*) Initiation of transcription

(*c*) RNA polymerase binding to DNA template

(*d*) Inhibition of the oxidation potential

1.21 The DNA polymerase responsible for semiconservative replication in *E. coli* is

(*a*) DNA polymerase I

(*b*) DNA polymerase II

(*c*) DNA polymerase III

(*d*) DNA polymerase IV and V

1.22 Subunit composition of *E. coli* RNA polymerase holoenzyme is

(*a*) αα'ββ'σ (*b*) αββ'σ (*b*) αα'βσ (*d*) αβγ

1.23 During protein synthesis in E. coli, aminoacyl tRNAs are bound to the A site. Following transpeptidation reaction the peptidyl - tRNA is moved to the ribosomal P site. Factor involved at the translocation step is

(*a*) EF - Ts (*b*) EF - Tu (*c*) EF - G (*d*) EF - lα

1.24 Shine-Dalgarno sequence found in the prokaryotic mRNAs facilitates ribosome binding by its interaction with the 3′ end of the

(*a*) 5S rRNA (*b*) 23S rRNA

(*c*) 16S rRNA (*d*) 18S rRNA

1.25 Diptheria toxin

(*a*) Acts catalytically

(*b*) Releases incomplete polypeptide chains from ribosomes

(*c*) Leads to misreading of mRNA

(*d*) Cleaves 16S rRNA into two fragments

M2. Answer the following:

(*a*) How are the P1 and λ phages different with respect to their transduction properties? (1)

(*b*) Which one of the two phages (P1 and λ) will be useful to transduce a marker linked to Tn10 in an unknown location on the E. coli chromosome? (1)

(*c*) An F^+ strain of E coli gave rise to Hfr progeny by random integration of the F factor into the circular chromosome at many, points such that the segregants transfer the genetic markers in different order. When six of the Hfr segregants were checked for the order of the marker transfer to a recipient by interrupted mating experiments, following results were obtained. What is the order of the markers? (3)

Hfr segregant	Order of marker transfer into an appropriate recipient
1	— PAQB →
2	— CZEF →
3	— EFBQ →
4	— FEZC →
5	— ZCWD →
6	— APDW →

M3. Extensive nuclease digestion of chromatin results in a 146 bp 'nucleosome core' particle. This core particle is linked with another unit through a linker of varying length. A eukaryotic organism contains a single chromosome of 2×10^8 bp. Given that the Avogadro's number is 6.02×10^{23}, answer the following. (1 × 5 = 5)

(*a*) What is the number of nucleosomes in this organism if the average linker length was 54 bp?

(*b*) Name the core histones.

(*c*) What is the number of core histone molecules present on the chromosome?

(*d*) If the volume of nucleus is considered to be 0.001μl, what is the concentration of each of the core histones.

(*e*) Which of the histones is not present on the nucleosome core particle?

M4. Organisms can utilize α-ketoglutarate, glutamate and aspartate to fix NH_3.

(*a*) What are the enzymes that utilize α-ketoglutarate, glutamate and aspartate to fix NH_3? (3)

(*b*) What cofactor (s) are used to fix NH_3, utilizing α-ketoglutarate? (1)

(*c*) How many molecules of NH_3 can be fixed during conversion of α-ketoglutarate to glutamine? (1)

M5. If Down syndrome occurs in 1 out of 700 births and the Turner syndrome occurs in 1 out of 5000 cases, what are the chances that the following will occur?

(*a*) Two cases of Down syndrome in one hospital on the same day. (2)

(*b*) If the number of births in a country is 35×10^6, how many cases of Down syndrome are likely to be recorded among the new1 borns? (1)

(*c*) If the Down and Turner syndromes are randomly distributed, what are the chances that a new born will be found with the Down syndrome and Turner syndrome (2)

M6. The following are the examples of host cell surface receptor proteins that facilitate virus entry into the host cell. Match the names of the viruses (panel A) with the names of the corresponding receptors used (panel B). (1 × 5 = 5)

Virus	Cell surface Protien
(*a*) Vaccinia virus	(*i*) Intracellur adhesion molecules on the surface of respiratory epithilial cells (ICAM)
(*b*) Rhinovirus	(*ii*) Receptor for C_3d complement protein on human B lymphocyte
(*c*) Epstein-Barr virus	(*iii*) CD4 protein on T-helper cells
(*d*) Herpes Simplex virus type I	(*iv*) Epidermal growth factor receptor
(*e*) Human immuno-deficiency virus	(*v*) Fibroblast growth factor receptor

(N) ZOOLOGY

N1. For each sub-question given below, four alternatives are provided of which only one answer is correct. Write the correct answer in the answer book by writing *a, b, c* or *d* along with the corresponding sub-question number. (1 × 20 = 20)

1.1 The line that divided oriental zoogeographic region from that of Australian zoogeographic region is known as

(*a*) Wallace line (*b*) Darwin line

(*c*) Lyel line (*d*) Smith line

1.2 The nematodes are

(*a*) Acoelomate organism

(*b*) Pseudocoelomate organism

(*c*) Coelomate organism

(*d*) Hemocoelomate organism

1.3 The origin of vertebrate during evolution occurred during

(*a*) Cenozoic era (*b*) Mesozoic era

(*c*) Paleozoic era (*d*) Archeozoic era

1.4 Dinosaurs first appeared and adaptive radiation of reptiles took place during

(*a*) Cretaceous period (*b*) Jurassic period

(*c*) Triassic period (*d*) Carboniferous period

1.5 The giant panda is a natural inhabitant of

(*a*) India (*b*) China

(*c*) Australia (*d*) North America

1.6 Anuran heart is divided into

(*a*) One chamber (*b*) Two chambers

(*c*) Three chambers (*d*) Four chambers

1.7 The antibody whose concentration is highest in human blood under normal condition is

(*a*) Ig M (*b*) Ig A (*c*) Ig E (*d*) Ig G

1.8 The prosthetic group in respiratory pigment hemocyanin is

(*a*) Iron (*b*) Copper (*c*) Mercury (*d*) Zinc

1.9 The phenomenon of MHC restriction was discovered by

(*a*) Doherty and Zinkernagel

(*b*) Medawar and Billingham

(*c*) Edelman and Porter

(*d*) Burnet and Nossal

1.10 Working principle behind DNA vaccine is believed to be

(*a*) Anti DNA antibody is produced in vaccinated individual

(*b*) The vaccine DNA codes for antibody directed against the pathogen

(*c*) The vaccine DNA codes for antigenic protein which is expressed in the immunized animal

(*d*) The vaccine DNA boosts the immune system of the animal

1.11 The RNA molecule often used to determine evolutionary relatedness is

(*a*) Messenger RNA (*b*) Transfer RNA

(*c*) Ribosomal RNA (*d*) Sn RNA

1.12 A post-pubertal human female would have more number of ova at the age

(*a*) 45 (*b*) 35 (*c*) 25 (*d*) 15

1.13 The precursor for coenzyme A is

(*a*) Niacin (*b*) Thiamine

(*c*) Riboflavin (*d*) Pantothenic acid

1.14 A major protein constituent of plasma membrane of erythrocytes is

(*a*) Haemoglobin (*b*) Glycophorin A

(*c*) Albumin (*d*) Actin

1.15 The codon for amino acid tryptophan is

(*a*) UAA (*b*) UAG (*c*) UGA (*d*) UGG

1.16 Beriberi is the result of deficiency of

(*a*) Vitamin B1 (*b*) Vitamin B2

(*c*) Vitamin B6 (*d*) Vitamin B12

1.17 The genes for T cell receptors were characterized by

(*a*) Tonegawa (*b*) Kabat

(*c*) Benaceraf (*d*) Jerne

1.18 The hormone secreted by adrenal cortex is

(*a*) Adrenaline (*b*) Corticosterone

(*c*) Prolactin (*d*) Vassopressin

1.19 The histone octamer associated with nucleosome contains
(*a*) $(H2A)_4$ $(H2B)_4$
(*b*) $(H3)_4$ $(H4)_4$
(*c*) $(H2A)_3$ $(H2B)_1$ $(H3)_1$ $(H4)_3$
(*d*) $(H2A)_2$ $(H2B)_2$ $(H3)_2$ $(H4)_2$

1.20 Which of the following is called "master gland of the endocrinc orchestra".
(*a*) Pituitary (*b*) Thyroid
(*c*) Thymus (*d*) Adrenal gland

N2. (*a*) Match the diseases in column A with their causative organism in column B. (1 × 3 = 3)

(*i*) Malaria	(*a*) Trypanosoma
(*ii*) Filaria	(*b*) Plasmodium
(*iii*) Sleeping sickness	(*c*) Wuchereria
	(*d*) Ascaris

(*b*) Match the class of animals listed in column A with the phyla in column B. (1 × 2 = 2)

(*i*) Arachnida	(*a*) Mollusca
(*ii*) Gastropoda	(*b*) Arthropoda
	(*c*) Annelida

N3. Define the following: (1 × 5 = 5)
(*a*) Telomere (*b*) Osmoregulation
(*c*) Climax community (*d*) Imprinting
(*e*) Aneuploidy

N4. (*a*) To which class and order the following animals belong: (1 × 3 = 3)
(*i*) mouse (*ii*) whale (*iii*) platypus
(*b*) Why is the basal metabolic rate higher in rodents compared to elephants. (2)

N5. (*a*) What are the conditions under which the frequency of dominant and recessive alleles in a population remain constant from generation to generation? (3)
(*b*) What are molecular chaperons? (2)

N6. (*a*) What is the function of homeotic genes in drosophila? What is the result of mutation in this gene? (2)
(*b*) What is the function of the protein P53? What is the consequence of mutation in P53? (2)
(*c*) What is the function of "checkpoints" in cell cycle? (1)

N7. (*a*) Where is Gahir matha beach located? What zoological phenomenon it is associated with? (2)
(*b*) What do you understand by the term "replicon"? (1)
(*c*) What is codon degeneracy? (1)
(*d*) Why lymphocyte are not suitable for animal cloning? (1)

ANSWERS

(H) CHEMISTRY

1.1 (*c*)	1.2 (*b*)	1.3 (*d*)	1.4 (*c*)	1.5 (*b*)	1.6 (*a*)	1.7 (*a*)	1.8 (*a*)	1.9 (*b*)	1.10 (*d*)
1.11 (*c*)	1.12 (*d*)	1.13 (*b*)	1.14 (*c*)	1.15 (*b*)	1.16 (*b*)	1.17 (*c*)	1.18 (*b*)	1.19 (*d*)	1.20 (*d*)
1.21 (*a*)	1.22 (*c*)	1.23 (*a*)	1.24 (*b*)	1.25 (*a*)					

(J) BIOCHEMISTRY

1.1 (*d*)	1.2 (*a*)	1.3 (*c*)	1.4 (*b*)	1.5 (*a*)	1.6 (*d*)	1.7 (*b*)	1.8 (*d*)	1.9 (*d*)	1.10 (*c*)
1.11 (*d*)	1.12 (*a*)	1.13 (*c*)	1.14 (*a*)	1.15 (*a*)	1.16 (*a*)	1.17 (*b*)	1.18 (*a*)	1.19 (*c*)	1.20 (*d*)
1.21 (*c*)	1.22 (*b*)	1.23 (*d*)	1.24 (*a*)	1.25 (*c*)					

(L) BOTANY

1.1 (*a*)	1.2 (*c*)	1.3 (*c*)	1.4 (*d*)	1.5 (*c*)	1.6 (*b*)	1.7 (*d*)	1.8 (*d*)	1.9 (*a*)	1.10 (*c*)
1.11 (*b*)	1.12 (*c*)	1.13 (*a*)	1.14 (*c*)	1.15 (*a*)	1.16 (*a*)	1.17 (*a*)	1.18 (*c*)	1.19 (*d*)	1.20 (*b*)
1.21 (*c*)	1.22 (*c*)	1.23 (*a*)	1.24 (*d*)	1.25 (*b*)					

(M) MICROBIOLOGY

1.1 (*c*)	1.2 (*b*)	1.3 (*d*)	1.4 (*a*)	1.5 (*b*)	1.6 (*b*)	1.7 (*c*)	1.8 (*b*)	1.9 (*a*)	1.10 (*d*)
1.11 (*c*)	1.12 (*b*)	1.13 (*b*)	1.14 (*c*)	1.15 (*a*)	1.16 (*c*)	1.17 (*d*)	1.18 (*d*)	1.19 (*c*)	1.20 (*c*)
1.21 (*c*)	1.22 (*a*)	1.23 (*c*)	1.24 (*c*)	1.25 (*a*)					

(N) ZOOLOGY

1.1 (*a*)	1.2 (*b*)	1.3 (*c*)	1.4 (*c*)	1.5 (*b*)	1.6 (*c*)	1.7 (*d*)	1.8 (*b*)	1.9 (*a*)	1.10 (*c*)
1.11 (*c*)	1.12 (*c*)	1.13 (*d*)	1.14 (*b*)	1.15 (*d*)	1.16 (*a*)	1.17 (*a*)	1.18 (*b*)	1.19 (*d*)	1.20 (*a*)

EXPLANATIONS

H : CHEMISTRY (COMPULSORY)

1. The ionic radius of the cesium ion is 1.88 Å and that of the chloride ion is 1.67 Å. In this case the cation is the larger ion, and the ratio of radii for the anion and cation is $r^-/r^+ = 1.67/1.88 = 0.888$. With a radius ratio of 0.888, the smaller ion (Cl^-) is expected to prefer a cubic hole. Both Cs^+ and Cl^- exist in a cubic coordination environment, thus CsCl has (8, 8)-coordination. So, each Cs^+ is surrounded by 8 Cl^- ions.
2. The complex reaction of the coordinate covalent compound Cr $(NH_3)_5Cl_3$ with $AgNO_3$ is a different reaction. This is because the correct representation of the complex is $[Cr((NH_3)_5Cl]Cl_2$ where $[Cr((NH_3)_5Cl]$ and Cl^- are the two ionisable parts of the compound. Hence its reaction would be as follows:

   $[Cr((NH_3)_5Cl]Cl_2 + 2AgNO_3$

   $\rightarrow [Cr((NH_3)_5Cl](NO_3^-)_2 + 2AgCl$

   So, it is clear that one mole of the compound consumes 2 mole of $AgNO_3$.
3. The most important properties of atomic and molecular structure may be exemplified using a simplified picture of an atom that is called the Bohr Model. The basic feature of quantum mechanics that is incorporated in the Bohr Model and that is completely different from the analogous planetary model is that the energy of the particles in the Bohr atom is restricted to certain discrete values. One says that the energy is quantized. But Bohr's Model could not explain the spectra of atoms containing more than one electron.
4. The oxygen atom in OF_2 undergoes sp^3 hybridization, much like the oxygen atom in water. The electron cloud geometry would be tetrahedral with a molecular shape of angular and a bond angle of around 104°.
5. Electronegativity is a measure of the ability of an atom in a molecule to draw bonding electrons to itself. The most commonly used scale of electronegativity is that developed by Linus Pauling in which the value 4.0 is assigned to fluorine, the most electronegative element. Lithium, at the other end of the same period on the periodic table, is assigned a value of 1. Electronegativity generally increases from left to right on the periodic table and decreases from top to bottom. Metals are the least electronegative of the elements. So the correct order is: $S < N < O < F$.
6. Nitrogen triflouride is the least basic compound amongst the halides of nitrogen. This is because fluorine is the most electronegative element in the periodic table and so any lone pairs of electrons that are present on the nitrogen atom are not easily available for donation which results in poor basicity of the compound.

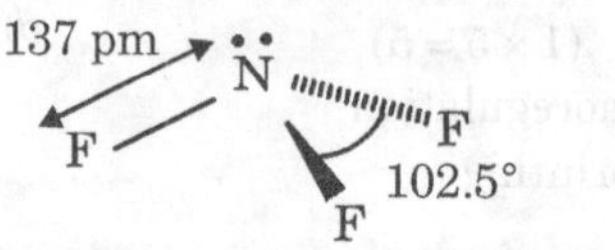

7. We know any kind of solution which is formed of a weak acid and a strong basic forms a solution which is highly basic in nature. NaCl and NH_4Cl are salts and so their pH is lower than the basic solutions that are formed on dissolving of CH_3COONa and NaCN.

   $CH_3COONa + H_2O$

   $\rightarrow CH_3COOH + NaOH$

   $NaCN + H_2O \rightarrow HCN + NaOH$

   In both the cases, same basic inorganic compound NaOH is formed. However, the pKa value of CH_3COOH is lower than that of HCN. Thus, pH of CH_3COONa will be higher.
8. In terms of electronegativity, Fluorine is more electronegative than oxygen. So, the reaction of a compound with an abundant supply of fluorine gas will liberate oxygen gas. So, the correct reaction which will give oxygen is:

   $4NaOH + 2F_2 \rightarrow 4NaF + 2H_2O + O_2$.
9. When 1-butyne is reacted with sulphuric acid in presence of mercuric sulphate as a catalyst, the stable product that is formed is a ketonic product butan-2-one.

   $CH \equiv C - CH_2 - CH_3 + \text{dil. } H_2SO_4 \rightarrow$ (in presence of $HgSO_4$) $CH_3 - CO - CH_2 - CH_3$; which is formed as a result of tautomerisation.
10. The haloform reaction is a chemical reaction where a haloform (CHX_3, where X is a halogen) is produced by the exhaustive halogenation of a methyl ketone (a molecule containing the $R–CO–CH_3$ group) in the presence of a base. The reaction can be used to produce chloroform ($CHCl_3$).

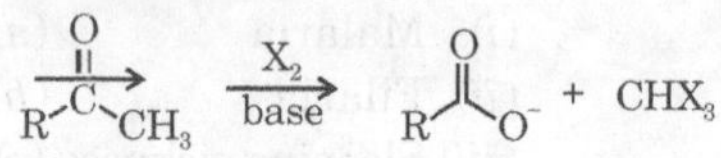

R = H, alkyl, aryl
X = Cl, Br, I

So, $R - C = O$ group is required for the formation of Chloroform. However, in case of propanol ($CH_3 - CH_2 - CH_2OH$), there is no $R - C = O$ group and so it does not produce any chloroform.

11. Cyanohydrins are more easily formed with aldehydes than ketones. HCN is formed from acid-base reaction of –CN with HCl. The reaction does not occur with HCN alone; cyanide is required. Thus, the reaction can be made to occur using HCN/catalytic base. Cyanohydrin formation can occur via the attack of cyanide to both aldehydes and ketones, usually in the presence of acid which protonates the resulting alkoxide to give the hydroxy group. The products of these reactions can also be called hydroxynitriles.

Aldehyde

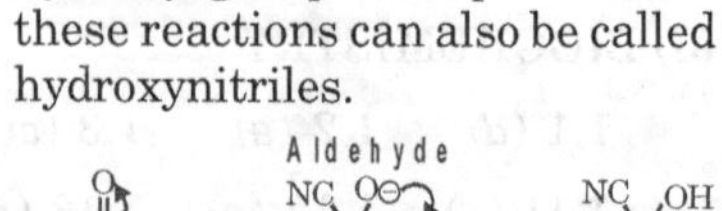

Ketone

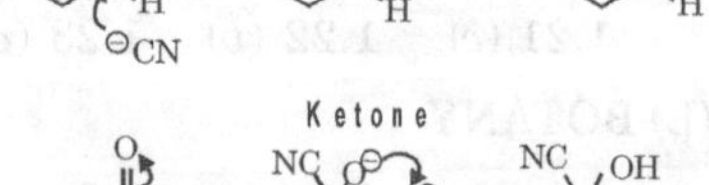

Since phenylacetaldehyde is an aliphatic compound having polarity, so it is the most reactive for the formation of cyanohydrins.

12. Acids include strong acids, which completely dissociate in water, and weak acids, which only partially dissociate. When an acid dissociates, it releases a proton to make the solution acidic, but weak acids have both a dissociated state (A^-) and

undissociated state (AH) that coexist. The Henderson–Hasselbalch equation mathematically connects the measurable pH of a solution, the concentration of hydrogen ions, with the pKa, the negative log of the acid dissociation constant, of the acid. Amongst all the phenolic compounds, NO_2, Cl_2 are electron withdrawing groups which decrease the basicity and increases the acidity of the phenols. However, CH_3 and OCH_3 are electron donating groups which increase the basicity of the phenoxide molecule. OCH_3 has a higher value of electron releasing than CH_3 because of the Oxygen molecule. So, *p*-methoxyphenol has the highest pKa value.

13. Industrially, alkyl groups can be substituted into a benzene ring using a variant on Friedel-Crafts alkylation. One possibility is that instead of using a chloroalkane with an aluminium chloride catalyst, they use an alkene and a mixture of aluminium chloride and hydrogen chloride as the catalyst. Benzene is treated with a chloroalkane (for example, chloromethane or chloroethane) in the presence of aluminium chloride as a catalyst.

$$CH_3CH_2Cl + AlCl_3 \longrightarrow CH_3CH_2^+ \; AlCl_4^-$$

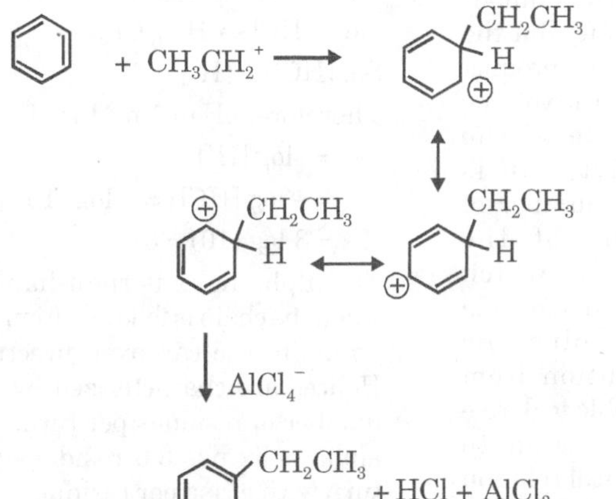

14. Nucleophilic substitution is the reaction of an electron pair donor (the nucleophile, Nu) with an electron pair acceptor (the electrophile). In the S_N1 reaction, a planar carbenium ion is formed first, which then reacts further with the nucleophile. Since the nucleophile is free to attack from either side, this reaction is associated with racemization. The more highly substituted is the incipient carbenium ion, the more probable that the reaction will follow an S_N1 pathway. The more non-reactive the nucleophile, the more probable it becomes that a reaction with secondary and tertiary electrophiles will follow an S_N1 pathway. A weaker nucleophile is not as effective in the backside attack, since this location is sterically shielded, especially in the case of tertiary substrates. Carbenium ions are planar and therefore less sterically hindered, and are naturally more reactive as electrophiles than the uncharged parent compound. The hydrolysis of tert-butyl chloride is a typical S_N1 reaction:

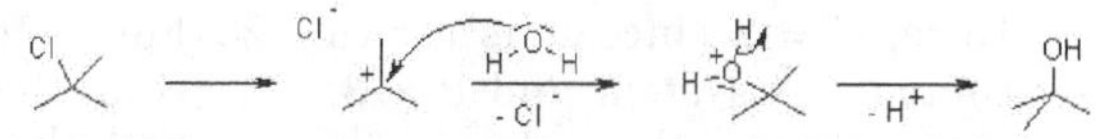

15. An Aldol condensation is an organic reaction in which an enolate ion reacts with a carbonyl compound to form a β-hydroxyaldehyde or β-hydroxyketone, followed by dehydration to give a conjugated enone. Aldol condensation often require low temperature (–78°C) for the formation of an enolate using an organic lithium derivatives and to avoid proton transfer.

$$CH_3CHO \xrightarrow[H_2O,\,\Delta]{\text{catalyst: } NaOH} CH_3CH = CHCHO$$

Since, in aldol condensation there must be α-hydrogen in the aldehyde or ketone, so phenyl acetaldehyde is the only compound which has the presence of α-hydrogen in it.

16. The Claisen condensation produces beta-ketoesters. These products may then be modified or enhanced by further reactions. It is a typical aldol reaction followed by reduction to a 1, 3-diol (2-ethyl-1, 3-hexanediol).

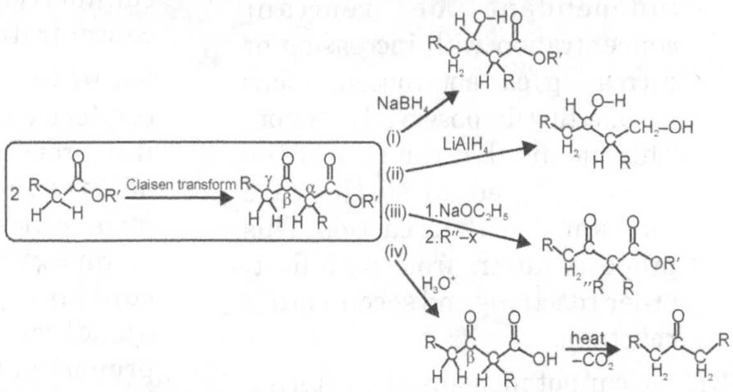

Here, $NaBH_4$ (Sodium Borohydride) reduces α-ketoester to produce a secondary alcohol.

17. When treated with Br_2 or Cl_2 radical substitution of benzylic-H generates the benzyl halide and HX. The benzyl radical is quite stable, so bromination will often be selective for the benzyl position. Only chlorination and bromination are useful in the laboratory. NBS is an alternate source for bromine.

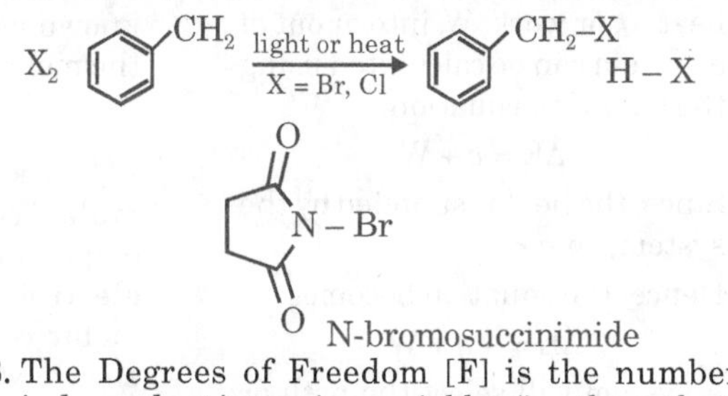

N-bromosuccinimide

18. The Degrees of Freedom [F] is the number of independent intensive variables (i.e. those that are independent of the quantity of material present) that need to be specified in value to fully determine the state of the system. The Phase Rule describes the possible number of degrees of freedom in a (closed) system at equilibrium, in terms of the number of separate phases and the number of chemical constituents in the system. The number of phases is represented in the relation by P. The Chemical Constituents are represented as C.

The rule is: F = C – P + 2.

$$CaCO_3\,(s) \Leftrightarrow CaO\,(s) + CO_2\,(g)$$

Here, C = 2 since it is a two component system and P = 3, since there are three phases

Therefore, F = 2 – 3 + 2 = 1 which is the number of degree of freedom.

19. In general, catalytic action is a chemical reaction between the catalyst and a reactant, forming chemical intermediates that are able to react more readily with each other or with another reactant, to form the desired end product. A catalyst enhances the rate of the reaction by decreasing the energy barrier and the activation energy of the system.

20. A zero-order reaction is a reaction that proceeds at a rate that is independent of reactant concentration with increasing or decreasing reactants concentrations not affecting the observed reaction. This means that the rate of the reaction is equal to the rate constant, *k*, of that reaction. This property differs from both first-order reactions and second-order reactions.

21. We cannot measure the internal energy in a system, we can only determine the change in internal energy, ΔE, that accompanies a change in the system.

$$\Delta E = E_{final} - E_{initial}$$

The change in internal energy that accompanies the transfer of heat, *q*, or work, W, into or out of a system can be calculated using the following equation:

$$\Delta E = q + W$$

Since, the heat is supplied by the system, so $q < 0$

Hence, the equation becomes:

$$\Delta E = -q + W$$

22. A system will select the path or assemblage of paths out of available paths that minimizes the potential or maximizes the entropy at the fastest rate given the constraints. So, when a drop of ink is put in a glass of water, the ink drop slowly spreads uniformly and mixes with time. So, the entropy increase with time and ultimately leads to maximization.

23. For isotonic solution, we have equivalent osmotic pressures for both the solutions

Therefore, $\pi_{sugar} = \pi_{NaCl}$

Now, we have π = iMRT, where i is Van't Hoff factor; M is the molarity; R is the gas constant; T is the thermodynamic (absolute) temperature

Thus, $\pi_{sugar} = \pi_{NaCl}$

$\Rightarrow i_{Sugar} M_{sugar} RT = i_{NaCl} M_{NaCl} RT$

$\Rightarrow 1 \times 0.2 = 2 \times M_{NaCl}$

$\Rightarrow M_{NaCl} = 0.1$

So, the concentration of common salt solution is 0.1 M

24. The molar conductivity of a strong electrolyte (Λ_m) is given as the ratio of measured conductivity (κ) to the molar concentration (c): $\Lambda_m = \kappa / c$.

On increasing the dilution, the conductivity (κ) does decrease as it is proportional to the number of ions in a unit volume. But the molar conductance is the product of Λm = κV where V is the volume containing one mole of the dissolved electrolyte. It is proportional to the number of ions in V volume of the electrolytic solution which includes all the ions in one mole of the electrolyte plus the additional contribution from water. Onsager was able to derive a theoretical expression to account for the empirical relation known as Kohlrausch's Law, for the molar conductivity, Λ_m.

$$\Lambda_m = \Lambda_m{}^0 - K\sqrt{c}$$

$\Lambda_m{}^0$ is known as the limiting molar conductivity, K is an empirical constant and c is the electrolyte concentration. So, molar conductivity of a strong electrolyte varies linearly with the square root of concentration of the electrolyte.

25. The name Gibbs-Helmholtz is usually associated with the equation:

$$H = G - T(\partial G/\partial T)_P$$

Where H is enthalpy, G is Gibbs free energy and T temperature, with the implied assumption that the differentiation is to be carried out at constant composition. The greatest utility of this equation lies in the presence of the temperature derivative of the Gibbs free energy. For example, the equilibrium constant in a chemical reaction is determined by the standard Free Energy change for the reaction. Thus, knowledge of the temperature derivative of the free energy provides information relating the temperature derivative of the equilibrium constant. The equilibrium constant, K, may be written as: $\Delta G^0 = -RT \ln K$, where ΔG^0 is the standard Gibbs free energy change for the reaction at temperature T and R is the universal gas constant. So, specific heat of the stable solid is positive.

(J) BIOCHEMISTRY

1. Given, concentration of HCl $= 1 mM = 10^{-3}$ M

We know, pH of a solution = $-\log [H^+]$

Here, $HCl \rightarrow H^+ + Cl^-$.

So, $[HCl] = [H^+]$

Therefore, pH of 1 mM HCl

$= -\log [H^+]$

$= -\log [HCl] = -\log [10^{-3}]$

$= 3 \log (10) = 3$

2. The alpha helix is right-handed when the chain is followed from the amino to the carboxyl direction. Helices are characterized by the number of residues per turn. An alpha helix has 3.6 residues per turn with a rise per residue of 1.5 Å. This means that every 3-4 amino acids in an alpha helix are on the same side of the helix, where they are positioned to interact with each other.

Given, number of amino acid residues in a polypeptide chain = 20

We know, rise per residue for an α-helix = 1.5 Å

Therefore, rise for 20 residues

$= 20 \times 1.5 = 30$ Å

Hence, the length of the α-helical section is 30 Å.

3. Amino terminal end of polypeptide chain determined by either of three methods namely Sangar method, Edman's method and Dansyl chloride method. In Sanger method, Fluorodinitrobenzene used. Polypeptide reacts with

FDNB to form Dinitrophenol complex with polypeptide. Subsequent analysis releases a colored dinitrophenol labelled amino terminal amino acid, which can be identified by its characteristic migration rate on thin-layer chromatography or paper electrophoresis. In Edman degradation method, Phenyl isothio cyanate (PIT) is used as reagent. First the polypeptide is reacted with phenyl isothio cyanate to forma polypeptidyl phenylthiocarbamyl derivative. Gentle hydrolysis releases the amino terminal amino acid as a phenylth-iohydantoin (PTH), which can be separated and detected spectrophotometrically. Dansyl chloride is also used to determine N-terminal amino acid. This method is more sensitive because of fluorescence measurement. Fluorodintrobenzene is used when the peptide concentration is very less in amount.

4. The most common method for quantifying DNA samples is by conventional absorbance measurements; nucleic acids have an absorption maximum at 260nm. Most samples contain contaminates such as proteins and single stranded DNA/RNA that absorb maximally at 280nm. The equation for calculating DNA in the presence of contaminates is: A [260] /A [280] = pure dsDNA. The higher the ratio, the more pure the DNA sample. It is acceptable to have a ratio between 1.8 and 2.0 for a cuvette spectrophotometer. When a DNA solution is heated enough, the non-covalent forces that hold the two strands together weaken and finally break. When this happens, the two strands come apart in a process known as DNA denaturation, or DNA melting. The temperature at which the DNA strands are half denatured is called the melting temperature, or Tm. The amount of strand separation, or melting, is measured by the absorbance of the DNA solution at 260nm. Nucleic acids absorb light at this wavelength because of the electronic structure in their bases, but when two strands of DNA come together, the close proximity of the bases in the two strands quenches some of this absorbance. When the two strands separate, this quenching disappears and the absorbance rises 30%–40%. This is called hyperchromic shift.

5. β-amylase acts on starch, glycogen and related polysaccharides and oligosaccharides producing beta-maltose by an inversion. The term 'β' relates to the initial anomeric configuration of the free sugar group released and not to the configuration of the linkage hydrolysed. The catalyzed reaction occurs through Hydrolysis of (1->4)-α-D-glucosidic linkages in polysaccharides so as to remove successive maltose units from the non-reducing ends of the chains. β-amylases are present in yeasts, moulds, bacteria, and plants, particularly in the seeds. They are the principal components of a mixture called diastase that is used in the removal of starchy sizing agents from textiles and in the conversion of cereal grains to fermentable sugars.

6. Gangliosides are the group of glycosphingolipids that show the greatest structural variation and also the more complex structure. This group includes molecules composed of ceramide linked by a glycosidic bond to an oligosaccharide chain containing hexose and N-acetylneuraminic acid (NANA, acidic sugar known also as sialic acid) units. They reside in the outer plasma membrane of animal cells and some intracellular membranes. They are the major constituents of neuronal cell membranes and endoplasmic reticulum. Gangliosides are thought to provide protection from harsh conditions, such as low pH and degradative enzymes, in the extracellular environment. They can help cells interact with extracellular matrices and other cells and serve as surface receptors for bacterial toxins and, perhaps, normal, endogenous extracellular molecules. Gangliosides are characterized by a high amount of stearic acid (C18, about 80%), the rest being C16, C20 and C22.

7. Given, Number of restriction sites for EcoRI in the gene = 1

   After digesting the DNA with EcoRI, the digested DNA was probed with labelled cDNA of the gene that has no repeats in the DNA, it occurs only once. Now, after southern hybridization of the template and the probe, autoradiography was performed. The resultant band in the autoradiogram would be only 1 because the DNA has only one site for cleavage and it belongs to E. coli. So the DNA is circular in nature and its single point cut would only give rise to a single digested fragment.

8. Nearly all of the energy needed by the human body is provided by the oxidation of carbohydrates and lipids. Whereas carbohydrates provide a readily available source of energy, lipids function primarily as an energy reserve. The amount of lipids stored as an energy reserve far exceeds the energy stored as glycogen since the human body is simply not capable of storing as much glycogen compared to lipids. Lipids yield 9 kcal of energy per gram while carbohydrates and proteins yield only 4 kcal of energy/gram. Excess lipids in the blood are eventually converted into adipose tissue. If lipid levels in the blood become too low, the body synthesizes lipids from other foods, such as carbohydrates, or removes lipids from storage. Abnormally high levels of triglycerides and cholesterol are thought to be involved in hardening of the arteries. Lipids may be deposited on the walls of arteries as a partial consequence of their insolubility in the blood. Thus, adipose tissue has the largest energy reserve in terms of kilocalories.

9. Replication occurs as the result of the enzyme DNA polymerase. As the DNA strands pull apart, the DNA polymerase moves along the template strand adding new base pairs to the strand being synthesized. When the strands

denature in a given segment of DNA, a replication bubble is formed, having two replication forks at the ends where the strands continue coming apart. The point where replication begins is also known as the origin of replication. However, in eukaryotic cells, there is so much DNA that many different origins of replication are needed to be able to replicate all the DNA in the necessary time frame. When a DNA from one origin catches up to the DNA from another origin, they are joined an enzyme called a ligase. Replication also contains built-in error checking. The frequency of errors is about 1 per 100 million bonds (1×10^{-8}). There are really only around three errors per replication because of DNA repair. If a repair enzyme finds a mistake, it can fix it, and it can tell which strand is wrong because it can tell which strand is the newly synthesized strand by at the extent of cytosine methylation.

10. Exocytosis is a general term used to denote vesicle fusion at the plasma membrane, and it is the final step in the secretory pathway that typically begins in the endoplasmic reticulum (ER), passes through the Golgi apparatus, and ends at the outside of the cell. Endocytosis refers to the recovery of vesicles from the plasma membrane. Exocytotic vesicle fusion involves the coalescence of vesicle and plasma membranes and allows the so-called fusion pore to form. The fusion pore is a channel that passes through the vesicle and plasma membranes and allows delivery of the vesicle contents to the extracellular compartment. Docking is the process by which the exocytotic vesicle is fixed beneath the plasma membrane before fusion. The fusion of secretory vesicles with the plasma membrane occurs in essentially all cells in the form of constitutive exocytosis that is required for the insertion of new cell membrane. In many cell types, a second pathway also exists in which exocytosis can be tightly regulated to allow the controlled release of vesicle contents or regulated insertion of new membrane components due to fusion of preformed secretory vesicles only in response to a physiological signal.

11. ELISAs can be performed with a number of modifications to the basic procedure. The key step, immobilization of the antigen of interest, can be accomplished by direct adsorption to the assay plate or indirectly via a capture antibody that has been attached to the plate. The antigen is then detected either directly (labelled primary antibody) or indirectly (labelled secondary antibody). The most powerful ELISA assay format is the sandwich assay. This type of capture assay is called a "sandwich" assay because the analyte to be measured is bound between two primary antibodies - the capture antibody and the detection antibody. A detection enzyme or other tag can be linked directly to the primary antibody or introduced through a secondary antibody that recognizes the primary antibody. It also can be linked to a protein such as streptavidin if the primary antibody is biotin labelled. The most commonly used enzyme labels are horseradish peroxidase (HRP) and alkaline phosphatase (AP). Enzymes provide a high turnover number for better observation of results.

12. Follicle Stimulating Hormone (FSH) is a glycoprotein hormone, produced in the anterior pituitary and released into the blood in response to GnRH (GnRH is released from the hypothalamus). Glycoprotein hormones are protein hormones with carbohydrate chains. This carbohydrate group protects the FSH molecule from rapid breakdown and metabolism. This shielding group adds to the hormone's half-life. The FSH is transported to the ovary, enters the developing follicle, and stimulates the granulosa cells to produce oestrogen. FSH is also responsible for growth of the follicle, involving both an increase in the number of granulosa cells and secretion of follicular fluid. As the follicle grows, the granulosa cells secrete a hormone called inhibin into the follicular fluid. This hormone is carried, through the vascular system, back to the anterior pituitary where it suppresses the secretion of FSH. Cyclic AMP responses to FSH in isolated Sertoli cells are observed at different stages of sexual maturation. So cyclic AMP serves as a second messenger to FSH.

13. The classical complement pathway is activated most effectively by IgM and the most abundant of the immunoglobulin, IgG. But, for activation to occur, antibodies must be bound to antigens (the antigen-antibody complex mentioned above). Free antibodies do not activate complement. To initiate the cascade, the first complement protein in the pathway, C1, must interact with a bound immunoglobulin. Specifically, C1 interacts with the tail of the Y portion of the bound antibody molecule-i.e., the nonspecific part of the antibody that does not bind antigen. Once bound to the antibody, C1 is cleaved, a process that activates C1 and allows it to split and activate the next complement component in the series. This process is repeated on the following proteins in the pathway until the complement protein C3-the most abundant and biologically the most important component of the complement system-are activated. The effectivity of IgM in complement activation is stronger than that in IgG because of the fact that IgM is a pentamer and IgG is a monomer. So, IgM is more capable of very strong opsonization of the antigen molecule.

14. Major histocompatibility complex (MHC) molecules serve as peptide receptors. The MHC gene complex encodes two major classes of molecules, MHC class I and class II, whose function is

to present peptides to CD8+ (cytotoxic) and CD4+ (helper) T cells, respectively. The genes encoding both classes of MHC molecules seem to originate from a common ancestral gene. Peptide antigens from these particles are preserved for presentation in association with major histocompatibility complex (MHC) class I or class II molecules in order to stimulate antigen-specific T cells. MHC I glycoproteins are present on almost every cell in the body, acting to present endogenous antigens that originate from the cytoplasm. MHC II glycoproteins are only present on specialised antigen-presenting immune cells, including macrophages that engulf foreign particles such as bacteria, dendritic cells that present antigen to T cells, and B cells that produce antibodies. MHC II proteins present exogenous antigens that originate extracellularly from foreign bodies.

15. RNA molecules can be 3′ end-labelled using [5′-^{32}P] pCp (cytidine-3′, 5′-bis-phosphate) and RNA ligase. The RNA to be labelled must have a 3′ hydroxyl, so most degradation products will not label with pCp (except the original 3′-end, of course). pCp end-labelling is the method of choice for end labelling stable RNAs because, in most cases, the 5′ ends of such molecules are hybridized the the 3′ ends of the molecules & are recessed, so that they label poorly with ^{32}P-ATP & polynucleotide kinase. T_4 Polynucleotide Kinase (PNK) catalyzes the transfer of the gamma-phosphate of ATP to the 5'-hydroxyl termini of DNA or RNA. This phosphate transfer is commonly referred to as a kinase or phosphorylation reaction ([γ -^{32}P] ATP is often used in the reaction). Nucleic acids with a 5′-hydroxyl (OH^-) group can be added directly to a kinase reaction. Nucleic acids with a 5′-phosphate should be de-phosphorylated (e.g., with Calf Intestinal Phosphatase) prior to labelling with PNK and [γ -^{32}P] ATP. Thus, for studying RNA synthesis mostly γ P^{32} ATP is used as substrate.

16. The codon CCC codes for the amino acid Proline (Pro). The codon AAA codes for the basic amino acid lysine (Lys). The codon TAC codes for the aromatic amino acid tyrosine (Tyr). Thus, the DNA sequence 5'-CCCAAATAC-3' codes for the tripeptide → Pro Lys Tyr.

17. Transposons are segments of DNA that can move around to different positions in the genome of a single cell. In the process, they may cause mutations or increase (or decrease) the amount of DNA in the genome of the cell, and if the cell is the precursor of a gamete, in the genomes of any descendants. There are two distinct types: Class II transposons (consist of DNA that moves directly from place to place) and Class I transposons (first transcribe the DNA into RNA and then use reverse transcriptase to make a DNA copy of the RNA to insert in a new location). All complete or "autonomous" class II TEs encode the protein transposase, which they require for insertion and excision. Class II TEs are characterized by the presence of terminal inverted repeats, about 9 to 40 base pairs long, on both of their ends. Unlike class II elements, class 1 elements—also known as retrotransposons—move through the action of RNA intermediaries. Because transposon movement can be destructive, it is not surprising that most of the transposon sequences in the human genome are silent, thus allowing this genome to remain relatively stable, despite the prevalence of TEs.

18. IgG antibodies are found in all body fluids. They are the smallest but most common antibody (75% to 80%) of all the antibodies in the body. IgG antibodies are very important in fighting bacterial and viral infections. IgG antibodies are the only type of antibody that can cross the placenta in a pregnant woman to help protect her baby (foetus). Since IgG is present in all body fluids, thus they can be easily transported across epithelial cells.

19. After the exhaustive dialysis of muscle extract with sodium phosphate buffer, it resulted in the loss of ATPase activity of the extract. Now, ATP is being provided in the extract. Hexokinase is an important enzyme that catalyses the ATP-dependent conversion of aldo- and keto-hexose sugars to the hexose-6-phosphate (H6P). The enzyme can catalyse this reaction on glucose, fructose, sorbitol and glucosamine, and as such is the first step in a number of metabolic pathways. The addition of a phosphate group to the sugar acts to trap it in a cell, since the negatively charged phosphate cannot easily traverse the plasma membrane. Since, H6P requires ATP as well as Mg^{2+} as its cofactor, so conversion of glucose to glucose-6-phosphate by hexokinase can be catalyzed in the presence of ATP and Mg^{2+}.

20. Dintrophenol is a potent non-selective inhibitor of oxidative phosphorylation, which results in increased metabolism and increased body temperature, and has been used illegally for weight control. 2, 4-Dinitrophenol (DNP) is reported to cause rapid loss of weight, but unfortunately is associated with an unacceptably high rate of significant adverse effects. It causes uncoupling of oxidative phosphorylation; the classic symptom complex associated with toxicity of phenol-based products such as DNP is a combination of hyperthermia, tachycardia, diaphoresis and tachypnoea, eventually leading to death. Thus, the temperature of the mouse increases when injected with dinitrophenol because DNP results in uncoupling reaction from oxidative phosphorylation.

21. Avidin is a glycoprotein consisting of four identical subunits. It is a minor constituent of the egg white of reptiles, amphibians, and birds. It binds the vitamin biotin with high affinity and is therefore thought to be a defence protein against biotin-requiring microbes. Pyruvate Carboxylase utilizes biotin as prosthetic group. Biotin has a 5-carbon side chain whose terminal carboxyl is in an amide linkage to the e-amino group of a lysine of the enzyme. The biotin and lysine side chains together form a long swinging arm that allows the functional group of biotin to swing back and forth between two active sites. Biotin carboxylation is catalyzed at one active site of Pyruvate Carboxylase. When Gluconeogenesis is active in liver, oxaloacetate is diverted to form glucose (via PEP). Oxaloacetate depletion hinders acetyl CoA entry into Kreb's cycle. The resulting increase in [acetyl CoA] activates Pyruvate Carboxylase to synthesize more oxaloacetate. Avidin, a protein in egg whites with a b barrel structure, tightly binds biotin. Thus, pyruvate carboxylase can be inhibited leading to no conversion of pyruvate to oxaloacetate and then to phosphoenolpyrivate.

22. Cyclic AMP is an important second messenger. It forms when the membrane enzyme adenylyl cyclase is activated (by the alpha subunit of a G protein). The cyclic AMP then goes on to activate specific proteins. Some ion channels, for example, are gated by cyclic AMP. But an especially important protein activated by cyclic AMP is protein kinase A, which goes on to phosphorylate certain cellular proteins. Protein kinase A (also known as the cyclic AMP-dependent protein kinase or A kinase) is an enzyme that covalently decorates proteins with phosphate groups. The unique characteristic of protein kinase A is that its activity is regulated by fluctuating levels of cyclic AMP within cells. Protein kinase A is ultimately responsible for essentially all of the cellular responses due to the cyclic AMP second messenger system. When cyclic AMP levels are low, catalytic subunits are bound to a regulatory subunit dimer and are inactive. As the concentration of cyclic AMP increases, it binds to the regulatory subunits, leading to an allosteric change in conformation which causes unleashing of the catalytic subunits. Free catalytic subunits are active and begin to phosphorylate their targets.

23. At pH optima of 4, the amino acid that could remain an active residue of the active site of an enzyme should be a polar and acidic amino acid. There are only two acidic amino acids out of the 20 amino acids → aspartic acid (aspartate) and glutamic acid (glutamate). At pH = 7, these amino acids have a negative charge on them leading to their acidity. They have an additional -COOH group present in their alkyl side chain. The catalytic triad of an enzyme, which is the active site, is mainly composed of amino acids which determine the pH optima for the particular enzyme.

24. Ion-exchange chromatography separates proteins based on molecular charge. Protein mixtures are applied to in oppositely charged, chromatographic matrix and the various proteins are bound by reversible, electrostatic interactions. The adsorbed proteins are eluted in order of least to most strongly bound molecules (by increasing the ionic strength or varying the pH of the elution buffer), collected as individual chromatographic fractions, and analyzed separately. Proteins carry both negatively and positively charged groups. The net charge of a protein is dependent on pH. At its isoelectric point (pI), the net charge of a protein is zero and no binding to any type of ion-exchange gel matrix will occur. Given, the pIs of the various proteins :

γ-globulin = 6.6,

Human serum albumin (HSA) = 4.9,

RNAse = 7.8 and

hen egg lysozyme (HEL) = 11

CM cellulose is a cation exchange resin. Since the pH gradient is constantly increasing starting from pH 7, the cation resin maintains its charge. So, amino acids having isoelectric points lower than that of the buffer/ salt pH will be positively charged and will bind to the negatively charged cation resin while those amino acids having isoelectric points greater than pH 7, will be negatively charged and will be repelled by the cation resin. So, the order of elution of the given proteins is:

HSA (pI = 4.9<7), γ-globulin (pI = 6.6<7), RNAse (pI = 7.8>7) and HEL (pI = 11>7).

25. DNA Polymerase I from E. coli was the first DNA polymerase characterized. There are approximately 400 molecules of the enzyme per cell. E. coli DNA polymerase I is abbreviated pol I. The enzyme is a single large protein with a molecular weight of approximately 103 kDa (103,000 grams per mole). The enzyme requires a divalent cation (Mg^{++}) for activity and has three enzymatic activities associated with it: 1) 5′-to-3′ DNA Polymerase activity, 2) 3′-to-5′ exonuclease (Proofreading activity), and 3) 5′-to-3′ exonuclease (Nick translation activity). DNA polymerase I require a primer from which to initiate replication and polymerizes deoxyribonucleotides into DNA in the 5′ to 3′ direction using the complementary strand as a template. Newly synthesized DNA is covalently attached to the primer, but only hydrogen-bonded to the template. Only the alpha phosphate of the dNTP is incorporated into newly synthesized DNA.

(L) BOTANY

1. Microtubules are obligate proteinaceous elements found in nearly all eukaryotic cells. The protein which is a major component of cytoskeleton is tubulin. Tubulin is the main component of

microtubule. It is a glycoprotein. The most common members of the tubulin family are α-tubulin and β-tubulin, the proteins that make up microtubules

2. The specialized tissue in the roots of epiphytic orchids is known as velamen. The velamen of an orchid is the white or silvery cover on old roots. This is a multilayered structure (multiple epidermis) of dead cells with special thickenings in the cell walls. The special thickenings seem to prevent cellular collapse and provide the root with some protection from mechanical injury. When the root is wet, the velamen fills passively with water, aided by perforations or tears in the walls from when the roots went through a drying cycle. While dry, the velamen may provide a barrier to water loss via transpiration from the wet, internal cells of the root.

3. Lenticel is a corky slash or spot appearing on plant bark, above the epidermal stoma, that allows for the exchange of gases between the atmosphere and inner tissue. Lenticels originate beneath stomata, simultaneous with the initiation of the first during first growing season. As the lenticels formation starts, the parenchyma cells found near substomatal cavity lose their chlorophyll content and irregularly divide in different plants giving rise to a mass of colourless, rounded, thin walled, loosely arranged cells called Complementary cells. Thus lenticels originate from complementary cells.

4. Plant cell suspension culture is easily initiated from a friable callus. A friable callus is a callus formation that has grown with the cells further apart. When a callus is not friable, it is dense and compact and when it is used to regenerate plant tissue, it grows into a lump and doesn't grow to a viable plant. A friable callus, however, allows the regenerating tissue to grow suspensions.

5. Porogamy is the usual route by which a pollen tube enters an ovule via the micropyle in the fertilization of angiospermous and gymnospermous plants. When the pollen tube penetrates the ovule by a different route, the process is called aporogamy (for example, penetration of the chalaza is known as chalazogamy and penetration of integuments is called misogamy).

6. Germplasm conservation through tissue culture is known as ex situ conservation. Ex situ conservation is the conservation and maintenance of samples of living organisms outside their natural habitat, in the form of whole plants, seed, pollen, vegetative propagules, tissues or cell cultures.

7. An endangered species/taxa is a species of organisms (whether plant or animal) which is facing a very high risk of extinction. According to the red data book maintained by IUCN it is the second most severe conservation status for wild populations, following Critically Endangered. Under the IUCN Categories and Criteria, endangered species is between critically endangered and vulnerable.

8. Biodiversity is the variety and differences among living organisms from all sources, including terrestrial, marine, and other aquatic ecosystems and the ecological complexes of which they are a part. This includes genetic diversity within and between species and of ecosystems. Thus, in essence, biodiversity represents all life.

9. The diploid number of an organism is given as 12. We know nullisomy = $2n - 2$.

   Therefore, nullisomy = $12 - 2 = 10$.

   Thus 10 chromosomes would be expected in its nullisomic.

10. According to relative position of xylem and phloem, the vascular bundles are classified variously. Vascular bundles are radial when xylem and phloem form separate bundles lying on different radii alternating with each other as in roots. The space between the phloem and xylem is filled in with either parenchyma or fibres, or both.

11. Given, average number of chiasma is one pair homologous chromosome = 1.4

    Then, total length of linkage group = average number of chiasma $\times$ 50 =1.4 $\times$ 50 = 70.

    Thus, total length (in map units) for the linkage group is 70.

12. A section of DNA that contains the genetic code for a single polypeptide and functions as a hereditary unit is known as cistron. It can include regions preceding and following the coding DNA as well as introns between the exons.

13. The nucleosome core particle is essential in the packaging of DNA in the chromosomes. It is able to condense a Eukaryotic genome into a cell's nucleus. The nucleosome core particle consists of fourteen turns of B-form DNA around an octamer of histone proteins. The octamer contains two copies each of four different proteins: H2A, H2B, H3, and H4. In vivo, the nucleosome core particle contains a fifth protein, H1. H1 helps to bind the DNA to the core particle such that the number of base pairs bound to the nucleosome increases from 146 to 166 with the addition of H1.

14. The plant which is a member of evergreen forest is cryptomeria. Cryptomeria is a monotypic genus of conifer in the cypress family Cupressaceae, formerly belonging to the family Taxodiaceae. It includes only one species, Cryptomeria japonica. It is endemic to Japan, where it is known as Sugi.

15. John Hutchinson proposed the phylogenetic system of classification in 1926. The families of flowering plants were arranged according to a new system based on their probable phylogeny. It counted as 328 families. It was a radical revision of the angiosperm classification system devised by Bentham & Hooker and by Engler & Prantl

16. Robert Koch's postulates pertain to the disease and causal organisms. He gave the germ theory of disease. Koch's postulates (1984) were as follows:
    i. The positive organism should be associated with every case of disease
    ii. Organism should be isolated and cultured
    iii. Disease must be reproduced when a pure culture is introduced into another host
    iv. Organisms must again be isolated from the exponentially infected host.
17. Aflatoxins are mycotoxins produced by two species of Aspergillus, a fungus particularly Aspergillus flavus, which is especially found in areas with hot and humid climates. Several types of aflatoxins are produced in nature. Aflatoxin B1 is the most common in food and amongst the most potent genotoxic and carcinogenic aflatoxins. It is produced both by Aspergillus flavus and Aspergillus parasiticus.
18. *Phytophthora infestans* is a devastating pathogen of critical food crops, causing late blight of potato and tomato. It is notorious as the causal agent of the Irish Potato Famine more than 150 years ago. Today, epidemics recur in disease conducive environments.
19. Bordeaux mixture which is a combination of copper sulfate, lime, and water, is an effective fungicide and bactericide that has been used for decades to control diseases of fruit and nut trees, vine fruits, and ornamental plants. These natural minerals, when mixed in the correct order, provide long-lasting protection to plants against diseases. Although there are many formulas for preparing Bordeaux mixture, generally a ratio of 10-10-100 works well for many disease-causing pathogens. It comprises of 10 pounds of copper sulfate, 10 pounds of lime, and 100 gallons of water.
20. Any chemical that is used in the fusing of two cells or protoplasts is called a chemical fusogen. Polyethylene glycol (PEG) is used as a fusogen in the formation of hybridomas, and sodium nitrate in the fusion of plant protoplasts in solution.
21. In glycolysis of cellular respiration, NADH produces 2ATP because one ATP is used to transport a molecule of NADH into the mitochondria and continue with aerobic respiration. However, in pyruvate decarboxylation and the Krebs cycle, each NADH yields 3ATPs. $FADH_2$ yields 2 ATPs. This is given by the chemiosmotic theory which suggests essentially that most ATP synthesis in respiring cells comes from the electrochemical gradient across the inner membranes of mitochondria by using the energy of NADH and $FADH_2$ formed from the breaking down of energy-rich molecules such as glucose.
22. The two currently accepted photosystem units are Photosystem II and Photosystem I, which have their own distinct reaction center chlorophylls, named P680 and P700, respectively. These pigments are named after the wavelength (in nanometers) of their red-peak absorption maximum.
23. In C4 plants the initial fixation of carbon dioxide from the atmosphere takes place in the densely packed mesophyll cells. After the carbon dioxide is fixed into a four-carbon organic acid, the malate is transferred through tiny tubes from these cells to the specialized bundle sheath cells. Inside the bundle sheath cells, the malate is chemically broken down into a smaller organic molecule, and carbon dioxide is released. This carbon dioxide then enters the chloroplast of the bundle sheath cell and is fixed a second time with the enzyme Rubisco and continues through the C_3 pathway.
24. Cycocel is a plant growth regulator for ornamentals, including bedding plants and herbaceous crops. It enhances the crop's aesthetic appeal and improves durability during post production shipping and handling. Treated crops are more compact with shorter internodes, stronger stems, and greener leaves. It is a gibberellin inhibitor and is known as antigibberellic acid compound.
25. Anemophily is a term which is used to refer to plants that are usually pollinated by wind. In most cases, these plants have generally very light and loosely attached pollen grains for easy transportation by air currents. In addition, their flowers are not scented and also not brightly coloured.

(M) MICROBIOLOGY

1. Mitochondria and Chloroplast shows autonomy because of their own genetic materials like DNA and can prepare their own required protein. DNA can decode into mRNA and mRNA will be translated into proteins that is why they are semi autonomous.
2. There are two kinds of microorganisms that are divided into prokaryotes and those include bacteria and archaea. Methanobacteria show a number of features that distinguish them from other bacteria, and are now classified as a separate group, the Archaebacteria. Methanobacteria are found in the anaerobic sediment. It shows archeal cell features like cell membrane contains ether linkages; cell wall lacks peptidoglycan; genes and enzymes behave more like Eukaryotes; have three RNA polymerases like eukaryotes; and extremophiles.
3. Pseudopeptidoglycan (also known as pseudomurein) is a major cell wall component of some archaea that differs from bacterial peptidoglycan in chemical structure, but resembles eubacterial peptidoglycan in morphology, function, and physical structure. The basic components are N-acetylglucosamine and N-acetyl-talosaminuronic acid (peptidoglycan has N-acetylmuramic acid instead), which are linked by β-1, 3-glycosidic bonds.

4. Chromatophores are pigment-containing and light-reflecting organelles in cells found in amphibians, fish, reptiles, crustaceans, cephalopods, and bacteria. These are photosynthetic membrane where light is converted to chemical energy in the form of ATP.

5. Aerobic respiration requires oxygen in order to generate energy (ATP).

$$C_6H_{12}O_6\,(s) + 6\,O_2\,(g) \rightarrow 6\,CO_2\,(g) + 6\,H_2O\,(l) + \text{heat}$$

$\Delta G = -2880$ kJ per mole of $C_6H_{12}O_6$

The product of this process is energy in the form of ATP (adenosine triphosphate), by substrate-level phosphorylation, NADH and $FADH_2$. The reducing potential of NADH and $FADH_2$ is converted to more ATP through an electron transport chain with oxygen as the "terminal electron acceptor".

6. Group I introns are large self-splicing ribozymes. They catalyze their own excision from mRNA, tRNA and rRNA precursors in a wide range of organisms. In Group 1 intron splicing branched structures are not formed like others splicing events.

7. Ribosomal frameshift function is to allow alternative translation of an mRNA sequence by changing the open reading frame. It is commonly found in viruses including barley yellow dwarf virus, potato leafroll virus and simian retrovirus-1. Bacteriophage lysis involves at least two fundamentally different strategies. Most phages elaborate at least two proteins, one of which is a murein hydrolase, or lysin, and the other is a membrane protein, which is holin. The available evidence suggests that holins oligomerize to form nonspecific holes and that this hole-forming step is the regulated step in phage lysis.

8. Streptococcus species like *S.pyogenes, S.pneumoniae,* Staphylococcus species like *S.epidermidis, S.aureus* and Neisseria spp. are common surface associated microorganism populated in URT.

9. Autoimmune diseases arise from an inappropriate immune response of the body against substances and tissues normally present in the body. In other words, the immune system mistakes some part of the body as a pathogen and attacks its own cells. Myasthenia gravis is a type of autoimmune disorders. In people with myasthemia gravis, the body produces antibodies that block the muscle cells from receiving messages (neurotransmitters) from the nerve cell. In this platelet cells of the body act as an antigen.

10. Delayed hypersensitivity reactions are inflammatory reactions initiated by mononuclear leukocytes. Delayed hypersensitivity is a major mechanism of defense against various intracellular pathogens, including mycobacteria, fungi, and certain parasites.

The pathophysiology of the Tuberculin reaction is explained thus: M. tuberculosis are engulfed by macrophages after being identified as foreign, but due to a self- preserving mechanism peculiar to TB it is able to block the fusion of the phagosome within which it is existing with the lysosome which would destroy it. So tuberculin sensitivity test (also known as Mantoux test, Mantoux screening test, Pirquet test, or PPD test for purified protein derivative) is a diagnostic tool for tuberculosis in response as Type 4 hypersensitivity by immune system.

11. DNA methylation is a biochemical process whereby a methyl group is added to the 5 position of the cytosine pyrimidine ring or 6 nitrogen of the adenine purine (DNA nucleotides). DNA methylation stably alters the expression of genes in cells when cells divide and differentiate from embryonic stem cells into specific tissues. The statement 'methyl groups are added predominantly to cytosines in bacterial cells and to adenine in eukaryotic cells' is wrong as adenine or cytosine methylation is part of the restriction modification system of many bacteria, in which specific DNA sequences are methylated periodically throughout the genome. Also, cytosine methylation is a common DNA modification found in most eukaryotic organisms including plants, animals, and fungi.

12. Eukaryotic ribosome synthesis is especially complicated, because the ribosomal proteins themselves are made by ribosomes in the cytoplasm (that is, outside of the nucleus), so they then must be imported into the nucleolus for assembly onto the nucleolus-derived rRNA. Once assembled, the nearly complete ribosomal subunits are then exported out of the nucleus and back into the cytoplasm for the final steps of assembly.

13. G_2 phase, or pre-mitotic phase, is the third and final subphase of Interphase in the cell cycle directly preceding Mitosis. It follows the successful completion of S phase, during which the cell's DNA is replicated. G_2 phase ends with the onset of prophase, the first phase of mitosis in which the cell's chromatin condenses into chromosomes.

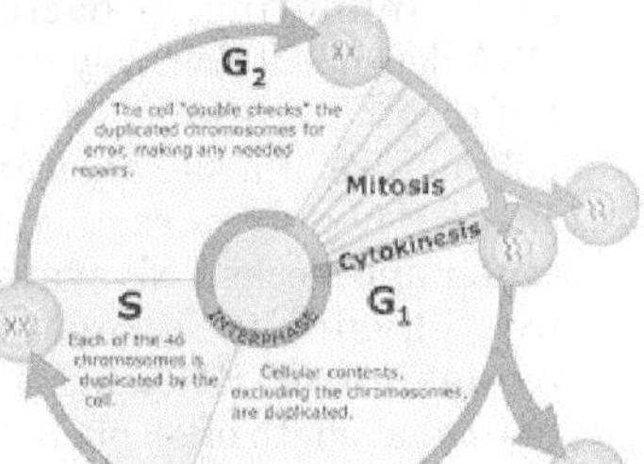

14. Brewing is the production of beer through steeping a starch source (commonly cereal grains) in water and then fermenting with yeast Malting is the process where barley grain is made ready for brewing. Malting is broken down into three steps in order to help to release the starches in the barley. First, during steeping, the grain is added to a vat with water and allowed to soak for

approximately 40 hours. During germination, the grain is spread out on the floor of the germination room for around 5 days to becoming dry.

15. Chargaff's rules state that DNA from any cell of all organisms should have a 1:1 ratio (base Pair Rule) of pyrimidine and purine bases.

16. Because heavy chain constant region is an unique character for all antibodies and it never changes.

17. The fragment antigen-binding (Fab fragment) is a region on an antibody that binds to antigens.

18. Batch (or "vat") pasteurization is the simplest and oldest method for pasteurizing milk. Milk is heated to 154.4 degrees Fahrenheit (63 degrees Celsius) in a large container and held at that temperature for 30 minutes.

19. Resolving power is the ability of magnifying instrument to distinguish two objects that are close together. The resolving power of light microscope depends upon the wavelength and the numerical aperture of the objective lens. The limit of the resolution is inversely related to the resolving power.

Thus, $d = 0.5\lambda/N \sin \alpha$

20. Rifampicin inhibits bacterial DNA-dependent RNA synthesis by inhibiting bacterial DNA-dependent RNA polymerase. Rifampicin binds to RNA polymerase at a site adjacent to the RNA polymerase active center and blocks RNA synthesis by physically preventing extension of RNA products beyond a length of 2-3 nucleotides ("steric-occlusion" mechanism).

21. DNA replication is semi-conservative; one strand serves as the template for the second strand. Primary enzyme involved with bacterial DNA replication is DNA Polymerase III (Pol III). DNA Polymerase III (Pol III) is the enzyme that performs the 5'-3' polymerase function.

22. When isolated from bacteria, prokaryotic RNA polymerase has two forms: The core enzyme and the holoenzyme. The core enzyme is a tetramer whose composition is given as $\alpha_2\beta\beta'$ (two α subunits, one β subunit, and one α' subunit). Core RNA polymerase is capable of faithfully copying DNA into RNA but does not initiate at the correct site in a gene. That is, it does not recognize the promoter specifically. Correct promoter recognition is the function of the holoenzyme form of RNA polymerase.

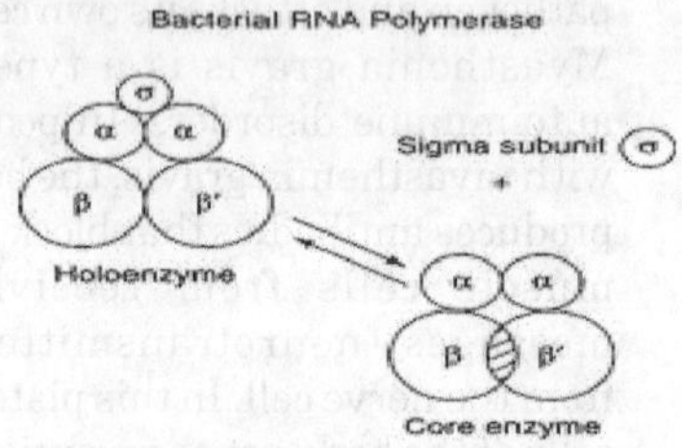

The RNA polymerase holoenzyme contains another subunit, σ (**sigma**), in addition to the subunits found in the core enzyme. Holoenzyme, $\alpha_2\beta\beta'\alpha$, is capable of correct initiation at the promoter region of a gene. σ thus must be involved in promoter recognition. σ subunits are related but distinct in different forms of RNA polymerase holoenzyme. These specialized δ subunits direct RNA polymerase to promoter sequences for different classes of genes.

23. EF-G or elongation factor G (historically known as translocase) is one of the prokaryotic elongation factors. The factor EF-G catalyzes the translocation of the tRNA and mRNA down the ribosome at the end of each round of polypeptide elongation. Homologous to EF-Tu + tRNA, EF-G also binds to the ribosome in its GTP-bound state

24. The Shine-Dalgarno sequence (or Shine-Dalgarno box), proposed by Australian scientists John Shine and Lynn Dalgarno is a ribosomal binding site in the mRNA. This sequence helps recruit the ribosome to the mRNA to initiate protein synthesis by aligning it with the start codon. The complementary sequence (CCUCCU), is called the anti-Shine-Dalgarno sequence and is located at the 3' end of the 16S rRNA in the ribosome. The eukaryotic equivalent of the Shine-Dalgarno sequence is called the Kozak sequence

25. Diphtheria and cholera toxins are released extracellularly from growing bacteria and cause host cell damage. Both of these toxins are A-B toxins, which have 2 fragments one of which is responsible for cell entry and the other of which is catalytically active.

(N) ZOOLOGY

1. Australian region zoogeography contains Australia, New Zealand, New Guinea and nearby Islands in the Pacific ocean Walice" includes Celebas islands in Australian region. The Oriental region comprises of the Indo-Malayan biogeographic regions. The line dividing the oriental and the Australian zoogeographic region is known as the Wallace line.

2. The body of a nematode is long and narrow, resembling a tiny thread in many cases. The epidermis (skin) of a nematode is highly unusual; it is not composed of cells like other animals, but instead is a mass of cellular material and nuclei without separate membranes. This epidermis secretes a thick outer cuticle which is both tough and flexible. The cuticle is a feature shared with arthropods and other ecdysozoans. Nematodes have worm-like appearance, simple structure of an internal body cavity called a pseudocoelom, and the lack of features such as cilia and a well-defined head that are found in most animals. This group is variously known as Aschelminths or Pseudocoelomata.

3. The first vertebrates were fish that appear in the fossil record 530 million years ago. This group evolved into lampreys, sharks, and bony fishes, eventually becoming amphibians. The origin of these groups is unclear. Palaeozoic Era began 542 million years ago with the Cambrian explosion which was an extraordinary diversification of marine animals, and ended 251 million years ago with the end-Permian extinction, the greatest extinction event in Earth history. The first vertebrates originated due to the Cambrian explosion.

4. Triassic Period, in geologic time, was the first period of the Mesozoic Era. It began 251 million years ago, at the close of the Permian Period, and ended 199.6 million years ago, when it was succeeded by the Jurassic Period. At the beginning of the Triassic, virtually all the major landmasses of the world were collected into the supercontinent of Pangea. At the end of the Triassic, however, plate tectonic activity picked up, and a period of continental rifting began. Reptiles increased in diversity and number, and the first dinosaurs appeared, heralding the great radiation that characterized the group during the Jurassic and Cretaceous periods.

5. The giant panda is a medium sized black and white bear that lives only in the mountainous temperate forests of southwest China. They have a diet of bamboo. The giant panda is one of the most endangered animals on earth. Only about 1600 of these rare bears are left.

6. Anurans are any of the vertebrates of the order Anura (or Salientia), characterized by absence of a tail and very long hind legs specialized for hopping: class Amphibia (amphibians). The group includes the frogs and toads. They are tailless stout-bodied amphibians with long hind limbs for leaping. They are semi-aquatic and terrestrial species. Since they belong to the class of Amphibia, they are having three chambered heart.

7. All IgG's are monomers (7S immunoglobulin). The subclasses differ in the number of disulfide bonds and length of the hinge region. IgG is the most versatile immunoglobulin because it is capable of carrying out all of the functions of immunoglobulin molecules. IgG is the major Immunoglobulin in serum'75% of serum immunoglobulin is composed of IgG. IgG is the major immunoglobulin in extra vascular spaces. IgG is the only class of immunoglobulin that crosses the placenta. Transfer is mediated by a receptor on placental cells for the Fc region of IgG.

8. Haemocyanin is a very large protein with 20-40 subunits and molecular weight of 2-8 million Daltons and having a characteristic cuboidal appearance under the electron microscope. These are respiratory proteins in the form of metalloproteins containing two copper atoms that reversibly bind a single oxygen molecule (O_2). Oxygenation causes a colour change between the colourless Cu (I) deoxygenated form and the blue Cu (II) oxygenated form. The copper atoms of haemocyanin are bound as prosthetic groups coordinated by histidine residues.

9. MHC or major histocompatibilty complex restriction means that different T-cells are restricted to either MHC class I or class II antigens. Cytotoxic T-cells are restricted to class I antigens present on nucleated body cells, thus play a role against virus-infected cells or cancerous cells. Helper CD4 T-cells are restricted to class II MHC antigens present on immune cells, thus play a role in increasing the humoral immune response. It was discovered by Doherty and Zinkernagel.

10. The DNA vaccine has proven to be one of the most promising applications in the field of gene therapy. DNA vaccines can circumvent the general re-infection danger because they contain only DNA and not infectious agents. It involves the direct introduction into appropriate tissues of a plasmid containing the DNA sequence encoding the antigen(s) against which an immune response is sought, and relies on the in situ production of the target antigen. This approach offers a number of potential advantages over traditional approaches, including the stimulation of both B- and T-cell responses, improved vaccine stability, the absence of any infectious agent and the relative ease of large-scale manufacture. As proof of the principle of DNA vaccination, immune responses in animals have been obtained using genes from a variety of infectious agents, including influenza virus, hepatitis B virus, human immunodeficiency virus, rabies virus, lymphocytic choriomeningitis virus, malarial parasites and mycoplasmas.

11. An important indicator of evolutionary relatedness is to determine: a) size of the ribosomes, b) size of the bacterial chromosome, c) nitrogen base sequence of rRNA d) size of the periplasmic space e) similarities of cell membrane proteins. The number and types of differences that accumulate between genes or proteins of two different species can be used to assess their evolutionary relatedness and the amount of time since they diverged from a common ancestor. Ribosomal RNA is used to measure the extent of evolutionary relatedness based on divergent or convergent evolution and substitution or mutation of the base pairs of rRNA.

12. In human females, due to the phase of post puberty, the number of ovum produced by them increases or becomes more from the age of 25. But after, a female has entered the late 30s; the number of ova produced decreases gradually and stops at the age of 45. This phenomenon is known as menopause. The fall in number of ova produced decreases from the age of 35 or above.

13. Pantothenic acid is a water-soluble vitamin. Animals require pantothenic acid to synthesize coenzyme-A(CoA), as well as to synthesize and metabolize proteins, carbohydrates, and fats. It is also known as vitamin B5. In its metabolically active form, vitamin B5 gets combined with another small, sulfur-containing molecule to form coenzyme A (or simply, CoA). This conversion allows vitamin B5 to participate in a wide variety of chemical reactions. When found in its CoA form, vitamin B5 plays a pivotal role in helping release energy from sugars, starches, and fats. Most of this energy release occurs in the energy production factories found in every cell called the mitochondria. Two basic types of fats - fatty acids and cholesterol - both require the CoA form of B5 for their synthesis.

14. The plasma membrane of the red blood cell (RBC) consists of a complex, ordered array of lipids and proteins stretched over the outer surface of the cell in the form of a lipid bilayer punctuated by penetrating or attached proteins. The most prominent component of the red cell membrane cytoskeleton, by molecular mass at least, is a fibrous polypeptide called spectrin. The spectrin tetramers are organized into a meshwork that is fixed to the membrane by the protein ankyrin. Ankyrin is itself connected to a transmembrane protein called 'band 3' or anion exchanger protein. Spectrin is also linked to a transmembrane protein called glycophorin C (25 kDa) by the protein known as 'band 4.1.' Glycophorin A (GpA) is a 131 amino acid protein that spans the membrane once and presents its amino-terminal end at the extra-cellular surface of the human red blood cell. Glycophorins A and B are major sialoglycoproteins of the human erythrocyte membrane which bear the antigenic determinants for the MN and Ss blood groups.

15. Tryptophan is one of the 10 essential amino acids that the body uses to synthesize the proteins it needs. It's well-known for its role in the production of nervous system messengers, especially those related to relaxation, restfulness, and sleep. Tryptophan has two important functions. First, a small amount of the tryptophan we get in our diet (about 3%) is converted into niacin (vitamin B3) by the liver. Second, tryptophan serves as a precursor for serotonin, a neurotransmitter that helps the body regulate appetite, sleep patterns, and mood. It is encoded in the standard genetic code as the codon UGG.

16. Beriberi is a neurological and cardiovascular disease. The three major forms of the disorder are dry beriberi, wet beriberi, and infantile beriberi. Thiamine or vitamin B1 deficiency commonly presents sub-acutely and can lead to metabolic coma and death. A lack of thiamine can be caused by malnutrition, a diet high in thiaminase-rich foods. Well-known syndromes caused by thiamine deficiency include beriberi, Wernicke-Korsakoff syndrome, and optic neuropathy.

17. The genes for T-cell receptors were characterised by Tonegawa. T-cell receptor α and β chains each consist of a variable (V) amino-terminal region and a constant (C) region. The organization of the gene segments is broadly homologous to that of the immunoglobulin gene segments. The TCR-α locus, like those for the immunoglobulin light chains, contains V and J gene segments (V_α and J_α). The TCR-β locus, like that for the immunoglobulin heavy-chain, contains D gene segments in addition to V_β and J_β gene segments. The T-cell receptor gene segments rearrange during T-cell development to form complete V-domain exons. T-cell receptor gene rearrangement takes place in the thymus.

18. Adrenal glands are triangle-shaped glands located on top of the kidneys. The outer part of the adrenal gland is called the cortex and produces steroid hormones such as cortisol, aldosterone, and testosterone. The inner part of the adrenal gland is called the medulla and produces epinephrine and nor-epinephrine, which are commonly called adrenaline and nor-adrenaline. The cortex contains cells that synthesize and secrete glucocorticoids, mineralocorticoids, and certain gonadocor-ticoids (sex steroid hormones that are also produced in the gonads). These steroids are all derived from cholesterol.

19. Histones are highly alkaline proteins found in eukaryotic cell nuclei that package and order the DNA into structural units called nucleosomes. They are the chief protein components of chromatin, acting as spools around which DNA winds, and play a role in gene regulation. Five major families of histones exist: H1/H5, H2A, H2B, H3, and H4. Histones H2A, H2B, H3 and H4 are known as the core histones, while histones H1 and H5 are known as the linker histones. Two of each of the core histones assembles to form one octameric nucleosome core particle, and 147 base pairs of DNA wrap around this core particle 1.65 times in a left-handed super-helical turn. The linker histone H1 binds the nucleosome at the entry and exit sites of the DNA, thus locking the DNA into place and allowing the formation of higher order structure.

20. The pituitary gland is a small endocrine organ that controls a multitude of important functions in the body. It is divided into an anterior lobe, intermediate lobe and posterior lobe, all of which are involved in hormone production. The posterior pituitary is composed of axons from the neurons of the hypothalamus. Blood vessel connections between the hypothalamus and pituitary allow hypothalamic hormones to control pituitary hormone secretion. The pituitary gland is termed the "Master Gland" because it directs other organs and endocrine glands, such as the adrenal glands, to suppress or induce hormone production. The pituitary gland actually functions as two separate compartments'an anterior portion (adenohypophysis-hormone producing) and the posterior gland (neurohy-pophysis).

■■

GATE-2000

XL : LIFE SCIENCES

Time : 3 Hours *Maximum Marks : 100*

(H) CHEMISTRY (Compulsory)

Useful Information:

Gas constant, R = 8.314 J mol^{-1} K^{-1}

Planck's constant, $h = 6.626 \times 10^{-34}$ Js

Mass of electrons, $m_e = 9.108 \times 10^{-31}$ kg

H1. For each subquestion or statement given below, four alternatives are given of which only one is correct. Write the correct answer in the answer book by writing *a, b, c* or *d* along with the corresponding subquestion or statement number. (25 × 1 = 25)

1.1 Which one of the following element has the largest atomic radius?

(*a*) Be (*b*) C (*c*) N (*d*) F

1.2 The valence-electronic configuration of Cr atom (Atomic Number 24) in its ground state is

(*a*) $4s^1 3d^5$ (*b*) $3d^5 4s^1$ (*c*) $4s^2 3d^4$ (*d*) $3d^4 4s^2$

1.3 The phosphorus atom in the molecule PF_3 is in the state of hybridization

(*a*) sp^2 (*b*) sp^3 (*c*) p^3 (*d*) *dsp*

1.4 The ionic compounds MgO and CaO have the same crystal structure except that the interionic distances are 2.10 Å respectively. The ratio the lattice energies, U(MgO)/U(CaO), is

(*a*) 0.766 (*b*) 0.875 (*c*) 1.143 (*d*) 1.306

1.5 The quantities K_c and K_p are the concentration equilibrium constant and the pressure equilibrium constant for a reaction in gas phase, which of the following relationships holds good, if there is no change in the number of moles due to the reaction?

(*a*) $K_p = K_c$ (*b*) $K_p > K_c$ (*c*) $K_p < K_c$ (*d*) $K_p = \frac{1}{2} K_c$

1.6 Let p_1 and p_2 be the vapour pressure of water at 372 K and 374 K respectively. Then

(*a*) $p_1 > p_2$ (*b*) $p_1 = p_2$ (*c*) $p_1 < p_2$ (*d*) $p_1 = 2p_2$

1.7 Which one of the following alcohols will react most easily with HBr to give the corresponding bromide?

(*a*) CH_3OH (*b*) $(CH_3)_3COH$

(*c*) CH_3CH_2OH (*d*) $(CH_3)_2CHOH$

1.8 During the nitration of benzene with concetrated HNO_3-H_2SO_4, the nitrating species is

(*a*) HNO_2 (*b*) NO_2 (*c*) NO_2^+ (*d*) NO_2^-

1.9 Which one of the following species is not isoelectronic with N_2?

(*a*) CN^- (*b*) NO (*c*) CO (*d*) CS

1.10 One of the given elements combines with hydrogen to yield an electron-deficient hydride. Identify it.

(*a*) Be (*b*) C (*c*) N (*d*) O

1.11 The oxidation state of Ba in BaO_2 is

(*a*) Zero (*b*) + 1 (*c*) +2 (*d*) + 4

1.12 One of the species given below is a Lewis acid. Which one is it?

(*a*) I (*b*) I^- (*c*) I_3^- (*d*) I_2

1.13 Identify the most stable species from the following divalent halides.

(*a*) CCl_2 (*b*) $GeCl_2$ (*c*) $SnCl_2$ (*d*) $PbCl_2$

1.14 Which of the following ligands causes the maximum crystal field splitting while forming a complex with Fe^{2+} ion?

(*a*) H_2O (*b*) NH_3 (*c*) CN^- (*d*) Cl^-

1.15 The formal oxidation state of Ni in $Ni(CO)_4$ is

(*a*) Zero (*b*) + 1 (*c*) + 2 (*d*) + 4

H2. For each subquestion or statement given below, four alternatives are given of which only one is correct. Write the correct answer in the answer book by writing *a, b, c* or *d* along with the corresponding subquestion or statement number. (10 × 1 = 10)

2.1 The largest ionization energy is found with

(*a*) alkali metals (*b*) alkaline earth metals

(*c*) halogens (*d*) inert gases

2.2 In Planck's hypothesis E = hv, E is the energy of

(*a*) a photon (*b*) a hydrogen atom

(*c*) one electron (*d*) one H_2 molecule

2.3 The most widely applicable condition for spontanerty of processes is

(*a*) $(\Delta E)_{S, V} \leq 0$ (*b*) $(\Delta S)_{E, V} \geq 0$

(*c*) $(\Delta A)_{T, V} \leq 0$ (*d*) $(\Delta G)_{T, P} \leq 0$

2.4 The unit of the rate constant for a second-order process is

(*a*) mol 1^{-1} s^{-1} (*b*) s^{-1}

(*c*) 1 mol^{-1} s^{-1} (*d*) mol 1^{-1}

2.5 The major product obtained from the reaction of 2-methyl-2-butene with 50% H_2SO_4 in water is

(*a*) 2-methyl-2-butanol (*b*) 3-methyl-2-butanol

(*c*) 3-methyl-1-butanol (*d*) 2-methyl-1-butanol

2.6 The correct decreasing order of nucleophilic character of the following species is

(*a*) $H_2O > Cl^- > NH_3 > OH^-$

(*b*) $NH_3 > H_2O > Cl^- > OH^-$

(*c*) $OH^- > Cl^- > NH_3 > H_2O$

(*d*) $Cl^- > OH^- > H_2O > NH_3$

2.7 Which of the following species is aromatic?

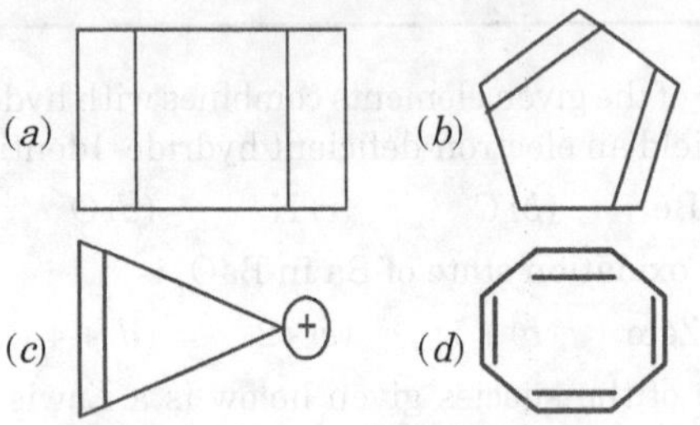

2.8 The reaction of 1-octyne with $HgSO_4$-H_2SO_4.H_2O will give

(*a*) octan-1-one (*b*) octan-2-one

(*c*) octan-3-one (*d*) octan-4-one

2.9 The correct order of decreasing rate of dehydrohalogenation of alkyl halides is

(*a*) RBr > RI > RCl > RF

(*b*) RI > RBr > RCl > RF

(*c*) RI > RBr > RF > RCl

(*d*) RI > RF > RBr > RCl

2.10 The reaction of sodiumphenoxide with CO_2 at high temperature and pressure followed by acidification gives

(*a*) *p*-hydroxy benzoic acid

(*b*) *m*-hydroxy benzoic acid

(*c*) *o*-hydroxy benzoic acid

(*d*) *p*-hydroxy sodium benzoate

H3. (*i*) Calculate the lattice energy of sodium chloride from the following data:

ΔH_{vap} of Na(*s*) = 101 kJ/M

$\Delta H_{dissociation}$ of $Cl_2(g)$ = 239 kJ/M

ΔH_f of NaCl (*s*) = – 411 kJ/M

Ionization energy of Na(g) = 494 kJ/M

Electron affinity of Cl(g) = 369 kJ/M

(*ii*) Find the speed of an electron that has a deBroglie wavelength of 1 nm.

H4. (*i*) The reaction $CCl_3COOH \rightarrow CHCl_3 + CO_2$ is first-order with rate constant $k = 6.7 \times 10^{-7}\ s^{-1}$ at 25° C. (3)

(*ii*) Write the electronic configuration of N_2^+, and find the N-N bond order in the same species.

H5. (*i*)

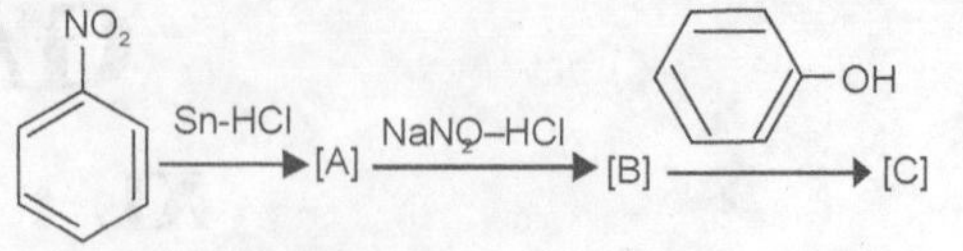

(*ii*)

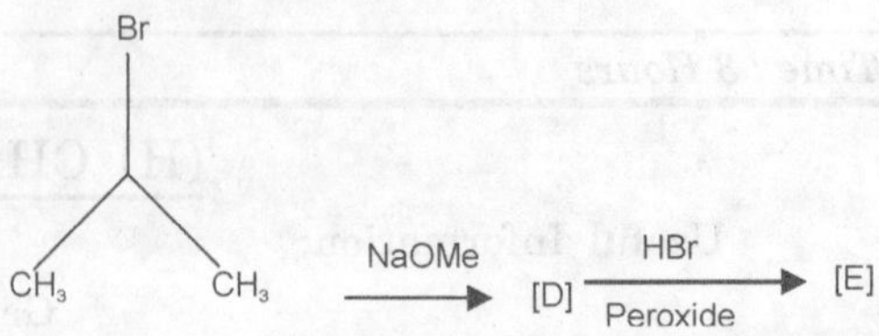

H6. (*i*) Draw the most stable conformation of each of the following compounds: (2)

(*A*) *cis*-1, 2-dibromocyclohexane,

(*B*) *trans*-4-*t*-butylcyclohexanol.

(*ii*) Nickel is estimated gravimetrically by using the reagent dimethylglyoxime. Draw the structures of the reagent and that of the precipated complex. Will the complex be paramagnetic? (2)

H7. (*i*) What is an icosahedron? For which element that is the most common structural feature?

(*ii*) Calcium reacts with nitrogen to give an ionic compound. A which on hydrolysis yields B and C. Identify A, B and C. (3)

(I) BIOCHEMISTRY

I1. For each sub-question given below, four alternatives are provided of which only one is correct. Write the correct answer in the answer book by writing *a, b, c* or *d* along with the corresponding sub-question number. $(20 \times 1 = 20)$

1.1 The properties of water include

(*a*) The ability to form hydrophobic bonds with itself

(*b*) A disordered structure in the liquid state

(*c*) A low dielectric constant

(*d*) Being a dipole, with the negative end at the oxygen atom

1.2 Deficiency of which one of these enzymes causes defect in the storage of glycogen?

(*a*) Lactate dehydrogenase

(*b*) Glyceraldehyde 3 phosphate dehydrogenase

(*c*) Phosphorylase

(*d*) Glycogen synthetase

1.3 The turnover number of chymotrypsin is $100\ s^{-1}$ and for DNA polymerase it is $15\ s^{-1}$. This means that

(*a*) chymotrypsin binds to its substrates with higher affinity than does DNA polymerase

(*b*) the velocity of the chymotrypsin reaction is always greater than that of DNA polymerase

(*c*) the velocities of reactions catalysed by both enzymes at saturating substrate levels could be made equal if 6.7 times more DNA polymerase than chymotrypsin were used

(*d*) the velocities of chymotrypsin reaction at a particular enzyme concentration and saturating substrate levels is lower than that of DNA polymerase reaction under the same conditions

1.4 Which of the following statements is true? Enzyme catalysis of a chemical reaction

(*a*) Increases the forward and reverse reaction rates
(*b*) Decreases ΔG′ so that the reaction can proceed spontaneously
(*c*) Increases the energy of transition state
(*d*) Decreases the entropy of reaction

1.5 Which of the following enzymes can be irreversibly inactivated with Diisopropyl-fluoridate (DIPF)?

(*a*) Carboxypeptidase A (*b*) Trypsin
(*c*) Lysozyme (*d*) EcoRI endonuclease

1.6 Histones have very high percentage of arginine and lysine residues (15-30%). For this class of proteins which of the following reagents would be a suitable choice for generating peptides in the determination of the amino acid sequence of the protein.

(*a*) Cyanogen bromide (*b*) Thermolysin
(*c*) Trypsin (*d*) N-bromosuccinamide

1.7 The half life of [^{32}P] phosphate is approximately 14 days. Forty two days after the purchase of a batch of [^{32}P], the radioactivity present was 1.25 mCi. The radioactivity on the date of purchase would be

(*a*) 5 mCi (*b*) 0.625 mCi
(*c*) 2.5 mCi (*d*) 10 mCi

1.8 A 100 ml of 0.1 M sodium acetate solution was mixed with 300 ml of 0.3 M sodium acetate. The molarity of the final solution would be

(*a*) 330 mM (*b*) 250 mM
(*c*) 200 mM (*d*) 400mM

1.9 A double stranded DNA has 30% Thymine. The percentage of Cytosine is

(*a*) 30% (*b*) 20% (*c*) 70% (*d*) 15%

1.10 The following type of interaction is mainly responsible for aggregation of proteins in dilute solutions

(*a*) Hydrogen bonds
(*b*) Hydrophobic interactions
(*c*) Disulfide bonds
(*d*) Peptide bonds

1.11 The isomerization of this chromophore by light is the first event in visual excitation

(*a*) Retinol (*b*) All-trans retinal
(*c*) 11-cis retinal (*d*) Retinoic acid

1.12 In the transaminases the cofactor is linked via Schiff base formed between the cofactors and the

(*a*) α-NH_2 group of N-terminal amino acid
(*b*) β-NH_2 group of asparagine
(*c*) ε-NH_2 group of lysine
(*d*) None of the above

1.13 An enzyme protein forms 0.001 % of the total soluble protein in a crude extract. The degree of purification required to obtain a homogeneous enzyme is

(*a*) 1000 fold (*b*) 100 fold
(*c*) 100,000 fold (*d*) 10 fold

1.14 A homogeneous protein of native molecular weight 100,000 gave a single band of molecular weight 50,000 on SDS - PAGE in presence of β-mercaptoethanol. N-terminal analysis gave two amino acids alanine and leucine in equal proportions.

(*a*) Protein is a homodimer
(*b*) Protein is contaminated with another protein
(*c*) Protein has two polypeptides linked by disulfide bridges
(*d*) None of the above

1.15 Cholecalciferol (vitamin D), in order to become biologically active undergoes hydroxylation at two positions in the molecule. Hydroxylation at the 25th position is done in the liver whereas hydroxylation at the 1st position occurs in

(*a*) Skin (*b*) Pancreas
(*c*) Intestine (*d*) Kidney

1.16 How many asymmetric carbon atoms are present in the compound whose structure is given below

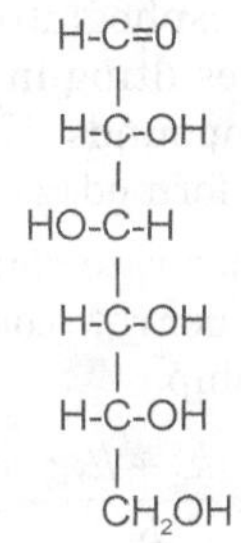

(*a*) 1 (*b*) 2
(*c*) 3 (*d*) 4

1.17 Diptheria toxin inhibits protein synthesis by

(*a*) causing formation of ADP-EF2 complex
(*b*) release of peptidyl-t-RNA from the 'P' site
(*c*) binding to factor EF-1
(*d*) inhibiting peptide bond formation

1.18 Antigenic peptides are presented to T cells by

(*a*) TCR/CD3 (*b*) CD 28
(*c*) CTL A4 (*d*) MHC

1.19 Which of the following statements about cyclic photophosphorylation is not correct?

(*a*) It does not involve NADPH formation
(*b*) It uses electrons supplied by photo-system II
(*c*) It involves a substrate level phosph- orylation
(*d*) It does not generate oxygen

1.20 Which of the following statements about biological membranes is not true?

(*a*) They contain carbohydrates that are covalently bound to proteins and lipids

(*b*) They are large sheet-like structures with closed boundaries

(*c*) They are symmetric because of the symmetric nature of lipid bilayers

(*d*) They contain specific proteins that mediate their distinctive functions

I2. Match the entries in column 1 with those in column 2 and write matching pairs in the answer book. $(5 \times 1 = 5)$

Column 1	Column 2
(A) Van der Waals bonds	(*i*) Spatial arrangement of amino acids that are near each other in the linear sequence
(B) γ- Globulins	(*ii*) Glycosylation inhibitor
(C) Tertiary structure	(*iii*) Cooperativity of oxygen binding
(D) Hill coefficient	(*iv*) Involves polarizable atoms
(E) Tunicamycin	(*v*) Immune protection

I3. (*a*) In the Entner - Doudoroff pathway, 2-keto-3-deoxy-6-phosphogluconate is acted upon by an enzyme resulting in the formation of two 3-carbon compounds. Name the enzyme and the products formed. (3)

(*b*) Two first order rate constants k_2 and k_3 and one second order rate constant k_1, define K_m by the relationship,

$$K_m = \frac{k_2 + k_3}{k_1}$$

By substituting the appropriate units for the rate constants in this expression, show that K_m must be expressed in terms of concentration. (2)

I4. (*a*) Arsenate, AsO_4^{3-} is an uncoupling reagent for oxidative phosphorylation but unlike dinitrophenol it does not transport protons across the inner mitochondrial membrane. How might arsenate function as an uncoupler? (3)

(*b*) Removal of the thymus gland from a young animal not only compromises the production of cytotoxic T cells, but also decreases antibody production by B cells. Why is this the case? (2)

I5. (*a*) Sketch the appropriate plots if the following variables are plotted. Assume that single Michaelis - Menten kinetics apply.

(*i*) v versus [S]

(*ii*) [S] versus time

(*iii*) [ES] versus time $(3 \times 1 = 3)$

(*b*) When lactose is used as an inducer, there is a lag before the enzymes of the lactose operon are synthesized. With IPTG there is no lag. Explain. (2)

I6. (*a*) The structure of a dimer of murein present in bacterial cell wall is represented below.

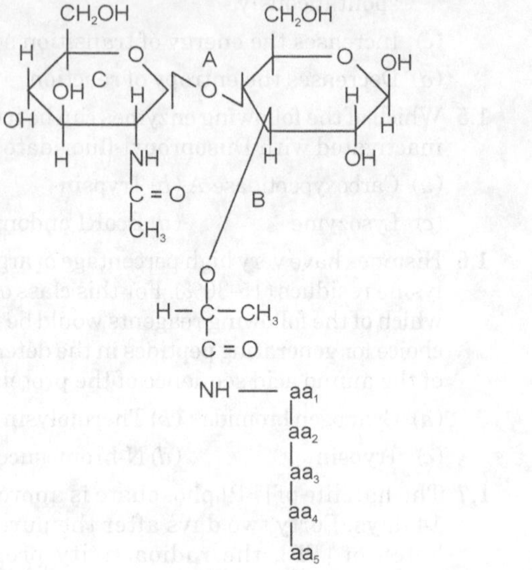

(*i*) Name the linkage at A

(*ii*) Name the linkage at B

(*iii*) Name the sugar at C (3)

(*b*) The DNA in a bacterium is uniformly labeled with ^{15}N and the organism is shifted to a growth medium containing ^{14}N - labeled DNA precursors. After two generations of growth, the DNA is isolated and is subjected to density-gradient equilibrium sedimentation. What proportion of light-density DNA to intermediate - density DNA would you expect to find? (2)

I7. (*a*) If $^{18}O_2$ were added to C_3 plants on a bright, sunny day, would you expect glycine subsequently isolated from the leaves to be labeled? Explain. (2)

(*b*) Early experiments on the problem of protein folding suggested that the native three dimensional structure of a protein was an automatic consequence of its primary structure. Cite an experimental evidence that shows that this is the case. (3)

(J) BOTANY

J1. For each sub-question given below, four alternatives are provided of which only one is correct. Write the correct answer in the answer book by writing *a*, *b*, *c* or *d* along with the corresponding sub-question number. $(25 \times 1 = 25)$

1.1 Microbodies found in cells of fat-rich endosperm are known as

(*a*) Peroxisomes (*b*) Glyoxysomes

(*c*) Lysosomes (*d*) Spherosomes

1.2 If glucose is the sole respiratory substrate, the respiratory quotient would be

(*a*) 0.36 (*b*) 0.80 (*c*) 1.00 (*d*) 1.30

1.3 What role does acetosyringone play in the *Agrobacterium* mediated gene transfer ?

(*a*) Induces expression of *vir* genes

(*b*) Attaches *Agrobacterium* to the plants

(*c*) Transfer T-strand to plant cells

(*d*) Induces site specific nicks in the bottom strand

1.4 The processes of guttation in plants usually takes place through certain specialized structures known as

(*a*) Hydathodes (*b*) Nectar glands

(*c*) Stomata (*d*) Trichomes

1.5 Which of the following amino acids is unable to form a proper peptide bond ?

(*a*) Valine (*b*) Cysteine

(*c*) Arginine (*d*) Proline

1.6 DMSO (Dimethylsulfoxide) is used as

(*a*) Osmoticum (*b*) Cryoprotectant

(*c*) Gelling agent (*d*) Chelating agent

1.7 Random change in gene and genotype frequencies in small population is termed as

(*a*) Genetic load

(*b*) Genetic advance

(*c*) Genetic equilibrium

(*d*) Genetic drift

1.8 Indicate the theory among the following, that relates to "ontogeny repeats phytogeny"

(*a*) Theory of clonal selection

(*b*) Theory of natural selection

(*c*) Theory of recapitulation

(*d*) Theory of speciation

1.9 The enzyme responsible for movement of genetic element around the genome is

(*a*) DNA helicase (*b*) Primase

(*c*) Transposase (*d*) Reverse transcriptase

1.10 Which of the following seed is used for commercial crop production ?

(*a*) Breeders seed (*b*) Certified seed

(*c*) Foundation seed (*d*) Registered seed

1.11 Food web is

(*a*) A series of producers

(*b*) A series of consumers

(*c*) A collection of producers and decomposers

(*d*) A matrix of food chain

1.12 A plant cell where nucleus is absent

(*a*) Sieve tube cell (*b*) Guard cell

(*c*) Cambium cell (*d*) Companion cell

1.13 Which of the following phytohormone induces fruit ripening

(*a*) Ethylene (*b*) Abscisic acid

(*c*) Zeatin (*d*) Gibberellins

1.14 Corn (*Zea mays*) has a diploid number of 20. The chromosome number in a microspore mother cell would be

(*a*) 10 (*b*) 20 (*c*) 30 (*d*) 40

1.15 Among the following which one is single membrane organelle

(*a*) Chloroplast (*b*) Nucleus

(*c*) Lysosome (*d*) Mitochondria

1.16 Which one of the following statements about hexose monophosphate shunt is not true?

(*a*) Major means in the cell by which reduced NADP is produced

(*b*) Major pathway by which necessary ribose and deoxyribose are supplied in the biosynthesis of nucleotides and nucleic acid

(*c*) This pathway takes place in cytoplasm and requires oxygen for its entire operation

(*d*) It leads to synthesis of 28 molecules of ATP

1.17 A mechanism that can cause a gene to move from one linkage group to another is

(*a*) Translocation (*b*) Inversion

(*c*) Duplication (*d*) Deletion

1.18 An amino-acyl synthetase is responsible for

(*a*) Formation of a peptide bond

(*b*) Binding of m-RNA to ribosomes

(*c*) Attaching an amino group to an organic acid

(*d*) Joining an amino acid to t-RNA

1.19 How many different kinds of matings can be made in a population containing two alleles?

(*a*) 4 (*b*) 6 (*c*) 8 (*d*) more than 8

1.20 Red rot of sugarcane is caused by

(*a*) *Claviceps purpurea*

(*b*) *Cochliolobus miyabeanus*

(*c*) *Colletotrichum falcatum*

(*d*) *Cercospora personata*

1.21 Mangroves are specially adapted to aquatic ecosystem because of the presence of

(*a*) Pneumatophores

(*b*) Distinct aqueous tissue in leaves

(*c*) Vivipary

(*d*) All of the above

1.22 Which one of the following should be considered a model plant for investigation in molecular genetics ?

(*a*) *Allium cepa*

(*b*) *Happlopappus gracilis*

(*c*) *Arabidopsis thaliana*

(*d*) *Rheo discolor*

1.23 The physiologically receptor state in which a bacterial cell is able to be transformed is called

(*a*) Lysogenic (*b*) Competent

(*c*) Sensitized (*d*) Inducible

1.24 The type of inflorescence found in *Ficus* species is

(*a*) Cyathium (*b*) Verticillaster

(*c*) Hypanthodium (*d*) Coenanthium

1.25 Photooxidation of chlorophyll is prevented by

(*a*) Carotenoid (*b*) Anthocyanin

(*c*) Phycobilin (*d*) Fucoxanthin

J.2 Mention the botanical name of the plants which yield the following products of economic importance

(*a*) Reserpine (*b*) Menthol

(*c*) Quinine (*d*) Vincristine

(*e*) Opium (5)

J3. (*a*) Enumerate three important advantages of liquid culture in micropropagation of plants. (3)

(*b*) List two factors that affect the extent of somaclonal variation. (2)

J4. (*a*) What is a maintainer line in hybrid seed industry ? (2)

(*b*) How does incompatibility differs from male sterility ? (3)

J5. (*a*) What are the differences in the mechanism of CO_2 fixation between most C_4 plants and those exhibiting Crassulacean acid metabolism? (3)

(*b*) What is Diffusion Pressure Deficit (DPD) and how it is expressed? (2)

J6. (*a*) DNA based molecular markers have acted as versatile tool in plant genome analysis. State three properties desirable for an ideal DNA marker. (3)

(*b*) The cloning vectors currently used have one component in common (in addition to origin of replication). Name the component and indicate its function. (2)

(K) MICROBIOLOGY

K1. For each sub-question given below, four alternatives are provided of which only one is correct. Write the correct answer in the answer book by writing *a, b, c* or *d* along with the corresponding sub-question number. (20 × 1 = 20)

1.1 Which one of the following statements is correct?

(*a*) Gram +ve bacteria lack peptidoglycan.

(*b*) Gram –ve bacteria lack peptidoglycan.

(*c*) Both Gram +ve and Gram –ve bacteria possess peptidoglycan and the outer membrane.

(*d*) Both Gram +ve and Gram –ve bacteria possess peptidoglycan but the Gram +ve bacteria lack outer membrane.

1.2 For infection of *Escherichia coli* with the lambda phage, the *E. coli* is usually grown in a medium containing maltose because

(*a*) Maltose is essential for the lysis of *E. coli.*

(*b*) Maltose serves as an important cofactor during the phage DNA replication.

(*c*) The presence of maltose induces maltose binding protein which is inhibitory to bacterial growth.

(*d*) The presence of maltose induces maltose binding protein which also serves as a receptor for the lambda phage.

1.3 Which of the following statements about the Archaebacteria group of organisms is incorrect?

(*a*) Archaebacterial initiator tRNA carries methionine instead of formyl methionine.

(*b*) Archaebacterial ribosomes, like the eukaryotic ribosomes, are sensitive to anisomycin but insensitive to chloramphenicol.

(*c*) Archaebacterial RNA polymerase is insensitive to rifampicin.

(*d*) Archaebacterial genomic DNA contain base modifications which make it refractile to cleavage with restriction endonucleases prepared from eubacteria.

1.4 Walking pneumoniae (atypical pneumoniae) affects human beings in the age group of 5 to 25 years. The main causative agent of this disease is

(*a*) *Mycobacterium tuberculosis*

(*b*) *Klebsiella pneumoniae*

(*c*) *Mycoplasma pneumoniae*

(*d*) *Streptococcus pneumoniae*

1.5 Which of the following bacteriophages is used for generalised transduction?

(*a*) φ × 174 (*b*) M13 (*c*) Lambda (*d*) P1

1.6 Which of the following statements is incorrect?

(*a*) During conjugation of an F^+ (donor) and F^- (recipient) *E. coli*, a copy of the F factor is almost always transferred to the recepient.

(*b*) Conjugation between Hfr strain and F^- strain leaves the recepient strain F^-

(*c*) Conjugation between Hfr strain and F^- strains results in high frequency of recombination and therefore the recepient become Hfr or F^+.

(*d*) Conjugation between F' and F^- strains results in the recepient becoming F'.

1.7 For which of the following property does the A-form double helix DNA not differ from that of B-form double helix?

(*a*) Appearance of the major and minor grooves

(*b*) Thickness of the helix

(*c*) Tilt of the bases

(*d*) Polarity of the two complementary strands

1.8 Organellar protein synthesis occurs
(*a*) Only in mitochondria
(*b*) In mitochondria as well as in chloroplast
(*c*) In endoplasmic reticulum
(*d*) In lysosome

1.9 Which of the following characteristics holds true for prokaryotes but not for eukaryotes?
(*a*) Motility by cilia
(*b*) Phospholipids in plasmamembrane
(*c*) Peptidoglycan in the cell wall
(*d*) DNA as the genetic material

1.10 Oncogenic retroviruses change normal mammalian cells into cancerous cells. This transformation is primarily associated with
(*a*) Release of numerous viral particles and concomitant death of the host cells
(*b*) Integration of the viral genome into the host nuclear DNA
(*c*) Presence of viral particles in the host cell membrane
(*d*) Efficient replication of the viral genomic RNA in the host cells

1.11 Which of the following is not a peptide antibiotic?
(*a*) Polymyxins (*b*) Gramicidins
(*c*) Chloramphenicol (*d*) Tyrocidines

1.12 The group of organisms which uses light as the energy source and CO_2 as the principal carbon source are called
(*a*) Photoheterotrophs (*b*) Chemoautotrophs
(*c*) Chemoheterotrophs (*d*) Photoautotrophs

1.13 Which of the following bacteria are capable of oxidizing nitrite to nitrate in the soil?
(*a*) *Nitrosomonas* (*b*) *Nitrobacter*
(*c*) *Nitrospira* (*d*) *Nitrosococcus*

1.14 Which of the following statements on photorespiration is incorrect?
(*a*) It occurs only in photosynthetic cells.
(*b*) NAD^+ is reduced to NADH.
(*c*) No ATP molecules are formed.
(*d*) H_2O_2 is formed.

1.15 How many ATP molecules are generated in complete biological oxidation of one molecule of glucose?
(*a*) 36 ATP (*b*) 12 ATP (*c*) 30 ATP (*d*) 38 ATP

1.16 Which of the following viral infection often leads to hepatocellular carcinoma in humans?
(*a*) Hepatitis A virus
(*b*) Hepatitis C virus
(*c*) Polio virus
(*d*) Human rhino virus

1.17 The replication of the polio virus positive strand RNA genome requires
(*a*) Virus encoded RNA dependent RNA polymerase
(*b*) DNA dependent RNA polymerase
(*c*) DNA polymerase
(*d*) Reverse transcriptase

1.18 The drug colchicine exerts its inhibitory action during which of the following phases of the cell cycle?
(*a*) G0 (*b*) Gl
(*c*) G2 (*d*) M

1.19 Which of the following statements is wrong?
(*a*) Lactic acid is produced by *Lactobacillus delbrueckii.*
(*b*) Bacterial amylase is produced by *Bacillus subtilis.*
(*c*) Citric acid is produced by *Rhizopus nigricans.*
(*d*) Gibberellic acid is produced by *Fusarium monoliforme.*

1.20 During DNA replication, the synthesis of the leading strand occurs in the 5′-3′ direction along with the movement of the replication fork . Which one of the following statements is true about the synthesis of the lagging strand?
(*a*) DNA polymerase II, which has an additional activity of polymerization in 3′-5′ direction, is utilized.
(*b*) DNA polymerase I is utilized which can carry out DNA synthesis in the absence of any primer.
(*c*) Synthesis of the lagging strand occurs in the small fragments by DNA polymerase in 5′-3′ direction using a *de novo* synthesized DNA primer.
(*d*) Synthesis of the lagging strand occurs in small fragments in 5′-3′ direction utilizing RNA primers.

K2. Write whether the statements made below are True or False. (1 × 5 = 5)
(*a*) T-helper lymphocytes secrete a factor which stimulates formation of other types of lymphocytes.
(*b*) T-suppressor lymphocytes cause lowering of the intensity of the immune response.
(*c*) T-cytotoxic lymphocytes recognise nonself antigens on cells and lyse them.
(*d*) B- lymphocytes develop into cells that secrete antibodies.
(*e*) Hypersensitivity to pollen can be cured by repeated injection with pollen in order to boost levels of IgG in the circulation.

K3. (*a*) Write the name of the enzyme involved in maintenance of chromosomal ends. What are the major components of the enzyme? (2)

(*b*) Chromosomes contain DNA folded into different order structures. The first order structure corresponds to formation of nucleosomes wherein about 200 bp are wrapped around the histones. The diameter of the nucleosomes is about 11 nm. The nucleosomes are folded further into a second order structure to form a super helix (solenoid) consisting of 6 nucleosomes per turn.

Calculate the total packaging ratio of DNA at the level of nucleosomes and the solenoid. Further if the genome size of a eukaryotic microorganism is 2×10^7 bp and the size of its chromosome is 4 m, what will be the final packaging ratio of DNA in the chromosome? (3)

K4. Match the function (panel B) of the enzymes listed in panel A. (1 × 5 = 5)

Panel A

(A) Reverse transcriptase

(B) DNA polymerase

(C) RNA polymerase

(D) Alkaline phosphatase

(E) DNA ligase

Panel B

(*i*) Joining of 5′-PO_4 with the 3′ OH in double stranded DNA

(*ii*) Synthesis of RNA using DNA as template

(*iii*) DNA directed DNA synthesis during DNA replication

(*iv*) Synthesis of complementary DNA from RNA

(*v*) Removal of phosphate groups from the terminii of DNA and RNA molecules

K5. (*a*) Mononucleotide, dinucleotide and trinucleotide fractions of an in vitro transcription reaction were purified. Predict phosphate to nucleoside ratios in these fractions. (3)

(*b*) What is the nature of sugar puckering at 2′/3′ position in A and B forms of DNA double helices? (2)

K6. Under laboratory conditions in a rich nutrient medium *E. coli* was found to have a doubling time of 20 min during the exponential phase of growth (Figure K 6(*a*)).

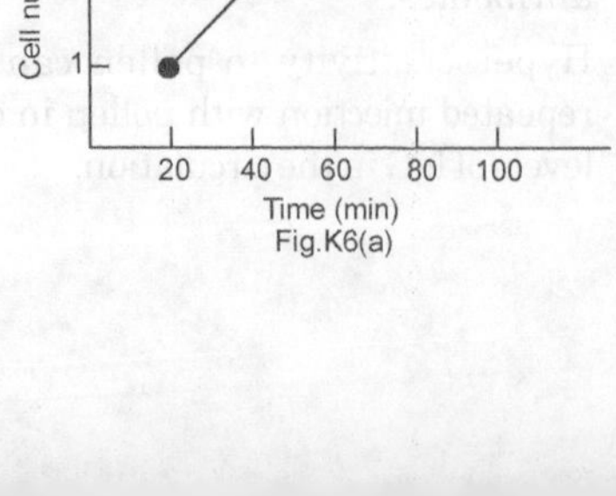

Fig.K6(a)

(*a*) What is the property of a synchronously growing culture? How would you determine if the growth curve shown in Figure K6(*a*) corresponded to a synchronously growing culture? (3)

(*b*) What is apoptosis and what will be the state of the chromatin in an apoptotic cell? (2)

K7. (*a*) Children are given triple antigen vaccine to protect them against certain bacterial diseases. Name the diseases and the corresponding causative bacteria. (3)

(*b*) What cell types does human immuno deficiency virus (HIV) infect? What receptor on these cells are used for the entry of this virus into these cells? (2)

(L) ZOOLOGY

L1. For each sub-question given below, four alternatives are provided of which only one is correct. Write the correct answer in the answer book by writing *a, b, c* or *d* along with the corresponding sub-question number. (20 × 1 = 20)

1.1 Glucagon is produced by

(*a*) Acinar cells of pancreas

(*b*) Alpha cells of the islets of langerhans of pancreas

(*c*) Beta cells of the islets of langerhans of pancreas

(*d*) All of the above

1.2 Sympatric populations show

(*a*) Populations whose geographic ranges overlap

(*b*) Populations showing similar adaptations

(*c*) Populations showing similar behaviour

(*d*) Populations at the verge of extinction

1.3 The cells that actively synthesize spongy bone are called

(*a*) Osteocytes (*b*) Osteoclasts

(*c*) Osteoblasts (*d*) Osteon

1.4 A dioecious, triploblastic, pseudocoelomate, bilaterally symmetrical animal with unsegmented body possessing mouth and anus and showing some degree of cephalisation at the anterior end belongs to the phylum

(*a*) Annelida (*b*) Nematoda

(*c*) Platyhelminthes (*d*) Mollusca

1.5 Which of the following is an example of transition mutation?

(*a*) A replaced by T (*b*) A replaced by C

(*c*) A replaced by G (*d*) A replaced by any base

1.6 During which one of the following periods, first mammals appeared on the earth?

(*a*) Devonian (*b*) Silurian

(*c*) Triasic (*d*) Jurassic

1.7 If a single strand of DNA molecule reads as 5′-ACCTAG-3′, which one of the following is the complementary RNA molecule?

(*a*) 3′-TGGATC-5′ (*b*) 5′-TGGATC-3′

(*c*) 3′-UGGAUC-5′ (*d*) 5′-UGGAUC-3′

1.8 A frog exhibits
(*a*) Cutaneons respiration only
(*b*) Buccal respiration only
(*c*) Pulmonary respiration only
(*d*) All of the above

1.9 The correct order for respiratory quotient for the following substrates is
(*a*) Carbohydrate > Protein > Fat
(*b*) Fat > Protein > Carbohydrate
(*c*) Protein > Carbohydrate > Fat
(*d*) Carbohydrate > Fat > Protein

1.10 Study involving DNA differences suggests that chimpanzees are more closely related to
(*a*) Humans (*b*) Gibbons
(*c*) Capuchins (*d*) Rhesus Monkeies

1.11 The kingdom protista contains
(*a*) Prokaryotic unicellular autotrophic organisms
(*b*) Eukaryotic unicellular photosynthetic organisms
(*c*) Prokaryotic multicellular heterotrophic organisms
(*d*) Eukaryotic multicellular heterotrophic organisms

1.12 There are five major classes of Immunoglobulin molecules. Which one of them is produced early during the immune response?
(*a*) Ig G (*b*) Ig A (*c*) Ig M (*d*) Ig D

1.13 A baby born to which one of these couples is most likely to suffer from hemolytic disease of the new born?
(*a*) Rh^+ mother and Rh^+ father
(*b*) Rh^+ mother and Rh^- father
(*c*) Rh^- mother and Rh^- father
(*d*) Rh^- mother and Rh^+ father

1.14 If a cell has no rigid cell wall, has no chloroplast or plastids, and the stored carbohydrate is glycogen, then the cell is from
(*a*) Plant (*b*) Fungus (*c*) Bacteria (*d*) Animal

1.15 In humans, the implantation of blastocyst occurs at
(*a*) Immediately after ovulation
(*b*) 1-2 days after ovulation
(*c*) 6-8 days after ovulation
(*d*) 2-5 days after ovulation

1.16 The pattern of growth in primate is
(*a*) Limited and allometric
(*b*) Limited and isometric
(*c*) Unlimited and isometric
(*d*) Unlimited and allometric

1.17 Homeotic mutations result in
(*a*) Loss of Homeostasis
(*b*) Loss of homing of proteins to their targets
(*c*) Deletion of body parts
(*d*) Conversion of one body part to another

1.18 Bacillary dysentery is produced by the organism belonging to the genes
(*a*) Bacillus (*b*) Shigella
(*c*) Mycobacterium (*d*) Clostridium

1.19 Mitotic spindle is formed by bundles of
(*a*) Microtubules (*b*) Microfilaments
(*c*) Microbodies (*d*) Intermediate filaments

1.20 Interpretation of behavioral data in terms of human experience is called
(*a*) Anthropocentrism (*b*) Anthropomorphism
(*c*) Teleology (*d*) Ethology

L2. Match the Scientists in Column I with their contributions in column II ($5 \times 1 = 5$)

Column I	Column II
(*i*) Berk and Sharp	(A) Reverse Transcriptase
(*ii*) Singer and Nicholson	(B) RNA dependent RNA polymerase
(*iii*) Harurna and Spiegelman	(C) Fluid-mosaic model
(*iv*) Alvarez and Alvarez	(D) RNA splicing
(*v*) Baltimore and Temin	(E) Polio vaccine
	(F) DNA is genetic material
	(G) Cretaceous mass extinction

L3. Define the following: ($5 \times 1 = 5$)
(*a*) Semispecies (*b*) Primitive streak
(*c*) Batesian mimicry (*d*) Cistron
(*e*) Paratope

L4. (*a*) Colour blindness is a sex-linked recessive trait in humans. A normal woman, who had a colour-blind father, marries a colour-blind man ($3 \times 1 = 3$)
(*i*) What is the probability that her sons will be colour-blind?
If the same woman marries a normal man
(*ii*) What is the probability of her having a colour-blind child?
(*iii*) What is the probability of getting a colour-blind daughter?
(*b*) What is autophagy and what is its function? (2)

L5. (*a*) What are oncogenes and Tumor suppressor genes? (2)
(*b*) Why would depletion of ozone in atmosphere lead to increased incidence of skin cancer? (3)

L6. (*a*) Cloning sheep Dolly proved that the somatic cells of animals are also totipotent: Explain. (3)
(*b*) Why one produces long term immunity against measles virus after single infection while no long term memory is produced against influenza? (2)

L7. (*a*) What is the consequence of haploid parthenogenesis in honey bee? (3)
(*b*) What is eutrophication of a lake ecosystem? (2)

ANSWERS

(H) CHEMISTRY

1.1 (*a*) 1.2 (*b*) 1.3 (*b*) 1.4 (*c*) 1.5 (*a*) 1.6 (*c*) 1.7 (*b*) 1.8 (*c*) 1.9 (*b,d*) 1.10 (*a*)
1.11 (*c*) 1.12 (*d*) 1.13 (*d*) 1.14 (*c*) 1.15 (*a*) 2.1 (*d*) 2.2 (*a*) 2.3 (*d*) 2.4 (*c*) 2.5 (*a*)
2.6 (*c*) 2.7 (*c*) 2.8 (*b*) 2.9 (*b*) 2.10 (*c*)

(I) BIOCHEMISTRY

1.1 (*d*) 1.2 (*d*) 1.3 (*b*) 1.4 (*d*) 1.5 (*b*) 1.6 (*c*) 1.7 (*d*) 1.8 (*b*) 1.9 (*c*) 1.10 (*b*)
1.11 (*c*) 1.12 (*a*) 1.13 (*c*) 1.14 (*a*) 1.15 (*d*) 1.16 (*d*) 1.17 (*a*) 1.18 (*d*) 1.19 (*b*) 1.20 (*c*)

(J) BOTANY

1.1 (*b*) 1.2 (*c*) 1.3 (*b*) 1.4 (*a*) 1.5 (*d*) 1.6 (*b*) 1.7 (*d*) 1.8 (*c*) 1.9 (*c*) 1.10 (*b*)
1.11 (*d*) 1.12 (*a*) 1.13 (*a*) 1.14 (*b*) 1.15 (*c*) 1.16 (*c*) 1.17 (*a*) 1.18 (*d*) 1.19 (*a*) 1.20 (*c*)
1.21 (*d*) 1.22 (*c*) 1.23 (*b*) 1.24 (*c*) 1.25 (*a*)

(K) MICROBIOLOGY

1.1 (*d*) 1.2 (*d*) 1.3 (*d*) 1.4 (*c*) 1.5 (*d*) 1.6 (*c*) 1.7 (*d*) 1.8 (*b*) 1.9 (*c*) 1.10 (*b*)
1.11 (*c*) 1.12 (*d*) 1.13 (*b*) 1.14 (*c*) 1.15 (*d*) 1.16 (*b*) 1.17 (*a*) 1.18 (*d*) 1.19 (*c*) 1.20 (*d*)

(L) ZOOLOGY

1.1 (*b*) 1.2 (*a*) 1.3 (*c*) 1.4 (*b*) 1.5 (*c*) 1.6 (*c*) 1.7 (*c*) 1.8 (*d*) 1.9 (*a*) 1.10 (*a*)
1.11 (*b*) 1.12 (*c*) 1.13 (*d*) 1.14 (*d*) 1.15 (*c*) 1.16 (*a*) 1.17 (*d*) 1.18 (*b*) 1.19 (*a*) 1.20 (*d*)

EXPLANATIONS

H : CHEMISTRY (COMPULSORY)

1. Atomic radius is generally stated as being the total distance from an atom's nucleus to the outermost orbital of electron. In simpler terms, it can be defined as something similar to the radius of a circle, where the center of the circle is the nucleus and the outer edge of the circle is the outermost orbital of electron. An atom gets larger as the number of electronic shells increase; therefore the radius of atoms increases as one goes down a certain group in the periodic table of elements. In general, the size of an atom will decrease as one move from left to the right of a certain period. So, Be has the largest atomic radii.

2. The electronic configuration of Chromium with atomic number of 24 is

   $_{4}Cr = 1s^2\, 2s^2\, 2p^6\, 3s^2\, 3p^6\, 3d^5 4s^1$

   $= [Ar]\, 3d^5\, 4s^1$

   So, the outer shell configuration of Cr is $3d^5\, 4s^1$.

3. In PF_3 the lone pair on the phosphorus pushes the P-F bonding electrons away from itself, resulting in F-P-F bond angle of 97.8°, which is appreciably smaller than the ideal bond angle of 109.5°. So, the phosphorus molecule has sp^3 hybridization.

4. The total potential energy of an ionic compound, which is often referred to as the lattice energy, UL per mole may be represented as the sum of the electrostatic and repulsive energy terms. Lattice energy is given by the Born Lande equation. Lattice Energy Formula per mole is represented as:

   $$E = \frac{N_A Mz + z^- e^2}{4\pi\varepsilon_0 r_0}\left(1 - \frac{1}{n}\right),$$

   Where, U_L is the equilibrium value of the lattice energy and r_o is the equilibrium value of inter ionic separation.

   In case of MgO and CaO, both have the same crystal structure and so all the parameters are equivalent except the inter-ionic distances;

   $r_{CaO} = 2.4$ Å

   and $r_{MgO} = 2.10$ Å

   Therefore, $E \propto 1/r_0$

   Hence, the ratio of lattice energies:

   $E_{MgO}/\, E_{CaO} = r_{CaO}/\, r_{MgO}$
   $= 2.4/\, 2.1$
   $= 1.1428$
   $= 1.143$

5. The relation between K_p and K_c is given as:

   $K_p = K_c(RT)^{\Delta n}$

   K_p = equilibrium constant in terms of partial pressures (atm)

   K_c = equilibrium constant in terms of concentrations (molarity)

   R = ideal gas constant (0.082 atm.L / K.mol)

   T = absolute temperature (700°C = 973 K)

   $\Delta n = \Sigma$n products – Σn reactants

   Given, there is no change in the number of moles due to the reaction. This means that $\Delta n = 0$

   Now, the equation becomes:

   $K_p = K_c\,(RT)^0 \Rightarrow K_p = K_c$

6. Vapor pressures are dependent only on temperature. The vapor pressure of a liquid does not depend on the amount on the liquid in the container, be it one liter or thirty liters; at the same temperature, both samples will have the same vapor pressure. Vapor pressures have an exponential relationship with temperature and always increase as temperature increases. It is important to note that when a liquid is boiling, its vapor pressure is equal to the external pressure. So, it is clear that higher the temperature, greater is the pressure. Therefore, vapour pressure of water at 374 K is greater than that at 372 K, i.e. $p_1 < p_2$.

7. When treated with HBr or HCl alcohols typically undergo a nucleophilic substitution reaction to generate an alkyl halide and water. Alcohol relative reactivity order is 3° > 2° > 1° > methyl in terms of stability of the carbocation that is formed in the reaction. Reaction usually proceeds via an S_N1 mechanism which proceeds via a carbocation intermediate that can also undergo rearrangement.

$$H-X-\overset{|}{\underset{|}{C}}- \xrightarrow[X = Br, Cl]{} -\overset{|}{\underset{|}{C}}-X \quad X-OH$$

So a tertiary alcohol will react most easily with HBr. The 3^0 alcohol would be $(CH_3)_3COH$.

8. In nitration of benzene, the use of HNO_3-H_2SO_4 results in the generation of the electrophile NO_2^+ which results in the nitration of the benzene ring. Thus NO_2^+ is the nitrating species.

9. Isoelectronic species are elements or compounds which have the same number of electrons present in them. Number of electrons in $N_2 = 14$

Now, $CN^- = 6$ of C + 7 of N + 1 $e^- = 14$

NO = 7 of N + 8 of O = 15

CO = 6 of C + 8 of O = 14

CS = 6 of C + 16 of S = 22

So, NO and CS are not isoelectronic with N_2.

10. Beryllium combines with hydrogen to form an electron deficit hydride (BeH_2). The overlap between the hydrogen-1s orbitals and the two lobes of the beryllium sp-hybrid orbitals constitutes the two Be—H "bonds" in BeH_2 molecule.

11. In BaO_2, oxygen is present as a peroxide ion (O – O) linkage. So, the oxidation state of each oxygen atom is -1. So, the overall oxidation state of peroxide ion is -2. Hence, the oxidation state of Ba is +2.

12. A Lewis acid is any substance, such as the H^+ ion, that can accept a pair of nonbonding electrons. In other words, a Lewis acid is an electron-pair acceptor. A Lewis base is any substance, such as the OH^- ion, that can donate a pair of nonbonding electrons. A Lewis base is therefore an electron-pair donor. Here, I_2 is the Lewis acid as it can accept an electron pair.

13. Inert pair effect may be defined as inertness of inner ns sub-shell towards chemical reaction. It is seen in groups 3A and 4A especially (5s and 6s electrons). Therefore Pb shows mainly +2 oxidation state frequently as compared to +4 oxidation state. Valence electrons in an s orbital penetrate to the nucleus better than electrons in p orbitals, and as a result they are more tightly bound to the nucleus and less able to participate in bond formation. A pair of such electrons is called an inert pair. So, $PbCl_2$ is the most stable because of lower oxidation state due to inert pair effect.

14. Crystal field theory is based on details of their symmetry lower in energy than the remaining two. The difference in energy between the two sets is denoted Δ and is called the crystal-field splitting energy (CFSE). This energy is the parameter that is used to correlate a variety of spectroscopic, thermodynamic, and magnetic properties of complexes. The Crystal Field Theory experiment illustrates the effects on a metal's d orbital energies of moving a set of negative point charges close to a metal ion. Stronger the ligand, higher and better is the splitting effect. Amongst the given ligands, the strongest is CN^-, so it splits Fe^{2+} ion while forming complex.

15. In $NiCO_4$ complex, the CO molecule does not carry any charge as it is neutral. Hence, the formal oxidation state of Ni in the complex is 0.

16. Ionization Energy can be defined as being the energy required to remove the outermost electron from a gaseous atom. It is possible to remove more electrons from most elements, so this quantity is more precisely known as the first ionization energy, the energy to go from neutral atoms to cations with a 1^+ charge. The second ionization energy is the energy that is required to remove a second electron, to form 2^+ cations from 1^+ cations. The ionization energy decreases from top to bottom in groups, and increases from left to right across a period. Thus, helium has the largest first ionization energy, while francium has one of the lowest. So, the inert gases have the largest ionization energies.

17. According to the Planck hypothesis, all electromagnetic radiation is quantized and occurs in finite "bundles" of energy which we call photons. The quantum of energy for a photon is not Planck's constant h itself, but the product of h and the frequency. The quantization implies that a photon of blue light of given frequency or wavelength will always have the same size quantum of energy. So, the equation is given by, $E = h\nu$ where E is the energy of the photon, ν is the frequency of radiation and h is Planck's constant.

18. A spontaneous process is a process that occurs in a system without any input of energy from the surroundings. We can combine entropy and enthalpy together to make a new quantity, the Free Energy which, under conditions of constant temperature and pressure, will determine the direction of spontaneous change. A reaction will proceed to decrease the free energy of the system. In other words, all spontaneous processes have a negative change in free energy. Therefore, $(\Delta G)_{T,P} \le 0$

19. For an nth order reaction, the unit of rate constant, k is given by $\{mole/L\}^{1-n} \times s^{-1}$

For 2nd order reaction, we have $n = 2$

Thus, Unit of k is $(mole/L)^{-1} s^{-1}$ or L/mole-s.

20. 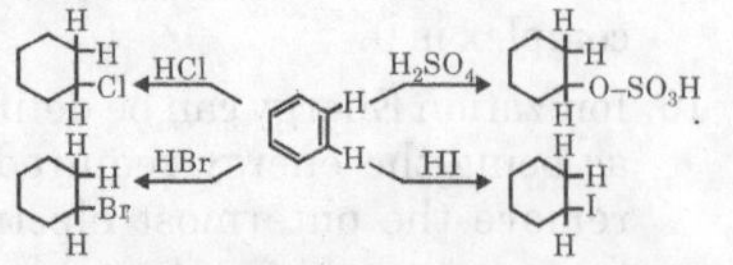

Strong Bronsted acids such as HCl, HBr, HI & H_2SO_4, rapidly add to the C = C functional group of alkenes to give products in which new covalent bonds are formed to hydrogen and to the conjugate base of the acid. Only one product is possible from the addition of these strong acids to symmetrical alkenes such as ethene and cyclohexene. However, if the double bond carbon atoms are not structurally equivalent, as in molecules of 1-butene, 2-methyl-2-butene and 1-methylcyclohexene, the reagent conceivably may add in two different ways. This is shown for 2-methyl-2-butene in the following equation.

$(CH_3)_2C = CHCH_3 + H\text{-}Cl$
$\rightarrow (CH_3)_2CH\text{–}CHClCH_3$
or $(CH_3)_2CCl\text{–}CHHCH_3$

2-methyl-2-butene
2-chloro 3methylbutane
or 2-chloro-2-methyl butane

So, the major product formed for 2-methyl-2-butene is 2-methyl-2-butanol.

21. Acids and bases exist as conjugate acid-base pairs. Every time a Bronsted acid acts as an H^+-ion donor, it forms a conjugate base. Conversely, every time a base gains an H^+ ion, the product is a Bronsted acid. Strong acids have a weak conjugate base and strong bases have a weak conjugate acid. So, the nucleophiles on their acidity are arranged as:

$$H_2O < HCl < NH_4^+ < H_3O^+.$$

These substances have their conjugate bases which are arranged in terms of basicity as:

$$OH^- > Cl^- > NH_3 > H_2O$$

22. In order to be aromatic, a molecule must have a certain number of pi electrons (electrons with *pi* bonds or lone pairs) within a closed loop of parallel, adjacent *p* orbitals. The *pi* electron count is defined by the series $4n + 2$ where n = zero or a positive integer (0, 1, 2, etc.). This is Huckel's Rule ($4n + 2$ rule). Amongst the given compounds, the aromatic compound which follows $4n + 2$ rule is:

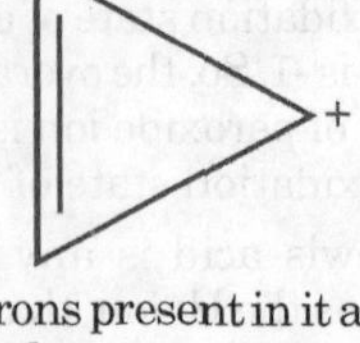

2π electrons present in it and follow $4n + 2$ rule

23. 1-octyne reacts with $HgSO_4$-H_2SO_4/ H_2O to give rise to octan-2-one, an aldehyde.

The reaction is as follows:

$CH_3(CH_2)_5C$
$\equiv CH \rightarrow HgSO_4/H_2SO_4\ (H_2O)$

After tautomerism, we have

$\rightarrow CH_3(CH_2)_5(C{=}O)\text{-}CH_3$

24. Elimination reactions are commonly known by the kind of atoms or groups of atoms leaving the molecule. The removal of a hydrogen atom and a halogen atom, for example, is known as dehydrohalogenation; when both leaving atoms are halogens, the reaction is known as dehalogenation.

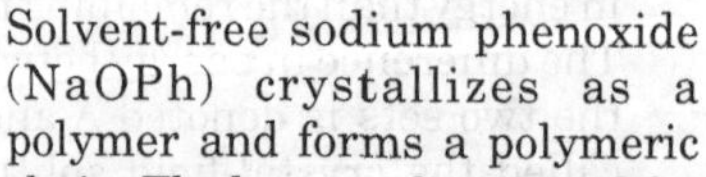

Alkyl halide relative reactivity order:

$$3° > 2° > 1°$$

Alkyl halide relative reactivity order:

$$I > Br > Cl > F$$

25. Solvent-free sodium phenoxide (NaOPh) crystallizes as a polymer and forms a polymeric chain. The low coordination of the sodium atoms, as evident in the crystal structure, is confirmed by the easy coordination of oxoligands (α-donors). Hence, the four-membered ring chain of the solvent-free sodium phenoxide is separated by oxoligands, and forms partial structures as the polymer fragments. Sodium phenoxide reacts with CO_2 under high temperature and pressure conditions. This reaction after acidification results in the formation of o-hydroxy benzoic acid.

(I) BIOCHEMISTRY

1. The odd shape of water molecule with both hydrogen atoms occurring on the same side of the oxygen atom gives water its ability to "stick" to itself and to other surfaces. The hydrogen atoms create a positive electrical charge while the oxygen atom creates a negative charge. The attraction to one another is what causes water to form droplets. This gives rise to a dipole in the water molecule with partial positive charge on the hydrogen ions and partial negative charge on the oxygen ions.

2. Glycogen is a polymer of glucose residues linked mainly by α (1, 4) glycosidic linkages. There are α (1, 6) linkages at branch points. Glycogen synthase (GS) is the enzyme responsible for the synthesis of -1, 4-linked glucose chains in glycogen. It is the rate limiting enzyme in the synthesis of the polysaccharide, and its activity is highly regulated through phosphorylation at multiple sites and also by allosteric effectors, mainly glucose 6-phosphate (G6P). The enzyme glycogen synthase is needed for the body to make glycogen. A deficiency results in very low amounts of glycogen stored in the liver.

3. Given, turnover number of Chymotrypsin = 100 s^{-1}

Turnover number of DNA polymerase I = 15 s^{-1}

This means that in 1 second, chymotrypsin can cleave 100 sites in a polypeptide molecule. Whereas in 1 second, DNA polymerase I can incorporate 15 bases to a newly synthesizing DNA strand. Thus, it implies that the velocity of action for chymotrypsin is almost 7 times that of the velocity of DNA polymerase I.

4. Enzymes are biological macromolecules that catalyze chemical reactions. They are fascinating molecules for several reasons. First, enzymes show high specificities toward their physiological substrates; compounds that differ only slightly from the natural

substrate are often not acted upon. Second, activity of many enzymes can be finely tuned, allowing the metabolism proceed at a rate optimal for the well-being of the organism. Third, is the fact that many enzymes bring about enormous rate accelerations. Enzyme catalysis decreases the activation energy of the substrate for its conversion into product. Enzyme catalysis leads to decrease in entropy of the reaction which results in the stabilization of the free energy change for the reaction. The involvement of enzyme leads to decrease and stability of energy of the enzyme-substrate transition state complex leading to spontaneous and stable product formation.

5. Irreversible inhibitors that covalently bond to the enzyme provide an alternative and often complementary means for elucidating functional groups at the enzyme active site because they modify the functional groups, which can then be identified. DIPF modifies only 1 of the 28 serine residues in the proteolytic enzyme trypsin, implying that this serine residue is especially reactive.

6. Mass spectrometry based proteomics almost invariably involves the enzymatic degradation of proteins to peptides by trypsin. This protease has high cleavage specificity, is very aggressive and stable under a wide variety of conditions. Most importantly, by cleaving C-terminal to arginine or lysine residues, it lead to peptides in the preferred mass range for effective fragmentation by tandem mass spectrometry and it places the highly basic residues at the C-termini of the peptides. Given, histones have very high percentage of arginine and lysine residues (15-30%). So, using trypsin for partial hydrolysis or cleavage of the histone protein, several peptides can be generated for the determination of the amino acid sequence of the protein.

7. Given, half life of ^{32}P molecule, $t_{1/2}$ = 14 days

Present day radioactivity of the molecule, N = 1.25 mCi

Days elapsed after the purchase of the molecule, $t = 42$

We know, $t_{1/2} = 0.693/\lambda$

$\Rightarrow \lambda = 0.693/t_{1/2}$

$\Rightarrow \lambda = 0.693/14$

$\Rightarrow \lambda = 0.0495$

Now, according to the law of radioactive decay, we have :

$$-dN/dt = \lambda N_0$$

$\Rightarrow \ln (N/N_0) = -\lambda t$

$\Rightarrow \ln N - \ln N_0 = -(0.0495 \times 42)$

$\Rightarrow \ln (1.25) - \ln N_0 = -2.079$

$\Rightarrow \ln N_0 = \ln (1.25) + 2.079$

$\Rightarrow \ln N_0 = 0.2231 + 2.079$

$\Rightarrow N_0 = \text{Antilog}(2.3021)$

$\Rightarrow N_0 = 9.995$

Therefore, the initial radioactivity of ^{32}P was 10 mCi (approx.)

8. Given, for solution 1 of Sodium acetate, volume (V_1) = 100 mL and molarity (C_1) = 0.1 M

For solution 2 of Sodium acetate, volume (V_2) = 300 mL and molarity (C_2) = 0.3 M

Molarity of the mixture of the two solutions will be :

$$C = \{(C_1V_1 + C_2V_2)/(V_1 + V_2)\}$$

$\Rightarrow C = \{(0.1 \times 100 + 0.3 \times 300)/(100 + 300)\}$

$\Rightarrow C = \{(10 + 90)/(400)\}$

$\Rightarrow C = 100/400$

$\Rightarrow C = 0.25$

The molarity of the final solution is 0.25 M or 250 mM.

9. Given, in a double stranded DNA, % of thymine = 30 %

According to Chargaff's rule, adenine (A) = thymine (T) and cytosine (C) = guanine (G).

Therefore, % of adenine in the dsDNA = 30 %

Now, according to Chargaff, for any species, (A + G)/ (T + C) = 1 or A + G = T + C. Now, for the purpose of equality, values of A + G and C + T must be = 100 %. Hence, % of guanine = (100 – 30) % = 70% and % of cytosine = (100 – 30) % = 70%.

10. Formation of aggresomes in cells is a general cellular response to the presence of mis-folded proteins when the degrading capacity of the cells is exceeded. There is role of aggresomes in disturbance of the proteosomal system operation and in cellular death, particularly in the so-called "protein conformational diseases". The main driving force behind the formation of aggregates in a dilute solution is the hydrophobic interaction of the non-polar residues of protein.

11. The light is mapped as an image along the surface of the retina by activating a series of light-sensitive cells known as rods and cones. The outer segments of the rods and cones contain a region filled with membrane-bound discs, which contain proteins bound to the chromophore 11-cis-retinal. When visible light hits the chromophore, the chromophore undergoes an isomerization, or change in molecular arrangement, to all-trans-retinal. In retina, absorption of a photon promotes a π electron to a higher-energy orbital (a π-π^*excitation). This excitation "breaks" the π component of the double bond, thus allowing free rotation about the bond between carbon atom 11 and carbon atom 12. Thus, when 11-cis-retinal absorbs a photon in the visible range of the spectrum, free rotation about the bond between carbon atom 11 and carbon atom 12 can occur and the all-trans-retinal can form.

12. Transaminases catalyze the transfer of $-NH_2$ groups from the amino acids, onto α-ketoglutarate. The prosthetic group of the transaminase enzyme is pyridoxal phosphate (PLP), a derivative of vitamin B_6. In the "resting" state, the aldehyde group of pyridoxal phosphate is in a Schiff base linkage to the ε-amino group of an enzyme lysine side-chain. The α-amino group of a substrate amino acid displaces the enzyme lysine, to form a Schiff base linkage to PLP. The active site lysine extracts a proton, promoting tautomerization (shift of the double bond), followed by re-protonation with hydrolysis. Several other enzymes that catalyze metabolism or synthesis of amino acids also utilize PLP as prosthetic group, and have mechanisms involving a Schiff

base linkage of the amino group to PLP.

SCHIFF BASE FORMATION

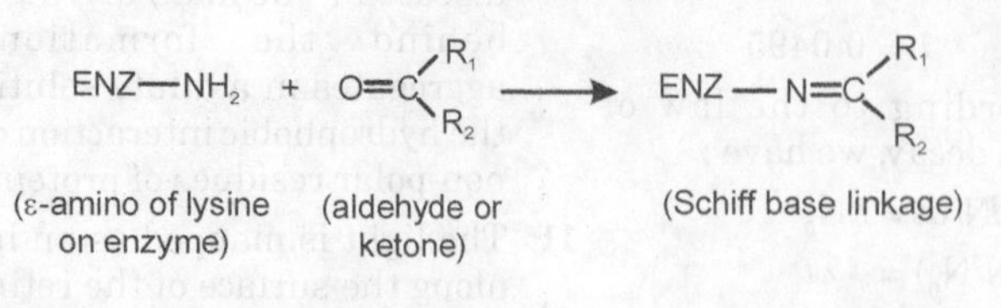

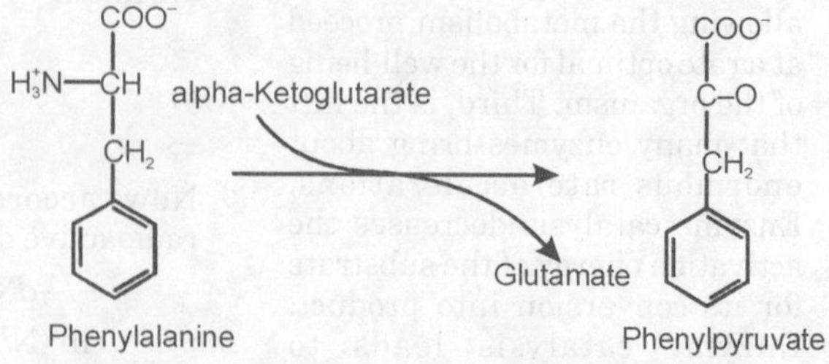

Transamination of Phenylalanine to Phenylpyruvate

13. Given, there is a crude extract of protein. The enzymatic portion of the protein accounts for about 0.001 % of the total crude extract. If crude extract is X mL, then the quantity of enzyme protein is: 0.001 % of X = (0.001 × X)/ 100 = X × 10^{-5} mL. So, for extraction of purification of the enzyme protein, the homogenate should be purified by a factor of 10^5 folds.

14. Most homodimeric proteins have symmetric structure. A dimer is something made up of two subunits. So a dimeric protein is made up of two individual protein chains. *n* the given homogenous protein (molecular weight =100,000) which gave only a single band on performing SDS-PAGE of molecular weight 50,000, it shows that the subunits of the protein are equal in weight. Also, on amino acid sequencing through N-terminal analysis, it was found that the protein was made up of 2 subunits each of alanine and leucine. So, it is very clear that the homogenous protein is homodimeric in nature with equal proportions of alanine and leucine.

15. Bioactive vitamin D or calcitriol is a steroid hormone that has long been known for its important role in regulating body levels of calcium and phosphorus, and in mineralization of bone. Vitamin D_3, also known as cholecalciferol is generated in the skin of animals when light energy is absorbed by a precursor molecule 7-dehydrocholesterol. Vitamin D is thus not a true vitamin, because individuals with adequate exposure to sunlight do not require dietary supplementation. Vitamin D transformation occurs in two steps: 1) Within the liver, cholecalciferol is hydroxylated to 25-hydroxycholecalciferol by the enzyme 25-hydroxylase and 2) within the kidney, 25-hydroxycholecalciferol serves as a substrate for 1-alpha-hydroxylase, yielding 1, 25-dihydroxycholecalciferol, the biologically active form.

16. An asymmetric carbon is a carbon atom attached to four functional groups or four different atoms. A carbon atom is asymmetric if it has four different chemical groups attached. Glucose, with six carbon atoms, has four asymmetric carbon atoms. The arrangement of the OH's and H's on these atoms is very important. Thus, there are four asymmetric carbon atoms (4 chiral centres) in the given molecule of glucose.

17. Diphtheria toxin is one of the most extensively studied and well understood bacterial toxins. Diphtheria toxin (DT) is an extracellular protein of *Corynebacterium diphtheriae* that inhibits protein synthesis and kills susceptible cells. The diphtheria toxin repressor (DtxR) is a global regulatory protein that uses Fe^{2+} as co-repressor. DT is a proenzyme that must be processed to activate its latent NAD: EF-2 ADPR-transferase activity. Treatment of DT with trypsin selectively cleaves the peptide bond located on the carboxyl-terminal side of the surface-exposed arginine (R) residue R190, R192, or R193 to generate an amino-terminal fragment A (DT-A) and a carboxyl-terminal fragment B (DT-B) that remain covalently linked by the disulfide bond between C186 and C201.

18. The basis for the immune response against intracellular pathogens is the recognition by cytotoxic T lymphocytes of antigenic peptides derived from cytosolic proteins, which are presented on the cell surface by major histo-compatibility complex (MHC) class I molecules. The structural basis for the specificity of peptide binding to MHC class I molecules and the identification of proteins encoded in the class II region of the MHC are putatively involved in the production of peptides and their transport into the endoplasmic reticulum, where they assemble with class I molecules.

19. Photophosphorylation is the process of creating ATP using a Proton gradient created by the Energy gathered from sunlight. The process of creating the Proton gradient resembles that of the electron transport chain of Respiration. But since formation of this proton gradient is light-dependent, the process is called Photophosphorylation. During Cyclic Photophosphorylation the electrons are recycled, hence the name cyclic photo-phosphorylation. The excited electrons resulting from the absorption of light in photosystem I are received by the primary electron acceptor and then transferred to the cytb6-f complex which acts as an electron transport chain. The electrons return back to the reaction center of Photosystem I, where the cycle is ready to start all over. The electrons are using to translocate Protons which the ATPase uses to synthesize ATP. No reduction of $NADP^+$ occurs in Cyclic Photophosphorylation. During the movement of electrons, H^+ moves across the membrane. These electrons don't generate NADPH, but the H^+ transport can produce ATP.

20. Biological membranes are dynamic structures composed of a diverse set of phospholipid molecules and proteins. Biological membranes are the structures that define and control the composition of the space that they enclose. The lipids making up components of membranes are of three major classes that includes glycerophospholipids, sphingolipids, and cholesterol. Biological membranes also contain proteins, glycoproteins, and lipoproteins. Proteins associated with membranes are of two general types: integral and peripheral. Integral membrane proteins (also called intrinsic proteins) are tightly bound to the membrane through hydrophobic interactions and are inserted into and/or penetrate the lipid bilayer. The lipid portion of a lipoprotein anchors the protein to the membrane either through interaction with the lipid bilayer directly or through interactions with integral membrane proteins. Lipoproteins associated with membranes contain one of three types of covalent lipid attachment. Although biological membranes contain various types of lipids and proteins, their distribution between the two different sides of the bilayer is asymmetric.

(J) BOTANY

1. Microbodies found in cells of fat rich endosperms are known as glyoxysomes.

   These are specialised peroxisomes that are found particularly in the fat storage tissue of germinating cells and also found in filamentous tissue. Thus glyoxysomes contain enzymes that initiates the breakdown of fatty acids and also help in synthesis of sugars by gluconeogenesis, which is used by seedlings as aenergy source until they come mature enough to produce energy themselves by photosynthesis.

2. If glucose is the sole respiratory substrate, the respiratory quotient would be 1.

   Respiratory quotient is a dimensionless number. The respiratory quotient is calculated by dividing the amount of CO_2 eliminated from the organism by the amount of O_2 consumed in respiratory process.

   $$RQ = \frac{\text{Volume of } CO_2 \text{ released}}{\text{Volume of } O_2 \text{ consumed}}$$

   For glucose,

   $$C_6H_{12}O_6 + 6O_2 \rightarrow 6O_2 + 6H_2O + \text{energy}$$

   $$RQ = \frac{6}{6} = 1$$

   When substrate is fats or protein then,

   $$RQ < 1$$

   When substrate is organic acids then,

   $$RQ > 1.$$

3. Acetosyringone is a phenolic compound that initiates Agrobacterium to infect plant cells. Agrobacterium have flagella that allow them to swim through soil towards photoassimilates that accumulate in the rhizosphere, some strains may chemotactically move towards chemical exudates such as acetosyringone. Acetosyringone is identified by the Vir A protein which is produced by the Vir A gene of Agrobacterium Ti plasmid. Thus helping Agrobacterium to attach itself to the plants.

4. Hydathodes is a type of secretory tissue in leaves usually of angiosperms that secretes water through pores in the epidermis or margin of leaves, typically at the tip of marginal tooth or serration. These are typically evolved from stomata and are involved in guttation process.

5. The amino acid which is unable to form a proper peptide bond is 'Proline'. This is because it does have a hydrogen on its amino group ($- NH_2$), so it cannot donate a hydrogen bond to stabilize any α helix or β sheet thus creating a kink in the structure.

6. DMSO (Dimethyl sulphoxide) is most often used as 'Cryoprotectant'. Cryoprotectant is a substance that is used to protect biological tissue from freezing damage, i.e due to ice formation.

7. Genetic drift is the change in the frequency of the gene variant (allele) in a population due to random sampling. The alleles in the offspring are a sample of those in the parents and a chance in determining whether a given individual survives and reproduce.

   When there are few copies of an allele, the effect of genetic drift is larger and when there are many copies the effect is smaller.

8. Theory that relates "ontogeny repeats phylogeny" is Recapitulation Theory.

   Recapitulation Theory also called as "Biogenetic Law or Embryological parallelism' is a biological hypothesis that is developing from embryo to adult animal go through stages resembling or representing successive stages in the evolution of their remote ancestors.

   It was proposed by Von Baer and late on modified by Ernst Haekel (1866) as Biogenetic law.

9. Transposase is an enzyme that binds to the ends of a tranposon and catalyses its movement to another part of genome by cut and paste mechanism. Thus helping in the movement of genetic material.

10. For commercial crop production certified seeds are used. The certified seeds are necessary because-

    (*i*) it maintains a pedigree on seed of a specific variety.

    (*ii*) The produced seed is assured of having adequate supply of a high quality, clean seed stock

    (*iii*) It has high nutritive value.

11. Food web shows how plants and animals are interconnected to each other that is showing a matrix of food chain.

    Example- trees produce acorns which act as a food for many insects and mice. Because there are many mice, insects so snakes have foods. The insects and acorns also attract birds. Birds also act as food for snakes. Thus all are interconnected.

12. Sieve tube is a characteristic element of phloem, which functions in the transport of food materials, such as sugars and proteins, synthesised within plant.

Sieve tubes are remarkable in that their cell lacks nuclei when mature. They are closely associated with parenchymatous companion cells with prominent nuclei.

13. Many climacteric fruits like banana, apple, tomato shows a strong increase in ethylene levels at a late green or breaker stage. As a consequence of high ethylene chlorophyll is degraded, and ripening of fruits takes place. Activity of many maturation related enzyme increases. Starch, organic acids in some cases are converted into sugars. Pectin, the main component of middle lamella are degraded thus fruits softens.

14. The chromosome number in a microspore mother spore cell also has the diploid nature (2*n*) where *n* = ploidy. Therefore, it will also contain 20 chromosome as that of the diploid corn.

15. Lysosome is a single membrane bounded cell organelle. Lysosome contain acid hydrolase enzyme that breaks down waste material and cellular debris. They are frequently nicked name as 'suicidal bags' due to their phenomenan of autolysis.

Chloroplast and mitochondria are also called as cell within cell so that more than one membrane is present.

16. The hexose monophosphate pathway is used for production of NADPH from NADP. This pathway takes place in cytoplasm and requires oxygen for entire operation. No ATP synthesis is involved in this process.

17. Translocation is a mechanism in which a part of one chromosome breaks and reattaches to a different chromosome. Chromosomal translocation can be detected by analysing karyotypes of effected cells.

18. Amino acyl synthetase catalyses a keyu reaction in protein synthesis. They match the 20 amino acids to genetic code by transferring them to tRNA. Reaction proceeds in 2 steps:

(*i*) Amino acid is first activated by ATP to form amino acyl adenylate.

(*ii*) Then it is transferred to the terminal ribose of tRNA.

19. In a population containing 2 alleles 4 kinds of mating can be made because 2 sexes of the organism with 2 alleles are present

For example: If 1 of the allele is T and other is t then for a population mating

Male = Tt, Female = Tt

Tt X Tt = TT, Tt, Tt, tt

20.

	Organism	Disease
(*i*)	Colletotrichum falcatum	- red rot of sugarcane
(*ii*)	Claviceps purpurea	- ergot disease of wheat, barley, triticales, rye etc
(*iii*)	Cochliobolus miyabeanus	- brown spot disease in rice
(*iv*)	Cercospora personata	- disease in groundnut

21. Mangroves are special type of xerophilous plant which grow on saline soils with high concentration of salts like NaCl, $MgCl_2$, and $MgSO_4$. Soils are physiologically dry. Their osmotic pressure values are very high. Therefore they have special adaptation to survive in these conditions. Most of them produce negatively geotropic root to encourage the entry of oxygen gas. They show vivipary that is germination of seeds before they shed from parent plant. Most of them are succulents their leaves are evergreen, then small and leathery with water storage tissues, thick cuticle and well developed palisade tissue.

22. Arabidosis thaliana is considered as a model plant for investigation in molecular genetics. The reasons are as follows-

(*i*) Very small genome (~115mb). Small genome make it easier to find mutations.

(*ii*) The genome was successfully sequenced in 2000 (AGI).

(*iii*) Self pollinating plant so maintaining genotype is easy.

(*iv*) Single pollinating plant produces 6000 seeds per generation which is critical when studying inheritance of complex traits.

(*v*) Very short life cycle (8weeks), size of the plant is also small. Short life span reduces time taken for experiment.

(*vi*) Can be easily transformed with A.tumificiens or any other mutagen.

23. Only competent bacteria can be transformed whether naturally or artificially. In transformation, exogenous genetic material is introduced in bacterial cells. This may be done by creating small hole in bacterial cell and injecting the external DNA into it.

24.

Inflorescence		Species
Hypanthodium	–	Ficus
Cyathium	–	Euphoria
Verticillaster	–	Ocium
Coenanthium	–	Dorstenia

25. Carotenoids can remove oxygen exited chlorophyll oxygen complex via a carotenoid epoxide cycle. This prevent photo oxidation or bleeching of chlorophyll which actually explains the protective action for chlorophyll done by carotenoids.

(K) MICROBIOLOGY

1. Both the Gram- positive and Gram- negative cell walls contain peptidoglycan, however, the cell wall of Gram-negative bacteria is much more complex than Gram-positive bacteria as Gram-negative bacteria also consist of an outer membrane which is absent in Gram-positive bacteria. Thus the Gram-positive cell wall is single layered while Gram-negative cell wall is double layered. Gram-positive bacteria have more peptidoglycan or murein layer (20-80 nm thick) as compared to Gram-negative bacteria (2-7 nm thick). Gram-negative bacteria possess an outer membrane which is 7-8 nm thick.

2. For infection of *Escherichia coli* with λ phage, the E. coli is usually grown in a medium containing maltose because the binding site for phage lambda is a maltose

transport protein in the *E. coli*. Thus *E. coli* cells used as a host for lambda must be grown in media containing maltose to induce expression of the lamB gene. Bacteriophage Lambda binds to an *E. coli* cell by means of its J protein in the tail tip. The J protein interacts with the maltose outer membrane porin (the product of the lamB gene) of *E. coli*, a porin molecule, which is part of the maltose operon.

3. Archaebacterial genomic DNA contain base modifications which make it refractile to cleavage with restriction endonucleases prepared from eubacteria is a wrong statement. A major difference between archaebacteria and eubacteria exists in the composition of their respective DNA-dependent RNA polymerase. Archaebacteria have only one type of DNA-dependent RNA polymerase. It is a multi-subunit complex that is more complex than the a2bb´s eubacteria enzyme and simpler than the RNA polymerases type I, II, and III of eukaryotes. The Archaeal RNA polymerase contains 8-10 different polypeptide subunits, thus resembling the eukaryotic enzyme.

4. Walking pneumonia, or atypical pneumonia, is a less serious form of the lung infection pneumonia. It's caused by *Mycoplasma pneumoniae*, which causes cold-like symptoms in addition to a low-grade fever and a hacking cough. Colds that last longer than 7 to 10 days or respiratory illnesses like respiratory syncytial virus (RSV) can develop into walking pneumonia.

5. Generalized transducing phages accidently package host DNA into a small fraction of the phage capsids produced during lytic infection. Phage P1 is a commonly used generalized transducing phage for *E. coli*. Any region of the bacterial chromosome can be transferred by a generalized transducing phage.

6. During conjugation, the Hfr bacterium would attempt to transfer its entire DNA to the F^- bacterium. However, since the mating bridge is structurally fragile the genetic transfer is often incomplete. Hence, the recipient bacterium may only receive a portion of, and rarely the entire, bacterial genome of the donor Hfr bacterium. The recombination frequency of conjugation between Hfr strain and F^- strain is high but the transfer of F factor is slow.

7. A form of DNA double helix does not differ from B form of DNA double helix in case of polarity of the two complementary strands. Both the A and B form of DNA are right- handed forms. The rest differences between the two are enlisted below:

	B-DNA	A- DNA
Helix sense	Right Handed	Right Handed
bp per turn	10	11
Vertical rise Angstrom per bp	3.4	2 . 5 6
Rotation per bp Degree	+36	+ 3 3
Helical diameter Angstrom	19	2 3

8. Organellar protein synthesis occurs in mitochondria as well as in chloroplast. Many mitochondrial and chloroplast proteins are imported into the organelles after their synthesis in the cytosol. Most chloroplast and mitochondrial proteins are synthesized outside the organelle on cytosolic ribosomes that are not bound to the rough endoplasmic reticulum.

9. Many kinds of prokaryotes and eukaryotes contain a structure outside the cell membrane called the cell wall. With only a few exceptions, all bacteria have thick, rigid cell walls that give them their shape. Among the eukaryotes, fungi and plants have cell walls. The cell walls of prokaryotes are generally formed of a different molecule (peptidoglycan) to those of eukaryotes (many eukaryotes do not have a cell wall at all).

10. Oncogenic retroviruses can be divided into two classes: acute and slow transforming viruses. Acute transforming retroviruses induce polyclonal tumours within 2 to 3 weeks after infection of the host. Transformation by these viruses is mediated by the expression of viral oncogenes. In contrast, slow transforming retroviruses induce mono- or oligoclonal tumors with a longer latency of 3–12 months. Tumor genesis caused by slow transforming retroviruses is not induced by the presence of a virally modified proto-oncogene in the virus but results from mutations caused by insertion of the proviral retrovirus into the host genome. Retroviral infection of cells is dependent on the binding of viral envelope proteins to cell surface receptors. After incorporation of the provirus into the genome, cells will start producing viral envelope proteins and cell surface receptors become occupied with these proteins, thus inhibiting reinfection of the cell. Many integrated proviruses appear to harbor defective envelope sequences allowing reinfection by the same virus. Thus oncogenic retroviruses integrate into the host nuclear DNA.

11. Chloramphenicol is known as a broad-spectrum antibiotic, which means it is effective against infections caused by a wide variety of bacteria. Chloramphenicol works by preventing bacteria from producing proteins that are essential to them. Without these proteins the bacteria cannot grow, replicate and increase in numbers. Chloramphenicol therefore controls the infection and remaining bacteria die or is killed by the body's immune system.

12. A photoautotroph is a living organism, typically a plant that obtains energy from sunlight to process inorganic materials into organic compounds. These organisms carry out the process of photosynthesis converting carbon dioxide, water and light into nutrition for the plant in which they live.

13. Nitrobacter is a bacterium which oxidizes nitrite to nitrate in the nitrogen cycle. Nitrobacter uses energy from the oxidation of nitrite ions into nitrate ions in soil. Nitrobacter have an

optimum pH between 7.3 and 7.5, and will die in temperatures exceeding 120 F (49°C) or below 32°F (0°C).

14. Photorespiration occurs when the CO_2 levels inside a leaf become low. If the plant continues to attempt to fix CO_2 when its stomata are closed, the CO_2 will get used up and the O_2 ratio in the leaf will increase relative to CO_2 concentrations. When the CO_2 levels inside the leaf drop to around 50 ppm, Rubisco starts to combine O_2 with RuBP instead of CO_2.

    There is no ATP production in photorespiration. Since there are no Carbon's being put into the Krebs cycle (O_2 is put in instead of CO_2 because RuBP has an affinity for both) in photorespiration, a carbon compound is not released.

15. One molecule of glucose oxidized by aerobic respiration in prokaryotes yields the following:

    Glycolysis

    2 net ATP from substrate-level phosphorylation

    2 NADH yields 6 ATP (assuming 3 ATP per NADH) by oxidative phosphorylation

    Transition Reaction

    2 NADH yields 6 ATP (assuming 3 ATP per NADH) by oxidative phosphorylation

    Citric Acid Cycle

    2 ATP from substrate-level phosphorylation

    6 NADH yields 18 ATP (assuming 3 ATP per NADH) by oxidative phosphorylation

    2 FADH2 yields 4 ATP (assuming 2 ATP per FADH2) by oxidative phosphorylation

    Total Theoretical Maximum Number of ATP Generated per Glucose in Prokaryotes

    38 ATP: 4 from substrate-level phosphorylation; 34 from oxidative phosphorylation.

    In eukaryotic cells, the theoretical maximum yield of ATP generated per glucose is 36 to 38, depending on how the 2 NADH generated in the cytoplasm during glycolysis enter the mitochondria and whether the resulting yield is 2 or 3 ATP per NADH.

16. Hepatocellular carcinoma (HCC) accounts for most liver cancers. This type of cancer occurs more often in men than women. It is usually seen in people age 50 or older. In most cases, the cause of liver cancer is scarring of the liver (cirrhosis). Cirrhosis may be caused by:

    - Alcohol abuse
    - Autoimmune diseases of the liver
    - Hepatitis B or C virus infection
    - Inflammation of the liver that is long-term (chronic)
    - Iron overload in the body (hemochromatosis)

    HCC is overwhelmingly related to chronic liver disease, particularly hepatitis B and hepatitis C; hepatitis C is the main causative agent in the U.S.

17. Viruses that replicate via RNA intermediates need an RNA-dependent RNA-polymerase to replicate their RNA. Poliovirus is a positive stranded RNA virus. In these viruses, the virion (genomic) RNA is the same sense as mRNA and so functions as mRNA. This mRNA can be translated immediately upon infection of the host cell.

18. Colchicine inhibits microtubule polymerization by binding to tubulin, which disrupts spindle formation during mitosis (M) phase of the cell cycle. Colchicine is an example of a mitotic inhibitor used in the treatment of gout. A mitotic inhibitor is a drug that inhibits mitosis, or cell division. These drugs disrupt microtubules, which are structures that pull the cell apart when it divides

19. Citric acid is a weak organic acid with the formula $C_6H_8O_7$. Citric acid is commonly associated with citric fruits; oranges, lemons, pineapples. Citric acid is produced by *Aspergillus Niger*. Cultures of *Aspergillus niger* are fed on sucrose to produce citric acid. After the mold is filtered out of the resulting solution, citric acid is isolated by precipitating it with lime (calcium hydroxide) to yield calcium citrate salt, from which citric acid is regenerated by treatment with sulfuric acid. Alternatively, citric acid is sometimes isolated from the fermentation broth by extraction with a hydrocarbon solution of the organic base trilaurylamine, followed by re-extraction from the organic solution by water.

    Thus citric acid is not produced by *Rhizopus nigricans*.

20. In DNA replication, the lagging strand is the DNA strand at the replication fork opposite to the leading strand. It is also oriented in the opposite direction when compared to the leading strand, with the 5' near the replication fork instead of the 3' end as is the case with the leading strand. DNA polymerase cannot build a strand in the 3' $\rightarrow$ 5' direction. This poses no problems for the leading strand, which can continuously synthesize DNA in a processive manner, but creates a problem for the lagging strand, which cannot be synthesized in the 3' $\rightarrow$ 5' direction. Thus, the lagging strand is synthesized in short segments known as Okazaki fragments. On the lagging strand, primase builds an RNA primer in short bursts. DNA polymerase is then able to use the free 3' hydroxyl group on the RNA primer to synthesize DNA in the 5' $\rightarrow$ 3' direction. The RNA fragments are then removed (different mechanisms are used in eukaryotes and prokaryotes) and new deoxyribonucleotides are added to fill the gaps where the RNA was present. DNA ligase is then able to join the deoxyribonucleotides together, completing the synthesis of the lagging strand.

(L) ZOOLOGY

1. Glucagon is a hormone produced in the pancreas. Glucagon is used to raise very low blood sugar. Glucagon has a major role in maintaining normal concentrations of glucose in blood, and is often described as having the opposite effect of insulin. That is, glucagon has the effect of increasing blood glucose levels. The major effect of glucagon is to stimulate an increase in blood concentration of glucose. The hormone is

synthesized and secreted from alpha cells (α-cells) of the islets of Langerhans, which are located in the endocrine portion of the pancreas.

2. Sympatric speciation is occupying the same or overlapping geographic areas without interbreeding. Although they share the same geographic range, sympatric populations of related organisms become isolated from each other reproductively. This can happen by the development of subpopulations that become dependent on distinct food sources or that evolve distinct seasonal mating behaviour. Flowering plants frequently become reproductively isolated through the development of polyploid hybrids (hybrids with three or more sets of chromosomes) that cannot backcross with either parent. The development of new species as a result of the reproductive isolation of populations that share the same geographic range is called sympatric speciation.

3. Spongy bone, also called cancellous bone, is light, porous bone enclosing numerous large spaces that give a honeycombed or spongy appearance. The bone matrix, or framework, is organized into a three-dimensional latticework of bony processes, called trabeculae, arranged along lines of stress. The spaces between are often filled with marrow. Cancellous bone makes up about 20 percent of the human skeleton, providing structural support and flexibility without the weight of compact bone. Cancellous bone can develop into compact bone through the action of bone-forming cells called osteoblasts. The osteoblasts deposit new bone matrix in layers around the trabeculae, which thus enlarge at the expense of the spaces between them. Eventually the spaces are eliminated, and immature compact bone is produced.

4. Nematodes are bilaterally symmetrical, worm-like organisms that are surrounded by a flexible non-cellular layer called a cuticle. A true coelom is lacking, instead, nematodes have a pseudocoel formed directly from the cavity of the blastula. The cavity of the pseudocoel is small, being mostly filled with intestine and oviducts or testes. Most nematode species are dioecious, with separate male and female individuals. Both sexes possess one or two tubular gonads.

5. Transition mutation is a point mutation involving substitution of one base pair for another by replacement of one purine by another purine and of one pyrimidine by another pyrimidine but without change in the purine-pyrimidine orientation. This means that if adenine is replaced by guanine or cytosine is replaced by thymine, then the type of point mutation due to change in the single nucleotide position is called transition mutation.

6. Triassic Period, in geologic time, is the first period of the Mesozoic Era. It began 251 million years ago, at the close of the Permian Period, and ended 199.6 million years ago, when it was succeeded by the Jurassic Period. Although reptiles ruled the Triassic, this period also saw the emergence of the world's first true mammals. While scientists continue to debate which mammals appeared first, weasel-like creatures, such as *Morganucodon watsoni* or *Gondwanadon tapani*, are likely candidates. It's believed these first mammals were small, nocturnal insect eaters. They were also warm-blooded and furry.

7. Given, Single strand read of a 5′ to 3′ DNA molecule = 5′-ACCTAG-3′. Therefore, the complementary RNA molecule is given as: 5′-UGGAUG-3′. This complementary RNA synthesis based on DNA molecule as the template is called transcription which occurs in the nucleus.

8. Frogs are the most familiar group of amphibians. The frog has three respiratory surfaces on its body that it uses to exchange gas with the surroundings: the skin, in the lungs and on the lining of the mouth. While completely submerged all of the frog's respiration takes place through the skin which is known as cutaneous respiration. A frog may also breathe much like a human, by taking air in through their nostrils and down into their lungs. So they also follow mode of pulmonary respiration. Frogs also have a respiratory surface on the lining of their mouth on which gas exchange takes place readily. While at rest, this process is their predominate form of breathing, only fills the lungs occasionally. This is because the lungs, which only adults have, are poorly developed. This mode is called buccal respiration.

9. Respiratory quotient (RQ) is the ratio of the volume of carbon dioxide given off by the body tissues to the volume of oxygen absorbed by them; usually equal to the corresponding volumes given off and taken up by the lungs. The respiratory quotient (RQ) is calculated from the ratio:

$RQ = \frac{CO_{2\ eliminated}}{O_{2\ consumed}}$ where the term "eliminated" refers to carbon dioxide (CO_2) removed ("eliminated") from the body. Respiratory quotients of certain substances are: Carbohydrate (RQ = 1), Proteins (RQ = 0.8 – 0.9), Triolein (fat, RQ = 0.7), Oleic acid (fat, RQ = 0.71), Oxalic acid (RQ = 4).

10. In terms of similarity or difference on the basis of DNA, humans are the most closely related to the chimpanzees. Humans (*Homo sapiens*) and chimpanzees (*Pan troglodytes*) last shared a common ancestor ~ 5 – 7 million years ago. Human and chimpanzee chromosomes are very similar. The primary difference is that humans have one fewer pair of chromosomes than do other great apes. Humans have 23 pairs of chromosomes and other great apes have 24 pairs of chromosomes. There are nine other major chromosomal differences between chimpanzees and humans: chromosome segment inversions on human chromosomes 1, 4, 5,9, 12, 15, 16, 17, and 18.

11. The protistans are conventionally divided into three categories: protozoans (animal-like), algae (plant-like), and slime molds (fungus-like). Characteristics of Protists are: a) mostly unicellular, some are multicellular (algae), b) can be heterotrophic or autotrophic, c) most live in water (though some live in moist soil or even the human body), and d) all are eukaryotic (have a nucleus). A protist is any organism that is not a plant, animal or fungus.

12. During immune response, the random gene arrangement of the variable heavy chains results in the formation of IgM at the beginning. This is because the immunoglobulin coding gene C_M is located in the first position in the heavy chain. So, after the process of random gene arrangement through RSS and recombination and splicing, IgM is first produced as the protein product. IgM is by far the physically largest antibody in the human circulatory system.

13. Haemolytic disease of the newborn (HDN) is an incompatibility of the Rh blood group between the mother and foetus. Pregnancies at risk of HND are those in which an Rh D-negative mother becomes pregnant with an RhD-positive child (the child having inherited the D antigen from the father). The mother's immune response to the foetal D antigen is to form antibodies against it (anti-D). These antibodies are usually of the IgG type, the type that is transported across the placenta and hence delivered to the foetal circulation. Thus, a baby born to Rh^- mother and Rh^+ father can have haemolytic disease.

14. If a cell has no rigid cell wall, has no chloroplast or plastids and the stored carbohydrate is glycogen, then the cell is from animal. Animal cells have a phospholipid bilayer of cell membrane with no rigid cell wall as in plants and fungi. Animals are heterotrophs and so they consume their food from producers and other sources. Thus, they do not require phostosynthetic molecules like chloroplast or plastids for entrapment of photons as energy to generate carbohydrate or starch in case of plants. So, the main storage molecule in animals is glycogen for residual energy. Glycogen is utilised as reserved source of energy by the process of glycogenolysis.

15. Implantation is the very early stage of pregnancy at which the embryo adheres to the wall of the uterus. The implantation stage begins with the deposition of the blastocyst at the uterine mucosa that normally is only formed in a region of the uterine wall.

    An implantation of the blastocyst outside this zone means an extra-uterine pregnancy with serious consequences for the person's health. The implantation stages of the blastocyst in the uterine endometrium can be seen as taking place in three phases: apposition, adhesion and the embedding in the endometrium. The stages of the implantation result in a cascade of molecular mechanisms. In humans, implantation of a fertilized ovum is most likely to occur about 9 days after ovulation, ranging between 6 to 12 days.

16. The fundamentals of growth and development are important in primate evolutionary studies. Allometric growth is the increase in size of different organs or parts of an organism at various rates. It is also called heterauxesis. Allometry literally means "different measure" and refers to the fact that allometric traits grow at a different rate than the body a whole. The growth pattern in primates and humans is of limited nature and it follows the principle of allometry.

17. Homeotic mutation is a mutation that causes tissues to alter their normal differentiation pattern, producing integrated structures but in unusual locations. For example, a homeotic mutation in the fruit fly, *Drosphila,* causes legs to develop where antennae normally form. Mutation in antennapedia hox gene results in the formation of a leg from the head of a fruit fly instead of the expected antenna. These are thus defined as mutations (defining genes) with a phenotype in which a given cell develops along a pathway normally followed by a different cell type.

18. Dysentery is any of a number of disorders marked by inflammation of the intestine, especially of the colon, with abdominal pain, tenesmus, and frequent stools containing blood and mucus. Any of various severe infections of the colon caused by microorganisms, especially of the genus *Shigella,* that result in abdominal cramping, fever, and passage of blood-stained stools or of material consisting of blood and mucus is called bacillary dysentery. Bacillary dysentery is the most common and violent form of dysentery. Ampicillin is the drug of choice for sensitive strains of *Shigella.*

19. The mitotic spindle is the macromolecular machine that segregates chromosomes to two daughter cells during mitosis. The major structural elements of the spindle are microtubule polymers, whose intrinsic polarity and dynamic properties are critical for bipolar spindle organization and function. In most cell types, spindle microtubule nucleation occurs primarily at two centrosomes, which define the spindle poles, but microtubules can also be generated by the chromosomes and within the spindle itself. Many associated factors help organize the spindle, including molecular motors and regulators of microtubule dynamics.

20. Ethology is the scientific study of animal behaviour, especially as it occurs in a natural environment.

    The modern science of animal behaviour, which we call 'ethology', has come a long way in the past few decades, from a largely observational, descriptive science to a modern, quantitative science based on solid foundations of evolutionary biology and quantitative methodology.

■■